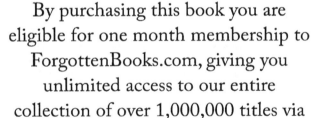

ISBN 978-0-260-13826-2
PIBN 10930127

THE

AMERICAN JOURNAL

OF THE

MEDICAL SCIENCES.

EDITED BY

FRANCIS R. PACKARD, M.D.

NEW SERIES.

VOL. CXXVII.

PHILADELPHIA AND NEW YORK:
LEA BROTHERS & CO.
1904.

DORNAN, PRINTER,
PHILADELPHIA.

THE

AMERICAN JOURNAL
OF THE MEDICAL SCIENCES.

JANUARY, 1904.

ON THE VISCERAL MANIFESTATIONS OF THE ERYTHEMA GROUP OF SKIN DISEASES.

[THIRD PAPER.]

BY WILLIAM OSLER, M.D.,
OF BALTIMORE.

ACCORDING to the classification of recent writers under the erythemas—les erythèmes of the French—are included simple erythema, erythema exudativum, herpes iris, erythema nodosum, certain of the purpuras, urticaria, and angioneurotic œdema. The essential process is a vascular change with exudate, blood, serum, alone or combined. While five or six of the affections just named are described usually as separate diseases they belong to one family, and are characterized by the similarity of the conditions under which they occur, the frequency with which the lesions are substituted the one for the other in the same patient at different times, the tendency to recurrence, often through a long period of years, and, lastly, the identity of the visceral manifestations. In the latter for some years past I have been particularly interested, and in 1895 I published a series of eleven cases,[1] and in 1900[2] a second series of seven cases. In this paper I shall give a third set of eleven cases, and shall consider the features presented by the entire group of twenty-nine cases.

Eight only of the patients were under ten years of age; thirteen were between the tenth and twentieth years. There were eleven females and eighteen males.

The seriousness of the condition is attested by the occurrence of seven deaths in my series—24.1 per cent.

[1] THE AMERICAN JOURNAL OF THE MEDICAL SCIENCES.

[2] Jacobi Festschrift and British Journal of Dermatology, vol. xii.

CASE XIX. *Onset, with erythema over cheeks and nose, in October, 1880; puffiness of one small joint, œdema of one eyelid; increase in the erythema and swelling of the face; marked puffiness and stiffness of the hands; recurring attacks of erythema of the face and local infiltrations in different parts of the body; slight fever; in March very high fever, to 105° F.; much swelling and infiltration of the face and neck; acute nephritis; persistence of œdema of face; death by uræmia May* 13, 1900.—Miss C., Pittsburg, Pa., aged fifteen years; seen January 9, 1900. Father neurotic. No rheumatic history in the family. She has been a very healthy girl; is well grown. She began to menstruate at fourteen years. Large framed; has developed rapidly. Late in October, one Sunday returning from church, an erythematous blush of both cheeks was noticed, extending to the bridge of the nose. It was thought to be due to the sun, as it was a very hot day. As the congested condition of the face did not disappear, a dermatologist was consulted, who pronounced it eczema and gave her an application. For two weeks subsequently she showed a slight puffiness over the tendon of the left metacarpal bone of the middle finger. This disappeared quickly, then followed a puffiness of the left eyelid, and in a few days of the right eyelid, the erythema of the face changing in appearance, at times nearly fading. The eyelids were infiltrated and œdematous (not red). The urine was repeatedly examined and was negative.

Just before Christmas the face became very much more swollen and the eyes were nearly closed. The erythema became much more intense. On Christmas-day the backs of both hands over the middle metacarpal regions were very puffy and œdematous (not reddened). There had been no itching or burning of the face or hands. She had one attack of pain under the left breast—pleurodynia, the physician thought—quite severe, relieved by three days' rest and local applications.

Present Condition. The patient looks remarkably well.

Face. There is a marked erythema, with swelling of both cheeks and the nose, and to a less extent over the chin. It had a purplish-red look as she came in from the cold air. After rest in a warm room it became of a brighter red. On the cheeks it extends to within about 1½ cm. of the angle of the mouth, a little more extensive on the left than on the right. The nasolabial fold, the whole of the under lip, and the greater part of the upper lip are uninvolved. The nose is involved, about the same color as the cheeks, and a slight extension can be seen over the supraorbital ridges, a swelling and a slight blush of redness. The eyelids are at present only a little puffy; the conjunctivæ are slightly congested; on the chin the patches are discrete; individual isolated spots, slightly infiltrated and a little raised, and extend under the chin and behind the ears. There is no ecchymosis. The tonsils and pharynx look natural.

The left hand feels stiff, and to make a fist is painful. On the back of this hand, during Christmas-week, there was a large serous infiltration of a few hours' duration. There is now only a slight patch of erythema over the second metacarpal bone of the middle finger. On the back of the right hand there are a few scattered patches. On the back of the fingers of the right hand there are raised reddened patches, the largest one on the index.

Dr. Duhring, of Philadelphia, saw the patient the next day, and regarded the rash as a peculiar form of erythema.

The subsequent history of the case is as follows:

On February 6th the doctor wrote: "The lobes of the ears have desquamated, leaving a normal appearance, except a little dry, thin scale, not yet loosened; the redness and puffiness of the lobes have disappeared. The upper outer angles of the redness of the cheeks show a tendency to desquamate; a little roughness of the skin; thin, scaly epidermis. The upper lip, which was blotchy, has desquamated, the base being still red. The contour of the face is improved; the general erythema of the cheeks varies. The œdemas and infiltrations change from point to point: upper eyelids slight, one elbow from time to time, both knees or one knee, a finger or the back of the hand. On Sunday afternoon it developed beneath the tendo Achillis of left foot; previous to that both ankles on their outer aspects; last night the left ankle, the right knee, with some pain, and the right elbow was so stiff that it was difficult for her to use her knife or fork with that hand at dinner. Occasionally, when the œdema is more prominent, there may be a feeling of heat to the touch, the temperature at bedtime ranging from 99.8° to 100° F., to 100.2° F., to 100.4° F.; at other times normal, morning and evening. The œdema lasts from twenty-four to thirty-six hours, the back of the left hand week before last proving to be the most persistent. This morning in bed she had free movement of all her joints, showing that the disturbance of yesterday was passing away. As a rule, toward each evening she feels stiff, it may be in the extremities or hands, but by morning, unless the œdema is prominent, the stiffness is not noticeable. The spaces beneath the quadriceps tendon, the tendo Achillis, and beneath the malleoli of the ankles, and the metacarpals are the points now where the swellings occur. The eyelids have never been so bad as during Christmas holidays. Locally the face looks badly enough. Physically, notwithstanding the recurring œdema, I consider her better than one month ago. In animation and general good spirits she is becoming more natural, though the going out among people requires some pluck and determination."

On February 19th I saw the patient in Pittsburg. She seemed somewhat better, but she had still the swelling of the face and of the ear, and occasionally erythematous patches over the nose. For a few days she had had a little fever, up to 100° F., and the day I saw her she was not feeling so well and the temperature had risen to 103° F. The spleen was palpable. Then for a month she had a very severe attack of extensive inflammation of the skin of the face. She had high, irregular fever, ranging to 105° F., and the doctor writes: "The force of the trouble, whatever the cause, expended its power on the face and neck. No clinical picture could compare with it in my experience, except that seen in erysipelas—I mean in dimension, appearance, and parts involved. The extremities have remained perfectly free. The submaxillary and sublingual glands—in fact, the entire circumference of the neck was distended. The infiltration was so extensive that on March 2d she complained of pain in the left ear, and on March 5th the right ear was in the same condition, marked dulness of hearing, and on March 14th paracentesis of the drum had to be performed. The drainage relieved her." The temperature did not begin to fall until after March 20th.

On April 10th the doctor wrote: "Her condition is not worse than when you last heard. The pathological process, whatever it is, is confined to the face and forehead. The rise and fall in the morning and evening temperature keeps about the same, varying from 99.8° to 100° F. The glands of the neck are not so large. There is some œdema of the parts. For several days in the late afternoon she is having a pretty severe frontal headache, which prostrates her. Her appetite is good, and she sleeps well. She sits up a little every day, but soon tires. She is taking a dessertspoonful of Basham's mixture with a sixtieth of strychnine. I have been hoping that no more serious complications might arise, but it is evident that we are not at the real cause of the trouble. The report of the urine is as follows: specific gravity, 1016; considerable amount of albumin, a few red blood corpuscles, hyaline and waxy casts.

"Since you saw her there has been but one outbreak of the œdema such as appeared at the beginning; it came on the back part of the left hand last week, and persisted for twenty-four hours."

On May 17th the doctor wrote: "During the latter part of March and the first part of April she was gaining. On Easter evening there was a rise of temperature, the albumin increased rapidly, and nausea and vomiting became very distressing. She had perforation of the drum of the right ear. The œdema of the face persisted. During the last week of life the left eye was closed entirely and the left half of the face was tense with œdema. The amount of urine diminished to two and a half ounces in the twenty-four hours. The mind kept clear. She died of uræmia on Sunday, May 13, 1900."

This case and No. XXVI., which presented many points of similarity, illustrate the very grave character of some of these obscure forms of erythema. Here was a healthy young girl of good family history who had a persistent erythema of the face and hands, with areas of angioneurotic œdema; then three months later a more severe attack, with fever and intense swelling of the face and an acute nephritis, which proved fatal seven months after the first appearance of the erythema.

CASE XX. *Attack of severe colic; admission to the surgical side for suspected appendicitis; a week before a purpuric eruption on the legs, with high-colored urine; rash of exudative erythema on the legs, with here and there purpura; no involvement of the joints; acute nephritis, abundant albumin, and blood casts, and a small amount of blood in the stools; recovery.*—This case is particularly interesting on account of the fact that he was admitted to the surgical side of the hospital with abdominal symptoms, which were suspected to be due to appendicitis.

Milton R., aged fifteen years, admitted March 14, 1900. He had been a healthy boy; never had rheumatism; no rheumatism in his family. He had never had similar attacks, though his mother said he had irregular, colicky pains at times, and once of such severity that he vomited with it.

Present Illness. About March 7th he noticed himself that the urine was very dark. He had had, a week or so before, some colicky pains in the abdomen.

With the highly colored urine there was no pain in the back, micturition was not painful, and there was no increased frequency. About the same time it was noticed that his legs were somewhat swollen and peppered with red spots, which continued to come out at intervals. The boy had been going to school and had seemed quite well up to this attack.

On admission he was a well-nourished, healthy-looking boy. There was no rash upon the face. Symmetrically arranged on the arms and elbows and about the wrists and hands were a few patches of a rash, chiefly discrete, consisting of papules 1 to 3 mm. in diameter, some distinctly raised, many of them capped with small vesicles, which in places were drying. About the elbows the patches were larger, more raised, and had a purplish-red color. They varied in size from a pin's head to 5 cm. in diameter. In the larger areas the centres were more yellowish in color, the periphery purplish red. The color did not entirely disappear on pressure.

On the legs there was an extensive symmetrical rash about the ankles and knees, the patches very diffuse, on the legs more discrete. On the outer sides of the legs there were patches 3 by 1.5 cm., slightly raised, and these presented three grades of color, the centre whitish, a reddish-brown staining, and then a zone of brighter red. Scattered between the larger areas were some distinct purpuric spots.

Heart. Apex-beat in fifth, 7 cm. from midsternal line, rather diffuse, no thrill, soft apex systolic murmur heard over the body of the heart.

The abdomen looked natural, soft to touch; liver not enlarged; spleen slightly enlarged, the edge distinctly palpable below costal margin. Slight general enlargement of lymphatic glands; reflexes normal.

The urine on admission was blood-red, specific gravity 1014; contained many granular casts, large and small, and some red blood casts; abundant albumin. I remarked to the class the first day how interesting it was to see a case of acute hemorrhagic nephritis without any diminution in the amount of urine, with no swelling of the face, and no trace of œdema. The temperature was 100.5° F.

Blood. Hæmoglobin, 60 per cent.; red blood corpuscles, 4,156,000; leukocytes, 6800; coagulation time, two minutes and a quarter. On March 3d blood cultures were taken, which were negative.

The rash gradually faded and no fresh spots of exudative erythema appeared, but on several days between the 18th of March and the 1st of April small purpuric spots appeared, some minute ones on the palms of the hands.

On March 18th the patient had a small stool containing clear mucus and bright-red blood.

The boy progressed very favorably. The urine on the 17th was 1720 c.c. The bright-red color persisted, and began to clear about March 22d. It remained smoky and had blood in it up to the middle of May. The albumin gradually disappeared. Red blood corpuscles, hyaline and granular casts were seen all through April.

On May 11th the condition was as follows: smoky, 1013; acid reaction, trace of albumin, granular casts, red blood corpuscles, red blood-celled casts. The patient was reported as quite well in the autumn.

CASE XXI. *Otitis; swelling of the hands and legs; extensive purpuric rash, in places papular; acute nephritis, with albumin, tube casts, and blood; cramps in the abdomen and vomiting; recovery; subsequent admission with meningitis from the otitis media; death.*—John D., aged twelve years; seen April 24, 1900. He complained of running from the left ear and swelling of the hands. His family history was good; no similar troubles that he knows of; no rheumatism. Except summer complaint when he was two years old, he has been an exceptionally strong, healthy boy; has had no acute infectious diseases. About two weeks before he applied at the Dispensary he had a running from the left ear. Five days before application his hands and legs became very much swollen, and he could not put on his shoes. The day before application a rash came out on the legs.

Present Condition. Fairly well-nourished boy, but he looked anæmic. The face and eyelids were somewhat puffy. Evidence of recent epistaxis about the nostrils. The hands looked swollen and œdematous. The pulse was rapid, regular. There was no enlargement of the heart. The first sound was rather thudding, and the second pulmonic was accentuated. Temperature, 101° F. The abdomen looked full; the spleen was easily palpable. The liver was not enlarged.

Below the knees the legs were much swollen, firm, and did not pit on pressure. There was an extensive petechial rash, papular in places, but nowhere with much swelling. The urine showed albumin and coarsely granular tube casts; no red blood corpuscles. He was ordered an iron mixture.

April 27th. The patient came again to-day; says he feels very much better. The œdema of the legs has almost gone and the rash has faded. The urine shows abundant albumin, numerous coarsely and finely granular and hyaline casts.

May 1st. Since the previous note the patient has had recurring attacks of severe cramps in the abdomen, with vomiting. The mother describes the material brought up as at first bloody, then black, and later yellow. The swelling of the face and feet is almost gone.

4th. Patient has vomited every evening since the last note; has not vomited to-day; does not complain of any pain.

10th. Patient began to vomit on waking, and continued to do so at intervals during the morning.

12th. He has had no nausea or vomiting since the last note. The legs are not œdematous. A few stains of the purpura remain.

14th. The urine is light colored, cloudy, 1 per cent. of albumin by Esbach, and contains a large number of red blood corpuscles, finely granular casts, and casts of red blood cells.

On July 30th the boy was admitted to the hospital with acute meningitis from the otitis media. He was removed by his parents on August 1st, and he died a few days later.

Case XXII. *Swelling of the legs, with purpura and pains in the knees and ankles; colic; acute nephritis, with blood, albumin, and tube casts in the urine; recurring attacks of purpura, with urticarial wheals; recovery.*—Edna C., aged six years; seen May 11, 1900, with Dr. Richardson, of Bel Air. Family history good. The child had been well and strong; never had rheumatism or chorea. Five weeks ago, about 4 P.M., the child complained of pains in the legs, and the mother noticed that they were swollen, and dark blotches came out. The legs became swollen as far as the knees, and it was difficult for her to move the knees and ankles. She has had for a year or so slight colicky pains in the stomach. On the following day Dr. Richardson found a good deal of albumin in the urine. On the day of the attack the urine contained blood. She has got pale, has had several recurrences of the blotches on the legs, and has with it much colic. Yesterday she had a very severe attack.

She is a fairly well-grown child; looks a little pale and brown, partly sunburn. Color of the lips pretty good. No swelling of the eyelids; no puffiness of the wrists. The tongue is clean; no swelling of the joints. There is a fresh crop of blotches, which came the night before last. The original crop was more than this. At present there are large areas 2 cm. across, slightly raised, evidently fading spots of urticaria, with purpura. Then there are in addition spots of simple purpura scattered between these large areas. The purpura extends as far as the hips. The spleen is not palpable, liver not enlarged. The apex-beat is within the nipple line, no thrill; heart sounds are clear. The urine has been albuminous at times.

The urine to-day had a specific gravity of 1024, clear, acid reaction; contained neither albumin, sugar, casts, nor red blood corpuscles.

March 13, 1903, the mother writes that there has been no recurrence of the purpura.

CASE XXIII. *History of attacks of pain in the knees; colicky pains, with nausea and vomiting and diarrhœa for many years, sometimes with swelling of the feet; enlargement of the spleen; recurring attacks of purpura, with abdominal pain and vomiting; outbreaks of erythema; recovery.*— Sarah E. W., aged fourteen years, admitted September 10, 1900 (Med. No. 11859), complaining of stomach trouble. Her mother had had rheumatism. She herself has an indefinite history of rheumatism, irregular pains, and has had three or four attacks in which her knees have been painful; no swelling, no redness, no fever. She had been subject to sore throat, especially three years ago. At times she has had attacks of vomiting. The child's mother states that she was well and natural until the attack of measles at her fourth month. Ever since she has had two serious troubles: first, attacks of abdominal pain, with nausea, vomiting, and diarrhœa; and, secondly, skin rashes, which come out suddenly and then fade away. They are usually symmetrical. With these attacks there is often swelling of the feet, which comes very rapi y.

For three weeks she has been having pains in the abdomen, and for five days past there has been much nausea and vomiting, and three days ago she had diarrhœa, five or six stools a day. She felt feverish, had some sweats at night, and loss of appetite. She has had to get up at night once or twice to pass urine. Eight days ago the feet and legs began to swell, and a red rash broke out on the skin. The knees were painful, and her eyes at the same time became puffy. The swelling of the legs has disappeared and she has been a good deal better.

On admission she was a small, pale, frail-looking child, not anæmic, eyelids slightly puffy. The temperature was 100° F.; pulse 116, slightly irregular. There was a somewhat diffuse heart-beat in third, fourth, and fifth; on palpation a systolic thrill; on auscultation a blowing systolic bruit transmitted to the axilla; accentuation of the pulmonic second. The abdomen looked natural; the liver was not enlarged; the spleen was fully 2 cm. below the costal margin. There was slight œdema of the feet and ankles, and there was a fading rash on the knees, elbows, over the clavicles and ankles. Some of these spots were distinctly purpuric. One above the left external malleolus was a bluish spot, looking like a bruise.

September 13*th*. Had an attack, with great coldness of the feet and a burning sensation in the pit of the stomach, which increased so that at 10 P.M. she had a great deal of abdominal distress. A fresh, brilliant-red rash in raised patches came out on both buttocks, extending down the thighs, and on both elbows. The abdominal pain persisted that night, and at 6 A.M. she vomited, at first curds, later a greenish fluid, and about 9 o'clock mucus mixed with blood.

14*th*. There is this morning an abundant purpuric rash over both buttocks, extending down the thighs, up the back on each side, over the elbows, and the upper arms. The rash is raised, and the individual spots have distinct margins. On the right elbow there is a bluish-red discoloration, which is painful to the touch. There is no pain or swelling in the joint itself. She had to have morphine. Throughout the day she vomited several times.

Blood. Red blood corpuscles, 3,680,000; leukocytes, 10,000; hæmoglobin, 75 per cent.; blood coagulation time, four minutes.

Urine. Specific gravity, 1012; no albumin, no blood, no tube casts.

15*th*. The rash is very extensive over the back. Some of the purpuric areas are infiltrated and raised and measure 5 x 3 cm. There is a little swelling in the left elbow-joint to-day. There are red blotches on the thumbs and over the knuckles. The spot where the hypodermic needle was inserted is surrounded by a hemorrhage.

16*th*. The swelling of the left elbow has disappeared. There is a fresh erythema on both forearms. From this time the patient improved. There was a good deal of pigmentation and staining left by the hemorrhages. She was discharged, feeling quite well, on September 24th.

CASE XXIV. *Erythema and purpura; acute nephritis; general œdema; persistence of the albumin for two months; gradual recovery.*—Morris S., aged three years, Hebrew; admitted December 20, 1900, with swelling of the face, abdomen, penis, and legs. There was nothing of any moment in his family history; no rheumatism. He was healthy as a baby; had a sore navel for some time. When two years old he had diphtheria, a severe attack, not followed by any swelling of the feet. With this exception the child has been very well. He has grown and thriven, eats heartily, and drinks three large cups of coffee in the day! Three days ago the father noticed some red spots on the back of the left hand, which looked like bites of insects. At the same time there was swelling of the wrists and back of the neck. That night the swelling became worse and the spots extended and formed large blotches. The father said the wrists looked as if they had been scalded. On the following day the spots appeared on the legs and body and became darker. The penis became œdematous.

I saw the child at my out-patient clinic and made the following note: There is well-marked purpura over the legs and around the crests of the ilia, and there is a general subcutaneous œdema of a brawny character. The skin of the penis is œdematous. The swelling and œdema which had been so marked on the wrists has disappeared and has left a brownish-red stain. The abdomen is large; there is dulness in the flanks; no percussion wave. Some œdema of the lower part of the back. On the outer surface of the skin of the right arm there are stains of a purpuric rash. Examination of the urine showed a large amount of albumin, but no tube casts.

The child was taken home by its father the same afternoon, but returned three days later with general anasarca and signs of slight fluid in the abdomen. The child looked very well. The face was only slightly swollen, the eyelids a little puffy. The urine had a specific gravity of 1023, dark yellow in color, and there were a few casts and much albumin. Throughout the month the dropsy persisted to a slight extent, but gradually disappeared. A very careful daily study of the urine was made, particularly with reference to the percentage of albumin and urea. The amount of albumin varied through January from 0.1 to 0.3 per cent. On the 17th, 18th, and 19th of February the amount increased rapidly, reaching on the 20th 1 per cent. There were no tube casts. On March 5th, for the first time, the urine was free from albumin. Then again, from the 25th to the 30th, the albumin returned, and reached on the 28th 0.5 per cent. From that time on the albumin was absent, and he was discharged April 21st in good condition. I heard on March 1, 1902, that the patient has remained perfectly well.

CASE XXV. *For the first six years of life recurring attacks like nettle-rash; then to the tenth year freedom; in tenth and eleventh years recurrence of the rash in larger blotches and much swelling of the face and eyes; recurring attacks of severe spasmodic croup, having no special relation to the skin rash; twice with these attacks there has been swelling of the throat; lately marked swelling of the soft palate and uvula; swelling of the feet and of the face; no nephritis.*—N. D. D., aged fourteen years, Lafayette, Ala.; sent May 6, 1901, by Dr. Love. When three weeks old red splotches came out all over him and itched like nettle-rash; lasted three weeks. It recurred periodically until he was six years old. He never passed six months without an attack; sometimes they would occur quite frequently. He had no pain in the abdomen with the attacks, no vomiting. From the age of six to ten years he was perfectly free from the attacks. At ten years the trouble reappeared, and recurred periodically until he was eleven years old. Good health until the thirteenth year, when the disease returned. The "splotches" were larger and there was swelling of the eyelids and face. About six weeks ago the inside of the throat began to swell, chiefly the uvula and the soft palate, and there was œdema of the outside of the neck. He has had one attack also in the left auditory canal. The last attack was ten days ago. The feet began to swell and he could scarcely get his boots on. The face was a little swollen in this attack.

The family history is good. The father has a quinine idiosyncrasy, and cannot take even a few grains without having a skin rash. An uncle also has the same peculiarity.

He is a healthy-looking boy, of good color. No swelling of the face to-day. The remnant of an urticarial spot just above the right eyebrow. The only eruption at present is above the popliteal space on the left side, where there is a large spot extending across the lower third of the thigh, measuring 8 x 10 cm. It is reddened, prominent, greatly infiltrated, the margins localized and distinct; a dusky red color, in places of a more vivid red; very hot. In one or two places the margins look a little less red. The hyperæmia is extreme, and pressure fills up at once. There is nothing at present in his throat; no other spots anywhere.

The heart sounds are clear; arteries not sclerotic. Pulse is good. Hæmoglobin, 80 per cent. Urine: no albumin, blood, or tube casts.

All through his life he has been subject in the winter to attacks of severe spasmodic croup, which have not apparently had any relation to the skin rash. It has recurred at intervals all his life, twice with marked swelling of the throat. It commences with difficulty in breathing, and lasts twenty or thirty minutes. He will call and say he is about to choke. Wet cloths about the throat relieve it. No cough with it.

May 8th. The swelling in the patch of the day before yesterday has subsided. There is left a bluish-green stain like a bruise.

I heard from Dr. Love on February 23, 1903. The boy is very much better. He has had no attack for two months. He took calcium chloride for a long time with benefit; recently camphor in three-grain doses four times a day, which seems to have had a very satisfactory influence.

CASE XXVI. *Onset in September, 1901, with erythema of the nose and cheeks; extension to the elbows and arms, usually in the form of wheals, but some spots purpuric; chill, followed by consolidation of the lower lobe of left lung; protracted fever; enlargement of the lymphatic glands; delayed resolution of the pneumonia; urine clear in the attack; gradual recovery; in May, 1902, onset of acute nephritis; uræmia; death in a convulsion.*—L. E., aged twenty-four years; seen at Pittsburg, Pa., on February 6, 1902, with Dr. Litchfield. Her family history was good; no rheumatism; no tuberculosis. She had been a very robust girl; no serious illnesses. Toward the end of the summer, when at the Thousand Islands, a rash began on the face, chiefly on the nose and cheeks. It looked, the doctor said, like lupus erythematosus. It persisted, and troubled her a great deal. Dr. Fox, of New York, who only saw her once, writes that he thought it looked like an acute lupus erythematosus. It spread in patches to the body, particularly about the elbows and on the arms. The patches were red, sometimes raised, and would, at times, come out like wheals. Before Christmas she had a very violent outbreak, and many of the spots became purpuric, and on the arm the doctor said there were spots which looked almost like the eruption of vaccinia. On December 27th she had a chill, and on the third day consolidation of the left lower lobe was found. The temperature was 104° F. From the fifth and sixth days there was a drop in the temperature. On the twelfth day it dropped to 98° F.; then it gradually rose, and from the twelfth to the twenty-sixth day it ranged to 105° F. Then the other lung became involved. There was very little cough, particularly after antipneumococcic serum was given. There were no true chills. The mind was clear, as a rule. For the past three weeks the temperature has ranged about 101° F., with no very great drops. The pulse has been from 112 to 120; respirations 22 to 40; mind clear; no delirium. The right lung has been clearing. The left lower lobe has been solid for some weeks. About two weeks ago the left leg became swollen, and she had a thrombus in the femoral vein. For ten days the lymphatie glands throughout the body have peen a little enlarged and tender.

At the time of my visit the patient looked thin and pale. There was no sign of any rash on the face, but there was erythema of the skin of the thighs, mottled and patchy, and in places a little raised. There was no purpura. The left leg was swollen, but was no longer tender. She had complete consolidation of the lower lobe of the left lung, with tubular breathing and a few râles. The fremitus was not very marked.

I put in a needle in two places, but got nothing. The Widal reaction was negative. The sputum was a little rusty, and I had some examined. There were pneumococci, but no tubercle bacilli.

The urine was examined repeatedly, and there was occasionally a faint trace of albumin, but nothing special. She was anæmic, and on January 29th blood count showed: red blood corpuscles, 3,310,000; hæmoglobin, 46 per cent.; leukocytes, 6000. The patient gradually improved through March and April, and seemed to be getting quite well. In May she went to Atlantic City, where she improved rapidly. Toward the end of the month an acute nephritis came on, without any special exposure; the urine was scanty, high colored, contained blood and tube casts and much albumin. There was fever, 101° to 102° F.; no skin rash. I saw her with Dr. Marvel shortly after she had had a uræmic convulsion. She died within a week of the onset of the nephritis.

CASE XXVII. *From infancy recurring attacks of colic, sometimes with vomiting; recurring attacks of blotches (erythema) on the skin of face and arms; at the time of examination a spot of erythema capped with blister.*—Dorothy B., aged thirteen years, referred to me by Dr. Charlton, of Savannah, Ga., June 18, 1902, for a peculiar trouble in her stomach. She was healthy when born, was a healthy child, and has grown and developed well. The family history is good; no special peculiarities. Since infancy she has had a peculiar stomach trouble, recurring attacks of nausea, and colic-like pain. The attacks recur at irregular intervals, a week or two apart, sometimes a number in succession, and then she will be free for several weeks. She will appear perfectly well, will eat a good meal, and an hour or so afterward will say: "May I go and lie down? I have a pain in my stomach." The attacks are chiefly in the morning. The abdomen seems tender and the colic at times has been severe enough to make her cry out. It has been a source of constant worry, and nothing has ever seemed to do her any good. At times she has had very obstinate vomiting with the attacks. Her mother says the pain is always in the pit of the stomach. When four or five years of age she had a very bad attack of "ivy poisoning." This spring some red spots came out on the neck, and she has had them recurring ever since. They occur on the face and arms as red blotches, and then become capped with little blisters.

The patient is a healthy-looking girl; color good; tongue clean. The abdomen is soft, natural looking; spleen not enlarged; stomach not dilated; no enlargement of the liver. No sensitiveness anywhere on pressure. The heart is not enlarged; the first and second sounds are loud. There is a soft systolic murmur at the base. The skin seems everywhere clear, except on the left foot, just above the middle toe. Here there is a raised, infiltrated, reddened spot about 5 x 5 mm., capped with a small, clear blister. This, her mother says, is the typical appearance of the rash. When the attacks are bad a number of these appear on the face and neck, and they come out on the extremities, looking at first like hives, and then are capped by the little blisters. The urine is clear; no blood.

A letter from her mother, March 22, 1903, states that the child has improved very greatly, and has been very free from that colic, and has had no return of the skin trouble.

CASE XXVIII. *For two years recurring attacks of purpura, chiefly on the legs; severe attack three months before admission, with colicky pains, vomiting, diarrhœa, and arthritis; in the last attack diarrhœa was a marked feature, with the passage of blood from the bowel.*—A. S. A., aged twenty-six years, white, single, lawyer, Montgomery, W. Va.; admitted February 12, 1902, complaining of skin disease and stomach trouble. No similar trouble in family; no purpura. Patient's father has chronic diarrhœa. Usual diseases of childhood. Typhoid fever in 1898, slight attack, but followed by a gastric (enteric?) trouble lasting about four months. Patient was in bed altogether about six months. He has had occasionally swollen and tender joints. One attack of swelling and pain about tendo Achillis. Appetite and digestion good prior to present illness. Tendency to constipation. Denies lues and gonorrhœa. Habits good. Average weight, 160 pounds. Present weight, 140 pounds. Patient first noticed the purpuric eruption on his legs in the spring of 1901, two years ago. At this time the spots were very small and situated only below the knees, especially about the ankles. At this time the patient had no nausea, vomiting, or diarrhœa; no arthritis. During the summer of 1901 the patient had indigestion and constant recurrences of purpura; no arthritis; some nausea, vomiting, and pain. At no time was he confined to his bed or compelled to give up his work.

In December, 1901, the patient had his first severe attack, which kept him in bed for about a week, and was soon followed by another of about the same severity and duration.

For eleven months, until November, 1902, the patient was well; then he had very severe abdominal pain, with diarrhœa, nausea, and vomiting, followed by arthritis and a hemorrhagic eruption on his legs. He was forced to give up work and go to bed, and until New Year's there were recurring attacks.. During the last month or six weeks he has been at work, but has been feeling badly, with arthritis and purpura, some "indigestion," and pain.

The attacks are all of the same character. The patient first noticed the purpura on his legs or arms (at first it was only on his legs below knees, but is now on thighs above the knees, and on hands and arms, particularly on extensor surfaces), accompanied with a mild arthritis. The joints are "sore and stiff," but he can use them. This is followed by a severe pain in his left side and left half of abdomen, passing over middle line in a narrow band. The pain is fixed, not radiating, and of a cramp-like character; sometimes requiring morphine by the mouth or hypodermically for relief. The pain usually lasts about two days. Following the pain the patient has diarrhœa and usually nausea and vomiting. The vomiting is the last event in the series, and about the time it begins the purpura fades, leaving brownish-yellow stains.

The joints attacked are usually the ankles and knees. In the last outbreak the left hand (metacarpophalangeal joints) was involved, and his wrists, never his elbows, shoulders, or hips. Last November the patient passed considerable blood per rectum of a very dark color. He has never had hæmatemesis or hæmoptysis. Slight epistaxis. No hæmaturia or bleeding from gums or mucous membranes. He has grown quite pale in each attack, and loses flesh rapidly, but regains it quickly.

Present Condition. Well nourished, but pale. Examination of heart, lungs, and abdomen negative. There is a purpuric eruption on back of hands and arms, more on right arm than on left, and on extensor than on flexor surfaces; same on feet and legs up to the groins. Tenderness and subjective feeling of stiffness in left hand (metacarpophalangeal joints) and right wrist. Blood pressure, 145 mm. of Hg. Red blood corpuscles, 4,280,000; leukocytes, 7600; hæmoglobin, 65 per cent. (von Fl.). Blood coagulation time, six and a half minutes. Urine negative.

On February 13, 1902, I made the following note: Patient is pale, sweating profusely. Tongue furred. Skin of face clear. Gums not swollen; a little red line; no blue line. There is a fading purpura on the arms; spots not raised, brownish, leaving stains, chiefly on flexor surface. No purpura on trunk and back. On the legs there are numerous stains of fading purpura over feet and extensor surfaces. The spots are larger on the legs. All are now fading. Joints nowhere red or swollen.

Circulatory System. Slight sclerosis of arteries. Apex beat visible in fourth left interspace, just inside nipple. Soft murmur at apex with first sound and over body of heart, not propagated to axilla.

Abdomen looks natural; nowhere painful; a little tender in spots over colon. Spleen not enlarged. Liver not enlarged. Appendix not palpable. Superficial glands not enlarged. He was ordered calcium chloride.

February 14th. Blood coagulation time, six and a half minutes.

16*th.* Purpura has almost disappeared. Patient has improved very rapidly. On his discharge a few days later the patient looked very well; blood coagulation time was three minutes.

CASE XXIX. *Acute otitis; arthritis; recurring attacks of colic, with occasional vomiting; hemorrhage from the bowels; purpura; acute nephritis; recovery.*—March 7, 1903, E. F., aged five years, seen with Dr. Hamburger, to whom I am indebted for the notes.

Personal History. He had a prolonged attack of summer diarrhœa two years ago. It followed an attack of otitis. For the past two weeks he has had pain in the ears. Last Wednesday (to-day being Saturday) there was a discharge from both ears. Fever has persisted off and on since the onset. This morning he was unable to stand on his feet because of pain. Temperature, 100.5° F. There is a purulent discharge from the right ear. Heart sounds are clear. Examination of the lungs negative. The spleen is not palpable. There is no tenderness in the abdomen. The dorsum of the right foot is swollen, not reddened, but very tender on palpation. There is some tenderness, but no swelling over the left foot.

March 8th. The patient had a restless night. His temperature rose to 102° F.; this morning it is 99.7° F.; pulse, 104. He has complained of pain in the wrists and in the interval between the thumbs and first fingers. He has pain in the abdomen, accompanied by vomiting of the milk. Heart sounds are clear.

9*th.* The patient was unable to retain food yesterday, and he has vomited this morning the nourishment, as well as some bile independent of taking food. Throughout the night he has cried because of intermittent pain in the abdomen, referred now to the left half and to the umbilical region. His temperature this morning is 99.6° F. The tongue is heavily coated. There is a decided fœtor oris. Every few moments he cries out with pain in the abdomen, which lasts a few minutes, then disappears, only to return in from ten to twenty minutes. He rolls over in the dorsal decubitus in these paroxysms. The joints are no longer sensitive. The abdomen looks natural. The left half is sensitive on palpation, particularly in the iliac region, while above in the upper half a fine gurgling can be detected. The abdomen is exquisitely tender during the painful period. Following an enema, a quantity of blood, sufficient to discolor the water a deep, dark red, was ejected with some fecal material. Early this morning he had a small movement (a couple of scybalæ) without blood. For the past four or five days the ears have been irrigated with 1.44 of bichloride of mercury to one quart of water three times a day.

10th. The boy had considerable pain during the night. Yesterday afternoon about 3.30 he passed about one ounce of pure blood. This morning he is comfortable. Pulse, 120; temperature, 98° F. The tongue is coated, but it is clearing at the tip and sides. There is no gurgling over the abdomen. There are no petechiæ. He is being fed on albumin water, and toward evening is given a starch and laudanum enema.

11th. The pain returned about noon yesterday. It was so intense that at 5.30 P.M. the starch and laudanum enemas were resumed. He had two stools, composed mainly of blood and in part of the enema. The night was restlessly spent in pain. Early in the morning he passed a bloody stool. The temperature this morning was 97.8° F.; pulse, 108. To-night the temperature is 98.6° F.; pulse, 93. The day was relatively comfortable and free from pain, but this afternoon about 6.30 the colic returned with such intensity that the patient cries out. There is no skin eruption. The starch and laudanum enemas are being discontinued and he is being given paregoric, half-ounce, every two hours.

12th. The colic continues this morning. He has had two stools to-day, one being composed of narrow, long casts, dark brown in color, evidently composed of changed blood. The other stool contains curded milk, blood, a little mucus and some fecal matter.

Urine acid, 1026, yellow, no albumin, no sugar.

13th. He had a great deal of pain during the night. This morning at ten he was given one-half ounce of castor oil. At 3.20 P.M. he had a stool approaching the normal. To-night another movement of blood and fecal matter. The day was quite comfortable, but beginning at about 8.30 the colic returned. Paregoric, twenty drops, and deodorized tincture of opium every two hours.

14th. The boy was very restless until 3 A.M.; from that time on he has been comfortable. He had a normal movement this morning and another this afternoon without blood. This afternoon he had very slight pain.

19th. Last night a slight eruption was noted. To-day, scattered over the legs, feet, and buttocks, are fine petechiæ, and on the calf of the left leg there is a bluish ecchymosis about 2.5 x 1 cm. in diameter. On both elbows there is an eruption formed by the coalescence of rose-colored, slightly raised papules. He has lost his appetite. The tongue is again lightly coated.

20th. The little fellow had an uncomfortable night, being restless and complaining of pain in the abdomen. This morning his appetite is poor. Temperature, 98.8° F. The petechiæ persist, and in addition he has a subcuticular steel-blue ecchymosis over the right hypothenar region. It is here that he complains of pain. The eruption on the right elbow has almost disappeared, leaving little brownish discoloration. On the left it still persists, although less evident. On pressure it is not entirely effaced, still leaving a brownish color. The urine is yellow and looks a little smoky; acid, 1009; moderate flocculent sediment, containing a few hyaline casts and red blood corpuscles; albumin is present. His diet is now again limited to soft food. Castor oil is administered, and calcium chloride, 10 grains, three times a day is being given.

24th. The boy is again comfortable. He is very hungry; he looks pale. The eruption has disappeared, with the exception of a bluish discoloration on the calf of the left leg, representing the old ecchymosis. The colicky pain during the foregoing illness occurred in paroxysms at intervals varying from five minutes to an hour. On the 12th the pain was almost continuous. Between the attacks the little fellow would fall asleep, only to be awakened by pain, which caused him to roll about in great discomfort. So severe was it that he would cry out. The left lateral decubitus and lying on his face were the favorite positions during the painful periods. The abdomen was exquisitely tender during the colic. Throughout the illness the abdomen was slightly distended. The spleen was not palpable. The constant feature was a fine gurgling detected by palpation of the left half of the abdomen, particularly in the upper quadrant. The days were relatively comfortable, with the exception of the 12th, when the pain was almost continuous. The colic appeared toward evening, increased in severity through the night, reaching its maximum between midnight and three o'clock; then a decrease in its intensity and a more comfortable morning.

April 7th. A specimen of the urine sent from Atlantic City, where the patient went March 28th, is pale yellow, with a moderate flocculent, grayish sediment, containing many red corpuscles, some round granular cells, and an occasional hyalogranular cast, 1008; albumin present, 0.5 per cent.

11th. The patient returned from Atlantic City, having gained weight and looking very well. Although the complexion is good, the conjunctivæ look a little pale. While in Atlantic City he once suffered from a little pain in his abdomen, and his mother noticed a few "spots" on his legs. The urine of to-night is pale yellow, acid, 1008; small flocculent sediment, containing many red blood corpuscles, a few hyaline casts. Albumin is present.

15th. The patient has been in bed and on strict milk diet, in spite of his dislike for this food. To-day he was much nauseated and vomited directly after taking food.

16th. The urine is brown and smoky and deposits a reddish-brown sediment containing blood, some round granular cells, and granular casts, 1024; contains much albumin. Very little fluid has been taken during the last twenty-four hours.

From the time he improved the albumin lessened. There were very few tube casts, and at the date of the last report, May 10th, he was doing well, though still kept in bed and on a milk diet as precautionary measures.

A criticism has been made on my previous papers that I had jumbled together a motley group of cases, some of purpura, some of angioneurotic œdema, others of peliosis rheumatica; others, again, of exudative erythema. I did so on purpose, for I was seeking similarities, not diversities, and I refrained as much as possible from the use of specific terms, often, indeed, not knowing what to call a case watched for a long period. What, for instance, shall we call Case II., which I studied at intervals for six years—purpura, erythema, angioneurotic œdema, or urticaria? The lesions varied from time to time, but there could be no question that all of them, with the extraordinary visceral symptoms, were manifestations of one and the same cause. Or Case XXVI., beginning with simple erythema, then crops of urticaria, and an exudative erythema with purpura and vesiculation? In Cases XIX. and XXVI. the most expert dermatologists were in doubt as to the nature of the lesions, and could only say that it was a peculiar type of erythema. On the other hand, the members of the erythema group have not all the same etiology, and, indeed, as is well known, the individual members have a very diverse etiology. For example, the urticaria of cholelithiasis, of an ague paroxysm, that caused by eating shell-fish or strawberries, the urticaria of hydatids, and an asthma attack has the same clinical and anatomical features, though caused by a variety of poisons —bacterial, protozoal, vegetable, and metabolic. It is not unlikely that the poison in itself, of whatever kind, is of less intrinsic importance than certain transient aspects of cell metabolism. In the first place, there is no constancy of action of the same poison in different persons, or even in the same person at different times. This is notoriously the case with the animal and vegetable substances causing urticaria. In the second place, the chronic forms of urticaria probably illustrate a morbid and persistent sensitiveness of the cutaneous vessels to poisons of either intestinal or tissue origin. And, thirdly, the importance of the local status is shown in that remarkable form of urticaria which comes on after exposure to cold. So long as the face is at a temperature above 60° F. the patient is all right; exposure at 40° F. is followed at once by an outbreak of urticaria. And, lastly, a peculiarity that may be transmitted through several generations, as in angioneurotic œdema, which is only urticaria "writ large," must either be a morbid susceptibility of tissue or an inherited peculiarity of metabolism, or both combined.

The relation of the erythemas to infective processes is interesting. Certain types of exudative erythema behave like an acute febrile disease, and Dühring, of Constantinople, has described an epidemic form. In many of the fevers—typhoid, pneumonia, rheumatic fever, etc.—there may be symptomatic erythemas. The severer forms of purpura urticans with arthritis and colic (Henoch's purpura and the peliosis rheumatica) may run an acute febrile course with heart complications. Many of the graver cases of purpura have followed an acute infection, puerperal fever, gonorrhœa, etc., and in No. V. of my series the patient had recently had gonorrhœa, and in Nos. XXI. and XXIX. there had been otitis media. The rheumatic poison is probably responsible for very many cases. But in a very large group the condition persists for so many years, as in Cases II., XIV., XV., and XXVII., that an infective process is out of the question.

The visceral lesions are most diverse in situations and form, and vary a good deal with the character of the eruptions. It has to be borne in mind that certain skin lesions are associated secondarily with diseases of the internal organs. Purpura of a severe type is very common in Bright's disease; urticaria and purpura in cirrhosis of the liver and cholelithiasis; urticaria in asthma, and all forms of erythema with the chronic valvular lesions of the heart in children. It may not always be easy to say, particularly in asthma, which is the primary, whether the urticaria has preceded the asthma, or *vice versa*.

The complications form two great groups—the angioneurotic and the inflammatory. To the former belong the swellings of the fauces, the œdema of the glottis, the changes in the bronchial mucosa, causing asthma, and the colic, which is probably due to localized œdema of the gastrointestinal walls; to the latter the more serious complications, endocarditis, pericarditis, pleurisy, pneumonia, and nephritis, but, as it is not easy to make a sharp distinction in all instances, it will be better to discuss the complications according to the organs attacked.

Cerebral. In two cases there were brain symptoms, active delirium in Case I. at the time of recurring attacks, while in Case XV. there were five or six attacks of aphasia and hemiplegia, and the cerebral and cutaneous manifestations lasted for thirteen or fourteen years! It seems not improbable that these transient attacks were due to vascular changes in the brain, the counterpart of those occurring in the skin. An analogous condition is met with in Raynaud's disease, of which I have reported a remarkable instance,[1] with repeated attacks of monoplegia, aphasia, and hemiplegia, alternating or occurring at the same time with the local syncope or asphyxia of the fingers and toes.

Respiratory. Swelling of the fauces and larynx may cause severe dyspnœa and attacks like croup. In the family I described with angioneurotic œdema two members died of œdema of the glottis. In Case XXV. of the series the lad had much swelling of the fauces and croup-like attack, twice accompanied with swelling of the throat and neck, evidently due to œdema.

The association of asthma with urticaria and other skin diseases of the erythema group has long been known, and one of the last papers of our lamented friend Dr. F. A. Packard dealt with this subject.[2] It seems to be most frequent with urticaria. There was no instance in my series, though in Case II. there was a persistent catarrh of the smaller tubes leading to emphysema.

[1] The American Journal of the Medical Sciences, 1891. [2] Ibid., 1896.

Three of the patients had severe pneumonia. In Case II. it occurred toward the close of the remarkable illness of five years' duration. In Case XI. the child died of croupous pneumonia a month after the onset of the third attack of purpura. It was impossible to say whether there was any connection between the two diseases. In Case XXVI. there was a protracted pneumonia following directly upon a severe outbreak of exudative erythema. It is likely that the recurring skin lesions, the pleuropneumonia, the phlebitis, the general glandular enlargement, and the fatal nephritis were due to one and the same poison.

Cardiac. Acute endocarditis seems a rare complication. I saw an instance in Philadelphia, and there are a good many cases in the literature, usually in the intense arthritic purpura (peliosis rheumatica). Only three cases in my series had heart murmurs, and in none of the patients was it likely that endocarditis existed. Pericarditis occurred as a terminal event in Case II.

Gastrointestinal Symptoms. One of the most constant features in this whole group, occurring in twenty-five of the cases, is the recurring attacks of colic, sometimes with vomiting, sometimes with diarrhœa, occasionally with the passage of blood. The association of attacks of colic with outbreaks of urticaria has long been known. Analyzing the series here reported there were eight cases in which the colic occurred alone with the outbreak of the skin lesions; in fifteen there were in addition gastric attacks, nausea and vomiting, and in five diarrhœa, and in eight blood occurred with the colic. The colic is severe, and the attacks may persist for an hour or more and may require morphine for relief. The diagnosis of renal colic was made in one case (II.), and in Case XX. the patient was admitted to the surgical ward for appendicitis. Two interesting associations of the colic may be referred to here. In certain cases of angioneurotic œdema, a malady which belongs to this erythema group, colic is a special feature, and in the family I reported almost all of the cases throughout the five generations had colic with the outbreaks of the œdema. Still more interesting is the relationship which this condition bears to those obscure cases of recurring colic and gastrointestinal crises in children, many of which I believe belong to this group. Take, for example, the following case:

Charles E. D., aged thirteen years, referred to me by Dr. Dick, of Salisbury, Md., on February 8, 1903, complaining of attacks of severe cramps in the abdomen, which have recurred at intervals for nine years. At first they occurred every month or two, and were associated with vomiting of green bile. Now he does not vomit. Of late years they have recurred with much greater frequency, so that now he never passes a week without an attack. So far as I can make out there is nothing in the diet which ever makes any difference. He is better in warm weather, and more often has the attacks in damp weather, in winter, and after prolonged exertion. He never has any diarrhœa. He has had swelling of the joints, occasionally has had growing pains and pains about the knees. The attacks begin abruptly. Occasionally he has a little premonition in the way of uneasy sensations. The doctor states that he writhes about the floor in the attack and doubles himself into a knot and squirms about the floor like a snake. As the father expresses it, the contortions are awful. Last week he had an attack every day, but not of great severity, and this is the rule. Attacks at long intervals are always more severe. The examination of the child was negative. The urine was negative, except that the morning specimen showed a slight trace of albumin. The child was not very well grown, and looked pale and delicate. The spleen was not enlarged.

Naturally I asked particularly about the occurrence of hives or of any other skin rash, or the occurrence of arthritis, but the history was entirely negative. What is particularly interesting about the case is the fact that his mother had similar attacks during her early life, which lasted until she reached puberty. The boy has three sisters, each one of whom suffered in early life severely with hives, but had no abdominal pains.

Cases XVIII. and XXVII. show the connection of this type of colic in children with the condition under discussion. For years there were attacks of colic of great obscurity. In the former case the child was admitted with a typical outbreak of purpura and erythema; in the latter the skin lesions have lately given a clue to the nature of the protracted abdominal attacks. In angioneurotic œdema the patients may have colic alone without the giant urticaria. In children recurring colic with nausea and vomiting may be sometimes a gastrointestinal counterpart or equivalent of a cutaneous attack, as they certainly are in angioneurotic œdema, and, as I think, we may take it for granted they were in Cases XVIII. and XXVII.

Renal. In fourteen of the cases there was acute nephritis, indicated by albumin and numerous tube casts, and in seven cases blood. In Case VII. there was albumin without any blood or tube casts. In two cases the picture was that of an acute nephritis with dropsy. The seriousness of the nephritis is shown by the fact that of the seven deaths among the twenty-nine patients five died of uræmia. The importance of the poisons causing the skin lesions of the erythema group is not sufficiently recognized as a cause of acute nephritis. Dickinson makes no mention of it in his article in Allbutt's *System*, and in most of the other systematic writers there is a corresponding silence on the subject. The nephritis, as a rule, comes on at the height of the skin lesion, or it may follow within a week or ten days, or even, as in Case XXVI., a couple of months after the subsidence of the skin lesion. There may be no dropsy even with an intense nephritis (Case II.). The œdema of the skin lesion may simulate the puffiness of the face in renal dropsy. This was very marked in Case XXV. The photograph sent by Dr. Love showed a typical renal facies, but in this boy the urine had never been albuminous. Five of the fourteen cases of nephritis died with uræmic symptoms. With reference to the skin lesions in the renal cases, in four purpura alone was present; in three, purpura and urticaria; in two, purpura, urticaria, and erythema; in one, purpura, erythema, and œdema; in one, at various times purpura, simple erythema, urticaria, and localized œdema were present; in one, œdema and erythema, and in two, purpura and erythema. Purpura was the most constant lesion, occurring in thirteen of the fourteen cases with nephritis. It is interesting to note that there was not an instance of nephritis with œdema alone, and I have never met with it in pure cases of angioneurotic œdema.

The morbid anatomy of this type of nephritis has not been very carefully studied, and I have no post-mortems on any of the fatal cases in my series. Dr. W. T. Watson,[1] of Baltimore, has reported a remarkable case in a girl, aged ten years, who had had for two or three months transient pains in the abdomen. On the evening of January 28th she had a chill, followed by vomiting and fever; on the 31st, patches of erythema and maculæ; on February 1st, arthritis; on February 2d, purpuric spots; on February 3d, acute nephritis. On March 1st there was an aggravation of the condition with blood in the urine. On March 5th there was almost complete anuria, followed by general anasarca and death on the 12th. There was no endocarditis. The spleen was enlarged and firm. The kidneys were immensely enlarged, measuring each 12 x 7 cm. The cortices were pale, the striations distinct, the glomeruli prominent as gray, translucent nodules, almost like miliary tubercles. There were some small hemorrhages. Dr. W. McCallum, who made the autopsy, reports that microscopically the kidney shows extensive degeneration in the renal epithelium. Many tubules are partly filled with desquamated and degenerated epithelial cells, while the lining of others is ragged and shows fatty change. The tubules contain, besides the desquamated cells, many hyaline casts, or are sometimes filled with red blood corpuscles. The glomeruli form the most striking feature in the section. The Malpighian tuft is in almost everyone much compressed by the new growth of a mass of cells in the area of the capsular space which forms a crescentic mass. These cells lie in a connective-tissue network, which is continuous with the connective tissue outside the capsule. They have often small, subdivided, capsular spaces lined by capsular epithelium, suggesting that

[1] Maryland Medical Journal, 1903.

the original capsular space was merely invaded by this new growth. Dr. McCallum tells me that the case belongs to a group which has been lately described under the name of adhesive glomerulonephritis, in which there is not only a proliferation of the epithelial cells, but also a new-growth of connective tissue in the capsules.

Arthritis or arthritic pains were present in seventeen cases. The joint lesions were slight, as a rule; in no case was there severe polyarthritis. The relation of the rheumatic poison to the arthritis and the other lesions is clear enough in some cases, but we cannot say that the arthritis is a hall-mark by which we can always recognize the rheumatic poison. A great many of the cases of arthritic purpura or the peliosis rheumatica have, I believe, nothing to do with the poison of rheumatism. On the other hand, erythema, with or without purpura and arthritis, may be in children, as are endocarditis, tonsillitis, and subcutaneous fibroid nodules, manifestations of the rheumatic poison—links in the rheumatic chain.

Hemorrhages from the Mucous Membranes. There may be recurring severe attacks of epistaxis, as in Case X.; more frequently they are slight. With the colic blood may be passed, usually in small amounts; it occurred in seven cases. Blood was passed with the urine in eight cases, in all in association with nephritis. In Case XIV., after outbreaks of urticaria for years, the final symptoms were those of a severe purpura hemorrhagica.

Lastly, it is of interest to tabulate the cases according to current nomenclature of skin diseases. In five purpura was the only lesion; in four, with arthritis; four, with fever. In seven there was the common combination of purpura with raised wheals—purpura urticans—which is the usual lesion of peliosis rheumatica. In five cases there was angioneurotic œdema, sometimes occurring alone, more frequently with other erythematous lesions, or alternating with them. Erythematous lesions occurred in fourteen cases, in only two alone, with swelling in the form of erythematous blotches, usually with purpura or urticaria, once only with vesiculation of an extensive character.

A word as to treatment. The very chronic cases with recurring colic for years may resist all measures. Alterative courses of gray powder, with careful dieting, may be helpful. With angioneurotic œdema nitroglycerin in full doses may be tried. Dr. Love writes that in his remarkable case (No. XXV.) camphor has done good. In such severe types as Case XIX. nothing seems to arrest the progress. The chief danger is from the kidneys, and in so frequently presenting this subject I have hoped to impress upon my colleagues the importance of recognizing this form of nephritis, and of taking early precautions to prevent its progress, against which I think protracted rest in bed and a milk diet are the best means at our disposal.

LIST OF CASES WITH VISCERAL LESIONS OF THE ERYTHEMA GROUP.

No.	Name.	Age and sex.	Skin lesions.				Fever.	Colic.	Vomiting.	Diarrhœa.	Hemorrhages.	Nephritis.	Albumin.	Arthritis or arthritic pains.	Endocarditis.	Enlarged spleen.	Other complication.	Mode of death.	Duration.	Remarks.
			Purpura.	Urticaria.	Œdema.	Erythema.														
1	B. L.	M. 27	...	...	...	1	1	1	1	...	....	...	...	...	...	1	....	....	6 yrs.	Delirium in attacks.
2	W. E. B.	M. 11	1	1	1	1	...	1	...	...	Nose.	...	...	1	...	1	Bronchitis, cough, emphysema, pneumonia.	Pericarditis.	5 yrs.	
3	I. W.	M. 6	1	1	...	...	...	1	...	1	Bowels.	1	1	1	...	...	....	Dropsy & uræmia.	10 wks.	
4	B. H.	M. 46	1	1	...	...	...	1	1	1	....	1	1	1						
5	J. D.	M. 28	1	1	...	1	1	1	1	...	Urine.	1	1	1	...	...	Gonorrhœa.	....	2 mos.	Came on after gonorrhœa.
6	W. L.	M. 9	1	...	...	...	1	1	1	...	Bowels.	1	1	1	...	...	....	Pneumonia.	Third attack.	Death from pneumonia a month after onset of third attack.
7	W. R.	F. 4	1	1	1	...	1	1	...	...	....	...	1	1	...	...	....	....	About 3 wks.	
8	O. L.	F. 5	1	...	...	...	...	1	...	1	Urine.	1	1	1	...	...	....	Uræmia.	......	General anasarca.
9	L. J.	M. 12	1	1	...	...	...	1	1	...	....	...	...	1	...	...	....	....	......	Remarkable case; symptoms like purpura hemorrhagica.
10	B. W.	M. 30	1	1	...	...	...	1	1	...	Nose, recurring attacks; gums.									
11	A. R.	F. 18	1	1	...	...	...	1	1	...	Stomach, bowels, lungs.	...	...	1	...	...	....	....	4 yrs.	Recurring attacks of great severity.
12	B. L.	F. 24	...	1	...	1	1	1												
13	R. B.	F. 49	...	...	...	1 exnd.	1	1	...	...	....	...	...	1	...	1				
14	A. D.	M. 57	1	1	...	...	...	1	1	...	Stomach, bowels, urine.	1	1	...	...	..	Bronchitis.	Uræmia.	27 yrs.	Extraordinary case; hemorrhages in final attack.

15	C. A. R.	M. 29	1	1	1	...	...	1	...	..	Urine.	1	1	...	...	...	Aphasia and hemiplegia, 5 or 6 attacks.	....	13 to 14 years.	Remarkable case.
16	H. L.	M. 11	1	...	...	...	...	1	1	...	....	...	...	1						
17	G. K.	M. 18	...	1	...	1	...	1	...	...	....	...	...	1	Apex mur.					
18	B. P.	F. 7	1	...	...	1	1	1	1	...	Bowels.	...	...	1	...	1	....	....	......	Remarkable case; recurring colic for five years; case like No. 26.
19	E. C.	F. 15	...	...	1	1	1	...	...	...	....	1	1	...	...	1	Otitis, enl. lymph glands.	Uræmia.	7 mos.	
20	M. R.	M. 15	1	1	...	1	...	1	...	...	Bowels. urine.	1	1	...	...	1	....	....	......	Admitted for appendicitis.
21	J. D.	M. 12	1	...	...	...	1	1	1	...	Urine.	1	1	...	...	...	Otitis.			
22	E. C.	F. 6	1	1	...	...	...	1	...	...	Urine.	1	1	1						
23	S. E. W.	F. 14	1	1	...	1	1	1	1	1	....	...	...	1	1 mur.	1				
24	M. S.	M. 8	1	...	...	1	...	..	...	...	....	1	1							
25	N. D.	M. 14	...	1	1	1	...	...	...	...	....	...	...	...	...	...	Swelling of throat, edema of face, spasmodic croup.	....	......	Remarkable case.
26	L. E.	F. 24	1	...	...	1	1	...	...	...	....	1	1	...	...	...	Pneumonia, thrombosis left femoral vein, enlargement lymphatic glands.	Uræmia.	8 mos.	Extraordinary case, like No. 19.
27	D. B.	F. 13	...	1	...	1	1	1	1	...	....	...	...	...	Syst. mur.	...	....	....	......	Colic from infancy.
28	A. S. A.	M. 26	1	...	...	...	1	1	1	1	Bowels.	...	...	1						
29	E. F.	M. 5	1	...	...	...	1	1	1	...	Bowels.	1	1	1	..	...	Otitis media.			

A CLINICAL AND PATHOLOGICAL STUDY OF TWO CASES OF SPLENIC ANÆMIA, WITH EARLY AND LATE STAGES OF CIRRHOSIS.

By George Dock, A.M., M.D.,
PROFESSOR OF INTERNAL MEDICINE IN THE UNIVERSITY OF MICHIGAN,

AND

Aldred Scott Warthin, Ph.D., M.D.,
PROFESSOR OF PATHOLOGY IN THE UNIVERSITY OF MICHIGAN.

(From the Laboratories of Internal Medicine and Pathology, University of Michigan, Ann Arbor.)

INTRODUCTION.

There is a growing belief in the existence of a disease described under many names—always a sign of ignorance—but at the present time called splenic anæmia more frequently than by any of the other synonyms. The term has been loosely applied, and, in fact, invites loose application, unless one has some acquaintance with the literature of splenic diseases and remembers "the good rule laid down by Socrates," as quoted by Osler. With that precaution, we think with Osler and Senator that splenic anæmia is a better word for the purpose than any other yet suggested. Since Banti showed the evolution of certain cases with enlarged spleen and anæmia into later stages with ascites and cirrhosis of the liver, his name has been used by some as a synonym, and, although Osler's suggestion that it be applied only to the later stages will doubtless have many followers, it will often be difficult to draw a line; for, though Banti thought he had discovered a disease distinct from splenic anæmia, he was aware of the difficulty of making a final conclusion. Even in the more recent literature, under the names splenic anæmia and Banti's disease, we find, besides some obviously faulty diagnoses, certain cases that differ from the generally accepted picture in some details. Senator, in adding greatly to our knowledge, showed that the symptomatology of the blood is not as Banti described it. Since not only this, but also many other allied topics in splenic pathology are only beginning to receive investigation, it is necessary to enlarge the casuistry and to collect and report as many cases as possible in which the clinical and anatomical features have been carefully studied. Banti's suggestion of extirpation of the spleen has already been of great benefit, not only as a therapeutic measure, but by increasing our knowledge of the changes in different stages, and should be followed in well-selected cases.

In the following we report two cases bearing upon the subject. One of these seems a good example of splenic anæmia in a comparatively early period. Clinically it is a good example of splenic anæmia in the old sense, but anatomically it shows changes in the liver that indicate the occurrence of cirrhosis of the liver had the condition gone on longer. The other has many of the features of Banti's late stage, but is complicated by an old and obscure peritonitis. Since this does not seem to have causal relations with the important changes in the liver and spleen, we report the case on account of the other changes. We do not intend to consider now the literature of the subject, reserving that for another time.

Part I. Clinical (Dr. Dock).

Case I. *Splenomegaly, anæmia; removal of spleen; death. Fibrosis of spleen; beginning fibrosis of liver; stenosis and calcification of the portal vein; hyperplasia of hæmolymph nodes; new formation of lymphoid tissue.*—I. T. A., aged forty-one years, was admitted to the University Hospital as an out-patient July 27, 1899.

Family History. Father died at seventy-two years, having had a cough for twenty years. Mother died at seventy-eight years, of pneumonia. Patient had six sisters and three brothers; two brothers and two sisters are alive. Two sisters died of consumption, one in childbirth, one of "stomach disease." One brother died of "brain disease." Patient has one daughter, aged ten years, in good health. (Though a strong and robust girl, she had extensive pharyngeal adenoids, besides enlarged tonsils, and some months after this underwent operation for appendicitis, when the lymphoid tissue of the appendix was found to show a marked hyperplasia without other signs of appendicitis.) The patient's wife died one year ago, of leukæmia. (She was treated as an in-patient and out-patient of the Medical Clinic for a year and a half, during which time the husband showed a great interest in splenic disease, bringing to the hospital several patients supposed to have enlarged spleens.)

Habits and Occupations. Patient lived on a farm in his youth; since the age of twenty-one years has been in mercantile business. Has worked hard and at long hours, but has not suffered from that, and has not been unusually exposed. Meals have been regular; food good. Appetite has always been good, but bowels irregular. Has used little tea and coffee for ten years; alcohol rarely; tobacco not at all.

Previous Diseases. Had the usual diseases of children; had a severe fever, probably typhoid, seventeen years ago, and a mild attack of influenza a few years ago. Had always been subject to sick headache, but in 1901 had rectal "polyps and ulcers" operated (by a notorious "orificial surgeon"), and headaches have been less severe since then. Most careful inquiry could elicit no history of venereal disease.

Present Disease. About a week ago first noticed a soreness in the left hypochondrium and uneasiness in the abdomen, and on feeling discovered a tumor in the left side. He had noticed a gradual enlargement of the abdomen for a year, but thought nothing of it.

Status præsens, July 27, 1899 (Dr. Arneill). Frame of medium size, rather slender; muscles small and soft; panniculus thin; weight, 126 pounds, the usual weight in summer. The bones and joints are normal;

the inguinal glands can be felt; the other superficial lymphatic glands are not enlarged.

The gait is normal, appearance somewhat cachectic, expression depressed, mind clear.

The skin is somewhat pale and sallow, the visible mucous membranes of fair color.

The teeth are artificial; the tongue is of medium size; has a thin, white, moist coat.

The thorax is of good size and shape; expansion moderate; percussion and auscultation of lungs negative.

The apex-beat is in the fourth interspace, one inch inside the nipple line; the dulness is not enlarged; the sounds normal; no murmurs.

The abdomen is an inch above the level of the ribs, larger in the left side. The liver dulness extends from the sixth interspace to the edge of the ribs; the thin edge can be felt an inch below the ribs in deep inspiration. The splenic dulness begins on the seventh rib, in the mid-axillary line; extends through Traube's space to the navel line in the left nipple line, and two inches below the navel in the middle line. On palpation a hard mass can be felt in this region, having a sharp angle two and a half inches below the navel. A sharp edge runs up one inch to the right of the navel, and shows a notch an inch above the navel.

The radial artery is somewhat tortuous, the pulse easily compressed, moderately full, tension medium, rate 90, regular. The veins of the thorax, especially on the right side and shoulder, are easily seen. The patient says this has always been so.

The urine shows a trace of albumin; no casts; otherwise negative.

The blood: red corpuscles, 4,480,000; leukocytes, 5857; hæmoglobin, 75.

July 29th. Test breakfast shows good digestion and motor power; Congo positive; Günzberg negative. The patient was ordered Fowler's solution and dilute hydrochloric acid.

August 29th. Patient returns for examination, saying he feels better at times. He complains of pain in the right side. The tumor is still present, the boundaries being the same as in the previous examination. Leukocytes, 6366.

September 20th. The patient is still sallow and cachectic, the spleen slightly smaller than at the last examination.

Examination of the stained blood taken at the early visits had shown red corpuscles of fairly uniform size, a few normoblasts, no megaloblasts or myelocytes. Returning from my vacation, I examined, with great interest, the specimens that had been preserved. Finding nothing essentially different from what is noted above, I sent for the patient, found the history and physical condition accurately described, and made further examinations of the blood.

22*d.* Differential count (Dr. Dock). Small lymphocytes, 32 per cent.; large lymphocytes, 5 per cent.; large mononuclear and transitional, 6 per cent.; polymorphonuclear, 52 per cent.; eosinophiles, 4 per cent.; degenerates, 1 per cent.; normoblasts, 4 to 100 leukocytes. The red corpuscles vary considerably in size and shape, but there are no very large or very small cells. Many cells show vacuoles. There are no polychromatophiles. The normoblasts have the usual characters well marked. Only one shows irregular staining of the nucleus. The polymorphonuclear leukocytes show a good many large ones, with small, deeply-staining nuclei. The lymphocytes are mostly very small, the nuclei staining deeply and showing fragmentation. The eosinophile cells are all of normal appearance.

The general appearance of the blood resembled that often seen in pernicious anæmia at times of comparatively good health. Numerous

Fig. 1.

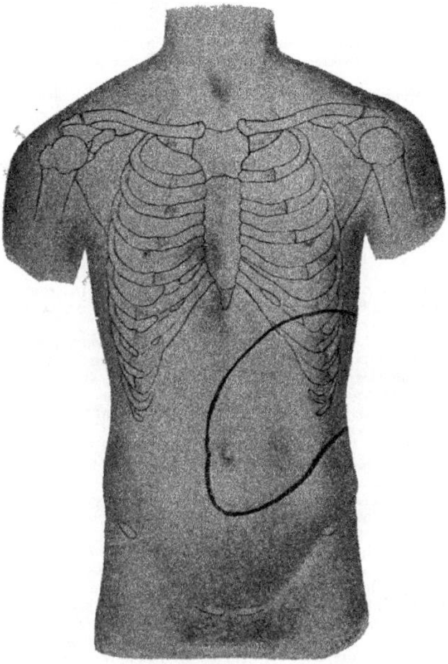

Case I.

examinations showed a total absence of megaloblasts and of Ehrlich's myelocytes, as well as of any other indication of bone-marrow disease. The diagnosis of leukæmia in the aleukæmic stage, such as the patient's wife had at one time, was ruled out, and as the result of a differential diagnosis not necessary to detail here, splenic anæmia was accepted. In view of the theory of Banti and of the operations based on it or a similar theory, I advised an attempt at removal of the spleen, which, after some consideration, the patient accepted. The advice was given on October 2d, but as the patient wished to arrange his affairs before the operation, he was examined at long intervals in the next month. In this period there was an interesting change in the proportion of the various forms of leukocytes, as appears best from the following counts, which include all up to the last day:

29th. Hæmoglobin, 60; red blood corpuscles, 3,640,000; leukocytes, 2037; normoblasts, 1 per cent.; small lymphocytes, 22.5 per cent.; large lymphocytes, 3.6 per cent.; transitionals, 1.5 per cent.; polymorphonuclears, 60.1 per cent.; eosinophiles, 5 per cent.; degenerates, 7.3 per cent.

October 2d. Hæmoglobin, 70; red blood corpuscles, 4,288,000; lenkocytes, 2546; normoblasts, 1 per cent.; small lymphocytes, 25 per cent.; large lymphocytes, 3 per cent.; transitionals, 3 per cent.; polymorphonuclears, 63 per cent.; eosinophiles, 3 per cent.

15th. Normoblasts, 1 per cent.; small lymphocytes, 15.5 per cent.; large lymphocytes, 5 per cent.; transitionals, 1 per cent.; polymorphonuclears, 75.5 per cent.; eosinophiles, 3 per cent.

November 1st. Hæmoglobin, 75; red blood corpuscles, 4,300,000; normoblasts, 0.9 per cent.; small lymphocytes, 18 per cent.; transitionals, 7.5 per cent.; polymorphonuclears, 78 per cent.; eosinophiles, 3.5 per cent.

3d. Normoblasts, 1.1 per cent.; small lymphocytes, 8.6 per cent.; large lymphocytes, 13.2 per cent.; polymorphonuclears, 76 per cent.; eosinophiles, 2.6 per cent.

4th. Leukocytes, 3056; normoblasts, 1 per cent.; small lymphocytes, 6 per cent.; large lymphocytes, 4.33 per cent.; transitionals, 2.66 per cent.; polymorphonuclears, 85.66 per cent.; eosinophiles, 1.33 per cent.

6th. During anæsthesia, leukocytes, 4909; small lymphocytes, 6 per cent.; large lymphocytes, 4 per cent.; transitionals, 4 per cent.; polymorphonuclears, 84.5 per cent.; eosinophiles, 1.5 per cent.

7th. Leukocytes, 18,080; normoblasts, 4 per cent.; large lymphocytes, 1.5 per cent.; transitionals, 4.6 per cent.; polymorphonuclears, 91.9 per cent.; degenerates, 1.9 per cent.

9th. Leukocytes, 21,000; normoblasts, 6 per cent.; large lymphocytes, 2.9 per cent.; transitionals, 4.6 per cent.; polymorphonuclears, 90.8 per cent.; degenerates, 1.4 per cent.

Not only were the small lymphocytes less numerous, but the most typical forms were even fewer than the figures indicated, because the small and large lymphocytes showed many intermediate forms. The nuclei stained less intensely, but clearly, resembling those of large lymphocytes. Degenerated leukocytes were usually numerous up to the time of operating, and were nearly all of the polymorphonuclear class. These cells, therefore, were more numerous than in the beginning of the observation, but showed an unusual tendency to break down. While they are largely artefacts as found in the preparations, the variable numbers are suggestive.

October 31st. Patient enters hospital. Appetite is good; general condition as before.

November 3d. The spleen extends from one and a half to two inches below the navel, in the middle and left parasternal lines. There is a palpable groove half an inch above the navel.

6th. The spleen was removed under ether anæsthesia by Dr. C. B. Nancrede. There was considerable distention of the intestines. The spleen had very few adhesions at the anterior surface, but there were many at the upper end. The upper end was unusually thick in proportion to the other dimensions, and this, with the adhesions and the great size of the vessels, made the removal unusually difficult. Slight symptoms of shock appeared as the vessels were being tied. The pulse and respiration were good all through, but perspiration became profuse just at the end. After the operation there was nausea, tympanites, freqnent and small pulse; the mind was clear. The patient, who had before looked on the operation with calmness, became very anxious, and on November 9th, three days after the operation, became collapsed, with cold skin, sweating, pallor, small and soft pulse of 88 beats to the minute, and died on November 10th, at 3.30 P.M.

CASE II. *Intestinal hemorrhage with diarrhœa; ascites; splenomegaly; fibroid tumors of uterus; laparotomy; removal of fibroids; discovery of cirrhosis of liver at operation; death from hemorrhage from varicose vein in stomach; sclerosis and calcification of portal vein; fibrosis of spleen and liver (atrophic cirrhosis); hyperplasia of hæmolymph nodes.*—Mrs. M. S., aged fifty-three years, housewife, born in Michigan, was admitted to the Medical Clinic of the University Hospital October 7, 1902. She had entered the Surgical Clinic for treatment of hernia, but was referred to the Internal Clinic on account of ascites.

Family History. Mother died at age of fifty-eight years, of "consumption." Father died at seventy-two of "heart disease." Four brothers and four sisters are in good health. Habits and mode of life have been good.

Previous History. Patient had whooping-cough, measles, and mumps in childhood, with good recoveries. Menstruation began at fourteen, stopped for a year, and was regular after that, lasting about three to four days, without unusual symptoms. At thirteen had an attack of "dysentery," in which she passed much blood. At nineteen was married. Has never been pregnant. (No reason for this could be discovered. Syphilis seems positively excluded.) Menopause in fiftieth year.

Six years ago the patient had "dysentery," and was confined to bed for six weeks. She passed large amounts of blood with loose and watery stools. Since then she has had similar attacks at intervals. A week before admission had a slight diarrhœa without blood in the stools. After the attack six years ago the abdomen gradually became larger, and at that time Dr. H. A. Shurtleff, of Partello, Mich., discovered free fluid in the abdomen, by physical signs. Soon after that œdema of the legs and ankles came on, lasting for two months. It has recurred at intervals since then, but less severely. The umbilical hernia appeared after vomiting, three years ago, and has grown larger; the inguinal hernia came on after coughing, one and a half years ago.

The patient now complains of constant soreness over the whole abdomen. She is constipated and has frequent desire to defecate, but bowels are moved with difficulty. Appetite fair, but patient eats sparingly on account of feeling of distention and sensation of weight in abdomen.

Status præsens, October 7, 1902. Medium height, slender frame; muscles small and soft; panniculus scanty; weighs 120 pounds; best weight, ten years ago, 150. The joints are normal, reflexes not altered, superficial lymphatic glands not enlarged.

The patient looks weak and cachectic, the expression is weary; mind clear.

The skin is pale, sallow, and inelastic; the visible mucous membrane pale; there is no œdema.

FIG. 2.

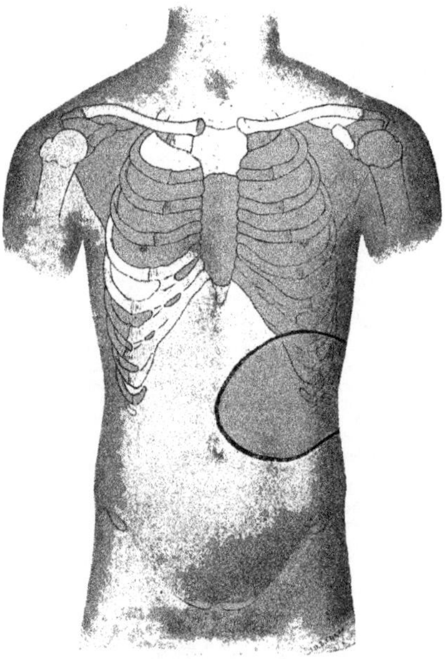

CASE II.

The teeth are artificial; the tongue is white-coated.

The thorax is broad, short, wide; epigastric angle wide and lower aperture of thorax distended. The expansion is fairly good, and symmetrical. The right lower lung border is on the sixth rib, the descent limited. Percussion of lung, front and back, negative. Auscultation reveals good vesicular murmur.

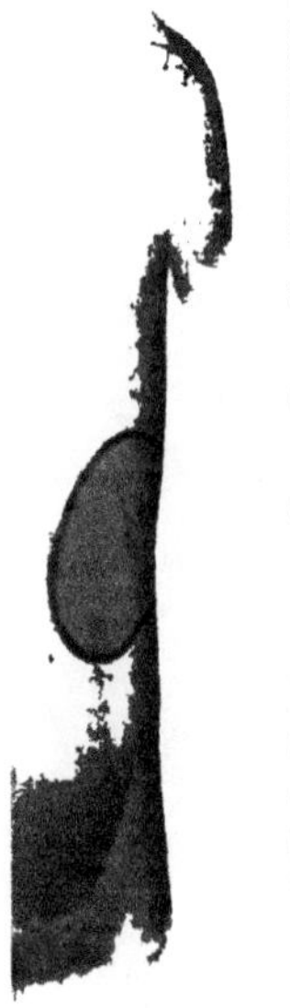

Heart. The apex-beat is indistinct, but can be felt in the fourth interspace, just inside the nipple line. There is a faint pulsation in the third left interspace. Cardiac dulness begins on the third rib, extends to within half an inch of the nipple line. Dulness under the sternum from the fourth rib down to the right of the sternum in the fifth interspace, one finger's breadth. The apex sounds are clear, the first accentuated. In the pulmonary area there is a short systolic murmur, followed by an accentuated second sound, lower than the aortic second. Radial pulse slightly tortuous, perhaps slightly thickened; rhythm regular, tension low.

The abdomen is enlarged, measuring thirty-seven inches at the umbilicus. It is bulging at the sides and flattened on top, with a prominence in the umbilical region. (During the examination this prominence subsided, leaving a slight depression in the same place.) The superficial abdominal veins are not enlarged. There are a few large venules over the anterior spines of the iliac bones. In the left side, above and below the iliac crest, some small veins are visible through the skin. On sitting up the protrusion reappears in the umbilical region, becoming larger than before. There is also a wide separation of the recti, permitting a great protrusion all the length of the abdomen. A large hernia also appears in the right inguinal region. The intestines can be plainly felt through the skin in the middle part.

Lying down, there is dulness on percussion in both flanks, almost to the nipple lines, and in front two inches above the pubes. The lines change quickly on change of position. Fluctuation is not distinct. Palpation of the lower abdomen is negative.

The liver dulness reaches to the margin of the ribs in the nipple line. Palpation is unsatisfactory on account of the distention.

Splenic dulness begins at the seventh rib, and is continuous with the dulness in the flank. The lower end can be felt about three inches below the edge of the rib.

Examination of the anus and rectum shows the small atrophic tags of old external hemorrhoids, and very small internal hemorrhoids, without evidence of hemorrhage. The mucosa shows a bleeding spot the size of a pinhead about six inches from the sphincter.

Examination of the pelvic organs (Dr. Peterson): negative.

Examination of urine: negative.

The blood flows freely; is thin; bright red. Red blood corpuscles, 2,800,000; leukocytes, 5857; hæmoglobin, 60 per cent. The differential count gave: small lymphocytes, 6 per cent.; large lymphocytes, 5.9 per cent.; large mononuclears and transitionals, 4.2 per cent.; polymorphonuclears, 81.7 per cent.; eosinophiles, 1.2 per cent.; degenerates, 0.6 per cent.; normoblasts, 3 per mille. The red corpuscles show very slight variation in size and shape.

October 21st. The superficial veins of the abdomen are slightly distended. Abdomen tapped in Monro's point and 3800 c.c. of fluid withdrawn. The fluid is clear, reddish-yellow; specific gravity, 1012. It contains a slight increase of red blood corpuscles. Differential count of the other cells: small lymphocytes, 53 per cent.; large lymphocytes, 8 per cent.; polymorphonuclears, 6 per cent.; large mononuclears, 33 per cent. The large mononuclear cells have the appearance of young endothelial cells; the lymphocytes partly that of endothelial cells, partly that of ordinary lymphocytes.

After tapping, the abdomen measures thirty-two and three-quarter inches at the umbilicus. The spleen can be easily felt three fingers' breadth below the ribs, and reaching to the median line. Liver dulness not quite to edge of ribs. Liver cannot be felt.

22d. Patient has been more comfortable since the tapping. There is gaseous distention in the right side. The spleen reaches the navel line in the nipple line and the middle line, four fingers' breadth above the umbilicus. The surface of the spleen is smooth, flat; the edge thick; there is a notch above the lower end, on the inner side.

24th. The abdomen is larger; thirty-four and a half inches. Signs of free fluid not so extensive as before the tapping. The ankles are slightly œdematous. The superficial abdominal veins are not enlarged. No murmur in the epigastric region.

Blood. Red corpuscles, 4,266,666; leukocytes, 7894; hæmoglobin, 70 per cent. Differential count: small lymphocytes, 3.4 per cent.; large lymphocytes, 6.4 per cent.; transitionals, 11.4 per cent.; polymorphonuclears, 77 per cent.; eosinophiles, 1 per cent.; degenerates, 0.8 per cent. No nucleated red cells found; a few poikilocytes.

30th. The patient has complained much of pain and soreness in the pelvis, which could not be explained by any of the manipulations practised upon her. Another consultation was held with Dr. Peterson, and an examination made under ether. A small, hard mass was found in front of the uterus, apparently a fibroid tumor.

Up to this time the diagnosis had not been sufficiently clear to offer a surgical operation to the patient, who was convinced that medicines would not relieve her. Cirrhosis of the liver, most likely at first glance, was made doubtful on account of the history, the long duration of ascites without more venous enlargement, and the relatively large spleen. A Talma operation did not seem warranted. A late stage of Banti's disease seemed ruled out also by the long duration of the ascites and relatively good condition of the blood. On the other hand, I presented the patient both in clinic and before the Medical Society as a possible case of late Banti, with a complication, perhaps in the pelvis, causing chronic peritonitis, and with the blood picture (polymorphonuclears increased relatively) obscured by the local conditions in the abdomen. Here, too, surgical intervention did not seem more promising than it did on the theory of cirrhosis, because if the case were one of Banti's it was probably past the aid of surgery; and my surgical colleague declined to explore in order to determine that point. Tuberculosis and malignant disease of the peritoneum were ruled out by the long duration and the character of the fluid, as well as other features not necessary to point out. Chronic peritonitis due to an undiscovered disease in the pelvis was a diagnosis I took up several times to explain the ascites as an associated phenomenon with the enlarged spleen, but up to the discovery of the fibroid this diagnosis did not lead to an exploration.

Although the fibroid could not be correlated with the enlarged spleen, or even the ascites, save as an exceptional condition, it gave us something to operate for, and so meet the pressing wishes of the patient as well as our own desires for an exploration. Accordingly, Dr. Peterson operated November 7th. A large amount of fluid having the same character as that previously examined escaped from the incision. An irregular, roundish tumor, one and a half inches in diameter, was found adherent to the lower and anterior part of the uterus. It proved to be a calcified fibromyoma. The uterus was very small, the fundus round and of stony hardness. It was found to be merely a shell around another calcified fibroid, and was removed. There was no distinct disease of the tubes and ovaries, but there were many adhesions around all the pelvic organs. The omentum was fastened low down by adhesions. The spleen was large, the lower surface uneven. The liver was also uneven to the touch, though as seen by light thrown into the abdominal cavity it showed only slight granular change. There were numerous adhesions around the liver and spleen.

The wound healed well at first, but left a small sinus. The ascites gradually returned, and on December 2 five litres of fluid were removed. Specific gravity, 1012.

December 6th. The patient returned to the medical ward. *Status præsens:* The patient looks tired and sleepy, and complains of feeling sick all over. She has had diarrhœa, with great pain. The stools were dark and watery, and contained fresh blood. The abdomen measures thirty-four inches. The abdominal veins are distinct, but not swollen. Palpation of the abdomen causes pain. The wall is soft in general. There is a flattened mass just above the navel line and two inches to the left of the navel, apparently adherent to the deep tissues. The spleen extends not quite two fingers' breadth below the ribs in the nipple line, three fingers' breadth in the parasternal line. There is a soft, blowing, systolic murmur over the base of the heart. A few crackling râles can be heard in the right axilla.

There had been leukocytosis ever since the operation. from 10,000 to 18,000 per cm., with increased percentage of polymorphonuclear cells and many degenerates.

Red blood corpuscles, 3,040,000; leukocytes, 17,200; hæmoglobin, 40 per cent. Differential count: small lymphocytes, 12.2 per cent.; large lymphocytes, 2.2 per cent.; transitionals, 1.1 per cent.; polymorphonuclear, 84 per cent.; eosinophiles, 0.45 per cent. No nucleated reds. Moderate poikilocytosis.

At 1.45 P.M. the patient vomited half a pint of blood, and twenty minutes later a similar quantity. The blood is bright red, alkaline; contains large clots. At 6.30 P.M. patient vomited about six ounces of bloody fluid. Pulse small and irregular. Patient feels weak, dizzy, and nauseated.

7th. Patient feels better. Has not vomited, but passed bloody fluid per rectum.

8th. Patient is weaker and in great pain. Retention of urine.

9th. Still passing bloody fluid per rectum. Cannot swallow.

10th. Incontinence of rectum.

11th. Died at 12.05 P.M.

PART II. PATHOLOGY (DR. WARTHIN).

CASE I.—Mr. I. A., aged forty-one years, American. Died November 10, 1899, at 3.30 P.M. Autopsy by Dr. Warthin, 7.30 P.M., November 10, 1899.

Autopsy Protocol. Body of average height and build. No anomalies or deformities. No signs of trauma. In the left hypochondrium there is a recent laparotomy wound, extending from the edge of the ribs to within three fingers' breadth above the iliac crest. It is covered with surgical dressings. On removing these the edges of the wound are found to be separated and a fold of intestine protruding. Edges of the wound are discolored (gray to black), but present no evidences of pus. Abdomen distended above the level of the ribs.

The skin is pale, sallow; there is slight hypostasis posteriorly; small boil on right forearm; teeth artificial; hair is negative. The panniculus is greatly decreased; no œdema; muscles are small and emaciated; rigor mortis is present throughout. The extremities are cold. There are no signs of decomposition.

Brain and *spinal cord* not examined. (No permission.)

Diaphragm at the fourth rib on the right; fifth rib on the left.

Position of thoracic organs is normal. Apex of heart in fourth intercostal space, just inside of the nipple line. The mediastinum is rich in fat; no enlarged glands. The thymus fat is in large amount, and in it there is found a pinkish lobulated body 3 cm. long by 1 cm. in diameter. There is no fluid in the pleural cavity. Both pleuræ are free; there are no adhesions.

The *pericardium* is lax; contains a very small amount of clear fluid. Subepicardial fat is slightly increased.

Heart weighs 320 grams; is about the size of cadaver's right fist. The auricles contain ante-mortem white clots; the ventricles are filled with fluid blood and currant-jelly clot. The heart muscle is firm, brownish-red; papillary muscles are prominent. The left ventricle wall measures 15 to 20 mm. in thickness. The endocardium is slightly thickened. The pulmonary, tricuspid, and aortic orifices and valves are normal. The mitral orifice is rather small; does not admit two fingers. Mitral flaps are slightly thickened and shortened. Coronary vessels are negative.

Right lung weighs 272 grams; *left lung* weighs 336 grams. Both lungs are partly collapsed. Pleuræ negative. Slight anthracosis. On section the parenchyma of lungs is grayish-pink; lower lobes slightly hypostatic; no airless areas; very slight exudate on pressure; bronchi are empty; mucosa pale; pulmonary vessels negative; bronchial glands moderately pigmented; on section negative. A number of enlarged glands along the thoracic aorta. On section they are red and spleen-like. The great vessels of the thorax and the thoracic duct are negative.

Mouth and *neck organs* were not examined.

Abdomen. The omentum is rolled up, greatly thickened, and moderately injected, and is adherent to the diaphragm and anterior abdominal wall in the splenic region, and to the peritoneal surface of the ileum by fresh fibrinous exudate. In the region of the spleen there is a large mass of fresh fibrinous adhesions, but no evidence of hemorrhage. Spleen (see below) is absent, having been removed at operation. Ligatures on stumps of splenic vessels are in position. Splenic vessel filled with fresh red thrombi.

The small intestine is greatly distended throughout. The serosa is cloudy, moderately injected, and everywhere covered with a fine fibrinous deposit. Many of the coils are adherent by coarser strings of fibrin, the adhesions being easily separated. The lower sixteen inches of the ileum lie in the left side of the abdomen, a portion of the ileum projecting through the laparotomy wound.. Coils of the ileum are adherent to each other by fibrinous exudate, the adhesions being firmer in neighborhood of wound. They are also adherent to the large intestine by a similar fresh fibrinous exudate. About two and a half inches above the cæcum there are several (six) dark patches in the intestinal serosa, covered with greenish-gray fibrin. These patches are irregular, not triangular in shape, and do not extend entirely around the bowel; some reach about two-thirds of the way. From the serosa these patches extend some little distance into the fat of the mesentery, which shows a superficial necrosis corresponding to the patches of fibrin. These areas have the appearance of having been cauterized; they are all on the upper surface of the mesentery.

The *stomach* is greatly distended, its wall very thin. It lies pressed against the anterior abdominal wall, and was cut during the median incision, letting out a large quantity of sour-smelling gas under high pressure. It contains about 500 c.c. of brown, bile-stained, sour fluid. The mucosa of the stomach shows slight post-mortem change. Veins of stomach wall are greatly distended. The large venous branches in the greater curvature contain fresh thrombi. Around the gastro-epiploica sinistra there is a ligature which includes the serosa of the stomach wall, but not the muscle coats. The coronary veins are greatly dilated, as are also the anastomoses with the œsophageal veins.

The *duodenum* is greatly distended with gas; it contains a small amount of grayish, slimy material. Its mucosa is injected and somewhat swollen. Bile passages are patent.

The *ascending* and *transverse colon* and *cæcum* are greatly distended as far as the splenic flexure, the descending colon being more moderately distended. They contain a small amount of formed feces and a large amount of grayish mucus. The sigmoid flexure and the descending colon are unusually pale and nearly white. The *appendix* is long and narrow, extends into the pelvis; no adhesions about it.

Liver weighs 1280 grams, measures 23 x 15½ x 8 cm.; is small; left lobe very atrophic; right lobe shows posteriorly a number of small anomalous lobules. Capsule is thickened, especially near the ligaments. Veins of capsule congested. Small cavernous angioma, size of a pea, on the upper surface of the right lobe. On section the blood-content is found to be fairly rich. In one of the larger branches of the portal there is a fresh but firm red thrombus. The cut surface of the organ is granular, in some areas markedly so; the granules slightly elevated. The largest granules are paler in color than the remainder of the liver parenchyma, which is of a pale-brown color. Outlines of the lobules are distinct over the greater part of the cut surface; they are smaller than normal. The peripheral zone of the lobules is more grayish, cloudy, and apparently swollen. The connective tissue is apparently increased. In some areas the tissue of Glisson's capsule is thickened, hyaline, and scar-like. In about the middle of the right lobe there is an area about 5 cm. in diameter, which is firmer and lighter in color than the other portions of the cut surface, and is slightly elevated and more distinctly granular. In this area the connective tissue seems to be increased to a greater extent, and the lobules are larger than elsewhere.

The *gall-bladder* is distended, containing about 200 c.c. of dark-brown fluid and three grayish cholesterin stones of small size. Its mucosa is very thin, the wall much stretched.

The *portal vein* is extremely distended, and is filled with a fresh but firm mixed clot. The lumen of the vein at its beginning, just above the union of the splenic and superior mesenteric veins, is irregularly narrowed and partly bridged off by fibrous, valve-like constrictions, which contain calcareous plates. The vein is divided by these fibrous bands into several sac-like spaces, the walls of all these showing calcification. The tortuous lumen barely admits the tip of a lead-pencil or large probe. The stenosis involves the mouth of the splenic vein, almost completely occluding it. The splenic and superior mesenteric veins back of the stenosis are enormously distended and filled with a soft red thrombus, which is continuous with the firmer mixed thrombus filling the portal. In the media of the portal vein at the point of constriction there are thin plates of calcification. The walls of the splenic and mesentery veins are greatly thickened, and present scattered patches of hyalin.

The *pancreas* is of normal size; on section apparently normal, save for congestion and small areas of hemorrhage. The splenic vein and its pancreatic branches are greatly distended, and are filled with firm red thrombi. In the neighborhood of the pancreas there are several glands resembling accessory spleens. They possess very thick capsules.

In the root of the mesentery, particularly near the portion of ileum showing the dark fibrin patches, the lymph glands are slightly enlarged and hyperæmic. Hyperæmic patches are scattered over the surface of the mesentery, in some cases grayish-black; these are covered with fibrinous exudate.

The *retroperitoneal lymph glands* are not enlarged, but are red, firm, and spleen-like. Abdominal aorta, iliacs, etc., negative.

Ureters negative.

Bladder empty, collapsed; mucosa pale.

Adrenals show post-mortem softening of medullary portion.

Kidneys. The fatty capsule of both kidneys is moderately rich in fat; the fibrous capsule strips easily and is not thickened. The right kidney measures 9½ x 5 x 3½ cm., and weighs 128 grams. The left kidney measures 10½ x 4½ x 3 cm., and weighs 112 grams. The surfaces of both kidneys are bright red, and the venæ stellatæ well marked. On section both kidneys are bright red. Cortex of each measures ½ to ¾ cm. Outlines between labyrinths and medullary rays not well defined; glomeruli not visible; consistence firm; bloodvessels engorged; pelvis of left kidney somewhat dilated, that of right negative.

Ureters and *bladder* negative.

Genitals. External genitals negative. Testicles and epididymis negative. Prostate and seminal vesicles not examined.

Aorta, iliacs, iliac veins, femorals, and *vena cava* negative.

Bones. Negative. Right tibia, fourth lumbar vertebra, and several ribs removed. Tibia split longitudinally. Slight hyperplasia of red marrow. Small lymphoid areas throughout the fatty marrow; the largest of these, in the middle of the tibia, measures ½ x ¼ cm.

Peripheral Glands, Nerves, and Vessels. Negative. (Material was taken from all parts and organs of the body, fixed in Flemming's solution, Müller's, mercuric chloride, alcohol and formalin, and embedded in celloidin and paraffin, and stained by ordinary and special staining methods.)

Microscopic. Heart. Sections show atrophy of heart muscle and slight increase of connective tissue.

Lungs. Sections taken from different portions show a number of small recent and old hemorrhagic infarcts. Many of the alveolar walls are thickened, and there is an increase of connective tissue about the larger vessels. In the lower lobes there is slight emphysema. The bloodvessels are congested, and many of the smaller arteries show sclerotic changes. A few organizing thrombi are found. Anthracosis is moderate. There is a slight œdema. In the capillaries there are found numerous emboli of bone-marrow giant cells, similar to those found in the spleen and liver. These are so numerous that three to six may be found in one field. In the small arterioles the protoplasm of the giant cell is preserved, in the capillaries only the deeply-staining knobbed and lobulated nuclei are visible. A few multinuclear giant cells are found in the arterioles.

Liver. In the sections taken from all parts of the liver, with the exception of the elevated area in the middle of the right lobe, the lobules

FIG. 3.

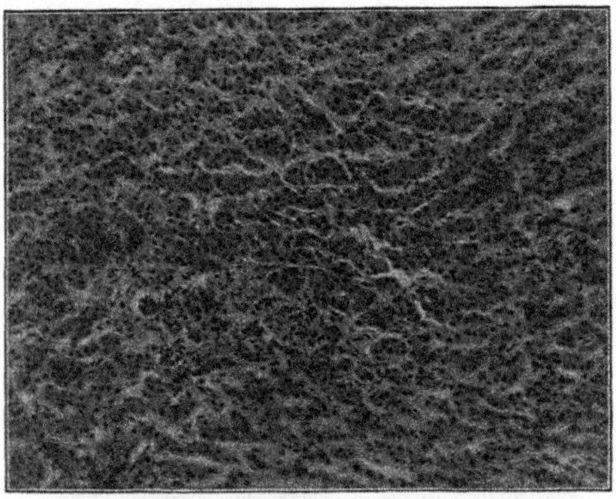

Liver of Case I. Intralobular increase of connective tissue. Early stage of diffuse interstitial hepatitis. Hyperplasia of intralobular reticulum. × 175.

are atrophic, the atrophy involving chiefly the central portions of the lobules. The central veins and capillaries are dilated, while the liver cells of the central zone are atrophic or in part necrotic, or show varying stages of fatty degeneration, cloudy swelling, and necrosis. In some lobules the liver cells of the central zone have completely disappeared. In the majority of lobules there is an endothelial or fibroblastic proliferation in the capillaries of the central zone. This is most marked in those areas showing the most pronounced atrophy or necrosis of the liver cells. The liver rods present a more decided radiating appearance than usual, and in many places appear as if elongated by pressure. The periportal islands of connective tissue are relatively increased in number, the connective tissue in the majority being of a hyaline character and presenting no infiltration. The fine reticulum of the lobules is everywhere increased, but particularly in the areas of most marked atrophy, where it replaces in part the liver cells. In many areas it is very cellular and presents an endothelial or fibroblastic proliferation. With Van Gieson's stain the greater part of the newly formed reticulum stains a light red. By the same stain heavier lines and strands of connective tissue may be seen in places extending into the lobule. Small focal necroses are found scattered throughout the sections; the necrotic areas showing the same endothelial or fibroblastic hyperplasia as seen in the central part of the lobules. Hypertrophic liver cells are also found throughout the lobules. The central veins and branches of the hepatic veins are greatly dilated and their walls thickened. Giant cells are found in the capillaries; they resemble bone-marrow giant cells and are similar to those found in the lungs and spleen, but are not nearly so numerous as in those organs. In many sections the only changes are those of a chronic passive congestion.

Sections taken from the yellowish, elevated area in the middle of the right lobe show that the liver-lobules are larger and the liver cells are increased in size, the blood capillaries being nearly obliterated. Many of the liver-cell nuclei are very large and stain deeply. In Glisson's capsule there is a marked small-celled infiltration and proliferation of the connective tissue and the smaller bile-ducts. The periportal connective tissue is somewhat increased and the finer reticulum of the lobule likewise shows an increase. The central congestion and atrophy are less marked in this portion.

The liver as a whole presents the picture of a chronic passive congestion and atrophy of the central portion of the lobule, with an increase of the reticulum of the lobules, chiefly central, but also periportal. This increase is in many places due to a fibroblastic proliferation. In some areas these changes are so marked as to warrant their interpretation as a beginning stage of cirrhosis, in part central and in part periportal.

Portal Vein. Sections of the wall show sclerotic changes and calcification, involving chiefly the media. No evidence of recent phlebitis. Branches of portal show similar conditions. Fresh thrombi in all branches.

Stomach and intestines present the picture of a chronic passive congestion with atrophy and chronic catarrhal inflammation.

Pancreas shows decrease in size of lobules and a moderate fatty infiltration. Near the middle of the body of organ a small adenoma the size of a pea was found. This consists of tubules lined with simple columnar cells, the majority showing mucoid degeneration. Pancreatic veins greatly dilated, and walls thickened.

Omentum. Congested and œdematous, and showing a marked small-celled infiltration and fibroblastic proliferation, hemorrhage, etc. Surface covered with a fibrinous exudate.

Mesentery. Peritoneal surface shows patches of fibrin. Very slight small-celled infiltration near surface. The necrosed patches on upper surface correspond to small areas of anæmic necrosis caused by the thrombosis of small mesenteric vessels. Mesenteric veins greatly dilated and sclerotic. Throughout the root of the mesentery are small calcareous nodules surrounded by areas of lymphoid cells. Other collections of lymphoid cells surround small concentric hyaline masses; others surround small arterioles showing hyaline thickening of the intima, sometimes arranged in concentric laminæ. As all stages of transition can be found between the calcareous and hyaline nodules and the hyaline vessels with proliferating endothelium, it seems probable that the former represent a latter stage of the process. The cells surrounding the masses are of the character of lymphocytes, they lie in a fine reticulum containing small bloodvessels, and some contain typical germ-centres. They are, therefore, regarded as representing newly formed lymphoid tissue. Similar formations are found throughout the retroperitoneal fat.

Mesenteric Glands. Atrophic, and contain hyaline areas, some of which show calcification. Vessels congested. Stroma increased. Few germ-centres seen. Numerous phagocytes in sinuses.

FIG. 4.

Spleen of Case I. Area showing advanced fibrous hyperplasia of reticulum of pulp. × 175.

Kidneys. Somewhat contracted, the number of glomeruli in a field being greatly increased. Many hyaline and calcified glomeruli are found, as well as numerous cystic ones. Connective-tissue stroma increased in areas. Many of the tubules contain hyaline casts. Bloodvessels congested. No giant cells found in kidney capillaries.

Retroperitoneal Glands. The red spleen-like glands on section are hæmolymph nodes, closely corresponding in structure to that of the normal spleen, and are of the type known as hæmal glands, possessing no lymph vessels or sinuses. They are surrounded by a very thick capsule from which trabeculæ containing unstriped muscle run into the gland. No definite blood sinuses are present; the greater part of the gland structure consists of a pulp-like reticulum and blood spaces lined by endothelium. Lymphoid cells lie in the meshes of the reticulum. Small scattered collections of lymphoid cells suggest follicles or germ centres, but these lack the true vascular relations of splenic follicles. The blood spaces are filled with blood, and occasionally bone-marrow giant cells are found. An unusual number of pigment-containing phagocytes are present in the larger blood spaces. With Mallory's reticulum stain the reticulum appears as a rather coarse, deeply-blue network enclosing spaces filled with blood. The resemblance to normal spleen is so close that the glands no doubt would be classed as accessory spleens. They resemble very closely the spleen-like hæmolymph glands of the hog. The ordinary lymphatic glands of this region are atrophic,

FIG. 5.

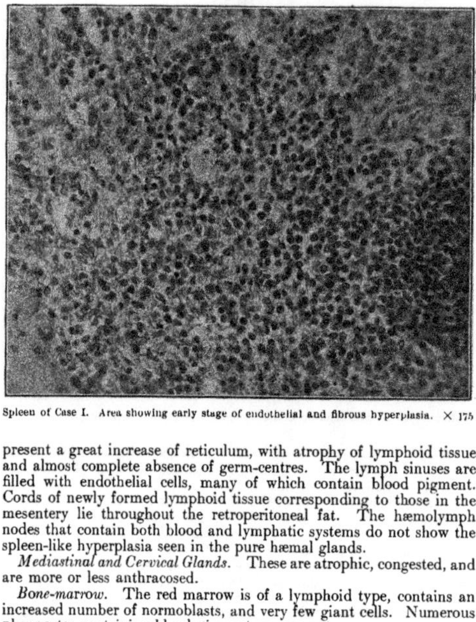

Spleen of Case I. Area showing early stage of endothelial and fibrous hyperplasia. × 175

present a great increase of reticulum, with atrophy of lymphoid tissue and almost complete absence of germ-centres. The lymph sinuses are filled with endothelial cells, many of which contain blood pigment. Cords of newly formed lymphoid tissue corresponding to those in the mesentery lie throughout the retroperitoneal fat. The hæmolymph nodes that contain both blood and lymphatic systems do not show the spleen-like hyperplasia seen in the pure hæmal glands.

Mediastinal and Cervical Glands. These are atrophic, congested, and are more or less anthracosed.

Bone-marrow. The red marrow is of a lymphoid type, contains an increased number of normoblasts, and very few giant cells. Numerous phagocytes containing blood pigment are present.

Spleen. (Removed at operation by Dr. Nancrede, November 6, 1899.) Nearly a perfect oval in shape. It measures 23 x 13 x 9 cm., and weighs 1536 grams. Its capsule is greatly thickened and covered with fine stringy adhesions which are more numerous in the region of the hilum. The enlargement of the organ is most marked in the upper two-thirds, the thickness diminishing below. On the anterior margin there are two notches at the lower third, the lower one of these extending almost through the lower part of the organ and forming a shelf-like depression. In the hilum there is a small accessory spleen. On section the spleen bleeds freely. The pulp is a pale red and of firm consistence.

FIG. 6.

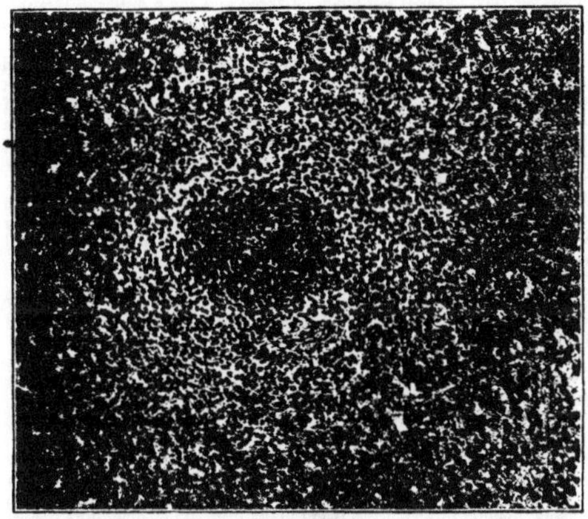

Spleen of Case I. Diffuse fibrous and endothelial hyperplasia of pulp. Hyaline mass in follicle. × 175.

The stroma is greatly increased. Splenic follicles cannot be seen. On exposure to the air no Charcot-Leyden crystals were formed on the surface.

The organ was received warm from the surgeon's hands. Portions were fixed at once in Flemming's solution, Müller's, mercuric chloride, alcohol, and formalin.

Microscopic. The capsule is greatly thickened, consisting of a rather dense hyaline connective tissue. It is covered with partially or wholly organized deposits of fibrin. The trabeculæ are thickened to a less extent and are much farther apart than normally. The lymphoid tissue of the pulp is scanty, the pulp being replaced largely by a dense fibrous network enclosing the enlarged blood spaces. These are lined and in many cases partly filled by large endothelial or reticular cells having one or more lightly staining nuclei, and in the majority of cases nucleoli. The fibrous tissue represents a hyperplasia of the reticulum of the pulp, the endothelial cells lining the blood spaces apparently taking part in the formation of the new fibrous tissue. In many places, particularly beneath the capsule, it is more dense and hyaline, and the blood spaces are smaller. In the denser areas the fibrous tissue stains deep red with Van Gieson's. In such areas the lymphocytes are very scanty and the endothelial cells are not so numerous. In other portions of the pulp the fibrous tissue is less dense, more cellular, stains lighter with Van Gieson's, and presents a more fibroblastic character. In such areas the blood spaces are much enlarged and the number of lymphocytes and endothelial cells much greater. The latter are found not only in the spaces, but also between the fibrillæ of the new connective tissue. Occasional giant cells resembling those of the bone-marrow are found in the blood spaces; they are similar to those found in the lungs and liver, and are probably to be regarded as emboli. There is no evidence of their origin *in situ*. Occasional nucleated red blood cells are found in the blood of the pulp spaces, but neither the ordinary stains nor the triacid stain, etc., show any peculiar cells, myelocytes, or other bone-marrow elements to be present. In the neighborhood of the trabeculæ there are found occasional small collections of densely packed lymphoid cells resembling follicles. A thickened hyaline arteriole may be seen in the central portion of some of these collections of cells; others surround small hyaline masses. The bloodvessels of the organ are very prominent, being greatly dilated and showing marked thickening of the walls. Small deposits of blood pigment (hæmosiderin) are found about some of the trabeculæ, and throughout the pulp spaces occasional endothelial phagocytes containing pigment are seen.

The study of many sections taken from different parts of the spleen leads to the conclusion that the conditions here represent a chronic passive congestion, with great enlargement of the pulp spaces, a coincident or secondary fibrous hyperplasia of the pulp reticulum dependent upon or associated with a hyperplasia of the reticular or endothelial cells lining the spaces. In connection with these changes there is a secondary atrophy of the lymphoid tissue of the pulp and of the follicles. As a result of such atrophy and destruction of the splenic parenchyma the splenic function of hæmolysis is gradually lost. The spleen-like hyperplasia of the hæmal glands, the new formation of lymphoid tissue throughout the root of the mesentery, and the retroperitoneal fat are regarded as compensatory in character.

Summary of Pathology. The most striking feature of the case is the marked fibrous hyperplasia of the spleen. That this cannot be secondary to the liver condition is shown by the marked differences in degree and character of the hepatic and splenic conditions respectively. The splenic condition is, without doubt, much the older condition, as seen by the greater abundance of the fibrous tissue, its greater density and more hyaline character, and its difference in reaction in areas to Van Gieson's stain; moreover, the atrophic condition of the splenic parenchyma is more marked than that of the liver. The process in the liver is interpreted as a chronic passive congestion and atrophy, followed, secondarily, by an increase of the finer reticulum of the lobules. In several areas, notably in the middle of the right lobe, there is also a beginning periportal increase of connective tissue with hyperplasia of the smaller bile-ducts. This beginning hyperplasia may be regarded as a very early stage or beginning of a cirrhosis, and is evidently of much more recent occurrence than the splenic condition.

In explanation of the congestion and fibrosis of the spleen, the stenosis and calcification of the portal vein may be regarded as an etiological factor. That the changes in the wall of the vein at the junction of the splenic and superior mesenteric veins represent an old and not a recent process is shown by the hyaline thickening of the wall and of the fibrous septa and the plates of calcification. These changes must be taken as evidences of an old thrombosis and pylephlebitis, with subsequent organization, contraction, stenosis, and calcification. It is possible that the stasis in the splenic vein and the damming back of the blood upon the spleen have caused the atrophy and the progressive fibrosis seen in that organ. On the other hand, it is also possible that the splenic condition is primary, and the condition of the portal vein may be purely coincidental or may result from a toxic condition of the blood in the splenic vein dependent upon the disturbed splenic function, or upon a general intoxication, or one affecting the portal area primarily. The changes in the hæmolymph nodes and the new formation of lymphoid tissue are regarded as compensatory for the lost splenic function. It is also probable that a similar compensation is present in the bone-marrow, as shown by the changes described above. The anæmia may be regarded as due either to an excessive destruction of red blood cells by the endothelial phagocytes of the portions of the spleen still exercising the function of hæmolysis, in connection with an excessive activity of endothelial phagocytes in the hæmolymph nodes and bone-marrow, or to a toxic hæmolysis, or to a disturbance of balance between the destruction of hæmoglobin and the elaboration of the products resulting from such destruction. From a careful study of the case we have arrived at the following:

Pathological Diagnosis. Fibrosis of the spleen (*splenomegaly*), with beginning fibrosis of liver (*early stage of Banti's disease*); stenosis and calcification of portal vein, with extreme passive congestion of radicles of portal, particularly of splenic vein; chronic passive congestion of gastrointestinal tract, lungs, etc.; compensatory hyperplasia of hæmolymph nodes and new formation of lymphoid tissue in retroperitoneal fat; increase of lymphoid marrow; acute fibrinous peritonitis following splenectomy; embolism of bone-marrow giant cells; general sclerosis and atrophy; secondary anæmia; cholelithiasis.

CASE II.—Mrs. S., aged fifty years, American, died 12.05 P.M., December 11, 1902. Autopsy by Dr. Warthin at 1.30 P.M., December 11, 1902.

Autopsy Protocol. Cadaver of slender build; no anomalies; no deformities. Right inguinal hernia. Abdomen on level of ribs. In the median line, between the umbilicus and pubes, there is a laparotomy scar 14 cm. long, which is entirely healed with the exception of a sinus about 1 cm. long at about the middle of the scar. Pus exudes from the opening, which communicates by a fistulous tract with an abscess cavity in the abdominal wall.

Skin is pale, hair negative, teeth artificial. Over the back there is pale hypostasis. Transfusion punctures in pectoral regions. The muscles are greatly emaciated; on section they are deep brown and dry. There is no rigor mortis. The panniculus is of a fair amount. Œdema is present over both ankles. Body heat is present.

Brain and spinal cord not examined.

The diaphragm is at the third intercostal space on both sides.

Mammæ atrophic. In the adipose tissue of the right there is a firm swelling about the size of a walnut, consisting of hyperæmic and œdematous fat tissue (transfusion area).

Apex of heart is behind the fourth rib, half-way between the left parasternal and nipple lines. The *mediastinal fat* is abundant and of an orange color; contains no enlarged glands. In the *thymus region* there is an abundance of orange-colored fat. No remains of thymus.

No fluid in *pleural cavities*. The left lung is adherent throughout, the adhesions being very dense over the base, where they have to be cut. Right lung is adherent by easily torn adhesions at apex and over the posterior surface and at the base; the adhesions here not so firm as on left side.

The *pericardial sac* is not tense; contains no fluid. Surfaces of pericardium are moist and shining.

The heart is much smaller than cadaver's right fist; weighs 272 grams, and measures 13 x 9.5 x 5 cm. There is a small, irregular, tendinous spot on the posterior wall of left ventricle; another near the apex, and one on the anterior wall of right ventricle. The subepicardial fat is increased. Heart muscle is pale brown, fairly firm. The right auricle contains currant-jelly and mixed clots and plum-colored fluid blood. The wall of the right ventricle measures 5 mm., 3 mm. of which are of fat. Right ventricle is empty. The left ventricle is empty, wall contracted; measures 20 mm. The left auricle contains plum-colored fluid blood and small red jelly clots.

The *mitral valve* barely admits two fingers. Circumference of orifice, 8 cm. Flaps are thickened along proximal edges. Tricuspid barely admits three fingers; orifice measures 11 cm.; flaps negative. Pulmonary barely admits thumb; orifice measures 6.5 cm.; flaps negative; aortic admits thumb easily; orifice 7 cm. in circumference; slight thickening of central segment.

The *aorta* shows beginning sclerosis, most marked about the coronary orifices. The descending branch of the left coronary artery is moderately sclerosed.

The *left lung* weighs 216 grams, and measures 17 x 13 x 3 cm. It is collapsed, pale, moderately anthracosed, and the pleura is covered with the remains of adhesions. On section the lung is pale, dry, almost bloodless, and yields almost no fluid on pressure. Beneath the pleura, particularly over the lower lobe, there are scattered a few dark areas of small size, which are firm on pressure.

The right lung is more voluminous and contains more air than the left. It weighs 256 grams, and measures 19 x 12 x 4 cm. On section it is more pink and moist over the middle and lower lobes; otherwise similar.

Bronchi negative. Bronchial glands moderately anthracosed. Pulmonary vessels contain large ante-mortem mixed clots and post-mortem jelly clots.

Thoracic aorta measures 5 cm. in circumference; contains small jelly and mixed clots. The azygos veins are greatly dilated.

FIG. 7.

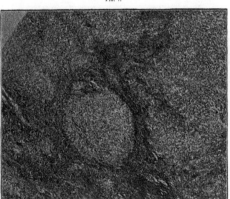

Low-power view of liver of Case II., showing picture of advanced cirrhosis. × 45.

Thoracic duct is distended with clear fluid.

Thoracic portion of œsophagus contains a brownish fluid. The lower third shows marked varices; the œsophageal veins and their anastomoses with the coronary veins of the stomach are markedly dilated. There are no evidences of hemorrhage from the œsophageal mucosa. No erosions of the varices.

Mouth, pharynx, and *larynx* not examined. The cervical portion of the œsophagus contains a brownish fluid. The thyroid is small and of firm consistence. On section it is pale and more brown than normal.

Cervical Hæmolymph Nodes. In the deep cervical tissues numerous reddish, spleen-like glands resembling hæmolymph glands are found. They are larger and appear much more numerous than normally.

Cervical vessels and nerves negative.

Abdomen. The *omentum* is adherent to the abdominal wall in the neighborhood of the umbilicus by easily torn adhesions, between which there is a fibrinopurulent exudate. The lower border is adherent to the anterior abdominal wall just above the pubes. The intestinal coils present scattered fresh fibrinous adhesions, particularly on the left side. From between the adhesions one and a half litres of turbid fluid containiug many fibrin flakes are obtained, the greater part being taken from the left side below the spleen. The adhesions are strongest in the neighborhood of the incision. In the abdominal wall at this point there is a fistulous tract extending through the rectus muscle as far as the pubes, and communicating with the external opening in the laparotomy wound. Between the adhesions there is a collection of pus. The intestines in this region are firmly adherent to each other and to the abdominal wall. In one of the loops there is a darkened, thin, and softened area, but no perforation. The pelvis is filled with coils of small intestine which are adherent to the sigmoid and rectum. Between these adhesions there are about 50 c.c. of fluid similar to that in the abdominal cavity, but more turbid, and containing more fibrin. The transverse colon and cæcum are moderately distended; the former is S-shaped, the lowest part two fingers' breadth above the umbilicus. The *liver* is high and very small, the lower edge in the right parasternal line being three finger breadths above the edge of ribs and just at the tip

FIG. 8.

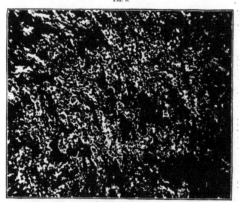

Spleen of Case II. Fibrous hyperplasia of reticulum, with hyaline change. Dark areas = hyaline area stained deep red with Van Gieson's. No follicles. × 175.

of the ensiform in the median line. The left border is two fingers' breadth to the left of the left sternal line. The *spleen* is greatly enlarged, filling in the entire left hypochondrium and projecting a hand's breadth below the edge of the ribs. It is adherent to the diaphragm by several easily torn adhesions. The lower border of the stomach is three fingers' breadth below the ensiform. There are easily torn adhesions between the stomach, omentum, and hilum of spleen. No accessory spleen found in gastrosplenic omentum.

Spleen weighs 944 grams, and measures 19 x 14 x 7 cm. It is triangular in shape, broader at upper pole, the enlargement involving chiefly the upper third. The upper pole is slightly recurved. There is one deep

FIG. 9.

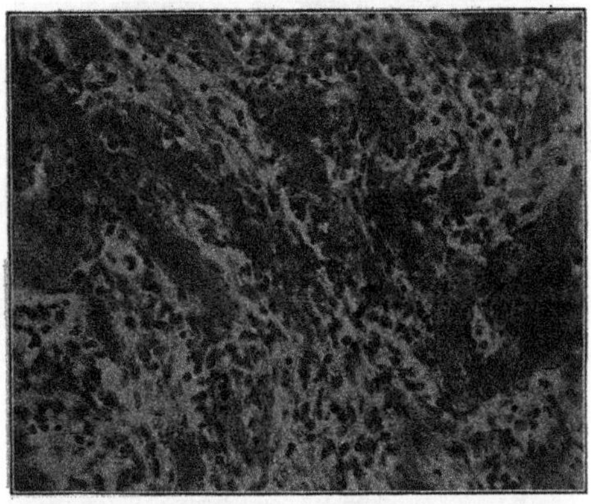

Spleen of Case II. Higher power view of Fig. 8. Fibrous hyperplasia of splenic reticulum, with hyaline change. Dark areas = hyaline areas staining deep red with Van Gieson's. × 350.

notch at about the middle of the anterior border, extending nearly halfway across the organ. The capsule is thickened, particularly along the anterior margin, where there are flattened hyaline thickenings and the remains of stringy adhesions. The organ flattens somewhat, but is of increased consistence. On section it is firm and tough, creaks to the knife, pale, grayish-blue red, almost homogeneous, and shining, semi-translucent, but slightly granular in areas. Contains but little blood. The follicles are greatly diminished in number and in size—only a few can be seen. There is a diffuse fibroid hyperplasia of the reticulum of the p[illegible]. The vessels at the hilum appear normal; veins collapsed.

Adrenals well preserved; no pathological changes.

Left Kidney. Fatty capsule very rich in fat. Fibrous capsule strips easily; shape about normal; less plump than the right one; weighs 120 grams; measures 10 x 6 x 3 cm. Small, yellowish areas on the posterior surface. These are neither elevated nor depressed. On section they are found to extend through the cortex and medullary pyramids. In other respects resembles right kidney.

Right Kidney. Fatty capsule very rich in fat. Fibrous capsule strips easily. Surface of kidney smooth, mottled brownish-red and yellow; weighs 104 grams; measures 8½ x 5½ x 3 cm. Several yellowish spots, size of a pea, seen over the surface. On section cut surface is pale brownish-red, containing small yellowish areas size of a pepper-corn,

FIG. 10.

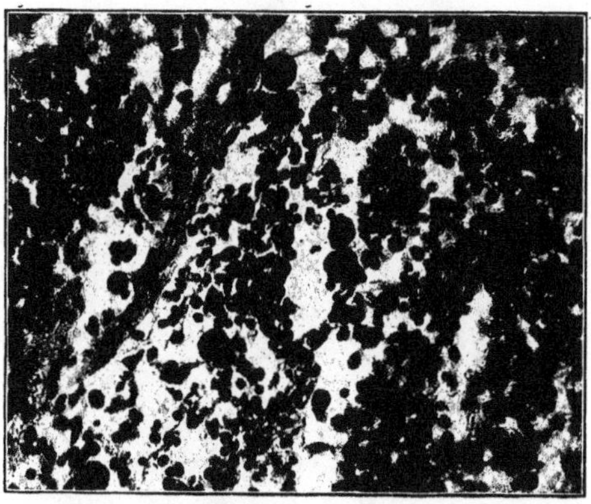

Portion of a sinus of retroperitoneal hæmolymph node from Case II. Large phagocytes filled with red blood cells, the outlines of the latter being just visible. Free blood cells in meshes of blood sinus. × 175.

and is more translucent than normal. Cortex measures 2 to 3 mm. Outlines of labyrinths and medullary rays well preserved. Vessels anæmic; consistence firm; subpelvic fat increased; pelvis negative.

Ureters negative.

Bladder distended with cloudy urine. Mucosa negative.

Duodenum contains plum-colored, bloody fluid, with strong odor of H_2S. In this fluid are four large currant-jelly clots, weighing 12.2, 10.8, 7.3, and 6.1 grams respectively. Mucosa anæmic, and presents no erosions or evidences of hemorrhage.

Bile Passages. Patent.

Small Intestine. The jejunum and ileum contain fluid similar to that found in duodenum, with yellowish clots. Toward the lower end of the

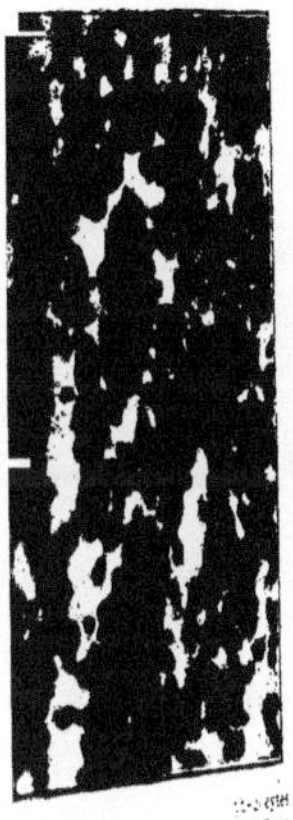

ileum the fluid becomes thicker and darker in color. The mucosa is very anæmic. No evidences of hemorrhage.

Appendix. Firm adhesions containing pus about the appendix. Lumen negative.

Large Intestine. Entirely filled with tar-like material. About the middle of transverse colon there is a small polyp. Mucosa is very anæmic. No evidences of hemorrhage. The *rectum* is filled with a black, tarry, tenacious material adhering to the mucosa. In the latter are the scars of healed ulcers. No evidences of hemorrhage. Hemorrhoidal veins greatly enlarged, but collapsed. No evidences of hemorrhage from these.

Stomach. Contains 750 c.c. of a thick, black fluid, composed chiefly of red blood cells and a few small red clots. The mucosa is thickened and covered with a thick, brownish mucus. About 14 cm. below the cardiac orifice there is in the posterior wall an erosion in the mucosa, having undermined edges, and about 3 mm. in diameter. Beneath this and under the neighboring mucosa there is a space about 2 cm. in diameter, filled with a fresh blood clot, and communicating with a ruptured vein in the posterior wall, a greatly dilated branch of the coronary veins. This is undoubtedly the source of the hemorrhage. All of the veins of the stomach wall are greatly dilated and tortuous, but are for the chief part collapsed and empty. The coronary veins in particular show a marked dilatation.

Liver. Small, about size of a child's head, nearly round, but irregular. Weighs 1856 grams; its greatest dimensions are 23 x 17 x 11 cm. It is adherent to the diaphragm by very firm and tough adhesions. The surface is very irregular and nodular, particularly along the lower edge and near the ligaments. It contains numerous small hyaline areas and small, translucent, glistening, brownish points, varying in size from that of a pinpoint to that of a pinhead. These are most numerous along the lower edge. Over the upper surface of the organ the capsule is 0.5 cm. thick, and firmly adherent to the diaphragm. The consistence is very firm; creaks on cutting. On section Glisson's capsule is greatly thickened in areas, the cut surface being mottled whitish and brown, the white areas corresponding to the dense hyaline connective tissue of the thickened Glisson's capsule. The increase of Glisson's capsule is, however, very irregular, being most marked in the central portion of the right lobe and beneath the external capsule. There appears to be a diffuse increase of connective tissue throughout the organ. The cut surface is slightly granular, the liver tissue showing as irregular islands surrounded by connective tissue. Surface is more translucent than normal. The outlines of the lobules cannot be made out. The branches of the hepatic vein are dilated, those of the portal nearly obliterated by the periportal increase of connective tissue. No icterus.

Gall-bladder is very small; size of a pigeon's egg. It is retracted above the edge of the liver. Tissues of the wall are thickened. It contains a very thick, glairy, brownish-like bile; no stones.

Portal Vein. Just above the junction of the splenic and superior mesenteric veins the wall of the portal vein is thickened and contains calcareous plates. The lumen is stenosed, barely admitting tip of lead-pencil. The wall is irregularly thickened and shows lines of contraction radiating from the areas of calcification. The lumen is filled with a recent mixed thrombus, chiefly white, firm in consistency, and extending to the portal of the liver and into the smaller portal branches within the liver. No evidences of organization of the thrombus. All the radicles of the portal are enlarged and show thickenend walls, the splenic vein in particular.

Pancreas. Smaller than normal. Lobules atrophic. Fatty infiltration between the lobules. Throughout the organ there are numerous whitish areas of fat-necrosis in the interlobular fat. These are most marked along the upper border. In the great omentum about a hand's breadth below the greater curvature there is a red body the size of a cherry, embedded in the omental fat. It is rather soft and fluctuating, resembling a congested hæmolymph node. On section it shows a small, firm, whitish nodule resembling epithelial tissue and suggesting pancreatic tissue, the remaining portion being made up of reddish, lymphoid tissue and a small abscess cavity containing a brownish, pus-like material. Small areas of fat-necrosis are found in the fat-tissue near by.

Mesentery. Mesenteric glands not enlarged. No hæmolymph nodes found except in root, where there is a great number of reddish and bluish glands embedded in the mesenteric fat, probably hæmolymph nodes.

Retroperitoneal Glands. Over 250 red, spleen-like glands found in the root of mesentery, retroperitoneal fat, about the renal vessels, behind and along the great abdominal vessels, and particularly along the brim of the pelvis. Along the left common iliac there is one 4 cm. long and as thick as a lead-pencil. A similar cord lies along the vena cava. The majority of the red glands are the size of a bean; others vary in size from that of a pinhead to that of a bean. On section they are firm, bluish-red, and spleen-like; only a few show dilated sinuses and a softer consistence.

External Genitals. Negative.

Uterus and Appendages. Absent. (Removed at operation.)

Site of operation covered with fibrinopurulent exudate. About 50 c.c. of turbid fluid in pelvis.

Bone-marrow. Tibias, opened longitudinally, show no lymphoid changes. Red marrow in sternum and ribs hyperplastic.

Peripheral Lymph Glands. Prominent, but not enlarged.

Peripheral Bloodvessels. Femoral veins filled with recent thrombi; the left completely occluded by a clot of firmer consistency than that found in the right femoral. Lumbar and azygos veins greatly enlarged. (Material taken from all organs and tissues fixed in Flemming's, Müller's, Zenker's, mercuric chloride, alcohol, and formalin. Embedded in paraffin; stained in ordinary and specific stains.)

Microscopic Examination. Heart. Sections of heart muscle show brown atrophy. Fatty infiltration of right ventricle.

Lungs. Sections show atrophy and sclerosis of bloodvessels. Great numbers of bone-marrow giant cells in capillaries.

Spleen. Marked fibrosis of the reticulum of the pulp, with hyaline change of the newly formed connective tissue, the blood spaces being outlined by hyaline cords of varying thickness. The process is fairly uniform throughout the entire organ, although denser and more hyaline areas, with wholly or partially obliterated blood spaces, are seen in portions, particularly near the external capsule. The blood spaces are very prominent, and many greatly enlarged, some areas being cavernous.

The lymphoid tissue of the pulp is very atrophic, and only small, scattered collections of cells resembling follicles are seen. The majority of these contain hyaline masses. The blood spaces are lined by large, hypertrophic, endothelial cells, but these do not show any evidences of hyperplasia into the spaces. A few giant cells resembling those of the bone-marrow seen in the blood spaces (embolism?); a few normoblasts are also found. No unusual forms of cells observed in sections stained by special methods (triacid, polychrome, methylene blue, etc.). All the bloodvessels of the spleen are enlarged and show marked sclerotic changes and numerous nodules of calcification. A deposit of lime-salts is also found in some of the hyaline masses of the follicles. Testing of many sections for iron with potassium ferrocyanide and hydrochloric acid entirely negative. No phagocytes containing blood pigment seen, and no free blood pigment.

Liver. Sections taken from different parts of the liver show that the greater part of the organ presents the picture of an atrophic cirrhosis. Glisson's capsule is greatly increased, and there is also a growth of connective tissue into the lobule. The periportal increase of connective tissue is, however, very irregular; in some areas it is very marked, in others it is but slight, small areas showing no cirrhotic changes. In other areas there is a central increase of connective tissue. The greater part of the lobules show central dilatation of the capillaries and atrophy of liver cells. Much of the connective tissue, particularly toward the surface of the organ, is hyaline and scar-like; in those areas showing less change the new tissue has more of a fibroblastic character and contains more small cells. There is a slight increase of the small bile-ducts. Liver cells are atrophic; those of the central portion of the lobule contain a very small amount of hæmatoidin. Iron test is entirely negative.

Pancreas. Sections show a fatty atrophy. Vessels are sclerosed. There is a small-celled infiltration of the interlobular fat, and localized areas of fat necrosis with small hemorrhages are present.

Body from Omentum. Sections show the red body found in the omentum to consist of three separate structures: A hæmolymph node showing great numbers of phagocytes containing red cells in its blood sinuses; an accessory pancreas containing all the characteristics of pancreatic tissue, acini, and areas of Langerhans. There is an increase of the stroma of the parenchymatous portion as well as of the islands, and an infiltration of fat-cells. No large duct leading from this accessory pancreas can be found, but a small duct can be traced leading into the third structure of the mass—an abscess cavity filled with a pus-like material, and having a wall of granulation tissue in which there are many large, thin-walled vessels. Small groups of necrosed fat-cells are found in the neighboring tissue.

Stomach and Intestine. Sections show a chronic passive congestion with catarrhal inflammation.

Kidneys. Sections show atrophy, sclerosis of vessels, and localized areas of interstitial inflammation. Convoluted tubules show moderate cloudy swelling. Iron test wholly negative.

Hæmolymph Nodes. These constitute one of the most interesting features of the case, judged from the pathological standpoint. The changes may be summed up as follows: All the red glands examined show the structure of hæmolymph nodes in varying stages of hyperplasia. They contain but few germ-centres. The blood sinuses are all very prominent and large, but the majority are only partly filled with blood. In some glands the sinuses are distended. They contain also great numbers of large hyaline cells having a y ish or brownish color, and staining deep red with eosin. Some of the sinuses are completely filled with these cells. With the higher powers these cells are found to be phagocytes completely filled with red cells, or with the products of the disintegration of red cells. The nucleus of the phagocytic cell is usually pushed to one side, and shows more or less karyorrhexis. The outlines of the red cells can be distinctly seen in the phagocytes, and in many cases appear unchanged. In other phagocytes only hyaline droplets staining deeply with eosin or a brownish pigment are seen. The majority of the cells give a strong iron reaction with ferrocyanide and hydrochloric acid. In some there is a yellowish pigment which does not respond to the iron test (hæmatoidin?). Great numbers of mononuclear eosinophiles are found in some of the glands. Normoblasts and giant cells resembling those of the bone-marrow are found in large numbers in the blood sinuses. With the triacid stain numerous cells resembling myelocytes (neutrophile granulation and large excentric nuclei) are also found in the blood sinuses. In many of the retroperitoneal hæmolymph nodes there are also large masses of hyalin which occupy the lymphoid areas between the blood sinuses. Many of these show calcification. Encapsulated caseous tubercle found in one gland. In the sections treated with ferrocyanide and hydrochloric acid the areas of calcification give a marked iron reaction, which is diffuse or very finely granular. A similar reaction is observed in many of the hyaline areas in which calcification has not taken place. The appearances suggest some connection between the hyaline masses and the blood destruction.

Lymphatic Glands. Atrophic; show marked hyaline change.

Bone-marrow. The normoblasts are increased, and the giant cells greatly diminished in number. The reticulum of the red marrow appears hyperplastic and the blood spaces smaller. In the blood spaces and in the reticulum are great numbers of pigmented phagocytes, as in the hæmolymph nodes. Free pigment is also present. The iron test shows the pigment to be hæmosiderin.

Tumor of Uterus (removed at operation). The tumor was found to be nearly completely calcified. After decalcification of portions sections were obtained showing it to be a myofibroma, with increase of the connective tissue, atrophy of the muscle, hyaline change, and calcification. Traces of atrophic muscle found throughout the dense hyaline tissue between the masses of calcification. Very few nuclei found in the hyaline connective tissue.

Summary of Pathology. The immediate cause of death is the anæmia resulting from the hemorrhage from the eroded varix in the stomach wall. The dilatation of the stomach and splenic veins is the result of the portal obstruction. For the latter two etiological factors are present, the stenosis and calcification of the portal vein and the periportal cirrhosis. It is impossible to decide the relative part played by these factors. The most important question is the relation of the splenic condition to that of the liver. It is, however, impossible to decide positively which is the primary condition, the splenic fibrosis or the cirrhosis of the liver. Because of the more advanced stage of the splenic fibrosis, the dense hyaline character of the new tissue formed in the walls of the pulp spaces, the areas of hyaline and calcification, the greater atrophy of splenic parenchyma, etc., it seems very probable that the splenic process is older than that of the liver. If this is the case the question also arises here as to the relationship between the changes in the spleen and those in the portal vein. Is the splenic fibrosis primary, or is it secondary to the disturbance of the splenic circulation following thrombosis and the resulting stenosis of the portal? This question, unfortunately, cannot be positively answered. The portal condition is, undoubtedly, the result of an old pylephlebitis and thrombosis, but it is impossible to determine if it preceded the splenic condition or is secondary to some toxic condition of the portal blood, dependent, possibly, upon a primary change in the spleen or upon a general toxæmia.

The changes in the hæmolymph nodes are to be interpreted as compensatory for the lost splenic function. The complete absence of blood pigment or of phagocytes in the spleen may explain the great excess of hæmolysis occurring in the hæmolymph nodes and bone-marrow. The evidences of phagocytic hæmolysis in the hæmolymph nodes presented by this case show a much greater blood destruction than that occurring in these glands in any of the cases of pernicious anæmia observed by the writer. In spite of so great a hæmolysis no hæmosiderin is found outside of these glands and the bone-marrow. Iron tests of liver, spleen, and kidneys do not show a trace of iron. The hæmolysis is therefore different from that occurring in pernicious anæmia, and is most probably not a *toxic hæmolysis*, but is to be interpreted as a *compensatory* one. The anæmia may then be explained as due to an excess of hæmolymphatic hæmolysis over that of the normal splenic hæmolysis, or to a disturbance in the elaboration of the products of blood destruction.

There is no histological evidence of a destruction of red cells in the general circulation, as is the case in pernicious anæmia.

From the study of the case we have arrived at the following:

Pathological Diagnosis. Splenic fibrosis with cirrhosis of the liver (late stage of Banti's disease), gastric hemorrhage, anæmia, stenosis, and calcification of portal vein, chronic passive congestion of portal system, ascites, peritonitis, hyperplasia of hæmolymph nodes with excessive hæmolysis, hyperplasia of red marrow, giant-cell embolism, general atrophy and sclerosis, tuberculosis of retroperitoneal gland, accessory pancreas, fat-necrosis.

Comparison of Cases. Both cases present the following common features:

1. Splenic fibrosis.
2. Hepatic fibrosis.
3. Stenosis and calcification of portal vein.
4. Chronic passive congestion of portal system.

5. Sclerosis of vessels, particularly of portal area.

6. A marked tendency to hyaline change and calcification throughout portal area.

7. Hyperplasia of hæmolymph nodes and bone-marrow and new formation of lymphoid tissue in retroperitoneal fat.

8. Secondary anæmia.

Comparing the two cases the splenic fibrosis in Case I. represents an earlier stage; that in Case II. a much more advanced stage. In Case I. the liver changes are relatively slight, a beginning fibrosis. In Case II. they are marked—an advanced cirrhosis, a cirrhosis, however, which does not present all the features of an ordinary atrophic cirrhosis. The changes in the portal vein in both cases were at the same site and of about the same degree. In Case I. the more irregular character of the vessel wall, the bridging strands of tissue across the lumen of the vein, might indicate a more recent process. The chronic passive congestion of the portal is more marked in Case II. than in Case I., as shown by the greater development of anastomoses and the pronounced varices in œsophagus and stomach leading to the fatal hemorrhage in the former case

In Case I. [illegible] perplasia of the hæmolymph nodes is not nearly so marked, [illegible] in these glands there are not the evidences of the pronounced hæmolysis seen in Case II. In Case I. the spleen contains some phagocytes and blood pigment. In Case II. none of these were found in the spleen. These differences may also be interpreted as indicat[illegible] early stage of the process in Case I. and a later stage in Case II. [illegible]he pathological findings, therefore, would appear to warrant the diagnosis of early and late stages of Banti's disease.

In both of these cases (unlike some others described under the head of splenic anæmia or Banti's disease) there is no clinical evidence and no positive anatomical proof of the existence of syphilis. On the contrary, the clinical history gave strong arguments against the possibility of this disease.

The important question as to the relationship between the splenic condition and the stenosis of the portal remains to be settled. Is the splenic fibrosis a distinct pathological entity or is it a secondary process? The changes in the spleens of the two cases do not represent any features that could not be explained by a chronic passive congestion of marked degree; that is, it is possible for such a hyperplasia of connective tissue to follow a severe and long-continued passive congestion, as is sometimes the case in the lung, liver, etc. This question, however, cannot be answered by these two cases. It can only be said that there is a possibility that the clinical picture of splenic anæmia or Banti's disease may be caused by a stenosis of the portal vein due to old phlebitis and thrombosis and the resulting stenosis.

On turning to the cases of splenic anæmia reported in the literature under such heading, we find that the condition of the portal vein is not mentioned at all, or so briefly as to convey the impression that the vessel had not been carefully examined. In the older literature there is, however, a number of very suggestive cases similar to the two described above, and reported under the head of "Thrombosis," or "Stenosis of Portal Vein, with Hypertrophy of the Spleen." The descriptions given of these cases, though incomplete and meagre, when judged from modern standpoints of diagnosis, suggest very closely the cases now described as splenic anæmia. Among these is one reported by Sir Andrew Clark (*Trans. London Path. Soc.*, 1867). The patient had suffered previously from "biliousness" and intestinal hemorrhages; died of gastric hemorrhage. Skin sallow, body very fat. Autopsy showed spleen to be three times normal size; liver "thinner" than normal; wall of portal vein contained calcareous plates; in the lumen there was a fresh thrombus.

It is possible that this and some of the similar cases reported in the literature, as well as some of the cases of cirrhosis with changes in the portal vein, may represent the same morbid processes as do our two cases and that they should be placed in the category of splenic anæmia.

CONCLUSION. The two cases reported above present, clinically and anatomically, the pictures of an early and a late stage of Banti's disease—an older fibrosis of the spleen with a more recent fibrosis of the liver. Both cases present also the condition of stenosis and calcification of the portal vein. Is the latter the primary condition, to which the splenic fibrosis follows secondarily, or is it the result of a portal or general intoxication, to which the splenic and hepatic fibrosis are also due? The solution of this problem must wait upon the observation and investigation of other similar cases. The two reported above, however, may be taken as further evidence in favor of the view that the symptom-complex of splenic anæmia represents a group of varying pathological conditions, the splenic condition being secondary.

DESQUAMATION OF THE SKIN IN TYPHOID FEVER.*

BY DAVID RIESMAN, M.D.,
PROFESSOR OF CLINICAL MEDICINE, PHILADELPHIA POLYCLINIC; ASSOCIATE IN MEDICINE, UNIVERSITY OF PENNSYLVANIA; VISITING PHYSICIAN TO THE PHILADELPHIA HOSPITAL.

DESQUAMATION of the skin of a pronounced character is rare in typhoid fever, and is mentioned by but few of the systematic writers

* Read before the Section in Medicine of the College of Physicians of Philadelphia, February 9, 1903.

upon the disease. The great Louis,[1] whom almost nothing escaped, refers to it in the following words: "Desquamation of the epidermis occurred to a greater or less extent in some of the grave cases of the typhoid affection that terminated favorably, even in persons that had no sudamina. Like the sudamina, this desquamation indicated a previous disease of the skin, and I regret very much that I did not look for it oftener." Elisha Bartlett,[2] the first American writer to recognize, in a systematic work, the difference between typhoid and typhus fevers, makes no mention of desquamation. Nothing is said about it in the majority of the French theses upon typhoid fever—and the number of these following Louis' publications is truly astounding. I find a brief reference in one of them, that of Macario,[3] who speaks of desquamation as following sudamina. Harley,[4] in Reynolds' *System*, says that roughness and desquamation of the cuticle, especially of that covering the abdomen, are observed after the cessation of febrile symptoms in severe cases, the desquamation occurring independently of the existence of sudamina, which alone is sufficient to produce it. This is practically a quotation from Murchison,[5] who notes desquamation, in the form of minute, branny scales, as either following sudamina or occurring independently during convalescence. Liebermeister[6] does not refer to desquamation; Dreschfeld,[7] in Allbutt's *System*, says that a desquamation of fine, branny scales is often observed toward the end of the fever or during convalescence. Hutchinson,[8] in Pepper's *System*, alludes to desquamation following sudamina, but makes no mention of its occurring in other circumstances. Strümpell[9] speaks of desquamation; and Osler,[10] in the last edition of his book, states that a branny desquamation is not rare in children, and that occasionally the skin peels off in large flakes. In his extensive observations on typhoid fever in the Johns Hopkins Hospital, Osler[11] noticed a distinct desquamation only four times. Wilson[12] states that slight desquamation is occasionally observed during convalescence; and Chantemesse[13] speaks of furfuraceous desquamation on the lateral aspects of the body, especially in children. In his elaborate monograph on the *Medical Complications of Typhoid Fever*, Hare[14] alludes to desquamation, and states that it is common and that he has frequently seen it. Brannan,[15] in *Twentieth Century Practice*, says that a desquamation of fine, branny scales may occur in typhoid fever independently of sudamina. Both he and Hare assert that the desquamation occasionally follows a scarlet rash or erythema that at times occurs in typhoid fever without any obvious cause.

One of the first to study the subject of desquamation specifically was Weill,[16] of Lyons, who, like myself, was struck with the paucity of references to it in literature, he having succeeded in finding but one, viz., in the thesis of Hutinel. Weill's studies were made principally upon children, and in 37 cases he found desquamation thirty-three times. He also observed it in adults, but not so frequently. In 1895 Coulon[17] reported a case of scarlatinous desquamation following typhoid fever in a girl aged eleven and a half years.

Stimulated by the observations of Weill, Comby,[18] the well-known French pediatrist, gave attention to the subject of desquamation, and found it in all of 18 cases of typhoid fever in children examined for it. He attributes it to antecedent sudamina. Weill, on the other hand, does not think that it has anything to do with sudamina, but looks upon it as the analogue of the alopecia and the ungual changes that are so common in typhoid fever.

The desquamation occurs on the trunk, the shoulders, and the hips. According to Weill and Comby, it is never observed on the face, the palms, or the soles. This, however, is not strictly correct, as will be seen in the history of my second case. The desquamation begins toward the end of the disease—as a rule, at the commencement of convalescence or a little later—and lasts from several days to several weeks. Weill believes that there is a relation between the form, intensity, and duration of the desquamation and the character of the fever, grave cases being usually accompanied by early, extensive, lamellar, and prolonged desquamation; while in mild types the desquamation occurs later, and is discrete, furfuraceous, and transient. As stated above, Comby considers the desquamation to be a sequel of the sudaminal eruption; he looks upon the latter—erroneously it seems to me—as a critical discharge in the typhoid fever of children, even going so far as to say that it is absent in patients that are going to die.

As in one of Osler's cases, the desquamation may at times be preceded by a diffuse, erythematous blush, the true nature of which is problematical. Very probably it is of septic origin. In the second of my patients, who was under continuous observation, such a rash was not noticed. The first patient was not seen until the stage of desquamation was well advanced.

The question of the infectivity of the scales might be raised; it is hardly likely, however, that they play any part in the epidemiology of the disease.

The possibility that vigorous sponging and the bath treatment may be provocative of desquamation suggests itself. I do not think, however, that the rare form presented by my two cases, in which desquamation occurred in large scales, is produced by this agency. In Case II. the desquamation was more marked on the limbs and the abdomen than on the chest, and was quite pronounced on the face—a part not subjected to special hydrotherapeutic measures. A limited furfuraceous scaling might follow in the wake of the bath-treatment, but Comby emphatically states that the desquamation observed by him bore no relation to bathing.

My own cases are two in number:

The first patient, J. S., aged seventeen years, had a typical attack of typhoid fever. He had been admitted into the inebriate ward of the Philadelphia Hospital and afterward transferred to the ward of Dr. Henry, where I happened to see him. My thanks are due to Dr. Henry for this privilege and for permission to make use of the case.

The patient was admitted on February 11, 1902, the abdomen showing at that time many rose-colored spots. The temperature reached normal on the 28th of the same month. During the height of the fever the patient received two tub-baths and nineteen antipyretic sponges. There are, unfortunately, no notes concerning the desquama-

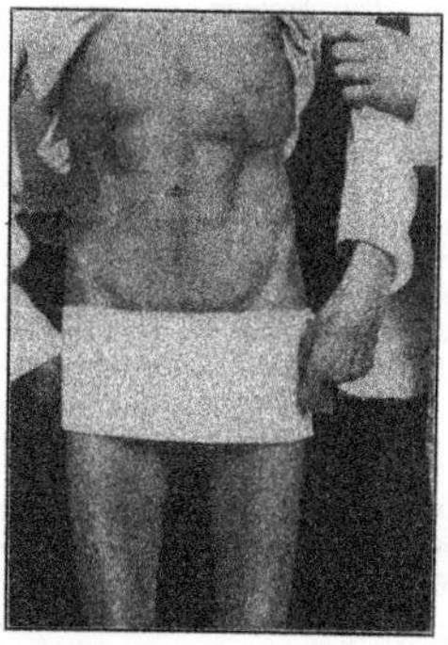

tion; but the photograph, here reproduced, which was taken during convalescence, shows clearly an extensive formation of fine scales over the abdomen, the thighs, and the upper parts of the legs.

The second patient, S. J. F., a native of Sweden, was admitted to the Philadelphia Hospital on January 23, 1902, in the service of Dr. Tyson, to whom I wish to express my thanks for the opportunity of studying the case. The symptoms were those of a severe type of typhoid fever. The characteristic eruption was present on admission, but was not unusually profuse. There was a marked bronchitis and a high degree of adynamia. Within a few days after admission the rash became more widespread, spots appearing on the arms, the face, and the thighs, and a few being seen also below the knees. The temperature, which had not been high at any time, reached normal on February 12th, about three weeks after the patient's entrance into the hospital, and probably four weeks after the beginning of the fever. Tub-baths were at no time required, and the patient was sponged for fever but once. The temperature remained normal until March 3d, when, after a severe chill, it rose to 106° F.; there being, at the same time, acute pain in the right side. The signs of pleurisy promptly appeared, and an effusion necessitating aspiration rapidly formed. The patient left the hospital in a fair state of health early in April.

The desquamation of the skin began during convalescence from the typhoid fever; but there is no record of the exact date. It was widespread and in the form of scales, some of which were fully a quarter of an inch long. On the chest and the abdomen the desquamation was most noticeable, but it was scarcely less pronounced on the extremities. It could also be seen distinctly on the forehead, the ears, the nose, the cheeks (especially the malar prominences), and the neck. There was no desquamation in the region of the hairy scalp; nor on the shoulders, the palms, or the soles. On the back it was slight. On the extremities the distribution of the scales was somewhat peculiar. Thus, on the arms it was disposed in the form of narrow, circular bands, from one-eighth to one-quarter of an inch in width. The desquamating circles were almost parallel, with zigzag borders, but in a few places the bands ran into one another. In the interspaces, which were about as wide as the bands themselves, the skin appeared to be normal. The desquamating areas were dead-white in color and somewhat crinkled. On the legs the desquamation was arranged in similar circular stripes, the scaling being just as pronounced there as on the arms. A photograph of this case was taken, but, unfortunately, it does not do justice to the condition.

The patient was exhibited to several sections of students, and all that saw him were struck with the appearance of the skin. I have here a few of the scales, taken at random. They will give an idea of the size. I firmly believe that anyone seeing the patient without knowing anything of his history would have concluded that he had passed through an attack of scarlet fever or of some other exanthem attended with pronounced scaling.

Conclusions. We may distinguish the following varieties of desquamation in typhoid fever:

1. That confined to the roseolar spots. In some instances each spot has a tiny vesicle upon its summit, which quickly passes into a thin, scale-like crust. I myself have never seen such vesicles, but they are mentioned by several good authorities. I have, however, noticed a tiny scale in the areas of the spots.*

2. That appearing as a sequel of sudamina. This is confined to the

* Since writing this I have had a patient at the Polyclinic Hospital in whom a few, but not all, of the rose-colored spots were each capped with a minute vesicle.

areas that have been the seat of the sudaminal eruption, although Louis states that the intervening skin may readily be peeled off. The desquamation is usually furfuraceous, but is sometimes scaly. It occurs upon the trunk and the proximal parts of the limbs, and is never seen upon the distal parts of the extremities or upon the face. It appears in the bathed and in the unbathed.

3. In some instances, as illustrated by the second case here reported, there is, in typhoid fever, an extensive, almost universal desquamation, either furfuraceous or lamellar, which seems to be independent of sudamina, and in all probability is a trophic change analogous to the shedding of the hair. It affects the trunk and the roots of the limbs, and, in rare instances, also the face and the distal parts of the extremities. Usually, but not always, the extent and the intensity of the desquamation bears a relation to the severity of the fever.

References.

1. Louis. Anatomical, Pathological, and Therapeutical Researches upon the Disease known as Gastroentérite, Putrid, Adynamic, or Typhoid Fever. Translated by Henry A. Bowditch, 1836, vol. ii. p. 209.
2. Bartlett. History, Diagnosis, and Treatment of Typhoid and Typhus Fever, 1842.
3. Macario. Des fièvres continues graves dites typhoïdes, Thèse de Paris, 1851, p. 23.
4. Harley. Reynolds' System of Medicine, 1868, vol. i. p. 584.
5. Murchison. The Continued Fevers of Great Britain, 1884, third edition, p. 517.
6. Liebermeister. Ziemssen's Cyclopedia of the Practice of Medicine, vol. ii.
7. Dreschfeld. Allbutt's System of Medicine, vol. i. p. 815.
8. Hutchinson. Pepper's System of Practical Medicine, vol. i. p. 275.
9. Strümpell. Specielle Pathologie und Therapie, twelfth edition, p. 30.
10. Osler. Practice of Medicine, fourth edition, 1901, p. 17.
11. Osler. Studies in Typhoid Fever, Johns Hopkins Hospital Reports, vol. iii. p. 426.
12. Wilson. Loomis-Thompson's American System of Practical Medicine, p. 197.
13. Chantemesse. Traité de médecine, p. 120.
14. Hare. The Medical Complications of Typhoid Fever, pp. 172 and 248.
15. Brannan. Twentieth Century Practice, vol. xvi. p. 629.
16. Weill. Gaz. des hôpitaux, 1896, p. 232; Congrès de médecine, Lyon, 1894, p. 373.
17. Coulon. Médecine infantile, January 15, 1895 (quoted by Comby).
18. Comby. Gaz. des hôpitaux, 1896, p. 315.

THE DIFFERENTIAL DIAGNOSIS OF TYPHOID FEVER IN ITS EARLIEST STAGES.[1]

By William Colby Rucker, M.D.,
ASSISTANT SURGEON UNITED STATES PUBLIC HEALTH AND MARINE HOSPITAL SERVICE.

Note.—In the following article the author has drawn extensively on many standard works and also upon the medical journals, both foreign and domestic. He is aware that too great an amount of medical

[1] Read before the Association of Military Surgeons of the United States, at the annual meeting, Boston, Mass., May 19, 1903, and awarded second prize by the Enno Sander Prize Medal Board of Award.

compilation and redundancy is being imposed daily upon the medical public as original work, and has endeavored as far as possible to assemble only those facts which bear directly upon the subject in hand. He has fused his own experiences with those of many other observers and tried to give an impersonal résumé of the whole, endeavoring to treat the subject in its entirety, rather than make the paper an excuse for a dissertation on one particular point.

In the list of references an attempt has been made to mention the name of every author whose work has been quoted, or from whom ideas have been borrowed for this essay. Experiments have not been quoted in detail, as they are at best uninteresting reading, and only the results of such work have been here recorded.

The term "earliest stages," while it limits in a measure the ground to be covered by this essay, is vague and indefinite, and may either include only the earliest prodromata or the first symptoms after the fever has commenced, or both. The author understands the term "earliest stages" to include the period of incubation and the first seven days of fever, and has, therefore, endeavored to eliminate diseases which complicate the diagnosis after this time only.

The differential diagnosis of a disease presenting such multiformity of aspect as typhoid fever is necessarily difficult, and especially is this true in its earliest stages, when few infectious diseases exhibit such great variations in their manner of attack and onset. The extreme variability of the clinical factors to be considered, the intensity of the infection, the resistance of the patient, the sanitary surroundings, all render it impossible to tabulate with any degree of accuracy the differences existing between the earliest manifestations of typhoid fever and those of diseases which may resemble it. Were it possible to demonstrate with ease and certainty the presence of the bacillus typhosus or its products at every stage of the disease, these difficulties would cease to exist, but, unfortunately, no satisfactory method has yet been brought forward which fulfils all these requirements ideally.

During the period of incubation no entirely satisfactory bacteriological method of diagnosis exists, and even clinical signs are hazy and uncertain. Not only is it practically impossible to determine exactly the time of the receipt of the contagium, but it is equally difficult to mark the dividing line between the period of incubation and the actual commencement of the disease.

Different organs may bear the brunt of the infection and consequently the manifestations of the disease may be extremely variable; certain symptoms commonly present may be replaced or masked by others referable to the lungs, kidneys, or to derangement of the mental functions. As Herrick has so truthfully remarked, typhoid fever is not only an imitator of other diseases, but many other diseases imitate typhoid fever. Even the length of the initial period is variable, occupying from one to three weeks, and at such times patients are rarely under observation.

The many forms which typhoid fever may assume also form an obstruction to early diagnosis. It may be abortive, mild, severe, hemorrhagic, renal, pneumonic, or ambulatory. It may be modified or masked by the strength of youth or the weakness of old age or childhood.

The ill-defined languor and indisposition, mental depression, headache, vertigo, sacral pain, anorexia, and irregularity of the bowels, in the absence of fever and physical findings, are in sharp contrast to the initial period of other febrile diseases, which during this stage generally present no manifestations. In those cases which come under close observation a careful examination of the temperature curve may show wide daily fluctuations of temperature, even though fever be absent. This taken into consideration with the symptoms will often put a careful clinician on the road to an early diagnosis. Pepper claimed to have been led to anticipate an attack of enteric fever by the unusual dulness of hearing and persistent occipital headache following a few days of malaise.

Epistaxis is of differential value simply as a part of the symptom-complex. It occurs, however, with far greater frequency in typhoid fever than in many other diseases, which are apt to be considered in the differential diagnosis. Its value is diminished chiefly by the fact that it also occurs early in cerebrospinal meningitis and in acute miliary tuberculosis.

The first febrile symptoms mark the actual commencement of the disease, the fever gradually increasing, and accompanied early by slight, oft-repeated chilly sensations. This occurs with such regularity that in cases ushered in by a hard chill and a sharp rise of temperature, typhoid fever is usually eliminated from the diagnosis at once. The temperature rises gradually with slight morning remissions and at the close of the first week usually reaches 40° C. The platted curve of these step-like gradations should be of great weight in the differential diagnosis. It should be mentioned in this connection, however, that while the gradually ascending temperature curve is typical of typhoid, there are cases occasionally in which there is a sharp initial rise in all respects similar to that of other infectious diseases.

Remittent malarial fever presents very irregular curves. Typhus, relapsing fever, scarlet fever, measles, and smallpox all exhibit a sharp initial rise of temperature. Intermittent malarial fever presents paroxysms of fever hardly to be mistaken for the steady progression of enteric fever. The disease presenting the febrile movement most closely resembling typhoid is Malta fever. If the history of exposure be elicited, the diagnosis can only be made by the clinical and bacteriological findings. A differential diagnosis of this fever is almost impossible in the majority of cases without the aid of the microscope and the serum test.

It will also be observed that the pulse rate of typhoid fever, while it exhibits a striking parallelism to the temperature curve, is relatively infrequent and does not attain the rapidity which we are accustomed to find in like degrees of fever. In no other febrile disease does this occur with such regularity.

By the fourth or fifth day the pulse is already dicrotic and usually remains so throughout the disease. This occurs more often in typhoid fever than in all the other infectious diseases put together, and, as will be shown, is of great differential value.

Oddo and Audibert, in the *Gazette des Hôpitaux*, under the title "Le dicrotisme dans la fièvre typhoïde," give some interesting facts illustrative of the character of the pulse of typhoid. They speak especially of the frequency with which dicrotism occurs during the initial period, stating that in the great majority of their cases it was present on the day of entry of the patient into the hospital. In a few cases this phenomenon was an early symptom only, disappearing in a short time. The authors accordingly recognize several types, dicrotisme ephemere, and dicrotisme persistent, the latter being subdivided into dicrotisme continu, dicrotisme secondaire, and dicrotisme intermittent. In all, fifty cases were examined. Thirty-four of these presented dicrotism. Of these thirty-four, six were ephemeral and lasted from ten to forty-eight hours, and thirteen were continuous. In five cases the dicrotism was continuous, but disappeared about the twentieth day and reappeared about the twenty-fifth, and continued until the close of the disease. This is the so-called dicrotisme secondaire. In thirteen cases the dicrotism was intermittent, continuing for two or three days, with an intermission of about the same length of time. From these cases, which were not selected, it would appear that the dicrotism, though valuable, is a variable sign and should be carefully searched for, even though absent when the patient is first examined.

The average pulse tension of typhoid fever is about 140. Just what diagnostic import is to be attached to this fact the author is not prepared to state. From his limited experience with the tonometer of Riva Rocca, he is led to believe that careful tabulation of the pulse tension in various diseases, together with the accurate recording of the various factors which may tend to raise or to lower pulse tension, will prove of considerable value in differential diagnosis.

Of great diagnostic significance are the roseola, which appear during the latter half of the first week, and are distributed upon the abdomen, chest, and back. The roseolous exanthemata of other infectious diseases in some cases resemble it, but rarely so closely as to deceive an experienced observer. Taken into consideration with the state of the spleen and the bowels, the time of the eruption and the subsidence of the rash, its succession of crops, its characteristic distribution and efflorescence, it is perhaps the most valuable single sign of the disease. Its value is enhanced by the fact that it is not preceded by an evanescent erythema as are most of the papular rashes of the acute exanthemata. Further, many reputable observers have recently determined that in the greater number of cases the blood obtained from the rose spots contains the bacillus typhosus.

The typhoid eruption appears later than that of any of the other exanthematous diseases; that of rötheln appearing on the first, scarlet fever on the second, measles and smallpox on the third, typhus on the fifth, and typhoid on the sixth or seventh day of the disease. The rash of rötheln is bright pinkish-red and lasts but two or three days; that of typhoid comes on in crops and the entire rash lasts much longer. Scarlet fever presents a subcuticular flush which may be so intense that the patient's skin may have the color of a boiled lobster, yet a noteworthy fact is the exaggeration of redness at certain points so that the skin has a mottled appearance. No rash like this occurs in typhoid. The eruption of measles is macular. The macules are dusky red and tend to coalesce and arrange themselves in crescentic areas. The typhoid roseola are papular, bright pinkish-red, and rarely coalesce. The papules of variola are shotty and do not disappear on pressure as do those of typhoid. Typhus presents a dusky subcuticular mottling. The typical typhoid eruption is raised above the level of the surrounding skin.

One of the most unique of recent diagnostic suggestions is that of Gibbes to recognize the rose spots by photographic processes before they are visible to the unaided eye. He uses an orthochromatic or non-halation plate, or, in the absence of one of these, a ray filter. Care is taken to focus exactly and the development is not pushed too far. A slow developer is used. By this means he has in several instances anticipated the roseola by several days.

In relation to the skin manifestations of typhoid, mention may be made of the drug rashes which may tend to cloud a diagnosis. Copaiba roseola are found most often on the extremities and do not possess the bright hue of those of typhoid. Furthermore, they appear suddenly, itch, and disappear on the withdrawal of the drug. The rash of quinine and atropine both resemble scarlet fever more closely than they do typhoid. Turpentine produces a blotchy rash, scarlatiniform in character, and only rarely resembling typhoid.

From the beginning of typhoid there is a progressive diminution in the number of the white blood corpuscles. There is usually also a reduction in the number of the red blood corpuscles and a corresponding decrease in the percentage of hæmoglobin. The red cells rarely exhibit marked changes in form, size, or color. The latter changes are found in most infectious diseases, but the absence of leukocytosis is of significance in the elimination of pneumonia, cerebrospinal meningitis, sepsis, and other diseases usually accompanied with an increase of white corpuscles.

Although enlargement of the spleen is observed in all infectious diseases, it is of special diagnostic significance in typhoid fever. There are reported cases in which it is demonstrable during the period of incubation, but it is very unusual to find this condition before the middle of the first week. In few other infectious diseases does the enlargement occur so early or persist so long, if we except Hodgkin's disease and malaria. Exception must be made in the case of typhus, however, in which the enlargement occurs during the first days of fever.

The stools of typhoid fever present no chemical or physical diagnostic peculiarities, if the presence of the bacillus of Eberth be excepted. However, their thin liquid, ochre-yellow, "pea-soup" character, penetrating ammoniacal odor, tendency to separate into two layers, and their relative infrequency will always call to the mind of the clinician typhoid fever.

The diazo reaction of Ehrlich may be found first occurring in typhoid from the fifth to the thirteenth days, and continuing while the disease is at its height. It is diminished in value by the fact that it may be found at times in pneumonia, scarlet fever, malaria, variola, measles, septic conditions and advanced malignant disease. Its absence in a case which otherwise closely simulates typhoid decides rather against the latter.

The negative rôle of profuse sweating, herpetic eruptions, jaundice, coryza, conjunctivitis, and vomiting is to be noted. Profuse sweating would point rather to acute tuberculosis, relapsing fever, pyæmia, acute ulcerative endocarditis, or acute articular rheumatism than to typhoid. Herpes occurs with frequency in malaria, pneumonia, epidemic cerebrospinal meningitis, and after the ingestion of salicylic acid, but very rarely in typhoid fever. Jaundice would indicate Weil's disease, remittent malarial fever, or acute yellow atrophy of the liver, rather than typhoid. Coryza and conjunctivitis at the onset would cause the diagnostician to incline more to the belief that measles or influenza existed; and vomiting would point to variola, typhus, or cerebrospinal meningitis, rather than to typhoid. "It must be emphasized that the ordinary symptoms of coryza—sneezing, increased secretion, conjunctival catarrh—are among the greatest exceptions, at least in moderately severe and severe cases of typhoid fever, and may be thrown in the balance against a diagnosis of typhoid fever. Severe infectious conditions with a predominating coryza generally have some other significance. Under such circumstances typhus fever and influenza especially would have to be considered."

Other symptoms referable to derangement of the respiratory organs have not uncommonly to be taken into diagnostic account. For the most part they obscure rather than aid in the diagnosis. Epistaxis has already been commented upon. It depends, as do most of the manifestations occurring in the upper air-passages in typhoid, upon the spongy hyperæmic condition of the mucous membrane. It is observed most frequently during the period of incubation and in the beginning of the febrile stage, and occurs in about seven per cent. of cases.

Tonsillitis and laryngitis occasionally occur early, and from the fact that the bacillus of Eberth has been repeatedly isolated from these locations, it would appear that in some cases, at least, the initial infection takes place in these organs. It may also be noted in this connection that the bacillus typhosus has been isolated from the sputum in the initial bronchitis sometimes met with. Just how much diagnostic weight is to be assigned to such findings it is hard to say, but with improved bacteriological methods it may be considerable.

The field which has long held forth the greatest promise of an infallible diagnostic method has been that of bacteriology. As has been stated, these expectations have in part to be fulfilled, but much has been already accomplished; the bacillus typhosus has been clearly differentiated from the colon bacillus; the specificity of the agglutinating action of immune serum has been demonstrated; cultures have repeatedly been made from the rose spots, urine, feces, sputum, and, what is of greater importance in the early diagnosis, from the blood itself.

Before considering the differences which exist between the bacillus typhosus and the colon bacillus, a brief description of the morphological and biological peculiarities of Eberth's bacillus will be à propos. The bacilli, as ordinarily seen, are short, thick rods about the length of one-third the diameter of a red blood corpuscle. The ends are rounded and their width is about one-third their length. They are actively motile and possess large numbers of flagellæ, which spring from the entire surface of the bacillus. In different environments the bacilli undergo various alterations in form, size, and arrangement. This has been the cause of many contradictory statements in regard to the biology of the organism. Undoubtedly there does exist a group of organisms which are intermediate in their biological manifestations between the typhoid and the colon bacilli. Whether these belong to the colon group or to the typhoid group or are in a separate division is a mere matter of nomenclature; the fact that they have been repeatedly isolated from the blood of patients, and the fact that these organisms display the Pfeiffer phenomenon with immune serum, is sufficient proof of their existence. They will be considered at greater length under the discussion of the elimination of paratyphoid fever from the diagnosis of typhoid fever.

The typhoid bacillus displays facultative anaërobiosis and grows readily upon the various culture media, especially the potato, at room temperature. The investigations of Gaffky into the cultural peculiarities upon the potato have been the nucleus from which have sprung many valuable methods for isolating the typhoid bacillus.

Of the special cultural and biological differences existing between the colon and the typhoid bacilli little need be said. The longer and more numerous flagellæ of the bacillus of Eberth, its greater motility, its cultural peculiarities on potatoes, litmus milk and glucose agar, and its specific reaction to the typhoid serum render its recognition comparatively easy.

The reaction of the colon bacilli to the serum of guinea-pigs immunized against it and the similar reaction of the paracolon group should be specially mentioned as differentiating them from the typhoid bacilli. To be sure, the typhoid bacillus also reacts to these sera, but only in the low dilutions, and therefore would not deceive a careful and experienced observer.

The Widal method of serum diagnosis has probably received more space in the typhoidiana of recent years than any other single sign of typhoid fever. As this paper includes the differential diagnosis of typhoid fever in its earliest stages only, any prolonged discussion of the methods and shortcomings of the agglutination test would be out of place.

The lysogenic action of the serum has proven in the hands of thousands of competent observers to be of inestimable value, but the statement of Widal that the reaction occurs as early as the end of the first week has been fulfilled only in the minority of cases. It is unfortunate for the early differential diagnosis that the occurrence of the reaction is usually delayed until the tenth day and may not present itself until late in the disease. It is equally unfortunate that the reaction occurs during health with the blood of individuals who have never had the disease; that it is found in the presence of other diseases, especially the acute infectious diseases; and that it sometimes persists for years after an attack of typhoid fever. It is to be remembered, however, that these errors are only apparent and that they occur only when the lower dilutions of the serum are used. With the higher dilutions and careful noting of the length of time elapsing before the reaction occurs, the liability to error will be greatly minimized.

Only very recently a method which combines the serum reaction of Widal and the culture of the bacilli from the stools, has been introduced by Wolff, of Hartford. It is very original and evidently practical, as will be seen by the following excerpts from Wolff's original article:

"The technique is very simple. A loop from the feces of the suspected case is smeared upon the surface of an agar slant in a prepared tube. . . . . From this first specimen one or more bouillon cultures are prepared. The bouillon must react from 1 to 2 per cent. *alkaline* with the $\frac{n}{10}$ acid, using phenolphthalein as the indicator. The infected bouillon is now incubated at the usual temperature for twelve hours, when we are ready to make the examination. A sample of the blood is taken at the same time the specimen of the feces is procured. This is mixed with the bouillon culture by the usual procedure and placed upon the stage of the microscope. If now there is sufficient agglutinative material present, the typhoid bacilli (if they exist in the culture) will very shortly form clumps in the fields, which will be observed full of colon bacilli in active motion; and if this reaction does occur, we can of course safely say that the case has advanced at least to the second week of the disease. Should no reaction occur, another sample of the bouillon culture is tested with the blood from an advanced case of typhoid fever, the agglutinative power of which has been tested by the ordinary method, with a pure culture of the bacillus of Eberth. Indeed it is necessary for the proper use of this test to keep in stock a number of specimens of blood from well-marked typhoid cases. These can be kept in a dry place, and they retain their power to produce a reaction with a pure culture, probably indefinitely. With this blood, if the feces contain any typhoid bacilli, a positive and distinct reaction will shortly occur, the clumps of typhoid bacilli being more or less numerous according to the number of typhoid organisms present; while the still motile colon bacilli occupy the rest of the field, and are seen to be in active motion. This indicates that the case is one of typhoid fever, and that the disease is in an early stage, at least from the middle to the end of the first week. By means of this simple method we are enabled, 'in my opinion,' to make an accurate diagnosis in the early stages of the disease when the other symptoms may be more or less masked, and thus remove many elements of doubt in a suspicious case."

Within the last two years blood cultural methods have been constantly brought forward which demonstrated the bacilli in the general circulation. Recently, however, the bacilli have been demonstrated prior to the occurrence of the Widal reaction and, in a few instances, before the enlargement of the spleen or the appearance of the roseola:

The method of Seeman for examining the blood obtained from the rose spots is perhaps the simplest. A drop of bouillon is placed over the sterilized skin and an incision made into the rose spot through the bouillon. A little of the blood from the rose spot is then squeezed out and mixed with the bouillon, which is examined by the ordinary cultural methods.

The examination of the blood obtained from the rose spots is not without limitations, especially in the early diagnosis. The spots do not appear before the sixth or seventh day as a rule, and in doubtful cases may be absent even then. To be of value the rose spots must be quite fresh, as the old bacilli are too weakened to grow well on ordinary media. Further, if the observer is competent to make a bacteriological examination of the fluid obtained from a rose spot, he is just as competent to examine blood obtained by venesection.

The technique of this method of investigation is comparatively simple and can be easily carried out in any fairly well equipped laboratory. The most important factor is the avoidance of contamination. To this end, the arm at the bend of the elbow is prepared by the usual surgical methods and a wet bichloride dressing allowed to remain until the time of taking the blood. The hands of the operator are prepared as for an aseptic operation. A constriction is placed above the patient's elbow to distend the veins and the skin is anæsthetized by pure carbolic acid or ethyl chloride. A solid metal or glass syringe, provided with a tight piston and a sharp needle, is boiled five minutes. The needle is passed directly into (not through) the vein, great care being taken not to contaminate it in any way during the procedure. Five cubic centimetres of blood are withdrawn and distributed equally between five Erlenmeyer flasks, each containing 100 c.c. of bouillon. These are well shaken to distribute the bacilli from within the clots, and incubated for twenty-four hours, when if a culture is apparent transplantations may be made on the various media. The original flasks may be incubated twenty-four hours longer and a stab culture then made on agar. If the hanging drop at this time shows a motile organism, a six-hour culture in bouillon is made and the Widal reaction tried with a known immune serum. The results of this method have proven very satisfactory, and its value in early diagnosis is shown by the fact that it occurs in about 87.5 per cent. of cases during the first week.

As an evidence of the high diagnostic value of blood cultural methods in diagnosing typhoid, may be quoted Schottmüller, who in his series of 119 cases discovered the bacillus of Eberth in the blood in 84 per cent. The earliest case in which it was possible to make an examination was on the second day of the disease, and the result was positive. In a great many cases typhoid bacilli were discovered before the Widal reaction occurred. These investigations must naturally alter our idea of the pathology of typhoid, in that they show that throughout the entire course of the disease the bacilli circulate in considerable number in the blood. This accounts for the occurrence of the roseola and remote inflammatory changes during the course of the disease.

Typhoid bacilli have been frequently isolated from blood obtained by splenic puncture. The date of their appearance in splenic blood is probably very early, and, from a diagnostic standpoint, very important. This has, in the past, led many "who rush in where angels fear to tread" to adopt this method of procedure, regardless of the very grave consequences which it may entail. The practice is now discountenanced by most investigators and has given way to the examination of the blood obtained from other sources.

Typhoid bacilli have long been known to exist in the stools and have been isolated in many cases, but only after the use of much difficult laboratory technique. The great objection to the bacteriological examination of the stools has been the extreme difficulty in separating the typhoid bacilli in pure culture uncontaminated with the colon bacillus.

The method of Remy has proven successful in the hands of several investigators. The principle underlying it is the use of a medium which endeavors to approximate the chemical constitution of the potato, and to this end definite amounts of asparagin and several of the inorganic salts are added. Just before using, a little milk-sugar and two drops of 1:40 solution of carbolic acid are added to each test tube. The feces are diluted about 1:8000 and plated with the melted medium. At room temperature colonies appear in forty-eight hours. The colonies are transplanted on bouillon and examined for motility and also cultivated to determine gas or indol production. By this method the bacilli have been found in several reported cases before the occurrence of the Widal reaction.

Several other equally good methods, each working on a different principle, have been introduced within the past two years. That of Hiss has met with considerable approval, and, as he has outlined his method with far more clearness than the author can, a portion of his original article on the subject is herewith inserted:

"Two media are used: one, for the differentiation of the colonies of the typhoid bacilli from those of the colon group, by plate culture; and one, for the differentiation of these forms in pure culture, in tubes.

"The plating medium is composed of 10 gm. of agar, 25 gm. of gelatin, 5 gm. of sodium chloride, 5 gm. of Liebig's extract of beef, 10 gm. of glucose, and 1000 c.c. of distilled water. The final titration of this medium should indicate the presence of about 2 per cent. of normal acid (1.8 per cent. to be exact), phenolphthalein being the indicator; and the medium should be brought to this acidity by the addition of normal hydrochloric acid solution.

"The growth of the typhoid bacilli in plates made from this medium gives rise to small light greenish colonies with irregular outgrowths and fringing threads. The colon colonies, on the other hand, are much larger, and as a rule are darker and do not form threads. This medium is practically solid and the differentiation seems to depend upon the fact that typhoid bacilli form threads in a medium of this acidity when peptone is absent.

"The tube medium contains 5 gm. of agar, 80 gm. of gelatin, 5 gm. of sodium chloride, 5 gm. of Liebig's extract of beef, 10 gm. of glucose, and 1000 c.c. of distilled water, and should react 1.5 per cent. acid, phenolphthalein being the indicator.

"In this semisolid medium the growth of the typhoid bacillus produces uniform turbidity at 37° C. within eighteen hours. The colon cultures do not give the uniform clouding and present several appearances, dependent upon differences in the degree of their motility, and upon their power to produce gas in the medium.

"The usual method of making the test is to take enough of the specimen of feces—that is, from one to several loopfuls—and transfer it to a tube containing broth, making the broth fairly cloudy. From this emulsion five or six plates are usually made by transferring one to five loopfuls of the emulsion to tubes containing the melted plate medium, and then pouring the contents of these tubes into Petri dishes. These dishes, after the medium has hardened, are placed in an incubator at 37° C. and allowed to remain for eighteen to twenty-four hours, when they are ready for examination. If typical colonies with fringing threads and outgrowths are found, the tube medium is inoculated from them and placed in the incubator at 37° C. for eighteen hours. If these tubes then present the characteristic clouding, our experience indicates that the diagnosis of typhoid may safely be made; for the bacillus of typhoid alone, of all the organisms occurring in feces investigated during these experiments, has displayed the power of giving rise both to colonies with fringing threads in the plating medium, and the uniform clouding in the tube medium, when exposed to a temperature of 37° C.

"A diagnosis may thus be made in thirty-four to forty-eight hours. If doubt is entertained as to the distinctiveness or value of these characters, the bacillus may be further tested against a dilution of typhoid serum."

Higley believes that the method of Hiss has given slightly better results in his hands than the Widal reaction. It has occurred in a few instances earlier by several days. The method is more difficult than the cultural examination of the blood. It remains to be seen if it is in any way superior to it, but this does not detract from its value as a link in the chain of diagnostic evidence.

It is doubtful if the bacillus typhosus occurs in the urine sufficiently early to be of material aid in the early diagnosis. In a few isolated cases they have been found as early as the sixth day, but this is very rare. Later they may occur in such enormous numbers as to cause a peculiar shimmer when the urine is shaken.

What has been said of the urine applies even more forcibly to the expectoration, sweat, and expired air. That the first may contain the bacillus of Eberth early in the disease is not to be denied; but this occurs most often in typhopneumonia, which is a rare early complication. The elimination of the bacilli in the sweat, tears, and expired air is too infrequent to entitle them to diagnostic importance.

The method of Moore acts upon the combined principles of the lysogenic action of the colon serum and the motility of the typhoid organism. In one arm of a W-shaped tube containing bouillon, to which has been added the serum obtained from a rabbit immunized to the colon bacillus, is planted a loopful of the culture from which it is desired to obtain the bacillus typhosus uncontaminated. The serum causes the Gruber reaction to occur with the colon bacilli and they are agglutinated and precipitated. The typhoid bacilli emigrate and may be obtained in pure culture in the other arm of the tube.

Still another method is that of Biffi, who also utilizes the agglutinating serum of the bacterium coli. Contrary to Cambier, he found that the colon bacillus would pass through an earthen filter quite as readily as the bacillus typhosus. He accordingly first introduces the substance to be examined into bouillon, to which has been added a serum which will agglutinate all the varieties of the colon bacilli. This is prepared according to the method of Pfeiffer for preparing typhoid agglutinating serum. The rabbit which is to furnish the serum should be injected with all the varieties of the colon bacilli, so that he shall be equally immune to all the varieties, and his serum able to agglutinate any species of the colon bacilli which may be present in the substance to be examined. This serum should be tested as to its agglutinating power and a quantity added to the bouillon proportional to its agglutinating ability.

The foregoing has considered the general data for diagnosis and has indicated their application in a few instances. The specific differences which exist between typhoid fever and the diseases which may resemble it must now be considered.

During the developmental period of the acute exanthemata they may present symptoms which will render difficult the differential diagnosis. This is especially true of measles, scarlet fever, variola, and typhus. The knowledge of exposure to any one of these diseases will of course aid materially, but the most reliance can be placed upon the initial symptoms. Perhaps the earliest manifestation of all the eruptive diseases occurs in the pharyngeal mucous membrane; such involvement is very rare in typhoid fever. The coryza and conjunctivitis of measles, the angina of scarlet fever, and the initial backache of smallpox are all in contradistinction to the onset of typhoid. Variola presents in addition an initial rash, which may be as diffuse and vivid as a true scarlatina. A careful observation of the wrists and hair line for shotty papules will usually prevent error.

Confounded and associated under the same name until the middle of the nineteenth century, it is not surprising that, even at the present time, some difficulty may exist in making an early and accurate diagnosis between typhus and typhoid fevers. Prior to the appearance of the eruption it may be almost impossible. The uneventful period of incubation, followed by a chill and an abrupt and rapid rise of temperature; the extreme rapidity of the pulse; the early vomiting and extreme prostration of typhus are in sharp contrast to the step-like gradations of temperature, slowness of the pulse, and absence of early vomiting and prostration of typhoid fever. Proportional to the rapid rise and severity of the fever are the profound disturbances referable to the derangement of the nervous system which occur earlier and with greater severity than in typhoid.

Not infrequently typhoid patients continue on duty during the first ten days of the disease, and delirium and coma do not occur until late. In typhus, on the other hand, they are prostrated at the very onset of the disease, and delirium, stupor, and coma may rapidly succeed one another.

The blood findings of the two diseases present marked differences; typhus showing a moderate leukocytosis, while in typhoid an actual diminution of the white cells occurs. Typhoid presents in the great majority of cases the specific bacillus before the expiration of the first seven days. Thus far no organisms have been found in the blood of typhus patients. Later typhoid blood shows the Widal reaction, which does not occur with typhus serum.

Far more important and readier of demonstration are the skin eruptions of the two diseases. That of typhus occurs earlier, and in typical cases presents such marked differences that the differentiation is easy for an observer of experience. It should be mentioned in this connection, however, that typhus cases do occur in which it is very imperfectly developed or entirely absent. The exanthem of typhus is distributed with uniformity over the trunk and limbs. It is neither well defined nor sharply limited. It is macular, hemorrhagic, and distinctly petechial. It appears in a single crop, a second eruption being practically unknown. It has a dusky red, coppery hue, and appears as if beneath the surface of the skin. The eruption of typhoid, on the other hand, usually involves the trunk alone. It is sharply defined, papular, and purely hyperæmic. It appears in crops, is bright pinkish-red and is slightly elevated above the surface of the skin.

The face of typhoid fever early exhibits bright eyes and slightly flushed cheeks, later a dull and apathetic countenance. Typhus, on the contrary, presents a swollen, livid-red appearance, with injected conjunctivæ, contracted pupils, and an agitated expression.

The disease which may occasion the greatest difficulty in early differentiation is acute miliary tuberculosis. Many cases are under observation for weeks before the diagnostician can arrive at a conclusion, and then perhaps only after the recovery or death of the patient. Both have this in common, that the manifestations of each are due to the action of similarly acting toxins. The initial malaise, headache, anorexia, and irregularity of the bowels is present in both. Each presents enlargement of the spleen, but it occurs earlier and more markedly in typhoid. Both present the Ehrlich diazo reaction and febrile albuminuria. The reddish spots which occur on the abdomen in miliary tuberculosis may cause confusion. They do not appear in crops and are much less abundant than the roseola of typhoid. Profuse sweating occurs much more often in miliary tuberculosis. An important difference occurs in the temperature pulse curve of the two diseases, the marked irregularity of temperature, with a proportionally rapid pulse, of acute phthisis being quite the opposite of the steady ascent and comparatively slow pulse of typhoid. Acute phthisis presents Kernig's sign; typhoid never. Dicrotism is rare in miliary tuberculosis. There may be, though unusually, a leukocytosis in acute tuberculosis, and the bacillus tuberculosis has been found in the blood of a few cases. The absence of leukocytosis would not necessarily decide in favor of typhoid, but the discovery of the bacillus of Eberth in the blood, or the occurrence of the Widal reaction, would. The relative increase in the large mononuclear leukocytes found in typhoid does not occur in acute tuberculosis. In the minority of cases the eye-grounds show choroidal tubercles. This is a decisive condition when present. Tubercle bacilli are rarely found in the sputum of an acute tuberculosis, and the lung findings may be exactly the same at the beginning of both diseases. There is, however, a greater tendency to respiratory frequency and slight cyanosis in miliary tuberculosis. Curschmann considers acute pulmonary emphysema "an especially decisive objective sign" never occurring "as the result of typhoid bronchitis."

In peritoneal tuberculosis the persistent abdominal pain and physical signs of effusion will make the diagnosis. Very early a decision will rest upon the physical findings indicative of tuberculosis of other organs.

When tubercular meningitis accompanies the general process, the diagnosis is rendered somewhat easier. The sudden onset with a convulsion, or severe headache and high fever; the agonizing pain; projectile vomiting; hydrocephalic cry, and contracted pupils go to make up a picture widely different from that of typhoid. The pulse of basilar meningitis is at first small and rapid. Subsequently it is as slow as in typhoid, but is irregular and rarely dicrotic. Quincke's lumbar puncture should never be omitted in doubtful cases. If the tubercle bacilli be present they will be discovered on centrifugalization of the spinal fluid, and will, of course, determine the diagnosis.

Cerebrospinal meningitis, however, is not so readily differentiated from those cases of typhoid ushered in by headache, photophobia, delirium, retraction of the head, twitching of the muscles, and even convulsions. It is easy to make a decision when an epidemic of one or the other is prevailing, but it is in sporadic cases that the chief difficulty lies. The irregular and variable temperature, the marked increase in the polynuclear leukocytes, and the profound psychical disturbances have no great resemblance to typhoid. The cutaneous symptoms of the two diseases are very different. Herpes occurs with great frequency in cerebrospinal meningitis, but almost never in typhoid. The rash of the first is petechial and is sometimes distributed over the entire skin. That of the latter is hyperæmic and usually limited to the trunk.

The examination of the fluid obtained by lumbar puncture for the diplococcus intracellularis meningitidis of Weichselbaum is the most reliable method of diagnosis. Blood cultures should also be made to determine the presence of the bacillus of Eberth, and with the newer bacteriological methods will prove of great value.

Meningitis or cerebral abscess from ear disease may sometimes resemble typhoid. The history of sudden cessation of a chronic ear discharge, followed by a rise of temperature, nausea, vomiting, and the symptoms of an acute septic infection engrafted on an existing chronic saprogenic suppuration, would certainly point to a purulent meningitis. The careful examination of the mastoid will sometimes render a decision.

Irregular forms of malarial fever, particularly when due to infection with the æstivo-autumnal parasite, may closely resemble typhoid fever. The onset of typhoid differs from that of remittent fever, in that that of the former is gradual and progressive, with slight chilly sensations and step-like gradations of temperature which rarely reach 40° C. before the fourth day; while the onset of remittent fever is generally intermittent, with severe chills and irregular remissions of temperature which may reach 40° C. in twenty-four hours or less. The temperature of malarial fever disappears under the use of quinine, while that of typhoid is not influenced by it. The grayish color of the face, the subicteric sclera, and the anxious, restless expression of remittent fever are all quite the opposite of the facies of typhoid, which early presents flushed cheeks, clear sclera, and an alert but not anxious countenance. Herpes is common in æstivo-autumnal fever, but rare in typhoid. Early delirium is rare in typhoid, but when occurring is persistent and variable only in degree. The delirium of remittent fever, on the contrary, may come on in the early days, is recurrent, and changes with the exacerbations of temperature and other symptoms.

An increase of the lymphocytes to 40 per cent. or over, without any increase in the large mononuclears, points to typhoid as against malarial fever. An increase in the large mononuclears to 12 per cent. or upward, especially during the remissions of temperature, indicates malaria rather than typhoid. The presence of myelocytes in any such number as from 1 to 5 per cent. indicates malaria rather than typhoid. A high degree of anæmia is more common in malaria. A very great reduction in the total leukocyte count is more frequently met with in malaria than in typhoid fever; while the proportion of white to red corpuscles in malaria is not infrequently less than 1 to 2000, which is rare in typhoid fever.

Finally, it is to be noted that cases have been reported in which typhoid fever is superimposed upon a malarial infection; and that, in these cases, the blood not only contains the bodies of Laveran, but also the typhoid bacillus. Fortunately such an occurrence is rare, at least it is rarely recognized; but the knowledge that such double infections do occur will sometimes call for more careful clinical and bacteriological examination.

Remittent fever presents no typical exanthem and the urticaria, which occurs not uncommonly, is very different from the roseola of typhoid. The early anæmia of æstivo-autumnal fever is not found in typhoid. The blood in the former shows leukocytosis, without diminution in the eosinophiles; that of the latter, no leukocytosis and marked diminution of the eosinophiles. Further, typhoid blood shows no malarial parasites or pigmented leukocytes, but, on the contrary, the typhoid bacilli and the Widal reaction.

Plague may occasionally be mistaken for typhoid fever, but the reverse will very rarely happen. The history of exposure to plague may be obtainable, though not commonly. The period of incubation of plague is much shorter than that of typhoid, nine days being the extreme limit. The prodromes may be entirely absent or at least of such mild character as to be unnoticed by the patient himself. Occasionally they may exactly duplicate those of typhoid, but pain and stiffness in the joints and tenderness in the groins or axillæ will be present also in the glandular type. The stage of invasion with chills, rigors, or sensations of heat is in sharp contrast to typhoid fever. In pestis siderans, the overwhelmingly sudden onset, with rapidly succeeding delirium, vomiting, hæmatemesis, hæmaturia, melæna, coma, collapse, and death, has no parallel in typhoid fever. The presence of the bacillus pestis in the blood and the reaction of the serum to Pfeiffer's phenomenon are final distinguishing points from typhoid.

Influenza of the gastrointestinal form may be readily mistaken for typhoid. The abrupt onset, early prostration, and multiplicity of symptoms found in typical cases of influenza are very different from the gradual onset of typhoid. The absence of splenic enlargement and the typical roseola in influenza should also be noted. In those typhoid cases in which the nervous element preponderates, examination of the blood may be necessary to make a diagnosis. The presence of an epidemic, the contagious nature of the affection, and the presence of Pfeiffer's organism all point to influenza.

Cases of typhoid presenting marked pulmonary symptoms at the onset may be readily confounded with lobar pneumonia. On the other hand, cases of pneumonia with insidious onset may be mistaken for typhoid fever. This is particularly true of the so-called senile pneumonias, and also of those cases in which the pneumonic process commences in the centre of the lung. Osler says, "Nervous symptoms are more frequent in pneumonia than in typhoid, and from the onset may so dominate that the local lesion is entirely overlooked." The absence of leukocytosis in typhoid and the presence of Eberth's bacillus in the blood and the dejections are of great differential value. The presence of the Widal reaction will, of course, be decisive. If the bacillus typhosus be found, the case may be considered pneumotyphoid. It should be mentioned in this connection that there occur, not infrequently, cases in which a diplococcus pneumoniæ is engrafted upon typhoid. It is not to these cases that the term pneumotyphoid is applied, but to those whose manifestations depend upon the bacillus of Eberth alone.

Pyæmia and other septic processes may sometimes require differentiation from typhoid fever. It is in such cases that the examination of the blood, with the view of determining the presence of Eberth's bacillus and the Widal reaction, and the absence of leukocytosis in typhoid, will prove of great value. In differentiating typhoid from puerperal septicæmia, the fact that pregnant women ill of typhoid usually abort may sometimes prevent error. The appearance of the roseola and the serum reaction will end all doubt in the matter.

Another pyæmic process which may occasion great difficulty is malignant endocarditis. Both diseases present enlargement of the spleen, abdominal tenderness, and diarrhœa; each shows delirium, stupor, and progressive exhaustion. If the heart was previously intact, symptoms referable to a cardiac lesion would be almost pathognomonic, as ulcerative endocarditis complicating typhoid usually occurs very late in the disease, at a time when the diagnosis has already been made. The temperature of ulcerative endocarditis is less regular in type than typhoid, and chills and sweats are far more common. Leukocytosis is marked in malignant endocarditis, but is absent in typhoid unless inflammatory complications occur. Furthermore, cardiac distress occurring in the course of typhoid is usually devoid of the extreme oppression and shortness of breath of endocarditis.

Infectious osteomyelitis, the "typhe epiphysaire" of Chassaignac, may simulate typhoid. The examination of the epiphyseal regions of the long medullated bones, and the inspection of the extremities for œdema, livid redness, and points of circumscribed tenderness will yield valuable information. Another diagnostic point is the presence of leukocytosis and the absence of the serum reaction and the specific bacilli from the blood in osteomyelitis.

As has been previously pointed out, Malta fever may very closely resemble typhoid. The temperature curves of the two diseases may be almost identical, and both give rise to headache, insomnia, and anorexia. The presence of the micrococcus melitensis in the blood, and the serum reaction with this germ would be diagnostic of Malta fever. Probably the micrococcus is present in all the dejections. It has been isolated from the urine and blood repeatedly. Sweating and violent joint pain are common and early symptoms in nearly all cases of Malta fever. Joint pain may occur early in typhoid also, but rarely with such severity as mentioned above.

Relapsing fever, at the onset or at the beginning of an epidemic, may be mistaken for an anomalous typhoid. The temperature of febris recurrens nearly always rises suddenly at the onset and remains in the neighborhood of 40° C. from three to seven days, when it suddenly falls by crisis. High initial temperatures are rare in typhoid, and a fall by crisis practically unknown. The presence of the spirillum of Obermeier in the blood of relapsing fever, and the bacillus of Eberth in that of typhoid, together with the rarity of relapsing fever, all aid in the diagnosis.

There are times when trichiniasis with predominant gastroenteric symptoms may closely simulate typhoid fever. Distinguishing points are the presence of vomiting, œdema of the face and eyelids, and extreme myositis in trichiniasis.

Trichiniasis rarely presents the characteristic typhoid roseola or the enlargement of the spleen. The flexor contractures of the arms and legs, the painful swelling and tension of the muscles, the profuse sweating and itching of the skin, all make a much different picture from typhoid. The marked leukocytosis, especially the extraordinary increase in the eosinophiles, is in strong contrast to typhoid. The examination of a portion of the pectoral muscles will render final decision.

"Trichinosis and typhoid fever have been frequently associated, but most commonly the trichinosis has been in the patient and the typhoid fever in the mind of the physician. The association in the patient of these two diseases appears to be exceedingly rare." There are only two reported cases to be found in the literature of the subject, and this extreme rarity would almost exclude such a condition from the diagnosis, but might, in some cases, require an examination both of the blood and the muscle section.

Weil's disease with marked gastrointestinal symptoms may sometimes simulate typhoid. Its mode of onset, the history of exposure to cold, and the fact that it occurs most often in brewers, butchers, and ice-plant laborers, are all diagnostic points. The jaundice is severe and early. As has been before pointed out, this occurs but rarely in typhoid. The temperature is high and remains so from the beginning of the disease. There is usually enlargement of the liver and subcutaneous œdema over the hepatic area. The blood may contain the bacillus proteus fluorescens, which is in marked contrast to the bacillus of Eberth.

Very mild cases of typhoid are apt to be diagnosed simple continued fever, in the early stages especially. The examination of the blood for Eberth's bacillus and the Widal reaction will settle the diagnosis.

During an epidemic of typhoid fever, catarrhal enteritis, especially in children, may give rise to symptoms like a mild or abortive attack of enteric fever. The absence of splenic enlargement, the rose spots, and the Widal reaction will usually determine the disease.

Papular syphilides may resemble the typhoid roseola. Usually they are easily differentiated, but Curschmann speaks of a case in which not only the eruption but also the general symptoms closely simulated typhoid. On the whole, a papular syphilide is of a darker and more coppery hue and more generally distributed. In these cases the history of a preceding initial lesion may aid materially.

Acute glanders with marked gastrointestinal symptoms may be suggestive of typhoid. However, the characteristic rash and the presence of the bacillus mallei will make a diagnosis. The use of mallein for diagnostic purposes is also of value.

Cases of prolonged appendicitis with slow onset will present differences which require careful investigation to be discovered. The pulse will be higher in proportion to the fever, and there will be much smaller remissions of temperature, and rarely roseola or the diazo reaction. There is marked leukocytosis.

Weiss, in his admirable paper read before the American Medical Association at the Chicago meeting in 1900, detailed a method for the staining of blood to determine the presence of suppuration in the body. The stain he used is as follows:

℞.—Iodi sublim.	1
Kali iodati	3
Aqua destil.	200
Gummi arab. q. s. ad consistentiam syruposam.	

A drop of blood taken from the lobe of the ear is carefully pressed between two cover-glasses so as to get as thin a smear as possible. This is air dried or fixed, after which a drop of the staining solution is then added to the slide, and the specimen is then ready for examination with the microscope. Blood from a perfectly healthy individual shows a dark yellowish staining of the red corpuscles. The nuclei of the white corpuscles take on a lemon-yellow colored, very glossy appearance, while the body of the cell is a slightly darker yellow. Normal blood also contains brown granules (extracellular glycogen).

The blood gives an altogether different reaction if suppuration be present. There is a great increase of extracellular glycogen, as shown by the large numbers of dark-brown granules present in the stained blood. The leukocytes assume a brownish hue, varying in intensity from reddish-brown to dark yellow. The polynuclear neutrophiles are almost exclusively concerned in this reaction, as it never appears in the eosinophiles.

The value of this method in eliminating suppurative appendicitis from the diagnosis is great. It is easy of application and in the hands of the author has proven very satisfactory.

An affection whose clinical manifestations may be identical with those of typhoid is paratyphoid fever. Since 1896, when Archard and Bensaude made their first report, eighty-four cases have been recorded; and, without doubt, many, which hitherto have passed as true typhoid, but which have presented no Widal reaction, except in low dilution, are to be classed under this head. The symptoms during the period of incubation are in most respects identical in the two diseases, headache, malaise, anorexia, irregularity of the bowels, rose spots, enlargement of the spleen, and a gradually ascending temperature being the rule. Epistaxis has been noted in a number of instances, and the diazo-reaction of Ehrlich may be given by the urine. In uncomplicated cases the blood shows no leukocytosis. On the whole, the paratyphoid is milder and rather shorter than true typhoid; but in the early stages a differential diagnosis may be almost impossible. In low dilutions of the serum, even the Widal reaction occurs positively.

The knowledge which we now possess in regard to this disease has been the result largely of the practice of making blood cultures, and this still remains the surest method of diagnosing the disease. Two species of paratyphoid bacilli are recognized. Buxton classifies them as the alpha and beta paratyphoids. The alpha produces less gas in glucose media and resembles the typhoid in its action on milk. It differs from the beta paratyphoid in that the acidity on litmus milk is persistent, while that of the beta paratyphoid is finally changed to alkalinity.

Both of the paratyphoid organisms present Pfeiffer's phenomenon with immune serum. As Pratt has clearly pointed out, the blood should be tested with both species of the paratyphoid bacilli whenever there is any doubt about the diagnosis. As an example of this he quotes a case in which the serum gave a negative reaction with the alpha paratyphoid in 1:10 dilution, but completely clumped the beta paratyphoid in as high a dilution as 1:500. There may possibly be cases in which typhoid and paratyphoid coexist. At least it would seem so from some of the recent bacteriological findings. Pratt cites an instance in which "Bain, working in Dr. F. C. Shattuck's wards at the Massachusetts Hospital, found a case of typhoid fever the blood of which agglutinated the bacillus paratyphoid immediately and completely in dilution of 1:10. In higher dilution up to 1:200 there was clumping without loss of motility. There was no reaction with the typhoid bacillus in dilution of 1:10. A culture from the blood, however, yielded a pure, abundant growth of the bacillus typhosus. The case died. Unfortunately no autopsy was held." Everything taken into consideration, the surest method of diagnosing paratyphoid from true typhoid lies in the cultivation of the bacillus from the blood of the suspected case.

There are times when the medical officer is called upon to make what might be called "a sanitary diagnosis," and to determine the presence or absence of typhoid fever.

The writer refers to those cases in which epidemics of disease occur—*e.g.*, during the Spanish-American war; and boards of officers are called upon to decide as to the nature of the infection. Under such circumstances they would be required to make the diagnosis of the disease in its earliest stages but very rarely; as in the great majority of instances cases in all stages could be seen, and by the averaging of the signs and symptoms in the various cases, and making close investigation into the food and water supplies, and the methods employed in the disposal of refuse, a diagnosis could be accurately arrived at.

Conclusions. 1. There is no single symptom on which alone an early diagnosis of typhoid fever can be made. It is only by careful consideration of the symptom-complex that a clinical diagnosis can be arrived at.

2. The most trustworthy, as well as the earliest, sign of typhoid fever is the presence in the circulating blood of the bacillus of Eberth.

3. The demonstration of the bacillus of Eberth in the blood is not beyond any fairly well equipped laboratory.

4. The bacillus of Eberth is found in the feces later than in the blood, but with comparative ease. The presence of the bacillus typhosus in the feces is of great value as a corroborative sign.

5. The presence of the bacillus typhosus in the rose spots is a trustworthy sign, but has no advantages over the examination of the blood from other localities.

6. The serum reaction of Widal is seldom demonstrable during the earliest stages of typhoid fever. It is of value only in the higher dilutions.

References.

Allen. The American Journal of the Medical Sciences, January, 1903.
Archard and Bensaude. Bull. et mém. de la soc. des hôp. de Paris, 1896, vol. xiii.
Biffi, V. La rif. méd., 1902.
Brannon. Twentieth Century Practice, 1899.
Busquet. La presse méd., Paris, 1902.
Cabot. Serum Diagnosis of Disease, 1898.
Coleman and Buxton. The American Journal of the Medical Sciences, 1902.
Courmont. Bull. et mém. de soc. méd. de Paris, 1902, vol. xviii.
Craig. The American Journal of the Medical Sciences, 1903.

Curschmann. Nothnagel's Encyclopedia, 1901.
Geddings. Public Health Reports (Surgeon-General U. S., P.H. and M.H.S.), 1900.
Gibbes. British Medical Journal, 1901.
Hare. Practical Diagnosis, 1899.
Higley. Medical News, New York, 1902, vol. lxxix.
Hiss. Ibid., 1901, vol. lxxvii.
Kerr and Harris. Chicago Medical Record, 1902, vol. xxiii.
McCrae. The American Journal of the Medical Sciences, 1902.
Moore. British Medical Journal, 1902, vol. ii.
Musser. Medical Diagnosis, 1896.
Oddo and Audibert. Gaz. de Hôp., Paris, 1902.
Osler. Practice of Medicine, 1901.
Pratt. Boston Medical and Surgical Journal, 1903, vol. cxlviii.
Remy. Annales de l'Institut Pasteur, 1900.
Richardson. Boston Medical and Surgical Journal, 1903, cxlviii.
Rogers. British Medical Journal, 1902, vol. i.
Sajous' Annual, article on Typhoid Fever, 1900.
Schottmüller. Münch. med. Woch., 1902.
Schumacher. Zeitsch. f. Hyg. u. Infect., 1901, vol. xxxvii.
Seeman. Berliner med. Woch., 1901.
Simon. Clinical Diagnosis.
Weiss. Journal of the American Medical Association, 1900.
Wolff. The American Journal of the Medical Sciences, 1903.

THE LOCALIZING DIAGNOSTIC SIGNIFICANCE OF SO-CALLED HEMIANOPIC HALLUCINATIONS, WITH REMARKS ON BITEMPORAL SCINTILLATING SCOTOMATA.

By Professor A. Pick,
of Prag.

A short time ago Jolly[1] proved that a form of excitation phenomenon in the hemianopic field of vision, viz., scotoma scintillans, has not its origin in the cerebrum, especially not in the cortex, but in the primary optical tracts. I concur with this observation and shall verify the same absolutely in the following: My aim, however, is to prove that more complicated phenomena than elementary light sensations, as characterized by the scintillating scotoma—*i. e.*, real hallucinations—may be produced in the hemianopic field of vision by localized focal or functional affections in the optic tracts. The commonly accepted idea, therefore, that such hallucinations are of value for the localization of the lesion in the occipital lobe, is not correct. The cases at my disposal, for the most part from private practice, have not been verified by autopsy, but the conclusions to be derived therefrom as to the site of the lesion are so clear, that even a hyperskeptical critic should have no doubt. This theory has already been exploited by Uhthoff,[2] by means of his own observations, by what he found in

[1] Berliner klinische Wochenschrift, 1902, Nos. 42-43.

[2] Monatschrift f. Psych. and Neurol., 1889, Bd. v. I must here remark that American authors, especially Seguin and Peterson, deserve a great deal of credit in this question.

literature, and also by the report of a case with autopsy; but the force of his conclusions is restricted by his own doubts, and perhaps this is the reason that the original theory still holds good. On this account it will not be superfluous to bring new material to clear up this question. On the subject of diagnosis, as to the site of lesion, I shall be as brief as possible.

Case I.—Bricklayer, aged sixty-two years, came into the clinic January, 1902. Had a purulent discharge from the ear as a child; since then hearing impaired on left side; had trachoma while a soldier, otherwise healthy. Suffers from trigeminal neuralgia since winter before last; impaired vision of five years' duration.

Six months ago he had a slight apoplectic seizure, a sudden feeling of weakness, causing him to drop an article, which he held in his hand, and fall to the floor. He was stunned but not unconscious; heard what was spoken, but could not understand all that was said. Spoke irrationally, disconnectedly, and knew that he did so, but could not help it. This condition lasted for from three to four hours, then he fell asleep. On awakening he felt much better, spoke again rationally and the general weakness gradually subsided. About a fortnight later he had a second attack, which took the same course as the first; only the patient observed, immediately after he was picked up from the floor, that the right half of the field of vision of both eyes had disappeared. These right halves of the visual field were represented by a black shadow divided from the left seeing halves by an exactly vertical line. This shadow slowly became paler without changing its form. Two weeks later he had another attack, the shadow moved still further into the field of vision, but returned to its former limit after a few hours. Three times more he had attacks, accompanied by the same phenomena—*i. e.*, general weakness, a faulty understanding of what was said to him, and an irresistible impulse to irrational, disconnected speech. Later he had a fourth, but lighter attack.

The somatic examination showed atheroma, vision reduced to 0.5 on both sides due to a commencing cataract, fundus normal, right homonymous hemianopsia, fields of vision as shown in Fig. 1.

Extrinsic ocular muscles normal, as was also the pupillary reaction. In the left eye accommodation was almost *nil*. No painful pressure points in course of left fifth nerve. The right corner of the mouth a little the lower, right palpebral aperture somewhat wider than the left; no other disturbances of motion except a slight paresis of the right leg; sensation normal; knee-jerks on both sides considerably increased. No Babinski reflex. Closer questioning shows conclusively that the disturbances of speech and writing following an attack were paraphasia and paragraphia. The patient himself cites the example that instead of saying "close the door," he said "close the closet," knowing full well that he spoke incorrectly. Even now symptoms of paragraphia can occasionally be demonstrated.

The patient, who calls at the clinic from time to time, told the following story January 15, 1903: About six months ago, while walking, he suddenly observed that everything on the right side of his field of vision was of a reddish color, changing later to green. Then he noticed for about half an hour at his right side a dog walking along with him, the dog always appearing on the side on which he usually saw nothing. It looked like a real dog, but he convinced himself that it was only a shadow. Another time a girl with a colored shawl on her head walked

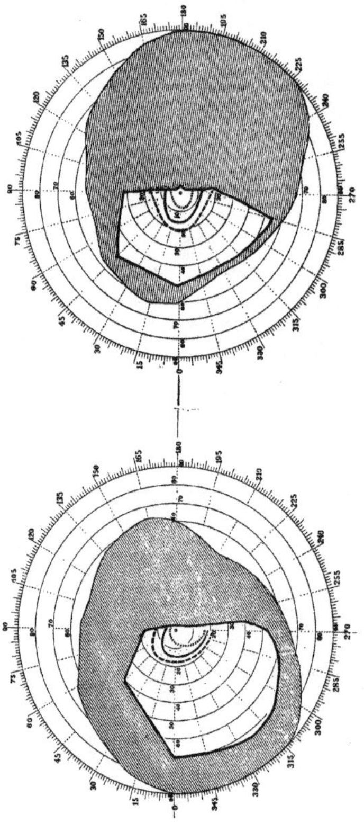

FIG. 1.

on his right side, but again he convinced himself that it was only a phantom. The color also was delusive. In general, he reports that occasionally he has slight attacks; as, for instance, on this day he had a feeling of chilliness and numbness in his left leg. Examination shows deviation of the tongue toward the right side, weakness of right arm, sensibility normal. It must still be remarked that the patient typically exhibited for a long time the faulty halving of horizontal lines, which phenomenon was first studied by Liepmann.[1] This symptom disappeared later, so that the patient now halves the lines correctly.

The phenomena described in the foregoing case and which presented themselves at first give rise to the assumption that we here have to deal with a focus of softening in the region of the left gyrus angularis, especially participated in by its medullary mass. The initial phenomena of paraphasia and paragraphia can be interpreted as neighboring symptoms, while the permanent hemianopsia is caused by the focus extending into the visual radiations of that locality. There is no reason to assume that there is a continuation of this focus toward the occipital lobe, as one would have to believe according to the older theory—as to the localization of the lesion in these cases of hemianopic hallucinations. Neither is there any reason by which a deeper disturbance of the functions of the occipital lobe, besides the optic tracts, could be demonstrated. Thus, this first case can only be looked upon as one contrary to the older theory.

Regarding hallucinations in general, it is now known that their provocation, and I emphasize provocation in contradistinction to the question as to the seat of the causative processes, can take place at any part of the visual apparatus, from the cornea to the cortical layer of the occipital lobe. Undoubtedly a similar theory, upon a broader basis, regarding hemianopic hallucinations will eventually be promulgated.

Case II.—Man, aged fifty-six years; always well; fell on his head from a sleigh about one year ago without any apparent harm. About four months before the first examination (February 16, 1902) he noticed that his left leg "went to sleep," also pains in left big toe; soon after a disturbance of vision toward the left was observed. Preceding the symptoms by two weeks he had occipital pains; other disturbances were not observed, especially no apoplexy. The patient afterward had a certain numbness in his left hand and for a few days after the disturbance of vision he noticed toward the left, in the blind half of the field of vision, all sorts of figures, or imagined occasionally somebody was sitting next to him. Dr. Bayer, oculist at Reichenberg, made the following examination under date of October 9, 1901:

"*Status Præsens.* Looking outward the right eye lags, pupils equally dilated, 3 mm. in diameter, illuminating right retina contracts slower than left (hemianopic pupillary reaction?), fundus normal. Binocular left-sided defect of field of vision with straight limitation, which only

[1] Liepmann and Kalmus. Ueber eine Augenmassstörung bei Hemianopikern. Berliner klin. Wochenschrift, 1900, No. 38.

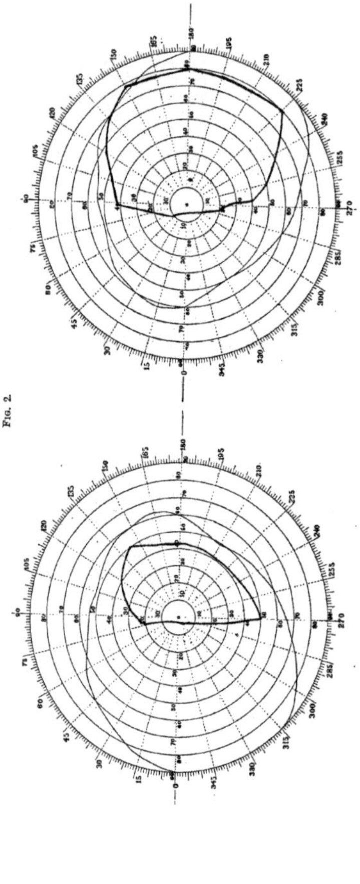

FIG. 2

toward the middle deviates slightly toward the left R. and L. 5/5 without correction, lead crust on his teeth, carotids feel somewhat harder than normal. Hemianæsthesia sinistra."

About one month later he had a seizure similar to an attack of Jacksonian epilepsy without loss of consciousness. Examination revealed, besides the hemianopsia, left-sided hemianæsthesia. My own examination on February 18, 1902, showed no disturbance of motion; the hand performs even the more delicate tests correctly. The sensibility of the hand seems slightly diminished, especially in fingers. Objects are not always definitely recognized. Sense of location undisturbed. Ophthalmological examination: Jaeger No. 1 can easily be read with glasses corresponding with his age. Insufficiency of right rectus internus; color sense normal. The right halves of both apillæ show changes in color Left homonymous hemianopsia with field of vision as seen in Fig. 2.

While the first case, when critically considered, admits of a possibility that the occipital lobe might be affected, in the second case this view must be altogether excluded, as moreover the provoking focus, producing the hemianopic hallucinations, is still further advanced and localized in the optic tracts. Looking at the symptoms of this case we will find only two localities by lesion of which the symptoms can be produced. We might consider the upper parietal lobe and the visual radiations running beneath it. But if we look upon the extent of involved territory, to make such extensive phenomena of hemianæsthesia and hemianopsia stationary, no apoplexy being present, we can only imagine that the latter were produced by one or several very small, very close foci of probable softening and we must look in another region. This we have in the posterior knee of the inner capsule, where the most posterior portion of the thalamus opticus meets the corpus geniculatum externum. In this region even a small focus can produce stationary hemianopsia or at first a complete and general, later incomplete and partial hemianæsthesia, as Henschen has demonstrated in a great number of cases.

Regarding the hemianopic hallucinations in this case, they present themselves as irritation phenomena, keeping step with the settling of the focus; while in the former case the identically localized hallucinations must be referred to some unknown irritative processes in the focus, the latter having existed for a longer period.

Case III. Woman, aged fifty-two years, has suffered for years from arteriosclerosis and cardiac disease, with frequent severe stenocardiac attacks with dyspnœa, pallor, and fainting. Had an apparently similar seizure, lasting for five minutes, on November 26, 1901, after which she suffered from a paresis of the left arm and left side of face. Disturbance on the left side of the field of vision was only noticed the second day and was then diagnosed by the attending physician as complete homonymous hemianopsia. Fundus normal. These attacks recurred several times, leaving a weakness of the former paretic muscles and occasional severe pains and paræsthesia in the left arm, left big toe, and the left side of the face. In addition she volunteered the statement, that for a few days after the first attack she suffered from an indefinable delirious condition, characterized by hallucinations, showing in

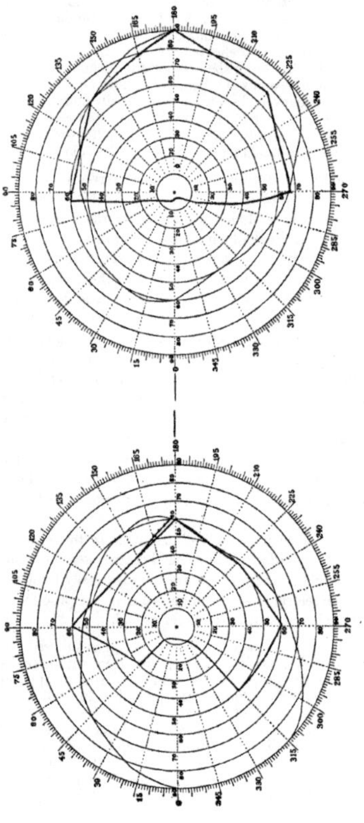

Fig. 3.

both the left blind halves of the field of vision all sorts of phantoms. She also asserted that at that time she had disturbances of smell and taste of a subjective nature, also sensations of coldness in the left half of the body. Urine was normal. Later had repeatedly pains in left arm, especially in the left index finger, and at the same time headache in the right side, dizziness, and feelings of anxiety. The left-sided homonymous hemianopsia remained stationary.

My examination on February 22, 1902, confirms the above-mentioned cardiac and arterial symptoms. Fundus normal. Complete left homonymous hemianopsia (Fig. 3). Sense of smell in left nostril diminished. Signs of paresis in the region of the left facial nerve, tongue not affected; slight evidences of paresis of the left hand, particularly of the thumb and index finger. Objectively no marked difference of motility of the legs, although subjectively complained of; sensibility in all qualities objectively quite normal; knee-jerk more pronounced in left than right. Subjectively, patient states that sense of touch and sensibility are diminished in the left hand.

The patient later complained of occasional headaches, accompanied by violent pains in the left index finger and left side of the neck, weakness of the left hand, which, however, disappeared after a few days. Later these attacks became less frequent. A subsequent examination showed the same picture of the field of vision. Liepman's disturbance still present.[1] Patient still complains of pain in the left upper extremity and a peculiar sense of dryness at the root of the tongue and at the palate.

Concerning this case I shall be very brief. The facts concerning localization agree so perfectly with Case II. that I should be forced to repeat. I believe, therefore, that according to all rules of localization the lesion should be considered as being in the most posterior part of the internal capsule, the optic thalamus, and perhaps also the corpus geniculatum externum. The hemianopic hallucinations here were also an expression of irritative processes produced by the focus, and later disappearing, when the irritation was removed. Hence this case also serves to strengthen the above cited theory of the localizing importance of hemianopic hallucinations.

I would call particular attention to two symptoms: 1. The evident "central" pains in the left arm. As early as 1879 Kahler and I[2] called attention to the relation of these pains to a focus in the region of the "Charcot carrefour sensitif." 2. Dryness of the mouth. Dejerine and Egger[3] have lately described a case of hemianæsthesia and concur with the investigations of Bechterew and Mislawsky, that the thalamus opticus exerts an influence upon salivation.

As an addition to the foregoing cases with stationary hemianopsia, I shall mention the observation of a case of scotoma scintillans bitem-

[1] I would here call attention to the first case. The man soon lost this disturbance and also understood how to correct his hemianopsia by holding the head properly, while this patient is as yet unable to do so.

[2] Beiträge zur Path. u. path Anatomie des Centralnervensyst., p. 42.

[3] Revue neurol., 1903, p. 402.

porale, justifying it for the reason that not only elementary light phenomena were present, but that the case progressed to real hallucinations. This case still further serves to strengthen the above theory.

CASE IV. Merchant, aged fifty-three years. Always healthy, except for "terrible" attacks of migraine, which lasted up to his thirtieth year and then disappeared. Strongly addicted to smoking, very moderate drinker. The somatic condition shows no abnormality of the nervous system, no evidences of alcoholism or pronounced atheroma. The eyes, frequently examined, are perfectly normal. Exposing himself to cold, he suffered from "rheumatism of the head," which nothing could alleviate. He felt "as if thousands of knives were in his head." As a last resort he wrapped his head in absorbent cotton, which made him feel very warm. In the evening of the same day, without any previous excitement, he noticed suddenly, without any pain and lasting for but a few seconds, on both external halves of the visual fields, peculiar phenomena, viz., colored lights, colored planes, figures, etc., while what really was in these halves of the fields he could not see. The line of demarcation between the lateral "blind" portions and the middle seeing ones was not sharp. As the patient happened to be in company, he did not pay any attention to these things, simply rubbed his eyes and everything vanished. On going to bed it suddenly returned so that on both temporal sides he noticed spots of soot which commenced to move; immediately after appeared numerous, rapidly moving objects of hallucinations, such as men, mice, serpents, birds. They were in all possible colors, blue, red, etc.

The very much frightened patient had sufficient presence of mind to observe the entire phantoms, and found just as before, that objects in the temporal fields of vision could not be seen and that, when trying to fix the phantoms, they immediately disappeared outward. Especially remarkable is the fact that he saw people of all shapes and sexes lying next to him.[1] He also observed that what he noticed in the temporal parts at times formed vertically running snake-like lines, so that, for instance, men in their upper parts moved in snake-like gyrations and in their lower parts formed into stationary curved lines. Closing the eyes did not change the phantoms. It then appeared to him as if he were looking into enormous mirrors. At one time he also observed that the real objects situated in the temporal fields of vision moved in the same snake-like lines. This all disappeared for a short time, but returned later and remained, without his being able to fall asleep, until the morning. He then undertook a journey to consult a specialist. But even then these strange visions did not disappear. While going to the station and throughout the journey he was accompanied by these hallucinations on the temporal sides of his fields of vision. "He lived in a panorama." The side cushion of the railroad car, on which he rested his head, changed into a human being, and later into a hundred other things. The figures appeared as a whole, but changed below into actively moving "fringes." Patient performed all his business obligations and consulted an oculist, who found the fundus normal and diagnosed "nerve trouble." Only toward evening, after having

[1] Compare Lauder Brunton (Journal of Mental Science, April, 1902, p. 253), Relations of Fairies and Other Visions to Scotoma Scintillans.

taken bromides, did the phenomena subside. Patient slept all night and the next morning the hallucinations still appeared, though less frequently and had lost their color, appearing black, and disappeared entirely during the day.

These observations during the attack of this very intelligent patient are so exact that nobody will fail to recognize the case as one of scotoma scintillans hemianopicum. But what makes the case in my opinion significant is the fact that we here have to deal with the bitemporal variety of that form, a variety which, as far as literature is concerned, I have not seen mentioned anywhere. Referring to the seat of the lesion provoking the process, I can only define one certain locality, viz., the chiasm. Although by reason of other observations there is no doubt in my mind that the phenomena of scotoma scintillans may be produced by exciting causes in the retina itself, there is no reason to assume that in this case an excitation in both temporal parts of the retina did take place; it is rather within the laws of scientific logic to assume that the phenomena were due to a lesion in one single locality. Lesion of the middle portions of the chiasm produce the now not quite so rare (*loc. cit.*) form of stationary bitemporal hemianopsia. Jolly has fully shown that the excitation provoking lesion for other forms of scotoma scintillans is to be looked for in the chiasm, and his view corresponds with this case. Whether we have to deal here with a hyperæmic condition of the hypophysis, the tumors of which especially produce acromegaly with stationary bitemporal hemianopsia,[1] it is hard to say. The possibility is also not excluded of having an abnormal vessel in the region of the circle of Willis. Weir Mitchell cites a case in which aneurism of an anomalous arterial branch produced stationary bitemporal hemianopsia.

A few more words in regard to the theory that we here have to only deal with a functional disturbance.

I believe there is no indication whatever of a localized basilar process, neither is there any reason to assume that the just mentioned causes, producing stationary bitemporal hemianopsia, can be applied to this case. We might still think of syphilitic basal meningitis, which has a predilection for just this locality and of which Oppenheim mentions bitemporal hemianopsia as an after-effect, but the etiology, the absence of any other endocranial disease, the sudden onset of the fully developed phenomena, above all absence of any ocular disease, all speak against it. There remains nothing, therefore, but the assumption of functional disturbance, which in this case is the migraine from which the patient suffered in former years. That he had no headache during or imme-

[1] Carven (Medical Chronicle, January, 1903) recently mentions a case of tumor of the hypophysis without acromegaly. This patient suffered from migraine a long time before and after the bitemporal hemianopsia had been demonstrated.

diately before the optical phenomena can not be considered here, as we know that frequently a typical attack of scotoma scintillans is unaccompanied by headache. Moreover, it is not clear in what relation the "rheumatism of the head" stands to this case. There is also absolutely no reason to believe that the phenomena were the premonitory symptoms of a subsequent paralysis or tabes.

In conclusion I would point out the transition of the elementary light phenomena of scotoma scintillans into real hallucinations, again confirming the afore-mentioned theory, that hemianopic hallucinations may be produced by a variety of localized excitations in the optical tracts and not in the occipital lobe only.

A CASE OF SPONTANEOUS PROLAPSE OF BOTH LACRYMAL GLANDS. REVIEW OF THE LITERATURE.

By Dunbar Roy, A.B., M.D.,
CLINICAL PROFESSOR OF EYE, EAR, NOSE, AND THROAT DISEASES IN THE ATLANTA COLLEGE OF PHYSICIANS AND SURGEONS, ATLANTA, GA.

The case here reported is anomalous in character rather than of any practical interest. In looking up the number of similar cases which had previously been reported, and also any other literature bearing upon the subject, I was surprised to find that spontaneous prolapse of the lacrymal gland could be placed in the category of rare affections.

Several cases of traumatic prolapse have been reported, as also one or two cases of spontaneous prolapse of one lacrymal gland, but nowhere can I find the report of a case where both lacrymal glands have become spontaneously detached.

Mary M., colored, aged twenty-seven years and unmarried, presented herself at the clinic of the College of Physicians and Surgeons in September, 1902. She came with the complaint that both upper eyelids remained swollen since an attack of bronchitis three weeks previously. There was no pain and no interference with vision; practically no discomfort from the present condition.

On casual inspection the upper lids gave all the appearance of œdema, especially on the temporal sides. By palpation I found a well-defined glandular body just beneath the border and at the outer edge of the supraorbital ridge. It was especially prominent when the patient looked down and held the head forward. Both sides had absolutely the same objective appearance and symptoms. It was freely movable under the touch, and could be pushed up underneath the orbital rim. The patient was perfectly positive that there was nothing wrong with the eyes up to three weeks previously. No enlarged glands could be found in any other portion of the body. As the condition was giving the patient no trouble, she refused any operative interference, leaving out the question of its own advisability. When last seen there were no changes visible.

I was very confident, as were my colleagues, that the bodies felt were the lacrymal glands, but we could in no wise account for this dislocation. There was no history of traumatism to which it could be traced, nor any severe straining on the part of the patient except the previous cough.

In this latter respect, as well as in several others, the case is similar to the one reported by Snell in 1881.

Anatomists tell us that the lacrymal gland is enveloped in a capsule which, by its attachment to the periosteum of the orbital cavity, is retained in place. In a case of this kind we can but surmise some anatomical malformation or some relaxation of the surrounding tissues as a cause of such a pathological condition.

In looking up the literature of this subject but few cases could be found recorded. For this reason I will give in detail a résumé of all cases of both spontaneous and traumatic prolapse of the lacrymal gland of which I have been able to find any report.

Case I.—In the *Ophthalmic Review* for the year 1881–82 we find a case reported by Simeon Snell, as follows:

On March 7, 1882, I was consulted by a tradesman, aged forty-five years, in consequence of a lump in the left eyelid. It had been observed first a week previous, and had been seen by Dr. Brook, who sent him to me. The swelling was distinctly visible, and particularly noticeable to the touch. Situated in the upper eyelid at its external part and coming from under the frontal bone, it was felt beneath the structures of the lid as about the size of an almond. It could be pressed between the fingers, but readily slipped back into the orbit. Its surface felt more smooth than irregular. Pressure causes it immediately to recede into the orbit beneath the frontal bone, but after depressing the head it was again found to be visible in the lid. This he had himself observed, and after several attempts to replace it he always found on bending the head downward that it had reappeared. He complained of it causing him discomfort, which was increased on manipulation.

On the night of the first appearance of the substance in the eyelid he had gone to bed in no wise ailing, and had detected it on rising in the morning. He had in the night been coughing a great deal. The same side of the head is marked by a large venous subcutaneous nævus which extends to the eyebrow and apparently passes into the orbit. The man is a free drinker, and is frequently laid up in consequence.

The question as to what the "lump" was did not present any great difficulty. Its situation, size, and feel suggested directly its being the lacrymal gland displaced, and this was the diagnosis also of the medical man who first examined the patient.

It was decided to try the effect of compression in keeping the gland in place. A few days later when the patient presented himself he desired to postpone the wearing of a "pad" for a short time. I, however, pressed the gland well back with my finger and kept it replaced. He left me without its having reappeared.

Being soon after laid up with one of his attacks of illness, he did not again see me until five or six weeks later. The swelling in the lid was then no longer visible, and he asserted that it had not appeared since his last visit, and that the sense of discomfort had gone.

Spontaneous displacement of the lacrymal gland must, I imagine, be a very rare condition. I cannot recall a recorded case like the one described. I remember the case of a man under treatment for keratitis some years since in whom the glands were distinctly visible and freely movable in the eyelids. The condition was congenital.

I am further reminded by a gentleman attending my clinic of another similar case which came under observation since the one just referred to.

It is worthy of mention that in the case of my patient, in his attacks of illness following his drinking bouts, he sometimes suffered from epileptiform convulsions, during which the large venous nævus at the margin of the orbit became greatly distended, looking as though it were ready to burst.

CASE II. Reported by Wm. George Syme from the hospital practice of Dr. Argyll-Robertson in the *Edinburgh Medical Journal*, 1887, vol. xxxiii.—J. C., a man aged thirty-six years, applied for treatment in May 1887, suffering from ptosis and a tumor situated in the right upper eyelid. The tumor extended along the whole length of the upper lid, from a point above the inner to a point above the outer canthus. By its weight it caused ptosis; the eyelids were nearly closed, and the upper lid could hardly be raised at all, the mass catching at once on the orbital edge. The skin over the tumor, though slightly congested, was not œdematous, and was freely movable over it. The tumor, which felt firm, lobulated, and glandular, was not attached to the deeper structures except about the middle for a distance of one-third of an inch, where it was moored to the orbital edge of the frontal bone.

It could not be reduced into the orbit. The ocular movements were in no way affected, and the vision in the two eyes was the same. The tumor was perfectly painless even on firm pressure; the neighboring lymphatic glands were not enlarged, and the patient seemed to be in perfect health. The history of this affection was that about the end of January of this year the patient had first noticed the swelling about the size of a bean in the upper eyelid. This was painless, but troublesome on account of the ptosis which it caused. At this time also he noticed that the right eye was more watery than the left—a condition which had not previously been present, and the swellings were larger in the mornings and became rather smaller in the day. He thinks that the tumor had suddenly attained the size of a bean, but is not quite certain; at any rate it had steadily increased in size from the time of its first appearance. In the winter of 1885 the patient had noticed a similar swelling in the same situation; this however had been much smaller, and caused no annoyance, and after a few weeks spontaneously disappeared.

Under these circumstances the diagnosis was made of a displaced and chronically enlarged lacrymal gland. On May 10 an incision was made over the tumor in the long axis of the upper lid, and the gland, which was lying immediately under the skin, was turned out. The accessory portion of the gland was found lying in the proper situation of the main part, and was left to carry on the usual functions of the gland. As soon as the swelling had subsided there was a marked diminution in the ptosis, which continued to improve until the patient left the hospital.

Case III. Reported by Dr. Henry D. Noyes and published in the *Transactions of the American Ophthalmological Society*, 1886-87.—Miss Carrie S., aged twenty years, of Paterson, N. J., presented herself February 8, 1887, because of the swelling under the upper lid of the right eye which had been growing for nine years. For the last few months it had been uncomfortable. It rested upon the eyeball at its superoexternal side, and reached within 6 mm. of the cornea. It was flattened, not lobulated, and nearly circular in outlines, and merged gradually into the surrounding conjunctiva. A few vessels coursed over it, and it had a faint yellow color. It was nearly three-fourths of an inch in diameter. It could be moved freely upon and also moved with the globe. It was very compressible and elastic. It seemed to have a capsule which at its lower border was densely white and firm; over the remaining surface it was thin and translucent, but with a yellow tinge. There had never been any blow nor sign of disease in this region, nor inflammation, nor serious pain. The progress had been very gradual and the cause unknown. The other eye had been lost sixteen years before by accident. This globe was atrophied, yet on lifting the upper lid a rounded mass, red and slightly lobulated, and a little larger than a cherry-stone, appeared at the upper and outer angle of the orbit, and was regarded as a part of the lacrymal gland which had become displaced.

Treatment. An incision was made obliquely across the tumor and the conjunctiva dissected off by the closed blades of curved and sharp-pointed scissors. Very little cutting had to be done, and the hemorrhage was moderate. When the mass was separated it proved to be normal lacrymal gland.

The conjunctival wound was stitched and a bandage applied. The healing was prompt and the reaction moderate. A wrinkled and swollen condition of the conjunctiva remained for a few weeks at the site of the operation. The prolapse seems to have been caused by simple laxity of the enclosing fibrous capsules, without any propulsion from behind.

Case IV. Reported by L. Mauthner in *Wien. med. Presse*, 1878, p. 110.—Man, aged twenty-four years, came to the clinic October 4, 1868, for inflammation of the eye of four weeks' standing, and for a tumor in the upper eyelid, first noticed a few days before. There was an injection of the conjunctiva palpebrarum et bulbi, ciliary injection, and diffuse coloring of the cornea; the upper lid was much thickened and drooping, and one feels in its lateral half a hard, movable, and slightly rough, painless tumor, not adherent to the skin, of size and form of the lacrymal gland. This showed no sign of an orbital tumor. By the use of atropine and compress bandage the inflammatory phenomena of the cornea disappeared in five weeks, but the tumor of the upper lid, which Jaeger thought might be the lacrymal gland, had not changed in spite of using iodide of potash and iodine salve. Jaeger operated November 11 1868; laid bare the tumor by section, from in and above outward and somewhat down in the direction of the length of the tumor; a small part removed showed nothing abnormal. The gland was replaced in the orbit and made fast by sutures, the patient being discharged sixteen days after operation. The gland was fixed to surrounding tissues and only a small tumor could be felt at the lateral upper orbital edge.

CASE V. Reported by S. S. Golovine, *Clin. Maitop.*, Mosk., 1895, vol. v. pp. 930–941.—A young man, aged eighteen years, admitted to the hospital July, 1893. The upper eyelids seemed swollen and slightly drooping. He carried his head erect, and even from time to time threw it backward, as if he wished thus to compensate for the fall of the eyelids; he instinctively contracted the frontal muscle; from this cause the skin above the brows was constantly wrinkled, and the face had a very strange expression. The skin of the eyelids was tense, very delicate, and formed a fold almost transversal which came down on the eye. This was not equally pronounced in its entire extent. The crease which one generally finds below the orbital edge was effaced. The skin, of normal color, was transparent and allowed subcutaneous veins to be distinguished. These phenomena were symmetrical, but more pronounced on the left eyelid. Below the skin one might palpate a hard compact lump, like a grape, ovular, 1½ cm. in diameter. It could be displaced in all directions and slid easily across the anterior surface of the cartilage. These movements seemed limited toward the interior by some adherences, although it was impossible to feel them. The movements were freer upward and outward. When the finger was raised the body came back little by little from the orbit, falling into the part of the cutaneous sac, which covered the external commissure. The elevation of the lid was hindered and the patient overcame this difficulty by contracting the frontal bones. It was very easy to turn the lid back, the mucous membrane of which was altogether normal.

The lacrymal conduits were normal, although latterly the tears were less abundant. Although the other organs were not changed, the general organism seemed much depressed and its development much retarded. The lids had been changing for the last three years.

There were two methods of treatment: 1. Total extirpation of the gland. 2. To bring the gland back to its place and fix it. Both methods were used.

The writer began by removing the right lacrymal gland.

The result of the operation was very satisfactory, the wound healing by first intention. Eight days later the other eye was operated upon, the lacrymal gland being replaced in the orbit and fixed with sutures. The result was very good, and three days later the cutaneous sutures were removed, and six days later those which held the gland in position. Two years later the writer received a letter from the patient, who expressed himself as well pleased with the result.

CASE VI. Reported by Briere in *Bull. et mém. de soc. de chir. de Paris*, 1876, vol. ii. p. 592.—Boy, aged eleven years. The affection began five and a half years ago. He struck his left temple against a nail. The wound suppurated and the external wall of the orbit began to necrose. The skin of the eyelid, temple, and brow, being drawn back by the cicatrix, was depressed to the walls of the orbit, which had become angular and unequal. The free edge of the eyelid, drawn more and more up and out, took progressively a form characterized by an elongation of the free edge, which measured 22 mm. more than that of the healthy lid. This deformity, produced by numerous cicatricial bands, had, as a secondary result, compressed the lacrymal gland. This gland was not protected by the bony depression in which it was normally lodged. The opening of the lid, increasing more and more, the lacrymal gland was soon exposed. The lobules, not being compressed from this period, became larger and formed a tumor the size of a large hazelnut, between the lid and the globe.

Operation August 10th under chloroform.

1. The writer took the exact length of the healthy right lid, and from the internal angle of the diseased eye he measured this length on the elongated lid.

2. Incision between lid and lacrymal gland to mobilize the upper lid.

3. Dissection of the upper lid 4 to 5 cm. as far as the middle of the forehead; considerable bleeding.

4. Curved incision, separating the outer side of the lacrymal gland from the superfluous part of the lid which was to be excised.

5. Incision at 2 mm. outside of the ciliary line and parallel to the preceding except at the upper part.

6. Excision of the whole flap.

7. Dissection of the temporal flap, the longest and most difficult part of the operation.

8. He assured himself that union would be possible by sliding the two flaps.

9. Before applying the sutures he put on a compress bandage and allowed the patient to revive from narcosis.

10. Twenty minutes later, when hemorrhage had stopped, the lacrymal gland was replaced in the cavity which had been made by the removal of the sequestra of bone.

11. Applied twisted sutures with fine pins.

The operation may be considered a mixture of that of Adams and Jaeger.

It is now eight months since the operation. The lid covers the eyeball except the parts nearest the external commissure, where there is a space of 2 mm. between the lids when the lids are closed. The lacrymal fistula has closed spontaneously; there only remains a slight depression of 2 mm. in length, the bottom of which is healthy looking.

Case VII. Reported by G. Ahlstrom, in *Centralbl. f. prakt. Augenhlk.*, 1898, vol. xxii. p. 300.—The patient, a boy aged twelve years, fell when he was three years old and struck his right eye upon a sharp-cornered block of ice. There was a bloody wound which soon healed. When first seen there was found to be quite a high-grade ptosis of the right eye, so that in looking straight out the upper lid covered half of the pupil. The ptosis had been caused by the thickness of the lid. The skin of the lid was normal, easily movable, and hung on the palpebral edge in the form of a fold a little below the edge; no scar was to be seen. By palpation one could perceive a tumor-like mass just below the skin, about the size of an almond. This was quite firm, somewhat ragged, showing no adherence with the deeper parts, but was easily movable under the skin, and could not be pressed into the orbit. The tumor was removed. It was found to be the lacrymal gland.

The ptosis became less immediately after the operation and the lid resumed its normal appearance.

CASE VIII. *Bericht d. k. k. Krankenh. in Wien*, 1889.—A very superficial mention is made of this case. A laboring man, aged forty-one years, was transferred to the ward. He had suffered from a scrofulous (?) conjunctivitis, and also had had an ulcer of the same nature on the upper eyelid. As a result of this latter there was a depression and strangulation of the lacrymal gland and ectropion, by which the upper lid adhered in about its middle to the edge of the orbital cavity as a part of the lacrymal gland, being in this way removed. The remainder of the gland is seen as a strangulated tumor. Separation of the adherence to the edge of the orbit, the transplantation of the flap from the temple region, resulted in a cure.

CASE IX. Reported by von Graefe, *Arch. f. Ophthalmol.*, 1866, vol. xii. p. 224.—Boy, aged ten years, was brought to Graefe on account of a wound of the upper eyelid, having been struck the day before by falling on a piece of glass. There was a wound 18 mm. long which passed through the whole thickness of the upper lid parallel with the edge of the orbit. From the wound there arose a reddish plug about the size and shape of a finger phalanx, which he recognized as the lacrymal gland. It hung down over the cleft of the lids, which it partly covered and was somewhat drawn in at its base, so that the physicians thought of removing the whole mass. The prolapsed lacrymal gland was held back by an assistant while Graefe closed the wound with four stitches and then applied a compressive bandage. There was a slight suppuration, and in the end there was left a fistula of the lacrymal gland.

CASE X. Mentioned by Panas in his *Lecons sur les Affections de l'appareil lacrymal*, Paris, 1877, p. 8.—A case similar to that of von Graefe was shown by Lariboisière at a clinical meeting. There was a deep contused wound in the left upper lid just at the external extremity of the orbital ridge, in which was seen a prolapsed lacrymal gland. A single stitch of metal suture was enough to keep the gland in place and bring on cicatrization of the edges of the wound, which was 2½ cm. long. When the patient left the hospital there was a slight induration of the gland which would probably disappear in time.

CASE XI. Reported by R. Rampoldi, *Ann. di Ottamol.*, Pavia, 1884, vol. xiii. pp. 68-70.—Boy, aged twelve years, admitted to the hospital in January, 1880, for grave ectropion of the upper lid. About a year before he had been struck by a stick in the left temporoparietal region, followed by pronounced exophthalmos. He was taken to an eye clinic, where a diagnosis of retrobulbar phlegmon was made, the abscess opened, and the exophthalmos thus much reduced. The vision was preserved intact, and the patient returned home almost completely cured. A slow process of the osteoperiostitis went on in the orbit, the drainage aperture becoming fistulous and discharging slowly disintegrated grayish pus, while the cicatrix adhering to the brow of the orbit turned back the aperture of the fistula and drew the lid strongly upward and outward, turning the free margin so that the externo-superior conjunctiva was all turned out. The patient, in a very anæmic state, was now admitted in the hospital. The exophthalmos was moderate and the bulb turned out in a limited degree only. The cicatrix was strongly adherent and had a tendency to invade the lacrymal fossa. A local treatment was used with disinfectants and the Paquelin cautery, supplemented with a liberal diet and tonics. After some time the patient left the hospital before it was thought best to attempt a radical cure.

In August, 1880, the palpebral ectropion was considerably increased, and at the site of the wound was seen a tumor of solid consistence of the size and shape of a wild mulberry, which was recognized as a dislocated lacrymal gland. As it was impossible to replace it, the tumor was destroyed with the needles of Boerelli.

CASE XII. Reported by R. Hilbert. *Klin. Monatsb. f. Augenheilk.*, vol. xxxviii. p. 478.—Boy, aged one and one-half years, was brought to the writer December 28, 1889, whose left eye was said to have been injured the day before by his falling on a beam. Close to the outer left lid commissure just under the edge of the orbit was a wound 1 cm. long, horizontal, and from which protruded a red roundish body about the size of an almond. The whole lid was black and blue. From the article of Ahlstrom the writer considered the tumor to be a lacrymal gland. He removed it with one stroke of the scissors, closed the wound with two stitches. Healing followed promptly; there was no ptosis, and the microscopic examination showed the correctness of the diagnosis.

CASE XIII. Reported by Goldzieher, *Jahresber. u. b. Leist. u. Fortschr. im Gebiete der Ophthal.*, Tübingen, 1878, vol. vii. p.466.—A child, aged one year, was wounded in the upper eyelid, which was followed by bleeding and the appearance in the wound of a dark-red, fleshy body. When the writer first saw the patient this body was the size of a hazelnut and completely filled the skin wound, which was 4 mm. long. This body was cut off with the scissors and the wound healed promptly. An examination of the growth removed showed it to be the lacrymal gland.

CASE XIV. Reported by Haltenhoff, *Annales d'oculistique*, 1895, pp. 319–321.—This was the case of a boy, aged two and one-half years, who fell forward in a road filled with broken stones. When he got up he could not open his eye, and in the lid appeared a wound from which protruded a solid bleeding mass. The upper lid was bandaged, and three days later was seen by the writer. The upper lid was found to be falling over, œdematous, tense, and quite ecchymotic. In its external third, several millimetres above the free border, there was a sort of fleshy protuberance of a livid grayish-red color and of a consistency which seemed to be firm for a simple clot. It adhered by a sort of pedicle to the bottom of a horizontal wound of the skin. The patient was etherized and the palpebral fissure opened enough to prove the integrity of the eyeball. It was then decided that it was a hernia of the lacrymal gland. The sharp edge of a broken stone had cut the lid wide open, penetrated obliquely from below upward through the wound. The three days' strangulation rendered it difficult to reinstate the protruded gland, so the author profited by the narcosis and cut it off from the lid. It was then noticed that at the bottom of the wound there were several grayish-red lumps, apparently lobules of the gland. They belonged to the palpebral portion which is formed by a mass of little isolated lobules with loose connections. The wound was united with two silk sutures, dressed with dermatol, the wound closing by first intention except at one small point. The recovery was perfect, and no difference was noticed in the appearance and moistening of the two eyes. Microscopic examination by Dr. Buscarlet confirmed the diagnosis.

CASE XV. Reported by L. Pistis in *Annales d'oculistique*, 1895, pp. 468–470.—J. D., aged one year. The child had fallen on her face in a road filled with stones, and the lid was cut near the external orbital border. The wound was on the upper lid of the left eye, and was œdematous and ecchymotic. The skin was intact only near the internal portion; the remainder was a bleeding surface with an almost triangular flap detached from the external third of the orbital border and turned downward. Through the lips of the wound, by a short pedicle, there appeared an oval gray mass. On raising the lid the writer found the cornea intact, and there was no exophthalmos. The gray mass was the orbital lacrymal gland. The writer reduced the prolapsed gland by suturing the lid in front of it, his observation differing in this point from that of Dr. Haltenhoff, who excised the protruding gland. Union took place by first intention, and as a result the child has only a slight prominence in this region as if the gland had not perfectly resumed its anatomical position.

CASE XVI. Reported by W. F. Mittendorf, in *Transactions of the American Ophthalmological Society*, 1901, p. 382.—A young lady, aged twenty years, in pretending to be hypnotized by her brother, fell forward and struck his hand in such a manner that his index finger struck the upper part of the outer corner of her left eye. The next day the young lady found that there was a swelling in the upper temporal part of the eyeball, which hardly showed with the lids in the normal condition, but became very apparent by raising the upper lid. As the swelling did not diminish, the patient consulted the writer. The eye showed apparently no injury except a slight scratch of the finger-nail near the inner corner, the rest being perfectly normal, and so was the vision of the eye, nor was the motility interfered with in any way. The tumor itself was slightly painful to the touch and could be pushed up a little, but descended immediately as the pressure exerted upon it was relaxed. The upper and the outer part of the orbit felt a little tender, but no perceptible difference of the two sides could be made out. The diagnosis of dislocation of the lacrymal gland was immediately suggested from these symptoms.

The treatment of the case was simply expectant, as pressure failed to replace the swollen part and as it caused no visible deformity. The swelling has remained practically the same now after a lapse of three months.

The diagnosis of these cases of dislocated lacrymal glands is apparently easy, and especially so when there is any incised wound permitting easy inspection in addition to palpation.

In all of the cases reported, except the one by Mittendorf and Noyes, the deformity was noted externally rather than internally beneath the upper lid. In my own case nothing abnormal could be seen by the closest inspection beneath the lid.

Cases of spontaneous dislocation of the gland will, of course, present but one or two symptoms which are found when the conditions are due to trauma. With the exception of the deformity due to swelling and a possible limitation in the raising of the lid, these spontaneous cases usually cause no inconvenience to the patient.

It is a noteworthy fact that in none of the cases recorded has the lacrymal function of the gland been impaired, for in my own case neither an increase nor a decrease of the moisture could be noticed. Another remarkable symptom mentioned only in the case reported by Haltenhoff, where even the greater portion of the gland was removed, was the fact that there was no difference in the moisture in the two eyes.

The question of treatment must of course vary according to the character of the case. In those dependent on traumatism, where there is a contused or incised wound complicating the condition, operative intervention must always be considered. In those cases where there is no wound, or in the so-called spontaneous dislocation, the question of operation must be decided by the character of the individual case.

Mechanical compression is difficult of application. If the deformity is not marked and there are no uncomfortable symptoms, I do not see why it is necessary to do anything whatever. If there is ptosis from the presence of the gland, or if the latter should be painful and of great discomfort to the patient, fixation should first be attempted, and if that failed, there is no reason why the gland should not be removed.

ACUTE SUPPURATIVE THYROIDITIS.

By Henry Roth, M.D.,
ASSISTANT ATTENDING SURGEON, LEBANON HOSPITAL, NEW YORK.

Acute suppurative thyroiditis is a very rare condition, and usually secondary to some infectious disease. As a primary condition it has only been recorded in a very small number of cases. A case belonging to this class came under the writer's observation and gave the following history:

F., aged forty years, a native of Italy, laborer by ocenpation, was admitted to the service of Dr. Parker Syms, at the Lebanon Hospital, on November 26, 1902. On account of the patient's inability to speak English, a good history could not be obtained. As far as could be learned, the patient was suddenly taken with a chill and high fever on November 23, 1902. He became gradually worse, and after two days was brought to the hospital. On admission his temperature was 103.2° F., pulse 128. He seemed in a state of profound sepsis, sweating profusely and being decidedly cyanosed. On examination, a diffuse swelling was found around the anterior portion of his neck, extending from the suprasternal notch to the upper border of the cricoid cartilage. There was some redness around the most prominent portion of this swelling, but no fluctuation. The mass was tender, and engorged venous channels could be seen around the shoulders. The patient was breathing badly and swallowing with difficulty. There seemed to be considerable difficulty, also, in moving the head. No other lesion could be found, and a diagnosis was made of acute thyroiditis of unknown origin. The patient's condition being very grave, an immediate operation was decided upon, and under chloroform anæsthesia an incision was made by the writer, extending in the median line from the thyroid cartilage to two and one-half inches below. The muscles were separated, and the thyroid, readily exposed, presented itself as a smooth, dark-blue body, with a dull capsule. On opening the left side a few drops of pus escaped, and on thorough exposure the gland showed areas of necrosis. Iodoform gauze drainage was established, and the operation quickly terminated on account of the desperate condition of the patient. The temperature rose higher and reached 107° F. In spite of active stimulation, the condition became worse, and the patient died on November 27, 1902. The writer is indebted to Dr. Edward Schnapper, pathologist to the hospital, for the following record of the autopsy:

November 30, 1902. Body well nourished; rigor mortis well marked; no external marks of violence. Incised wound, two and one-half inches long, in median line of neck and leading down to thyroid gland.

Pleural Cavities: Normal, no fluid or adhesions.

Lungs: Right lung, upper lobe congested, middle and lower lobe congested and œdematous; left lung, congested and œdematous.

Heart: Left ventricle, wall thickened, myocardium pale in color, soft and flabby; cavity small. Right ventricle, wall thin, cavity slightly increased in size; mitral valve thickened and has small fibrinous nodules upon its edges. Aortic valves show moderate atheromatous changes. Pulmonary and tricuspid valves normal. Aorta shows here and there slight atheroma.

Abdomen not distended, and contains no fluid.

Omentum not adherent and contains a moderate amount of fat.

Intestines normal.

Appendix normal.

Liver moderately enlarged, its outer surface appears opaque, grayish-yellow, lobules indistinct.

Spleen enlarged, soft, Malpighian bodies prominent.

Right kidney enlarged, soft, capsule not adherent; cortex pale, swollen, pyramids congested. Both kidneys alike.

Bladder distended and normal.

Teeth and Gums: No pathological condition found.

Tonsils normal.

Tongue normal.

Œsophagus normal.

Stomach shows some post-mortem changes, otherwise nothing abnormal.

Pharynx normal.

Thyroid Gland: Both lobes enlarged and swollen; the right lobe is enlarged to a greater degree, firm, but in places there are areas of softening. In the right lobe there is an incised wound leading into a small irregular cavity.

Microscopic Examination of the Thyroid Gland. The connective tissue was found infiltrated with large numbers of leucocytes, the polynuclear predominating. By this marked infiltration of cells the colloid containing acini are obliterated. In places there are areas of necrosis and abscesses. Inoculations upon agar from the thyroid gland showed a growth of pure streptococci.

From a study of the history and post-mortem record we are led to consider this case as one of primary suppurative thyroiditis. Inflammation of the enlarged thyroid is not at all uncommon, and cases of strumitis are seen comparatively often. Simple thyroiditis is occasionally observed, and the writer recalls seeing two cases belonging to this class; both of them occurred in women, were associated with constitutional symptoms, and terminated in resolution.

Suppurative inflammation of the thyroid, on the other hand, is a rare disease, and when it does occur it is usually secondary to one of the infectious diseases, or it may be due to an injury and consequent infection. Inasmuch as the thyroid is not frequently the seat of injury, the cases belonging to this class are of passing interest only. Ransohoff[1] calls attention to the fact that the thyroid has no excretory duct, being surrounded by a firm capsule, and is well protected against infection. It is most likely invaded by microbes through the blood circulation. According to Mygind,[2] quoted by Robertson in a paper on "Thyroiditis Complicating Typhoid Fever,"[3] the condition is most common in females between the second and third decades, rarely in previously healthy persons, or as a result of traumatisms, but most frequently during or following an attack of typhoid fever, acute articular rheumatism, diphtheria, influenza, malaria, erysipelas, puerperal fever, sepsis, orchitis or prostatitis. It may occur during or following scarlet fever, pneumonia, and pyæmia. According to Robertson, thyroiditis is most common after rheumatic or typhoid fever, and the first case supervening on rheumatism was reported by Molière, of Lyons. As a complication or sequel to typhoid, it usually terminates in suppuration, and this may be caused entirely by the Eberth bacillus. Thyroiditis may terminate in resolution, suppuration or necrosis. The simple form usually terminates in recovery; where gangrene occurs the condition is more grave, the symptoms being very marked, and this is usually due to a streptococcus infection.

In the subject of this report the infection was due to streptococcus, but the source of the infection remains undetermined after a careful autopsy which included a very careful examination of the mouth and pharynx. Rheumatism may be excluded because none of the joints showed any evidences of it during life, nor did the patient complain of

[1] Transactions of the American Surgical Association, 1894, p. 275.
[2] Journal of Laryngology, Rhinology, and Otology, 1895, vol. ix. p. 181.
[3] The American Journal of the Medical Sciences, 1902, vol. cxxiii. p. 67.

any pain. It seems worth noting that the right lobe of the thyroid was involved more than the left. It would be difficult to draw a clinical picture from the study of a single case, and the writer will not attempt to do more than point out that in his case the symptoms of sepsis were pre-eminent. The local signs might have been those of an ordinary phlegmon, but the constitutional symptoms were too severe. These might possibly be attributed to interference with the thyroid secretion. Dyspnœa, dysphagia, the movement of the swelling with the trachea, are usually present at some stage of the disease. In primary suppurative thyroiditis, early incision and drainage is imperative. That it was of little benefit in the writer's case can be accounted for by the very profound state of sepsis at a comparatively advanced stage of the disease.

A CASE OF COMPLETE BILATERAL DUPLICATION OF THE URETERS.

By Henry B. Decherd, M.A., M.D.,
DEMONSTRATOR OF ANATOMY, UNIVERSITY OF TEXAS.

(From the Anatomical Department, University of Texas.)

The following case of double ureters was first noted in November, 1902, but many things prevented its being recorded at that time.

The subject was W. T., male, negro, who died at Sealy Hospital of amœbic dysentery. Strongyloides were also found in his stools. Acute nephritis was present; but in this regard the double ureters, of course, had no clinical significance. However, had catheterization of the ureters or operative interference upon them been demanded, the double condition might have caused considerable embarrassment.

The kidneys measure 13 x 6½ x 4 cm. (right) and 11 x 6 x 4½ cm. (left). The left ureters are 25 cm. in length, and the right are 24 cm. All four are about the same size, and each is almost as large as an ordinary single ureter. Their relations to the vessels at the kidney hilum and to structures elsewhere in their course are normal. The bladder orifices, two on each side, are 1 cm. apart; the mesial (adjacent) ones being 2½ cm. apart. Dissection of the pelves and calices show that the upper ureter drains the upper third of the kidney, while the lower one drains the lower two-thirds. Fig. 2 is a tracing from a skiagraph of another kidney. It shows a bifid pelvis and the part of the kidney drained by each half; this resembles rather closely the condition found in each of the kidneys under consideration. The difference was that there were two pelves in each kidney, and one ureter from each pelvis. Moreover, the upper ureter drained rather less of the kidney than the upper segment of the bifid pelvis in Fig. 2. The two upper ureters open into the bladder by the two mesial orifices, the two lower ones by the two external.

It would have been interesting to have injected the infundibula and calices with bismuth and have taken skiagraphs, but the subject was

FIG. 1.

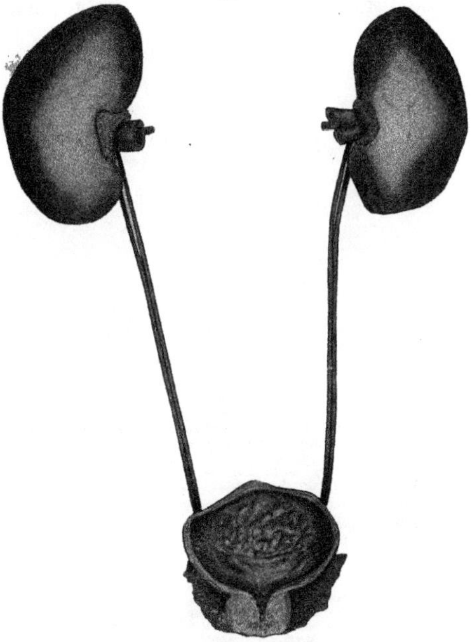

Shows kidneys, ureters, and bladder, some fat about the hilum on each side; one vein and one artery on the right, and two veins and two arteries on the left. The four bladder orifices are seen lying on a line slightly curved, with its convexity toward the urethral orifice. Surrounding the neck of the bladder is the prostate gland; and on each side of it is seen a mass of fatty tissue. (Drawn to scale from specimen.)

used in the dissecting-room, where the kidneys were too mutilated to admit of such measure.

Since it is the purpose of this paper merely to report this case, discussion of the embryological fault responsible for the abnormality is not entered into.

The rarity of complete bilateral duplication is shown by A. H. Gould, of Harvard (THE AMERICAN JOURNAL OF THE MEDICAL SCIENCES,

FIG. 2.

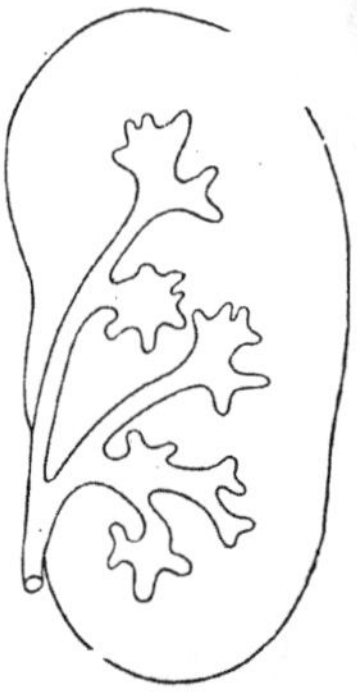

Tracing from skiagraph of another kidney injected with bismuth, showing bifid type pelvis and usual arrangement of calices.

March, 1903). He reported two cases, and found only eight others in the literature. Unilateral duplication, partial duplication on both sides, and bifid kidney pelvis are not uncommon findings.

BIBLIOGRAPHY.

See Gould's paper.
P. Rayer. Traité des Maladies des Reins, Paris, 1837.
Juetting. Double Bladder. Inaug. Diss., Berlin, 1838.
De Font-Reaulx. Bull. Société Anat. de Paris, 1865, 2d Ser., T. x. p. 645.
Coyene. Ibid., 1868, 2d Ser., T. xiii. p. 55.
Bachhammer. Two cases. Archiv f. Anat. und Physiol., 1879, p. 139.
William Ewart. Trans. Path. Soc. of London, 1880, vol. xxxi. p. 188.
T. C. Janeway. New York Medical Record, March 29, 1902.
A. H. Gould. THE AMERICAN JOURNAL OF THE MEDICAL SCIENCES, March, 1903.
In addition to these, I find a reference to two cases of "Complete Double Ureter" reported by Adami and Day (Montreal Medical Journal, 1893-94). Having no access to this journal, cannot verify the last reference.

THE PRESENT STATUS OF PSEUDODIPHTHERIA BACILLI.

By Thomas W. Salmon, M.D.,
BACTERIOLOGIST, NEW YORK STATE HOSPITALS.

A committee was appointed in July, 1900, by the Massachusetts Association of Boards of Health to investigate the occurrence of diphtheria bacilli in well persons. It was found at the outset of their work that there existed such a wide divergence of opinion as to the identity of diphtheria-like bacilli that it became necessary, in collecting data, to make use of an arbitrary classification which included many doubtful types.

A glance backward will show that this uncertainty as to the precise status of diphtheria-like organisms has existed since the discovery of the specific cause of the disease. In his second communication on the etiology of diphtheria, Loeffler described the pseudodiphtheria bacillus as a non-pathogenic organism, interesting chiefly for its resemblance to B. diphtheriæ. Von Hofman, Vincent, Roux and Yersin, and others subsequently found it in the throats of healthy children and of those ill with measles, scarlet fever, nasal catarrh, and laryngitis. A controversy arose as to whether the organism was a distinct variety with no relation to B. diphtheriæ or a variant of it, lacking virulence, but in other respects identical. A few investigators took the latter view, notably Roux and Yersin, who supported it in a paper published in 1890. They defended this position with much force, pointing out that less difference existed between diphtheria bacilli and pseudodiphtheria bacilli than between virulent and attenuated anthrax bacilli obtained from the same source.

At the present time bacteriologists are divided into three groups by their opinions on this question.

1. Perhaps the greater number in this country believe that the term pseudodiphtheria bacilli should be applied only to that group of non-virulent organisms which resemble diphtheria bacilli very closely, but which may be distinguished from them by certain cultural or morphological characteristics. They regard diphtheria bacilli which produce toxin and those which do not as variants of the same organism.

2. A lesser number of bacteriologists in America and many Continental observers, including Roux and Yersin and Behring, believe in the identity of diphtheria bacilli and the so-called pseudodiphtheria bacilli, and regard the latter solely as varieties of B. diphtheriæ. Dr. F. F. Wesbrook, of Minnesota, divided all diphtheria bacilli into granular, barred, and solid forms, according to their appearance when grown on blood serum and stained with Loeffler's methylene blue. These forms he has further divided into types with reference to their shape and size.

The drawings which he presented with his descriptions leave no doubt that he considers several forms often classed as pseudodiphtheria bacilli undoubted diphtheria bacilli. His classification was that adopted by the committee of the Massachusetts Association of Boards of Health in the investigation previously referred to.

3. A few observers still apply the name pseudodiphtheria bacilli to those which are identical with diphtheria bacilli, with the single exception of being non-virulent, as well as to those which show cultural differences.

As might be expected, many methods have been devised to separate true diphtheria bacilli from those resembling them. A few biological differences have been observed. In glucose bouillon one distinction was found by some to be constant. All virulent diphtheria bacilli and some non-virulent ones are said to produce acid when grown in this medium, while pseudodiphtheria bacilli either produce no acid or produce it after a few hours' growth, and then rapidly produce alkali. The experience of different observers has differed greatly as to this, and it has been pointed out that their technique has been too dissimilar for a fair comparison of their results, and that, moreover, avirulent diphtheria bacilli cannot in many cases be distinguished from pseudodiphtheria bacilli by this means.

Neisser's method of staining the polar granules was hailed as a certain means of identifying true diphtheria bacilli, but it has been shown that not all virulent diphtheria bacilli possess polar granules, and that many avirulent diphtheria bacilli are without them, staining solidly. Furthermore, some pseudodiphtheria bacilli, even when grown less than twenty hours, have polar granules which stain beautifully by Neisser's method. Pioskowski's method is open to the same objection.

It has been noticed that these polar bodies develop more rapidly in true diphtheria bacilli than in the bacilli which most resemble them. The character of the emulsion resulting from mixing a colony with a few drops of water and several other apparently distinctive features have been described, but they have not been found equally reliable by different experimenters. And so we are obliged to say to-day that there are no methods of identifying true diphtheria bacilli which are regarded as trustworthy by all those who have devoted special attention to the subject.

The matter is not one of importance to laboratory workers alone, but has serious bearing on the control of diphtheria. One of the most vexing questions which confronts public health officers is the proper disposal of well persons infected with diphtheria bacilli, and this uncertainty about a matter so fundamental complicates it exceedingly. At present there is little difficulty in isolating persons who have had diphtheria until the bacilli can no longer be found in cultures from their throats.

In some cities a more or less successful attempt is being made to detain or throw some safeguards about those who have been directly exposed to the disease and who have infected throats, but no one has yet ventured to suggest that those well persons who carry diphtheria bacilli and who have not been directly exposed to the disease should be detained until their throats are free from infection. If we are to believe that all the so-called pseudodiphtheria bacilli are variants of true diphtheria bacilli, we must regard so large a part of the population infected that it is unfair to detain the few whom our bacteriological examinations detect, and it may even be held by some, as it is said to be by Behring, that it is unjustifiable to isolate even those suffering from the disease. It may be urged that the non-virulent forms may be disregarded, but even if it were practicable to test all cultures for virulence, animal inoculations afford us no positive assurance that, transferred to the throat of a non-resisting person, the bacilli might not cause disease. On the other hand, if such well-defined differences are observed in the growth or morphology of the organisms that it may be demonstrated that they constitute two or more distinct varieties, bearing no relation to each other, the problem of dealing with persons infected with B. diphtheriæ will be immensely simplified. It will then be entirely practicable to isolate all well persons in infected families who bear the germs and to compel others to take reasonable precautions against spreading the disease.

The matter is of so much importance that every effort should be made by bacteriologists to meet upon common ground in classifying diphtheria-like bacilli. Reports on cultural peculiarities should be so complete that one who has used somewhat different methods, and thereby failed to arrive at a similar result, should not be at liberty to deny the validity of another's conclusions.

As none doubts that if the organisms are identical all varieties must have had their origin in cases of clinical diphtheria, investigations should be made in places where diphtheria has not recently prevailed. Too many such examinations have been made in cities where diphtheria is endemic, and in jails, schools, and asylums, and too few in those country hamlets remote from railways, where, as far as the memory of the oldest physician serves, no case of diphtheria has occurred.

Careful observation of the morphology of diphtheria-like bacilli will probably be of greater value than a study of cultural differences. Dr. Wesbrook's classification, if enlarged to include a few types which cannot be conveniently grouped with any of his, forms a most admirable basis for comparison, and the water-colored drawings which accompanied his original article may well serve as models of accuracy.

In examinations made for the diagnosis of diphtheria it is rarely that the decision depends upon differentiating diphtheria bacilli and pseudodiphtheria bacilli; but when we are called upon to determine the presence of diphtheria bacilli in well persons the difficulty is often insurmountable.

It is because any data, however fragmentary, which bear upon an important subject have a certain value that I present a few observations on the morphology of a single variety of pseudodiphtheria bacillus.

Diphtheria has prevailed at the Willard State Hospital since 1899. In the management of the epidemic it is considered of much importance to isolate all well persons among the inmates in whose throats or noses diphtheria bacilli may be found. To this end as great a number of cultures as the facilities of the laboratory permit are taken from the 2700 employés and patients residing in the institution. In 17,509 cultures from 1423 well persons which I have examined during the last year, undoubted diphtheria bacilli were found in 189 cases. The cultures were all grown overnight on blood serum. The large number of cultures does not permit plating each "suspicious" one or close study on different media, and so it has been necessary to adopt some rather arbitrary method of deciding which organisms found are diphtheria bacilli and which are not. As absolute uniformity in the conditions of growths exists, this plan has been followed by more success than might be imagined. In all cases in which considerable doubt is felt, another culture is taken and some special methods of growth employed, but in the vast majority of cases the decision is made from the morphology of the organisms present in the first cover-slip preparation.

The fact which, after this number of examinations, seems most prominent is that there is one variety at least of the diphtheria-like bacilli which possesses a constancy of form and distribution which entitles it to separate consideration. To avoid confusing it with a form to which several names have been applied, it may be termed, for the moment, "type a."

Occurrence. It has been found at the Willard State Hospital so frequently in the nose that it has come to be regarded as a normal inhabitant of that part. In a series of 100 cultures from the nose it is very common to find it in 25, and sometimes in 60, in most cases predominating in numbers over all other bacteria present. In a few cases I have found it in cultures in which were undoubted diphtheria bacilli, but all of these were from well persons, and I have not yet seen it in cultures taken from those suffering with diphtheria. It has been found in the throats of those in whose nose cultures it was present the same day and on other days, and, in somewhat less than 1 per cent. of all cultures examined, it has been found only in the throat. In many instances a culture from the nose shows no other organism; in a large number of cultures, staphylococci and "type a" are present together. In certain persons this organism is so constantly present that in cultures taken months apart it is possible to predict the finding with certainty, while many individuals have had cultures taken repeatedly and "type a" never found.

VIRULENCE. I have inoculated only a few guinea-pigs and no other laboratory animals with cultures of this bacillus. None of the animals inoculated with pure cultures which died showed evidences of illness or of local reaction.

MORPHOLOGY. This bacillus shows less variation in size, shape, and staining than any other of the non-pathogenic bacteria found in the throat or nose. Whether the culture be from the nose, or the throat the morphology is the same. It is a moderately thick bacillus usually composed of two deeply stained segments separated by an unstained portion. The entire bacillus commonly forms an elongated ellipse. The segments are joined base to base, and each is spade-shaped rather than lancet-shaped. The segments are apt to be equal in length, although often one is longer than the other. When this is the case the shorter one is usually thicker than the other. The unstained portion is

FIG. 1.

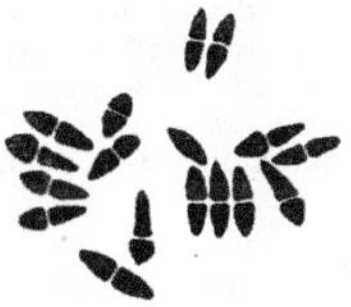

FIG. 2.

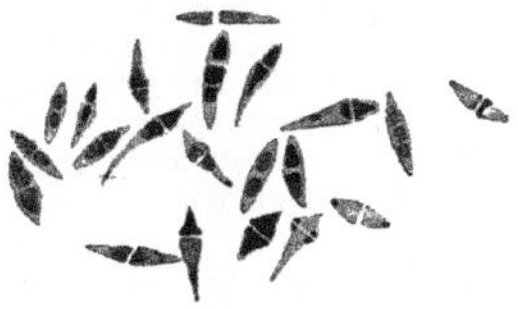

just perpendicular to the long axis of the bacillus, and narrow and uniform in width. In some cultures about every eighth or tenth bacillus does not present this segmented appearance, but forms an evenly stained ellipse. In cultures which have grown longer than eighteen hours there is a tendency for the ends to take the stain a trifle more intensely than other portions, but after twelve or fifteen hours the bacillus stains deeply and evenly with Loeffler's alkaline methylene blue. The arrangement is not quite as irregular as that of B. diphtheriæ, four or five bacilli often arranging themselves like the spokes of a wheel. Fig. 1 shows "type a" drawn from a cover-slip preparation. It is exceedingly common to find diphtheria bacilli, even in initial cultures from clinical cases, which resemble this bacillus closely, and yet, in the greater number of such instances there is enough difference in the morphology to distinguish between them. When such bacilli occur in pure cultures of B. diphtheriæ they resemble the forms shown in Fig. 2, which is drawn to a smaller scale. The inequality in the two segments is greater, the ends are more pointed, the sides are more concave, and the stain is rarely taken as evenly as by "type a."

This is not a complete description of the morphology of this type, but a few observations concerning a bacillus well known, often encountered, and variously named. If it can be generally agreed that this is a distinct variety, bearing no relation to B. diphtheriæ, and a distinctive name is given it, a great deal will be gained in classifying diphtheria-like bacilli, for it is certain that this organism is responsible for more difference of opinion in the examination of cultures from well persons than any other of the pseudodiphtheria bacilli.

A REPORT OF THREE MEDICOLEGAL CASES INVOLVING THE DIAGNOSIS OF CHRONIC DELUSIONAL INSANITY.[1]

BY SANGER BROWN, M.D.,
OF CHICAGO.

MY present purpose is not to discuss *in extenso* chronic delusional insanity, but merely to report briefly three medicolegal cases encountered in practice during the past year, in which the diagnosis mainly involved a consideration of that particular form of alienation, and, finally, to enunciate certain diagnostic criteria deducible from the histories presented.

CASE I.—B. C. (seen at Detention Hospital), aged forty-two years, married, coal-dealer; correct habits, general health and family history good; came to Chicago from Germany at the age of fourteen, and soon after twenty started in business successfully for himself and proposed marriage to a former schoolmate, who accepted his offer, coming from the old country to consummate the ceremony. The union was a fruitful and happy one. Both were active and consistent church members, their clergyman often citing theirs as the model family of his rather large congregation.

About two years prior to the date of my visit B. C. returned home, not by design, but quite unexpectedly, however, and found D. alone in the family bedroom with his wife; the children all on the floor below by order of the mother, and she sitting on the bed, which had the appearance of having been used; D.'s clothing was disarranged. Now, D. had gone to school in the old country with both B. C. and his wife, and had accompanied the latter on her voyage to this country, and B. C. had given him work some years before, which threw the suspected parties much together, as B. C.'s residence stood in the yard where D. was employed. B. C. said he could have killed D. then and there, but refrained from making a scene on account of his family. D. never came to the house again, though he had formerly been a frequent visitor there.

[1] Also sometimes designated monomania, paranoia, and reasoning insanity. Read at the Illinois State Medical Association, April 29, 1903.

After this B. C. frequently upbraided his wife for her frailty, but did not speak of it to a third party until over a year later, when on the occasion of a social gathering at their home he chanced to discover her in the arms of F. in a stairway, whereupon he shortly afterward confided his trouble to his clergyman, and subsequently the wife confessed. All was peaceful until a few days later, when she told B. C. that the confession was a bogus one, and that she made it at the instigation of his mother and the clergyman in order to placate B. C.'s "fixed idea." This the clergyman denied *in toto*, at least in so far as his connivance was concerned.

Now, B. C. became more demonstrative than ever, at times loudly taunting and denouncing his wife before the children, even insinuating to her that one of them, differing in appearance from the others, was the offspring of D., and that possibly their illicit relations had begun as they voyaged together to this country, and he likewise recalled incidents which he thought gave support to this hypothesis. Finally, his fellow-deacons tried to heal the breach, but without success. The congregation divided on the subject, and B. C. was summarily arrested while at work and taken to the Detention Hospital.

The hearing in court developed no material facts in addition to those stated. I felt warranted in testifying that the charge of insanity had not been sustained,[1] because, even though B. C.'s conclusions might have been unwarranted, his accusations were based wholly upon and never extended beyond the two incidents above named. No evidence was forthcoming—and I sought carefully for it—of any vague or general suspicions either before or after these occurrences. B. C. was acquitted, has since lived apart from his wife, but contributes fairly to the support of her and their children, and attends to business as formerly; but his opinion regarding his wife's infidelity remains unchanged.

Case II.—G. H (seen at a private sanitarium, where he was in custody pending trial), aged fifty-four years, married, practical mechanic, inventor, and manufacturer; correct habits, general health and family history good. Married happily in early life, and has three married children. Though they have lived in amity, his wife states that she has always had to reckon with his excessive jealousy in her social relations.

Two or three months prior to the date of my visit G. H. conceived the idea that his wife was practising masturbation, observed her narrowly, and thought her attitudes and movements, especially in bed, proved his suspicions; would lie awake in an adjoining room at night listening; secured a powerful flashlight, which he turned upon her frequently while she slept, in order to take her unawares and define accurately her position. Finally, he told her he was certain she was a confirmed and almost constant masturbator, and begged her to go to a sanitarium for treatment.

Several weeks were consumed up to this point, at which time he likewise confided his suspicions to one of his sons-in-law, and added he was certain his wife was also having sexual intercourse with her house dog. Matters went on thus till about a week previous to my visit, when, at their summer home, where she was staying with her children, he accused his wife of criminal intimacy with K., a gentleman neither he nor she had ever met, and cited certain noises he heard about the house at night as confirmation of the charge. He shortly told his son-in-law he

[1] This diagnosis may seem to contradict the title of the paper.

was certain by the way his wife looked at men generally and the way her glances were returned that her sexual irregularities and marital infidelity were commonly known; he was greatly exasperated when his confidant ridiculed his stated convictions.

Finally, a day or two later, the family having assembled in the sitting-room, he appeared at the door with a loaded pistol in each hand and opened fire, saying excitedly that he would "compel them to listen to him." He did not appear to be actuated by anger against his wife, and did not aim at her particularly. Fortunately, he was overpowered before anyone was hurt, though one of the bullets passed through the sleeve of a member of the group. After his arrest, which immediately followed, he made several conflicting statements regarding his purpose in shooting. To me he admitted it was very foolish, but firmly maintained the correctness of the convictions above expressed.

Obviously here the delusive conceptions and conclusions germinated and flourished altogether upon a pathological activity of certain cerebral neurones or essential cerebral elements. In other words, they rested entirely upon a subjective basis; hence a diagnosis of insanity might be confidently pronounced.

Incidently, pending the legal proceedings, G. H. had a large and painful hemorrhoid removed—he had been troubled with piles more or less for many years—and on recovering from the anæsthesia his delusions appeared to have vanished. He apologized to his wife, who was present, and three weeks subsequently the legal proceedings were dismissed, no recurrence of his delusive ideas having been manifested in the meantime.

Case III.—L. P. (appeared in court as defendant in a charge of insanity preferred by the members of his immediate family), aged fifty-four years, merchant, married, three grown children; habits correct, general health and family history good, except that two maternal uncles became insane after middle life.

In his early twenties he married a charming and estimable young lady of distinguished family, and lived happily with her until about three years prior to the above date, when the shadow about to be described first fell across their path.

L. P. developed the idea, without any alteration of conduct on her part, that his wife was unfaithful to him; that she kissed her brother-in-law, a venerable clergyman, in a suggestive manner and quite unlike she had done before; and that further she lodged him in their house on an occasion when he paid them a visit, as he frequently did, with a view to having illicit sexual intercourse with him; that generally she admitted men surreptitiously and indiscriminately to the house for the same purpose, even specifying mechanics who were making repairs; and that his daughter, a girl of eighteen, and his mother-in-law, a lady nearly eighty, who lived in his home, were cognizant of his wife's transgressions, and aided and abetted her in them. After he had pledged them to secrecy, the coachman and housemaid were offered a large sum if they could furnish conclusive evidence of his conviction, and he showed them how to spy unobserved into certain rooms where he suspected his wife habitually participated in illicit sexual orgies. Later he confided his conviction to his grown son, and asked him to carefully watch the rear of the house at night to see if men—no particular man—did not surreptitiously enter. He smelled his wife's menstrual napkins to determine whether or not he could determine an odor of semen upon them, claiming that he could do so—thus to his own mind conclusively confirming his suspicions. In company with his wife they met a mutual friend at a golf club, and he knew by the glances exchanged that they would remain at the club-house and cohabit while he was out on the course playing.

Afterward he sent a telegram to a favorite relative living a thousand miles distant to meet him half-way, as he had something of vital importance to communicate. At the meeting he related the above and much more of a similar nature as facts about which there could be no doubt. His relative accompanied him home, and, with the co-operation of others, succeeded in getting him to retract his charges, become reconciled to his wife, and take a trip for his health. This partial remission of his delusions occurred about eight months from the date of their first appearance. He returned home after about two months' absence, having, while away, however, occasionally thought he was being watched by detectives. A few weeks after his return his delusions recurred with full force, and continued up to the time of the trial. In the meantime he made several extended trips abroad, at times thinking he was in imminent danger of arrest and incarceration, sometimes even disappearing and concealing his whereabouts for several weeks together. Finally, shortly before the hearing, he ordered the proper allowance he had formerly made his wife reduced to a mere pittance, and stipulated further that she might only receive this on conditiou that she take up her residence outside the city limits, asserting that her conduct justified him in forcing this humiliation upon her.

Many business acquaintances testified that they had known L. P. for many years; had met him during the period covered by this investigation, and had never seen anything in him indicating insanity. And, indeed, it may here be stated that in none of the three cases under discussion was there anything in the demeanor, deportment, or general conversation suggestive of mental derangement. To the casual observer there was no noticeable impairment of judgment or of any of the mental faculties. Hence it not infrequently happens that a petition for the application of legal restraint to such patients is denied by a jury, which thus, perhaps, unwittingly, permits the perpetration of a terrible but preventable tragedy.

For the reasons stated in the preceding case I had no hesitation in testifying that L. P. was insane, and, further, that his expressed attitude relative to the reduction of his wife's allowance afforded ample ground for apprehending that he might make a homicidal attempt upon any of the parties concerned in his morbid convictions. The jury disagreed, and, after a few weeks, L. P. in the meantime having made a division of his income satisfactory to his family, the legal proceedings were dropped. He, however, still retains his delusions as before.

The essential diagnostic problem in these cases was whether the particular ideas in question were conceived and elaborated on a basis of objective data, denoting cerebral reactions not inconsistent with those natural to the individual, or whether they were wholly or essentially subjective, the product of autogenous pathological cerebral activity. In either case the conclusions reached might be ever so erroneous—delusions, indeed; only in the latter, however, could they properly be designated as insane delusions. If these criteria are kept clearly in view, the difficulty of reaching a correct diagnosis in these cases may, I think, be to some extent simplified.

Though Cases II. and III. are clearly illustrative of the inception and early course of chronic delusional insanity, and happen to exhibit many singular similarities, it would be erroneous to infer that they represent the most usual type of that disorder. It commonly commences in early life, even during adolescence, and, while the delusions frequently involve some phase of the sexual sphere, this is by no means constant. Indeed, the range and strength of the delusions present almost infinite variations when a large number of cases is examined. All, however, and I think this may be applied to insanity generally, exhibit in common the criterion cited above. That is, to repeat, the delusions rest upon a subjective basis, represent a morbidly autogenous manifestation of cerebral energy. In fact, the cerebral disturbance may be so great as to give rise to hallucinations of the special senses, morbid activity of the cortical centres related to the organs of special sense being erroneously accepted by the patient as the normal exercise of these organs.

The character of the delusions and the temperament of the individual in which they occur determine his conduct. Some of the subjects of this disorder, after having learned by experience that assertion of their peculiar convictions means deprivation of liberty, are able to repress them and live at large, sometimes even conducting an extensive business successfully; while others comprise the most dangerously homicidal patients ever encountered in the wards of a hospital for the insane.

Though subject to some fluctuations, or even complete remissions in its early stages, when the disease is once fairly seated permanent recovery is exceedingly rare.

MERCURIAL NEPHRITIS.*

By John M. Swan, M.D.,

DEMONSTRATOR OF OSTEOLOGY, UNIVERSITY OF PENNSYLVANIA; PATHOLOGIST TO ST. MARY'S HOSPITAL; INSTRUCTOR IN CLINICAL MEDICINE, PHILADELPHIA POLYCLINIC.

(From the Chemical Laboratory, Medical Department, University of Pennsylvania.)

In the concluding paragraph on the subject of mercury, H. C. Wood[6] says that "it appears to be established that certain disagreeable and perchance serious effects may be produced by mercurials when freely and continuously used in the treatment of syphilis, against which the practitioner must be on his guard. The most important of these is nephritis, with its consequent albuminuria."

* Read before the College of Physicians, Philadelphia, November 4, 1903.

The case which serves as the basis of this study illustrates in a striking manner the serious results of the overadministration of mercury:

The patient is a widow, aged thirty-one years.

Family History. Her father is living, at the age of seventy-four years; he complains of symptoms that point to the disturbances due to the uric acid diathesis, and recently has shown the early indications of posterior spinal sclerosis; at the age of thirty years he had an attack of psoriasis. Her mother is living and suffers from chronic gastric disturbance. One brother died of cholera infantum. Two sisters are living and in good health. One of these sisters has four daughters, each of whom suffers from periodic attacks of psoriasis. Her paternal grandfather died at the age of forty-two years, of cerebral hemorrhage; her paternal grandmother died at the age of eighty-seven years, of an unknown cause. Her maternal grandfather died at the age of fifty-two years, of cerebral hemorrhage; her maternal grandmother died at the age of thirty-seven years, of enteritis.

In April, 1898, the patient noticed an eruption, which first appeared on her arms and face, but which disappeared under treatment in about four months. In February, 1900, a similar eruption appeared, first on her face, whence it spread until it involved her entire body. At that time the eruption was associated with gastric pain and she was put on a restricted diet, so that in six months the eruption disappeared. A similar eruption appeared again in February, 1901. The eruption, at this date, first made its appearance on her face and then spread until it involved her entire body. The eruption persisted until October, 1901, at which time she consulted a dermatologist in another city, who told her that it was due to syphilis. She was then put upon a mixture containing $\frac{1}{32}$ grain of mercury biniodide and 15 grains of potassium iodide, which she took three times a day. In addition to this she took $\frac{1}{4}$ grain of the yellow iodide of mercury four times a day, and 2 drachms of mercurial ointment by inunction daily. The first prescription she used during October and November; the others she used during October, November, December, and January. During the time she was on this treatment she complained of soreness of the teeth, salivation, running at the nose, pains in the legs and in the abdomen, nausea without vomiting, and occipital headaches. Her bowels were loose and she passed two semisolid, fetid stools daily. The pains in her legs were cramp-like and deep-seated; they were paroxysmal in character and worse at night. These symptoms came on about four weeks after treatment was begun, which was then stopped for a week. At the end of this time the symptoms had disappeared and she began to take the medicines again and continued taking them for about three weeks longer, until the same symptoms reappeared. The administration of the medicines was again stopped until the symptoms disappeared, after which she was told to begin taking them a third time. On February 23, 1902, she began to complain of œdema of the feet, legs, and thighs, of occipital headache, and of pain in her eyes when they were exposed to the light. At that time she noticed that she was frequently passing a small quantity of urine at short intervals. About one week later she began to complain of dyspnœa and precordial pain. This pain was stationary, and was increased by movement and by deep inspiration. In January, 1902, she was confined to bed for a week on account of universal pains, suppression of urine, and vomiting.

On March 2, 1902, the patient returned to her home in Philadelphia on account of dyspnœa, pain in the precordium, œdema of the lower extremities, and partial suppression of urine. She then had an eruption of small, scaly patches, most marked on the back; but also visible on the thorax and abdomen, the arms, the legs, and the face. Her pulse was 96 per minute, small, weak, but regular. Her heart action was rapid, the sounds were deficient in muscular quality, but no murmurs could be detected. Her urine was acid in reaction; had a specific gravity of 1014, and contained 1.4 per cent. of albumin by the Esbach method. Microscopically, the urine was found to contain large numbers of hyaline casts, renal epithelium, and leukocytes. The examination of the other organs showed no evidences of disease.

On account of the fact that a dermatologist in another city had diagnosed the skin eruption of which the patient complained as syphilis, I thought that the renal condition was due to syphilis. Cases of syphilitic nephritis have been reported, particularly one recently by Hoffmann and Salkowski,[1] which was cured by mercurial inunctions; and one reported by Mühlig,[14] which was cured by hypodermic injections of mercuric chloride. Hoffmann and Salkowski have no doubt that the syphilis caused the nephritis in their patient, which was indicated by urine containing hyaline casts and 7 per cent. of albumin. They also believe that the mercury cured the kidney condition; in fact, their patient, five months later, had a return of his syphilitic eruption and albuminuria with casts, which was again apparently cured by mixed treatment. Waldvogel[3] has also recently reported a case of nephritis due to syphilis which was cured by mercurial inunctions. This author, however, points out the difficulties in demonstrating absolutely that nephritis is due to syphilis in a given case.

In 1901 Ferras[18] published a thesis entitled "Studies on the Nutrition in Syphilitics by the Chemical Analysis of the Urine." Out of nineteen cases studied in preparing this thesis, one patient presented a serious albuminuria complicating a malignant syphilis. This patient passed 3300 c.c. of urine in twenty-four hours, which contained 16 gm. of albumin. After an exclusive milk diet for eight days it was found that the albumin remained stationary, that the general condition of the patient was not ameliorated, and that the urine had diminished to 1500 c.c. The author, therefore, concluded that the nephritis was dependent upon the syphilis and not on some cause existing before the syphilis was acquired. In spite of mercurial treatment, the albumin excreted increased to 40 gm. in twenty-four hours and the patient died of uræmia.

Believing that my patient was suffering from a nephritis due to the syphilitic poison, I put her upon treatment with ¼ grain of the yellow iodide of mercury three times a day, increasing 1 grain daily; in conjunction with 2 drachms of infusion of digitalis and 1 drop of spirits of glonoin every four hours. After taking the yellow iodide of mercury for twenty-four hours the patient began to complain of sleeplessness and nausea without vomiting. At that time she was passing from 2000 to 2500 c.c. of urine in twenty-four hours, which had a specific gravity of 1021, and which contained hyaline and granular casts, renal epithelium, and leukocytes, and 0.7 per cent. of albumin by the Esbach method. The administration of digitalis was discontinued, but the mercury was continued until she had been taking it for five days. As the symptoms did not improve, but rather seemed to be aggravated, the administration of mercury was stopped. At that time she was taking 2 grains of the yellow iodide of mercury daily. After an interval of a week, treatment with mercurial inunctions was begun, 1 drachm daily, and after three days this was stopped because the patient complained of nausea, insomnia, occipital headache, foul breath, œdema of the feet, the legs, and the thighs. The eruption during this mercurial treatment showed no signs of improvement. The feet, the legs, and the thighs were painful as well as œdematous. There was a red line on the gums and the tongue was thickly coated. It then appeared plain that the eruption was not due to syphilis, and, in consultation with Dr. Jay F. Schamberg, a diagnosis of psoriasis was made. During this time the patient passed from 1500 to 2750 c.c. of urine in twenty-four hours, which contained from 0.35 per cent. to 0.6 per cent. of albumin, as determined by the Esbach method, as well as hyaline and granular casts.

It now appeared as though the nephritis from which the patient was suffering was due to the large quantities of mercury that she had taken. Her urine was examined for mercury according to the method of Almén, as given by v. Jaksch.[2] To 300 c.c. of urine a little sodium hydroxide and some saccharose were added and the mixture boiled. After boiling, the precipitate was allowed to settle and the fluid was decanted. The precipitate was then dissolved in hydrochloric acid and the resulting solution was diluted with six volumes of water. A small piece of thin, polished copper-foil was then placed in the fluid, which was maintained at a moderate heat for an hour and a half. The copper-foil was then removed, boiled in alkaline water, washed with alcohol and ether, dried and heated in a Reinsch tube to sublime the mercury. By this process mercury was obtained as small globules, the finding being confirmed by Dr. John Marshall.

This process of detecting mercury in the urine is very tedious, requiring about three hours, and Dr. Marshall suggested the following method as being simpler and more rapid, requiring only about one hour to complete the process. To 600 c.c. of urine 100 c.c. of strong hydrochloric acid are added, together with 0.5 gm. of potassium chlorate.

The mixture is heated to the boiling-point in a porcelain dish, and is then, while hot, transferred to a funnel provided with a cock in which a folded filter has previously been placed. The end of the funnel is placed in the wide portion of a thistle tube, the end of which has been fused so that it should have a small outlet, into which at the outlet a piece of bright copper-foil, rolled in the shape of a spiral, has previously been placed. The rate of passage of the hot filtrate through the thistle tube is regulated by the stop-cock in the funnel so that about 100 c.c. pass over the copper-foil in about seventy seconds. The liquid which has passed through the thistle tube is collected in a suitable receptacle, kept hot, and while hot passed over the copper-foil repeatedly until the entire amount of the fluid has passed over the copper-foil six times. The copper-foil is then washed in water, alcohol, and ether, and, when dried in the air, is heated in a Reinsch tube to sublime the mercury. This method was first applied on April 2, 1902, mercury having been detected in the urine by the process of Almén on April 1, 1902, and the patient's urine since then has been examined at intervals, first of one month, and later of two weeks. Mercury was found in all the specimens examined until April 16, 1903. From April 2, 1903, until April 16, 1903, the amounts obtained by sublimation in the Reinsch tube were very small. The last dose of mercury, 1 drachm of mercurial ointment, was administered to the patient on March 18, 1902. The patient had been eliminating mercury, therefore, for one year and twenty-nine days since the last dose was administered.

The œdema from which the patient suffered was deep-seated and, over the internal surface of the tibia, appeared to be situated beneath the periosteum. On one occasion I examined the urine for albumose, thinking some subacute inflammatory lesion of the bones might be present which would cause this substance to appear in the urine, but no albumose was found.

During the course of the treatment the patient was given hot salt-water baths, with the hope of increasing the elimination of mercury through the sweat glands. This produced a profuse red rash, somewhat similar to the rash of scarlet fever, and, as the lesions of psoriasis were also still present, the latter eruption formed circular, pale areas in the midst of the diffuse redness. As Hoffmann[12] reported two cases of mercurial dermatitis in which eosinophilia was present in the blood, a blood examination made during the persistence of this eruption gave the following result: erythrocytes, 4,840,000; leukocytes, 11,200; hæmoglobin, 100 per cent. Differential count: polymorphonuclears, 65 per cent.; lymphocytes, 24 per cent.; transitionals, 6 per cent.; eosinophiles, 5 per cent. It will be noted that there was a slight eosinophilia. Further, the granular degeneration of the erythrocyte, described by White and Pepper[13] in chronic lead poisoning, was looked for, but not found.

During the progress of the case the patient had several acute exacerbations, which were characterized by a diminished excretion of urine, increase of œdema, nausea and vomiting, and headache. Rest in bed, hot baths, and liquid diet controlled these in a day or two.

On July 1, 1903, the patient's condition was as follows: She had been teaching school for seven months, part of the time both day and night school. She feels tired and complains of pains around her heart, particularly at night; she is a little short of breath at times, usually in the evening. Her vision is good. There is probably slight œdema of the ankles in the morning. She has headache occasionally, when she is unusually tired. Her appetite is good, her bowels are regular, and she sleeps fairly well; little noises keep her awake, but if she is not disturbed she sleeps all night. She passes about 1500 c.c. of urine daily; an examination of the morning specimen gave the following result: color, amber; reaction, acid; specific gravity, 1010; sediment, slight; microscopic examination—few granular casts, large quantities of epithelium, leukocytes; chemical examination—albumin, 0.025 per cent. by the Esbach method; no sugar. She does not complain of palpitation, of nausea or vomiting, nor of indigestion. Her psoriasis is worse than it has ever been.

Her eyes are prominent; the pupils react both to light and distance. The mucous membranes are of good color. The tongue is clean and moist. Pulse 90 per minute, regular, small volume, artery normal.

Heart. Apex neither visible nor palpable. Dulness third interspace, midsternal line, midclavicular line, fifth interspace. The sounds are heard most distinctly in the fifth interspace just outside the midclavicular line. There are no murmurs. The muscular quality of the systolic sound is deficient. The diastolic sound at the base is accentuated.

The lungs are normal except for cog-wheel inspiration in the left axilla. The thyroid body is distinctly palpable.

Blood Examination. Erythrocytes, 4,500,000; leukocytes, 10,800; ratio, 1:416. Hæmoglobin, 82 per cent. Differential count: polymorphonuclears, 70.6 per cent.; lymphocytes, 24.6 per cent.; transitionals, 3.2 per cent.; eosinophiles, 1.6 per cent. There was no granular degeneration of the red cells.

She is taking ten drops of tincture of digitalis and one glass of lithia water daily. On account of having just got her system rid of one metallic poison, I did not feel warranted in giving her arsenic for the psoriasis, so put her upon 5-grain doses of potassium acetate three times a day.

Dr. Marshall's procedure for the detection of mercury in the urine is based on the theory that mercury is eliminated in the urine in some organic combination. The addition of hydrochloric acid and potassium chlorate to the urine breaks up the combination and converts the mercury into a soluble chloride. Metallic mercury is then deposited from the hot acid solution on the copper-foil by electrolysis, so that, by sublimation in the Reinsch tube, it redeposits on the walls of the glass tube and can be detected as small globules adhering to the walls of the capillary portion of the tube, with a low power of the microscope. When Dr. Marshall suggested the process he thought it was original, but subsequently he found essentially the same process described by Witz,[5] except that Witz used potassium permanganate instead of potassium chlorate to assist in the decomposition of the organic mercurial compound.

The accumulation of mercury in the tissues, its subsequent elimination, and its possible deleterious effects are subjects of considerable importance to the physician, particularly so to the genito-urinary specialist and the syphilographer. White and Martin[7] point out that lesions of the kidney particularly predispose to the development of hydrargyrism and say that the drug should be used with caution in cases in which there are crippled kidneys.

V. Jaksch[20] says that when the diagnosis has been correctly made the administration of mercury in syphilis has never done permanent evil, although individuals that are afflicted with nephritis tolerate the drug badly. The urine in such cases contains albumin, casts, and renal epithelium. Cornil[21] says that mercury has a profound action on the kidneys. It is, in the first place, an irritant to these organs and causes a swelling with fatty degeneration of the epithelium of the tubules.

According to Wood,[6] mercury has been found in the blood, the urine, the serum of ulcers, the saliva, the feces, the pus from ulcers, the semen, the milk of nursing women, and in every conceivable secretion and in every tissue. It has been demonstrated that a single dose of mercury does not remain in the system, but when the drug is administered constantly for a length of time, elimination does not keep pace with absorption, so that the drug accumulates in the tissues. There appears to be no limit of time during which stored-up mercury may remain in the body. All the probabilities point to the possibility of mercury being deposited in the tissues in such form that it is practically inert and exerts no effect on the system; liable, however, under certain agencies to be set free and exert its power upon the general nutrition. Wood refers to Klemperer's conclusions* that the changes in the kidneys due to mercury are: excessive hyperæmia, parenchymatous nephritis, hemorrhagic nephritis, widespread degeneration of the epithelium, and deposits of chalky material. My patient has apparently reached the condition of parenchymatous nephritis with widespread degeneration of the renal epithelium, which, I fear, is permanent.

Hare[4] says that there are three theories concerning the absorption of mercury: 1. The theory of Miahl, that the mercurial preparations are transformed in the stomach and intestines into the bichloride, which, in turn, unites with the sodium chloride in the blood and circu-

* Virchow's Archiv, cxviii., 1889.

lates as a double chloride of mercury and sodium. 2. Henoch's theory that the metal forms an albuminate of mercury. 3. Voit's theory that a chloro-albuminate is formed. Hare also says that mercury is climinated as an albuminate by every excretion of the body. A single dose is rapidly eliminated, but large doses frequently repeated show a cumulative action, and the mercury is so slowly eliminated as to remain for indefinite periods. He refers to the work of Balzer and Klumpke, which shows that mercury can be eliminated by the kidneys for many weeks when the body is saturated with the drug in doses of $\frac{1}{16}$ grain daily.

The literature, besides that referred to by Wood and Hare, contains a few reports of cases of nephritis due to the ingestion of mercury and of the finding of mercury in the urine. These cases are usually instances of poisoning by a single large dose of some preparation of the metal. For instance, Benham and Hendly[8] report the case of a girl, aged twenty years, who took ninety grains of red oxide of mercury and ammoniated mercury. After the symptoms of acute poisoning had passed off the urine became scanty and contained a large amount of albumin and casts. By the test with a piece of bright copper-foil, mercury was found in the urine, saliva, and the stools. The patient presented a vivid-red rash, like the rash of scarlet fever. The girl recovered after a miscarriage, but there is no note concerning the ultimate condition of the kidneys.

Axenfeld[9] reports the case of a man who presented the symptoms of chronic mercurial poisoning from using acid nitrate of mercury in the preparation of rabbit skins. The urine of the patient was normal in quantity and did not contain albumin. A quantity of urine, evaporated to a small volume, was decolorized with a hypochlorite and a portion then treated with hydrogen sulphide; a black precipitate of mercuric sulphide was produced. Another portion of the liquid treated with potassium iodide gave a red precipitate of mercuric iodide. Mercury was also obtained as a whitish-gray deposit on a strip of gold wrapped around a layer of tin (Smithson's pile) from another portion of the liquid. Mercury was found in the saliva by the same reaction.

Seguin[10] reports the case of a boy who took red iodide of mercury and potassium iodide for a cerebellar tumor. The symptoms of the disease improved under the treatment; but on examining the urine it was found to contain hyaline and epithelial casts, but no albumin. The administration of mercury was stopped and the renal condition improved. Then the symptoms of cerebellar tumor returned and mercury and potassium iodide were again given. This time the urine contained albumin, hyaline and granular casts, and free renal epithelium. He also notes a case the particulars of which were given to him by

Kinnicutt. The patient was taking mercury biniodide for secondary syphilis. He also had a urethritis. The urine contained albumin, leukocytes, and hyaline casts. The leukocytes and the albumin were due to the urethritis and disappeared with that lesion, but the casts persisted. The casts disappeared when the iodide was stopped, although the administration of mercury was continued.

Bouchard[14] reports the case of a man who was suffering from secondary syphilis and who had had an attack of lead poisoning eight months before. When first seen he had no albumin in his urine. After he had been treated with mercurial inunctions for five days he began to complain of swelling of his gums, and in spite of stopping the use of the mercurial ointment a sharp attack of stomatitis developed. Under the influence of this intoxication, seven days after the beginning of the stomatitis, the urine showed marked changes. The total quantity in twenty-four hours was 150 c.c.; specific gravity, 1017; albumin and traces of sugar were present, and the urea content was 3.6 gm. per litre.

Holle[15] quotes a fatal case of nephritis, reported by Riegel, in which the patient died from injury to the kidney and general poisoning after the prolonged administration of calomel. He also refers to a case reported by Pel in which the patient died soon after the administration of calomel, which had not produced diuresis as had been hoped. In this case it was found that there were large deposits of mercury in the kidneys.

Chauffard[16] reports the case of a young woman who took 5 gm. of mercuric chloride followed by 10 c.c. of laudanum. Among the symptoms referable to the kidneys in this case were complete anuria for five days, after which the patient began to pass 70 c.c. of albuminous urine in twenty-four hours containing an abundance of granulofatty casts and epithelial cells. The patient died from the effects of a complicating pericarditis twenty days after taking the poison. No mercury was found in the urine, and at the autopsy the kidneys were found to belong to the class of large white kidneys.

Chauffard and Gouraud[17] report a case of syphilitic nephritis in a man, aged forty-seven years, who had had scarlet fever at the age of six years. In spite of energetic mercurial treatment the patient died. At the autopsy it was found that both kidneys were swollen; the convoluted tubules were most affected and their lumina were filled with albuminous coagula. The glomeruli were not congested, but were surrounded by the same albuminous exudate, which, in certain places, half-filled the capsules of Bowman. The authors hold that the large quantity of albumin found in their case, 55 grams to the litre, argues in favor of the syphilitic origin of the nephritis, and say that this condition is quite the contrary in cases of mercurial nephritis. It seems to me more probable that this was a case in which kidneys injured by scarlet fever were put into active inflammation by their efforts to eliminate the mercury administered for the treatment of the syphilitic infection than that it was one of syphilitic nephritis as claimed by the authors.

Cornil[19] reports the case of a hatmaker, who had been under the toxic influence of mercurial vapor for seven years. He died soon after he was admitted to the hospital suffering from clonic convulsions. He had neither alcoholism nor syphilis. At the autopsy a fatty degeneration of nearly all the striped muscles of the body was found. Mercury was found in the brain. The liver and the kidneys showed a fatty degeneration analogous to that observed in intoxication.

References.

1. Erick Hoffmann and Salkowski. Berliner klin. Woch., February 10 and 24, 1902.
2. Rudolf v. Jaksch. Clinical Diagnosis. English translation of fourth German edition, 1897, p. 387.
3. Waldvogel. Deutsch. med. Woch., October 30, 1902.
4. Hobart Amory Hare. A Text-book of Practical Therapeutics, eighth edition, 1900.
5. Witz, quoted by Dragendorff. Die Gerichtlich-Chemische Ermittelung von Gifteng, fourth edition, 1895, p. 434.
6. Horatio C. Wood. Therapeutics: Its Principles and Practice, tenth edition, 1897.
7. J. William White and Edward Martin. Genito-urinary Surgery and Venereal Diseases, fifth edition, 1902.
8. R. F. Benham and H. Hendly. British Medical Journal, 1885, vol. i. p. 484.
9. Axenfeld. Gaz. d. Hôp., March 1, 1870, p. 97.
10. E. C. Seguin. Arch. Med., N. Y., 1879, p. 332.
11. Bouchard. Comptes Rendus de la Soc. de Biol., vol. v., Series 5, p. 227.
12. Erick Hoffmann. Berliner klin. Woch., October 6, 1902.
13. C. Y. White and William Pepper. The American Journal of the Medical Sciences, September, 1901.
14. F. Mühlig. Münch.-med. Woch., March 24, 1903.
15. August Holle. Therapeutic Monthly, June, 1902.
16. A. Chauffard. Le bull. méd., 1899, No. 12, p. 129.
17. A. Chauffard and F. X. Gouraud. La presse méd., July 5, 1902.
18. Jean Ferras. Recherches zur la Nutrition chez les Syphilitiques par l'Analyse Chimique des Urines. Paris Thesis, 1901, No. 51.
19. V. Cornil. Jour. de l'anat. et de physiol., 1868, p. 214.
20. R. v. Jaksch. Nothnagel's Spec. Path. u. Ther., Wien, 1897, vol. i.
21. V. Cornil. Des Differentes Especes de Nephrites, Paris, 1869.

THE CARDIOSPLANCHNIC PHENOMENON.

By Albert Abrams, A.M., M.D.,
San Francisco.

To my knowledge this is a heretofore undescribed phenomenon as far as its clinical manifestations are concerned. The facts, however, up to the point of its clinical identification, have been fully established by the physiological investigations of others. These facts are correlated to intra-abdominal tension and the effects of such tension on the circulation. It may be apposite before describing the phenomenon in question to succinctly review a few essential points on the subject of intra-abdominal tension. In the norm the latter is greater than the atmospheric pressure, and its positive pressure is exerted on the viscera, which in turn press on the abdominal parietes, causing them to bulge. Should a reverse condition of things prevail, the abdominal walls would become retracted. Positive intra-abdominal pressure is subject to two chief conditions, viz., atmospheric pressure upon the yielding abdominal walls and the contraction of the abdominal muscles. Therefore, intra-abdominal pressure is most pronounced in individuals with well-developed musculature and least evident in multiparous women with flaccid abdominal walls. Clinicians recognize the secondary effects of low intra-abdominal tension in conducing to splanchnoptosis, for with relaxation of the abdominal walls the support to the underlying tissues becomes defective and ptosis of the viscera is the likely result. The effects of reduced intra-abdominal tension on the circulation has received but scant consideration from clinicians—a most lamentable fact, considering the gravity of the issues involved.

Hall and Barnard[1] have contributed exhaustively to this important subject which has been practically elaborated in the excellent work of Campbell.[2] They have demonstrated that there is a tendency of the blood to accumulate in the splanchnic area, with consequent syncope. Like the generality of veins, the great splanchnic veins are very susceptible to pressure, and the amount of blood within them is greatly influenced by pressure on the abdominal walls. Mere pressure of the latter suffices to squeeze out of them a large quantity of blood. Thus, gravity, posture, the accoutrements of dress and other facts greatly influence the amount of blood contained in the splanchnic area. More blood accumulates in the splanchnic veins in the erect than in the recumbent posture, and it is not an uncommon observation for syncope to occur in bedridden patients who are suddenly constrained to leave the bed. The removal of stays in women often induces a feeling of faintness, and the same symptoms may occur when a large quantity of ascitic fluid is removed and in susceptible individuals when the bladder is emptied or feces discharged. There are some subjects who experience a sensation of faintness even in health when much pressure is brought to bear by the abdominal muscles in the evacuation of the bowels, and it is not an uncommon observation to note, when the patient is very ill, that the administration of a purgative may be followed by symptoms of collapse. In all these instances there is a determination of blood to the splanchnic area with consequent brain anæmia. The sensation of faintness or syncope is much accentuated when the abdominal walls are flaccid. Three factors enter into consideration in the mechanism of blood supply to the splanchnic vessels, viz.:

(1) contraction of the abdominal muscles, (2) respiration, and (3) the regulating vasomotor action of the splanchnic vessels. The first factor is an important one, the transversales maintaining the anterior and posterior abdominal walls in fairly close contact, preventing in the erect posture the gravitation of blood to the splanchnic area. The second factor concerns the diaphragmatic descent and pulmonary suction. Each time the diaphragm descends the intra-abdominal vessels are compressed, and the action thus exerted is less evident in the firm arteries than in the flaccid veins, the blood being squeezed from the latter into the right heart. De Jager[3] has shown that even strong pressure upon the abdomen has little or no effect on the arteries, but serves to express a large amount of blood from the splanchnic veins. Hill has also shown that in consequence of some failure in certain compensatory mechanisms the blood gravitates into the splanchnic veins from the right heart, and that abdominal compression will send the blood back from the veins to the right heart, thus re-establishing the circulation. Such compression not only augments the input into the right heart, but likewise increases, according to some observers, the systemic arterial pressure by increasing the peripheral resistance in the splanchnic area. Pulmonary suction refers to the large quantity of blood drawn into the lungs with each inspiration, and this physiological process has not been inaptly compared to a species of dry cupping. Chapman[4] avers "that if at the termination of expiration the quantity of blood in the lungs is from $\frac{1}{15}$ to $\frac{1}{18}$ of the total quantity of blood in the body, at the termination of inspiration it will be from $\frac{1}{12}$ to $\frac{1}{13}$." The pulmonary vessels expand with each inspiration and contract during expiration, the results being an increased flow of blood from the right heart and the lungs; the dilated vessels, as Campbell[5] puts it, "actually suck the blood out of the right heart." The final factor, the splanchnic vasomotor mechanism, in preventing the gravitation of blood into the splanchnic veins, is an important one. Hill and Barnard[6] have demonstrated that the splanchnic vasomotor mechanism suffices to combat this contingency, but when this mechanism is inhibited, as occurs when the splanchnic nerves are cut, a second mechanism is brought into prominence, viz., expiratory compressions of the abdomen occurring simultaneously with inspiratory thoracic suctions, the former squeezing and the latter sucking the blood out of the splanchnic pool. The latter mechanism compensates ineffectually in carrying on the circulation, and is referred to by Campbell[7] as the "respiratory mechanism." That the latter is not as efficient as the vasomotor mechanism is evidenced by the fact that the effects of gravity may be entirely compensated after the injection of curare, which paralyzes the muscles. Both mechanisms may be inhibited by division of the spinal cord at the first dorsal vertebra, and if the animal operated on be held with

the head up all the blood accumulates in the splanchnic veins and the empty heart ceases to beat; if, however, the abdomen of the animal is compressed, the blood is expressed into the heart and the circulation is restored. With the foregoing facts at our command, we will be able to appreciate what I have called the cardiosplanchnic phenomenon. If the lower sternal region—*i. e.*, the sternum contiguous to the heart—is first percussed in the standing and then again in the recumbent posture, one may appreciate a decided alteration in the percussion tone; in the former attitude it is resonant or even hyperresonant, in the latter it is dull or flat. This is the cardiosplanchnic phenomenon. It may be elicited, but less effectively, when the patient is in bed and sits up. Vigorous compression of the abdomen will exaggerate the phenomenon in all instances. Not infrequently the relative cardiac dulness will extend beyond the right border of the sternum. In no instance was this percussional phenomenon absent, although hundreds of individuals were examined. In a few instances the phenomenon was only feebly expressed by mere attitudinal changes, yet reinforcement by abdominal compression made its elicitation easy. A few forced inspirations at once dispelled the phenomenon, and it could likewise be made to disappear by the application of a vacuum cup to the abdomen. If the liver and spleen are percussed, first in the erect and then in the recumbent posture, a decided variation in regional percussion is obtained. In the former attitude the area of dulness is increased; in the latter it is diminished, and the splenic area of normal dulness may completely disappear. Abdominal compression exaggerates the results just as it does in increasing the sternal dulness. These conditions are superadded to the cardiosplanchnic phenomenon. Primarily it is necessary to adjust the discrepancy of my observations with those already accepted, and then to analyze the manifestations which give genesis to the phenomenon. Theoretically, one could assume at the outset that the situs of the heart more nearly approaches the anterior chest wall in the erect than in the recumbent posture, and, indeed, it is not only assumed but accepted by clinicians, that in the latter posture the heart falls away from the thoracic wall. Kingscote[8] perpetuates a similar error by assuming that the predominance of asthmatic seizures at night was caused by the posture of recumbency, the dilated heart in this position causing it to impinge on the vagi. I have shown elsewhere[9] the fallacy of this contention. With the aid of the Roentgen rays the triangular spaces in front and behind the heart are clearly defined in forced inspiration, and the rays give undeniable demonstration that change of posture only slightly modifies, if at all, the spaces in question; in fact, it may be observed that in not a few instances the anterior triangle is diminished and the posterior triangle is increased in recumbency. The foregoing facts contravene the contention that posture influences the relation of the heart to the chest wall. Again, percussional results are often influenced by the prejudiced preconceived ideas of the clinician. The skilled clinicist in his interpretation of percussional phenomena is guided not so much by the ear as by the *tactus eruditus;* thus, palpatory percussion will often yield results which would wholly escape the observer who is influenced only by what he hears and not by what he feels. In the elicitation of the cardiosplanchnic phenomenon, palpatory percussion must be our chief mentor. Others may contend that my lung reflexes (that of contraction and dilatation) and heart reflex may account for the phenomenon in question, but these reflexes have been assiduously eliminated and play no rôle in the cardiosplanchnic phenomenon. It is true that in recumbency the splenic and hepatic areas of dulness become diminished; this is in accordance with the well-known fact that postural changes influence the position of the lung borders, the so-called passive mobility of the lung borders. In recumbency the lower lung border descends about one-half inch lower than in the erect posture. The decrease in hepatic and splenic dulness as associated signs of the cardiosplanchnic phenomenon takes into consideration only the deep or relative hepatic dulness, together with the additional fact that the areas under consideration are diminished to an extent not to be accounted for by mere passive mobility of the lung borders. The cardiosplanchnic phenomenon permits of simple explanation. In the erect posture the blood leaves the right heart, which topographically is beneath the lower sternum, and tends to accumulate in the splanchnic area, whereas recumbency opposes this influence of gravity. Abdominal compression, which in some instances must be vigorous, assists still further in expressing the blood from the splanchnic veins and sending it back to the heart. The same factors prevail with relation to the liver and the spleen, the quantity of blood in the latter viscera being in direct proportion to the amount of blood contained in the splanchnic veins, and in inverse proportion to the amount of blood contained in the heart. Forced inspirations hasten the output of blood from the heart, hence the almost immediate evanescence of the cardiosplanchnic phenomenon after vigorous breathing. To those who seek the elicitation of the phenomenon care must be bestowed on the fact to counsel the subject to conduct superficial breathing, but not to suspend it, for otherwise this manoeuvre alone will cause the blood to accumulate in the right heart. Exhaustion of air by means of a vacuum cup to the abdomen will decrease intra-abdominal tension and increase in consequence the quantity of blood in the splanchnic veins. After the latter manœuvre, the right heart chambers will become depleted. I have endeavored by means of the Roentgen rays to determine whether any of the manœuvres already suggested for provoking the cardiosplanchnic phenomenon in any way influence the cardiac diameters, and my investigations show that they do not. If the latter observation is correct, how then are we able to account for the increased dulness of the lower sternum, the necessary concomitant of the cardiosplanchnic phenomenon. The sternum contiguous to the right cardiac ventricle in the norm yields percussional resonance which is caused in the main by the transmission of the percussion blow to the neighboring lung tissue. A percussion blow is propagated from one and one-half to two and one-half inches on the surface, and to a depth of about two and one-half inches. It is evident, then, that in the normal subject the dulness of the right ventricle is not sufficiently pronounced to dampen the sound obtained from the vibration of air within the lung alveoli. It is, however, possible to conceive that if the right ventricle were sufficiently filled or even overfilled with blood—and this is capable of fulfilment without any increase in the dimensions of the cardiac chambers—the normal resonant sound of the lower sternal region would become dull or even flat. Our final endeavor is to show the value of the phenomenon in diagnosis and treatment. In estimating the size of the liver or spleen by percussion we are constrained to regard three factors, viz., position of the patient, the amount of blood in the right heart, and the vigor of respiration. The liver size is normally dependent, in part on the amount of blood which it contains, and this has been estimated by Foster[10] to be equivalent to one-quarter the amount of blood contained in the body. The skilled diagnostician will not find it a difficult task to demonstrate reduction in hepatic and splenic dulness after repeated forced inspirations. Such reduction cannot wholly be accounted for by the opening up of atelectatic lung areas, for in the case of the liver my investigations only refer to the deep or relative hepatic dulness. Supposing the object of our examination is an enlarged liver or spleen, and that we desire to know how much of the enlargement is due to hyperæmia and how much to tissue hyperplasia? Percussion in different attitudes, repeated inspirations, and abdominal compression, if necessary, will solve this question. If a crucial test is to be applied, all that is necessary is to apply a vacuum cup to the abdomen, and then, in accordance with the facts already established, the liver and spleen would still further show augmentation in size by percussion. Of course, each observer must estimate for himself to what degree the normal liver or spleen will enlarge under such conditions.* Supposing a patient complains of sternal pressure, which, if dependent on a

* Since writing the above I have directed attention to the "liver reflex" (Occidental Medical Times, September, 1903). This reflex is readily available for diagnostic purposes. It consists essentially of retraction of the lower liver border from a half-inch or more as determined by percussion, after irritation of the skin contiguous to the lower liver border. The liver reflex is pronounced in enlargement of the liver dependent on hyperæmia, and slight or absent, if due to connective-tissue hyperplasia.

dilated heart, would disappear on application of a vacuum cup to the abdomen, the blood would be expressed from the heart to the abdomen and the sensation of pressure would disappear at once. Let us further assume that we are confronted with an abdominal neoplasm and the question arises, are we dealing with a growth connected with the liver or spleen, the application of the vacuum cup may solve the problem, for the latter viscera would show augmentation in size and conversely they would show diminished size were the abdomen compressed. The elicitation of the cardiosplanchnic phenomenon would prove valuable

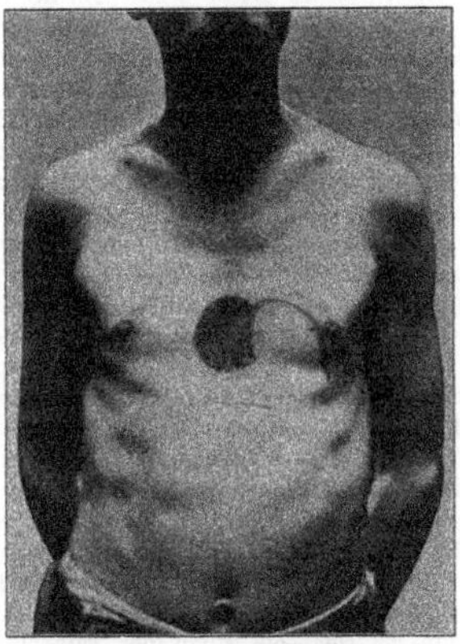

The cardiosplanchnic phenomenon. The shaded area is the circumscribed patch of dulness elicited after vigorous compression of the abdomen; the contiguous area is the superficial or absolute cardiac dulness.

in the differential diagnosis of a dilated heart from a pericardial exudate; in the latter affection it would not be elicited. Idiopathic syncope and vertigo and the vertiginous attacks of Glénard's disease may be attributed to a defective splanchnic vasomotor mechanism. Now, in the average normal subject the cardiosplanchnic phenomenon is fairly evident, but in the conditions just cited it would be exaggerated. In other words, the more perfect the mechanism, the less pronounced the phenomenon. A large number of respiratory affections owe their dyspnœa to an overtaxed right heart, and this is notably the case in asthma. While I do not agree with Kingscote," that a dilated heart is the invariable concomitant of asthma, yet I do contend that an enlargement of that viscus is operative in predisposing to a paroxysm and augmenting its severity. In a severe asthmatic attack which resisted the conventional remedies, a vacuum cup to the abdomen arrested the attack. In this instance, suggestion probably played no rôle, insomuch as the relief of the paroxysm coincided with the disappearance of substernal dulness.

It is unnecessary to adopt the theory of Kingscote that a dilated heart striking the vagi is responsible for nocturnal exacerbations of asthmatic paroxysms, for an overburdened right heart is a sufficient explanation. Indeed, the predominance of dyspnœic attacks at night in cardiorespiratory affections can be explained by the augmented blood supply to the right ventricle, the mere result of recumbency. In my opinion the upright posture instinctively assumed in orthopnœa is not only due to the fact that the extraordinary muscles of respiration may work to better advantage, but also for the additional reason that the blood from the right heart is enabled to gravitate to the splanchnic veins. In dyspnœa from any cause the implication of the heart in this symptom may be gauged by expressing blood from the right heart by means of the vacuum cup applied to the abdomen; if the dyspnœa is relieved we have reasonable assurance that it is caused by an overburdened heart. Many other instances could be cited to show the importance of this phenomenon in diagnosis, but the examples already mentioned will suffice. In treatment, the phenomenon suggests many possibilities in the direction of re-establishing the circulation and in relieving the heart when it is overtaxed. While the estimation of blood tension is a reliable gauge in estimating the value of any therapeutic method which has for its object cardiac stimulation, yet we cannot deny the fact that cardiac activity may be awakened without any corresponding increase in blood tension, just as we may awaken the respiratory centre by cutaneous stimulation without any necessary increase beyond the normal in the number and depth of the respirations.

My own observations show that the elicitation of the cardiosplanchnic phenomenon is unattended by any increase in the blood tension. Our only guide in estimating the amount of blood which is diverted to the right heart is the cardiosplanchnic phenomenon, not only the phenomenon *per se*, but the degree of its demonstration. The precordial dulness is, as has already been intimated, not so much dependent on the approximation of the heart to the chest wall, but rather to the amount of blood contained in the cardiac chambers. The following manœuvres in order of citation will express the largest amount of blood to the right heart: 1. Suspension by the feet, a method easy of execution in children. 2. Inversion of the patient. 3. Compression of the abdomen. 4. Recumbency. Inversion or suspension of the subject by the feet accentuates the dulness to the left of the lower sternal region and diminishes it over the latter area. In syncope it appears to me that the object achieved is not so much the determination of blood to the anæmic brain as it is to the determination of blood to the heart. To effect compression of the abdomen in acute conditions demanding cardiac stimulation, paroxysmal abdominal compression will suffice; in chronic conditions a firm cushion applied to the abdomen and secured by a rubber bandage or broad strap which permits of any degree of traction will prove serviceable. The objection to continuous abdominal compression is the respiratory embarrassment often experienced by the patient. An overtaxed right heart is present in so many cardiorespiratory conditions that it may be apposite to select croupous pneumonia as a paradigm. There are so many indications and contraindications cited by writers for venesection in this affection that it is really problematic whether bleeding is beneficial or harmful; at any rate, it is an empirical practice. It appears to me that in pneumonia our object should be to preserve the quantity of blood, for it is the chief stimulus for maintaining the cardiopulmonary circulation and furnishes the leukocytes, which do so much in conducing to a favorable issue. Instances do occur when bleeding is justifiable, and it would prove more effective if the patient were bled into his own vessels. The application of a vacuum cup to the abdomen meets the emergency and should be employed, if only as a tentative measure, should an overburdened heart with its consecutive phenomena warrant its employment. If this manœuvre is effective, it may be repeated any number of times, as it is a method harmless and painless if the exhaustion of the cup is not executed beyond a reasonable degree. It may be remarked in conclusion that alterations in blood tension do not synchronize with the intensity of the cardiosplanchnic phenomenon. This may be explained by the fact that the great amount of blood which is expressed into the right heart makes the latter unable for the time being to disburden itself of this large access of blood. The condition thus induced is somewhat similar to that when the breath is held, and Marey has shown, by tracings of the right ventricle when breathing is suspended, that its beats become slower and that it manifests an increasing difficulty in emptying itself, the amount of residual blood increasing with every beat.

BIBLIOGRAPHY.

1. Journal of Physiology, vol. xxi. p. 323.
2. Respiratory Exercises, 1898, p. 12.
3. Journal of Physiology, vol. vii. p. 202.
4. Lancet, 1894, vol. i. p. 587.
5. Ibid., p. 86.
6. Journal of Physiology, vol. xxi. p. 323.
7. Ibid., p. 14.
8. Gaillard's Medical Journal, January, 1901.
9. American Medicine, January 3, 1903.
10. Text-book of Physiology, 1893, p. 71.
11. Asthma: Recent Developments in its Treatment.

THE ETIOLOGY, PATHOLOGY, AND DIAGNOSIS OF ADRENAL HEMORRHAGE.

By Leonard S. Dudgeon, M.R.C.P. Lond.,
Superintendent of the Clinical Laboratory, St. Thomas' Hospital, London, etc.; Late Pathologist to the East London Hospital for Children, London.

In this paper I have recorded four cases of hemorrhage into the adrenal glands, and also entered into a short discussion on the subject.

Case I. *Thrombosis of the superior longitudinal sinus and the cerebral and cerebellar veins; pin-point hemorrhages in the cerebellum; extensive purpura; hemorrhage into the left adrenal gland and left kidney; thymic abscess; staphylococcus aureus and albus cultivated from the heart blood.*—Annie M., aged two years and eight months, admitted December 12, 1902, under the care of Dr. Eustace Smith, to the East London Hospital for Children.

The child was obviously rickety, and is said to have been delicate from birth. There was no evidence of congenital syphilis. She had been vaccinated successfully.

The present illness commenced on December 3, 1902, with pain in the head and general weakness. On December 6th a "swelling" was noticed at the angle of the jaw, on the left side. The child had frequent screaming fits, but no true convulsions.

On admission to the hospital the infant appeared to be very ill. She lay in an apathetic state, but occasionally put her hands to her head and screamed, as if she suffered great pain. Temperature was 101° F. The veins of the scalp were greatly distended, especially on the right side, and there was also a very prominent vein about the middle of the forehead. A large abscess was found on the left side of the neck, and a smaller abscess was situated in the lower part of the left pectoral region. The knee-jerks were brisk. Kernig's sign was absent. There was double otorrhœa. There was nothing else abnormal noted in any other part of the body.

December 13th. Infant was worse. The face was a pale leaden color. There was slight cyanosis. Temperature was 103° F., and the child was semicomatose. Respiration was rapid. Pulse was rapid and running. A small patch of purpura appeared on the outer side of the left knee, and gradually spread over the rest of the limb. Toward the end of the day the right foot became similarly affected, and the purpura gradually spread upward. There was swelling of the limbs but no pitting on pressure. There were no convulsions. Death occurred on December 14th.

I performed the post-mortem examination sixteen hours after death. Nutrition was fairly good. There was a large abscess on the left side of the neck beneath the lower jaw, which contained about half an ounce of thick yellow pus. There was no communication between this abscess and the pharynx. Another small abscess was found in the seventh intercostal space which contained about a drachm of pus. This had no connection with the ribs, thorax, or abdomen. It was situated between the skin and the chest muscles. There was deep-red staining of both legs and considerable swelling of the right thigh; but when one cut into these tissues they appeared to be normal. There were no abnormal changes found in the femoral artery or vein. All the thoracic viscera were normal, except the thymus gland, which was enlarged, owing to an abscess in the right lobe, which contained thick yellow pus.* The left kidney contained about a dozen "black spots," which were situated in the cortex, and were found to be hemorrhagic. Capsule stripped readily. No other naked-eye changes observed. Right kidney appeared to be normal. Bloodvessels were normal.

Left Adrenal Gland. This was simply a "coffee-colored" hemorrhagic mass, which was quite obvious through the capsule of the gland. There appeared, however, to be a small covering of apparently normal cortex, which formed a wall for the blood clot lying in the medulla. I regret that I failed to notice the condition of the suprarenal vein. There were no hemorrhages into the surrounding tissues.

Right adrenal gland was apparently normal. Mesenteric glands were normal.

Brain. There was complete thrombosis of the superior longitudinal sinus, the superior and middle cerebral veins, and a slight extension of the clot into the right lateral sinus. The cerebellar veins were also completely thrombosed. The clot was tough, pale red, and firmly adherent to the vessel walls. Pinpoint hemorrhages were visible in the gray matter of the cerebellum, but none elsewhere. There was no evidence of meningitis, but some œdema of the pia mater. There was no excess of fluid in the ventricles. There was softening of the brain in the region of the thrombosed vessels. Cranial bones were normal. Mastoids were normal.

Bacteriology. A pure culture of the staphylococcus aureus was obtained from both subcutaneous abscesses; and both the staphylococcus aureus and albus from the blood of the right ventricle.

Microscopic Examination. There were numerous scattered hemorrhages all through the medulla of the left adrenal gland, and in some places the hemorrhages occupied quite a large area of the gland tissue. The capillaries were overdistended, and in many places the walls of the bloodvessels had ruptured. Large, prominent, and distended capillaries were also seen between the columns of cortical cells, but otherwise the cortex was normal. The parenchyma of the medulla was unaffected except in the hemorrhagic areas. Here, many of the adrenal cells were destroyed, others had undergone "a granular degeneration"; a few apparently consisted of little more than a nucleus. Sections of the gland were stained by Gram's and Pappenheim's methods for microorganisms, but with negative results.

The renal epithelium of both kidneys had undergone a considerable degree of cloudy swelling. Many of the glomeruli of the left kidneys were injected, and a few large scattered hemorrhages were seen in the cortical tissue.

The walls of the superior longitudinal sinus were injected and showed small-celled infiltration, while the lumen was filled with fibrin, and blood corpuscles, leukocytes, and endothelial cells.

The right adrenal gland was normal.

* Unfortunately no bacteriological examination was made.

Case II. *Extensive burn; large hemorrhage into the right adrenal gland, associated with symptoms which rather pointed toward an acute lesion in the abdomen.*—Rose S., aged six years, admitted January 22, 1903, under the care of Mr. Keetley into the West London Hospital, Hammersmith. The child had burns of the first and second degree on her face, back, and both forearms. Temperature was 96° F. Boric acid fomentations were applied.

On January 24th the child was very restless and vomited during the night. Temperature was 99.8° F. January 26th she was restless and suffered from frequent vomiting. She is said to have complained of pain in the abdomen, but it moved well on respiration, and there was no localized tenderness. Pulse was 110. Temperature was 98° F.

January 27th. Abdomen moved well on respiration. Vomiting had stopped. Extremities were cold. Pulse was 140. Temperature was 98° F. Urine contained no albumin. Death occurred in the evening of January 27th.

Post-mortem examination was performed about twenty-four hours after death. There was very little found at the autopsy. All the thoracic organs were normal. The mesenteric glands were calcified. The right adrenal gland was very much swollen, of a deep-red color, and there was a very large hemorrhage into the medulla of the gland which so distended the cortex that it formed a sort of capsule. Left adrenal gland was normal. All the other abdominal viscera were normal. Brain was normal.

Microscopic Examination. Through the kindness of Dr. A. E. Russell, I was able to examine the suprarenal gland and to prepare specimens for microscopy.

The whole of the medulla of the gland was composed of blood clot. There was no parenchymatous tissue left. The cortex was very vascular and contained numerous vessels engorged with blood, but there were very few hemorrhages, and the parenchyma was apparently normal. No micro-organisms were seen in any of the specimens.

Case III. *Gangrenous varicella; tubercular mesenteric glands; tubercular ulceration of the intestines; double adrenal hemorrhage; pure culture of the pneumococcus isolated from the heart blood and from the adrenal glands.*—Beatrice G., aged one year and ten months, admitted March 5, 1903, under the care of Dr. Coutts, to the East London Hospital for Children, with the following history:

Child had been restless, and had loss of appetite for about a fortnight before admission to the hospital. Typical varicella rash appeared on Monday, March 2d. Papules rapidly became vesicles, and as some of these spots subsided others appeared. On Wednesday, March 4th, some of the spots rapidly spread, and tended to form "large spreading sores." On March 5th the child vomited twice and was so ill that the mother brought her to the hospital.*

On admission. The trunk, head, and limbs were covered with bluish-black "ulcers" which varied greatly in size. The large ulcers were confined to the back. The floor of the ulcers was dry and glazed, and

* Three other children in the family had gangrenous varicella about the same period. Two recovered, but the third has since died in the East London Hospital from bronchopneumonia. The adrenals were healthy and there was no tuberculosis.

the edge was in some places serpiginous. Some of the small varicella spots were in the same condition. Several ulcers were present on the scalp. There were no purpuric spots. There were no physical signs in the lungs or other viscera. Pulse was extremely rapid, 200 per minute, and the respiration was also very rapid. Throat was normal. Child was almost comatose, and died within twenty-four hours of admission to the hospital.

Post-mortem examination was performed on March 7th. Body was well nourished. Skin covered with ulcers, as already described. There was well-marked evidence of rickets. Throat, larynx, trachea, and pharynx were normal. Pleuræ were covered with numerous hemorrhages, but there was no fluid in either sac.

Lungs. There were numerous dark-red hemorrhagic areas about the size of a pin's head, or a little larger, in the left lower lobe, otherwise there was no consolidation of either lung. Tracheal and bronchial glands were normal. Heart was normal. Epicardial and pericardial hemorrhages were found. Right lung was normal. Mesenteric glands were pale and about normal in size, and most of them contained small caseous masses.

Intestines. Lower end of the ileum and colon contained large tubercular ulcers, with localized tubercles on the peritoneal surface of the gut. There were no adhesions and no free fluid. Both adrenal glands were swollen and of deep purple color, but the bloodvessels were normal. There were no lesions elsewhere in the abdomen. Brain was normal. Bones were normal.

Bacteriology. A pure culture of the pneumococcus was isolated both from the heart blood and from the adrenal glands, but no confirmatory inoculation experiments were made.

Microscopic Examination of the Adrenal Glands. The whole of the parenchymatous tissue of the glands was almost entirely replaced by blood clot. Some of the cells of the zona glomerulosa and fasciculata appeared to be normal, but the great majority were destroyed. The capillaries were engorged with blood. No organisms were detected in any of the microscopic specimens.

CASE IV. *Bronchopneumonia; sudden death; double adrenal hemorrhage.*—Charles M., aged fourteen weeks, was seen by Dr. Jordan Harvey (to whom I am indebted for the notes of the case), on Thursday, January 23, 1903, just before death.

The child had been delicate from birth, otherwise there were no special points of interest in the case until the morning of the above date, when the mother noticed that the child's breathing was labored. The dyspnœa rapidly increased until death, which occurred at 11 P.M. on the same day. There had been no vomiting, diarrhœa, abdominal pain, convulsions, or any purpuric spots.

Post-mortem examination was performed by Dr. Jordan Harvey within twelve hours of death.

The body was pale and flabby, and weighed twelve and one-half pounds. The anterior fontanelle was greatly depressed. There was a patch of eczema over the left ear.

Chest. The pleural sacs were normal. The upper lobe of the right lung was solid from confluent patches of bronchopneumonia, and the lower lobe of the left lung was in a similar condition. The other thoracic organs were healthy.

Abdomen: Adrenal Glands. Both glands were deep purple in color and distinctly swollen. The cortex and medulla appeared to be equally affected. The bloodvessels were not examined. All the other abdominal organs were healthy. Brain was normal.

No bacteriological investigation was made.

Microscopic Examination. The whole of the medulla of the glands was composed of blood clot. A few scattered nuclei seen here and there in the various sections, and some cells which had no nuclei and stained in an irregular manner proved to be the only evidence of any parenchymatous tissue. The capillaries in both the medulla and cortex were greatly distended with blood.

Numerous isolated hemorrhages were seen in the cortical portion of the glands, but there was less destruction of the parenchyma than had occurred in the medulla. No abnormal changes were seen in the walls of the bloodvessels. No micro-organisms were found in any of the specially stained sections.

The Clinical Aspects of Hemorrhage into the Adrenal Glands.

Adrenal hemorrhage is generally a complication of various maladies, but occasionally there are symptoms which appear to be somewhat characteristic and lead to the diagnosis of a separate and possibly distinct disease. It has generally been found that other clinical phenomena have been sufficient to attract the entire attention of the observers, and the condition of the suprarenal glands has never been referred to.

As already stated, the clinical aspects are various, and have been considered from many standpoints by such writers on the subject as Arnaud, Still, Graham Little, and others. The first named has contributed the most valuable monograph on the subject, both from a clinical and a pathological standpoint. He gives the following classification: (1) the asthenic type; (2) peritoneal; (3) nervous. This classification is to my mind incomplete. The most interesting group is omitted. I should therefore add to Arnaud's classification:

1. Cases with a very acute onset and many symptoms which lead one to suspect an acute specific fever.
2. Cases with severe skin lesions, purpura, etc., but not suggesting an acute specific fever.
3. Those cases in which the adrenal hemorrhage occurs as a complication of some pre-existing disease, and is only recognized at the autopsy.
4. Hemorrhage in the newborn.

Possibly this classification is inadequate, but it will be found to meet the large majority of cases.

The most interesting group (No. 1 in my classification) has been fully dealt with by former writers on the subject. The chief points of interest in these cases are briefly as follows: A very acute onset, generally in infants who previously are said to have been healthy. There are one or more convulsions, vomiting, diarrhœa, and within a few hours from the onset of the illness a petechial or purpuric eruption appears, which may spread diffusely all over the child. Pyrexia varies from 101° to 105° F. Collapse rapidly supervenes, and death takes place within twelve to forty-eight hours. The diagnosis of a specific fever has been made in many of these cases, and more especially variola, chiefly from the fact that the infants have generally been *unvaccinated*. Dr. Voelcker[1] describes a case in the *Pathological Reports of Middlesex Hospital for* 1894, of a well-nourished child, aged two years, who was admitted in November, 1894, into the Middlesex Hospital with a history of a severe illness of twenty-four hours' duration. The child was *unvaccinated*. There were vomiting, marked prostration; temperature 105° F., and an extensive petechial eruption which extended over the whole body. The case terminated fatally within forty-eight hours from the onset. It was recorded as doubtful variola. *Post-mortem* evidence showed hemorrhage into both suprarenal glands. Dr. Andrews[2] in the *Transactions of the Pathological Society of London*, reports a similar case to the above, in a well-nourished female child, aged one year and three months, who was *unvaccinated*, and where death also occurred within forty-eight hours. Both suprarenals were hemorrhagic. A. E. Garrod and J. H. Drysdale,[3] in the same *Transactions*, refer to the case of an *unvaccinated* female child, aged four months, who was brought to the hospital dead, covered with a blotchy purpuric eruption. Both adrenals were deep purple in color, and were found to be hemorrhagic. Dr. Batten,[4] also in the same *Transactions*, describes the case of a male child, aged two and a half years, which had been attending the outpatient department at Great Ormond Street Hospital for some time, suffering from lichen urticatus. The child was taken suddenly ill with vomiting and diarrhœa. Temperature was 102° F. Knee-jerks were exaggerated. Temperature rose to 106° F. before death, which occurred within forty-eight hours from the onset of the attack. The right adrenal was found to be hemorrhagic, but the left was normal. Eustace Talbot[5] reported two cases in the *St. Bartholomew's Hospital Reports* for 1900.

CASE I.—A well-nourished child, aged five months, *unvaccinated*, was brought to the hospital suffering from severe abdominal pain, vomiting, and convulsions of a few hours' duration. Temperature was 101° F. There was no rash, but the child was not admitted, as it was thought that the case was probably infectious. About four hours later the mother returned to the hospital with the child moribund, and death rapidly supervened. *Post-mortem:* There was double suprarenal hemorrhage.

CASE II.—A well-nourished child, aged five months, *unvaccinated*, was suddenly seized with vomiting, abdominal pain, convulsions, and a temperature of 101° F. There was no rash. Death occurred within twenty-four hours from the onset of the illness. Double adrenal hemorrhage was found at the autopsy.

Clive Riviere*[6] recorded four cases in the *Transactions of the Pathological Society of London*. The children were all under the age of twelve months. *Three were unvaccinated*. One had been vaccinated and showed two good scars. There were vomiting, diarrhœa, and pyrexia, and death supervened within forty-eight hours; in one case within twelve hours. In every case there was hemorrhage into the suprarenal gland.

Graham Little,[7] in the *British Journal of Dermatology*, has referred to the case of a child, aged four months, which was admitted to St. Bartholomew's Hospital under the care of Sir Dyce Duckworth, suffering from a purpuric eruption all over the trunk and limbs. There was some pyrexia. The child was rickety and was *unvaccinated*. Death took place within twenty-four hours from the onset of the illness. Both suprarenal glands were found to be deep purple in color.

Another case of great interest is also quoted by Graham Little.[7] A male child, aged thirteen months, was admitted to the Royal Free Hospital, under the care of Dr. Sainsbury. There was a diffuse purpuric eruption on the arms, legs, and face; also conjunctivitis, vomiting, convulsions, cyanosis, and pyrexia which reached 108° F. just before death, which took place within twenty-four hours from the commencement of the illness. There was a large hemorrhage in the right suprarenal gland. The left contained numerous hemorrhages.

This practically completes the list of these extremely interesting cases in which the diagnosis has caused such great difficulty.

What is the nature of these cases?

First and foremost, are they examples of fulminating smallpox? This diagnosis has been made in some cases, in others strongly suspected.

Fox,[8] in his article on hemorrhagic fulminating smallpox, says: "It runs its course precipitately and at times most unexpectedly, sometimes killing the patient in a few hours, in other cases not completing its career until the fourth or fifth day." There seems to be an entire absence from the literature of smallpox of cases similar to those recorded above, and at such an extremely early age. It is stated that infants are not so susceptible to smallpox as children and adults, but this is doubtful. Cases of fulminating smallpox often have extensive purpura, but present none of the characteristic features of variola, because death occurs at

* These cases have also been recorded by Graham Little in the British Journal of Dermatology, and by Blaker and Bailey in the British Medical Journal.

the commencement of the disease. Practically the only strong evidence in favor of smallpox in the cases under discussion rests on the fact that so frequently the children were unvaccinated (nine cases out of twelve recorded). It would be interesting to know, however, the exact percentage of *infants* who are brought to the various hospitals *unvaccinated*. There is nothing else in the clinical history of the cases which is not perfectly in accordance with an acute bacterial infection, fulminating scarlet fever, or measles, etc.

A most interesting case is recorded by Fox,[8] of an adult male, who died within twenty-four hours from the commencement of an illness which was considered to be hemorrhagic scarlet fever. This diagnosis was afterward found to be incorrect, as a friend who had occupied the same room developed smallpox within a fortnight. This is one of the few recorded cases in adults which resembles in many ways the cases described above, but this proved to be infectious, while every case I have collected failed to convey infection. This is most remarkable when we consider the overpopulated districts in which most of these children lived. MacCombie,[9] in his article on smallpox in Allbutt's *System of Medicine*, says: "I have not seen this fulminating form, which is characterized by its extreme rarity, rapid onset and termination, and by high temperature, delirium, coma, and collapse, rapidly terminating in death after a few hours' illness. No skin hemorrhages are seen, only visceral." In the recorded cases, however, skin hemorrhages have usually occurred. Lastly, physicians of such experience as Osler[10] and Immermann[11] do not refer to cases similar to those recorded in this paper in their various contributions to the literature of smallpox. It is extremely probable that we are dealing with an acute toxæmia of unknown origin, quite apart from any acute specific fever.

As already stated, the cause of the disease is unknown. In one case, however, the child had been given "some sausage" prior to the onset of the illness. This suggests the possibility of a gastrointestinal origin in some cases.

What Arnaud describes as the "peritoneal" type closely resembles the cases recorded above, except that the children were older, some had been vaccinated, and there was no purpura. In fact, in most examples of this class, the diagnosis has been made of an acute lesion in the abdomen.

About two years ago I was called to see a little boy, aged three years, who died with symptoms common to both types now under discussion. As far as I can remember the history was as follows: A woman took her two little boys for a day's excursion into the country. The mother and one of the children ate a pork pie on the journey home. Within a few hours both mother and son were seized with vomiting, diarrhœa, and acute abdominal pain. When I first saw the child, about twelve hours after eating the pie, he had a high temperature (the vomiting and diarrhœa had now stopped), and he was covered with a diffuse purpuric eruption. Death supervened within twenty-four hours from the onset of the illness. A post-mortem examination was not allowed. The mother recovered after a long illness. The other little boy, who did not take any pie, was unaffected. Without the history of a gastrointestinal infection this case would no doubt be classed, by some people, among those resembling an acute specific fever. To my mind it serves to illustrate that we are not always dealing with one class of cases, but only with various clinical phenomena dependent on one main pathological lesion, adrenal hemorrhage.

A history of food poisoning only rarely presents itself in our cases. In ptomaine poisoning diffuse purpura appears to be a very rare occurrence, although visceral hemorrhages have frequently been recorded.

Goodhart and Still[15] report cases in infants of a week old, who have died quite suddenly with severe abdominal pain and collapse. At the autopsies hemorrhage has been found in one or both suprarenals, which have ruptured, allowing extravasation of blood into the surrounding tissues and peritoneal cavity.

Graham Little[7] has recorded cases which he has collected from the literature associated with purpura, but where the symptoms in no way resembled an acute specific fever.

Perhaps the most interesting case has been described by Arnaud.[12] A man, aged thirty-six years, was admitted to hospital in a state of coma. Cerebral hemorrhage was diagnosed, and all "other causes" were excluded, so far as it was possible to do so.

Post-mortem Examination: Both suprarenals were practically destroyed by an extensive hemorrhage into the gland tissue. All other organs were found to be normal. This case is the best example in the literature of adrenal hemorrhage presenting such symptoms that even in competent hands a diagnosis was made of a lesion of the central nervous system.

I can find no certain examples in the literature of the asthenic type of Arnaud, and cases which belong to class 4 (of my classification) will only be considered from a pathological standpoint.

Etiology. 1. In most cases the term "idiopathic" might justly be applied.

2. A gastrointestinal infection.

3. Very common occurrence in the newborn.

4. In both acute and chronic lung and cardiac disease, and in convulsions; in fact, any disease which is known to produce stagnation of

the blood in the veins or a marked increase of blood pressure may be associated with adrenal hemorrhage.

5. Septicæmia, pyæmia, acute miliary tuberculosis,* and the toxæmia from severe burns, etc.

6. Congenital syphilis. It would have been a matter of some surprise if congenital syphilis had been omitted from the list of causes, but there is very little to substantiate the opinion held by some observers as to the importance of this factor in adrenal hemorrhage.

7. Blows in the back, fracture of the spinal column, and severe abdominal lesions, such as ruptured liver, etc.

8. The so-called blood diseases—*e. g.*, scurvy, etc.

9. Lastly, adrenal hemorrhage is sometimes found at the autopsies on chronic diseases of the nervous system—*e. g.*, general paralysis of the insane.

PATHOLOGY. *Experimental Evidence on Animals.* Roux and Yersin,[14] by injecting diphtheria bacilli under the skin of rabbits, guinea-pigs, and pigeons, induced general dilatation of bloodvessels, congestion of the intestines and kidneys, and, almost constantly in guinea-pigs, congestion, and less often hemorrhage of the suprarenal glands.

Various other organisms appear to produce the same result—*e. g.*, Gaertner's bacillus, bacillus pyocyaneus, bacillus mucus capsulatus, pneumobacillus, streptococcus pyogenes, and the bacillus pestis, etc.

BACTERIOLOGY. Considerable importance has been placed by some observers on the fact that an organism has been found in the blood or tissues after death, and therefore that organism has produced the disease in question. To say the least, such a statement is likely to lead to a difference of opinion. In one of my cases the staphylococcus pyogenes aureus and albus were cultivated from the heart blood. In another case I obtained the pneumococcus in pure culture both from the heart blood and also from the suprarenal glands. Drysdale found the "streptococcus" in one of Talbot's cases. Riviere isolated the bacillus coli communis from the splenic blood and a saprophyte from the heart blood in one of his cases. Riesman found at the autopsies on six newborn children who had adrenal hemorrhage the staphylococcus aureus and albus in the spleen and right suprarenal of one case; and in three of the other cases he cultivated the staphylococcus albus and aureus from the adrenal glands. In every other recorded case of adrenal hemorrhage, from which a bacteriological examination was made, the results proved to be negative. It is possible that the streptococcus found in one of the cases, and the pneumococcus in

* Still reported a case of a male child, aged fourteen months, who died of acute miliary tuberculosis and hemorrhage into the left adrenal gland. There was no purpura.

another, may have had some important bearing on the causation of the disease, but the results are not by any means proof positive.

When we consider the numerous organisms which produce adrenal hemorrhage experimentally in animals, it is not unlikely that we shall find a parallel in the human subject.

Lately I have examined carefully the condition of the adrenal glands in several cases of bronchopneumonia and general pneumococcic infection in children, but have not found a single example of adrenal hemorrhage. Congestion might be described in one or two cases, but when we consider the delicate structure of the medulla of the suprarenal and the congestion likely to result from the mechanical effects due to consolidation of the lungs, absolutely no importance can be placed on such results. Again, a boy was admitted to the East London Hospital for Children with infective periostitis of the left radius and tibia, due to the staphylococcus aureus. At the autopsy pinpoint abscesses were found in practically every organ, and the staphylococcus aureus and albus were obtained from the heart blood, spleen, and kidneys. The suprarenal glands appeared to be fatty to the naked eye, otherwise normal. Microscopically two small hemorrhages were seen in one of the adrenal glands, and both glands would possibly be described by some writers as congested, but there was no fatty change. Undoubted adrenal hemorrhage was seen in two cases which died with marked cyanosis from cardiac disease, but this is probably a very common occurrence, and of no interest.

Two cases have been already reported of adrenal hemorrhage associated with burns. The first case was described by Churton,[16] of double adrenal hemorrhage which followed on a severe burn. The other, by Arnaud,[17] of a girl, aged seventeen years, who was found to have a large hemorrhage into the medulla of the right gland, but the left gland was normal. There was no bacteriological examination made in either case. The last-named writer also refers to two cases of liver abscess, one due to a suppuration of a hydatid cyst, the other post-dysenteric, associated with adrenal hemorrhage. In the latter case there was also phlebitis and thrombosis of the left suprarenal vein.

Morbid Anatomy. The following is probably the most suitable classification:

1. The whole gland or glands are converted into "blood sacs," with occasional extravasation into the surrounding tissues.*

2. A hemorrhage may occupy the medulla of the gland, but the cortex is spared, except for a few red corpuscles scattered between the columns of adrenal cells.*

* Thrombosis of the adrenal vein may be met with in either class of cases.

3. Scattered hemorrhages into the gland substance, chiefly in the medulla, with little destruction of the parenchyma.

I have not referred here to congestion of the adrenal glands. There is no doubt that it is very hard to decide what should be justly termed congestion. The medulla has such a rich blood supply, and the vessels are only, so to speak, blood spaces, that anything and everything may lead to what is termed congestion. It is quite certain that it occurs very often and is a very much commoner lesion than we are led to suppose. Arnaud[12] fully justifies my remarks; he says: "The frequency of vascular lesions of the suprarenals is difficult to estimate, as unless there is bronzing of the skin the examination of the capsules is generally neglected. It would certainly be found to be less rare if a systematic examination was made." In a hundred post-mortem examinations he found from personal observation three cases which showed large hemorrhages into the adrenal tissues; eight cases with smaller hemorrhages which were identified by the microscope, and lastly, hyperæmia and congestion in eighteen cases.

Post-mortem Appearances of the Adrenal Glands. They are either swollen and deep purple color, or there is one large hemorrhage visible to the naked eye, such as one sees in any other part of the body. In some cases the medulla is a very dark red and entirely composed of blood clot, while the cortex is apparently normal.

Thrombosis of the adrenal vein or veins has been noted in some cases, but it is important to examine the vessels in every positive or suspected case. This can be readily accomplished by putting the tissues on the stretch, when the bloodvessels will be plainly seen.

From the recorded cases the right gland appears to be more often affected than the left. Mattei[17] considers that this may be due to either of two causes: (1) that the right adrenal vein opens directly into the inferior vena cava, or (2) that the gland is compressed between the liver and the vertebral column.

Lastly, what is the relation of adrenal hemorrhage to Addison's disease?

When we come to think of the extremely high death rate which is probably associated with the former disease, it is unlikely that there are many cases of Addison's disease which are primarily due to a vascular lesion of the adrenal glands apart from tubercle. There is only one place where we are able to diagnose adrenal hemorrhage with any degree of certainty, viz., the post-mortem room.

Pigmentation is one of the cardinal signs of Addison's disease, and purpura is very commonly associated with adrenal hemorrhage; possibly purpura stands in the same relation to acute destruction of the adrenals, as pigmentation does to chronic. These two clinical phenomena seem to me to be the most important points in the association of the two diseases.

Rolleston,[18] in Allbutt's *System of Medicine*, says: "Suprarenal hemorrhage has been associated with Addison's disease." Again, Hektoen[15] remarks: "The substitution of the blood clot by connective tissue might lead to induration and contraction, with atrophy of the medulla, which, if bilateral, might suspend the internal secretion and lead to Addison's disease." There may be a very slow destruction of the glands by hemorrhage, and, as a result, fibrosis, with the production of Addison's disease; but if this rarely does occur, it must be very rare. Everything tends to show that the large majority of cases of adrenal hemorrhage are very acute, and terminate fatally long before there is time for true Addison's disease to develop.

In conclusion, my best thanks are due to Drs. Eustace Smith and Coutts for the loan of their cases, and also to Mr. Keetley for permission to make use of the notes of the case which had been under his care.

References.

1. A. F. Völcker. Pathological Report. Middlesex Hospital Reports, 1894–95.
2 F. W. Andrews. Transactions of the Pathological Society of London, 1898, vol. xlix.
3. A. E Garrod and J. H. Drysdale. Ibid.
4. Frederick Batten. Ibid.
5. Eustace Talbot. St. Bartholomew's Hospital Reports 1900, vol. xxxvi. pp. 209–211.
6. Clive Riviere. Transactions of the Pathological Society of London, 1902, vol. liii.
7. E. Graham Little. British Journal of Dermatology, 1901, p. 451.
8. George Henry Fox. Smallpox, Part I., 1902.
9. MacCombie. Allbutt's System of Medicine, vol. ii. p. 204.
10. Osler. The Initial Rashes of Smallpox. Montreal, 1876.
11. Immermann. Variola. Nothnagel's Encyclopædia, American Translation, 1902, vol. ii.
12. François Arnaud. Les Hemorragies des Capsules surrénales. Archives Générales de Médecine, 1900.
13. Goodhart and Still. Diseases of Children, 1902.
14. Roux and Yersin. Annals de l'Institut Pasteur, Juin, 1889, p. 273.
15. Ludvig Hektoen. Hektoen and Riesman's Pathology, 1901, vol. ii. p. 920.
16. T. Churton. Lancet, 1886, vol. i. p. 248.
17. Mattei, quoted by G. S. Hamil. Archives of Pediatrics, February, 1901, vol. xviii.
18. H. D. Rolleston. Allbutt's System of Medicine, vol. iv. p 568.
19. G. F. Still. Transactions of the Pathological Society of London, 1898, vol. xlix.

REVIEWS.

A SYSTEM OF PHYSIOLOGIC THERAPEUTICS. Edited by SOLOMON SOLIS COHEN, A.M., M.D., Professor of Medicine and Therapeutics in the Philadelphia Polyclinic; Lecturer on Clinical Medicine at Jefferson Medical College; Physician to the Philadelphia Hospital and to the Rush Hospital for Consumptives, etc. Vol. IX. Hydrotherapy, Thermotherapy, Heliotherapy, and Phototherapy. Illustrated, pp. 570. Philadelphia: P. Blakiston's Son & Co., 1903.

THIS volume contains also special chapters on Balneology and Crounotherapy, notes on American Springs, Classification and Distribution of Mineral Waters in the United States, Saline Irrigations and Infusions, and on cognate subjects. The Physiologic Basis of Hydrotherapy in four chapters, with a brief exposition of the fundamental principles and practical applications of heliotherapy and phototherapy is from the pen of Professor Wilhelm Winternitz, than whom no one has enjoyed a larger experience with or greater enthusiasm for the use of water as a therapeutic agent. We may accept this as an exposition of his matured experience and as the strongest argument for the use of these physical agencies which can, at this time, be presented. While the practitioner of a broader experience may admire the thoroughness of his work in the study of the physiological facts, and may assent to their application in therapeutics, yet he may differ as to their applicability to the needs of daily practice. Moreover, he may find that other methods will more speedily, more pleasantly, and more surely yield better or at least equally good results. Should he reach this conclusion, then physical agencies will still find a place in his therapeutic equipment but as adjuvants. This position is still tenable and in consonance with a thorough appreciation of the valuable work which the author has done. To say that this section is the most forcible presentation of the subject, from the philosophical standpoint with which we are familiar, is but to give the author his just due. Dr. Alois Strasser presents the technique and methods of hydrotherapy in a thoroughly practical manner and with painstaking detail: a fitting sequence to Winternitz. Special hydrotherapy by Dr. B. Buxbaum considers symptoms and diseases, how these methods must be varied, and offers some statements as to the results which may be expected.

He is optimistic, as an advocate should be; dogmatic even to the point of compelling attention. To this section supplemental chapters by Dr. T. H. Kellogg on "Heliotherapy, Phototherapy, and Thermotherapy," and by Dr. Harvey Cushing on "Saline Iufusions and Irrigations," are added. Of the first we may say that it is interesting, instructive, and, based on the great opportunities to be found in a large and favorably known institution, thoroughly practical. Of the last so much has been done in this line, both at home and abroad, that a thorough acquaintance with the literature, which is here shown, has entailed an enormous demand upon the author's time and patience. We believe that the physician and surgeon will find this the best presentation of the subject, and we have in mind the excellent work of both Kemp and Dawbarn.

"Balneology and Crounotherapy" is written by Professor E. Heinrich Kisch. This section has for its introductory chapter a dissertation on the "Classification of Mineral Waters," by Dr. Albert C. Peale, which leads to a more intelligent understanding of what may be anticipated and as well a broader view of this rather neglected subject. In order that resources at our doors may receive proper attention the services of the well-known writer, Dr. Guy Hinsdale, have been levied upon. The result of these combined efforts is in the highest degree satisfactory, and, whether in enumeration or in claimed efficiency, nothing to be desired is left for the most patriotic reader, and yet foreign-bath methods and drinking-cure plans are fully presented. If our nosological catalogue may seem unduly long, certainly the list of places and resources can rival it. In fact, this section compares favorably with works especially devoted to this particular subject. The translation is satisfactory, and to Dr. Augustus A. Eshner much credit is due. That such words as "explicable" (p. 149) have crept into the text is pardonable when the peculiarities of idiom are at times perplexing. In this volume the editor is more in evidence. First he very properly objects to the hybrid "Crounotherapy" and suggests "Loutrotherapy" as an improvement, and with this we agree. Secondly, in the Appendix he offers "Additional Methods of the Therapeutic Use of Water, Heat, Cold, Light, and Mineral Baths." This adds much to the value of the book, and could readily have been made still more indicative of what has been accomplished in this country in the way of simplification and adaptability. Others, whose work is not mentioned, have made important contributions, and even if their writings lack dogmatism their influence has been none the less important. Of volumes presenting much excellence we would single out this as one which has impressed itself upon us, not from the importance of the subject, but rather from the thoroughness with which the methods are illustrated and the ability shown in its presentation.

R. W. W.

HYPNOTISM: ITS HISTORY, PRACTICE, AND THEORY. By J. MILNE BRAMWELL, M.B., C.M. London: Grant Richards, 1903.

WHATEVER one's opinion concerning the usefulness of hypnotism may be, this is a very interesting book. It is, of course, written by a man biased in favor of his subject, but that is characteristic of the majority of the books written on the subject. Judicial calm is not to be expected, or at least is very rarely met with, in the discussion of a matter like hypnotism. Much less claim of its therapeutie value is made in this book than in many others. The historical chapter is very entertaining and contains quite a number of facts not mentioned in other historical sketches. For example, it is not commonly known that Herbert Spencer published in *The Zoist* essays "On the Situation of the Organ of Amativeness" and "A Theory Concerning the Organ of Wonder." This, to be sure, was a long time ago, and proves only that even geniuses may sometimes jump the wrong way. In Bramwell's opinion, "the evidence as to the production of blistering and changes of temperature by suggestion is by no means conclusive." All experiments on clairvoyance that he has seen he regards as valueless, an opinion in which most sober-minded men will agree with him. He has found nervous, ill-balanced, and hysterical people the most difficult to influence by hypnotism; healthy people who possessed the power of mental concentration the easiest. He thinks that apparent hypnosis in animals is often if not always really a willed simulation of death for purposes of protection. He believes the greatest therapeutie use of hypnotism is in functional nervous diseases. There is a quite long chapter on the theories of hypnotism. Everyone interested in the subject should read this book. C. W. B.

PROGRESSIVE MEDICINE. A Quarterly Digest of Advances, Discoveries, and Improvements in the Medical and Surgical Sciences. Edited by HOBART AMORY HARE, M.D.; assisted by H. R. M. LANDIS, M.D. Vol. III., September, 1903: Diseases of the Thorax and its Viscera, including the Heart, Lungs, and Bloodvessels; Dermatology and Syphilis; Diseases of the Nervous System; Obstetrics. Philadelphia and New York: Lea Brothers & Co., 1903.

THIS issue of this valuable quarterly contains four most important sections, namely, those on Diseases of the Thorax and its Viscera, including the Heart, Lungs, and Bloodvessels, by William Ewart, M.D., F.R.C.P.; that on Dermatology and Syphilis, by William S. Gottheil, M.D.; on Diseases of the Nervous System, by William G. Spiller, M.D., and on Obstetrics, by Richard C. Norris, M.D. The volume, as usual, is very much more than a mere year book of medical literature. Those in charge of its various departments are qualified to write *ex cathedra* on the subjects committed to them. Instead of taking all the current articles as they appear, and making abstracts of them, the editors confine their attention to the most important contributions which have appeared during the year, and discuss them in such a way as to present what is really valuable in them to the reader in an available form. There is no medical publication which has more thoroughly earned the respect and confidence of the medical profession, and which more thoroughly deserves its support than this periodical, which has so long maintained its pre-eminence among all the innumerable year books, epitomes, and annuals, which have recently endeavored to compete with it.

These four volumes practically constitute a text-book of medicine and surgery, appearing revised up to date each year. They are not only invaluable for reference to those who wish to write, but they furnish the practising physician with information on all subjects upon which he may desire a guide. J. H. G.

DISEASE OF THE PANCREAS: ITS CAUSE AND NATURE. By EUGENE L. OPIE, M.D., Associate in Pathology, Johns Hopkins University; Fellow of the Rockefeller Institute of Medical Research. Philadelphia and London: J. B. Lippincott Co., 1903.

THE author has devoted this book almost entirely to the study of the conditions peculiar to the pancreas, and has omitted the forms of disease common to many other organs. Thus he avoids descriptions of acute suppurative lesions, tuberculosis, malignant growths, etc., but carefully considers hemorrhagic and gangrenous pancreatitis, hyaline degeneration with and without involvement of the islands of Langerhans, fat-necrosis, the relation of pathological change in the pancreas to diabetes, hæmochromatosis, diabète bronzé. The author goes at length into the anatomy, both gross and histological, and discusses the various anomalies of the pancreas, showing the relation that the anatomy and even the anomalies may have to disease, especially to the acute forms of pancreatitis.

Acute pancreatitis is divided into two forms, acute hemorrhagic and gangrenous, but the author very clearly points out that these forms are merely different degrees of the same process, with the same etiological factor at work. Of special interest is the ingenious theory in regard to the production of acute pancreatitis by the injection of bile into the greater pancreatic duct.

The mechanism of this process is explained and illustrated by a diagram. The author considers acute pancreatitis as secondary to biliary stone. The gallstone is passed through the common duct, arrives at the duodenal opening, and is there arrested temporarily or permanently. In those cases where the stone is of such size that it blocks the duodenal opening without blocking either the common biliary duct or the pancreatic duct, it is possible for bile to flow or even be forced directly into the pancreatic duct with resulting hemorrhagic or gangrenous pancreatitis. So many correlating conditions must be fulfilled to produce this result that the theory amply accounts for the rarity of the disease.

Of the chronic forms of inflammation of the pancreas, two are recognized, namely, the interlobular and interacinar, while the author gives a separate chapter to a chronic hyaline degenerative process confined to the islands of Langerhans, resulting in the production of an unknown substance, and associated with diabetes in a very large percentage of cases. The weight of argument backed by post-mortem findings tends to prove that whatever impairs the health of the islands of Langerhans produces diabetes mellitus; that the interlobular form is to a less extent a factor, as there is in this type of inflammation small tendency until late in the disease to involve the interacinar islands. The interacinar form ranks next as a causative power, while hyaline degeneration primarily attacking the islands has the highest percentage of associated diabetes. The author recognizes that in more than half of all cases of diabetes the cause lies in a destructive lesion of the pancreas.

The volume shows evidence of much work carefully done, and the author's conclusions are arrived at by solid reasoning from experiments and symptoms.

J. N. H.

A NURSES' HANDBOOK OF OBSTETRICS, FOR USE IN TRAINING SCHOOLS. By JOSEPH BROWN COOKE, M.D. Philadelphia: J. B. Lippincott Co., 1903.

THIS is without question one of the most satisfactory books for nurses yet published. As the author remarks in his preface, there is no dearth of small volumes upon this subject, but most of the writers have attempted to speak in such a way that they might appeal to the patient herself even more than to the nurse. On the other hand, the present volume keeps its intent, as expressed in its title, consistently in remembrance, and addresses a trained audience exclusively. It is most clear, yet concise, and though at first sight there may be a feeling that the author has gone a little too deeply into the subject, we feel sure that consideration will compel agreement with his belief, that the more intelligent the nurse is theoretically, the greater aid she will be to the physician and the safer guardian to the patient.

An underlying aim, and one with which we have the most hearty agreement, is noticeable throughout the book, namely, to prepare the nurse to cope with the complications which may arise in the absence of the physician. Let it not be understood that any encouragement is offered to influence the nurse to assume undue responsibility, since in no instance is this true, the intent merely being to furnish intelligent "first aid" while awaiting the doctor's arrival. The book is well illustrated, and this fact, together with the appended glossary, enhances its value.

One of the noteworthy features is the chapter upon the preparation of the patient for labor, together with its armamentarium as well as the directions for the preparations of instruments, dressings, etc., for major obstetrical operations.

Throughout the book the necessity for asepsis is emphasized, though the value of the rubber glove is not dwelt upon.

We can most heartily recommend the book to the attention of all superintendents of training schools. W. R. N.

The Practical Medicine Series of Year Books. Edited by Gustavus P. Head, M.D., Professor of Laryngology and Rhinology, Chicago Post-Graduate Medical School. Vol. VIII., pp. 326. Chicago: The Year Book Publishers, 1903.

This volume has for its subjects Materia Medica and Therapeutics, Preventive Medicine, Climatology, Suggestive Therapeutics, and Forensic Medicine; and for authors George F. Butler, Henry B. Favill, Norman Bridge, Daniel R. Brower, and Harold N. Moyer. Over other Year Books this series presents the advantage of small size and more frequent appearance, containing about the same material, the value of all consisting in careful selection, accurate perspective, and judicial comments. For convenience of reference it would be well if the year could be gathered into one volume with an accurate and complete index; for reading perhaps the present is more advantageous. The collaborators have attacked their task with commendable thoroughness, and, while the careful reader will find but little with which he is familiar, perhaps repetition will fix it more indelibly upon his memory. The sub-editor's judgment may not always accord with that of the reviewer as to the importance of work, and he might even suggest that it be brought down to a later date. However, the results are good, and as a review it may take its place with others and find its sphere of usefulness. As we recall some of the earlier volumes, the presswork and paper have improved to the point where, like the contents, they are satisfactory. R. W. W.

A MANUAL OF OBSTETRICS. By A. F. A. KING, A.M., M.D., Professor of Obstetrics and Diseases of Women and Children in the Medical Department of the Columbian University, Washington, D.C., and in the University of Vermont. Ninth Edition. New York and Philadelphia: Lea Brothers & Co., 1903.

A REVIEW of this well-known work seems hardly to be required. Few, if any, students are unacquainted with the work, and its popularity is evidenced by the appearance of this, the ninth edition since 1882. Its size has been gradually enlarged until at present it comprises a volume of over six hundred pages, an increase of two hundred pages since the fourth edition was published. The advance in medical science during the past twenty years has compelled the introduction of considerable new material as well as the practical rewriting of the chapter on Puerperal Septicæmia. We can, from our own personal experience as a student, most heartily recommend the work.

W. R. N.

INTERNATIONAL CLINICS. Edited by A. O. J. KELLY, A.M., M.D., of Philadelphia, Pa., U.S.A., with the collaboration of Collaborators and Correspondents. Vol. II., pp. 311. Thirteenth Series. Philadelphia: J. B. Lippincott Co., 1903.

THE present volume opens with an excellent symposium on the Summer Diarrhœas of Children, in which the subject is presented from the viewpoints of bacteriology, pathology, symptomatology, and therapeutics. It is well balanced, temperate in statement, instructive, and comprehensive, well worthy of the names it bears: Conn, Hand (Jr.), Cotton, Westcott, Nicoll (Jr.), and Marfan. Disease of the Pancreas, of which the medical aspect is taken up by Opie and the surgical by Deaver and Muller, is creditable to the authors. Here we find well-known opinions reiterated, but in condensed form, and yet from both sides the facts as presented are easily grasped and the importance of a comparatively new subject demands its acquisition. Treatment is introduced by Levi on Trunecek's Serum in Arteriosclerosis. Although his claims are perhaps too much tinged with enthusiasm, yet the insidious character of the condition, its widespread and unfortunate results when fully developed, and its baneful effects as a complication urge the fullest investigation of any method which may promise anything of arrest or mitigation. Gaston's short "Practical Notes on the Prophylactic and Curative Treatment of Influenza, Malaria, Erysipelas, and Ozena" are correctly entitled. Bouchard pleads for local, when possible, in contradistinction to general medication, and cites numerous instances in which normal tissues may be spared inundations of active medicaments. His list might be advantageously further extended. Taylor recapitulates the indications for and conduct of the rest treatment. Even if verbose, this is a good presentation of the subject, and for those to whom the master's writings are not familiar its study is to be commended. In the "Etiology, Prevention, and Treatment of a Common Cold" Haig adjusts his theories to a practical end, although certain difficulties in the way of full acceptance suggest themselves. The remainder of Medicine is devoted to the heart, and Bishop, Poynton, and the always instructive Satterthwaite present excellent papers. Surgery covers Hemorrhoids (Gay), Abdominopelvic Diagnosis (Bishop), and Traumatic Epilepsy (Roncali), each adequately presented, although containing nothing of novelty. Hamilton traverses the question of "Cirrhosis of the Liver in Children," insisting upon the rôle of certain infectious diseases as causative agents. With his opinions we are in accord, and would suggest a reading of the remarkable work of Boix in this connection, which demonstrates the influence of other agents, some of which may come into the life-history of the child. In Obstetrics and Gynecology Goffe on "Sterility," Lockyer on "Ectopic Gestation," and Palmer on "Cervical Lacerations" are particularly satisfactory. The single paper on Ophthalmology is by Landolt on "Surgical Intervention in Paralysis of the Ocular Muscles."

We have noted the articles in this volume *in extenso* because all possess so great merit that omission would be unjust to author and editor. The standard, high as it was, set by the new editor is fully maintained, and we trust that others will find the same pleasure and profit in its reading which we have experienced and gained.

R. W. W.

The Medical Epitome Series. Medical Jurisprudence: a Manual for Students and Practitioners. By Edwin Waller Dwight, M.D., Instructor in Legal Medicine, Harvard University. Series edited by V. C. Pedersen, A.M., M.D. Philadelphia and New York: Lea Brothers & Co.

The difficulties of preparing a brief manual which rises above the level of a quiz compend, yet answers the same purpose, and in which the essential facts concerning the subject are stated shortly and intelligently, are manifest; but notwithstanding these difficulties the present number of the Epitome Series fulfils the required conditions and fully realizes the editor's hopes. The text is continuous, but so paragraphed that any division of a subject may be readily referred to; while at the end of each chapter is placed a series of questions, thus rendering the book suitable for quizzing. The volume opens with a short chapter on the general principles of medical jurisprudence, after which follow chapters on special divisions of the subject. Whenever it has been possible, tables have been inserted. Although many tables and much space have been devoted to the distinguishing features between human and animal blood, no mention is made of the newer methods for diagnosing human blood by the action of the anti-bodies. W. T. L.

THE MEDICAL EPITOME SERIES. MICROSCOPY AND BACTERIOLOGY: A MANUAL FOR STUDENTS AND PRACTITIONERS. By P. E. ARCHINARD, A.M., M.D., Demonstrator of Microscopy and Bacteriology, Tulane University of Louisiana, Medical Department. Series Edited by V. C. PEDERSEN, A.M., M.D. Philadelphia and New York: Lea Brothers & Co.

IN a book of this size and scope it is scarcely possible and indeed hardly desirable to do more than state the essential facts and accepted doctrines concerning the subject. The present work, therefore, represents in a way an abstract of the larger and standard text-books upon bacteriology and furnishes the outlines for a more extended and precise study of the subject. The first part of the book is devoted to a short review of the fundamental principles of bacteriology and to a description of the more common technical procedures, under which are included the preparation of media, sterilization, and a few staining methods; the later portions, on the other hand, deal with the morphological and physiological characteristics of most of the important pathogenic bacteria. The B. dysenteriæ receives due recognition. At the end of each chapter is appended a series of questions, which adapts the book for quizzing. There are 74 illustrations, among which are a few borrowed from Abbott's excellent plates. W. T. L.

A MANUAL OF BACTERIOLOGY. FOR STUDENTS AND PHYSICIANS. By FRED. C. ZAPFE, M.D., Professor of Histology in the College of Physicians and Surgeons, and Professor of Pathology, Bacteriology, and Hygiene in the Illinois Medical College, Chicago. Lea's Series of Pocket Text-books, edited by BERN. B. GALLAUDET, M.D.

THE selective faculty necessary in the preparation of as condensed a manual as the members of this series necessarily must be has been on the whole judiciously exercised in the present instance. Methods of sterilization and its surgical importance, the preparation of culture media, staining and culture methods, and the technique of animal inoculation and post-mortem examination are treated with sufficient detail; and the description of bacteria, particularly those which are clinically most important, leaves nothing to be desired, while the plates and engravings are excellent and well chosen. Theoretical questions, on the other hand, are put off in a most cursory fashion, the section devoted to such a subject as immunity, for example, being little more than an expanded glossary of technical terms, or at best a suggestive list of subjects for the student's guidance. In the discussion of antitoxins and other bacteriological products employed for therapeutic purposes the author strikes a conservative note; diphtheria is still, in spite of much good experimental work that has been done in this line, the only disease in which positive results can be expected from the use of antitoxin.

The text contains certain discrepancies that cannot fail to perplex the student and seem to call for some explanation. Thus on page 274 we read that "thus far it has been impossible to produce typhoid fever experimentally in animals," and later, on page 282, under immunization, that "it is possible to immunize animals against typhoid." Again, the assertion on page 256 that "cholera is pathogenic for men only" does not harmonize with the statement that "the serum of the blood of animals that have recovered from cholera contains a substance which has decided bactericidal properties." We assume that in each case the identical disease is meant, and if so, the statements either require revision or they are to be taken in a relative sense only. Perhaps the looseness of statement may be partly accounted for by a similar laxity in the use of words revealed, for example, in the case of "tubercular" and "tuberculous," which occur synonymously—sometimes in the same sentence —yet the distinction between the two is clear and, one would think, ought to appeal with special force to a pathologist. "Postmortemed" may be convenient, but is scarcely musical, and is certainly an avoidable barbarism that ought to be relegated to the laboratory, where it was presumably evolved. R. M. G.

Ambulance Work and Nursing. A Handbook on First Aid to the Injured, with a Section on Nursing, etc. Chicago: W. T. Keener & Co.

No pains have been spared to make this work attractive, as it is handsomely bound in cloth and gilt, and there are many illustrations, for the most part from photographs. Particularly good are those showing the different methods of bandaging. It is written for lay readers, and for such should prove of interest and value, though for the professional man there is little to be gleaned from its pages. The book consists of some chapters on anatomy for beginners, sections on first aid in all emergency cases, bandaging and rules for transporting patients, including the litter drill as used in England. The work is evidently intended for English readers, in fact, and the section on nursing is in many respects not applicable to conditions existing in America. G. M. C.

ADENO-MYOME DES UTERUS: AUS DEM PATHOLOGISCH-ANATOM. ARBEITEN. Herrn. Geh. med. Rath DR. JOHANNES ORT zu Feier seines 25 jährigen Professoren-jubiläums gewidmet von den Göttinger Assistenten, Schillern und Freunden. Von THOMAS S. CULLEN, M.D., Hülfsprofessor der Gynäkologie au der Johns Hopkins Universität.

IN a carefully worked out and excellently illustrated monograph Cullen discusses the pathological histology, etiology, and symptomatology of adenomyoma of the uterus. The work is based on an exhaustive and accurate study of 19 cases of this affection which occurred at the Johns Hopkins Hospital among 700 instances of myomata of the uterus.

The class of tumors under discussion is divided into three groups:

I. Adenomyomata with preservation approximately of the normal shape of the uterus.

II. Subperitoneal or interligamentary adenomyomata.

III. Submucous adenomyomata.

The tumors in general consist of a growth of smooth muscle fibres arranged in bundles, between which are scattered glands and ducts embedded in a stroma exactly like that of the normal uterine mucosa. The glands are also identical with the glands of the mucous membrane lining the uterine canal. In the first class of cases, where the growth extends diffusely through the uterine wall, the muscle bundles of the tumor fuse imperceptibly with the muscle bundles of the wall of the uterus, and a direct connection is often to be made out between the glands embedded in the growth and the glands of the uterine mucosa. Frequently several glands or a single gland can be traced as it makes its way down from the mucous membrane between the muscle bundles into the adenomyomatous growth; and in such cases a small amount of the normal stroma of the mucosa surrounds the gland and isolates it from the muscular tissue.

Occasionally small cystic spaces are seen which are lined by what appears as a mucous membrane indistinguishable from the normal uterine mucosa, while in the subperitoneal tumors very large cysts may occur, the cavities of which are filled, as a rule, with bloody or chocolate-colored fluid. The origin of the bloody fluid is explainable on the supposition that the mucous membrane lining the cysts undergoes much the same alterations during menstruation as the mucous membrane lining the uterine cavity, and at these periods blood escapes into the cyst. The tumors may be found in the wall of the cervix as well as in the wall of the uterus.

The origin of the glandular portion of the growth can be directly traced to the mucous membrane of the uterus, and whether the tumors are submucous, subperitoneal, or ligamentary in position, the glandular portion arises from some part of the Müllerian duct. The older theory, advanced by von Recklinghausen, that the remains of the Wolffian body furnish tissue from which the glands may spring, is no longer tenable, and the author's view is upheld both from a study of his own cases and of those reported recently by others. The etiological factor concerned in the production of the tumors is uncertain, but it would at least seem that the myomatous portion of the growth develops first, just as adenocarcinomata may arise from normal uterine mucosa, so they may take their origin from the glandular islands or cysts of the adenomyomata; but the tumors themselves are essentially benign, as can be demonstrated both from a histological standpoint and from clinical observations. The symptomatology is dependent in large part upon the size and position of the tumors. Menorrhagia and pain in the back are frequently noted. Other symptoms may arise from pressure produced by the tumors. The condition was found oftenest in women between the thirtieth and sixtieth years of life. The prognosis is good even after partial myomectomy. W. T. L.

"Golden Rules" Series. For Diseases of Children. By George Carpenter, M.D. Of Hygiene. By F. J. Waldo, M.D. Of Aural and Nasal Practice. By P. R. W. de Santi, F.R.C.S. Of Refraction. By Ernest E. Maddox, M.D. Bristol: John Wright & Co.

This series of little books, none of them exceeding a hundred pages in length, is an attempt to present in the most concise form some of the more important principles of the different branches of medicine and surgery whereof they treat. Their authors are all men of experience and standing in the profession, and they have succeeded in condensing in these little volumes what may be described (as the title of the series would indicate) as the absolutely essential rules of practice in the different specialties. It may be truthfully said of them that while much is left out that might with value have been put in, there is nothing inserted which should have been left out. They are, therefore, of much more value to the student than is the general run of such vest-pocket companions. F. R. P.

PROGRESS

OF

MEDICAL SCIENCE.

MEDICINE.

UNDER THE CHARGE OF

WILLIAM OSLER, M.D.,

PROFESSOR OF MEDICINE IN THE JOHNS HOPKINS UNIVERSITY, BALTIMORE, MARYLAND,

AND

W. S. THAYER, M.D.,

ASSOCIATE PROFESSOR OF MEDICINE IN JOHNS HOPKINS UNIVERSITY, BALTIMORE, MARYLAND.

On the Production of Specific Cytolytic Sera for Thyroid and Parathyroid, with Observations on the Physiology and Pathology of the Parathyroid Gland, especially in its Relation to Exophthalmic Goitre.—In 1902 GONTSCHARUKOV claimed that he had been able to produce a specific antithyroid toxin by the injection, at intervals of four weeks, of an emulsion of dog's thyroids into the subcutaneous tissue of a sheep. By the injection of the blood serum of this sheep, which died during the experiment, into the circulation of other dogs certain tetanic symptoms resulted which he thought indicated the existence of a specific antithyroid toxin.

W. G. MACCALLUM (*Medical News*, October 31, 1903, p. 820) conducted a series of experiments to control these results. He points out first that the destruction of the thyroid alone produces disturbances of metabolism, which appear slowly and are characterized by the symptoms known as myxœdema. Destruction of the parathyroid alone, on the other hand, produces the acute rapidly fatal nervous phenomena which have so long been thought to be due to the extirpation of the thyroid. These phenomena are tetany and polypnœa. Until recent years the early fatal results following thyroidectomy had been attributed to the extirpation of the thyroid, while in reality they were due to removal of the parathyroid glands, which are small and inconspicuous and usually embedded in the tissue of the thyroid.

In his investigation MacCallum made repeated injections of an emulsion of dog's parathyroids into the peritoneal cavities of geese. At intervals the centrifugalized serum from the defibrinated blood of these geese was injected into the peritoneal cavity of dogs. The symptoms produced in these dogs were not at all striking. Emaciation and a cachexia developed in a number of them. These symptoms, however, occurred also in dogs injected with normal geese serum. In one case convulsive twitching of the muscles resulted without dyspnœa. After the injections a large number of the dogs were killed at varying intervals and their thyroids examined histologically. In none of the cases could a microscopic change be made out. The writer therefore concludes that the attempt to produce a cytotoxin capable of destroying the cells of the thyroid glands *in situ* has not been successful. He believes, however, that a material was probably produced in the blood of the geese capable of combining with the normal secretion of the dog's thyroid or parathyroid and neutralizing it, thus allowing the symptoms which ordinarily follow extirpation of these glands to occasionally appear in a mild degree. MacCallum thinks that his experiments throw considerable doubt on Gontscharukov's results, at least on the interpretation of them, for one would not expect tetanic contractions as an effect of the destruction of the thyroid by a specific serum.

The writer was led by the above work to carry on some investigations with the view of determining the rôle of the parathyroid glands under normal conditions and in disease. Dogs were used in the experiments. The parathyroids were removed in a number of animals. The symptoms of the parathyroidectomized animals were briefly as follows: After symptoms of unrest, with slight twitchings of the muscles, the animal rapidly develops violent tetanic spasms. It experiences difficulty in walking and periodically falls to the floor in an epileptiform convulsion. There is marked trismus, and the eyes appear to project owing to retraction of the upper lid. The respirations are greatly increased, even up to 200 to 250 per minute, but there is no cyanosis. There was no specially increased heart action. The animal may die at the height of the attack, or the convulsions may gradually become less violent, death resulting from exhaustion.

Three problems present themselves: (1) Are these symptoms due to absence of some necessary secretion of the parathyroid? (2) Are they due to some poison produced somewhere in the body and circulating in the blood, but which, in the normal animal, would be neutralized by the parathyroid cells themselves or by their secretions? (3) Is this poison absorbed from the intestine; is it the result of metabolism of certain groups of cells, or is it the product of muscle or nerve metabolism? As a result of some ingenious experiments the writer concludes that while it seems improbable that the parathyroids secrete a necessary material which is circulated in the blood, the lack of which produces the disturbances described, it does seem probable that they produce a material which neutralizes poisons produced elsewhere, poisons which if not so neutralized may be mechanically washed out with the relief of the symptoms.

The parathyroids were shown to have no influence on nitrogen metabolism, whereas it was demonstrated that the nitrogen output was markedly affected by removal of the thyroids.

There is no very convincing evidence advanced by the writer to show that the parathyroids are in any very close way associated with the etiology of exophthalmic goitre. Parathyroidectomy is followed by muscle spasms, and muscle tremor is a symptom of exophthalmic goitre. Occasionally there is slight prominence of the eyes following the operation. Further than this there is no particular resemblance. It is worthy of note, however, that an examination of the parathyroids embedded in the excised thyroid glands of exophthalmic goitre patients all showed atrophy, and in two instances the glands showed very distinct degenerative changes in the parenchyma cells with overgrowth of connective tissue.

The Thick-film Process for the Detection of Organisms in the Blood.—RONALD ROSS (*Thompson Yates and Johnston Laboratories Report*, 1903, vol. v., part I., p. 117) uses a very large drop of blood in this method, and does not attempt to spread the blood out in a thin layer on the cover-glass. No attempt at fixing the hæmoglobin is made. The thick film of blood on the slide is merely dried, and then very gently washed with water until all color has disappeared. For staining purposes only aqueous solutions of the stains are used. Ross now uses the following stock formulæ for staining: (1) Eosin, 1 gram; water, 1000 c.c. (2) Medicinal methylene blue, 10 grams; sodium carbonate, 5 grams; water, 1000 c.c. After washing out the hæmoglobin as described above, a drop or two of the eosine solution is now placed upon the cover-glass without previous drying, and allowed to remain for one minute. Then a drop or two of the methylene blue solution is run on and allowed to remain for fifteen to thirty seconds. Finally the cover-

Ross uses this method for detecting the presence of malarial organisms where they are very few, and also for trypanosoma. In one case of malaria where only one parasite could be found in a field by the old method, by the new one as many as eighty could be found. The malarial parasites stain blue and the nuclear chromatin a distinct red. The red cells are unstained, owing to their hæmoglobin being washed out. Bell and Laing advocate the use of this method for the detection of plague bacilli in the blood.

The Tendo-Achilles Jerk and Other Reflexes in Diabetes Mellitus—WILLIAMSON (*Review of Neurology and Psychology*, October, 1903, p. 667) states that in diabetic mellitus, as in locomotor ataxia, the tendo-Achilles jerks may disappear before the knee-jerks are lost. His results in the examination of these reflexes in 50 diabetics was as follows: (1) In 19 both Achilles-jerks were absent. In these cases both knee-jerks were present in 8; one present and one absent in 3; both absent in 8. (2) In 2 cases one Achilles-jerk was absent and one present. In these cases both knee-jerks were present. (3) In 29 cases both Achilles-jerks were present. In this series both knee-jerks were present in 28, and one knee-jerk present and one absent in one.

The writer points out that the knee-jerks are much more likely to be absent in hospital than in private cases, in which the conditions of life are better. Thus, in the former he found both knee-jerks absent in 49 per cent. of the cases, while in the latter both were absent in only 12 per cent. He finds that the wrist-jerks are usually absent where the knee-jerks are absent. The causes for the disappearance of the deep reflexes are not discussed. The superficial reflexes—plantar, abdominal and epigastric—are present in practically all cases. It is stated that in the severest cases the abdominal and epigastric reflexes are usually much increased. The plantar reflex is of the normal type.

SURGERY.

UNDER THE CHARGE OF
J. WILLIAM WHITE, M.D.,
JOHN RHEA BARTON PROFESSOR OF SURGERY IN THE UNIVERSITY OF PENNSYLVANIA; SURGEON TO THE UNIVERSITY HOSPITAL,
AND
F. D. PATTERSON, M.D.,
SURGEON TO THE X-RAY DEPARTMENT OF THE HOWARD HOSPITAL; CLINICAL ASSISTANT TO THE OUT-PATIENT SURGICAL DEPARTMENT OF THE JEFFERSON HOSPITAL.

The Diagnosis of Bone and Joint Tuberculosis.—Ludloff (*Centralblatt für Chirurgie*, September 5, 1903) states that in the treatment of bone and joint tuberculosis, the choice between resection and iodoform injections remains still but a matter of personal desire. The *x*-ray picture plays a large rôle, especially in cases of beginning tuberculosis, where one should try to recognize the trouble early enough to prevent its extension into the neighboring structures. The author reports in detail three cases in which an early diagnosis was made by means of the *x*-rays. Every case when seen early should be studied first in regard to its etiology, and the first question to be determined is, Was the synovial membrane infected secondarily from a lesion in the bone, or *vice versa;* or were both infected at the same time from the same place? It is to be remembered that the epiphysis is the point of entrance for the numerous nutrient bloodvessels into the bone, and that this point lies just on top of the synovial membrane. For a solution of these questions more accurate examination of the epiphysis and synovial membranes are necessary. It is still to be determined whether iodoform injections are of the same value on the bone as they are on the membrane near an enlargement of the bony parts of a diseased joint by reason of multiple deposits. If resection is not done, the only other method of any value whatever consists in iodoform injection.

A New Operation for the Relief of Wryneck.—Ullstein (*Centralblatt für Chirurgie*, August 15, 1903) sums up his remarks by placing the greatest importance on the following questions, which he asks and answers as follows:

1. How much of the muscle should be shortened? Of course, this varies with each particular case, and must be graduated according to the previous differences in length, and, as a rule, it will vary from 4 cm. to 8 cm.

2. In which part of the muscle should shortening be made? The shortening should be made in the upper portion above the entrance of the nerve supply. As to the best method, simple resection of the muscle is not satisfactory, for the reason that if this be done the muscle lacks the ability to contract, and for that reason it is essential to do resection, which not only does not interfere with the continuity of the fibres, but also does not interfere with the nerve supply. A bandage should be retained in place for about twenty days after the operation, at the end of which time it may be safely removed, and, as a general rule, the results are satisfactory.

New Method of Treatment for Backward Dislocation of the Hip.—Elgart (*Centralblatt für Chirurgie*, August 22, 1903) states that the method consists in anæsthetizing the patient, who is then placed upon the floor, and then the operator should get down on one knee and place the dislocated limb over his thigh, and then, while an assistant securely holds the patient's pelvis, the operator should grasp the ankle with one hand and make traction, while with the other hand clasped on the thigh, the femur should be rotated inward and the leg pressed outward. In a bad case of backward dislocation this was followed on the first trial by perfect reposition. The method differs from Kocher in that, by placing the dislocated limb over the operator's thigh, much more pressure can be brought to bear, and, as a result, the rednotion becomes easier.

The Lotheissen Method of Radical Cure for Femoral Hernia.—Gilli (*Centralblatt für Chirurgie*, August 8, 1903), after giving in detail the method employed, states that his experience has shown that the separation of the falciform process and of Poupart's ligament in these cases of irreducible hernia distinctly simplifies the condition of the hernial sac, as well as shortens the time of operation. The technique consists in making an incision parallel to Poupart's ligament, then exposing the sac of the hernia, which should be separated from its attachments at the edge of the ring. Then the aponeurosis of the external oblique should be separated and a Kocher sound should be passed between the sac and the falciform process until its tip appears at the abdominal side of the inner crural ring. The inguinal ligament and the falciform process can then be separated on the sound. After this separation the sac of the hernia may be easily isolated. The advantages of the method are: 1. That the separation is accomplished under the eyes of the operator, and there is no necessity for blind, uncertain work with a hernia knife, and any bleeding which may occur can be easily controlled. 2. In case of bad strangulation, the contents of the hernia are exposed to full view and can be thoronghly inspected before being replaced within the abdominal cavity. Experience has shown in cases where general anæsthetics are contraindicated that this method may be used with great satisfaction under local anæsthesia.

THERAPEUTICS.

UNDER THE CHARGE OF

REYNOLD WEBB WILCOX, M.D., LL.D.,

PROFESSOR OF MEDICINE AND THERAPEUTICS AT THE NEW YORK POST-GRADUATE MEDICAL SCHOOL AND HOSPITAL; VISITING PHYSICIAN TO ST. MARK'S HOSPITAL,

AND

SMITH ELY JELLIFFE, M.D., Ph.D.,

PROFESSOR OF PHARMACOGNOSY AT THE COLLEGE OF PHARMACY; INSTRUCTOR IN MATERIA MEDICA AND THERAPEUTICS (COLUMBIA UNIVERSITY), NEW YORK.

Physostigmine in the Treatment of Intestinal Atony.—Guglielmo Curlo concludes from his laboratory and clinical experiments that this substance (1) manifests an excitant action upon the intestinal muscles which results in spasm with increased peristalsis, (2) it is especially indicated in all forms of coprostasis due to intestinal atony, being contraindicated in spastic conditions, acute and chronic intestinal catarrh, and mucomembranous enterocolitis. (3) On account of its spastic action in increasing the tone of the intestinal muscles it is an excellent remedy for meteorism. (4) The maximum daily dose which can be given without symptoms of intolerance is from $\frac{1}{16}$ to $\frac{1}{13}$ grain, but the usual dose is one-half of this quantity. (5) Myosis and salivation mark the point of tolerance of the remedy. (6) The preferable salt is the salicylate, and it is best administered as a pill.—*La Riforma Medica*, 1903, No. 37, p. 1009.

Action of Hæmolytic Sera.—DR. ROBERT MUIR discusses this question from several points of view, detailing a number of experiments and methods of experimentation from which he derives the following conclusions: (1) Immune body and the complement differ markedly from each other in their mode of combination and in the firmness of their union. (2) Immune body can be in part separated before hæmolysis from red corpuscles containing multiple doses. (3) When red corpuscles containing multiple doses of immune-body are hæmolyzed by the minimum dose of complement the surplus molecules of immune-body remain attached to the receptors of the red corpuscles and can be in part separated. (4) Complement either after its union directly with cells or indirectly through the medium of an immune-body cannot be separated again. (5) Each dose of immune-body taken up by red corpuscles, in addition to the hæmolytic dose, leads to the taking up of an additional amount and corresponding amount of complement necessary for hæmolysis may be used up. (6) When red corpuscles containing multiple doses of immune-body are fully saturated with complement, immune-body can still be separated. The immune-body thus obtained comes off alone and not in the combination I. B. + C.—*Lancet*, 1903, No. 4172, p. 451.

Nauheim Treatment in Chronic Affections of the Heart.—DR. LESLIE THORNE, basing his conclusions on an experience with the Nauheim methods during the past seven years in London, divides his cases of heart disease into four groups: (1) those who will be cured; (or) benefited very greatly by the treatment; (2) those which cannot be cured, but can be greatly benefited; (3) the doubtful cases, and (4) unsuitable cases. Of the cases which will be cured or benefited very greatly by the treatment, the dilated, enfeebled, and irritable heart, a sequela of influenza, is one of the most promising, and it is also one that, in many instances, resists treatment by drugs, rest, or change of air, so that the unfortunate sufferer often becomes a chronic invalid with nothing but a broken and almost useless life to look forward to. He believes it no exaggeration to say that the Nauheim treatment often gives a new lease of life to these cases, though if they are of a severe type they may require two, or even three courses, at intervals of nine months to a year to restore them to health. Another class of cases which belong to the first group is that of the dilated and enfeebled heart produced by the raised arterial tension present in the circulation of patients suffering from rheumatic or gouty diatheses. This slowly but continuously acting pressure produces in time an overloaded and overworked heart, and thereby an increasingly impure blood supply and a progressive weakening of the cardiac systole. It is almost impossible to cure these cases absolutely and permanently; the very fact that the poison is manufactured in the system and can be eliminated only by a careful diet and well-regulated life often leads to a recurrence of the heart symptoms in time and makes it almost a necessity that the patient should undergo a course of treatment regularly every twelve months for two or three years, and then perhaps every second or third year. He says there is no greater mistake than to lead these people to believe that one course will cure them completely, though young patients suffering from mild forms of rheumatic and gouty hearts, without valvular disease, will often remain in good health for several years after a single course, especially if a careful dietary and habit of life are followed. Cases of cardiac enfeeblement from excessive smoking and prolonged illness, such as typhoid fever and malaria, belong also to this group, the Nauheim treatment being in these cases a most valuable aid to such methods of cure as rest, tonics and change of air, and producing a much more rapid return to health than could otherwise be expected. (2) In this group he ranks those cases of both rheumatic and gouty origin in which the valves have been permanently injured, and signs of commencing cardiac failure, such as headache, shortness of breath, palpitation, cyanosis, and pain, are present. It is self-evident that patients of this class cannot be cured and that one course of baths will not produce a permanent improvement, but it will undoubtedly produce a much more lasting and satisfactory one than any other treatment. (3) Authorities differ greatly as to the nature of the cases that should be included in this group. The author's experience of the treatment has led him to believe that unsuitable patients are those who are, and have been, habitually heavy drinkers, those whom one believes to be suffering from syphilitic affection of the heart, those suffering from marked degeneration of the vessel walls, those exhibiting typical symptoms of aortic regurgitation, and very old people. The chronic heart case usually met with in hospitals, broken down by a long struggle to work when unfit and accustomed to bad and even insufficient food, is also one of the most unsatisfactory for the Nauheim treatment.—*Lancet*, 1903, No. 4168, p. 153.

Sublamine in the Treatment of Parasitic Scalp Diseases.—DR. WILLIAM S. GOTTHEIL, in reporting an extensive experience in ringworm in a large institution, finds that this remedy was more rapid than the bichloride because of its greater penetration and because it can be employed in stronger solutions, being less irritant. The solutions employed were 1:750 or 1:1000.—*The Medical News*, 1903, vol. liii. p. 735.

Sciatica; its Nature and Treatment.—DR. WM. BRUCE contributes some revolutionary ideas to the etiology and pathology of sciatica, based on deductions of some 418 cases which have been under his observation during the past thirteen years. He believes that, after all, sciatica is a disease of the hip-joint and not a neuritis of the sciatic nerve, and that it is connected with the gouty or rheumatic diseases, and may be called a monoarticular rheumatic arthritis of the hip. The reasons for his deductions he presents, and his conclusions lead him to a modification in the treatment. Rest of the joint is one of the most important features. Blisters may be of some service, and sedative lotions and fomentations are sometimes valuable. Massage and electricity are contraindicated. Antigout and antirheumatic remedies are recommended. Turpentine has proven of benefit when taken internally.—*Lancet,* 1903, No. 4173 p. 511.

The Treatment of Puerperal Sepsis.—DR. HIRAM N. VINEBERG employs the ointment of colloidal silver (unguentum Credé) in cases when he can find no lesion which demands surgical intervention, believing that it is of some service either in aiding the system to eliminate the toxins produced or in some way counteracting their deleterious influence. It is certain that several desperate cases, in which this silver was employed by inunction, ended in recovery.—*Journal of Obstetrics,* 1903, No. 9, p. 325.

DR. H. FEHLING believes that this substance intravenously employed in sterile 2 per cent. solutions, 2 to 5 drachms for a dose, is of great value.—*Münchener medicinische Wochenschrift,* 1903, No. 33, S. 1409.

Treatment of Chorea by Ergot.—DR. EUSTACE SMITH calls attention to the use of ergot as a sedative in nervous diseases. He says in children particularly it acts as a very valuable sedative, believing this is an action due to its influence on the blood supply, on the nerve tissues in the spinal cord in part, or perhaps a direct sedative. No ill effects have ever been observed by him, although he gives doses of a drachm every hour for three weeks for children seven or eight years of age and doses of 20 drops or more for many months at a stretch. In chorea its action is not as reliable as Fowler's solution, but often arsenic is not well borne by many patients. Ergot acts more quickly than arsenic. He states a number of cases, saying that it is sometimes necessary to push the doses of the remedy, boys seemingly requiring larger doses than girls.—*British Medical Journal,* 1903, No. 2220, p. 133.

Aspirin in Chorea—DR. R. T. WILLIAMSON has recently been prescribing aspirin in thirty-five consecutive instances of chorea. Inasmuch as the mild forms of the disease have a tendency to recover without treatment in from six to ten weeks, his conclusions are given with a certain amount of reserve. In mild cases the aspirin has seemed to be of service, but other drugs have proven equally valuable. In severe cases he believes that the drug in from 10 to 15 grain doses, given three or four times a day, is of value. Aspirin cannot be considered as a specific of chorea, but it is well worth trying, particularly in severe cases. It is best given in powders in water to which a little lemon juice has been added.—*Lancet,* 1903, No. 4173, p. 526.

Antitoxin in Hay Fever.—DR. FELIX SEMON gives his impressions on the efficiency of Dunbar's antitoxin in hay fever, some preliminary results of which he published in 1903. He bases his remarks on the observations of eight hay fever patients whom he has personally treated. These cases have been under his direct supervision and the patients themselves have not had charge of the treatment. Thus far he has not met with any untoward by-effects of any kind in his limited experience, and he thinks it reasonable that patients may be trusted with the self-administration of the drug. In his trials he has used proportions of 1:500 antitoxin with equal quantities of normal horse serum. He has found that a single application will not ward off or cure the disease for any prolonged period and he says that he unfortunately cannot say that the remedy has in any sense acted as a cure in any cases.—*British Medical Journal*, 1903, No. 2220, p. 123.

Ichthyol in Pulmonary Disease.—DR. THOMAS BURNETT has been using ichthyol extensively in pulmonary tuberculosis, in bronchitis, acute and chronic, and in pulmonary fibrosis. In 6 of the cases of tuberculosis he found that at the end of the first month of treatment the cough was less harassing, while in 5 others there was no improvement. At the end of the second month all of the patients, 13, showed distinct improvement with reference to cough, while in 8 expectoration was either less in amount, or both less in amount and easier in expulsion. By the end of the third month 7 of the patients were so far improved that no night-sweating was noted, and at the end of four months night-sweating was entirely absent in every case, while only a slight cough remained. Toward the end of the fifth month all of his cases showed a continued improvement, and at the end of the six months every one had gained in weight to the extent of from three to seven pounds, the average gain in weight being a pound a month. These 13 cases referred to were all of pulmonary tuberculosis. Ichthyol also relieved 2 of the patients with chronic bronchitis, and was very valuable in bronchiectasis. With reference to doses, the amount given was from 8 to 20 grains, four times a day, in capsule form, each capsule containing 4 grains of ichthyol. As a rule, the initial dose consisted of two capsules given four times a day, which was gradually increased until five capsules were taken four times daily. After a short time the patients became habituated to these large doses.—*Lancet*, 1903, No. 4171, p. 384.

Intravenous Injections of Iodoform in Advanced Phthisis.—DR. T. W. DEWAR presents a short preliminary report on the treatment of patients with advanced pulmonary tuberculosis by intravenous injections of an ethereal solution of iodoform. Apart from certain difficulties in the mode of injection, he has been able to throw from 5 to 45 minims of an ethereal solution of iodoform into the veins. Each injection should be prepared from fresh solutions. Frequently, following the use of a large dose, 20 to 25 minims, momentary unconsciousness may result. The method is still under experimentation, and the details are promised at a subsequent period.—*British Medical Journal*, 1903, No. 2238, p. 1328.

Radioactive Substances.—DR. WILLIAM ROLLINS says that for the present, when using radioactive substances in internal therapeutics, the substances themselves cannot be employed on account of their high price. Advantage can be taken, however, of radium salts, which, when dissolved in water, give off emanations. These can be collected in air in a gas-holder over mercury and used in internal medicine. When radium is dissolved 75 per cent. of its radioactivity is at once liberated, but 25 per cent. remains, consisting, for the most part, of A particles. When the first rush of liberated active substances is over, radium in solution constantly gives off more emanations, which can be used in therapeutics. In using radioactive substances in disease of or near the skin, the depth of the diseased tissue to be affected must determine the distance at which the radiosubstance is placed upon the surface of the patient. The correct manner for treating a skin disease with these substances is to consider to what depth it is desirable to confine the activity. If to a slight depth, the radium should be almost in contact with the skin; the duration of the application always being shorter than when at a greater distance.—*Boston Medical and Surgical Journal*, 1903, vol. cxlix. p. 542.

Strychnine in Degenerative Diseases of the Nervous System.—DR. G. M. HAMMOND discusses the action of massive doses of strychnine in the treatment of tabes, optic nerve atrophy, progressive muscular atrophy, and pseudomuscular hypertrophy. In tabes he reports four cases in which, under doses of from 1 to 3 grains daily, gradually administered, improvement in gait was readily marked. Of optic nerve atrophy, three cases are reported, in which doses of from $\frac{1}{2}$ to $\frac{3}{4}$ of a grain of strychnine a day arrested the degenerative process. In three cases of progressive muscular atrophy, one improved, one was held stationary, and the third was unmodified. In one case of pseudomuscular hypertrophy, a decided improvement was noted. His practice is to begin treatment with a moderate dose, usually $\frac{1}{40}$ to $\frac{1}{30}$ of a grain, three times a day, and to increase the daily dose by about $\frac{1}{500}$ of a grain. If symptoms of toxæmia develop, the dose is diminished. Doses of $\frac{1}{4}$ to $\frac{3}{8}$ of a grain, three times a day, are well borne by this gradual development in dosage.—*Boston Medical and Surgical Journal*, 1903, vol. cxlix. p. 228.

PEDIATRICS.

UNDER THE CHARGE OF

LOUIS STARR, M.D.,

OF PHILADELPHIA,

AND

THOMPSON S. WESTCOTT, M.D.,

OF PHILADELPHIA.

The Relation of the Thymus Gland to Marasmus—At the recent meeting of the British Medical Association, JOHN RUHRAH (*British Medical Journal*, August 29, 1903, p. 455) reported the conclusions of his study of the post-mortem findings in eighteen cases of marasmus. He states that the most characteristic lesion of marasmus, except the wasting of fat and muscles, is not mentioned in any of the text-books on diseases of children—this is a wasting of the thymus gland. There are two conditions in which there is atrophy in infants—the primary cases, in which the cause is as yet unknown, and those that follow definite pathological conditions, or the secondary cases. The dividing line cannot at this time be definitely drawn. For the present, he thinks, the cases should be divided on a pathological basis into those where there are lesions of definite diseases and those where there are no special and constant lesions, except the wasting of the muscles and the body fat, and, as he now points out, of the thymus gland as well.

After referring to the various theories that have been advanced by Baginsky, Bendix, Heubner and Rubner, Czerny, and French writers, he thinks we may safely assert that the trouble is not due to the amount of food ingested nor to the amount absorbed from the intestinal tract, but that it is due to the malassimilation of the food material in the body.

Whether the thymus gland has anything to do with assimilation or not, he is not prepared to say, but it is certain that the thymus bears a direct relation to the state of the nutrition of the body, as pointed out by Herard, Friedleben, and more recently by Mettenheimer. It increases in size until about the second year, when it remains stationary, growing relatively smaller, when compared with the size of the growing body. At puberty, when the body growth is largely over, it begins to atrophy, and at about twenty-five years of age, when the body has attained its full growth, it is gradually replaced by fatty and connective tissue.

The thymus gland weighs about twelve grams at birth. Histologically, it consists of a connective-tissue framework holding up a parenchyma consisting of a cortex and medulla, which are similar in structure, but the cortex contains normally many more cells than the medulla. The parenchyma consists of a network of endothelial cells resembling the reticular spaces of the lymphatic structures. This space is filled with lymphoid cells and also with a few neutrophilic and eosinophilic leukocytes, and with a few giant cells. Here and there in the structure are little islands of epithelial cells, with a peculiar concentric arrangement—the so-called Hassall bodies. They are the remains of the epithelium which forms the principal part of the thymus gland during embryonal development.

In his eighteen cases the average weight of the gland was twenty-two grams. Excepting the lesions of the terminal infection, the atrophy of the thymus was the only lesion found in any of the necropsies. In these specimens the fibrous capsule of the gland is thicker than normal, and the trabeculæ are also greatly thickened, the increased interlobular tissue frequently cutting the lobules into irregular masses. Sometimes there is more fibrous tissue than lymphoid structure, and in well-marked cases there is more reticular tissue than lymphocytes and leukocytes. In most of the cases there was an increase in size and a hyaline degeneration of the Hassall bodies.

A microscopic examination of the thymus gives a clear indication of the state of nutrition of the infant. In normal infants the structure of the thymus is unaltered; in moderate atrophy the cortex and medulla are not easily distinguished, while in severe atrophies the changes mentioned above are plainly seen. In secondary atrophy the change is one of degree, and the average weight of the gland was 3.41 grams. Administration of thymus gland in tablet form produced no appreciable changes.

In the discussion of this paper the question of "thymus death" was mentioned. Ewart considered that the enlargement of the gland was not the only cause. Some other factor, such as pulmonary congestion or gastrointestinal distention, of a more sudden nature, must be admitted. But the chief factor, in his estimation, was an individual cardiac weakness, which, in the adult, showed itself in the tendency to fainting and to sudden death. CARPENTER did not believe in thymic asthma or sudden death from an enlarged thymus. He believed death in these cases, in many instances, was in reality due to spasm of the larynx, which did not relax. Thymus death was often death from laryngismus stridulus. More attention should be paid to the nasopharynx, and thymic asthma would be a less fashionable explanation.

The Prophylactic Use of Diphtheria Antitoxin in School Children.—AUGUSTUS CAILLE (*Archives of Pediatrics*, October, 1903, p. 748) advocates an immunizing injection of diphtheria antitoxin for young children once or twice during the school year—for instance, in November and February—with the hope of preventing infection from primary diphtheria or croup; and, furthermore, with the hope of lessening the mortality of the severe forms of scarlatina and measles, a large percentage of such cases being complicated by diphtheria from the beginning or in the course of the disease.

It is well known that cases of scarlatina which show a complicating diphtheria from the onset are of a very grave type, showing an overwhelming sepsis, with delirium and circulatory failure. In measles, diphtheria is an early or a late complication, but the most serious form is diphtheritic croup. The mortality from scarlet fever or measles complicated by diphtheria is quite high, and the author's clinical experience suggests that this mortality can be markedly reduced by means of protective inoculations of diphtheria antitoxin.

During the past two years he has practically followed out this line of thought, and has immunized about twenty children twice during the school year. As far as figures can be of value, it can be stated that not one of these children contracted primary or secondary diphtheria, and in no case was there the least unpleasant or unfavorable reaction after the injection. The parents readily accepted the "protecting vaccination for diphtheria." Dr. Caillé has every confidence in the feasibility of this plan for communities in which diphtheria is endemic or epidemic.

Contribution to the Study of Scarlatinal Infection.—SZEKELY (*Jahrbuch für Kinderheilkunde*, 1903, Bd. vii., S. 789) reports a curious case of scarlatinal infection. In a family consisting of father, mother, and two sons, the elder boy, aged eleven years, developed scarlatina. The younger boy, three years old, was at once removed to the house of a friend, and was kept there nine weeks without having any communication, directly or indirectly, with his home. After the complete recovery of the older brother, following a rigorous disinfection of the house and its contents, the child was brought home. Ten days later this boy developed sore throat, fever, and a scarlatinal eruption which presented no peculiarity other than in beginning on the back of the right thigh. The disease pursued a normal course, was very benign, and ended in desquamation.

The interest in the case centred in the avenue of the infection, and a careful inquiry established the following facts: The older boy had presented during his illness some excoriations of the skin, which had been treated with an ointment of oxide of zinc. It was discovered that some days after returning home the younger boy had developed a small eruption of vesicles on the right thigh, which had been smeared with the ointment which had been used for his brother, and which had not been destroyed at the time of the disinfection. Two days later the child had become ill with scarlatina, and, as already noted, the rash had begun upon the right thigh.

The author, therefore, asks if this case should not be considered as one of surgical scarlatina, the vesicles having served as a point of entry for the scarlatinal virus; and since the evolution of the disease was quite mild, he inclines to think that it proved to be, in effect, a sort of vaccination with a scarlatinal virus attenuated by its exposure to the mild antiseptic action of the zinc ointment.

Congenital Torticollis.—MAASS (*Zeitschrift f. Orthop. Chirurgie*, 1903, Bd. xi.) concludes from a study of forty cases of congenital torticollis, nearly all the subjects at the time of observation being under three years of age, that torticollis of intrauterine origin (due probably to lack of amniotic fluid) is rare; that the condition arises most frequently during birth, not as the result of tearing of the muscle, as Stromeyer contends, but from a traumatic necrosis of the muscle which has healed by formation of cicatricial tissue. This lesion, which is found principally in breech or forceps cases (80 per cent. in Maass' statistics), is due less to direct pressure upon the muscle than to its hyperextension.

When the distortion is too great to hope for regression, binder, massage and moist heat, Maass has recourse to Mikulicz's operation (partial resection of the muscle). With older children a post-operative orthopedic treatment should be continued for a long time, in order to correct secondary deformities of the vertebral column.

Polymyositis in Children.—SCHULLER (*Jahrbuch für Kinderheilkunde*, 1903, Bd. viii., S. 193) reports the observation of a child who, in the course of whooping-cough, was seized with fever, chills, headache, and dyspeptic symptoms. These phenomena, which lasted four days, during which the kinks were in abeyance, were replaced by swelling of the eyelids and a painful induration of the muscles of the face and neck. This rigidity, in turn, invaded the muscles of the thorax, back, abdomen, and, finally, those of the limbs. At the end of three weeks these painful contractures began to subside, and two months later the child was completely well.

In studying the features of this case, the author arrives, by exclusion, at a diagnosis of polymyositis, in favor of which he offers the following: The affected muscles were hard, infiltrated, both painful and tender, and were clearly outlined under the skin. The contractures persisted during sleep. Direct stimulation of the muscles by the faradic current produced slow contractions, while rapid contractions were produced by the indirect faradic or the galvanic current.

Five other cases of polymyositis in children have been found in the literature, and are abstracted in the paper.

Paralysis of Accommodation and of the Uvula following Mumps.—MANDONNET (*Annales d'oculistique*, 1903, No. 2) reports a case of this rare sequel of parotitis. The patient was a child aged nine years, who, during convalescence from an attack of mumps, complained of dimness of vision, especially for near objects. Externally the eyes showed no abnormality except a slight dilatation of the pupil which could scarcely be called mydriasis. Both eyes, the right especially, were hypermetropic; vision was $\frac{1}{3}$ in the right eye, $\frac{2}{3}$ in the left, but correction of the hypermetropia of the right eye restored normal vision for distance. Near vision was very poor, the child being incapable of reading even the large characters, but was restored at once by the use of a + 4 D. spherical lens. The integrity of the eye-grounds being shown by the ophthalmoscope, the diagnosis of paralysis of accommodation following mumps was made. Paralysis of the uvula was also present, confirming the diagnosis.

Diphtheria Antitoxin in the Treatment of Aphthous Stomatitis.—Influenced by several suggestive experiences of Sangiovanni, Gaspardi, and Santi, Del Monaco (*Revue Mensuelle des Maladies de l'Enfance*, August, 1903) was induced to use diphtheria antitoxin in the treatment of an infant one year old affected with a grave aphthous stomatitis which had produced a marked cachexia. The injection was promptly followed by a sensible amelioration in the general state, while at the same time the sublingual swelling, which had been unaffected by lotions of permanganate of potash and nitrate of silver, rapidly disappeared.

OBSTETRICS.

UNDER THE CHARGE OF

EDWARD P. DAVIS, A.M., M.D.,

PROFESSOR OF OBSTETRICS IN THE JEFFERSON MEDICAL COLLEGE; PROFESSOR OF OBSTETRICS AND DISEASES OF INFANCY IN THE PHILADELPHIA POLYCLINIC; CLINICAL PROFESSOR OF DISEASES OF CHILDREN IN THE WOMAN'S MEDICAL COLLEGE; VISITING OBSTETRICIAN TO THE PHILADELPHIA HOSPITAL, ETC.

Excessive Distention in the Wall of a Bicornate Uterus.—In the *Zentralblatt für Gynäkologie*, 1903, No. 45, Jurinka reports the case of a woman, aged thirty-two years, who complained of severe pain in the right lower portion of the abdomen. This pain increased greatly in severity.

On admission to the hospital the uterus was found to be anteflexed and rotated somewhat to the left, while upon the right side, and posteriorly, a tumor as large as an orange was present. This tumor was exceedingly painful on palpation. The left tube and ovary were normal, and the right tube and ovary could be distinctly palpated. Interstitial pregnancy was diagnosed, and the patient's intense and constant pain and the danger of uterine rupture made operation necessary. Accordingly, the abdomen was opened in the median line; the uterus, the tumor, and right tube and ovary were removed with the left tube, and a strand of iodoform gauze was carried through the stump of cervix for drainage. The patient made an uninterrupted recovery from the operation.

On examination pregnancy in the right cornu of a bicornate uterus was present. A fourteen weeks' ovum had developed, and a placenta was attached to the uterine wall. Especially noteworthy was the difference in the thickness of the uterine wall upon the two sides. Upon the right side the wall of the womb was 20 mm. in thickness, while on the left side, where the pregnancy existed, the wall of the uterus was but 3 mm. to 5 mm. in thickness. On microscopic examination the muscular tissue of the right side of the womb was much diminished in quantity and development, although the muscle cells and bloodvessels showed no especial irregularities. There was no hemorrhage.

A Case of Puerperal Tetanus.—WURDOCK (*Prager medicinische Wochenschrift*, 1903, Nos. 9 and 10) describes a case of tetanus in a woman, aged forty-two years, a multipara, who was delivered in Rubeska's clinic of a macerated and decomposed fœtus. Three hours afterward the placenta was manually removed and the uterus washed out. Fever developed for four days, but gradually disappeared, and the patient was discharged on the tenth day. On the next morning she could not open her mouth, had pain in the back and cramps in the back and neck, and these symptoms rapidly increased. Tetanus antitoxin was at once injected and urethan given by mouth. On the sixth day of her disease the patient died. A diagnosis of tetanus was made upon the clinical symptoms only. The bacteriological examination and the inoculation test upon animals both remained negative.

The Mechanical Sterilization of Rubber Gloves and Their Value in Practice.—This interesting subject receives attention from WANDEL and HOEHNE, in the *Münchener med. Wochenschrift*, 1903, No. 9. These observers found that vigorous washing of rubber gloves with soap and water sufficed to remove from the outer layers of the gloves bacteria. Simple washing with soap and water was not sufficient for this purpose. After the gloves have been used they should be washed while still upon the hands with soap and water. They should then be turned, again washed, and tried by filling them with fluid to detect a tear or perforation. They should then be powdered with sterile powder and kept in gauze or linen. Gloves so treated can usually be used five or six times.

Acute Contagious Pemphigus in the Newborn.—Before the Obstetrical Society of London, at its meeting on November 4, 1903, MAGUIRE read a paper upon this subject (*British Medical Journal*, November 14, 1903).

Most authorities consider pemphigus in the infant usually the result of syphilis. He reported the cases of eighteen infants suffering from acute contagious pemphigus, among whom eight deaths occurred. From the study of these cases, he concluded that a common contagion of unknown septic origin was conveyed from case to case by a certain midwife. The contagiousness was proved when the number of cases infected from each infant was ascertained. In two of the cases bacteriological examinations revealed the presence of the staphylococcus pyogenes aureus. The secondary symptoms were those of acute toxæmia, the infection having gained entrance through the unhealed umbilicus. The writer concludes that while this comparatively rare disease usually attacks the newborn, it may also be found in older children and adults. The eruption was bullous, variable in distribution and extent, and the specific germ was found in the contents of the vesicles. In mild cases no other symptoms than the eruption were present. In grave cases there was a general infection, with an acute toxæmia, which invariably ended fatally. The unhealed umbilical scar gave access to the poison in these cases. No method of treatment employed influenced the course or termination of the disease.

In discussion, Cullingworth had seen a case in an adult when it was very difficult to recognize the source of infection.

Dickinson referred to an epidemic of fourteen cases in the Foundling Hospital at Parma. Most of these cases were fatal, and an examination of the blood showed a marked leukocytosis caused by this specific organism. Syphilis had nothing to do with it. He did not believe that infection through the umbilicus was the cause of the toxæmia, as cases in adults could not be explained in this way.

MacLeod had observed the increasing rarity of this disease, and believed it due to the general use of antiseptic precautions in maternity hospitals. He believed that the streptococcus was the cause of the infection. In determining the germ he has used the method of Sabouraud, of Paris, who aspirated the bullæ into a sterile pipet containing acetic fluid. By this means MacLeod obtained streptococci in pure culture in a fatal case. He referred to the close resemblance of the disease to impetigo, whose cause had been found to be streptococcus pyogenes. He described a case in which an abrasion of the skin at the lip had been the point for the entrance of infection. He thought that usually a diagnosis could be readily made between this disorder and syphilitic pemphigus. A form of hereditary pemphigus, the result of vasomotor disease, might occasion difficulty in differential diagnosis.

Gonorrhœa during Pregnancy and the Puerperal State.—FRUEHINSHOLZ (*Zentralblatt für Gynäkologie*, 1903, No. 45) finds that gonorrhœa occurs among pregnant women in from 20 cent. to 25 per cent. of cases. The presence of an acute gonorrhœa does not prevent conception. Pregnancy causes latent symptoms of gonorrhœa to develop. Gonorrhœa does not, as a rule, bring on abortion, although, when abortion occurs in patients suffering from gonorrhœa, gonococci are often found in the decidua and placenta.

During the puerperal period gonococci increase rapidly in number, are found in the vaginal secretion, and often become abundant in the lochia. Puerperal infection is undoubtedly caused in some cases by gonococci. Cases of so-called puerperal rheumatism are most frequently the result of gonorrhœal infection.

Ectopic Gestation; Removal of Living Fœtus by Section, with Persistence of Secondary Hemorrhage—In the *Journal of Obstetrics and Gynecology of the British Empire*, November, 1903, MALCOLM reports the case of a patient, aged twenty-three years, previously healthy, who was seized with severe pelvic pain, followed by vomiting, nausea, and shock. The pain soon passed away and was followed by irregular menstruation. A second attack of severe abdominal pain, with vomiting and nausea, occurred, followed by what was apparently a menstrual discharge, and shortly after this a short attack of pain and vomiting. After a fourth attack of pain a slight rise of temperature was observed.

The patient was examined two and a half months after the first irregularity of menstruation. There was a mass, about the size of a three months' pregnant uterus, in the pelvis, extending more to the right than to the left. The lower border of this mass was below the os uteri and very firm. The cervix was high up, close to the pubic bones, a little to the left of the median line. The body of the uterus was attached to the left side of the abnormal mass. Its cavity was three inches deep. The patient's color was sallow, the breasts showed no sign of pregnancy, and the pulse was good. Immediate operation was declined. After a fifth attack of pain, the abnormal mass had increased in size, and great tenderness was present. The temperature was 101.5° F.; the pulse was 90; the complexion more sallow. There was frequent vomiting. On operation a sac filled with pus was found outside the peritoneal cavity. This sac contained a living fœtus. The placenta had a large attachment upon the right side of the pelvis and was allowed to remain. The amniotic sac was washed out and packed with iodoform gauze. The patient did well after the operation until the fifth and sixth days, when, upon changing the packing, a very free hemorrhage occurred from the cavity, which was controlled by firm packing. Changing of the dressing was invariably followed by hemorrhage. Two weeks after the operation the placenta was seen in the wound looking healthy and evidently well nourished. The cord had sloughed away. An attempt to separate the placenta was followed by profuse bleeding. The second effort to remove the placenta succeeded in bringing away a small piece, followed by copious hemorrhage. After this hemorrhage ceased the p a a evidently died, suppuration increased, and the placenta had to be removed by the finger. This was accompanied by an offensive discharge, by prostration, and free sweating on the part of the patient. Gradually the temperature dropped, the discharge ceased, and the patient made a good recovery. The placenta had been adherent over the right side of the pelvis nearly as high as the brim, over a portion of the left side of the sacrum and the left side of the pelvic floor. After the removal of the placenta a drainage-tube was introduced into the sinus. The patient had occasional attacks of pain, with increase in fever, and passed mucous casts from the intestine. She finally made a complete and satisfactory recovery. It is probable that in this case the Fallopian tube burst into the cellular tissue between the layers of the broad ligament, the placenta becoming attached to the wall of the pelvis in such a position that it did not involve any portion of the intestine. The gestation sac gradually raised the peritoneum out of the pelvis. Hemorrhage into the tissues had not occurred at any time. This case is also interesting from the fact that it occurred in a woman previously perfectly healthy and soon after her marriage.

Twin Pregnancy in Utero, with Ruptured Tubal Gestation.—In the *Journal of Obstetrics and Gynecology of the British Empire*, November, 1903, Marshall reports the case of a patient who had had four children with easy labors and good recoveries. Recently she had suffered from pain in the lower abdomen, slight vaginal discharge, and occasional faintness. She considered herself three months pregnant. She had had several attacks of severe pain, with collapse, vomiting, and great thirst. On admission to the hospital the patient had evidently had severe hemorrhage. The temperature was subnormal and the pulse very rapid. The abdomen was much enlarged, with dulness over the lower part and in the flanks. An ovoidal tumor, the uterus, extended upward to within three inches of the umbilicus and deviated to the right. On the left side there was a cystic partially fixed tumor lying deep in the pelvis, and very tender to the touch. It was evident that intrauterine and extrauterine pregnaney were both present.

On operation the abdomen was found full of fluid blood. A large ruptured ectopic gestation sac was found on the left side of the pelvis, from which a well-developed three months' fœtus was removed. As hemorrhage was active, the ovarian artery was ligated; the placenta was removed without injury to surrounding organs. As hemorrhage could not be checked without ligating the ovarian and uterine arteries, the uterus was removed. The oozing from the sac practically ceased, and the cavity was firmly tamponed with sterile iodoform gauze, the ends being brought into the vagina. The abdomen was closed with silkworm-gut suture. Under free stimulation the patient reacted, and forty-eight hours after the operation the clamps, which had been placed upon the broad ligaments and the gauze packing, were removed. There had been no hemorrhage. The pulse remained fuller and better. Secondary collapse came on; the patient complained of pain in the abdomen; the pulse became rapid and feeble, and death followed.

Upon autopsy the wound was clean and there were no signs of peritonitis or hemorrhage. Death was due to excessive loss of blood. The uterus contained a twin pregnancy at three and a half months. In this case the fetal sac had evidently ruptured slightly on several occasions, the last and possibly the largest rupture being caused by an enema administered when the patient entered the hospital.

GYNECOLOGY.

UNDER THE CHARGE OF

HENRY C. COE, M.D.,

OF NEW YORK,

ASSISTED BY

WILLIAM E. STUDDIFORD, M.D.

Disadvantages of Trendelenburg's Posture.—Franz (*Zentralblatt für Gynäkologie*, 1903, No. 32) after reviewing the cases reported by Kraske, Trendelenburg, and others, in which serious circulatory disturbances followed operations in the elevated position, states that in 745 abdominal sections he did not observe a single case. Studies of the pulse and respiration-curves led him to conclude that with the pelvis elevated the abdominal breathing is constantly diminished, while there is only a slight, if any, compensatory increase in the thoracic.

As regards the effect of anæsthesia, the writer noted in 825 cases of ether narcosis in the dorsal position 19 (2.3 per cent.) cases of bronchitis, while in 493 in which the pelvis was elevated there were 44 cases (8.9 per cent.); 150 chloroform narcoses with the patient in the dorsal position were followed by 4 (2.7 per cent.) cases of bronchitis, and 233 in Trendelenburg's posture by 9 (3.9 per cent.), showing that with the latter anæsthetic the difference is much less marked than when ether is used. The writer explains the frequency of bronchitis after operations in the elevated position as due to the escape of the infection mouth-contents into the bronchi after the patient is lowered, and suggests the advisability of carefully cleansing the mouth before the change is made to the dorsal posture.

He further emphasizes the fact that the diminished oxygenation, which is undoubtedly present when the patient is in the elevated posture, probably influences unfavorably the central nervous system, and that many disturbances which are referred to opening the abdomen are really due to this cause, since they are more often absent when the vaginal route is adopted.

The Abdominal and Vaginal Routes.—ERYSTROM (*Zentralblatt für Gynäkologie*, 1903, No. 32) compares his mortality after abdominal section (2.6 per cent.) with Dührssen's after vaginal operations on the adnexa (2.8 per cent.), and draws the following conclusions: The results of laparotomy for diseased adnexa are as good as those following vaginal section, but the former operation is more severe and the convalescence is longer. While the abdominal wound may be the cause of subsequent complications, the vaginal is not seldom a source of trouble. By the abdominal route the exact nature of the lesion can be better ascertained and repaired. The writer would by no means abandon vaginal section, but he believes that each case should be carefully studied and the indications clearly noted.

Development of Cancer from Mucous Polypi.—OPITZ (*Zeitschrift für Geb. u. Gyn.*, Band xlix., Heft 2) reports two cases, the first of which presented unusual features. The patient, aged fifty-seven years, had passed the menopause seven years before. On account of persistent hemorrhage, exploratory curettement was performed and the diagnosis of adenocarcinoma was made. After removal of the uterus a polypus was found near the fundus that had undergone sarcomatous degeneration. Cancerous nodules were scattered over the endometrium, and the gland near the surface of the tumor presented the typical structure of adenocarcinoma. In the second case a polypus was removed from the cervix of a patient fifty-eight years of age who had had hemorrhages and a foul discharge for several months. As the growth proved to be cancerous, vaginal extirpation was performed subsequently. The tumor showed a connective-tissue stroma with large cancerous alveoli, the cells being continuous with the squamous epithelium in the surface. Normal glands were present between the alveoli.

Endothelioma of the Cervix Uteri.—KIRCHGESSNER (*Zeitschrift für Geb. u. Gyn.*, Band xlix., Heft 2) adds the following case to the eight already reported. The patient, a young multipara, had suffered for a year and a half with a bloody discharge. On examination a flat, irregular growth the size of a walnut was seen on the anterior lip of the cervix, the posterior lip being normal, and the uterus and adnexa non-adherent. The patient died of peritonitis four days after removal of the uterus. Microscopically it appeared that the neoplasm had developed from the endothelium of the lymphatics and lymph spaces of the portio.

Etiology of Adenocystoma of the Ovary.—Walthard (*Zeitschrift für Geb. u. Gyn.*, Band xlix., Heft 2) as the result of his studies of serial sections of eighty normal ovaries from subjects of all ages, rejects the term "germ-epithelium" in favor of ovarian or surface-epithelium. In the ovaries of the newborn the follicular epithelium appears sometimes in solid masses and sometimes in the form of glandular pouches. The latter may develop into the primary follicles or may persist in the form of pouches or retention-cysts lined with flattened cells.

The writer believes isolated groups of cells found throughout the stroma subsequently form the surface epithelium. These cells may at any time after birth form glandular ingrowths from the surface, or may give rise to adenomatous growths within the stroma. Small collections of pavement epithelium are seen in the stroma or on the surface of the ovary which may separate in their centres and then form cysts.

Similar islands of ciliated epithelium among the surface cells may give rise to pouches lined with ciliated cells. Similar pouches are formed by masses of cubical cells, which are sometimes seen in the stroma as well as on the surface, and appear to be entirely independent of the ovarian epithelium. In all these pouches it is possible to trace two processes, either degeneration or proliferation, to the glandular type.

The remains of the primordial kidneys can be readily recognized in the hilum. The canals are greatly dilated and are lined with flattened epithelium. The writer was never able to find any trace of adenomatous structures in these. The pavement, ciliated, and cubical (or goblet-shaped) cells in the ovary are not derived, he thinks, from the surface or follicular epithelium, or from the remains in the hilum, but they are to be regarded as congenital cell-nests.

Treatment of Inversion.—Fresson (abstract of monograph in *Annales de Gynécologie et d'Obstétrique*, October, 1903) lays down the following rules: 1. Manual reduction should be attempted in every case of inversion, whether acute or chronic. 2. Bilateral incision of the cervix is applicable to all acute cases, and to those chronic cases in which the obstacle to reduction is demonstrated to be a constricting ring. 3. In others colpohysterotomy is the operation of election. 4. Vagiual hysterectomy is indicated only in the presence of intractable hemorrhage, infection, or when the irreducible uterus has been so injured that there is no probability of its regaining its functional integrity. 5. Hæmisection is the most rapid and convenient method of extirpating the organ.

Vulvovaginitis in Children.—Berkenheim (*Wratsch; Zentralblatt für Gyn.*, 1903, No. 32) reports the results of observations extending over ten years, from which he infers that 75 per cent. of the cases of vulvovaginitis in little girls is due to gonorrhœa. The relatively mild course of the inflammation is due to the shortness of the vagina in children, the absence of folds and glands, and the slight development of the vessels. The absence of such disturbing factors as coitus, menstruation and pregnancy favors the rapid cure. The average duration of the affection is eight weeks, but one-third of the cases become chronic.

Painful urination, local hyperæmia and leucorrhœa are the common symptoms. Complications are rare, especially peritonitis, urethritis, cystitis; arthritis and conjunctivitis are more common. Arthritis generally affects single joints, and the prognosis is favorable.

The writer recommends vaginal injections of solutions of sulphate of zinc, boric acid, permanganate of potash, protargol, and ichthyol, although he has never seen a case aborted by the use of these remedies. It is important that the patient should not be allowed to use the same vessels or towels as the other children.

The Normal and Diseased Peritoneum.—Clairmont and Haberer (*Wiener klin. Wochenschrift*, 1902, No. 45) conducted a series of experiments on rabbits to determine the absorptive power of the peritoneum. He followed the suggestion of Schnitzler and Ewald, injecting a 2 per cent. solution of iodide of potassium and noting its appearance in the urine. He adduced the following: Increased peristalsis increases absorption, while the introduction of air has no effect whatever. Sterile urine or intestinal contents do not, as a rule, hinder absorption.

In the early stage of peritonitis peritoneal absorption is increased, but later it is diminished. The latter result is also observed after abdominal sections in which dry sponging is employed, the converse being true when the wet method is adopted. In general, absorption is differently affected by different anæsthetics; transudation is not much affected by laparotomy.

A marked diminution of the power of absorption is noted after removal of the peritoneal covering of the diaphragm.

Treatment of Hæmatocele.—Bongle (*Arch. gén. de Méd.*, 1903, No. 3) believes that many small retrouterine hæmatoceles are absorbed without treatment. Large circumscribed ones may be incised and drained per vaginam, especially if suppuration is suspected. If it is inferred that several small collections are present, especially if the patient's menstrual period is due, vaginal incision may be attended with profuse hemorrhage, requiring immediate abdominal section. In other cases, in fact in the majority of hæmatoceles, laparotomy is the preferable procedure, above all when active bleeding is suspected.

Pigmentations of Genital Origin.—Dalche and Fouquet (*La Gynécologie*, 1903, No. 2) believes that certain pigment changes in the skin (chloasma, vitiligo, etc.) are of reflex uterine or ovarian origin, possibly due to disturbances in the so-called internal secretion of the ovary. They recognize several varieties, viz.: pigmentation attending menstrual disturbances, that due directly to organic utero-ovarian disease, and a third form which appears in connection with chlorosis, Raynaud's disease, etc., which may also be referred to some pelvic trouble.

As regards local treatments the authors recommend various ointments. The general treatment consists in the relief of amenorrhœa and dysmenorrhœa, or the removal of diseased organs. Oötherapy is also advised.

OPHTHALMOLOGY.

UNDER THE CHARGE OF

EDWARD JACKSON, A.M., M.D.,
OF DENVER, COLORADO,

AND

T. B. SCHNEIDEMAN, A.M., M.D.,
PROFESSOR OF DISEASES OF THE EYE IN THE PHILADELPHIA POLYCLINIC.

Corneal Ulceration Treated by Exclusion of Actinic Light.—W. Lowe (*Intercolonial Medical Journal of Australasia*, March 20, 1903) reports a case of ulceration of the cornea of two years' duration treated by exclusion of actinic light. The patient had intense intolerance of light, and was confined to a darkened room. Every form of treatment was tried without avail, until, acting on the theory that the actinic rays were keeping up the trouble, the patient was placed in a room the windows of which were covered with red photographic tissue paper. The effect was most remarkable. The intolerance to light and pain disappeared, while the injected cornea blanched as if adrenalin had been applied. The next morning lacrymation and discharge ceased, and on the third day the patient could read and sew. No sign of ulceration could be seen. The next day she went out of doors protected with ruby glass goggles.

The writer thinks that the red rays may have some germicidal action, or they may act by allaying inflammation.

Glaucoma.—Wahlsfors (*Arch. of Oph.*, November, 1903) insists that the conception of glaucoma, which goes back to von Graefe as being one with increased tension, is false. The attempt to differentiate certain cases of so-called simple glaucoma without increased tension from true glaucoma is a mistake. They are both essentially the same disease. We see simple glaucoma pass into inflammatory, and *vice versa*. He argues that the increase in tension is something accidental, and not even essential to glaucoma.

As regards the opinion now largely prevalent, that the cause of glaucoma lies in closure of the channels of exit, the writer asserts that while this may play an important role in inflammatory glaucoma, it is not applicable in simple glaucoma, where the increase in tension is quite subordinate and sometimes even absent. The latter class is very important in the explanation of glaucoma, as showing that this disease may exist without tension and without retention, thus proving that retention is not the cause of glaucoma. The writer calls attention to the variations in the fields. The defect may be central, peripheral, or irregular, or sector-like. There is no typical glaucomatous field. Excavation appears as a rule as a late sign. He insists upon the importance of one symptom as a true indication of the nature of the fundamental cause. This is reduction of the light-sense first, noticed by Forster, and emphasized by Mauthner. Hemeralopia may be the first and only symptom present for a long time, perhaps even overlooked by the patient, if confined to the periphery. The cause of hemeralopia is functional disturbance of the rods and cones in consequence of imperfect nutrition, the cause of which must lie in the inner layers of the choroid, whose vessels supply the outer layers of the retina. In the choroid, then, we must seek the cause of simple glaucoma. The choroidal lesion is an atrophy. The functional disturbances in simple glaucoma—diminution of the light-sense, narrowing of the field of vision, and diminution of central vision—may readily result from the atrophic process, which does not at once extend over the entire choroid, but begins usually in the periphery and gradually extends toward the centre, although the reverse is sometimes observed. The sector-like defects of the field depend upon limited layers of atrophy. The excavation of the nerve head is also best explained when the resistance is diminished by preceding inflammatory process, such as sclerochoroiditis. A normal disk possesses sufficient resisting power to withstand not only the normal tension, but considerable increase, as may often be observed in adherent leukoma, where we find a normal disk, with considerable increase in tension for years. Where the tissues of the disk (lamina cribrosa, in the formation of which the choroid takes some part) have lost their resistance, excavation may come on independent of increased tension, which should, therefore, not be designated pressure excavation.

The increased tension may also be explained as the result of the choroidal atrophy. Normally the choroid exerts pressure upon the liquid contents of the eyeball, as is shown by Donders' observation, that when all the coats of the eye are divided together the choroid retracts from the margin of the wound and leaves the sclera exposed. This contractility is doubtless due to the numerous muscular fibres which accompany the larger vessels and to Bruecke's muscle, which acts as a tensor. Such a muscular network acts as a restrainer of tension, not only by its direct resistance to the pressure of the contents, but also increases the lymph circulation (the currents of liquids) through the pressure it exercises. In glaucomatous increase of tension three factors are at work—paralysis of the muscular network of the choroid, causing a slowing of the currents of liquid; the channels of exit in consequence of the retarded flow become blocked and cause a retention of the ocular liquids, and finally, the venæ vorticosæ, which are compressed by the increased tension, lead to a venous stasis with all its results. As the disease process is due to choroidal atrophy, the prognosis of glaucoma in general must be considered bad, as we have no remedies to act on this process. The writer thinks that repeated injections of strychnine prevent the spread of the atrophy. He believes that an injection per day for ten or twenty days, repeated three or four times a year, has enabled him to preserve the vision for many years in simple glaucoma, with little or no increase in tension.

In simple glaucoma iridectomy is useless as a curative, but valuable as a prophylactic measure against acute attacks. Where the tension is increased iridectomy remains the sovereign means of reducing it, but its action is not understood; Exner's explanation that the short arterial twigs proceeding from the major arterial circle of the iris form direct anastomoses with the corresponding venous twigs, without having to pass through the capillary network, is probably the best. Iridectomy thus works, as Knapp expresses it, as a safety-valve. As, however, the atrophic process continues, central vision becomes poorer, the field contracts, and the disk becomes excavated.

Sclerotomy, both anterior and posterior, as long as the wound is not thoroughly healed, is useful in giving time for the circulatory disturbance to pass off. Eserine reduces tension in fresh cases of acute congestive glaucoma, through causing contraction of the tensor of the choroid and probably of its muscular network. In simple glaucoma eserine is only valuable so long as the atrophic process has not entirely paralyzed the muscular network and the tensor.

Some Modern Views on Primary Glaucoma.—Elliot, I. M. S. (*Ind. Med. Gaz.*, July, 1903), gives a résumé of the above subject, based on a review of the opinions of leading authorities as found in the literature of the subject, as well as from personal interviews. He sums up that under the term simple glaucoma have been in the past included: (1) cases in which the prime factor was disease of the optic nerve; (2) cases in which the triad of symptoms alone occur—*i. e.*, cupped disk, retracted field, and diminution of visual acuity, and (3) a long series of cases passing insensibly from the last class and merging at the opposite end of the scale into well-marked congestive glaucoma. Atrophic cases should be carefully distinguished and placed apart. Classes 2 and 3 may be separated from each other by advancing knowledge, which may lead to a better comprehension of their pathology, a result greatly to be desired, establishing more exact indications for operation. As respects treatment of glaucoma, there is no divergence as to the rational and medical measures—myotics and general hygiene.

Of surgical operations, sclerotomy and iridectomy, the writer concludes that the modern ophthalmologist undertakes iridectomy with a much more expectant heart than that with which he performs sclerotomy. Many operators prefer sclerotomy (1) in early cases where there is considerable doubt, (2) in late cases where it is employed as a *dernier ressort*, (3) in desperate cases where iridectomy has failed, and (4) in simple glaucoma where any operation is doubtful, and, therefore, the procedure of least magnitude is chosen, although the balance of safety does not lie wholly with the latter operation. Sympathectomy finds its rôle according to Abadie, in those cases in which the triad alone is present, which do not yield to medicinal and rational treatment.

The Wearing of Artificial Eyes over an Eyeball in Situ and after Abscission of Staphyloma.—F. A. Müller's Sons (*Klin. Mon. f. Augenheilk.*, October, 1903) call attention to the impracticability of fitting the ordinary shell, which answers well enough in cases like phthisis bulbi, to the full eyeball, or such as are but slightly shrunken, the thickened spot convex posteriorly in the region of the iris of the shell, exerting undue pressure if applied to a full globe and preventing perfect apposition. The perfectly flat shells still found in the shops are entirely worthless. They propose to meet the cases in question by giving the prosthesis a smooth concavo-convex form to permit perfect apposition.

The writers also criticise the horizontal cicatrix with its angular edges, which results from the usual mode of abscising staphylomata (a horizontal elliptical section with vertical sutures). These edges enormously increase the difficulty of prosthesis and quite destroy the cosmetic effect, for the reason that the bridging of these edges requires the shell to be broader horizontally, so that the artificial eye seems longer and larger than the sound one. To obviate this the writers raise the question whether the wound of excision for the staphyloma should not be given a vertical direction. The edges would then come to be beneath the lids, at which points the shell could be easily cut out to correspond; the horizontal meridian, which is the most important, would then furnish a stump of suitable convexity. A more symmetrical result might conceivably be secured by a triangular section with a purse-knot suture. The writers do not venture to offer an opinion whether this is a practicable procedure.

PATHOLOGY AND BACTERIOLOGY.

UNDER THE CHARGE OF

SIMON FLEXNER, M.D.,

DIRECTOR OF THE ROCKEFELLER INSTITUTE FOR MEDICAL RESEARCH, NEW YORK.

ASSISTED BY

WARFIELD T. LONGCOPE, M.D.,

RESIDENT PATHOLOGIST, PENNSYLVANIA HOSPITAL.

The Reactions of the Blood in Experimental Diabetes.—SWEET (*Journal of Medical Research*, 1903, vol. v. p. 255) says the fact long known to clinicians and students of immunity, that the diabetic organism is abnormally susceptible to infectious processes suggested the experiments which are the subject of this communication. Studies were made upon the hæmolytic and, to a less extent, the bactericidal power of the serum of rabbits suffering from phlorizin and adrenalin glycosuria, and of the serum of dogs which were the subjects of true diabetes mellitus caused by total extirpation of the pancreas. After subcutaneous injections in rabbits of an alcoholic solution of phlorizin, the serum showed a slight though readily demonstrable increase in the hæmolytic complement for bovine erythrocytes. This increase in complement is to be explained as an occurrence coincident with the inflammatory reaction of the organism to the injection. Such injections of phlorizin produced no effect upon the amboceptor for bovine erythrocytes. Intraperitoneal injections of adrenalin chloride were followed by much the same results as regards the serum reactions of the rabbits as was noted in the experiments with phlorizin. The only change exhibited by the serum was a slight increase in the hæmolytic complement, which occurred in certain animals that developed an inflammatory reaction following the intraperitoneal injections. Although injections of both phlorizin and adrenalin chloride give rise to a glycosuria, the condition cannot be considered as a diabetes mellitus, and therefore to reproduce this disease in animals as nearly as possible excision of the pancreas was resorted to; dogs were used for this purpose. Fourteen dogs were operated upon, and of this number two recovered completely from the operation, dying subsequently of a true diabetes mellitus. Following upon the diabetes produced by complete removal of the pancreas, the hæmolytic activity of the dogs' serum was markedly decreased for both rabbit and guinea-pigs' erythrocytes. There is, besides, what was interpreted as a complete loss of the normal bactericidal property of the serum for such bacteria as B. coli communis, B. typhi abdominalis, and B. dysenteriæ, while somewhat less conclusive was the decrease of bactericidal power of the blood for staphylococcus pyogenes aureus, since the serum of the normal dog has very little if any bactericidal effect upon this organism. The decrease in the hæmolytic action of the serum of the diabetic dog was, furthermore, shown to be due to a loss of hæmolytic complement, and from analogy the loss of bactericidal power was believed to be dependent upon the loss of bacteriolytic complement. Unless the pancreas was completely removed the above phenomena did not occur; consequently the author believes that extirpation of the entire organ is as necessary for the loss of complement as it is for the production of diabetes. In diabetic dogs the organism had not entirely lost its power of reacting to inflammatory processes by an increase of complementary substances. With these changes in the complements no disturbance of the normal relation of the receptors of the erythrocytes to specific hæmolytic amboceptors could be demonstrated. The author believes that the loss of the complementary substances in diabetes mellitus points conclusively to the fact that there is no relation between the leukocytes of any type and the production of the complements. During the experiments it was discovered that secondary infections were not accompanied by a decrease in the glucose excreted by the diabetic organism.

Contribution to the Physiological Study of Glycerin.—Nicloux (*Journ. de Phys. et de Path. Gén.*, 1903, T. v. p. 527) has found that under normal conditions glycerin is present in the blood of dogs and rabbits, 2 to 2½ mgr. of glycerin occurring in 100 c.c. of blood from dogs and 4 to 5 mgr. in rabbits' blood. The ingestion of fats does not appear to alter the proportion of glycerin in the blood. After an intravenous injection of glycerin this substance disappears rapidly from the blood and the relative proportion of glycerin in the urine is much increased above the amount found before the intravenous injections. Since the same relative increase of glycerin occurs in the urine after ingestion of glycerin, the author believes that the cells of the kidney possess a peculiar selective function for the excretion of this substance.

The Experimental Production of Uncompensated Heart Disease, with Especial Reference to the Pathology of Dropsy.—Charles Bolton (*Journal of Path. and Bact.*, 1903, vol. ix. p. 67) says three distinct theories exist at present to explain the primary factors concerned in the pathology of the dropsy of venous stagnation: 1. A secretory theory, of which Hamburger is the chief exponent, and according to which the capillary endothelial cells are believed to have a specific secretory function increased in dropsy. 2. A theory originated by Lazarus-Baslow which explains the œdema by assuming that an accumulation of waste products occurs in the tissues. 3. A mechanical and physical theory, according to which the œdema depends upon increased venous and capillary pressure, together with an alteration in the vessel wall. Cohnheim and Starling are among the main supporters of the mechanical theory. Cohnheim found that when oil was allowed to flow into the

In a

ments the pericardium was constricted and an

blood pressure in the peripheral arteries as well as in the inferior vena cava, portal vein, and peripheral veins before and at different periods during and after the operation. Upon constricting the pericardium there resulted immediately a considerable decrease in the arterial pressure and a rise of pressure throughout the entire venous system; but, whereas the arterial pressure remained low for some hours after the operation, the venous pressure gradually fell to normal. If the constriction was now relieved the arterial pressure rose to normal or rose slightly above normal, while the venous pressure dropped below normal. By intravenous infusions given while the pericardium was constricted the arterial pressure could not be elevated to its normal range, nor could the high level of the venous pressure be maintained. Cohnheim's experiments were repeated, and it was shown that when the pericardium is distended with oil the heart gradually tends to fail owing to the lack of blood supply, which is cut off by the pressure of the oil upon the thin-walled inferior and superior vena cava at their entrance into the auricle. Thus the condition brought about by Cohnheim's experiment is essentially different than that of the author's experiment, where the action of the heart as a force pump alone is interfered with and conditions are much the same as are produced by an adherent pericardium. Finally a third group of experiments demonstrated that when the animals were allowed to live after constriction of the pericardium until the onset of œdema, the arterial pressure gradually rose but never reached the normal level, while the venous pressure remained stationary. Bolton concludes that in uncompensated heart disease, such as is imitated by the present experiments, the capillary pressure is of necessity low, and he agrees with Starling in adopting the mechanical theory as an explanation for the development of œdema.

Leukæmia.—HANS LUCE (*Deut. Arch. f. Klin. Med.*, 1903, Bd. lxxvii. p. 255) records a peculiar form of lymphatic leukæmia for which he has suggested the name of "leukanæmia." A woman, aged forty years, developed a simple anæmia following an attack of acute tonsillitis. After six months' time the blood picture changed and assumed the characters of a typical lymphatic leukæmia. The anæmia increased with the appearance of a hemorrhagic diathesis until at the end of three and a half months the histological blood picture was typical of both lymphatic leukæmia and pernicious anæmia. For two mont preceding the patient's death this condition remained more or less constant. At autopsy all the organs showed an extreme grade of anæmia, while an extensive fatty degeneration was noted, especially of the heart muscle and liver. The bone-marrow was red. Microscopically there was leukæmic infiltration of the liver, kidneys, and heart muscle, with lymphadenoid hyperplasia of the spleen and cervical lymph glands, and almost complete lymphadenoid metaplasia of the bone-marrow. But the bone-marrow showed, besides, the histological elements characteristic of pernicious anæmia. The complete absence of siderosis throughout all the organs examined was noteworthy. This case together with those of Körmiöczi and Leube form a small group for which the author believes the term leukanæmia suitable—instances where the blood pictures of lymphatic leukæmia and pernicious anæmia are combined. The condition is looked upon as a disease of the bone-marrow, and the anæmia is considered to be of myelogenic rather than hæmatogenous origin, a view which is strengthened by the fact that there was no pigment in any of the organs. It has been shown that in certain cases of lymphatic leukæmia the lymphoid tissue of the bone-marrow is the seat of extensive hyperplasia. In instances such as the present it is probable that the lymphoid metaplasia takes place at the expense of the erythroblastic tissues, and thus there results an anæmia comparable in many respects to the aplastic forms of pernicious anæmia described by Ehrlich.

A New Cholera Vaccine, and its Method of Preparation.—STRONG (*Amer. Med.*, 1903, vol. vi. p. 272) has found that he can produce a cholera vaccine which contains free receptors, and has the power of building both uni- and amboceptors (agglutinins and bacteriolysins) in a cholera immune serum, by autolytic digestion of cholera spirilla in aqueous solution. When injected into rabbits this vaccine gives rise to the appearance of bactericidal and agglutinative substances in the blood sera of these animals which equal or exceed those obtained from inoculations of virulent living cholera vibrios. One advantage gained by the use of the vaccine instead of the living or dead bacteria is the absence of local reaction following the inoculation. The vaccine filtrate may be evaporated to a powder which when redissolved in water and injected into animals is capable of giving rise to an immunity. The author suggests that free receptors obtained by autolytic digestion and filtration of other bacteria may be used as a vaccine in diseases such as typhoid fever and dysentery.

Notice to Contributors.—All communications intended for insertion in the Original Department of this Journal are received only *with the distinct understanding that they are contributed exclusively to this Journal.*

Contributions from abroad written in a foreign language, if on examination they are found desirable for this Journal, will be translated at its expense.

A limited number of reprints in pamphlet form will, if desired, be furnished to authors, *provided the request for them be written on the manuscript.*

All communications should be addressed to—

DR. FRANCIS R. PACKARD, 1831 Chestnut Street, Philadelphia, U. S. A.

THE

AMERICAN JOURNAL

OF THE MEDICAL SCIENCES.

FEBRUARY, 1904.

GASTROENTEROSTOMY.[1]

By John B. Deaver, M.D.,

SURGEON-IN-CHIEF, GERMAN HOSPITAL, PHILADELPHIA.

Gastroenterostomy at the present day has a definite position in surgery, with a constantly widening of its field of usefulness in the treatment of lesions of the stomach or duodenum.

Twenty-two years ago Wolffler performed the first operation upon a patient where pylorectomy was impossible, and in 1900 Mayo Robson tabulated 1978 cases reported. At the present time gastroenterostomy is performed many times as a routine procedure in certain gastric diseases without much more comment than a cholecystostomy for a diseased gall-bladder.

During these twenty years, however, while the indications for the operation have become more definite, the method of operating and the technique of operation have been the subject of spirited debate. To overcome the confliction of the direction of peristalsis was the first important step, and many modifications in the original operation were made.

Gastroenterostomy was performed at first for the relief of the starvation in obstructive carcinoma of the pylorus, and then, as has happened so often in surgery, a palliative measure was broadened in scope until it became a valuable method of treatment. The one great indication for gastroenterostomy is found in all lesions of the stomach where the contents of the latter are not evacuated. Whether this is due to a malignant or benign obstruc-

[1] Read by title before the Southern Surgical and Gynecological Association, Atlanta, Ga., December, 1903.

tion, an inflamed or ulcerated pylorus, or atony of the gastric muscle, the retained stomach contents must be provided for by an anastomotic opening.

When carcinoma of the pylorus has progressed so far that its removal is impossible, the last months of the patient may be made more restful by the cessation of vomiting and the ability to assimilate food. In obstruction of benign origin usually consequent upon the healing of an ulcerated area of the pyloric mucous membrane, pyloroplasty is sometimes combined with gastroenterostomy, especially in those cases where a gastric pouch has formed, with loss of the muscle power of the stomach. Where the latter complications do not exist gastroenterostomy is not required, and if performed, soon loses its intended purposes and merely aids in the formation of adhesions.

Bleeding from acute or chronic ulceration of the wall of the stomach frequently offers a positive indication for gastroenterostomy, in order to place the mucous membrane in the region of the pylorus, the most frequent site of ulceration, in a state of partial rest, at least. In acute ulcers the excision of the bleeding point would seem to be the ideal operation, but the consensus of opinion of those of large experience in this work favors a simple gastroenterostomy.

A gastroenterostomy with correct technique will keep the stomach empty, and with the aid of careful feeding sufficient rest can be obtained to enable the ulcerated area to heal.

When a considerable area of mucous membrane surrounding an ulcer is the seat of marked inflammation, or in large erosions or in multiple ulcer direct treatment cannot be done, gastroenterostomy offers by far the best method of procedure. A chronic ulcer, especially in the neighborhood of the pylorus, requires the exercise of great discrimination as to whether a pylorectomy is necessary.

The literature of instances where malignant disease has developed upon the site of a chronic ulcer is increasing rapidly, and such a termination must always be considered and its likelihood an indication for the excision of the pylorus. Gastroenterostomy is too often considered a last resort for a carcinoma of the pylorus causing obstruction, whereas the lesion should have had surgical interference at a time when a cure was possible. But, on the other hand, it must be admitted that in many cases believed at the time of operation to be malignant by reason of enlarged inflammatory lymph nodes, induration about the ulcer, etc., gastroenterostomy has cured the condition and disproved its malignancy.

The various contractions consequent upon chronic gastric or duodenal ulceration may obstruct the stomach and require gastroenterostomy. In hour-glass stomach it is preferable to divide the wall of the organ in the long axis and close in the opposite dircetion, but when this is deemed inadvisable gastroenterostomy may be performed. In those cases of hour-glass stomach when the constriction is near the middle, and two large pouches are formed, a gastrogastrostomy at the most dependent portion of the pouches gives better results than gastroenterostomy.

In cases of extensive dilatation of the stomach with loss of motor power consequent upon a strictured duodenum, the result of ulcer, the anastomotic opening is required. The stomach lessens in size to an extent which will depend entirely upon the contractile power of the muscular coat. When the condition of dilatation has lasted for a long time and has appeared gradually, it is questionable whether there will be any actual lessening in the size of the stomach after operation; but if dilatation has come on very rapidly it will be readily seen that the muscular tone has not been overtaxed, and, therefore, the organ should regain its normal size in a comparatively short time. I would lay stress upon the careful examination of cases of dilated stomach. In some instances this condition is caused by kinking of the pylorus from the downward displacement of the organ due to peritoneal relaxation. In gastroptosis with dilatation of the stomach better results are obtained, in my opinion, by a gastroplication and a gastroenterostomy than by the other methods sometimes used.

In some cases of fistulæ between the biliary tract and the stomach where the extent and density of the adhesions may prevent the separation of such adhesions and the repair of the fistula with safety, gastroenterostomy gives good results. Even where gastrolysis can be performed and the fistula closed, the rest and drainage which gastroenterostomy affords gives additional security to the perfect healing of the stomach. In addition, adhesions are likely to reform, and in such an event the artificial opening prevents the dilatation and other symptoms incident to pyloric narrowing.

In those intractable cases of chronic gastritis where multiple erosions of the stomach are present at the pyloric region, with the mucosa in the neighborhood of the erosion deeply hemorrhagic, and with the occasional "occurrence of profuse or even fatal hemorrhage" (Osler), gastroenterostomy, by placing the pylorus at rest, may cure the condition.

A secretory neurosis of the stomach, with hypersecretion of hydrochloric acid, known in Germany and France as "Reichman's disease," is frequently rebellious to internal medication. In this disease, while the irritation of the highly acid gastric juice induces pyloric spasm at first, yet in most instances atony and dilatation of the stomach occur, and the pylorus becomes eroded and fissured. In these cases gastroenterostomy places the organ at rest and prevents the accumulation of the intensely acid gastric juice with its severe symptoms.

Mayo Robson suggests that, in acute dilatation of the stomach, after lavage has failed, the abdomen should be opened, the stomach emptied and connected with the jejunum, and Weir advises the same operation in tetany, which is often associated with a dilated stomach and may be caused by it.

The methods most often used at the present time for performing gastroenterostomy are: (1) the anterior operation; (2) the posterior operation, through the transverse mesocolon; (3) opening the gastrocolic omentum above the colon and anastomosing the jejunum to the posterior wall of the stomach; (4) the Roux Y operation, a modification of Wolffler's second method; (5) Kocher's operation.

The anterior operation is now usually performed by bringing the jejunum, not the duodenum, up over the great omentum and transverse colon and suturing to the stomach near its dependent portion. While in the hands of some good results are obtained, yet I believe that it entails greater risk from adhesions and intestinal obstruction than is the case in the posterior operation. Another objection is that the site of anastomosis is made too far above the greater curvature and not at the most dependent portion of the stomach, so essential where the stomach no longer possesses much muscular power. If care is taken, however, the anterior opening can be made nearly as low as the posterior, and, at any rate, it is usually believed that the traction of the small bowel brings the anastomosis to the lowest level, finally. After performing the gastroenterostomy the proximal and distal ends of the loop of the small bowel should be stitched to the stomach, the former at a point higher and the latter at a point lower than the anastomotic opening, preventing, to a great extent, any tendency toward spur formation.

The posterior operation is performed by making an incision in the transverse mesocolon, vertical in direction, to avoid interference with the blood supply of the colon, through which the posterior wall of the stomach is delivered and to which the jejunum is to be attached. The jejunum can always be readily found by passing the hand behind the coils of bowel to the left side of the second lumbar vertebra, where the duodenojejunal junction is grasped. I make it the rule to allow free play of the jejunum by leaving sixteen to eighteen inches of bowel between the anastomosis and the junction with the duodenum. This is done for several reasons: it prevents any kinking of the ligament of Treit, tends to prevent spur formation, and, most important of all, if any subsequent procedures are to be employed, such as enteroenterostomy or Roux's operation, sufficient bowel is left for such operations.

In incising the stomach, as well as the intestine, the incision should first be carried down to the mucous coat, which will then protrude, when, with a pair of tissue forceps, it is grasped and separated at the margin of the wound for some distance from the submucous coat (Robson and Moynihan). The mucous membrane is then cut away to the extent of the length of the wound and about one-half to three-quarters of an inch in width. This prevents the mucous membrane from pouting into the anastomotic opening and lessening its size, which might interfere during the repair of the wound with the emptying of the stomach, unless the opening is made liberally large. To prevent the slipping of a knuckle of bowel between the margin of the opening made in the transverse mesocolon and the wall of the stomach and consequent intestinal obstruction, as well as to prevent the circular compression of the afferent and efferent loops of the jejunum close to the anastomosis, the margins of the opening made in the transverse mesocolon should be stitched to the stomach wall at one or more points and about one inch away from the anastomotic opening.

The supracolic method merely consists of opening the gastrocolic omentum by a vertical incision, bringing up the jejunum over the omentum and transverse colon and suturing to the posterior wall of the stomach. It has no advantages over the anterior operation and is exposed to the same risk of adhesion formation.

Roux advocates an operation which seems to offer many advantages. The jejunum is divided, 20 to 40 cm. (eight to sixteen inches) below the point where it passed beneath the transverse colon and the distal end implanted into the stomach, the proximal end being sutured into an opening made in the descending limb, which has been sutured to the stomach and about four inches below the latter. It can readily be seen that the "vicious circle" cannot occur, as the bile and pancreatic secretion by the force of gravity will not return to the stomach, unless there is regurgitation of the intestinal contents. The objection that has been raised to this operation is the small opening afforded from the stomach by the rather narrow diameter of the jejunum. Such opening is not smaller, however, than that obtained by the use of the Murphy button or Mayo Robson bobbin, and not any less than the normal pyloric orifice. I have performed the operation without any disagreeable sequelæ at all, but as I have had like results from the same number of anterior and posterior anastomosis, I have not been able to draw any deductions regarding its greater value than the other operations. Roux's method requires some judgment in its use, and, unless performed with great care, subjects the patient to more risk than the simple posterior operation. Roux indicates its use in benign stenosis, gastroptosis, and gastrectasis. As will be seen later, the operation is of great value when the vicious circle has already occurred.

Kocher endeavors to avoid the return of intestinal contents into the stomach and their resulting decomposition and absorption by bringing the jejunum vertically upward, incising it at right angles to its long axis and suturing to the stomach, so "that the proximal portion of the loop passes vertically upward and the distal portion vertically downward, the former opposite to the stomach. A flap is also formed from the intestine to prevent regurgitation into the stomach." I do not believe, however, that the valve persists for any length of time, nor does the operation prevent the overfilling of the duodenum any better than the posterior operation.

In all of these operations various mechanical devices are used to perfect the anastomosis, of which the Murphy button is, doubtless, the most popular. Personally, I use simply a needle and thread, though in certain cases I have used both the Murphy button and the Mayo Robson bone bobbin. The great advantage of the needle-and-thread operation is that the materials are always at hand, the opening can be made of any length, thus lessening the tendency to subsequent contraction, which may close the opening. The objections to the mechanical devices are the rather small opening allowed and the subsequent contraction of the opening, particularly when the Murphy button or Senn's plates have been used. If too large a button or bobbin has been used, pressure necrosis of the bowel and perforative peritonitis may result.

Of the various other methods of performing the anastomosis, I have had no experience. I do not use the elastic ligature, because I see no advantages to be derived from its use, and it has the objection that we can never be absolutely sure that the ligature will cut through and establish the opening. The Connell suture has also been recommended, but I have never used it, nor do I use the clamps for the stomach and intestine. By the proper disposition of gauze the portion of bowel to be anastomosed, brought out of the abdomen, can be so compressed against the margin of the abdominal wound that no escape of contents occurs when it is opened. There is no danger of bleeding if the coats are well sutured, and if such is feared, Down's instrument could be used in making the openings. Personally, I do not use the cautery knife, believing it to be cumbersome and tending to a needless multiplicity of instruments.

The prevention of vomiting after operation from the formation of the vicious circle has occasioned much thought upon the part of many surgeons. Some deny that they have ever had to deal with this distressing complication, and it is fortunate that this vomiting is not frequently met with; yet that it does occur, even with perfect technique, cannot be disputed. The term vomiting from the vicious circle is applied to that condition where the gastric contents pass into the proximal or afferent limb of the loop, become mixed with the bile and pancreatic secretion and are returned to the stomach. Reflux vomiting (Fowler) is due to the passage of the secretions alone into the stomach, through the new opening, or backward through the partially permeable pylorus. The cause of such severe vomiting has not been determined, some observers having shown that the secretions of the liver and of the pancreas can be led directly into the stomach without impairing digestion or causing vomiting. Fowler[1] believes that the symptoms arising from the vicious circle

[1] Annals of Surgery, November, 1902.

are due either to "the passage of food into the duodenum and its more or less prompt reflux into the stomach, followed by its injection by vomiting, or from distention of the duodenum and a relative stagnation of the stomach contents from motor insufficiency." To correct these conditions after performing the usual posterior anastomosis, Fowler performs enteroenterostomy between the afferent and efferent portion of the loop of jejunum, and, finally, passes a No. 20 silver wire two or three times around the afferent loop between the two points of anastomosis and drawing upon the turns tightly enough to occlude the lumen of the intestine without strangulating its wall. This absolutely prevents the duodenal end of the loop from communicating directly with the stomach.

The question as to whether the enteroanastomosis should be performed in every case must be answered in the negative. I formerly used such a procedure, but at the present time believe that the simple posterior gastrojejunostomy is more rapid, safer, and perfectly efficacious in the great majority of cases, reserving subsequent operative procedures in the event of the establishment of severe vomiting.

The following case illustrates the few points that I particularly wish to emphasize:

Miss M. J., aged twenty-four years, was admitted to the German Hospital on July 7, 1903. Her family and previous personal history presented nothing of interest, nor did her occupation, that of tobacco stripper, have any influence on her condition.

Three years before the first symptoms of gastric trouble appeared with a gradual failing of the appetite, eructations of gas and fulness and distress after taking food. A year later she began to vomit after eating. The vomited material was quite sour, the sourness increasing when the food was retained for a while before the vomiting. There was never any hematemesis. The gastric distress increased and was soon accompanied by a burning pain in the epigastrium, just above the umbilicus, and referred along the costal margins of both sides. This pain was not relieved by eating or drinking. The bowels, which had been regular during the earlier months, became constipated. There was never any diarrhoea.

Her treatment had consisted, after a course of the various stomachics, of lavage practised every alternate day since December, 1902. When the stomach washing was practised in the morning remains of food eaten the night before were found, together with much mucus.

Upon admission nothing of moment was observed by a physical examination. There was tenderness of the abdomen 1 cm. above the umbilicus and over an area 3 cm. in diameter, and also a tender point over the twelfth rib, posteriorly. The stomach capacity was 1500 c.c., the lower border reaching to 1 cm. above the umbilicus when distended.

Operation, July 8, 1903, under ether anæsthesia. An incision five inches long was made through the right rectus, the peritoneum was opened and the stomach appeared immediately below the wound. Numerous adhesions, fibrinous in character, were found around the neck of the gall-bladder and duodenum. The gall-bladder was normal and slightly distended. The stomach was then carefully examined and observed to be slightly enlarged, rather low in position, and the pyloric opening somewhat thickened, otherwise negative.

The intestines were walled off with gauze pads, the transverse colon and mesocolon delivered out of the wound and protected with gauze. The transverse mesocolon was incised and the posterior surface of the stomach exposed and brought out of the wound; a loop of the upper portion of the jejunum was delivered and brought up to the posterior wall of the stomach, to which it was stitched by a continuous Lembert suture, introduced for a distance of about two and a half inches. An incision was then made into the jejunum, about two inches in length, through the serous and muscular coats, and the protruding mucous membrane excised. A similar procedure was performed upon the stomach. The free edges of the stomach and jejunal wounds were united with through-and-through silk suture. The Lembert suture was then continued anteriorly, completing the peritoneal apposition. The abdomen was closed with tier suture.

The patient reacted well from the operation, was free from vomiting until July 13th, when 700 c.c. of dark-green bile was vomited. General condition good.

July 15th. Patient vomited bile during the night. Appetite good; feels better than she has in years. Stitches removed. Incision healed by first intention.

17th. Patient vomited bile, with small portion of fecal matter.

18th. During the early morning the patient vomited; vomitus stercoraceous in character, about 300 c.c., and an intestinal obstruction was believed to have taken place, necessitating a second operation.

When the abdomen was opened the omentum was found adherent to the old scar. These were separated, and the omentum and transverse colon turned upward. This reflection upward carried several coils of small bowel along, and it was found that the proximal and distal limbs of the anastomosed loop were firmly adherent to the posterior layer of the transverse mesocolon, interfering to a marked degree with the peristalsis of the bowel. The adhesions were all separated and such bowel surfaces as were denuded by the separation were sutured with silk or covered with cargile. The gastroenterostomy was apparently perfect. An enteroenterostomy was then performed, 15 cm. (six inches) below the anastomotic opening, in the usual manner. The abdomen was closed by tier sutures. There was some vomiting of a green material upon the two days following operation, which stopped upon the use of lavage.

25th. Stitches removed; wound healed by first intention.

26th. Patient vomited twice about 300 c.c. of light-greenish material. Wine of ipecac, 10 drops every hour, was given.

27th. No vomiting.

31st. Ipecac stopped.

August 2d. Vomited 300 c.c. of light-green material about 10 P.M. Vomiting cannot be attributed to anything eaten. Placed upon ipecac wine 10 drops every two hours during the day.

7th. Vomited small quantity of yellow material. Ipecac stopped.

12th. Discharged; condition fine. Is gaining weight, and has not vomited since August 7th.

On September 14, 1903, this patient was readmitted to the German Hospital. She stated that on August 16th, four days after her discharge, vomiting had recommenced, at first of bile and later of food and bile. When admitted she vomited everything given by the mouth, and large quantities of thick, ropy, dark-green material, with a very strong odor. Feeding by rectum was begun, but notwithstanding this, the patient continued to vomit the thick, dark-green material, containing large quantities of bile. On washing out the stomach large quantities of the same material were obtained. It was evident that the biliary and pancreatic secretion were regurgitating into the stomach and causing the vomiting.

Her nourishment was good, notwithstanding the vomiting, proving that the food must be digested in great part, especially as the patient does not seem to have lost much weight. Eyes examined by Dr. W. T. Shoemaker, with no abnormal findings. By a rectal examination the pelvic organs were apparently normal; there were no symptoms or signs of locomotor ataxia.

Operation was performed on September 19th. When the peritoneum was opened the omentum was found universally adherent and there were dense adhesions between the coils of bowel. The gastroenterostomy was exposed and the opening found to be freely open. The enteroenterostomy was exposed, some difficulty being encountered in distinguishing the parts of the anastomosis by reason of the numerous adhesions. When these were separated the anastomosis was found to be in perfect condition, with some sacculation. Adhesions were further separated throughout the abdominal cavity. The entire omentum was ligated and cut away. The gall-bladder was found normal in size, numerous adhesions found around it; stomach normal in size. By means of a pedicle needle a piece of silver wire was passed around the pylorus and tied. Parts were then returned. Abdominal cavity filled with normal salt solution and the abdomen closed by tier suture. The patient was shocked, the pulse barely perceptible at the close of operation. An intravenous injection of salt solution was given before leaving the operating room.

September 20th. Patient has vomited bile several times during the day.

22d. Buttermilk ordered. Patient feels somewhat distressed in the epigastric region. No vomiting.

23d. Patient feels well; no epigastric distress.

29th. Ate light diet. No nausea or distress.

October 10th. Patient vomited after breakfast.

11th to *15th.* Vomited several times each day; complained of abdominal pain; there was some tympanites. The fourth operation was, therefore, performed, and a coil of small intestine found closely adherent to the parietal peritoneum. The intestines were found universally adherent to each other and to the remains of the omentum, binding together the transverse, ascending, and descending colon and sigmoid flexures and various loops of small intestine, one to another. No portion of the bowel, excepting about five feet of ileum, was free from adhesions. The adhesions were separated, bleeding points ligated, and all denuded surface covered with cargile. The enteroenterostomy and gastroenterostomy were examined and found patulous. At no portion were the intestines collapsed or unduly distended. The abdomen was closed by through-and-through sutures of silkworm gut.

17th. Much vomiting.

19th. No vomiting.

29th. Stitches removed; wound healed without inflammation.

November 2d. Patient allowed to sit up in a chair; no vomiting; feels strong.

9th. Patient walking about.

13th. Discharged.

The patient was home for ten days, when she again began to vomit as before, in the morning bile, later in the day particles of food; would vomit two or three times every day.

On readmission the patient's nutrition is good. On abdomen two scars of former operations; slight distention of the stomach.

The fifth operation was performed December 7, 1903. An incision seven inches long was made dissecting out the last cicatrix, peritoneum opened, and many adhesions found between intestines and under-surface of incision. Universal adhesions were present throughout the intestinal canal; these were carefully dissected free and two holes in the intestine, which were accidentally made, were closed by sutures of silk. Abdomen was filled with salt solution and the wound closed by through-and-through sutures of silkworm gut.

January 19, 1904. Patient apparently entirely well.

This unfortunate woman has, therefore, undergone five operations, one after the other, for the relief of severe vomiting. An enteroenterostomy and occlusion of the pylorus have both failed to relieve her condition. The etherization in each operation has been easy of accomplishment. Every cause for vicious circle or for jejunal reflux seems to have been eliminated, except the influence of adhesions, which have been met at each operation. The patient gained in weight, even while vomiting, indicating that the digestive power was unimpaired.

From this case and two former ones requiring reoperation I must believe that the formation of adhesions plays the chief part in favoring severe vomiting, by the inhibition of the normal peristalsis and the retention of the bile and pancreatic secretions in the loop of the afferent limb of the jejunum. This limb must be a loop, as we cannot make a rigid tube from the duodenum to the entero-anastomosis, and in the absence of sufficient muscular tone or the presence of obstructing adhesions the secretions must accumulate. The effect of food, the exciting agent of the flow of these secretions, causing vomiting an hour or so after eating, also would seem to indicate the influence of retained secretions. The sagging of the jejunum from the weight of the secretions dragging upon the efferent loop may also have an influence upon the stomach.

My future procedure will be to perform the posterior method of anastomosis or the Roux Y operation, and in the event of vomiting following the former method I will reoperate, divide the afferent limb just below the stomach, and implant it, as in the Roux Y, into the efferent limb some 10 or 15 cm. (four or six inches) below the stomach, closing the shallow sac above close to the anastomotic opening.

The after-treatment of a patient upon whom gastroenterostomy has been performed is of the greatest importance. Shock, vomiting, and pneumonia should be guarded against at the time of operating. I use a hot-water bed, hot bottles, and a cotton jacket during the operation, and have the anæsthetic administered with the greatest care. The arms should never be folded across the chest, thereby impeding respiration.

If shock occurs the usual remedies are administered, and, above all, saline solution by the bowel, at first combined with whiskey, and later intravenously, if the condition of the patient should demand it.

Vomiting is greatly to be feared, and while I usually allow liquid food eighteen hours after the operation, the occurrence of nausea is an indication for its discontinuance, substituting rectal feeding. If vomiting does occur, the best treatment is, undoubtedly, gastric lavage, using small quantities of water at a time, 200 to 300 c.c., and giving absolutely nothing by the mouth.

Peritonitis is unavoidable if the anastomosis gives way, but by the careful use of the needle-and-thread method the danger is minimized and far less liable to happen than with the use of mechanical appliances. Upon the onset of peritonitis, a reoperation is imperatively demanded, the anastomosis strengthened, and the peritoneum washed out. If the shock does not prove fatal, such a patient should usually recover, as the infection from the fasting stomach is not of a very virulent type.

THE NERVOUS COMPLICATIONS AND SEQUELÆ OF SMALLPOX.*

By Charles J. Aldrich, M.D.,

LECTURER ON CLINICAL NEUROLOGY AND ANATOMY OF THE NERVOUS SYSTEM, COLLEGE OF PHYSICIANS AND SURGEONS, CLEVELAND; NEUROLOGIST TO THE CLEVELAND GENERAL HOSPITAL AND DISPENSARY; NEUROLOGIST TO THE CITY HOSPITAL, CLEVELAND, OHIO.

Smallpox, like other infectious diseases, may present various nervous complications and sequelæ. Indeed, almost the first effect of the variolous poison is observed in the violent frontal headache, which constantly is an early symptom. Sharply contrasted with the many other complications and sequelæ of variola, the affections of the nervous system are not strictly confined to certain stages of the disease itself, not necessarily immediately sequential, nor are they at all related to the severity of the infection. It seems that the variolous process possesses, in a marked degree, the power to awaken latent predispositions to nervous disease, as well as to independently disorder function and create anatomical alterations in the various nervous structures of the body. These affections may be gross anatomical, purely functional, or both. Many cases present a varied clinical picture, which leaves us in doubt as to the exact nature of the lesion, and until further post-mortem examinations and other investigations have bettered our present knowledge, we must be content with collecting the rare and interesting cases for the literature and for future investigations and diagnosis. These complications and sequelæ invade all possible provinces of the nervous system—the brain, spinal cord, and peripheral nerves. Truly, the nervous complications and sequelæ of this loathsome disease offer a most fruitful and little-worked field for research.

Convulsions are often seen in children, and usually precede the eruption. They are mentioned by Trousseau,[1] who endorses the belief of Sydenham,[2] that they possess diagnostic value, especially in the young. Sydenham[3] states that convulsions occur more frequently in smallpox than in any of the xanthematous diseases.

Smallpox often exerts a profound effect upon the pysche.

In order of frequency, as a cause of the febrile deliria and psychoses, smallpox is placed sixth by Berkley.[4] Kraeplin,[5] who is, perhaps, the greatest authority upon this subject, also places variola in the same causative relation.

We may recognize at least four types:

1. Initial delirium.
2. Febrile delirium.

* Read before the Clinical and Pathological Section of the Cleveland Academy of Medicine, October 2, 1903.

3. Collapse or exhaustion delirium.
4. True postvariolous insanity.

The occurrence of initial delirium is quite constant, usually appearing toward the evening of the second or third day; the mind wanders, the speech becomes incoherent, and a true confusional condition develops. Throughout the attack there is much sleeplessness and great disquietude. . This delirium differs entirely from that with specifically colored delusions and accompanied by tremors, the delirium alcoholicum, which commonly occurs in inebriates attacked by smallpox.

Seppilli and Maragliano[6] reported three cases of acute mania occurring in smallpox. Two recovered and one remained incurably insane. Trousseau[7] referred to the case of a woman who was seized with an acute mania during the progress of a mild attack of smallpox. She had never before shown any symptoms of mental disturbance. Corlett[8] records the occurrence of an acute mania in the course of a discrete smallpox. The sufferer remained violently insane for six days, when death came.

Grave changes in the mental state, with peculiar speech disturbances, have been observed to follow variola by Welch,[9] Westphal,[10] Otto,[11] Foville,[12] Jaccoud,[13] Riva,[14] Quinquaud,[15] Leudet,[16] Whipham and Myers,[17] Pforzheim,[18] Béhier and Lionville,[19] Long,[20] the writer,[21] and others. These mental changes seem to be a part of widespread changes in the nervous system, and yet sufficiently uniform in their symptom groups and their pathological pictures to deserve separate and detailed description, which will be given later, in connection with two personally observed cases.

The occurrence of true dementia paralytica has been observed to follow variola by Mabille[22] and others. In fact, the writings of Hoppe,[23] Lagardelle,[24] Berthier,[25] Kiernan,[26] and many lesser known observers show that smallpox is a fruitful cause of mental alienation.

Meningitis, fortunately, is a rare complication. It is usually purulent, and probably a metastasis from the skin lesions. Gregory[27] states that it is most liable to occur in children and during the period of suppuration and beginning desiccation.

Reiner[28] has recorded a severe meningitis of the convexity occurring as a variolous complication.

The occurrence of paralysis in smallpox has been commented upon since that exanthem's history passed from tradition to record. Indeed, literature bears out the statement of Landouzy,[29] that "of all the eruptive fevers smallpox is, without contradiction, the one in which paralysis most frequently occurs, either at the onset, in the course of, or at the decline." How frequently it occurs, unfortunately, we have no means of ascertaining. That smallpox is less liable to cause the complication than typhoid fever seems to be the opinion of Landouzy,[30] but from a limited personal observation and an extensive search of the literature, I question the statement.

The nature, origin, and seat of the various paralytic affections attending and consequent to variolá are so varied that classification is most difficult. That they may originate in the brain, spinal cord, or peripheral nerves is certain. It is also positive that we may have a combination of two or more of these forms.

Paralysis may occur at the very onset of the infection, at any time during its course, or at any period of convalescence.

The majority of the paralytic affections are, as in other acute infections, of neuritic origin. Landouzy[31] believed that paraplegia was most frequent. I believe, however, that he included the cases of brachial paraplegia, as well as the crural monoplegias, in his consideration. Rejecting these as most likely peripheral neuritides, we place paraplegia of spinal origin farther down in the list of nervous complications and sequelæ of variola.

All are agreed upon the rather fortunate outcome of most of the paralyses of variola.

E. Wagner[32] has observed, on post-mortem examination, evidences of localized non-purulent encephalic disease. And that we may have a non-purulent meningoencephalitis of a simple character complicating variola, I believe, the first case to be reported in this paper will fully demonstrate.

Areas of simple softening and blood extravasations may occur in the brain and produce aphasia, monoplegia, or hemiplegia. According to Immermann,[33] such lesions may remain latent throughout life and be discovered only at autopsy.

Reiner,[34] Landouzy,[35] Edes,[36] Osler,[37] and many other writers mention and some relate personally observed variolous hemiplegias, but if the meagreness of the literature is an index of their infrequency, then they are rare, indeed.

Clinicians have long been aware of the relative frequency of cord affections in variola. The severity of the infection appears to have little to do with their occurrence, since they appear to develop with equal frequency in varioloid. The observed cases have been usually paraplegia, of the motor type, developing in any stage of the disease from the prodromal to a far-reaching period of convalescence. Leroy d'Etiolles[38] has recorded the occurrence of such affections in the stage of incubation before the proper beginning of the variola.

Trousseau[39] observed in cases where severe lumbar pain was complained of in the initial stage that a slight degree of paraplegia was often present. It was manifested by subjective numbness, tenderness, and loss of power. Occasionally the bladder was involved, producing difficult micturition and occasional retention. These symptoms usually disappeared with the appearance of the eruption, but in rare cases remained to the middle of the second week.

Henderson,[40] Westphal,[41] Kahler and Pick,[42] and others state that rarely acute ataxias have been observed to follow variola. It is quite probable that these cases of ataxia are ataxic forms of neuritis, although many of the cases of pseudomultiple scleroses manifested some ataxia. Henderson's[43] case of postvariolous ataxia presented numbness and tingling of the legs and hands. The skin reflexes and deep tendon reactions were all absent. The patient later recovered his power and station. In the discussion which followed Dr. Henderson's report, Dr. Whipham[44] referred to two similar cases, which, I presume, are embraced in the report of Whipham and Myers.[45] These cases have been looked upon as pseudotabes, the so-called ataxia variolique, but more likely belong to a class of disseminated focal inflammations scattered throughout the brain and spinal cord.

Peter Marie,[46] Sottas,[47] Long,[48] Charcot,[49] and others have observed typical examples of disseminated sclerosis following smallpox. The case of Sottas is quite typical, but it appears from the reports of most of these cases that, while for a time they presented an array of symptoms much like true disseminated sclerosis, they later slowly grew better, thus making a marked departure from the ordinarily progressive course of that disease.

Enough knowledge of the pathological changes has been found at the root of the disorder to demonstrate that we have disseminated encephalomyelitis which, although followed by a sequential sclerosis, has little or no tendency to extend or multiply itself. This subject will again be adverted to.

Westphal[50] recorded a case which was followed by paralysis of the legs and bladder that was due to disseminated foci of inflammation involving the gray and white matter of the spinal cord. Foci of softening in the structures of the cord have been described by Damaschino[51] and Joffroy,[52] Hayem[53] and Landouzy.[54]

Fiessinger[55] remarked the occurrence of acute myelitis appearing as a complication and disappearing with the disease.

Steven Mackenzie[56] has reported a case of poliomyelitis anterior as a sequel of variola. Damaschino and Roger[57] and Landouzy[58] record acute monoplegias in children presenting the clinical picture of acute inflammation of the cells of the anterior horns of the cord.

Although Huchard[59] observed not more than ten paraplegias in 2000 patients affected by smallpox, yet Landouzy[60] states that paraplegia is the most frequent form of variolous palsy.

A rapidly ascending myelitis presenting clinical symptoms of Landry's paralysis has been recorded by a number of authors: Marinesco and Oettinger,[61] Gubler,[62] Leyden,[63] Gros,[64] Chalvet,[65] Marie,[66] Bernhardt,[67] Gros and Beauvais.[68] These cases, as a rule, are rapidly fatal.

F. W. Goss[69] observed a typical case of acute ascending paralysis occurring early in a mild varioloid. It proved so quickly fatal that the patient died four days after the first paralytic symptoms.

Dr. M. Friedrich[70] personally related to me the details of a rapidly fatal case of undoubted ascending or Landry's paralysis, appearing in the stage of desquamation in a comparatively mild case of smallpox during our late epidemic in Cleveland.

It would appear from Oettinger and Marinesco[71] that the pathological picture of Landry's paralysis may exist in variola in combination with the disseminated myelitis described by Westphal. Indeed, a recent communication appears to have firmly established this fact.

Cases have been described by Vulpian[72] and others of acute ascending paralysis from variola in which a most careful search failed to show a myelitis. It seems reasonable to believe that these cases are polyneuritic in origin.

A careful examination of the literature convinces me that we have occurring as a complication or sequel of smallpox a disseminated encephalomyelitis, which possesses clinical features and pathological changes clearly entitling it to be recognized as a clinical entity, and which occurs with sufficient frequency to demand our special consideration and study. It occurs in other infectious diseases, as the case reported by Ebstein[73] conclusively proves. Ebstein's case is quoted particularly because it complicated typhoid fever and the symptom-complex was identical with that of the variolous cases, and the post-mortem disclosures were more complete and in keeping with the clinical findings.

I believe that these cases have in time past been described as and believed to be the disease which was named by Charcot disseminated sclerosis. Some of the reported cases bear a very close resemblance, but the majority are but coarse imitations. In this connection it is not thought wise to discuss the pros and cons of the question, but to report two personal observations.

I have been able to find fifteen cases in the literature, all presenting:

1. More or less ataxia in the four extremities, usually most marked in the legs.
2. Slowness and awkwardness of movement.
3. Slow, monotonous, explosive manner of speaking.
4. Faulty articulation.
5. A varying degree of mental degradation.
6. A decided tendency toward recovery.

The following personal observations are added to the literature:

To the courtesy of Dr. Martin Friedrich I am indebted for the privilege of examining and reporting this case:

Case I.—E. L., male, white, aged thirteen years, was normally born in the United States, and of German parents. He had never suffered any severe illness and was considered a large, well-developed boy. His father and mother are strong, healthy people, each giving a good family history. There are four other children in the family, all of whom are well. There have been no deaths in the family, nor history of miscarriages or stillbirths.

Edward was taken sick the last of June, 1902. The family attendant, Dr. Christian Sihler, was called and found the boy's temperature to be 103° F., from which it shortly rose to 104.5° F. Nothing could be found to account for the temperature, and because of numerous cases in the neighborhood, smallpox was suspected. On the fourth day an eruption appeared, and Dr. Martin Friedrich was called in consultation and made the diagnosis of discrete smallpox.

The temperature immediately fell on the development of the eruption, but little secondary fever developed, and the boy was not thought to be very ill. There had been no convulsions or other disturbances of the nervous system, either in the prodromal period or immediately following the eruption. He was sent to the Detention Hospital, where, for the first ten days, he was at no time confined to bed. He ate well, slept well, and did not complain. During the first week in the hospital an abscess developed on the right leg, which, although quite large, caused him little discomfort. He was homesick and anxious to go home, but was put off from time to time and felt very badly about the delay. On July 15th, and on the thirteenth day of his residence in the hospital, his father came to take him home, when the boy was discovered lying on the bed in a stupid condition and could not be aroused. It was thought, perhaps, that he was soundly sleeping, and the father went home without him. The attendant, failing to arouse the boy, informed Dr. Friedrich of his condition, who finally succeeded in awakening him, telling him to undress and get into bed. The boy recalls this and also that the nurse helped him to remove his clothing.

Dr. Friedrich states that his breathing was normal, but the pulse was very slow; the body was limp, with diminution of the reflexes. There were no changes in the pupils. The boy appeared dazed and his speech was slow and hesitating. The next day he was taken home. The stupor continued without any additional symptoms, except the advent of a temperature of 103.5° F. The abscess had been opened several days before this time and was discharging freely, but giving no pain. He remained in a stupor for a period of four or five days, during which time it was almost impossible to feed him; attempts to swallow were accompanied by choking, and it was necessary to feed him liquids with a spoon. From the hesitating speech he passed into a condition of complete aphasia, at the end of four days being unable to speak a word. The neck was stiff and the head slightly retracted; pulse very slow, rarely going above 60. There were no signs of ocular or other paralyses. The pupils were equal, of normal size, but reacted very slowly to various stimuli. The nose, larynx, and retinæ were carefully examined by Drs. Friedrich and Lenker and nothing abnormal discovered. No signs of thoracic or abdominal disease could be demonstrated.

His temperature continued irregularly elevated for a period of two weeks. His aphasia remained complete during this time, but he seemed able to understand everything that was said to him; could read print and writing, but he was not asked to attempt writing. There was no numbness, or paræsthesia, or loss of sensation. Before his aphasia became marked he complained bitterly of headache, and later, for a period of two weeks, by gestures continued to attempt to convey to his attendants the idea that the ache continued. If he attempted to get up on his feet he would fall, and he also fell out of bed and was unable to get up when down. After he was up and about his gait was markedly ataxic; he staggered like one intoxicated.

He cried a great deal, especially at the end of the second week, and seemed to be very much excited because he could not make his attendants understand what he wanted. Discovering that he cried because of hunger, his attendants began to feed him, when he developed almost a mania for food; would eat until they were afraid to feed him so much, and then shriek with rage and disappointment because he was not given more.

He was aphasic for a period of five weeks, and when speech returned by slow degrees it was distinctly scanning, slow, and thick. His parents relate that he was very much irritated by the presence of other children in the room and would usually order them out, speaking in a manner that was illustrated by the mother as follows: "You-u g-get r-i-i-ght o-u-ut—of-dis- ro-o-o-m—he-e-r-r"—this being the first formula which he seemed able to enunciate. The parents' and physician's account of this peculiar enunciation fits the apt description of Westphal, who said his patient's words came out as though each syllable was "squeezed out." His speech seemed to return rather rapidly; in fact, he soon insisted upon talking most of the time, but it was very hard to understand him, because of his enunciation being so thick, slow, and scanning.

I examined him in the following November: He is a large, well-developed boy, with hydrocephalic type of head. His eyes are prominent, pupils wide, vision normal; no nystagmus, ocular palsies, or pupillary disturbance; palpebral apertures are wide, showing the sclera above the cornea. His gait is peculiar. He walks like a boy who has on a pair of shoes that are too small for him. His station is not good. His parents state that if he receives a slight push he is unable to recover himself and falls. Knee-jerks are quick, no ankle clonus, no Babinski's sign. Left wrist-jerk and elbow-jerks are more marked than the right. His left hand is the seat of a peculiar movement resembling very closely an athetosis; this is particularly marked while walking. Indeed, his gait is worthy of attention and study. The legs are brought forward awkwardly and stiffly; the toes of both feet turn in, which his parents assure me was not the case previous to his illness. The toe of the left shoe is worn more than the right, and it is believed, when not on exhibition, that he drags this foot a little. The right hand hangs normally at his side, while the left is held partially behind him, the palm directed backward and on a line with the middle of the thigh, and at every step is the seat of a distinct athetoid movement involving the wrist and fingers. His parents inform me that this peculiar movement of the hand is often present while sitting still. All characteristics of chorea are absent, and I believe the movement to be an uncontrollable or athetoid movement consequent upon pathological alterations of the brain cells. He occasionally complains of headache.

There are now but few pits to be seen upon the face or body, and in a few months little will remain to show that he has suffered from smallpox. The only evidence of his aphasia at present is a certain thickness of speech and a tendency to stumble over syllables; in fact, he stumbles over the syllables in "United Irish Constabulary" as badly as a well-developed case of paresis. There appears to be, however, a slow and continuous improvement. His parents say that he seems to be as bright in school as before, but that his disposition has changed; that he is cranky and irritable. His father states that when children tease him about his tripping speech he weeps, "instead of punching them," as he formerly did when plagued.

There are some rather novel features in this case; some, indeed, suggesting hysteria; and were it not for the slow pulse, high temperature, and bulbar symptoms, one would be justified in suspecting a neurosis. The headache, slow pulse, and stupor point to an intracerebral pressure, probably due to a simple effusion. Assuming an intracerebral pressure, we have an explanation of the bulbar symptoms.

The aphasia, which was complete, and has left its mark in a halting speech, and an athetosis, point to an undoubted lesion of cerebral tissue, possibly hemorrhagic, or to areas of localized softening. The spinal symptoms of the case are as clearly marked as in Westphal's cases, and the clinical ensemble is certainly of that type.

Case II.—A healthy young woman was taken sick with smallpox the last of May, 1902, and was removed to the Detention Hospital. While there she was under the care of Drs. A. B. Spurney and M. Friedrich, to whose courtesy I am indebted for most of the data of the case. She had a good family history and had been quite healthy herself, with the exception of frequent attacks of night terrors, which still continue.

After the usual prodromal symptoms the eruption appeared at about the fifth day, and, although discrete, was widely disseminated and the pocks large and close together. The secondary fever was not high, but the third day following the eruption she became very delirious. The delirium was not entirely characteristic of the ordinary febrile delirium, since it largely partook of the type of religious mania. Shortly after this delirium manifested itself she lost her speech, swallowing became difficult, and she lay helpless in bed; all four extremities were limp and perfectly useless. The urine and feces passed uncontrolled into the bed. Dr. Spurney states that the deep reflexes were absent at this time. Quite a number of abscesses developed, some of which persisted long into her convalescence. Her speech was almost entirely absent for a period of over three weeks, when it began to slowly return and had the same characteristics of the preceding case.

It was found when she was able to get out of bed that she was markedly ataxic, so much so that she reeled and staggered like a drunken person, and continued to do so for a period of about three months. The speech gradually returned, but her mental degradation was marked and interesting. She appeared and acted like an imbecile. She did not know enough to go to bed, but when sent to her room would lie down on the floor. She did not even know enough to dress herself, and had to be watched closely to prevent her undressing in public. She remained practically in this condition for two months, when a slight improvement began and continued progressively until one day, while in the chapel at prayers, she seemed to rather suddenly acquire her orientation, and from then on began to gain so rapidly that one month later she was able to go out to the Smallpox Hospital in Newburg and aid in the care of patients. Her improvement has been steady since then, and at the present time she has practically recovered all her faculties.

Examination. A recent examination reveals practically nothing, except, perhaps, a slight increase of the knee-jerks, a little slowness and tendency to syllabication of words. Her gait is not as good as before; a slight ataxic condition still obtains. The special senses are normal.

There seems to be evidence that peripheral neuritis occurs in smallpox with greater frequency than heretofore believed. It was formerly supposed that the few cases observed were of very limited extent and probably related to gross anatomical lesions of contiguous structures. Postvariolous paralysis of the soft palate and structures of the pharynx quite similar to the more frequent diphtheritic affections of those parts have been noted by Curschmann,[74] Leyden,[75] and others.

Combemale[76] has collected ten cases of peripheral neuritis occurring as complications or sequelæ of variola. In all of his cases some speech disorder was remarked, which he evidently believed to be due to palatal paralysis, or paralysis, or ataxia of the organs of phonation. Limited cutaneous anæsthesia and paralysis of single muscles, like the case of paralysis of the deltoid reported by Curschmann,[77] may rarely occur, and are certainly due to peripheral neuritis. Of great interest in this connection is the case of serratus magnus paralysis occurring during a variola observed by James J. Putnam.[78] This was undoubtedly due to a neuritis of the posterior thoracic nerve. Atrophy followed, and there was no recovery.

Vulpian[79] reported a case of paralysis and anæsthesia of the right circumflex, with weakness in the distribution of the same nerve on the opposite side.

. Hitzig[80] has observed a case of double brachial neuralgia, with considerable loss of power; also neuralgia of one arm and shoulder, followed by paralysis of the deltoid alone. All of these cases appeared too early in the disease to be attributed to exhaustion or pressure from decubitus.

Eulenberg[81] has reported a case of partial paralysis of the left facial and both median nerves. The electrical reactions were little changed and recovery ensued.

Rosenblatt's[82] case of crural monoplegia was undoubtedly of peripheral origin, and, as before stated, it is my belief that Charcot's case of right brachial monoplegia, followed by permanent atrophy of the muscles, was also peripheral neuritis.

I find but one case of multiple neuritis following variola in which a post-mortem examination demonstrated conclusively the correctness of the diagnosis; it is reported by P. Grocco,[83] of Milan. The patient, a young man, six weeks after convalescing from smallpox developed all the symptoms of a multiple neuritis, later pneumonia, and finally died.

Gower[84] mentions a case of polyneuritis following varioloid. The patient died of pneumonia six months later, and the purely neuritic character of the paralysis and atrophy was demonstrated. Since he gives no reference to this case, I believe it to be the one reported by Grocco.

Joffroy[85] observed a patient who, while convalescing from a grave confluent smallpox, developed violent pains in the left arm and shoulder, which was followed by loss of power and muscular atrophy. Pulmonary tuberculosis supervened; the patient died, and a careful pathological and histological examination revealed a parenchymatous neuritis.

Charcot[86] has recorded a case of atrophy involving the muscles of the right arm consecutive to smallpox. It is possible that this case was a brachial plexus neuritis. Rosenthal,[87] of Vienna, reported a case of true progressive atrophy that appeared six weeks sequential to variola.

Indeed, the variolous poison or the combined infections which are so violently manifested in this disease may produce disturbed functions and actual degeneration of any part of the nervous system.

Functional nerve disturbances are not uncommon sequelæ to smallpox. They are commonly severe and persistent, but usually recover.

Epilepsy following variola has been mentioned by Bierlingus[88] as early as 1679.

Osler[89] states that rarely epilepsy appears during convalescence from smallpox.

H. E. Armstrong[90] relates a case of "catalepsy," with waxy mobility and afterward rigidity of the limbs and continuance of consciousness, followed by ecstasy, passing into obscene delirium," finally terminating in unconsciousness and death. The patient was a woman, aged twenty-four years, and in the tenth day of a severe variola, with confluent, crystalline eruption.

Dreyfus-Brisac[91] observed an hysterical hemiplegia and hemianæsthesia of the right side disappear at the time of the efflorescence of a varioloid.

To illustrate the profound effects which smallpox may exert in the production of neurasthenia, the following case is related:

CASE III.—W. S., an unmarried policeman, born in the United States thirty-two years ago, gives a good family history, excepting the pertinent fact that he was born when his parents were at an advanced age. He states that his mother was fifty-four years old and his father sixty-four years old at the time of his birth. The patient suffered a sunstroke at sixteen years, and from that time has been troubled with frequent headaches. He says that while he has been physically strong, yet has had little endurance. He experienced a severe attack of measles at twenty-two years, and at twenty-eight years a violent attack of *la grippe*, and since has been visited by yearly attacks of the affection at about the same time each year.

Three and one-half years ago he suffered a violent attack of confluent smallpox, and is very badly pitted as a result. He was completely disabled for two months and then returned to light duty, but caught cold and was laid up two months longer, suffering at this time rheumatic pains and remaining unexplainably weak. He again returned to work, when he suffered further relapse of pain and weakness and general indisposition. From then until two years ago, when the final collapse came, he was rarely able to be on light duty more than a week at a time. Shortly before this collapse he had an attack of severe pain in the left upper chest, which extended down the arm to the tips of the fingers and also across the chest. He suffered from several like attacks, but has had none during the past year. At the time of these attacks he was using a large amount of tobacco, but has not used any during the past year. He dates his complete disability to a time when on his "beat" he was seized with a sudden, unreasoning, and uncontrollable fear—a fear that he was going to die, or something terrible was about to take place. He immediately collapsed and was taken home in a carriage, since which time he has been completely disabled. He began losing flesh, became afraid to walk on the street, was unable to ride on the street car. He waxed irritable, restless, and sleepless; hands became unsteady and trembled, gait became reeling, and heart palpitated violently on exertion, and, in fact, without exertion. His condition became so pitiable and his emaciation so extreme that the medical police official and the medical head of the Health Department in the city in which he was an officer decided that he was permanently and totally disabled. He was retired and placed on the pension roll for life.

EXAMINATION. The patient is a strongly built man, and has so far recovered his former weight that he now registers 175 pounds, instead of 130 pounds, at which weight he was retired. His complexion is florid, hair reddish-brown, and face deeply pitted from smallpox. He is extremely nervous and walks with a peculiar, uncertain, reeling gait, typically and picturesquely neurasthenic. His ears are well placed, eyes on a level, features symmetrical, tongue protruded straight, palate highly arched, with torus; palpebral aperture on the left slightly larger than the right, and the pupil of the right eye is slightly smaller than the left. There is no nystagmus, and, to rough test, no ocular palsies. The pupils react to light and accommodation and consensually. The patient states that, although his vision is good, when he reads a short time he becomes mentally confused. He is slightly short-sighted. Knee-jerks rather weak, but equal; wrist-jerks are normal; a slight jaw-jerk is present. No Romberg. Although he reels in walking, it is not a true ataxia. He appears weak in the knees. The hand grasps are interesting. The right at first registers seventy-five, second attempt sixty, third sixty, fourth fifty-five, fifth and sixth attempts fifty. After an interval of about three minutes the best he can do is fifty-five. The heart muscle is normal; pulse rapid. Thoracic and abdominal viscera normal; urinary examination negative.

Among the functional disturbances we are, perhaps, warranted in placing the isolated cases of diabetes mellitus observed and reported by Freiberg,[92] v. Frerichs,[93] and others.

The occurrence of aphasia, with or without associated paralysis as a complication and as a sequel of smallpox, has been observed. Arnaud,[94] Combemale,[95] Saint-Phillippe,[96] Jaccoud,[97] Curschmann,[98] and Myers and Whipham[99] have reported such cases. Whether these aphasias are due, when alone, to actual destruction of the brain tissue is doubtful; that they are purely functional exhaustion or intoxication of the cortical cells of the speech centres seems more probable. Breganze's[100] case of aphasia, which occurred at the height of a variola and was complete until he made a single application of electricity, when speech returned, but remained stammering, is both puzzling and unique. He considered the loss of speech due to a cerebral atony from exhaustion of the nutrition of the cells. Notwithstanding the behavior of the speech in returning very like hysteria, we must consider the vocal halt which remained as confirmatory to his idea of its pathology, adding, perhaps, to his hypothesis the suggestion of a toxic exhaustion of the cells of the cortex presiding over emissive speech.

The following personally observed instance of aphasia in an otherwise uncomplicated case of smallpox in a boy, aged seven years, was recently reported at length:[101]

CASE IV.—E. M., white, was born in the United States, and possesses a good personal and family history. When first seen he had a temperature of 103.5° F., some coryza, a slight diarrhœa, and had vomited. There was no history of exposure to acute infectious disease, and, being informed by the parents that the child had been eating a large amount of sweets on the preceding day, I took the case to be a gastrointestinal disturbance, and treated it accordingly. On the following day the child suddenly went into violent convulsions and was more or less convulsed for an hour. The temperature was 103.8° F.; on the next day the temperature remained above 103° F., the child was stuporous, with a coated tongue and flushed face. The respiration was regular. The neck was slightly rigid, but no Kernig's sign was present. There was no rash upon the body, nor could the most careful examination disclose other signs of disease. He was thought to be in a state of meningismus of gastrointestinal origin. His condition remained unchanged, running a temperature of from 103° F., to 105° F., until the morning of the fourth day, when the characteristic eruption of smallpox appeared upon the face and calves of the legs. The eruption was discrete, frank, and classical. The temperature immediately fell and the child became conscious, but it was observed that he did not talk. He appeared to understand, but could not or would not speak. A very slight secondary fever followed, and the patient made an uninterrupted recovery. For a period of over three months the child never spoke a word. He seemed to have forgotten all the language he had ever learned. His hearing was perfect; the movements of his tongue, palate, and vocal cords were normal. He learned readily enough, and in the course of six months was speaking with almost as much fluency as before. It was impossible for obvious reasons to classify his aphasia.

BIBLIOGRAPHY.

1. Trousseau. Clinical Medicine, 1873, vol. i. p. 65.
2. Sydenham. Works of Thomas Sydenham, 1848, vol. ii. p. 252.
3. Sydenham. Quoted by Trousseau, loc. cit.
4. Berkley. Mental Diseases, New York, 1900, p. 338.
5. Kraeplin. Einfluss acuter Krankheiten, etc., Archiv f. Psych. u. Nervenkr., 1882.
6. Seppilli and Maragliano. Della Influenza del Vajuolo sulla Pazzia, Milano, 1878.
7. Trousseau. Quoted by Corlett. A Treatise on the Acute Infectious Exanthemata, Philadelphia, 1901, p. 66.
8. Corlett. A Treatise on the Acute Infectious Exanthemata, Philadelphia, 1901, p. 66.
9. Welch, Wm. M. American System of the Practice of Medicine, Philadelphia, 1897, vol. i. p. 540.
10. Westphal. Ueber eine Nervenaffektion nach Pocken, eine eigenthümliche Sprachstörung und Ataxie der Extremitäten zur Folge habend. Verhandl. d. Berl. med. Gesellsch. (1869–71), 1872, vol. iii. pp. 170–172.
11. Otto. Allgemeine Zeitsch. f. Psych., 1872–73, Band xxix. pp. 335–356.
12. Foville, S. Achille. Ann. méd. psych., 1873, p. 40.
13. Jaccoud, S. Sur un cas d'ataxie verbale suite de variole, Leçons de clinique méd, 1884–85, Paris, 1886, pp. 305–321.
14. Riva, Gaetano. Alterazioni gravi dei centri nervosi consecutive a variolo, Annali univ. di med., Milano, 1873, vol. ccxxiii. pp. 294–299.
15. Quinquaud, E. Sur quelques troubles nerveux consécutifs à la variole (fausse ataxie), l'Encéphale, Paris, 1884, pp. 33–47.
16. Leudet. Arch. gén. de méd., 1881, p. 641.

17. Whipham and Myers. Transactions of Clinical Society of London, 1886, vol. xix. p. 164.
18. Pforzheim. Schmidt's Jahrbücher, 1878, No. 1.
19. Béhier and Lionville. Sur les paralysies consécutives à quelques maladies aiguës, Thèse de Bailly, Paris, 1872.
20. Long. Landouzy, Des paralysies dans les maladies aiguës, Paris, 1880, p. 185.
21. Aldrich. Aphasia in Acute Disease, with Report of a Case Complicating Smallpox. The American Journal of the Medical Sciences, March, 1903.
22. Mabille. Démence paralytique à la suite d'une variole, Ann. méd.-psych., Paris, 1883, 6 S., vol. x. pp. 226-227.
23. Hoppe, A. Ueber Psychose nach Variolois, Greifswald, 1874.
24. Lagardelle. La variole et aliénation mentale pendant la guerre, Moulins, 1872.
25. Berthier. De l'influence de la variole sur l'aliénation mental, Gaz. méd. de Lyon, 1860, vol. xii. p. 465.
26. Kiernan, J. G. Variola and Insanity, Amer. Journ. Neurol. and Psychiat., New York, 1883, vol. ii. p. 365.
27. Gregory. Vorlesungen über die Ausschalgs-fieber (German by Helfft), Leipzig, 1845.
28. Reiner. Variola; meningitis convexitatis, Jahrb. f. Kinderk., Leipzig, 1876, x. p. 29.
29. Landouzy. Loc. cit., p. 174.
30. Landouzy. Loc. cit., p. 174.
31. Landouzy. Loc. cit., p. 177.
32. Wagner. Archiv der Heilkunde, 1872, Bd. xiii., S. 107 ff.
33. Immermann, H. Nothnagel's Encyclopedia of Practical Medicine, Amer. ed., 1902, p. 93.
34. Reiner. Variola vera; Apoplexia cerebri, loc. cit., pp. 25-27.
35. Landouzy. Loc. cit., p. 178.
36. Edes. A System of Practical Medicine, Philadelphia, 1886, vol. v.
37. Osler. Practice of Medicine, New York, 1895, 2d ed., p. 59.
38. Leroy d'Étiolles. Des Paralysies de membres inférieures, etc., Paris, 1856, T. ii. p. 93, ss.
39. Trousseau. Clinique de l'Hôtel-Dieu, T. i. p. 4.
40. Henderson, G. C. Lancet, London, December 24, 1881, p. 1089.
41. Westphal. Ueber eine Nervenaffektion nach Pocken, eine eigenthümliche Sprachstörung und Ataxia der Extremitäten zur Folge habend. Verhandl. d. Berl. med. Gesellsch. (1869-71), 1872, vol. iii. pp. 170-172; Archiv f. Psychiatrie und Nervenkrankheiten, Bd. iv. S 335 ff.; and Ueber Nerven affectionen nach Pocken, Berliner klin. Woch., 1872, No. 1; also Ueber eine Rückenmarkserkrankheit bei Paraplegie nach Pocken, ibid., No. 47.
42. Kahler and Pick. Ueber ataxie und ataxie nach acuten erkrankungen, Prager Viertel-jahrschrift f. d. Prakt. Heilkund, 1879.
43. Henderson. Loc. cit.
44. Whipham. Lancet, London, December 24, 1881, p. 1089.
45. Whipham and Myers. Loc. cit.
46. Marie, P. Sclerose en plaques et maladies infectieuses, Progrès méd, 1884, vol. xii.
47. Sottas. Un cas de sclerose en plaques dans la convalescence de la variole, Gaz. des Hôp. Avril 12, 1892, p. 405.
48. Long, quoted by Gower. Diseases of the Nervous System, Philadelphia, 1893, vol. ii. p. 898.
49. Charcot, quoted by Gower. Ibid.
50. Westphal. Ueber eine Rückenmarkserkrankheit bei Paraplegie nach Pocken, Berliner klin. Woch., 1872; No. 47.
51. Damaschino, quoted by Gower, loc. cit.
52. Joffroy. Ibid.
53. Hayem. Ibid.
54. Landouzy. Loc. cit., p. 182.
55. Fiessinger. La myelite aiguë curable dans la variole, Méd. mod., Paris, 1898, vol. ix. p. 341.
56. Mackenzie, Steven. Quoted by Corlett, loc. cit., p. 67.
57. Damaschino and Roger. Recherches anatomo-pathologiques sur la paralysie spinale de l'enfance, Gaz. méd. de Paris, 1871, p. 505.
58. Landouzy. Loc. cit., p. 184.
59. Huchard. Quoted by Landouzy, loc. cit., p. 174.
60. Landouzy. Loc. cit., p. 175.
61. Marinesco and Oettinger. Semaine médicale, 1895, No. 6.
62. Gubler. Archives générales de médecine, 1860, T. i. p. 537, ss.
63. Leyden. Klinik der Rückenmarkskrankheiten, Bd. ii. S. 201, ff.
64. Gros. De quelques accidents nerveux compliquaint la variolie et la varioloïde, Alger méd., 1883, vol. xi. pp. 328, 353.

65. Chalvet. Gaz. des hôpitaux, 1871, Nr. 93: also Paralysie ascendante aigué, Thèse de Paris, 1871,
66. Marie, P. Loc. cit.
67. Bernhardt. Berliner klin. Wochensch., 1871, No. 47, S. 561, ff.
68. Gros and Beauvais. L'Un. méd., 1894, No. 131.
69. Goss, F. W. Boston Med. and Surg. Journ., vol. lxxxviii. p. 464.
70. Friedrich, M. Personal communication.
71. Oettinger and Marinesco. Loc. cit.
72. Vulpian. Arch. de physiologie normale et pathologique, January, 1873.
73. Ebstein, W. Deuts. Arch. f. klin. Med., 1872, vol. ix. 528; vol. x. p. 595.
74. Curschmann. Wiesbadener Congress fur innere Medicin, 1886, S. 469, ff.
75. Leyden. Loc. cit.
76. Combemale. Archives générales de médecine, June, 1892.
77. Curschmann. Loc. cit.
78. Putnam, James J. Nervous Disorders Occurring during Variola. Boston Med. and Surg. Journ., vol. lxxxix. p. 125.
79. Vulpian. Analyse du mémoire de Westphal, in Arch. de physiologie, 1873, p. 95.
80. Hitzig. Quoted by Putnam, loc. cit., p. 127.
81. Eulenberg. Functionelle Nervenkrankheiten, Berlin, 1871.
82. Rosenblatt, E. Porazénie miesni podudzia prawego po,ospie (Paralysis of the Muscles of the Leg after Smallpox), Przegl. lek. Kranków, 1883, vol. xxii. p. 521.
83. Grocco, P. Milano, Centralbl. f. med Wissen., 1885, p. 693.
84. Gower. Diseases of Nervous System, third edition, Philadelphia, 1899, vol. i. p. 148.
85. Joffroy. Obs. II., du mémoire de Joffroy. De la névrite parenchymateuse spontanée, Arch. de Physiol., 1879, No. 2, p. 177.
86. Charcot. Amyotrophie du membre superieur droit consécutive à la Variole chez un fellah, N., incog. de la Salpêtrière, Paris, 1898, vol. xi. p. 57.
87. Rosenthal. Nervenkrankheiten, Erlangen, 1870.
88. Bierlingus. Epilepsia et paralysis ex variolis Advers. curios. cent. I., Jenæ, 1679.
89. Osler. Loc. cit.
90. Armstrong, H. E. British Medical Journal, November 11, 1871, vol. ii. p. 558.
91. Dreyfus-Brisac. Landouzy, loc. cit., p. 187.
92. Freiberg. Menschenblattern und Schutzpockenimpfung, Erlangen, 1874.
93. Frerichs. Ueber die Diabetes, Berlin, 1884, S. 222.
94. Arnaud. Troubles de la parole consécutifs a la variole, Marseille méd., 1896, vol. xxxiii. pp. 129–40.
95. Combemale. Loc. cit.
96. Saint-Phillippe. Quoted by Combemale, loc. cit.
97. Jaccoud. Loc. cit.
98. Curschmann. Loc. cit.
99. Myers and Whipham. Loc. cit.
100. Breganze. Allgem. med. Central-Zeitung, December 7, 1872.
101. Aldrich. Loc. cit.

A CASE OF TYPHOID FEVER PRESENTING AN ARTERIAL COMPLICATION—PROBABLY AN ARTERITIS.

BY WALTER R. STEINER, A.M., M.D.,
OF HARTFORD, CONN.,
FORMERLY HOUSE MEDICAL OFFICER, JOHNS HOPKINS HOSPITAL.

AMONG the protean complications and sequelæ of typhoid fever, those connected with the circulatory system are of great interest. They were recognized at least as long ago as 1806, when Hildenbrand,[1] in an epidemic of typhoid at Cracow, observed some cases in which

[1] Ueber den austeckenden Typhus, etc., 8°, Wien, 1810, p. 310.

gangrene of both extremities resulted. Since that time similar cases have been reported and have been explained as due to venous thromboses or emboli. In 1851 Fabre[1] suggested that autochthonous arterial thrombosis might account for some of these instances, and subsequently different observers, especially the French, have described the symptoms of thromboses of this variety. Some of the apparent cases, however, occurred in young individuals in whom a complete recovery of the affected part ensued. The following case is one of this nature. In these instances it is suggested that an arteritis only existed, which caused the pulse to be so much obliterated that it was merely not felt. A subsidence of the arteritis restores the patulency of the bloodvessels' lumen and the volume of the pulse is consequently increased, returning generally to its former condition.

The symptoms presented by these cases have been especially well given by Bariè,[2] Potain,[3] and Sallès,[4] but the recent publication of Thayer's[5] article renders a detailed discussion of this subject unnecessary. The symptoms in brief are those of "pain, heat, tenderness, swelling, and even resistance in the course of the artery, with diminution or disappearance of the pulsations and coldness or blueness of the extremity." A complete recovery may be noted in a few weeks, "with the disappearance of all symptoms and return of pulsation, not only in the peripheral, but in the affected vessels."

Typhoid fever; severe infection; two relapses; an arterial complication in the right upper extremity on the forty-first day of the disease; gradual recovery, with complete return of pulsation in the affected bloodvessels.—P. B., aged nine years, was first seen by me December 2, 1900. He complained at this time of headaches and general weakness. His family history was negative. He had never been a strong child, had suffered much from asthmatic attacks since infancy and was very susceptible to colds. The winter previous he had spent in California without apparent great benefit. Of the ordinary diseases of childhood he had had measles, mumps, and whooping-cough. He thought his present illness began two weeks before I saw him, when he first complained of headaches on coming home from school. Nothing especial, however, was thought of this symptom, and he still kept up and about, although three days ago he said he felt quite weak. One day ago he went to bed, at which time his mother said

[1] Cas de gangrène et séparation complète du pied dans le cours d'une fièvre typhoïde, Abeille méd., Paris, 1850, vol. vii. pp. 242, 243; and Gaz. méd. de Paris, 1851, 3 S., vol. vi. pp. 539–540.

[2] Contribution à l'histoire de l'artérite aiguë consécutive à la fièvre typhoïde, Rev. de méd., Paris, 1884, vol. iv., 1, pp. 124–149.

[3] De l'artérite et de la gangrène sèche dans la convalescence de la fièvre typhoïde, Gaz. d. hôp., Paris, 1878, vol. li. pp. 537–539; and De l'artérite transitoire des membres inférieurs dans la convalescence de la fièvre typhoïde. Bull. méd., Paris, 1890, vol. iv. pp. 845, 846.

[4] Note sur un cas d'obstructions artérielle au cours d'un cas de fièvre typhoïde chez l'enfant. Lyon méd., 1893, vol. lxxii. pp. 77–82.

[5] On Arteritis and Arterial Thrombosis in Typhoid Fever. New York State Journal of Medicine, January, 1903.

he seemed quite feverish. He had had no epistaxis, nausea, vomiting, or diarrhœa.

On examination he was a rather weakly developed and poorly nourished boy. The lips and mucous membranes were of a good color; the tongue was coated with a thick white fur; the temperature was 101.8° F., while the pulse was 100 to the minute, regular in force and rhythm, and of good volume and tension. The lungs were negative on examination. At the apex of the heart a soft systolic murmur was audible, which was not transmitted outward, but was heard with increasing intensity on passing upward, being loudest at the pulmonic area. The abdomen was not distended, and no rose spots were observed, but on palpation pain was complained of, not localized, but general over the entire abdomen. The spleen was not palpable. A dried blood specimen was obtained for a Widal reaction.

On the following day the report from the Widal was negative. The pain over the abdomen still continued, but was, as before, not localized. Some distention was now first noted, which subsequently proved very obstinate in not yielding to the various means employed for its relief. Because of these abdominal symptoms, leukocyte counts in the morning and evening were taken. They resulted in readings of 7800 and 7400, respectively. No rose spots were seen until the next day, and the spleen was not palpable until December 12th. The patient was ordered cold baths first, but as he resisted the taking of them so strenuously, cold sponges were next given every three hours if his temperature was over 103.5° F. These also had to be abandoned for a like reason, and cold packs were then tried. If they failed to bring about a satisfactory reduction of the temperature, cold sponges were resorted to and generally proved effectual.

In the matter of feeding great difficulty was encountered, as he objected to taking anything, and the nurses had many a struggle to get him to swallow even a small quantity of liquid nourishment. At one time milk, which was first given him, had to be entirely substituted by broths and egg albumen, as he had a tendency to vomit curdled milk and pass curds in his stools, even with the milk greatly diluted with lime-water. On December 22d, the twenty-second day of his illness, the temperature, which had been gradually falling, reached 99.2° F., and we hoped for a speedy recovery, but a relapse set in, with a temperature of 103.8° F., at 8 P.M., on December 24th, and a subsequent new crop of rose spots. The spleen was not apparently palpable, but he did not permit us to make a satisfactory examination. With the relapse he had a marked bronchitis—sibilant, sonorous, and coarse moist rales being heard everywhere over both lungs, especially the right. During this attack warm packs were tried, as he struggled and resisted so against the cold ones, and was frequently quite exhausted after one had been given him. As they seemed beneficial in lowering the temperature, they were continued throughout the course of the disease.

His condition remained satisfactory until January 5th, the fourteenth day of his relapse, when he became quite delirious. At this time his pulse was very small in volume and thready, 124 to the minute. On an examination of his lungs there was slight relative dulness from the angle of the spine of the right scapula, and the breath and voice sounds were here somewhat harsh. Under the stimulation of whiskey and strychnine, the pulse became again full and strong, and later the delirium left him, and the lung symptoms cleared up. The temperature reached normal on the thirty-ninth day of the disease and the eighteenth of his relapse. Two days later, on the evening of the forty-first day, he complained of numbness and tingling of the right index finger. The right radial was of the same force, rhythm, volume, and tension as the left radial, and no swelling or tenderness could be made out along the course of the right radial, brachial, or axillary arteries. There was no stiffness of the right index finger, and movement of the arm did not cause the slightest pain. Uncertain as to what this symptom exactly foreboded, I ordered the arm to be immobilized, and left the patient, thinking the outcome would be a neuritis or an arterial thrombosis. On the following day, January 11th, the right radial pulse was distinctly smaller in volume than the left, but differences between the axillaries and brachials could not be made out. The numbness and tingling had now been transferred mostly to the elbow, and there was also some pain radiating up and down the course of the brachial artery. There was no swelling or sensitiveness to pressure anywhere in the arm. The next day, January 12th, the pulse was wanting in the right radial, brachial, and axillary arteries, which, on account of the patient's emaciation, could be well felt. The skin overlying them was somewhat swollen and looked red and inflamed. Much pain was complained of on palpation, and the axillary and radial arteries had a hard, cord-like feel. The right upper extremity was distinctly colder than the left, and there was some blueness of the finger-nails. The patient's condition otherwise was good. In twenty-four hours the hand became still colder and had a mottled and cyanotic appearance. Dr. William Porter, Jr., of Hartford, who saw the case frequently in consultation with me, and I now became very apprehensive lest gangrene might set in. On January 14th we could get the axillary pulse, but could not feel any pulsation in either the brachial or radial arteries.

For two days his condition remained about stationary, during which period his temperature more nearly approximated the normal, there being but a slight evening rise. But at the end of this time, on January 16th, his temperature rose from 98.2° F. at noon to 100.8° F. at 4 P.M., while his pulse rate increased from 80 to 90 per minute. Coarse mucous rales were heard on this day over the entire right lung, and over the cardiac area a loud, blowing, systolic murmur was plainly audible, being loudest at the aortic area, where it almost completely obliterated the first sound. On examining the abdomen the superficial veins seemed especially prominent. There was much distention and tympanites, which prevented the spleen being palpated for. The arm was extremely cold and the finger-nails intensely cyanotic. A fresh crop of rose spots were visible on the following day.

The next few days he grew gradually worse, and soon became intensely delirious. The temperature on January 18th and 19th reached 105.2° F., but thereafter fell slowly until it was 103.5° F., on January 20th at 8 P.M. From this time on until January 22d the temperature was not taken, on account of his extreme delirium and restlessness, which nothing at our command could entirely control. On January 21st the emaciation was so marked, the weakness so intense, the delirium so extreme, and the pulse so small, irregular, and thready that dissolution seemed imminent. The respirations were Cheyne-Stokes in character, the urine was passed involuntarily, and the abdomen was extremely distended. The bowels had not moved for three

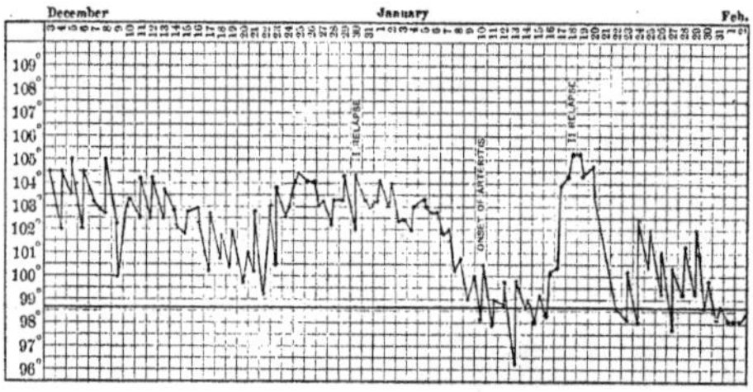

days. Under stimulants he rallied somewhat, but the delirium remained. In the next twenty-four hours his condition, though desperate, was a trifle improved, as the pulse was then more regular, and there was no longer Cheyne-Stokes respiration. Food of all kinds was refused, and he was occasionally with difficulty kept in bed. His mouth was dry and parched, sordes covered his lips and tongue, and his breath was foul. There was no change in the arm, save that the cyanosis had disappeared and the difference in temperature, as compared with the left arm, was almost unappreciable. On January 23d, the following day, his delirium ceased, he was able to take some food, and an enema was slightly effectual, much gas being passed. The prognosis became decidedly more favorable.

From this time on his improvement was rapid. The symptoms in the right lung cleared up, and his pulse became good and strong and much reduced in frequency. There was still no pulsation in the right radial and brachial arteries. He was seen on Jannary 26th by Dr. E. G. Janeway, of New York, who expressed a most hopeful prognosis. The patient's subsequent history was one of rapid progress. On January 31st his temperature became practically normal. Four days later I placed him on a soft diet, and on February 13th, thirty-five days after the onset of the arteritis, I first noted a return of pulsation in the right radial and brachial arteries. The pulse in each was slightly weaker and a trifle slower than in those of the left arm, but in three days I could detect no difference between the two sides. On this day he was placed on solid diet and was allowed to sit up. Shortly thereafter he was permitted to get up and walk about, and I released him from my care.

The urine examinations were negative throughout the course of the disease. I very much regret that I was unable to have another Widal reaction taken.

In considering this case, it seems best to regard the arterial complication as one of the so-called peripheral arteritides, as the symptoms so nearly correspond to those of this nature. The disappearance of the axillary pulsation and its speedy subsequent return may, however, be taken as an indication of the displacement of an axillary thrombus and its later lodgement in the bloodvessels of the brain. This would account for the extreme delirium, but the complete re-establishment of the radial and brachial pulsations is against the view of thrombus formation, and the symptoms of delirium may be well explained by the occurrence of his second relapse.

THE OCCURRENCE OF CELLS WITH EOSINOPHILE GRANULATION AND THEIR RELATION TO NUTRITION.[1]

By Eugene L. Opie, M.D.,

ASSOCIATE IN PATHOLOGY, JOHNS HOPKINS UNIVERSITY; FELLOW OF THE ROCKEFELLER INSTITUTE FOR MEDICAL RESEARCH.

(From the Pathological Laboratory of the Johns Hopkins University and Hospital.)

Many facts are known concerning the activities of the various wandering cells of the blood, yet the significance of few phenomena which they exhibit is clearly understood. Since Cohnheim showed that the polynuclear leukocytes migrate from the bloodvessels, numerous observations have demonstrated how important is the part played by these cells in the inflammatory changes which follow the invasion of bacteria. Nevertheless, we are ignorant of what they accomplish in resisting invasion of the body. Metschnikoff and his pupils believe that the polynuclear leukocytes with neutrophile granu-

[1] The present investigation has been conducted with the aid of a grant from the Rockefeller Institute for Medical Research.

lation resist the infective agent by ingesting and destroying it, while other observers, notably Büchner, maintain that the leukocytes furnish something to the fluids which destroys the micro-organism before it is engulfed. The functional significance of the peculiar granules which stud the protoplasm of these polynuclear cells is obscure. Much less is known concerning the activities of a second type of granular leukocyte, the so-called eosinophile cell, and almost nothing is known of its functions. A short survey of its occurrence in various vertebrate species will furnish some indication of its importance.

It is well known that the studies inaugurated by Ehrlich have demonstrated in the leukocytes of the blood distinctive granules which exhibit peculiar affinities for certain dyes or for a whole group of chemically related dyes. Those dyes of which the staining principle is a base distinguish the granules which are characteristic of certain cells. Another kind of granule is stained only by acid dyes. Neutrophile granules, according to Ehrlich, are stained by the neutral mixture of an acid and a basic stain. By the size of the cell, the shape of its nucleus, and the character of the granules scattered in its protoplasm, the various cells of the blood are classified.

By the microscopic study of fresh blood, Wharton Jones[1] was able to distinguish cells with coarse refractive granules, which many subsequent observers believed to be droplets of fat. These coarse granules occupied the attention of Ehrlich[2] at the outset of his studies upon the staining reactions of protoplasmic granulation. He demonstrated that they are readily stained by all acid dyes, but have such a marked affinity for eosin that when treated with various mixtures of this stain with other acid dyes, they take up it alone. In human blood these so-called eosinophile cells contain a polymorphous nucleus and are actively amœboid, resembling in these characters the more numerous leukocytes, which contain finer neutrophile granules. Eosinophile leukocytes were found by Ehrlich not only in the blood of man and other mammals, but in that of the frog as well, while subsequent studies have demonstrated that they are very widely distributed in the animal kingdom.

ZOOLOGICAL DISTRIBUTION OF CELLS WITH EOSINOPHILE GRANULATION. Comparative studies of Hirschfeld[3] and others have shown that two types of leukocyte with polymorphous nucleus, are present in the blood of all mammalian species. That variety which in almost all mammals constitutes a majority of the white corpuscles and migrating from the bloodvessels plays a very important part in inflammatory processes is provided with relatively fine granules, which exhibit an affinity for acid dyes. Since the common polymorphonuclear leukocytes of human blood contain granules which ex-

[1] Philosophical Transactions, London, 1864, p. 63.
[2] Verhandlungen der physiologischen Gesellschaft, Berlin, 1878-79, No. 20.
[3] Virchow's Archiv, 1897, vol. cxlix. p. 22.

hibit a peculiar reaction to a mixture of certain acid and basic dyes, but have a well-marked affinity for acid stains, they have been designated by Kanthack and Hardy[1] finely granular acidophile or oxyphile leukocytes. The amphophile granules of Ehrlich present in the polynuclear leukocytes of rabbits are stained by both acid and basic dyes. According to Hirschfeld, the more common polynuclear leukocytes of one mammal, the white mouse, exhibit no granulation, but Ehrlich and Lazarus[2] are inclined to doubt this statement.

Common to all mammalian species examined by Hirschfeld are leukocytes with coarse, acidophile granules. These granules usually exhibit an especial avidity for eosin and are stained by it alone when treated with mixtures containing other acid dyes. Hirschfeld has found that the coarse, acidophile granules of a few animals exhibit a slight modification of this reaction. In the dog and in the cat they take a mixed tint when treated with eosin and aurantia, while in the horse they are stained by eosin and indulin in combination.

Grünberg[3] and Meinertz[4] have studied the white corpuscles of birds, reptiles, amphibia, and fish by the methods introduced by Ehrlich. Small mononuclear cells, with basophile protoplasm free from granules, the lymphocytes of mammalian blood, occur in the various species examined, and forms with polymorphous nucleus are almost constantly found. The latter often contain granules which exhibit an affinity for acid or basic dyes. Cells with acidophile granules are very widely distributed, and in some birds and reptiles constitute a majority of the white corpuscles present in blood. In birds occur two varieties of acidophile granules, both of which show a strong affinity for eosin: (*a*) round or oval bodies, and (*b*) peculiar, elongated, spindle-shaped, or crystalloid particles. The latter occur in all birds and in certain reptiles. In the frog the greater number of polynuclear leukocytes are free from granulation, but a minority are studded with round, eosinophile bodies; crystalloid forms are absent. In fish the characters of the white corpuscles and of the granulation they exhibit are very variable. Acidophile granules are frequently found, but often differ in size, shape, and staining reaction from those of higher species. Certain Teleostean fish, for example, Gobio fluviatilis (Mesnil)[5] and Perca fluviatilis (Mesnil and Meinertz), possess no granular leukocytes.

The constant presence among mammals of two types of polynuclear leukocyte, one type being constantly more numerous than the other, suggests the possibility that each form has a peculiar functional significance. In lower vertebrates, namely, in birds, reptiles, amphibia, and fish, this constantly recurring relation is not present.

[1] Journal of Physiology, 1894, vol. xvii. p. 81.

[2] Normale und pathologische Histologie des Blutes, Nothnagel's spec. Path. u. Ther., 1900, Bd. viii. Teil, 1.

[3] Virchow's Archiv, 1901, vol. clxiii. p. 303.

[4] Ibid., 1902, vol. clviii. p. 353.

[5] Annales de l'Inst. Pasteur, 1895, vol. ix. p. 301.

Moreover, the color reactions first described by Ehrlich, being doubtless dependent upon certain chemical or physical peculiarities of the specific granulations, afford no proof that structures in widely separated species are anatomically or functionally homologous.

Hence, while the eosinophile cells of mammals, bearing a constant relation in different species, are, doubtless, analogous structures, even though they occasionally present slight variation in their staining reactions, they are not necessarily comparable in function, and other characters to the cells with acidophile or eosinophile granules of lower vertebrates. Such assumption seems to have been made by several writers, who have studied, experimentally, the activities of certain granular leukocytes in frogs and in fish.

Cells with eosinophilic granules form in man a small proportion of the total number of leukocytes; their relative number has been found somewhat variable. Ehrlich[1] has stated that they usually constitute from 2 per cent. to 4 per cent. of the leukocytes, and rarely reach as much as 10 per cent. The figures given by other observers vary within these limits. Zappert,[2] who has very carefully counted the eosinophile leukocytes of healthy individuals, finds the proportion noted by Ehrlich, but, preferring to estimate their absolute number, states that 50 to 250 are usually present in one cubic millimetre of blood, though they may reach 700. In children he found that they are usually more numerous than in adults.

In certain mammals the numerical relation of the eosinophile leukocytes to other forms varies within wider limits. In few species has the proportion been accurately determined. Nevertheless, in two widely separated mammals, namely, in the rabbit and in the dog, accurate counts have been made in the course of repeated experimental studies. Kanthack and Hardy found 1 per cent. to 2 per cent. of eosinophile (oxyphile) cells in the blood of the rabbit; Tallqvist and Willebrand,[3] 0.5 per cent. to 2.8 per cent.; Brinkerhoff and Tyzzer,[4] 0.5 per cent. to 1 per cent. The proportion of eosinophile cells in the dog's blood shows greater variation, and the normal average is higher. In fifteen animals, counts made by Tallqvist and Willebrand varied between 0.2 per cent. and 8.1 per cent., the average being 5.3 per cent. In ten animals Dawson[5] found a minimum count of 2.6 per cent. and a maximum of 21.6 per cent. The individual counts which Dr. Dawson has kindly placed at my disposal are as follows: 6.6 per cent., 12.2 per cent., 3.2 per cent., 2.6 per cent., 21.6 per cent., 4.6 per cent., 5 per cent., 10.8 per cent., 9.4 per cent., 2.6 per cent.

In several instances the count is so much above that obtained from the other animals and from those studied by Tallqvist and Wille-

[1] Charité-Annalen, 1888, vol. xiii.
[2] Zeit. f. klin. Med., 1893, vol. xxiii. p. 227.
[3] Skandinavisches Arch. f. Phys., 1900, vol. x. p. 37.
[4] Journal of Medical Research, 1902, vol. vii. p. 173.
[5] American Journal of Physiology, 1900, vol. iv.

brand that the presence of some pathological process to explain the apparent eosinophilia has been suspected. The frequency with which dogs are infected with animal parasites is well known, and uncinaria caninis is found with great frequency in the small intestine. With these facts in view, I have studied the blood of ten apparently healthy dogs, and have subsequently examined the intestines and other organs.

TABLE I.

No.	Leukocytes in 1 c.mm.	Eosinophiles in 1 c.mm.	Parasites in small intestine.
1	15,100	1208 = 8.0 %	U. caninis (3), tænia cucumerina (10 grm.).
2	22,350	939 = 4.2 "	U. caninis (25 to 50) and several tapeworms.
3	16,600	880 = 5.3 "	U. caninis (3), ascaris marginata (1), and small tapeworms in large numbers.
4	15,800	632 = 4.0 "	U. caninis (12) and several tapeworms.
5	10,700	567 = 5.3 "	T. cucumerina (large amount), A. marginata (3).
6	15,400	493 = 3.2 "	T. serrata (large amount).
7	14,200	454 = 3.2 "	Several small tapeworms.
8	16,400	328 = 2.0 "	A. marginata (10) and two tapeworms.
9	19,700	197 = 1.0 "	U. caninis (3).
10	5,800	24 = 0.5 "	

The figures are inconclusive, since in no instance does the proportion of eosinophile cells equal that noted by Dawson. Nevertheless, they afford a basis for further comparison and suggest, at least, that the absolute number of eosinophile cells bears some relation to the number of animal parasites within the intestinal tract, especially when it is noted that the smallest number of eosinophile cells was found in two animals, one of which contained three parasites (No. 9), while the other (No. 10) was free from infection.

METHODS. Few observations have been made upon the occurrence of eosinophile leukocytosis in lower animals, and while in a few instances experimental eosinophilia has been produced, the progress of the phenomenon has seldom been recorded by repeated differential counts, which are very laborious and time-consuming. In order to avoid, in some part, this difficulty, and at the same time to obtain a great number of observations upon the behavior of the eosinophile cells under a considerable variety of conditions, I have adopted the simple method of counting the leukocytes in fresh blood. Hardening and staining being obviated, the results are of necessity obtained without delay.

A drop of blood is allowed to spread between cover-slip and slide and is immediately examined with the oil immersion lens ($\frac{1}{12}$ obj.). Certain precautions are essential in order to make the white corpuscles so conspicuous that none are missed in counting. Of first importance is the use of artificial illumination, preferably that from the so-called Welsbach burner, since by this means the refraction of the corpuscles is increased and the characters of their granulation and of their nuclei become evident. A diaphragm with a rectangular opening is so inserted into the eye-piece of the microscope that the upper and lower segments of the field are obliterated and the count, performed with the aid of a mechanical stage, is confined to a somewhat narrow equatorial zone. It is obviously necessary to use only those specimens in which the blood is spread into a moderately thin layer, and to make the count immediately after the blood is drawn.

If these precautions are taken, on the one hand, few, if any leukocytes, are omitted from the count, while, on the other hand, the individual forms, notably the highly refractive eosinophile cells, are recognized with ease and their relative number noted. In most instances this percentage count was limited to the eosinophile cells, since they alone occupied attention and numerous observations, consuming much time, were necessary. As a routine the number of eosinophile cells in 300 or 400 leukocytes was determined. The character of the charts, which will be subsequently described, sufficiently vindicate the accuracy of the method and show that, even though it may not be absolutely exact, it gives an adequate presentation of the changes which the eosinophile leukocytes undergo. For comparison, I have counted by both methods specimens from five guinea-pigs and from five healthy men.

	Fresh specimen.	Hardened specimen.[1]
From guinea-pig	15.3	14.0
" "	8.7	10.2
" "	6.7	5.0
" "	1.7	3.0
" "	1.3	0.5
" healthy man	10.0	8.4
" "	3.3	3.2
" "	2.7	2.7
" "	2.0	2.6
" "	1.3	3.7

The proportion of eosinophile cells noted in the fresh specimen is not with constancy greater or less than that obtained from the hardened film. Doubtless the ordinary method of counting hardened and stained specimens is accurate only within certain limits. Thus, Boycott and Haldane,[2] making for the sake of comparison successive differential counts of 1000 cells in the same film, found in two cases the following figures for the neutrophiles in four successive thousands of white corpuscles:

59.2	55.5	55.2	53.6 %
35.8	32.7	38.7	34.8 "

For the purpose of certain experiments not included in the present paper, the guinea-pig was found more available than either the rabbit or the dog. Blood can be repeatedly obtained from the peripheral circulation by puncturing the skin of the ear or by nicking with sharp scissors the edge of the ear after clipping the hair.

[1] For assistance in counting these specimens I am indebted to Dr. Ernest Cullen.

[2] Journal of Hygiene 1903, vol. iii. p. 95.

It was soon found that the number of eosinophile leukocytes was so variable that a preliminary study of the conditions which influence them was necessary. Even though the facts concerned refer to a single species, they are, I believe, of sufficient general interest to justify a detailed study.

EOSINOPHILE CELLS OF THE BLOOD. The white corpuscles of the guinea-pig, which have been the subject of special study by Kurloff,[1] present several noteworthy peculiarities. In briefly describing the various types, I will mention characteristics observable in the freshly drawn blood. The following forms occur:

1. Polynuclear leukocytes with fine acidophile granulation constitute, Kurloff states, 40 per cent. to 50 per cent. of the total number of white cells. According to Ehrlich and Kurloff, the granulation is of the pseudoeosinophile or amphophile type, but Hirschfeld denies this statement and claims that the granules stain only with acid dyes, and, preferably, with indulin.

2. Eosinophile cells are readily recognized in fresh blood by their coarse, round, or oval, very refractive granules of somewhat greenish tint; they are very actively amœboid. In stained specimens the nucleus is often found to be horseshoe-shaped or trilobed, while all transitions between the two occur.

3. Basophile cells can be identified in the fresh specimen. They are filled with coarse, oval granules, which are easily distinguished from those of the eosinophile cell, being of greater size and only slightly refractive. These cells are actively amœboid at temperatures approximating that of the body.

4. Lymphocytes resembling those of human blood constitute, according to Kurloff, 30 per cent. to 35 per cent. of the total number of white corpuscles. Large and small mononuclear cells occur. I have frequently observed amœboid movement, but it is much less active than that of the forms previously mentioned. A short protrusion of the protoplasm occurs at one point. The projection becomes larger and knob-like, constricted where it joins the remainder of the cell. This constriction persists and passes like a wave from one side of the cell to the other as the projecting protoplasm increases at the expense of that which remains.

5. Vacuolated cells peculiar to the guinea-pig have been described by Kurloff and represent a considerable proportion of the mononuclear leukocytes. Within the protoplasm are one, or, occasionally, two globules, which, in fresh specimens, have a homogeneous, greenish color, and are more refractive than the cell protoplasm; the globule is frequently larger than the nucleus of the cell. Such vacuolated cells are inactively amœboid.

In order to obtain a basis for comparison, the occurrence of eosinophile leukocytes in the blood of normal guinea-pigs has been studied

[1] Quoted by Ehrlich and Lazarus.

and their distribution in the internal organs has been observed. Kurloff states that eosinophile cells constitute only 1 per cent. of the white corpuscles of the blood; Kanthack and Hardy give the proportion as 2 per cent. to 3 per cent. Finding these figures much exceeded in many apparently healthy animals, I have been inclined to suspect the presence of some latent pathological process. Post-mortem examination has failed to confirm this suspicion, though the possibility cannot be excluded with certainty. The intestine of the guinea-pig is subject to infection with several protozoan parasites, which apparently produce no noteworthy alteration of health. In the small intestine one not infrequently encounters the flagellate parasite, megastoma entericum, while in the cæcum infusoria are almost constantly present, often in considerable number. No relation was established between the presence of these protozoan forms and the occurrence in the blood of eosinophile leukocytes in unusually large numbers. The frequency with which eosinophile cells are found in the lungs, and notably in the wall of the bronchi, has directed especial attention to these organs. The relation of the eosinophile cells in the blood to those of the bronchi will be considered later.

Animals with high eosinophile count have been often found to be especially large, healthy specimens, and, indeed, a relation between the number of eosinophile cells and the weight of the animal is readily established. In the following table, in which the animals are ranged according to their weight, is recorded the preliminary count made upon many healthy animals previous to performing various experiments:

TABLE II.

Wt.	Eo. %	Wt.	Eo. %	Wt.	Eo. %	Wt.	Eo. %	Wt.	Eo. %	Wt.	Eo. %
299	0.6	398	0.0	481	1.3	546	16.0	667	2.3	785	19.3
287	0.0	363	0.3	436	0.3	509	0.0	615	1.5	788.	15.0
		309	0.0	400	1.5	501	1.0	653	3.3	718	8.7
		385	0.3	454	0.3	556	1.3	622	4.0		
		366	1.7	423	1.3	597	20.0	649	15.3		
		345	1.7	418	0.0	567	5.7	665	9.0		
				494	0.0	586	6.7	622	36.3		
				497	0.0	578	5.7	604	10.3		
				406	0.5	532	9.7	650	7.3		
				415	0.0	588	6.8	625	24.3		
				487	5.7			672	1.5		
								697	15.0		
								641	18.0		
								604	8.3		
Mean,	0.3		0.6		1.1		8.2		11.2		14.3

In the foregoing table certain facts are noteworthy. In animals weighing less than 500 grams the proportion of eosinophile leukocytes rarely exceeds 2 per cent., and agrees approximately with that found by Kurloff and by Kanthack and Hardy; but in animals of greater weight a much higher percentage is almost constant. Even where the animal weighs more than 500 grams the proportion is occasionally less than 2 per cent., but the mean for animals of this weight is much higher. The averages have been calculated from the figures in the various columns of the table, each of which, from left to right, represents an increase of 100 grams. After a very slight gradual increase in the proportion of eosinophile cells, reaching 1.1 per cent. for animals weighing from 400 to 500 grams, there is a sudden rise to 8.2 per cent. in the next column, followed by a more gradual increase in the columns containing guinea-pigs of greater weight. The animals, which in almost every case had been obtained from dealers only a short time before examination was made, had doubtless been subjected to varying conditions of nutrition. This fact, as will be subsequently shown, may account for some variation in the percentage of eosinophile leukocytes.

The great variation to which the number of eosinophile leukocytes in the blood of apparently healthy guinea-pigs is subject is further shown by the following table, in which in ten instances their number in one cubic millimetre of blood has been calculated from the total number of leukocytes:

TABLE III.

No.	Weight.	Leukocytes in 1 c.mm.	Eosinophiles in 1 c.mm.
1	454	8,100	24 = 0.3 %
2	521	8,700	1479 = 17.0 "
3	532	10,600	1028 = 9.7 "
4	556	16,600	249 = 1.5 "
5	578	24,200	1379 = 5.7 "
6	625	8,500	2916 = 34.3 "
7	650	12,500	913 = 7.3 "
8	690	15,700	1649 = 10.5 "
9	695	13,900	2127 = 15.3 "
10	718	10,800	940 = 8.7 "
Mean		12,960	1270 = 11 0 "

The total number of leukocytes varies within such wide limits that the proportion of eosinophile cells allows only a rough estimation of their absolute number. Nevertheless, if the figure which represents the percentage count is multiplied by 115 (the mean number of eosinophile leukocytes in one cubic millimetre of blood divided by the mean percentage count), a figure approximating the absolute number of eosinophile leukocytes is obtained. Hence the facts demonstrated by Table II. are applicable to the absolute as well as to the relative number of these cells.

EOSINOPHILE CELLS IN THE TISSUES. The distribution of eosinophile cells in the organs of the guinea-pig still further indicates that they play a very important part in metabolism. Heidenhaim[1] has shown with what frequency these cells are found in the mucosa of the dog's intestine, while Teichmüller[2] has emphasized

[1] Pflüger's Arch. f. Phys., 1888, vol. xliii. Suppl. Hft.
[2] Deutsches Arch. f. klin. Med., 1898, vol. lx. p. 576.

their abundance in the lungs. Their distribution in the organs will be briefly described.

Throughout the gastrointestinal tract eosinophile cells occur in great abundance and are most numerous in that part of the mucous membrane which is between and immediately below the tubular glands. They are readily recognized in sections stained with eosin by their large, oval, brilliantly red granules. They do not differ from the eosinophile leukocytes of the blood and are provided with nuclei which are trilobed, bilobed, or horseshoe-shaped.

In the superficial part of the gastric mucosa eosinophile cells are scant, but are very numerous between the ends of the glands and in the narrow zone between the glands and the muscularis mucosæ. In the submucosa immediately below the muscularis mucosæ they are again abundant, but elsewhere in the connective tissue of the gastric wall are rarely found.

Throughout the mucous membrane of the small intestine eosinophile cells are found between the bases of the glands of Lieberkühn, in the subglandular tissue which lies between these glands and the muscularis mucosa, but are scant in the villi and in the submucosa. Such cells are especially numerous in the mucosa overlying the Peyer's patches. In the guinea-pig a diverticulum of the superficial epithelium extending downward is situated just above each constituent follicle, and in the lymphoid tissue lying between two such diverticula eosinophile cells are not infrequently so numerous that they give a red color to the tissue examined with the low power of the microscope. In the mucosa of the large intestine, and especially in the cæcum, cells with eosinophile granules are numerous between the bases of the glands.

In the walls of the trachea, the bronchi, and the subdivisions of the latter eosinophile cells are found in considerable number; in the connective tissue surrounding the bronchi and the bloodvessels similar cells occur, while not infrequently they are present in the interalveolar walls outside the capillary vessels.

Of considerable interest is the readily demonstrable fact that eosinophile cells penetrate through the epithelium into the lumen of the small bronchi. Scattered in the loose areolar tissue of the mucosa may be found cells with eosinophile granulation, and between the columnar cells of the epithelium similar eosinophile cells are easily recognized, while others have made their way into the lumen of the bronchus. Cells with scant, partially disintegrated protoplasm, containing a somewhat irregular nucleus, are usually more numerous in the same situation. The possibility that some of these nuclei represent the remains of eosinophile cells altered by the bronchial secretions has occasionally suggested itself, but the occurrence of such transformation has not been demonstrable.

Eosinophile cells are at times even more numerous in the fibrous tissue external to the muscle than in the mucosa. Should a small nodule of lymphoid tissue occur in this situation, eosinophile cells show an especial tendency to accumulate in the part of the nodule which is next the lumen of the bronchus and in the tissue immediately overlying. Throughout the external coat of connective tissue eosinophile cells are numerous. A specimen in which eosinophile cells were particularly numerous has served to explain the origin of these cells, for in the small bloodvessels of the bronchial wall they are very numerous, probably held here by some chemotactic influence. They doubtless emigrate not only from the small veins of the connective tissue, but from the alveolar capillaries in the immediate neighborhood of the bronchus, for in these vessels they are present in much greater numbers than in the interalveolar capillaries more distant from the bronchus.

The passage of eosinophile leukocytes into the bronchi probably exerts an influence upon the number of eosinophile cells in the blood. Examination has not been made in a sufficiently large number of animals to determine the relation of the process to the eosinophilia noted in apparently normal guinea-pigs. In six of nine animals I have found eosinophile cells within the lumina of the bronchi; the weight and proportion of eosinophile cells in the blood were as follows: (1) 650 grams, 7.3 per cent.; (2) 625 grams, 24.3 per cent.; (3) 622 grams, 36.3 per cent.; (4) 604 grams, 8.3 per cent.; (5) 556 grams, 1.5 per cent.; (6) 521 grams, 17 per cent. In the three remaining animals no eosinophile leukocytes were found within the bronchi; their weight and percentage of eosinophile leukocytes were as follows: (7) 643 grams, 5.7 per cent.; (8) 454 grams, 0.3 per cent.; (9) 390 grams, 0.5 per cent.

In large, apparently healthy animals eosinophile cells migrate from the bloodvessels into the bronchi, and there is, as far as I have found, no additional evidence that the bronchi are the seat of a pathological process. The significance of this migration is not apparent.

Below epithelial surfaces other than those of the intestine and air-passages, eosinophile cells are rarely found. They do not accumulate below the squamous epithelium of the normal skin, nor of the tongue, in the mucosa of the bladder, nor in the walls of the ducts of the liver, pancreas, or testicles.

Kanthack and Hardy claim that the connective tissue is the especial habitat of the coarsely granular oxyphile cell, yet only in certain localities are they constantly present in considerable number. Cells with eosinophile granulation are infrequently observed in the subcutaneous areolar tissue, in the fascia and septa of muscles, and in the connective tissue of the liver, kidneys, adrenal glands, pancreas, thyroid, and testicles. In the serous membranes, the omentum and the mesentery, on the contrary, eosinophile cells are fairly numerous and are distributed in greatest number along the course of the small bloodvessels. Within the serous cavities, as Kanthack and Hardy have shown, these cells are constantly present and constitute from 30 per cent. to 50 per cent. of the total number of cells in the peritoneal fluid of the normal guinea-pig.

Little attention has been paid to the intimate relation which exists between the lymphatic apparatus and the eosinophile cells. Their abundance in the lymphoid tissue of the gastrointestinal mucosa has already been noted and attention has been directed to their accumulation in the Peyer's patches of the small intestine and in the lymphoid follicles of the bronchi. Their presence in the serous cavities is noteworthy. They are, moreover, constantly present in the lymphatic glands, not only in those at the base of the mesentery, but in the peripheral glands, such as those in the inguinal region as well. Eosinophile cells are not found within the follicles which occupy the cortex of the gland, but are fairly abundant at the periphery of the follicles, near and at times within the peripheral sinus. Within the sinuses of the medulla eosinophile cells occur in small numbers, but in the medullary cords they are more numerous and are not infrequently ranged along the margins of the sinuses.

In the connective tissue in the immediate periphery of the lymphatic glands eosinophile cells are often found in abundance, and their number diminishes as the distance from the gland increases. In one specimen, by a fortunate accident, I obtained evidence that these cells are derived not from the gland, but directly from the blood. Cells with eosinophile granulation were here numerous, both in the tissue and in the small veins, and had been actually fixed in process of migration from the latter. In several instances elongated eosinophile leukocytes had partially penetrated the endothelium of the vessel, part still remaining within the lumen.

In the bone-marrow cells, with coarse eosinophile granulation, are more numerous than in any other organ of the healthy animal. Here alone are found the large mononuclear eosinophile cells described by H. F. Müller and Rieder.[1] They are analogous to the myelocytes of Ehrlich, which are essentially cells of the bone-marrow and only in leukæmia find their way into the general circulation. The myelocyte with eosinophile granulation is considerably larger than the eosinophile leukocyte, and is provided with a large round or oval, often irregularly indented nucleus. In sections of marrow hardened in Zenker's fluid the nuclear membrane stains deeply with hæmatoxylin, giving a vesicular appearance to the nucleus, but chromatic substance is not abundant, so that the nucleus, particularly in dried preparations, stains palely. Müller and Rieder have shown that these cells are capable of little if any amœboid movement.

In addition to myelocytes with eosinophile granulation, smaller eosinophile cells with polymorphous nuclei are present in the bone-marrow. Many of these are identical with the eosinophile

[1] Deutsches Arch. f. klin. Med., 1891, vol. xlviii. p. 47.

leukocytes of the blood and are capable of amoeboid movement. Cells of the same size may contain a rounded nucleus, which is usually kidney-shaped as the result of an indentation at one point. Other small eosinophile cells have a nucleus which has the form of a bent rod; constrictions at intervals so divide the rod that it is transformed into the lobed nucleus which is found in the eosinophile leukocytes of the circulating blood.

Mitotic division of eosinophile cells in mammals was first described by H. F. Müller,[1] though similar observations had been made by Flemming[2] and Dekhuysen[3] in amphibia and birds. Such division in the guinea-pig takes place only in the bone-marrow and occurs in cells which are usually so large that they are recognized as myelocytes.

Corresponding to the varying number of eosinophile cells in the circulating blood of guinea-pigs, the bone-marrow exhibits variations which help to explain the origin of these cells. In animals of which the blood during life contains approximately 1 per cent. of eosinophile leukocytes fat is very abundant and the cells of the marrow occupy the interstices between the fat-cells. Eosinophile cells of the characters already described occur in moderate numbers scattered among the other cellular elements. In animals with a larger proportion of eosinophile cells in the blood, similar cells are more numerous in the marrow, but in guinea-pigs in which the eosinophile cells of the blood reach the proportion of from 15 per cent. to 30 per cent. the bone-marrow presents a characteristic appearance. The fat is in great part or wholly replaced by myeloid tissue, which is largely composed of cells with eosinophile granules. Myelocytes are particularly numerous, but smaller cells with polymorphous nucleus are not wanting. Eosinophile cells in process of mitotic division are readily recognized by the hyperchromatic condition of the nucleus, and never in large numbers, are much more numerous than usual; the so-called diaster stage of mitosis is not infrequent.

In the pulp of the spleen eosinophile cells are found in considerable number, and are more abundant the greater the number in the circulating blood. They are absent within the Malpighian corpuscles, but are particularly abundant in the pulp at their periphery. Eosinophile myelocytes do not occur and mitotic figures are not demonstrable.

Relation of the Eosinophile Cells to Nutrition. In apparently healthy guinea-pigs weighing more than 500 grams, eosinophile leukocytes, as it has been shown, not infrequently form from 15 per cent. to 30 per cent. of the total number of leukocytes, and in the greater number of instances constitute 8 per cent. to 14 per cent. In this animal, more readily than in man, where the eosinophile cells rarely exceed 4 per cent., it is possible to deter-

[1] Arch f. exper. Path. u. Phar., 1892, vol. xxix. p. 221.
[2] Arch. f. mik. Anat., 1891, vol. xxxvii. p. 249.
[3] Anat. Anz., vol. vi. p. 220.

mine the conditions with which these cells are diminished, as well as those with which they are increased.

It was considered desirable to make a preliminary study of the changes to which the eosinophile leukocytes may be subject under ordinary conditions. For this purpose the blood of guinea-pigs supplied with abundant food and water were examined repeatedly for a considerable period of time, and variations in the number of eosinophile cells were noted. The animals were allowed to feed at will and no allowance was made for a possible leukocytosis of digestion. The records which follow indicate that such leukocytosis is not an important disturbing factor. The weight of the animal serves as the best indication of its condition and has been recorded in conjunction with the count of eosinophiles.

CHART 1.

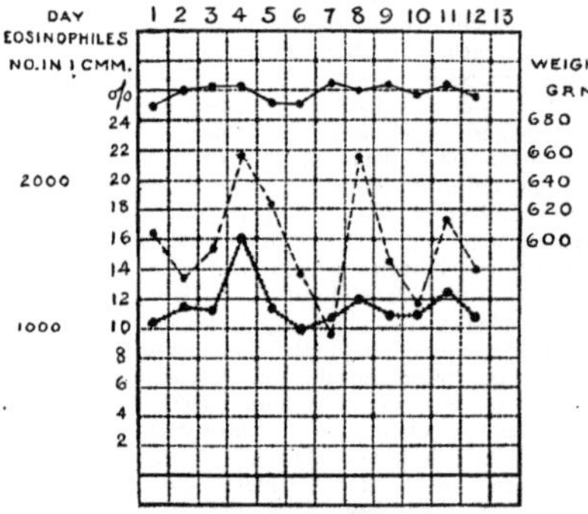

In this and in the charts to follow the percentage of eosinophile cells is represented by a dotted line, their number in one cubic millimetre of blood by a broken line. The weight of the animal is represented by a black line.

In Chart 1 are recorded the weight of the animal, the proportion of eosinophile cells in the blood, and their absolute number in one cubic millimetre of blood, calculated from the total number of leukocytes, which have been estimated daily by means of a Thoma-Zeiss apparatus. During twelve days the weight has varied little, ranging from 690 to 705 grams. The proportion of eosinophile cells exhibits slight variations, which correspond fairly well to much more marked alterations of their absolute number. At intervals of several days there is a recurring increase in the number of these cells, as though many were rapidly thrown into the circulation. The sudden elevation of the curve is followed by a somewhat more gradual fall.

In Chart 2 only the weight and proportion of eosinophile cells are recorded.

CHART 2.

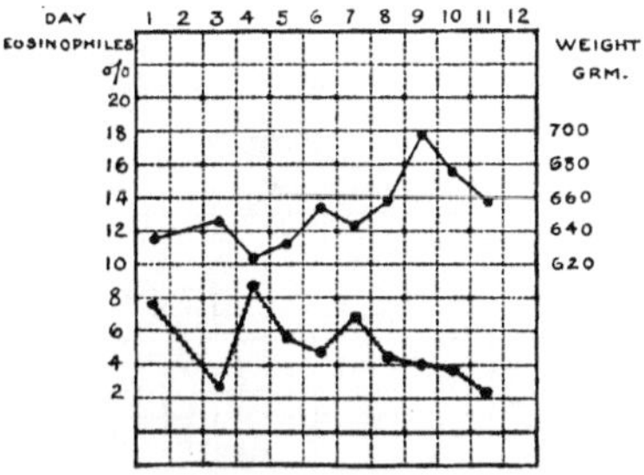

The weight of the animal varies within wider limits than that recorded in Chart 1, and, as in the previous instance, the proportion of eosinophile cells alternately increases and decreases. A comparison of the two curves suggests that the number of eosinophile cells bears a relation to changes in the weight of the animals, for repeatedly an increase in weight is accompanied by a fall in the proportion of eosinophiles, while a decrease of weight is accompanied by an increase in the number of these cells, so that the two curves tend to vary in opposite directions. This phenomenon is not constant, for on the tenth and eleventh days, though the weight has fallen, the eosinophiles do not rise. Doubtless, conditions other than those which affect nutrition exert an influence on the proportion of eosinophile cells, and in Chart 1, though the number of eosinophile leukocytes varied considerably, the weight changed little.

A relation between variations in weight and proportion of eosinophile cells is even better indicated in the following curve, where the eosinophile leukocytes rose gradually during a period of nearly three weeks. Alterations of the number of eosinophile cells, with much constancy, take an opposite direction from those of weight, and at times these contrary variations extend over a period greater than a week.

There was reason to suspect that the animal of which the number of eosinophile cells is recorded in Chart 3 had received, just before these observations were begun, an insufficient amount of food. The possibility has suggested itself that the food supply may exert an influence upon the eosinophile leukocytes of the blood.

By the use of Ehrlich's triple stain somewhat modified Heidenhain demonstrated the existence of cells with deep-red granules, undoubtedly eosinophile cells, in the villi, and still more abundantly in the subglandular layer of the dog's intestinal mucosa, and studied

CHART 3.

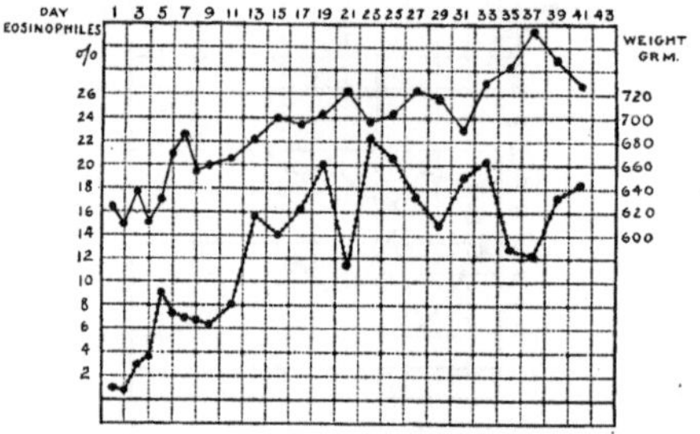

these cells under varying conditions of nutrition. If animals were starved during from four to seven days and then killed, eosinophiles disappeared from the villi and their number in the subglandular layer was diminished. Considerable variation was noted in individual cases, and in one instance eosinophile cells were numerous even after some days without food. Abundant feeding produced the opposite condition; if a dog receiving an ordinary diet was given a large meal of meat and was killed fourteen to sixteen hours later eosinophile cells were found in very large numbers, both in the villi and in the subglandular layer. Sugar in large amount had the same effect as proteid diet. Continued overfeeding diminished rather than increased the number of cells with eosinophile granulation.

Teichmüller repeated with guinea-pigs some of the experiments of Heidenhain. He found that starvation causes the number of eosinophile cells in the intestinal mucosa to diminish, but thought that the number in the spleen was increased. If, however, the animal was killed by starvation, eosinophiles were diminished in the intestine, spleen, and bone-marrow. Hence, he reached the conclusion that starvation causes a temporary increase of eosinophile cells, followed by diminution of their number.

As far as I have been able to determine, observations upon the eosinophile cells of the blood during starvation have been made only by Tanszk,[1] who observed the fasting juggler Succi. An increase in the proportion of eosinophile leukocytes was noted.

[1] Wiener klin. Rundschau, 1896, No. 18. Quoted by Teichmüller.

Following the suggestion offered by Chart 3, I have studied the effect which withdrawal of food exerts upon the eosinophile leukocytes of the circulating blood. The consequent changes are well shown in the following chart.

CHART 4.

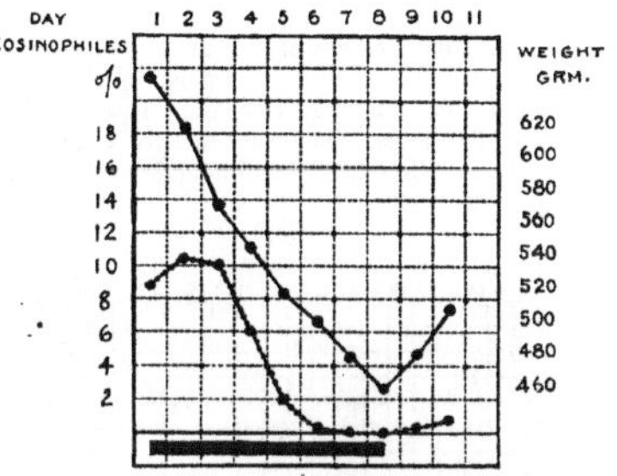

In this and in the charts to follow the period during which the animal received no food is indicated by a broad black line at the bottom of the chart.

Though the weight diminished continuously from the beginning of the experiment, there was a primary increase in the proportion of eosinophile leukocytes, but after the third day they also decreased in number, and on the seventh and eighth days none were found in the specimens of blood which were examined. Estimation of the total number of leukocytes in conjunction with the proportion of eosinophile cells in two animals from which food was withheld has shown that diminution of the absolute number of eosinophile cells is accurately represented by the preceding chart, which records only their relative number.

GUINEA-PIG A.

Day.	Weight, grm.	Leukocytes in 1 c.mm.	Eosinophiles in 1 c.mm.
1st	712	11,900	1428 = 12.0 %
2d	677	8,600	1075 = 12.5 "
3d	645	14,200	2087 = 14.7 "
4th.	619	10,600	1325 = 12.5 "
5th.	594	15,500	852 = 5.5 "

GUINEA-PIG B.

Day.	Weight, grm.	Leukocytes in 1 c.mm.	Eosinophiles in 1 c.mm.
1st	650	7,900	869 = 11.0 "
2d	615	12,900	1741 = 13.5 "
3d	579	12,000	840 = 7.0 "
4th.	550	17,500	787 = 4.5 "
5th.	526	10,900	414 = 3.8 "

In both experiments an increase in the relative and in the absolute number of eosinophile leukocytes preceded the fall, which began on the fourth day of starvation.

If food is withheld during several days, the animal may loose in weight 100 or more grams, and, gradually recovering, regain its former size only after several weeks. With the administration of food there is a sudden increase both of weight and of eosinophile leukocytes, but the increase of neither is uninterrupted. In the experiments recorded by the accompanying chart, withdrawal of food on two occasions, namely, from the first to the fifth days of observation, and again from the twenty-seventh to the thirty-third day, has been followed by a fall of eosinophile leukocytes to less than 1 per cent.

CHART 5.

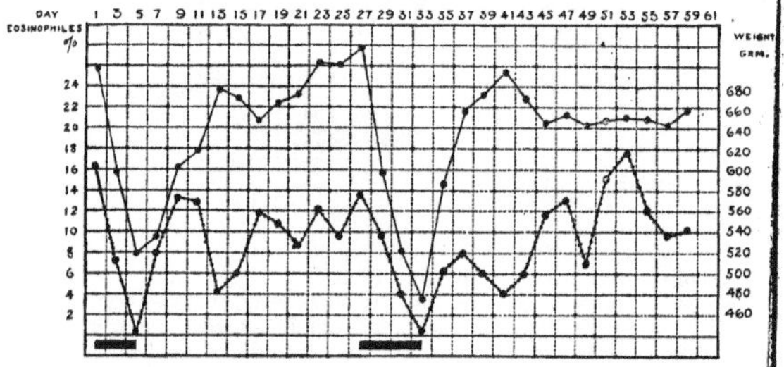

During the period which follows the administration of food the chart exhibits the phenomenon which has been noted in the normal animal. Increase in the proportion of eosinophile leukocytes is not continuous, and after two or three days their number falls, even though the weight, which is yet far from normal, continues to rise. Soon the increase of weight is interrupted, and with a fall in the curve of weight there is an increase in the proportion of eosinophile cells. This phenomenon is conspicuous during the first ten days or two weeks after starvation, but may be subsequently absent.

In the experiment recorded in Chart 6, an animal was employed of which the blood contained eosinophiles in the unusual proportion of 34 per cent.; the total number of leukocytes was, however, somewhat less than usual.

In this experiment the eosinophile leukocytes did not fall to 1 per cent. until the seventh day after food had been withdrawn; the weight diminished during this time 140 grams. The subsequent rise and fall of the curves representing weight and eosinophile cells show the remarkable relation previously observed, though the falls in weight on the nineteenth and again on the twenty-fifth day, with which in each case corresponds a sudden rise in the proportion of eosinophile cells, are so slight that they may be regarded as interruptions of the gradual return to normal. The total number of leukocytes was estimated at intervals, in order to determine the absolute number of eosinophile cells in one cubic millimetre of blood, but no important difference between the proportion and the absolute number of eosinophile leukocytes was observed. Particularly noteworthy is the fact that variations affecting the proportion of eosinophiles, and

CHART 6.

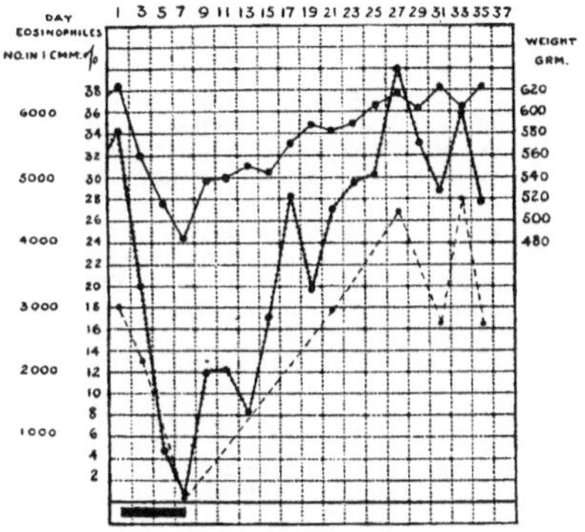

occurring between the thirty-first and thirty-ninth days, when the animal's weight had become normal, correspond to inverse variations of weight, and represent the absolute as well as the relative number of eosinophile cells.

In three animals I have studied in sections from tissues hardened in Zenker's fluid the effect of starvation upon the distribution of the eosinophile cells. The weight, the percentage of eosinophile leukocytes at the beginning of the experiment, and the date of death were as follows:

No. 1.	Weight, 385 grm.	Percentage of eosinophiles, 0.3.	Killed on the 5th day.
" 2.	" 712 "	" " " 12.0.	" " 6th "
" 3.	" 650 "	" " " 11.0.	" " 8th "

Except in the animal killed on the eighth day of starvation, there was no noteworthy diminution in the number of cells with eosinophile granulation in the wall of the small intestine, and especially in the Peyer's patches. On the eighth day, however, their number had appreciably diminished. In the mesenteric lymph glands and in the connective tissue of the mesentery and omentum, on the contrary, few such cells were found in any of the animals examined. The same statement can be made concerning the lungs where eosinophile cells are usually so abundant. The number in the spleen was much diminished, and, as usual, was in close relation with the number present in the blood.

In order to determine what changes have taken place in the bone-marrow, it is necessary to recall the fact that the number of eosinophile cells here present is variable and has a relation to the proportion of eosinophile leukocytes in the blood. In no case was a noteworthy diminution observed in this organ. In the animal killed on the fifth day, in which the eosinophile leukocytes at the beginning of the experiment numbered only 3 per cent., eosinophile cells were fairly abundant in the marrow and were, in great part, of small size, with polymorphous nuclei; myelocytes were not numerous. In the animals killed on the sixth and eighth days eosinophile cells were still present in great abundance, and smaller forms, resembling those usually found in the circulating blood, were far more numerous than myelocytes with eosinophile granulation. Particularly noteworthy is the fact that the eosinophile cells of the bone-marrow do not show the marked diminution which occurs in other organs.

Origin of the Eosinophile Cells. Ehrlich has maintained that a sharp distinction can be drawn between the lymphocytes and the granular leukocytes; the former have their origin in the lymphatic glands and in other tissues which form part of the lymphatic system, while the latter are derived wholly from the bone-marrow. The great number of eosinophile cells present in the bone-marrow furnishes evidence, Ehrlich has maintained, that they here undergo multiplication. Other observers (Müller and Rieder) have suggested that their presence may be explained by supposing that the bone-marrow is a storehouse for eosinophile leukocytes.

Max Schultze, who, almost forty years ago, classified the leukocytes observable in fresh blood studied upon a warm stage, reached the conclusion that the amœboid cells containing coarse granules are derived by gradual transition from the amœboid leukocytes with fine granules and many subsequent writers, including Ouskow,[1] Zappert,[2] Müller and Rieder,[3] Gulland,[4] and Van der Stricht,[5] finding in human blood what they believe to be transitional stages, have maintained that leukocytes with eosinophile granulation are derived from those with fine neutrophile granules. The transformation, they think, occurs either in the bone-marrow or in the circulating blood.

[1] From the Russian. Quoted by Ehrlich and Lazarus and others.
[2] Loc. cit.
[3] Loc. cit.
[4] Journal of Physiology, 1896, vol. xix. p. 385.
[5] Arch. de biol., 1892, vol. xii. p. 199.

To many observers the number of eosinophile leukocytes in the circulating blood has seemed too small to explain the large accumulations not infrequently noted in various organs. Ehrlich, indeed, reached the conclusion that the eosinophile cells of the frog are, in part at least, transformed cells of connective tissue. The presence of eosinophile cells in certain skin lesions has suggested to Neusser[1] and others that these cells in man may be formed in connective tissue. Certain writers, including von Leyden,[2] Schmidt,[3] and Grouven,[4] who have studied the eosinophile cells in the sputum and blood of patients suffering with asthma, claim that they are formed in the bronchial mucosa. Stutz[5] thinks that they may be formed in the intestinal mucosa as well. Howard and Perkins[6] believe that eosinophile cells are formed in various organs, especially in the lymphoid tissue of the gastrointestinal mucosa and in various exudations, from lymphocytes and from plasma cells, and state that transitions from one to the other may be observed.

According to another view, the eosinophile granules are formed from material ingested by leukocytes. In many instances this belief has had its chief support in the fact that the material supposed to form eosinophile granules stains deeply with acid dyes. Klein[7] thinks that neutrophile leukocytes take up hæmoglobin derived from extravasated red blood corpuscles and are transformed into eosinophile cells; Sacharoff[8] holds a somewhat similar view. Tettenhamer[9] has described the formation of eosinophile cells in the degenerate testicle of the salamander; acidophile substance formed from nuclei undergoing degeneration is ingested by phagocytes. In human muscle infected with trichinæ T. R. Brown[10] found both neutrophile and eosinophile leukocytes in contact with the substance of much-altered muscle fibres. Finding, in addition, what he regarded as transitional stages between the two varieties of cell, he thought it probable that the neutrophile leucocytes form eosinophile granules by ingesting material derived from the degenerate muscle fibres. He supported this view by observations upon the relation of the eosinophile and neutrophile cells of the circulating blood. When with trichinosis the eosinophile cells in the blood were very greatly increased, the neutrophile leukocytes had undergone a corresponding diminution in number.

Metschnikoff[11] and Mesnil[12] also believe that eosinophile cells may be formed by a process of phagocytosis. Metschnikoff has seen spirilla of cholera ingested by leukocytes of the guinea-pig become so

[1] Wiener klin. Woch. 1892, vol. v. pp. 41, 65.
[2] Deutsche med. Woch, 1891, vol. xvii. p. 1085.
[3] Zeit. f. klin. Med., vol. xx.
[4] Inaug. Diss., Bonn, 1895.
[5] Ibid.
[6] Johns Hopkins Hospital Reports, 1903, vol. x. p. 249.
[7] Cent. f. innere Med., 1899, vol. xx. pp. 97, 121.
[8] Cent. f. Bakt. u. Par., 1897, vol. xxi. p. 265.
[9] Anat. Anz., 1893, vol. viii. p. 223.
[10] Journal of Experimental Medicine, 1898, vol. iii. p. 315.
[11] Annales de l'Institut Pasteur, 1894, vol. viii. p. 58.
[12] Ibid., 1895, vol. ix. p. 301.

altered that they stain readily with eosin, while Mesnil maintains that anthrax bacilli are transformed into eosinophile granules by leukocytes of the lizard.

SUMMARY AND CONCLUSIONS. The opinions which have just been cited will not be discussed in detail. I will merely review certain facts which I believe serve to explain the origin of the eosinophile cells. In various tissues of the guinea-pig, notably in the mucosa of the gastrointestinal tract, in the mucosa of the air-passages, in the lymphatic tissue, and in the spleen, occur eosinophile leukocytes which are identical with those present in the circulating blood, and, like them, are provided with polymorphous nuclei. In the bone-marrow alone occur large mononuclear cells with eosinophile granulation. These cells of the bone-marrow undergo mitotic division and form daughter cells, which resemble in size the eosinophile leukocytes of the blood, while cells in which the nucleus presents varying irregularity in shape may be regarded as transitional forms. In the blood and in various organs the eosinophile cells give no evidence of multiplication.

The myelocytes with neutrophile or amphophile granules are analogous to the myelocytes with eosinophile granulation, resembling them in size and in the character of their nuclei. Muir[1] found that when the amphophile leukocytes in the blood of the rabbit undergo continued increase as the result of repeated bacterial infection, the myelocytes of the marrow are increased in number and mitotic division proceeds actively. An analogous phenomenon has been noted in those guinea-pigs of which the circulating blood contains a very large proportion of eosinophile leukocytes. The number of eosinophile cells is far greater than usual, while particularly abundant are the large eosinophile myelocytes. Mitotic division of these cells is observed much more readily than in the marrow of animals in which the blood contains few eosinophile leukocytes.

In certain instances in which eosinophile cells have accumulated in the tissues it has been possible to demonstrate their abundance in the bloodvessels of the part, and in one case the process of migration was actually demonstrable in sections of the hardened tissue. In apparently healthy guinea-pigs eosinophile leukocytes have been shown to migrate from the bloodvessels into the wall of a small bronchus, and hence through the epithelium into the lumen. Eosinophile cells manufactured in the bone-marrow reach the tissues by way of the bloodvessels.

The number of eosinophile cells in one cubic millimetre of blood is found to vary from day to day, and at intervals of three or four days undergoes an increase. It is not improbable that the number of eosinophile cells which the bone-marrow discharges into the circulation is subject to periodic variation. Complete withdrawal

[1] Journal of Pathology and Bacteriology, 1901, vol. vii. p. 161.

of food is followed by a decrease both in the proportion and in the absolute number of eosinophile leukocytes in the peripheral circulation. Disturbance of nutrition acting doubtless on the bone-marrow affects the multiplication of the eosinophile cells more readily than that of the polynuclear leukocytes with fine granulation. Diminution in the number of eosinophile cells is preceded by a temporary increase, which may be explained by supposing that ripe eosinophile leukocytes already stored in the marrow reach the circulation, and, perhaps, are no longer diverted to the intestinal mucosa. With the administration of food the eosinophile cells of the blood gradually increase in number, but neither the weight of the animal nor the eosinophile leukocytes increase continuously. That there exists a close relation between the nutrition of the animal and the eosinophile cells is shown by the fact that variations in weight and in the number of eosinophile cells take with much regularity opposite directions, so that a temporary fall in weight is accompanied by a rapid increase of the eosinophile leukocytes, while a rise in weight tends to retard this increase.

CIRCUMCORNEAL HYPERTROPHY (VERNAL CONJUNCTIVITIS) IN THE NEGRO.

By Swan M. Burnett, M.D., Ph.D.,
of Washington, D. C.

It would seem from a report of the discussion of a most carefully prepared paper on "Vernal Conjunctivitis," read by Dr. W. C. Posey[1] at the last meeting of the American Medical Association, at New Orleans, that opinion is far from being settled as to the peculiar manifestations of this singular affection in the negro in this country. As some statements of mine in a paper published in Knapp's *Archives* in 1881, in which the phases of the disease as it appears in the negro were first brought to the attention of the profession, have apparently not been clearly understood or not confirmed by other observers, it may not be without interest to revert to the subject again in an endeavor to harmonize views and clarify some seeming obscurities.

It appears to be a question with some whether the appearances described in that paper, and also in my chapter on "Diseases of the Conjunctiva" in Norris and Oliver's *System*, are not those of phlyctenular conjunctivitis, instead of that distinct form of disease now generally denominated as "spring catarrh" of the conjunctiva.

A rather extensive study of the disease (principally by Europeans) since Sämisch first reported upon it in 1876 has not added greatly to

[1] Published in Journal of the American Medical Association, July 25, 1903.

our very limited knowledge of the cause and pathology of the affection. The clinical characteristics of that feature of the disease manifest on the globe are so distinctive that it seems quite impossible that anyone who has once seen a pronounced case could be mistaken in the diagnosis, so utterly unlike any other known condition is it. The above-mentioned opinion of some well-known and accurate observers that it may be a form of phlyctenular disease leads me to think that they have never seen a typical case of circumcorneal hypertrophy; from which we may infer that the affection is much more frequent in some sections than in others, a fact that may be found of no small etiological importance, and give a clue which should be assiduously followed up. Those of us whose work lies in localities where the negro abounds are well aware of the great frequency of scrofulous or strumous affections of the cornea and conjunctiva in that race, and can confirm Dr. Bruns' statement as to its frequent cause of blindness and greatly impaired vision. But there is no manifestation of this diathesis, either on the cornea or conjunctiva, which at any stage bears any resemblance to the ocular form of circumcorneal hypertrophy as found in the negro. The clinical features of scrofulous conjunctivitis are marked by certain constant and well-recognized characteristics. When it appears under the distinctly phlyctenular form the elevations are discrete, though they may be several in number. Whether the inflammatory symptoms are slight or severe, the natural history of the phlyctenula is the same; its wall bursts, its contents are discharged, and an ulcer results, which heals, as we know, with a very greatly varying rapidity. Photophobia and lacrymation are rarely absent, and may be present in the intensest degree. When the manifestation is on the cornea itself the exudate is still more or less circumscribed and small, with a very variable amount of destruction of tissue and cicatricial formation as a result. On the other hand, the distinguishing mark of circumcorneal hypertrophy is that it is *not destructive*. It is a true hyperplasia, and it was with a view of making this essential feature prominent and descriptive in nomenclature that I adopted the name "circumcorneal hypertrophy" as the best English synonym of the "hypertrophie perikeratique" of Desmarnes and the "gallertige Verdickung des Limbus" of Gräfe. This hyperplasic character of the pathological condition has been confirmed by all examinations of the tissue that have been made. Scheile has shown that the principal change in the circumcorneal form is in the epithelial layer, manifested by a largely increased number of the cells with invaginations, constituting the so-called "cancroid formations," together with some increase in the connective tissue. A drawing representing these appearances is given in my chapter on "Diseases of the Conjunctiva" in Norris and Oliver's *System*. Some more recent investigations made by de Schweinitz and Shumway, and published in the *University of Pennsylvania Medical Bulletin* for June, 1903, reveal identical changes in the conjunctiva of the lid. Everywhere there is hypertrophy and nowhere a destruction of tissue.

There has not been a season since the publication of my paper in 1881 in which I have not observed cases of this disease—sometimes in considerable numbers—and not once have I observed any tendency toward destructive ulceration. If there is a destructive process, it is not circumcorneal hypertrophy. On the subsidence of the hypertrophy during the winter there seldom remains any sign of its former presence.

There are cases in which the symptoms of irritation are considerable. In the bulbar form, when the conjunctiva of the lid is but little involved, these symptoms are confined to a slight hyperæmia of the conjunctiva of the ball, but more often there is no complaint of photophobia or lacrymation. In the palpebral form, especially where there are large hard excrescences which rub on the cornea, the irritation may be quite marked, as indicated by a congested state of the conjunctiva of the globe and some photophobia. There is, however, never an involvement of the cornea aside from the hypertrophy. The usual, and, indeed, the characteristic complaint is not of pain, but of an intense itching of the eyes and sometimes of a "burning sensation," quite distinct from the subjective symptoms of phlyctenulæ.

It is the objective appearance, however, which is so strikingly distinctive, especially in the bulbar form. The dirty gray elevations at the base of the cornea bear no resemblance whatever, when they are at all marked, to any other pathological condition found there. It must be remembered in this connection that the circumcorneal epithelial changes vary enormously in degree. Sometimes they are so slight as to escape detection unless carefully sought for. It may be that there is manifest only a macerated condition of the cells, with some slight increase in number, and confined to a very limited portion of the corneal circumference. Even in pronounced cases the hypertrophy may not go entirely around the cornea. I believe that in every case, even where the changes are supposed to be limited to the conjunctiva of the lid, a careful examination will reveal some changes at the limbus. I have one such case, in a negro girl, aged nine years, under observation at my clinic now, in which the palpebral changes in the form of granulations are typical, but the circumcorneal alterations could easily be overlooked if particular care were not given to finding them. This child has been subject to the disease since she was three years old, the symptoms beginning in March and continuing until October. In her the rubbing of the cornea by the granulations gives rise to some lacrymation, but the irritative symptoms are slight.

At other times the alterations around the cornea are so striking that when seen fully blown, for the first time in the negro, they are likely to confound even an experienced diagnostician in eye diseases.

I remember such an experience with one of my associates in a hospital in this city. He was a man trained to careful observation, and had followed some large eye clinics in a neighboring city in the South, where the clientèle of negroes was large. He asked me to see a case of peculiar corneal disease, the exact nature of which he was unable to determine. As soon as the patient, a negro boy, aged eight years, entered the door of the clinic room I turned and asked him if he had ever seen such a condition before, recognizing, as I did, even at that distance, what the disease was. He was greatly surprised to find that it was a typical case of circumcorneal hypertrophy in the negro, a condition with which he was entirely unfamiliar, though he had seen the disease in the white race. Thereafter there was never any difficulty in his diagnostication of even slight forms of that disease, for it is a fact that one familiar with its appearances in the negro can easily make the diagnosis across the room. There is an aspect of the eyes, due to the peculiar appearance of the palpebral aperture, which, once seen, cannot be taken for anything else. The "white" of the eye in the negro, especially in the young, is very clearly marked, often brilliant, in contrast with the surrounding dark skin. In circumcorneal hypertrophy this is changed. The palpebral aperture has a dull, soggy look, and a dusky appearance, as though it had been smoked. This "smoked" look is not always of the same intensity, but even in mild cases is sufficiently pronounced to be recognized at a distance of many feet. In no other affection of the eyes in the negro have I encountered this singular look of the palpebral aperture. A closer examination shows the cause of this "smoked" appearance to be a pigmentation of the conjunctiva, which is more or less thickened and easily thrown into folds with the movements of the ball inward or outward. The epithelium has some of that lack-lustre look which is seen in a greater degree in xerosis of the conjunctiva. The smoky look is confined almost entirely to the space exposed by the palpebral fissure. The parts usually covered by the lids are not affected. The pigment is usually in very small, dot-like points, to be differentiated only under a magnifier, but toward the base of the cornea it may be in quite large masses, some of which measure a quarter of a millimetre in diameter. This smoky look of the palpebral aperture disappears with the subsidence of the disease during the colder months, when the eyes return to approximately their normal appearance; not always, however, for there are occasional cases which continue, with all the characteristic appearances, during the winter months, though commonly with diminished intensity. The statistics at my clinic and also, I learn, from my confrères, at the other eye clinics in Washington, show that the negro in this section is much more prone to the disease than the white race. At my clinic it is rare to see a case among the white patients. Of thirteen cases of the disease recorded during the last eighteen months all were colored.

Opinions differ as to the relative frequency of the bulbar and palpebral forms. My own belief is that they both exist together, but one may be so slight as to escape detection unless carefully looked for. I also think that the same patient may have one or the other form more pronounced at different seasons.

A typical but extremely pronounced case of the disease in the negro is shown in the accompanying drawing. The patient was a negro boy, not perhaps of full blood, but quite dark, who at the time the drawing was made (1899) was sixteen years old. The dull, "greasy," gray hypertrophy, which was elevated 0.5 mm. to 1 mm. above the surrounding tissue, was irregular as to surface, and not only occupied the conjunctival tissues in the vicinity of the cornea, but invaded the corneal surface so far as to leave less than one-half of the iris exposed to view. Both the internal and external edges of the elevation were irregular in outline. The cornea inside the inner border was perfectly clear and the vision was not materially affected. The conjunctiva visible within the palpebral fissure was dark brownish in tinge, and there were many points of pigment in the vicinity of the elevation arranged, as they usually are, in the form of triangles, with their apices toward the canthi. The conjunctiva of the lids presented an appearance quite different from that usually seen in such cases, in so far as there was not that distinctly granular aspect which is commonly regarded as characteristic. The tissue was much thickened and lined with many furrows, undoubtedly an exaggeration of the same pathological changes that produce the excrescences—namely, a large proliferation of the epithelial structure. Both eyes were affected and practically to the same extent. The final issue of the case, which I followed for several years, I am not able to give, as the patient disappeared from view soon after the drawing was made.

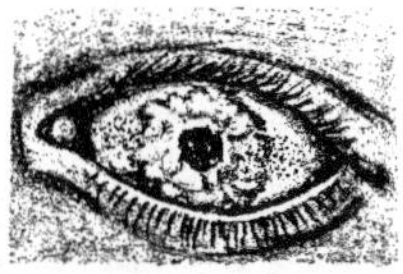

That the disease is the manifestation of a dyscrasia seems certain, but it is not so certain what that dyscrasia is. Of course, we can never exclude what we call scrofula in any patient of the colored race, and yet there is nothing about the appearance of the condition itself or in the patients which would justify the acceptance of any such stigma as a cause. It occurs often in the most robust-looking, with none of the usual signs of deficient nutrition. I have looked in vain for some connection of inherited syphilis with the disease. In my experience the male and female sexes are about equally represented; and while principally an affection of childhood, the adult is by no means free. I have seen one pronounced case in a mulatto woman aged thirty years. Both eyes are affected, but not always at the same time nor in the same degree. As is well known, the disease is most prevalent during the hot months, and so far as a seasonal nomenclature is applicable, "summer conjunctivitis" would be the more nearly appropriate. Strictly speaking, however, the affection is not a conjunctivitis at all, taking conjunctivitis to mean an inflammation of the conjunctiva. It is not only not confined to the conjunctival tissue proper, but there are none of the clinical characteristics of conjunctival inflammation, there being seldom any increase in the conjunctival secretion, either mucous or purulent. The term "catarrh" may be accepted in the conventional meaning of that term as applicable to all alterations in the mucous tissues.

The possible relation of the disease to trachoma has naturally attracted attention, since the granular condition of the lids suggests in some instances the appearances in trachoma. The similarity, however, is only superficial, for the essential nature of the two conditions is diametrically opposite. In trachoma the action is destructive, whereas in this disease it is purely hyperplastic, and when the affection subsides for the winter the conjunctiva assumes an almost if not quite normal appearance. There is an observation in this connection, however, which is not only interesting in itself, but may prove of value in making our final judgment as to the pathology of the disease, which should be noted, and this is the almost total absence of circumcorneal hypertrophy in Russia, where trachoma is so rampant. According to Natanson,[1] the "flying column" of 100 oculists, which was sent throughout the provinces of Russia from 1893 to 1897 to look after diseases of the eye among the peasantry, did not meet among 168,618 patients, a large percentage of whom were trachomatous, with a single case of vernal conjunctivitis. Of course, it may be said that only the severely affected applied for treatment, and, circumcorneal hypertrophy being a practically painless disease, the stoical peasants paid no attention to it. But the reports from the clinics at St. Petersburg, Moscow, Kiew, and other Russian cities show the same practical immunity of the Russian from this affection.

This fact, taken in connection with the other fact that the negro in this country is practically immune from trachoma and is very liable to circumcorneal hypertrophy, offers a suggestion as to an antagonistic character in the diseases which, if followed up, might lead to some more definite knowledge of both affections. It would be instructive to know how such countries as Ireland and Southern Italy, as well as other localities where trachoma prevails, stand as to the percentage of circumcorneal hypertrophy. At any rate, these facts, as well as others, point most strongly to a racial influence, and a dyscrasic nature for both affections. Temperature, humidity, and

[1] Klin. Monatsbl. f. Augenheilk., April, 1900.

elevation do not seem to be controlling factors to any great degree according to Natanson.

In regard to therapeutics, the indications, in view of what we know of the pathology, are for palliative local measures. Operative procedures, such as excision of the masses, expression, etc., have been recommended and practised, but evidently are not advisable. Attention to the nutrition and an improvement in the general condition are more properly called for. Arsenic administered in some form meets with the approval of most of those who have written upon the subject.

A CASE OF SEBORRHŒA NIGRICANS (BLACK MASK OF THE FACE).

By Arthur Van Harlingen, M.D.,
of Philadelphia.

I am obliged to my friend Dr. J. S. Bethune, of Baddeck, C. B., for the opportunity of seeing this extraordinary affection of the skin and also for some notes of the history of the case.

Maggie McL., aged twenty-three years, comes of a neurotic family. Some members of the family are said to have suffered from mental alienation, and her father is a man of marked peculiarity of temper and disposition. Until her nineteenth year the patient enjoyed fair average health. She was brought up in the salubrious atmosphere of Cape Breton, but had lived out as a domestic, in Boston, I think, for a short time.

At this age she began to fail in health, although an exact statement of the symptoms could not be obtained. She was obliged to relinquish domestic service, returned home, took to her bed, and had remained there for four years up to the time of my examination. This scanty history was all that I could get of the patient's previous condition. It was, however, stated that soon after she took to bed a discoloration began to appear upon the face, which gradually spread and grew deeper in color until the entire visage was covered with a thick black mask.

Within the past few months the area of discoloration diminished until it had shrunken to the dimensions about to be noted. When I first saw her the patient was lying in bed in a small one-room cottage within a few feet of the cook-stove. She had been bedridden for several years, but, although somewhat emaciated, did not seem particularly ill. The limbs could be moved without much difficulty, though each movement and even a touch excited complaints of pain. She usually lay with her eyes shut, the lids twitching, and seemed to be suffering from photophobia. The face was flushed and mottled, the skin dry and scaly. The lips were dry and the skin immediately circumjacent covered with a yellowish sordes or crust, vesicular or seborrhœic in character, which surrounded the whole mouth. Her tongue was parched, red, and slightly fissured. It was said that this eruption about the mouth was accustomed to run a course of several weeks, turning black and falling off, to be succeeded by a fresh outbreak. The forehead and nose were covered with a most extraordinary mask or crust more than a quarter of an inch thick, resembling a rind of ham—soft, greasy, sharply defined about the edges, and rounded. It could be easily broken off, and the forceps could be thrust into it at any point as if the crust were comprised of soft fat. The color of the crust was exteriorly of an inky blackness and tolerably smooth. The appearance of the face was as if a mask or vizard were worn over the upper part.

The patient's general condition was that of an hysterical person. The shrinking from light, the groans and complaints on the slightest attempt at moving her, or even touching any part of the body, were highly characteristic. Trials at various points of the surface with a sharp object failed to disclose any areas of insensibility; in fact, the tactile sense appeared normal. Exception should be made of the scalp, which was certainly hyperæsthetic.

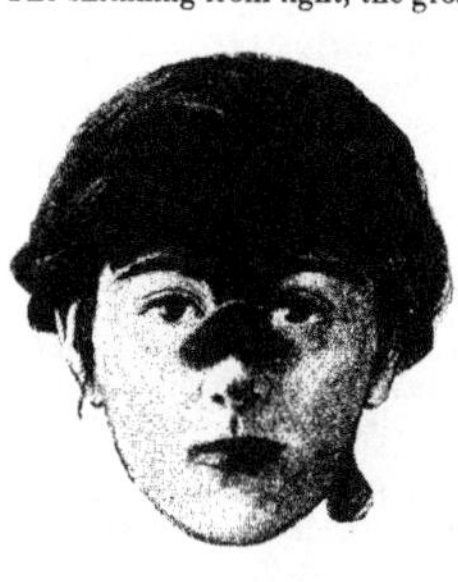

She had complained for some weeks of extreme sore throat, but seemed able to swallow without much difficulty. It was said she had taken nothing in the way of food for some weeks, but only an occasional drink of water. Her comparative lack of emaciation and the fact that the evacuations by the bladder and rectum were regular seemed to militate against the accuracy of this statement.

The attendants were supplied with a solution of sapo viridis in water and directed to endeavor to loosen the mask by daily washings. At the end of a week, however, when I saw her for the second time, the mask had not been at all cleaned off. It was loosened, however, and I had no difficulty in stripping off the entire coating. It came away like a thick crust of fat, tearing here and there, where undue traction was made. The outer surface was smooth, rather dry, and black, with bits of wool, hair, etc., matted in it. The internal surface was of a whitish color, soft and very greasy, showing numerous conical elevations, corresponding to the openings of the glands. The skin underneath was washed clean of the mask-coating, and then appeared moist and oily, the epidermis rather sodden and in places slightly abraded. The process of removal was in no way painful. The parts affected were ordered to be washed daily with a watery solution of green soap and powdered with a mixture of aristol and boric acid. A week after this I saw the patient again for the last time. The skin of the face was dry, red, and slightly scaly, the powder having dried it off. The washing having been very imperfectly performed, some greasy patches were still left of the mask. Also along one side of the nose there was a greenish crust, evidently seborrhœic in character. The skin being abnormally dry, it was decided that while continuing the daily washing with soap and water a dilute oxide of zinc ointment should also be employed. I preserved a portion of the greasy mask-like crust, which dried up gradually and shrunk, but retained a most offensive odor. Treated with ether a portion of the crust separated into various and heterogeneous components; there were fragments of wool and hair, granular débris, probably dust and grime, and whitish soft bits of tissue, which, picked out, treated with a solution of caustic potash and glycerin and examined under the microscope, were found to be composed of epithelial scales, with fine granular oil globules. The epithelial scales seemed dry and were not in a state of fatty degeneration. There were some few lanugo hairs.

The conclusion reached was that we had to deal in this case with a severe case of oily seborrhœa, giving rise to a dusky secretion upon the surface, which had been allowed to accumulate for several years, and which had, perhaps, been added to by the inunction or application of ointments and dressings of various kinds, together with accretions from the surrounding apartment, dust, flakes of soot, the sweepings of the carpet, etc. Most patients suffering from such affections are cleansed more or less frequently, and it is only by long-continued neglect that such extraordinary results are reached.

We have become familiar of late years with that form of chromidrosis which occurs in a black circle about the orbit or in rarer cases upon the forehead of certain hysterical women. In these cases the oily secretion from the coil glands is changed in color and consistency, and forms the discolored crust. In some cases, however, the sebaceous glands play the most prominent part, and such, I think has occurred in the case reported. As I believe this to be unique, I have not given any reference to the cases of chromidrosis recorded. A complete account of the latter affection is given in my article in the *Twentieth Century Practice of Medicine*, vol. v. p. 539, where the symptoms are fully described.[1]

[1] Since these notes were written I have received a letter from Dr. Bethune. He says: "The patient complains of a great deal of pain all over the face and head. The skin in patches over the face looks very red. She says it burns. This very likely is caused by the too frequent use of the sapo viridis, so I ordered it used less frequently. There is no sign of the mask, nor is there any sebaceous matter about the sides of the ala nasi. Her general condition is about the same as when you saw her (three months ago)."

A REPORT OF TWO CASES OF ECTOPIC GESTATION AND A CASE OF INTESTINAL OBSTRUCTION DUE TO MECKEL'S DIVERTICULUM.

By Harold H. Heyer, M.D.,

and

H. M. Lee, M.D.,

of New London, Conn.

Case I.—Mrs. X., white, American, aged twenty-six years; married in June, 1902. Housewife by occupation, presented herself at the office of my colleague, Dr. Heyer, on May 6, 1903, complaining of what she considered a prolonged menstrual period, and also of some slight pain and tenderness in the lower abdominal region

Family History. Negative.

Personal History. Had never had any illness she could remember except an attack of peritonitis (so-called) when eleven years of age.

Menstrual History. Commenced menstruation at the age of twelve years, and except on a few occasions had menstruated regularly. The average duration of her periods was five days—menstruating at an interval of twenty-eight days.

Since marriage her menstrual periods have appeared with regularity and without pain. She had never been pregnant.

Present History. On April 18th the patient was exposed to cold and wet, being alarmed thereby, because she expected her menstrual period to appear on April 19th. This, however, did not occur until April 22d, hence was delayed three days. From this time, namely, April 22d, to time she sought counsel, May 6th, she had flowed irregularly, the flow appearing suddenly and copiously at times, with some clots and of a dark color; then abating from a few hours to a few days. Pain, referred to the lower right abdominal region, and at times radiating downward over the anterior surface of the thigh, accompanied these periods of flowing. On several occasions faintness was marked. The patient was about during this time. The above irregular discharge and general condition continued up to May 12th, when she again consulted Dr. Heyer, her family physician. The patient was ordered to bed to insure rest and quiet, and, abortion being suspected, examination per vagina was made, with negative evidence. No sign or symptom of pregnancy could be adduced by a general physical examination. Throughout the whole vaginal vault tenderness was elicited upon pressure, more particularly on the *left* side. No tumor mass was detected, in fact, except for tenderness, this careful general examination was entirely negative. With conditions as above stated the patient remained in bed for the most part, when, during the night of May 19th she was seized with a very sudden sharp pain in the lower right abdominal region, accompanied by faintness and nausea. In the afternoon of May 20th Dr. Heyer was summoned, and upon examination a tumor was discovered occupying the lower right abdominal region. I was requested to see the patient in consultation, and at 6 P.M. found the following condition to exist:

The patient was in bed lying upon her back, with knees drawn up. Expression anxious and face pinched. Paleness of mucous surfaces quite marked. Mind clear and mental faculties fully acting. Temperature, 99.5° F.; pulse, 100, regular in rhythm, but irregular in volume, soft, small, rather pronounced upstroke. Respirations 30, shallow and thoracic in character. The patient complained of a tense dull pain in lower part of abdomen; slight headache; faintness, and no appetite. Thirst was not marked.

Physical Examination. Chest: Lungs normal. Heart rapid, regular, decreased muscular sound; valvular sounds normal.

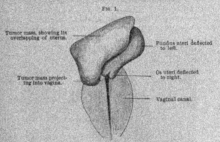

FIG. 1.

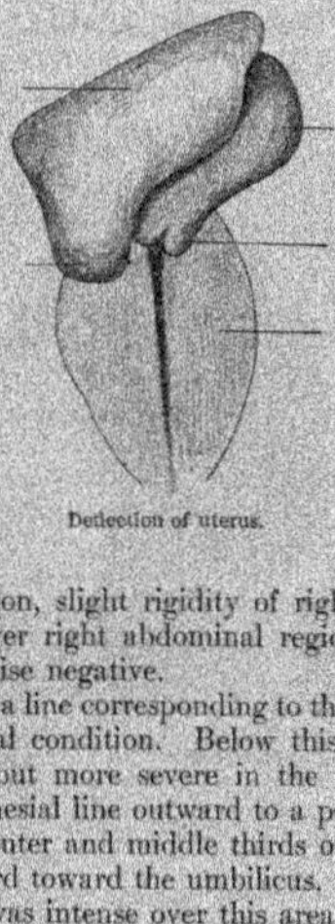

Deflection of uterus.

Abdomen: Inspection, slight rigidity of right rectus muscle and some bulging in lower right abdominal region apparent on deep inspiration. Otherwise negative.

Palpation. Above a line corresponding to the umbilicus palpation revealed no abnormal condition. Below this line tenderness was manifest generally, but more severe in the lower portion of the abdomen from the mesial line outward to a point corresponding to the junction of the outer and middle thirds of Poupart's ligament, and extending upward toward the umbilicus.

Pain on pressure was intense over this area, and produced faintness. A tumor was readily detected. The tumor mass was resistant and firm, the outer and upper border being sharply outlined.

Percussion. The percussion note over the various regions of the abdomen was normal, except over the tumor mass, where a dull note was elicited.

FIG. 2.

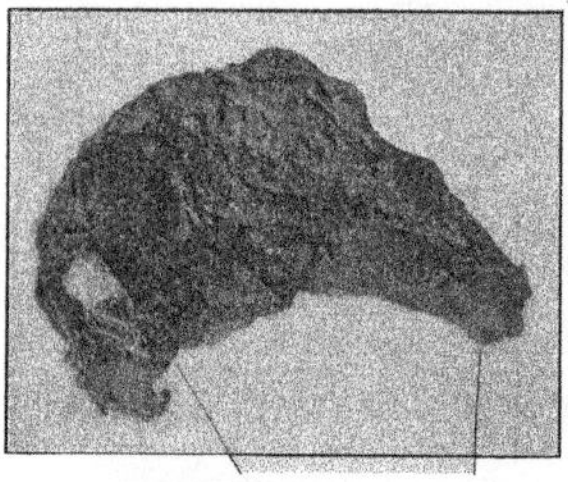

Sac. Tube.

Sac, with cotton placed in it.

FIG. 3.

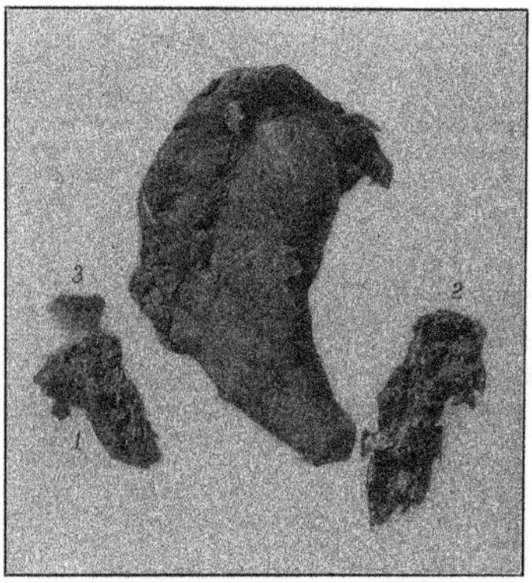

Other side of tube. Extent to which ovary was encroached upon in the sac formation. 1, 2, 3. Membrane and villi.

Vaginal Examination. The examining finger at once encountered a tumor mass projecting downward into the right side of vaginal canal, reaching below the cervix. The cervix was soft, and the os slightly dilated, discharging a dark bloody flux. Intense pain was elicited upon pressure throughout the vaginal vault. Cervix directed toward the right side. (See Fig. 3.)

Bimanual Examinations. Fundus of uterus deflected toward the left side. (See Fig. 3.) Uterus very slightly movable and perceptibly enlarged. Left ovary and tube readily felt and apparently of normal size. The tumor mass was very tense, immovable, and its upper borders sharply defined. The inner border seemed to merge into the body of the uterus and embrace that organ. (See Fig. 3.) However, it was apparent that there was no direct connection between the tumor and the uterus. This mass filled the pelvis on that side and was triangular in outline (see Fig. 2), extending upward in the mesial line two-thirds the distance from the symphysis pubis to the umbilicus and outward to a point corresponding to the junction of the outer and middle third of Poupart's ligament.

The right ovary and tube could not be made out. A dark thick discharge filled the os, and blood clots were quite numerous in the vagina. Examination of this discharge failed to reveal any membrane. During the examination the patient complained of increased pain throughout the entire pelvic cavity.

A diagnosis of rupture of an ectopic gestation sac was made, and operative interference was advised at once. The patient was admitted to the hospital on May 21st, and I operated on her the afternoon of that day.

On examination of the pelvic cavity it was found that the rupture of the gestation sac had taken place into the broad ligament, and dissected along between the layers of that structure close up to the body of the uterus. The reason of blood escaping as the peritoneal cavity was entered is explained by the fact that I either opened the wall of the hæmatoma, or else from the pressure alone it ruptured. The tube and ovary were now extirpated, and one litre of salt solution put into the cavity of the abdomen and the wound sutured in layer except at the lower inch, through which gauze drains were placed. The patient withstood the operation well, and her recovery was uneventful. Primary union was obtained and the drainage removed on the third day. At the end of two weeks the patient was allowed the liberty of moving about in bed, and on the sixteenth day, a tight-fitting support being applied to the abdomen, she sat up. At the end of three weeks she was discharged from the hospital.

Examination of the extirpated tube and ovary shows the gestation to have been of the so-called tubo-ovarian variety. It seems to me quite remarkable that this variety of ectopic gestation should have ruptured into the broad ligament. (See Fig. 2.)

The sac occupied quite a portion of the ovarian tissue, as shown in Fig. 3, which also shows the fetal membrane in part.

At the present writing the patient is enjoying as good health as ever, and the only discomfort from her serious difficulty and severe ordeal is a feeling of stiffness in the right groin, only evident after indulging in rather excessive exercise, and on becoming fatigued. However, the patient tells me that this feeling is gradually disappearing.

CASE II.—Mrs. Y., aged twenty-nine years; weight, 119 pounds; height, five feet two inches; American born of Scotch descent. Was married in June, 1898; housewife by occupation; was never pregnant.

Family History. Negative.

Personal History. As a child was not particularly strong. Never had any severe illness except an attack of diphtheria six years ago, and was not in her usual health for about a year thereafter.

Menstrual History. The patient commenced menstruating at the age of twelve years, and so far as she can remember was regular, and did not suffer at these times. The usual interval between the periods was twenty-five days, and the periods, as a rule, lasted five days. For three years after marriage there was no interference in the normal course of her menstrual history, but for the past two years she had suffered pain at these times on the first and second days.

This painful menstruation increased in severity as time went on, and in March, 1903, the patient consulted her family physician in regard to this, with the hope of obtaining relief. In conversation with Dr. H. W. Nichols, of Brooklyn, he told me that he found Mrs. Y. had a retroflexed and retroverted uterus. The patient was under his care about three months, and was then discharged, her trouble having been overcome, and the parts maintained in normal relations by a pessary. During the time under treatment the dysmenorrhœa abated.

I saw the patient for the first time on July 4th, and found her in bed suffering from pain in the lower abdominal region. At this time the patient's temperature was normal, pulse 80, and respiration 20. She did not feel sick, and only complained of pain which she described as being sharp and not constant. This pain was assumed by the patient to be due to the fact that she was menstruating. Inquiry into this menstrual period elicited the following facts: The patient menstruated on May 11th, the correct date for that function to appear, and this period was in every respect normal. However, she did not menstruate again until June 19th, and then only had a very slight show, darker in color than ever before, and not accompanied by pain. This slight discharge kept up until June 25th, on which day she was seized with intense pain in the lower left abdominal region, and became faint at the same time. She was compelled to remain in bed for a few hours until the pain and faintness abated, when she was up and around again as well as ever. The slight flow continued irregularly until June 28th, when pain and faintness again came on, but this time was only transitory. From this time until July 3d she was free from pain, and enjoyed her usual health. The slight flow continued, however, during this time.

On July 3d, in the night, after an active day, the pain came on again with great intensity, and I saw the patient at 6 A.M. July 4th.

Physical Examination. Chest negative. Abdomen: Inspection negative. Percussion note normal over the various regions of the abdomen, but elicited tenderness over the left lower abdominal region. On palpation tenderness was evidenced in the lower abdominal region over the uterus and its appendages, especially marked on the left side. No tumor mass could be made out.

Bimanual Examination. The pessary was removed, causing sharp pain. Cervix soft and slightly dilated. Uterus soft, movable, and enlarged perceptibly. The right tube and ovary easily felt and apparently normal. The left ovary apparently normal in size. The left tube was enlarged to about the size of a hen's egg, very tender, tense, and pulsating. This tumor mass was slightly movable and not directly connected to the uterus. Pressure about the vaginal vault elicited tenderness and caused severe pain. There was a rather foul odor to the discharge, which was dark in color and contained many clots. No membrane could be found, though the flux was carefully examined for such.

I strongly suspected I had a case of ectopic gestation, and explained to the patient's friends that operation was the best procedure, and advised the same. Under the circumstances, however, it was reasonable perhaps to have such advice received dubiously, and I was forced to leave the patient, with orders to remain in bed, to be quiet, and confine herself to liquid diet.

Owing to the press of other work I did not see the patient again until 8 P.M. At that time she was in intense pain and had been so for several hours.

Repeating my advice for operation, I summoned counsel, and at 10 P.M. Dr. Heyer and I returned to the patient. Her condition was most serious. She was not in pain, but anxious and very restless, and showed marked evidence of profound hemorrhage. Pulse 148, small, irregular, both in force and volume. Respiration 36, shallow. The thermometer did not register. The mucous surfaces were exceedingly pale, patient gasping and unable to speak aloud, complaining of suffocation, and asking for more air. Skin dry and cold. Heart very rapid and first sound exceedingly weak. Inspection, palpation, and percussion of the abdomen negative.

Strychnine and nitroglycerin were used subcutaneously; large amounts of normal salt solution introduced into the rectum, and hot applications externally. Without any means at hand for opening the abdomen we continued symptomatic treatment, and the patient began to respond slowly.

Operation was now demanded, but with no one at hand who had the power to give consent to such procedure, and expecting the arrival of the patient's physician at any time, I could only continue measures against shock and hemorrhage.

Upon the arrival of Dr. H. W. Nichols, of Brooklyn, we found the patient in much better condition. Temperature 100°, pulse 120, very weak and irregular. Respiration, 30.

The patient was removed to the hospital, and I operated upon her, opening the abdomen in the median line from the umbilicus to the pubes.

Upon entering the peritoneal cavity a great amount of fluid blood and blood clots escaped.

The tube was quickly found, tied off with a silk ligature, and extirpated. Search for fresh hemorrhage was made but none found. The abdomen was cleansed of the contained blood by flooding with normal salt solution in great amounts until it returned comparatively clear. The cavity was now partially dried, and search for the ovary made. This organ was found on the posterior surface of the broad ligament, and extirpated. The other pelvic organs were in good condition apparently. One litre of normal saline solution was now run into the abdominal cavity slowly, drainage established, and the wound closed by suture in layers. The patient acted fairly well under the anæsthetic, except on two occasions, when she became very weak. However, she left the table in far better condition than when I commenced the operation. Large amounts of saline solution were introduced per rectum, and this was kept up for thirty-six hours, almost all of it being retained, its administration taking place every four to six hours. The beneficial effect of this was very gratifying indeed. On the fourth day after operation the patient developed a sympathetic inflammation of the left parotid gland. No attention was paid to this, except wet dressings of a 5 per cent. solution of aluminum acetate were applied, and the inflammation disappeared in two days. Liquid foods were given in small doses frequently, as the stomach would allow, and champagne, brandy, with carbonated water, were given freely. Though these liquids were given very soon after the patient was returned to her room, yet they were borne exceedingly well and seemed to do much good. The patient made speedy progress toward recovery.

On the fourteenth day after operation, the wound having united throughout, she was allowed the liberty of moving about in bed, and on the eighteenth day she was sitting up in a wheel chair. At the end of three weeks the patient was up and about, a tight-fitting belt being used to support the abdominal wall. At the present writing the patient is practically a well woman, feeling in good health and showing only some anæmia, which is fast disappearing.

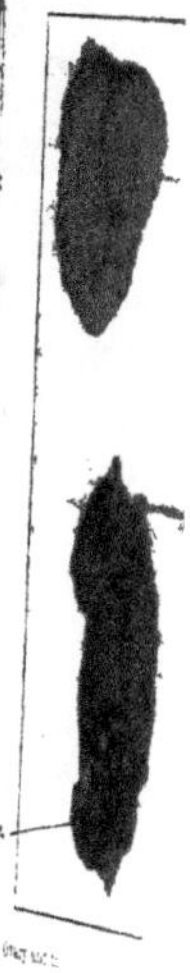

Examination of the tube shows this to have been a true tubal pregnancy.

The tube shows gross evidence of pathological change, it being thickened and tortuous, and a small cyst appeared at the extremity nearest the uterus. (See Figs. 4, 5 and 6). These are photographs of the tube and ovary, showing the gestation sac and point of rupture.

FIG. 4.

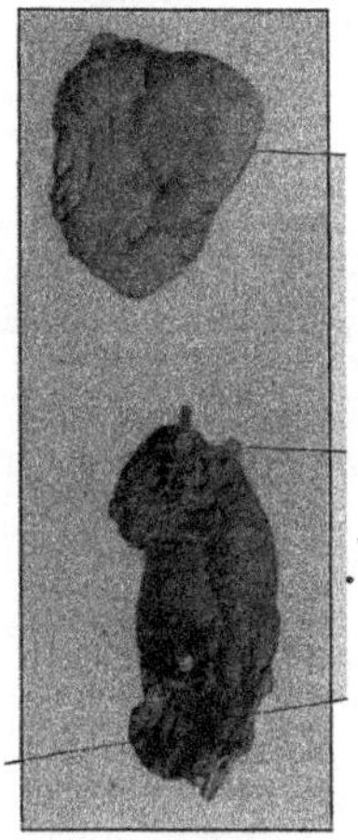

Sac.

Ovary and tube, showing sac and point of rupture.

FIG. 5.

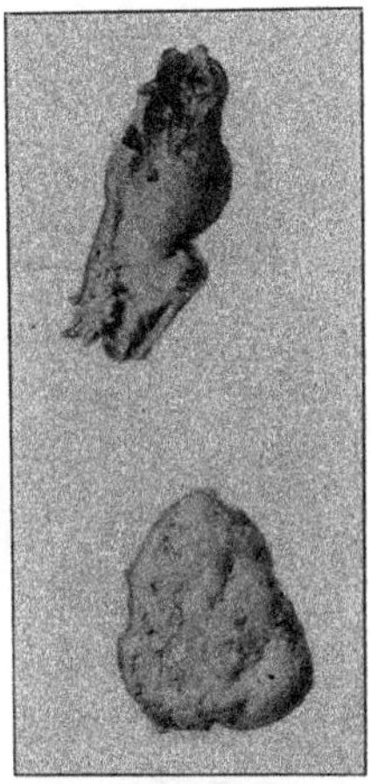

Same as Fig. 4, with tube turned to side, showing size of gestation sac.

CASE III. *A Case of Intestinal Obstruction due to Meckel's Diverticulum.*—Infant A., male, aged seven months; white, American. Father and mother living and in good health. No family history of tubercular disease nor of any abnormal growths or deformities.

Mother had no difficulty with this the first child. Child breast-fed, never had any other food but mother's milk until six months old, then had been given water freely and dry bread-crusts occasionally, but apparently never swallowed any amount of bread. Since birth the child had suffered from constipation at times, but had never had an attack of diarrhœa. The child had been under the care of two physicians at its home in Philadelphia for what seemingly were attacks of constipation. The child's bowels moved naturally twice daily on an average. However, a day or two before these attacks, which grew more frequent from birth until one week was the rule, the child's bowels would not move copiously as was the custom, and only once in twenty-four or thirty-six hours.

FIG. 6.

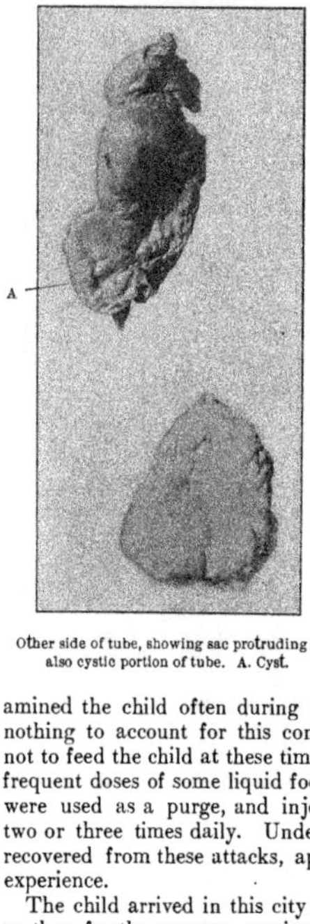

Other side of tube, showing sac protruding; also cystic portion of tube. A. Cyst.

Then the attacks of constipation came on, never lasting over thirty-six to seventy-two hours. The mother noticed that the movements were not at any time hard, but rather soft, and always free from undigested food.

Pain seemed to be the first evidence of trouble, and the child would cry out from time to time, drawing up its knees and straining quite violently without result. If the attacks lasted some few hours, vomiting occurred, generally of a bilious character. No temperature accompanied these attacks. The child would lie quiet when free from pain, oftentimes showing a desire for food. These attacks have never lasted over forty-eight hours, and the termination was signified by a movement of the bowels, never constipated in character, giving a very evident relief to the child, which seemed as well as ever as soon as the bowels moved. Such is the history I obtained from the mother on the day of my first visit. Her physicians had examined the child often during these attacks, but evidently found nothing to account for this condition. The mother was advised not to feed the child at these times, except giving it water and small, frequent doses of some liquid food. Castor oil and a laxative tablet were used as a purge, and injections of hot water administered two or three times daily. Under such care the child had always recovered from these attacks, apparently none the worse for such experience.

The child arrived in this city on June 25th, with the father and mother, for the summer, coming from Philadelphia. At the beginning of the trip the child was well, but during the ride on the train became somewhat fretful and cross, acting in the same manner as it had always done previous to one of these attacks of constipation. The bowels had not moved throughout that day until after its arrival in this city, when a very small movement occurred, accompanied by pain and considerable straining. The movement was soft in consistency and contained no undigested particles.

Throughout the night of the 25th the child was comfortable, and the bowels not moving on the morning of the 26th, the mother used the laxative tablet and enema without result. Throughout the day and night of the 26th the bowels did not move and the child lay quiet, taking little notice of surroundings, crying out with pain from time to time, and straining violently. The morning of the 27th there was no change, and vomiting of a bilious character began. The mother again used enemas, without result.

I was summoned to see the child at noon of the 27th, and found the following conditions to exist: Child well nourished and nicely proportioned, lying upon its back with legs extended. No temperature. Pulse 130, good quality. Respiration a little quickened. Examination of chest negative. Examination of abdomen: On inspection abdomen flat, no distention, no rigidity. Abdominal respiratory movement evident. Palpation: Abdomen flaccid, no point of tenderness, no pain caused by examination.

Low down in the abdomen, evidently in the sigmoid, a mass about the size of a pigeon egg was detected, giving the sense to the touch of fecal matter. Throughout the rest of the abdomen palpation was negative. The percussion note was normal throughout the various regions of the abdomen. Examination by rectum revealed nothing. The tongue was slightly coated and the vomitus without any odor.

With the history of the case as above written I felt that I was probably dealing with a case of temporary obstruction due to fecal matter in an abnormally long sigmoid flexure. Such was the diagnosis, and a high enema of oil followed by water was used without any result except a discharge of mucus and gas. The child was kept quiet, and egg albumen in water with small amounts of brandy given hourly. The mother was instructed to give enema of oil and glycerin every four hours.

The child remained in this condition without any change throughout the rest of the day.

At 8.30 in the evening I again saw the child, and found upon examination no change in any respect. The child was quiet except when crying out with abdominal pain. I next saw the patient the following day at noon, and found the child had had no movement of the bowels and also was decidedly sick, lying in a somewhat stupid condition, but easily aroused; on examining the abdomen a tumor mass of intense firmness was found lying in the mesial line between the umbilicus and the pubes, the long axis inclined from above downward and to the left.

This mass was about the size of a hen's egg, and the percussion note over it dull.

Realizing the gravity of the situation and fearing a permanent obstruction had taken place I requested counsel.

At 1 P.M. Doctor Heyer and myself found the patient in this same stupid condition, and at this time the tumor mass described had increased in size to that of a small orange, was evident on inspection, easily palpated, movable, and dull on percussion.

Believing a volvulus had occurred, about a quart of oil and glycerin was run into the rectum slowly. No result upon the tumor mass was made, and no gas or fecal matter escaped. There was no peristaltic movement felt or seen to take place around the tumor mass. The child was vomiting greenish fluid in small quantities frequently at this time. About one-half hour after using the high enema, while we were watching the abdomen, the child gave a sharp cry, and immediately we saw swelling take place over the site of the tumor mass described, which increased in size steadily until it was as large as a large orange and bulged forward to a considerable extent.

Upon laying my hand over this tumor the peristaltic movements of the intestine could be felt, and upon percussion a distinct tympanitic note was heard. Operation was advised immediately, and the patient was taken to the hospital.

When seen at the end of another hour the child was vomiting fecal matter very often and seemed in a moribund state, temperature subnormal, thermometer in the rectum did not register. Respirations 40. Pulse very rapid and weak. The tumor mass appeared no larger to the eye, but on palpation a perceptible increase in size was evident.

Operation. The abdomen was entered by an incision in the median line from the umbilicus to the pubes. Upon opening the peritoneal cavity a white, glistening mass was seen lying against the abdominal wall, looking much like a distended portion of the intestine. On putting the fingers into the cavity this mass was pushed aside and the fingers swept about it. No adhesions being encountered, the mass was delivered from the cavity of the abdomen and with it a large proportion of the intestinal tract. This tumor mass was pear-shaped, about six inches in length, and some three and one-half inches across in the largest portion, firm to the touch and distended with fluid. (See Fig. 7.)

The wall was smooth and shining and covered with distended veins of large size. It was absolutely free from adhesions and was connected to the under surface of the ileum, some sixteen inches from the ileocolic junction, by its upper and smaller extremity through the medium of loose connective tissue for about three-quarters of an inch. (See Fig. 7.)

The ileum had looped itself around the upper extremity of the tumor, and was then turned four times upon itself from left to right around the tumor mass, leaving a loop of gut some six inches long free and distended enormously with gas.

FIG. 7.

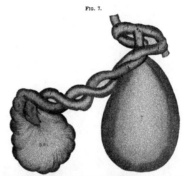

Tumor mass and volvulus. Sixteen inches from ileocolic junction. A. Attachment of tumor to ileum. D.P.I. Distended portion of ileum. I. Ileum. K. Neck of tumor. T. Tumor mass, 6 x 3¼ inches.

The volvulus was reduced without difficulty. An incision was then made into the tumor mass, and some eight or ten ounces of a clear serous fluid escaped. The incision was now carried along the tumor down to its attachment to the intestine, and, no communication being detected between the cavity of the cyst and the intestine, the wall of the cyst was excised close to the gut. On account of the exceedingly precarious condition of the patient no time could be given to dissecting the tumor from the gut. The gut was in good condition, and circulation was well established in a few minutes by the use of hot towels. The gut as it was returned was run through the hand as a matter of precaution; incidentally the appendix which was abnormally long, was removed and the wound closed. The operation occupied some fifteen minutes. The patient rallied well from the operation, the fecal vomiting ceased, the bowels moved freely, and large amounts of gas escaped per rectum.

The aspect of the patient improved remarkably in a few hours. Though the operation was followed by almost unlooked for relief in every particular, yet no hope was entertained for recovery, and about ten hours after operation, as the child was moved upon its pillow, it suddenly collapsed and died in a few minutes thereafter. Examination of the wall of this tumor mass showed it to be of intense toughness and very elastic, about one-eighth of an inch in thickness. (See Fig. 8.)

FIG. 8.

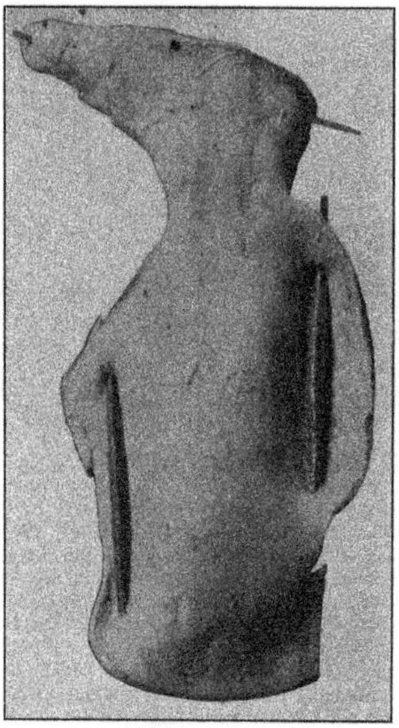

Wall of tumor mass.

The neck of the sac presented grooves from the pressure of the intestine as they were twisted about it. This tumor was suspected to be an intestinal diverticulum, possibly Meckel's, and the report of the pathologist to the Hartford Hospital, Hartford, Conn., prooves it to be such.

Dr. Walter R. Steiner, Pathologist to the Hartford Hospital, Hartford, Conn., furnished me with the following pathological report of the case:

The tissue coming from the wall of a cyst connected with the intestine was hardened in graded alcohols, embedded in celloidin, and the sections when cut were stained in hæmatoxylin and eosin.

The specimens on cross-section are seen to be composed of four layers or coats. The inner layer is made up of fibroelastic tissue, loosely compacted together and containing bloodvessels and lymphatics. In places there is a considerable amount of round-cell infiltration, especially about the bloodvessels. The next two layers are composed of muscular tissue—an inner circular layer and an outer longitudinal layer. The inner (circular) layer is the more compact of the two. The last or outer layer is fibrous in character and fairly vascular.

Diagnosis. From the location of the specimen and its structure (as seen on section), it seems probable that the cyst owes its existence to an intestinal diverticulum, which subsequently did not communicate directly with the intestine, but remained connected with it by adhesion (pedicle). The coats of the cyst correspond to the submucosa, the two muscular coats and the serosa, of the intestine. There are, however, no evidences of a mucosa. The location of the cyst with reference to the cæcum suggests strongly the possibility that it is a Meckel diverticulum.

The enormous size of this process in this case led me to make the above report, for I have been unable to find the history of its parallel. To theorize, perhaps, concerning this tumor mass we might say in the first place that it seems most plausible that the attacks of so-called constipation were in reality referable to this diverticulum, possibly by a temporary looping of the gut about it or by pressure of the structure upon a portion of the gut.

I cannot believe in the face of the history of the case and after the careful examination of the abdomen, made by several physicians in the course of the infant's life, that such a tumor of the size described could have existed all this time without detection. And again, as I have already stated, the tumor I felt on June 28th steadily grew in proportions, making one strongly incline to the theory that by a constriction at the neck of the tumor a passive congestion took place and serum continually escaped from the very numerous vessels in the wall of the cyst, causing the tumor to enlarge. That the volvulus was of short duration, I am positive, for I could almost see it develop, so to speak. A post-mortem could not be obtained, but I have every reason to believe that the contents of the abdomen were in good condition after operation, and that shock was probably the chief factor in the cause of death.

The enormous size of Meckel's diverticulum and the interest which surrounds the life-history of this little patient, evidently referable to that structure, and the rarity of ectopic gestation have led me to report these cases to my colleagues.

I am sure we may truthfully say that three desperate cases confronted us, two of which are able to pay their tribute to the art of surgery.

I want to call attention to the use of saline solution in the peritoneal cavity as a means of counteracting shock and supplying the body with fluid material.

In these two cases of ectopic gestation both patients had lost a great amount of blood, one being nearly exsanguinated. Upon the table both cases became in desperate condition, one particularly so. The opening of the peritoneal cavity, though occupying perhaps two minutes, with the loss of the contained blood, impressed both patients very markedly, but very soon after the saline solution was run in the peritoneal cavity—and this was the next step in the operation after securing the tube by ligature—the beneficial effect was observed both in the circulation and in the general appearance of the patient. In fact, it was not perceptibly longer than has been the case where I have used salines intravenously. So marked was the good result that the patients in both instances were kept upon the table some forty or fifty minutes, whereas the operation could have been completed in fifteen or twenty minutes. This solution was not only absorbed rapidly, but its effect was most marked, and it cleansed the cavity effectually, doing away with having to use so foreign a substance as the operator's hands or instruments among the intestines and against so sensitive a membrane as the peritoneum. Also the edges of the wound were insured against injury.

A rather significant fact is this: that no atony of the intestinal tract followed these operations.

In the case of the infant the beneficial effect of the saline, though used, was not so noticeable; but here no loss of blood had occurred. I feel certain, however, that the element of shock was at least mitigated. We know the peritoneum has a most wonderful capacity for absorption, and my experience in these and other cases has led me to use the abdominal method of administering salines in cases of abdominal surgery, where from loss of blood or from shock such would be indicated.

A case of double ovariotomy illustrates this practice well. The patient lost no blood, but owing to adhesions I had spent some thirty minutes before I could extirpate the tubes and ovaries. About this time the patient showed marked evidence of shock and collapse. I ceased further manipulation, and ran into the peritoneal cavity some three pints of salt solution. It was only a short time when the patient rallied, her pulse came up, and the operation was then completed without any further difficulty. She made an uneventful recovery. Owing to oversight on the part of a nurse no stimulation was at hand, and when ready was not needed.

LUDWIG'S ANGINA.

REPORT OF A CASE.

By Gwilym G. Davis, M.D.,

SURGEON TO EPISCOPAL, ST. JOSEPH'S, AND ORTHOPEDIC HOSPITALS, PHILADELPHIA.

Ludwig's angina is an infectious inflammation of the cellular tissue in the floor of the mouth, beneath the jaw, also behind it and down the neck as far often as the clavicle and sternum. The following case illustrates its pathology and treatment. It is often fatal.

C. R., male, aged twenty years, had had a bad tooth in the lower jaw, right side, for some time. A week previously the neck began to swell and later rapidly increased, until on admission he was only able to part the jaws less than a centimetre; the tongue was thick and filled the mouth, and it was also pushed upward by the swelling on the floor of the mouth. The neck was enormously swollen, the swelling extending from the zygoma above to the clavicle and sternum below, and from the edge of the trapezius muscle on one side to beyond the median line on the other. He had stertorous breathing, difficulty in swallowing, and could only talk in a whisper. Under primary anæsthesia an incision was made in the line of the anterior edge of the sternomastoid muscle and two rubber drainage-tubes passed parallel to the jaw and brought out near the median line. Only a very small amount—a few drops—of pus was obtained. The temperature was 101° F.; pulse 120; respiration 24.

The case is interesting for several reasons. The photograph, which was taken about the second or third day after operation, shows the swelling extending up to the zygoma. The swelling around the lower part of the neck is not shown, having disappeared, owing to the drainage.

The fact that the patient could only speak in a whisper and the noisy respiration showed that there was œdema of the larynx and probably compression of the trachea. That the œsophagus was compressed was shown by the trouble in swallowing. The greatest swelling was between the jaw and the clavicle. Immediate relief was required. While there was a feeling of fluctuation, no collection of liquid was found on operating. It was decided to place the incision some distance below the angle of the jaw, so as to avoid any superficial veins, for there is not infrequently a communication between the external and internal jugulars at this point, or the temporomaxillary and facial veins may there be encountered. As soon as the deep fascia was opened a closed hæmostat was pushed ahead into the tissues and opened. In this way two passages were tunnelled upward to beneath the lower jaw; also two across the neck, one curving upward toward the jaw and the other downward toward the clavicle and sternum. Drainage-tubes were placed in each. No distinct collection of pus was found. The tubes were surrounded with gauze. A culture showed an unmixed growth of virulent streptococci. The symptoms improved slightly by the next day, but not to the extent desired, and as there was practically no discharge from the tubes, the gauze dressing was removed and substituted by a flaxseed poultice. I thought that any further infection could only be for the better, and the poultice, I felt sure, would hasten and favor resolution. This it apparently did, for the next day the discharge of pus began, and the temperature had reached normal. On the fifth day after operation the discharge of pus was more free and the patient was taking solid food. He was dismissed on the tenth day, with the discharge almost stopped, and his general and local conditions excellent.

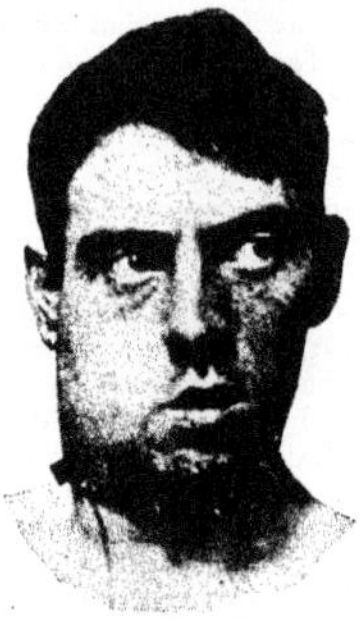

Some authors regard the disease as resembling erysipelas. This seems to me to be so only to a small extent. I believe it to be a distinctly local condition, propagated by travelling by direct continuity of tissue and capable of being relieved by free opening of the infected area. The safest way of making this opening is by pushing the nose of a hæmostatic forceps carefully into the tissue and opening the blades and so working one's way onward. The large bloodvessels of the neck did not appear to be pushedup near the surface by the effusion, but lay probably close to their normal position posteriorly. There was a direct causal relation between the diseased teeth and the onset of the inflammation. This fact, together with the prompt subsidence of both local and constitutional symptoms, as the result of local treatment alone, all point to the disease as being a distinct local infection and not erysipelatous in character. Complete anæsthesia is dangerous in these cases, and the safest course would be to use local anæsthesia or none. In this case it was simply used to deaden the skin incision.

A FATAL CASE OF POISONING WITH OIL OF GAULTHERIA.

BY J. WOODS PRICE, M.D.,

AND

EDWARD M. L'ENGLE, M.D.,

RESIDENT PHYSICIANS, POLYCLINIC HOSPITAL, PHILADELPHIA.

THE rarity of cases of fatal poisoning with oil of gaultheria makes the case we are about to report of some interest. It occurred at the Polyclinic Hospital in the service of Dr. McKee, through whose courtesy we are enabled to report it.

The patient, Fannie H., a child, aged two years, was brought to the hospital about 9.30 A.M., on April 18, 1903, by its mother, who said that it had swallowed the contents of a bottle, which she brought with her. As the bottle had been bought by the patient's father at the pharmacy in the hospital, it was easy to determine that it contained commercial oil of wintergreen, which is in reality oil of birch. It was estimated that the child had taken a drachm of the drug. The child had vomited several times before being brought to the hospital, and continued to do so until lavage could be done. Examination showed a temperature of 98.6° F.; pulse 100, regular, and of good volume; respirations 26, and regular.

There was nothing abnormal in the child's appearance, and it showed no evidences of suffering pain. There were no further symptoms for two hours, when the patient seemed to have pain in the abdomen, was drowsy, and complained of great thirst. The pulse rate increased to 150, and within an hour the child's face became flushed, the respirations were somewhat labored and irregular, and there were evidences of impaired hearing and some hallucinations of vision. The temperature was not increased, but there were slight twitchings of the hands and the muscles of the neck, and at this time delirium was first noticed. There was diarrhœa and a strong odor of oil of gaultheria in the stools.

At 3 P.M. the temperature was 99.4° F.; pulse 132, and of good volume; respiration regular, but somewhat labored. At 3.30 P.M., seven hours after the drug had been taken, the child had a general convulsion, in which the arms and legs were extended, eyes rotated upward, head thrown back, neck rigid, but there was no arching of the back. The pupils were equal and were moderately dilated. This tonic spasm lasted about half a minute and recurred at frequent intervals. The pulse was of fair volume, but was slightly irregular, and the respirations were deep, labored, and gradually decreased in rate to four or five per minute. These symptoms increased until, finally, the child died of respiratory failure at 6.30 P.M., ten hours after the ingestion of the poison. About three hours before death the child was catheterized, and salicyluric acid was found in the urine. An autopsy was not obtained.

In view of the frequent use of oil of wintergreen as a therapeutic agent and the comparative rarity of poisoning by this drug, it may be of interest to note that von Rottenbiller[1] believes that the poisonous effects are due to impure preparations, the result of imperfect methods. He cites cases of poisoning by oleum ricini, due to ricin in impure preparations, and thinks poisoning by oleum gaultheriæ analogous to these.

Hare and Wood,[2] from experiments on dogs, concluded that oil of gaultheria acted as a respiratory and vasomotor stimulant. While this result is verified by the reports of some who have observed cases of poisoning in man, it will be seen that in the case reported above there was at no time any evidence of respiratory stimulation, the only effect observed being depression, which became so marked as to be the immediate cause of death.

Gallaher[3] reports the case of a boy who after taking half an ounce of oleum gaultheriæ had marked gastrointestinal symptoms and an inordinate appetite, but no nervous symptoms. He recovered in two weeks, under a treatment which consisted of bleeding, leeching, and cupping.

Hamilton[4] reports a case in which there was almost entire absence of gastrointestinal symptoms. In his case a young woman took half an ounce of oleum gaultheriæ after having swallowed an equal amount of oleum morrhuæ. She had hallucinations of hearing and vision, extreme stupor, rapid pulse and respirations, and left hemiparesis. She recovered.

Pinkham[5] reports a case which lends added interest to the subject in showing its medicolegal importance. A woman took one ounce of oleum gaultheriæ to produce abortion. She died in fifteen hours, after showing symptoms of gastrointestinal and nervous disturbance.

Jewett,[6] Halderman,[7] and Pillsbury[8] report fatal cases following the ingestion of from three drachms in Halderman's to two ounces in Pillsbury's case. In the latter case an unusual symptom was erythema and an intense itching of the skin.

Abel[9] reports a case seen by Dr. Ott in which the symptoms resembled those seen in acute alcoholism. The patient was a child aged three years, who died eighteen hours after taking one-half pint of oil of birch.

Van Wagenen[10] saw two fatal cases, one in a boy, aged two years, who died twenty-four hours after taking one drachm.

Beck[11] mentions a fatal case, and also refers to the cases of six soldiers who were made ill after drinking a tea which contained, among other ingredients, some oil of wintergreen. They all recovered.

Potter[12] refers to a case which is probably the same one mentioned by Beck, but he gives no reference.

REFERENCES.

1. Von Rottenbiller. Klinisch-Therapeutische Wochenschrift, Mai, 1900.
2. Hare and Wood. Therap. Gaz., 1873-78.
3. Gallaher. Medical Examiner, June, 1852.
4. Hamilton. New York Medical Journal, 1875.
5. Pinkham. Trans. Massachusetts Medical Legal Society, Boston, 1878-87.
6. Jewett. New York Medical Gazette, 1867-68.
7. Halderman. Lancet-Clinic, 1886.
8. Pillsbury. Medical Record, New York, 1900.
9. Abel. Medical Gazette, 1885, p. 299.
10. Van Wagenen. Philadelphia Medical Journal, 1900; Medical Record, New York, 1868.
11. Beck. Medicine and Jurisprudence, vol. ii. p. 933.
12. Potter. Materia Medica, Pharmacology and Therapeutics, p. 326.

THE SIGNIFICANCE OF URINALYSIS IN PREGNANCY, WITH ESPECIAL REFERENCE TO ECLAMPSIA.

BY ROBERT N. WILLSON, M.D.,
OF PHILADELPHIA.

OPINIONS are so various at the present time with regard to the significance of urinary conditions during pregnancy, and especially with regard to the presence or absence of glucose or albumin, that a few pertinent cases in the experience of the writer have led him to briefly discuss the following questions:

1. What are the customary findings of urinalysis during a (clinically) normal pregnancy?

2. What variations from the normal may be noted, and what is their significance?

3. What dependence can be placed upon urinalysis as a warning of impending eclampsia?

The first question is by no means the most easily answered of the three, if one bases his reply upon the statements gathered from the current discussion of the subject by those who do purely obstetrical work. There seems to be as much diversity of opinion as to whether albumin or glucose may be found in the urine of a strictly normal pregnancy as there is with regard to the origin of these substances. One author states that a trace of either albumin or glucose has no significance, while another assures the student that the appearance of either renders the prognosis grave for the mother and child.

It may be stated as a general working rule, none the less, that the urinary picture which is normal for the ordinary conditions of life is also indicative of normal conditions in pregnancy. Just how far this principle will maintain itself will be discussed at a later point.

Question 1 then narrows itself down to the subquery: Can there be variations from the ordinary normal urinary picture which will still admit of a clinically normal labor?

The answer must be a prompt one in the affirmative. Not only do parturient women sometimes give normal birth to healthy children in spite of urinary conditions indicative of possible misfortune; but sometimes the urine in such cases appears of such a character chemically and under the microscope as to promise a rapid fatality if the labor be not at once terminated.

The specific gravity may be constantly depressed, the quantity of urine may be large or small, the excretion of urea may be diminished or increased; or there may be albumin, glucose, or both, present in large or in small quantities; and still the labor may be an easy one, and clinically normal for mother and child in every other respect.

A more frequent picture is that of a pregnancy during which (especially when the gravid womb is occupying considerable space in the abdominal cavity) a so-called trace of glucose or of serum albumin is detected by the ordinary tests. Still more frequent, and such a common occurrence as to cause no surprise when noted, is the presence of delicate quantities of serum albumin, detected only by careful methods and confirmed by control tests.

In a series of nearly 1800 urinalyses, made by the writer during the past two years, a considerable number of the examinations were in the cases of women in the later stages of pregnancy. Of the entire number of specimens of urine obtained from parturient women, only a comparatively small percentage (22 per cent.) were entirely free from albumin and sugar, while in no case in which glucose was noted was albumin absent. In nearly 60 per cent. at least a trace of albumin could be detected. In many of the cases the albuminuria began to manifest itself about the fifth month. In some it was not present until the last days before delivery. In a few it became evident directly before the appearance of active labor pains, its presence being discovered at times only by accident, if the term may be fairly employed.

When glucose appeared in the urine of a subject known to have not previously shown glycosuria, the occurrence, as a rule, took place at some time between the beginning and end of the last month of pregnancy. Occasionally there was a trace of glucose present throughout the pregnancy, often disappearing completely after the birth of the child. In no case in which, in the absence of other indications of acute or permanent renal change, small quantities of either serum albumin or glucose (not evident previously) were found present during pregnancy did the urine fail to regain its normal character shortly after the birth of the child except in the few cases in which fatal eclampsia supervened.

In the majority of cases the urea elimination was that of the normal woman under ordinary circumstances other than those of child-bearing. Its excretion varied with the individual, and especially in relation to the diet and exercise. Occasionally the quantity excreted appeared persistently high, and just as often exceedingly low; but with no evident bearing upon the otherwise normal outcome of the case.

When the microscopic sediment indicated positive renal change the beginning of this change almost invariably appeared to have antedated the pregnancy, and, as a rule, continued after the puerperium as a permanent condition. Exceptions were noted even to this rule, however, and the following case furnished rather a striking example of the kind:

Mrs. W. E. T., aged twenty-one years, was seen by the writer in her seventh month of pregnancy on March 19, 1901. Her father had died of trauma, and the condition of his kidneys was unknown. Her mother had chronic nephritis, and died from acute meningitis.

The patient had always been strong and well except for two attacks of pneumonia, followed on both occasions by a complete recovery. Since then she had always been active. Menses regular; no leucorrhœa. She had been married one year, her last menstrual flow having occurred seven months before. No headaches or dizziness; no swelling of the face, feet, or hands. On physical examination she was found well nourished, her skin healthy, no jaundice or œdema. Chest absolutely negative; heart sounds all clear and regular; arteries soft. The abdomen was that of advanced pregnancy. On examination the gravid uterus was found to contain a living fetus in the L. O. A. position. The pelvic measurements were all ample and normal.

The *urinalysis* on March 21st resulted as follows: 1011, acid, pale straw in color, slightly turbid, sediment scanty, white, and flocculent; albumin none, sugar none; microscopically, full of squamous and cylindrical cells, no casts, few leukocytes, no mucus, no crystals.

A request was made during the following week that another specimen be sent, for the reasons that the specific gravity was so low and because there was doubt in the writer's mind as to the estimated time of the pregnancy.

On March 26th the *urinalysis* was 1013, acid, pale straw in color, albumin a decided trace, sugar none; microscopically, much squamous and cylindrical epithelium, many leukocytes, no casts, much mucus, no crystals.

An *examination* the following day (March 27th) showed 1027, albumin none, sugar none, heavy phosphatic clouding with heat; microscopically, full of uric acid crystals; no casts, much squamous epithelium, few leukocytes, considerable mucus.

The patient felt at this time strong and well. Fetal movements distinct. During the next month the urine remained negative except for a very high specific gravity, a urea output of 2.8 to 3.6 gm. per 100 c.c., occasional showers of uric acid crystals in the freshly voided urine, and once a heavy sediment of calcium oxalate crystals. No albumin; no casts. On April 15th the patient's feet began to swell. Although requested, the urine was not obtained until ten days later, when the urinalysis showed 1030, albumin, 6.6 gm. per litre; sugar none; urea, 2.51 gm. per 100 c.c. Microscopically, full of small hyaline and hyalogranular casts, many leukocytes, no renal epithelium, no crystals.

On the following day the albumin still measured over 6 gm. per litre, and there were present many granular casts and much renal epithelium, although the patient had been in bed and on a liquid diet for two days. Periodical pains began to be evident during the early evening of this day, gradually increasing, and after a labor of twelve hours the head of the child was on the perineum, and was delivered naturally, with a slight laceration. The latter was repaired at once, and both mother and child advanced through a normal puerperium and adolescence.

At no time in this case was there a suspicion of renal involvement up to the time of the single appearance of albumin in quantity, one month before term, and followed by its complete disappearance. Its reappearance at some time during the last ten days before the birth of the child; its presence in large quantities, and above all the indication by the microscopic sediment of serious renal change, all made labor a dangerous prospect and raised the question as to the best course to pursue. The event proved that sometimes Providence allows us to rush on in safety, when in a different mood we would counsel prompt artificial termination of the dangerous condition.

This will be recognized as a case in which every feature of the urinalysis indicated danger of the much-dreaded eclampsia, and as one which, none the less, passed on to a normal labor and delivery. The urine one month later was nearly free from albumin (faintest trace) and casts, but unfortunately the patient has moved away from this vicinity and has disappeared from view.

It may be briefly stated that cases have been noted in which the urine has contained as much as 4 per cent. or 5 per cent. of glucose during pregnancy, and yet the woman has gone safely through to term and a successful delivery. The same must be said of such instances as of the case just cited, that the probabilities are all against a favorable outcome. We are, however, more intimately concerned with the subject of albuminuric eclampsia, and will pass over other considerations for the present. It will be sufficient to say that cases are constantly being noted in which albumin is present throughout the course of the pregnancy; others in which it appears early or late in its course; and in one or both, or neither, there may be casts and renal epithelium in abundance; and still there may be no departure from the normal in the labor.

In concluding his comment on this question, and partly by way of discussing Question 2 (What variations from the normal may be noted, and what is their significance?), the writer would simply say that most cases of pregnancy present minute traces of serum albumin in the urine, and that these can be detected if sufficient care be devoted to the search. Probably these traces are the result of pressure by the gravid uterus and of the consequent congested state of the kidneys. Sometimes there seems to be actual renal disease, and the ultimate cause may never become evident. Such cases must be placed in the category with those other problems that are too deep for our understanding; and when they go on to normal labor we should be thankful for the occurrence and content to accept the gift of Providence. Too often the urinary indications of renal involvement are verified by the dreaded onset of eclampsia, and too often, also, in such cases the opportunity is afforded on the autopsy-table to ascertain the extent of renal damage.

Much stress has been laid by some writers upon a diminution in the elimination of urea in certain cases of pregnancy, both as an indication of impaired renal activity and of the danger of eclampsia. Certain it is that in most pregnant women the specific gravity of the urine is high (1025 and upward), and the urea output correspondingly large; or, to state the sequence of affairs more accurately, the urea is excreted in abundant quantities, and the specific gravity is correspondingly high. The true significance of the variations in the elimination of urea must be estimated as in all other conditions —viz., when the kidneys are doing their proper share of work they will excrete a normal amount of urea; when hampered or diseased, their urea output is diminished and sometimes becomes exceedingly scanty. The doubtful claim that a decided fall in the amount of excreted urea is ever a dependable indication of oncoming eclampsia will be referred to again in connection with the cases cited under Question 3. The highest importance must always be attached to the presence of renal epithelium in quantity; also to tube casts, especially when in large numbers, and when of the granular, blood, or epithelial varieties. Normal urine always contains a few hyaline casts,. which may be found if looked for with care. No normal urine contains many of the latter, however, and normal kidneys are never responsible for casts of the granular or epithelial types. The microscopic sediment in the majority of instances furnishes our most accurate guide as to the condition of the renal apparatus, and its critical study should never be omitted from the urinary examination.

It remains to recall the fact that sugar (glucose, lactose, etc.) may often appear in small quantities, and that when confined to such inconsiderable amounts it has little or no practical significance, at least in the light of our present knowledge. When glucose is present in pathological or in permanent form it is interesting to note that there is present also, with few exceptions, some indication of renal change. We have yet to discover the real cause of the appearance of glucose, even in diabetes, but we have learned clinically that diabetic glycosuria is usually accompanied by renal sclerosis, and that its urine contains a renal sediment; and we have learned that the association is such a close one as to be valuable clinically for diagnostic purposes. The rule holds equally well in the pregnant woman and the non-pregnant diabetic. The presence of glucose, as already stated, is in itself by no means a grave sign, and in small quantities unattended by signs of renal incompetency can usually be ignored as far as concerns the outcome of the pregnancy. When it represents a diabetic condition, however, it assumes a new importance, furnishing the picture of a subject of a cachexia undergoing the greatest strain imposed by nature upon woman's vitality. Pregnancy under such conditions becomes a dangerous and questionable duty, instead of woman's trying but precious privilege.

In conclusion, Question 3 (What dependence can be placed upon urinalysis as a warning against impending eclampsia?) raises again an all-important and much-mooted discussion. The writer has already cited a case in which the urinary condition indicated serious renal change, and yet in which labor was carried on with entire exemption from eclampsia. He remembers with vividness a second case in the hands of a prominent obstetrician in which the urine had always been found normal prior to the pregnancy. Unfortunately, the urinalysis was omitted during the course of the pregnancy owing to confidence in the integrity of the renal function; and this case died in eclamptic convulsions. A third case is still under the care of the writer, and is interesting in that it presents the picture of a urine absolutely normal on the evening prior to the beginning of labor, a total absence of a history of nephritis, and yet a series of convulsions beginning while the fetal head was on the pelvic floor and continuing into the post-partum stage after an instrumental delivery. The following presents merely an outline of the case:

Mrs. J. F. E., aged twenty-six years; family history negative. One child living and well; forceps delivery after a long but otherwise uneventful labor. Seen for the first time by the writer on March 14, 1903, at which time the patient considered herself six months pregnant. The abdomen was very large, but the patient stated that this was also true of the first pregnancy. The right leg was swollen, also the right labium, the veins of which and of the right vaginal wall were swollen and tortuous. This condition was greatly relieved in the recumbent posture, and was evidently due to pressure in the abdominal cavity. The vertex was distinctly felt on vaginal examination, approximately in the L. O. A. position. Pelvic measurements were all normal.

The urine at that time was examined and showed, A. M.: 1010; albumin, faint trace; sugar, none; urea, 1.22 gm. per 100 c.c.; microscopically, full of squamous cells, no renal sediment, few leukocytes, no crystals; P. M.: 1020, acid, etc.; albumin, faint trace; sugar, none; urea, 2.80 gm.; no renal sediment, full of squamous cells.

From this time until May 18th, inclusive, the urine was examined weekly. On the latter date both the morning and evening specimens were examined. At no time during this period could albumin or sugar be detected. No casts and no renal epithelium were present. The urea averaged 2 gm. per 100 c.c., and on the last examination before labor began was 2.18 gm. On May 19 the writer was called because of colicky pains over the abdomen. There was some headache, and it was learned that the bowel had not been emptied for two days. At this time the patient was supposed to be about one month from term, but the abdomen appeared so large that oncoming labor was suspected, and the vaginal examination showed the cervix already dilating. After a long, slow labor of twelve hours the vertex was on the perineum. Convulsions suddenly supervened, following the second of which forceps delivery was carried out with the assistance of Dr. W. A. N. Dorland, and without injury to mother or child. The placenta was at once delivered with the hand in the uterus. An hour later a third convulsion took place, followed by a fourth, fifth, and sixth. The urine drawn by catheter showed the following: 1012, acid, etc., strong odor of decomposition; albumin, 1 gm. per litre; sugar, none; urea, 1.18 gm. per 100 c.c.; considerable number of hyaline and hyalogranular casts; no blood; considerable renal epithelium.

The patient was bled, and then transfused into a vein with normal salt solution. She was then kept in a steam bath almost continuously for six hours, when the kidneys again began to take up their share of the work. Consciousness was not fully regained for thirty-six hours, though no convulsions occurred after transfusion.

The urine rapidly cleared up, until at the present time it is perfectly normal, and the patient free from evident impairment of the renal functions, and with no recollection of the ordeal.

Dr. Dorland has informed the writer of a case of eclampsia, recently seen by him, in which the urine was examined immediately before labor, and found to be normal, but in which convulsions appeared and death ensued before morning.

We have studied cases, therefore, which have presented urinary pictures of seemingly grave import, but in which labor has followed a normal course; and, on the other hand, cases of dangerously obstinate, and even fatal eclampsia occurring in spite of kidneys in which, up to the moment of labor, were supposedly healthy. As a result of our study we are confronted with the question: Can eclampsia be accurately foreseen and avoided by the careful attendant upon the case; and does albuminuria, or even a renal sediment, predict with any degree of accuracy parturient or puerperal eclampsia? By way of answer the following conclusions seem warranted at the present time:

1. Careful urinalyses should be carried out in all cases of pregnancy at frequent intervals, and with increased frequency as term is approached.

2. The most dependable indications of impaired renal function and of probable eclampsia have been shown by general experience to be the presence of decided quantities of serum albumin, the diminution of the eliminated urea, and the presence of a microscopic renal sediment (casts, renal epithelium, blood, etc.). The character of the latter, when accompanied by the well-known clinical signs of nephritis, always constitutes a working basis for an estimate of the probability of imminent danger.

3. Even if the urine appear perfectly normal the possibility of eclampsia must be considered, especially in young women. Eclampsia in such cases is of equal severity with that of cases in which the urine has given due warning of impaired renal functions.

4. When eclampsia supervenes upon labor in a subject with previously (apparently) healthy kidneys, the tendency subsequently is toward a return to normal renal functions if the patient survives. This circumstance would seem to indicate still more strongly that the kidneys may actually have been normal up to the time of a temporary embarrassment and suspension of function.

5. Until the nature and ultimate cause of uræmia and eclampsia are more thoroughly understood, it would appear that urinalysis, though not an unerring guide, is our most valuable index of the condition of the kidneys and our most trustworthy source of information as to danger from such forms of toxæmia.

6. The prognosis seems to be vastly improved if eclampsia be combated by generous bleeding, followed by venous transfusion with normal salt solution. These measures reduce and dilute the poison in the circulation, and relieve the cardiac distress. Free diaphoresis and purging are of course indicated.

A NEW METHOD OF GASTRIC PROTEOLYSIS.[1]

By A. L. Benedict, A.M., M.D.,

OF BUFFALO, NEW YORK.

The essential chemical function of the stomach is the digestion of proteids. While digestion of fats has recently been shown to take place in the stomach, as well as in the intestine, it is always insignifi-

[1] Presented in abstract to the American Gastroenterological Association, 1903.

cant quantitatively. Digestion of (cooked) starches occurs within but not by the stomach, and may be very considerable, although no complete systematic study of this phase of digestion has been made as yet, and it is obvious that this phase of gastric digestion must be extremely variable. The method of gastric analysis submitted by the writer in 1900 to the Prize Committee of the American Medical Association, and published in the *Journal* of that body March 27-30, 1901, differed from the various clinical methods in vogue, in attempting to investigate directly the actual amount of digestive function performed, instead of measuring the acid, ferment or other potential energy remaining after the extraction of the stomach contents.

On account of the small quantity of raw material available in practical gastric analysis, the necessity of performing many manœuvres upon the clear filtrate, which seldom exceeds 50 per cent. of the total quantity extracted, and the necessity of using separate portions of the filtrate for other methods of examination, as those for acidity, peptic strength, and qualitative composition, it became evident to the writer, very early in his preliminary study of the problem, that exact scientific analysis of proteids was out of the question, even if it could be adapted to the use of the clinician. For this reason it was decided to employ the general method of centrifugal precipitation, and to throw out of solution the various proteids in successive groups corresponding to the degree of peptonization, and employing as precipitants substances which should produce fairly bulky precipitates, which should not precipitate non-proteid ingredients of chyme, nor result in confusing mutual reactions. By consulting the qualitative tables of proteid precipitants collated by Ewald, Gamgee, and others, some idea may be formed of the very considerable amount of preliminary study required, as, for one or other of the reasons mentioned, most of the reagents suggested were found inapplicable to the problem propounded.

Anyone who has used the centrifuge to any extent in clinical estimations of any kind, will assent to the statement that the only safe rule is to base a volumetric reading on the minimum obtained after several successive centrifugalizations at a considerable speed. Whether the hand, water, or electric centrifuge is employed, the maximum speed obtainable for tubes of considerable size, without great risk of breaking the glass and spoiling the result, is 2000 to 2500 revolutions per minute. The writer has obtained identical results with the hand and water instruments, and has always centrifugalized until the precipitate suffered no further diminution in volume. Usually three centrifugalizations of two minutes or more each have been used.

As originally reported, three precipitates were compared, dealing in all instances with an investigandum of 10 c.c. of clear filtrate from chyme, and using graduated tubes, which enabled the readings to be made directly in percentages of this amount. These precipitates were, successively: soluble albumin,[1] precipitated by heat alone; syntonin and albumoses, precipitated by saturation with ammonium sulphate; peptones, purin bodies, amido-compounds, etc., precipitated by phosphomolybdic acid.

From an investigation of about twenty normal cases and over one hundred abnormal ones the following data have been obtained:

	Minimum.	Average or normal.	Maximum.	
Albumin . .	trace.	2–4 per ct.	7 per ct.	
Albumose . .	trace.	½–1 "	3 "	(faint cloud always remained in suspension.)
Peptone . .	5 per ct.	20–30 "	47 "	

With regard to the last line, it should be said that less than 15 per cent. is rarely found, except some hours after a meal, or unless evidence of low peptic and acid power is forthcoming. The maximum precipitate given includes albumoses, the highest precipitate found for peptone alone being 36 per cent., and, otherwise, the highest for peptone alone or albumose and peptone together—albumose never being sufficient to increase the precipitate materially—being 33 per cent.

The albumose precipitate being always scanty and inconclusive for practical purposes, I have for some time followed the suggestion of Dr. G. H. A. Clowes, and have simplified the procedure so as to precipitate soluble albumin by heat and then all further products by phosphomolybdic or phosphotungstic acid. On account of the sharp demarcation between these two precipitates, it is unnecessary to decant from the former, but the volume of the second precipitate may be read beginning at the top of the first. The weight of the second will, however, compress the first considerably, say from 2 per cent. to 1 per cent., or from 4 per cent. to 2 per cent. For comparative purposes, the first reading is taken without this compressive effect.

It is of interest to translate these readings by volume into percentages by weight. The volume of albumin represents about one-fifth as much by weight. The volume of "peptone" by phosphomolybdic or phosphotungstic acid represents about four times the bulk obtained by tannin, in those instances in which the absence of starch—which is also precipitated by tannin and which may be present when the qualitative test for erythrodextrin masks it—allows a comparison to be made. The tannin precipitate, in turn, represents about the same exaggeration of the percentage by weight as in the case of albumin. Thus, the volumetric percentage of peptone represents an exaggeration of the weight percentage by about 20. However, these statements are not intended in an accurate quantitative sense, but merely to afford a general idea of the magnification, so to speak, obtained from this method. Like other clinical methods, it

[1] In the original report this was called *acid albumin* or *syntonin*. Although after the ordinary test meal all soluble albumin has become so through the action of acid, it is not *acid albumin* in the technical sense until it becomes uncoagulable by heat.

is intended only for comparative use, and must not be interpreted in too literal a sense.

So far as I am able to learn, there are no conditions liable to be encountered in stomach contents, obtained in the usual way and examined with a fair degree of promptitude, which interfere with or notably diminish the precipitates mentioned. Obviously, if the albumin precipitate were allowed to stand for a long time in either an acid or alkaline medium, resolution would occur, but no notable diminution of bulk can occur during the test as ordinarily performed. Nor, on the other hand, is there any extraneous precipitate obtained by boiling the acid filtrate, which can add to the apparent bulk of albumin. It may be remarked here that the properly prepared filtrate is almost absolutely free from mucin.

The precipitate by phosphomolybdic or phosphotungstic acid certainly does not consist of pure peptone. It was formerly taught that gastric digestion ended with the formation of peptone, but we now know that amido-compounds—using the word in a rather loose chemical sense—are formed, as in pancreatic digestion. I have noticed that in comparing the "peptone" precipitate of the same filtrate, before and after standing at room temperature for a day or two, a considerable diminution in volume may occur, which is probably due to chemical change beyond the stage of peptones proper. If so, the volume of the "peptone" precipitate is probably not materially exaggerated by the progress of digestion beyond the nutritive stage.

The lower proteids having been already removed, the "peptone" precipitate of filtered chyme may theoretically include peptones proper, amido-derivatives of proteids, amido-acids of bile, ammonium salts, alkaloids, and purin bodies. Any considerable admixture of bile spoils the sample for any kind of systematic analysis. Moreover, bile acids would be precipitated by HCl and excluded from the investigandum, unless there existed an absence of free HCl. Ammonium salts do not interfere materially, for even a 10 per cent.—practically a saturated—solution of ammonium sulphate yields less than 1 per cent. volumetric precipitate with phosphomolybdic acid, and an amount of ammonium demonstrable by the ordinary rough tests is almost never found in chyme. Alkaloids are, of course, never present in any appreciable quantity. In my report in 1900 the statement was made that phosphomolybdic acid did not precipitate with normal urine, although a blue color was produced. This statement is incorrect, as a small (usually 1 per cent. to 4 per cent.) but perfectly distinct precipitate is produced. The experiment was repeated several times, so that the discrepancy cannot be ascribed to a single exceptional urine, and the observation is so simple that the personal equation need not be considered. Doubtless, there was some imperfection in the reagent obtained for the control experiments with urine.

I have noticed a peculiar reaction with starch. Phosphomolybdic acid does not precipitate with a solution of HCl corresponding to the ordinary maximum in gastric juice, nor with a concentrated solution of starch. When, however, phosphomolybdic acid is added to a concentrated solution of starch, also containing hydrochloric acid in gastric strength, a precipitate up to 4 per cent. by volume may be obtained. This reaction well illustrates a possible fallacy in dealing with complex mixtures of organic and inorganic substances, for, aside from mutual reactions to produce insoluble substances, which form an important part of inorganic analysis, a genuine precipitation may drag down other substances in a mechanical way, or various changes of conditions may influence the solubility of certain substances. It is obvious that the method of analysis described follows the plan of successive precipitation and removal which characterizes the "wet method" of inorganic analysis. It is equally obvious that organic substances do not interact with the same definiteness as inorganic and that the conclusions drawn cannot be so absolute. Nitrogen estimations have naturally suggested themselves as a means of gastric analysis, and have been employed in different ways by various chemists. Unfortunately, the estimation of nitrogen does not afford a clue to its source from this or that proteid or proteid-derivative, and the nitrogen percentage of albumin, albumose, and peptones in the generic sense is nearly the same, while, on the other hand, nearly or quite as great variations of nitrogen percentage may occur within each of these groups. It is theoretically possible to analyze quite accurately the various proteids of chyme. The process is, however, altogether too difficult for ordinary clinical use, and I am informed that it is impossible, even for an expert chemist, to make such an analysis with the small quantity of investigandum available —usually less than 20 c.c. of filtrate, after allowing for the ordinary acid titrations.

In order to determine how far the so-called peptone precipitate might be increased by the reaction with purin bodies, the following experiment was applied to a number of cases—about ten in all. The liquid above the strata of albumin by heat and remaining proteids, etc., by phosphomolybdic acid was decanted and the precipitates dissolved, so far as possible, by liquor potassæ. The remaining sediment was again centrifugalized and was found to amount to about 0.5 per cent. (taking the 10 c.c. as 100 per cent.) by volume of a beautiful, navy-blue pigment. I am informed by chemists that this is a reduction product of molybdenum, of unknown constitution. It is, however, probable that the potassium hydroxide redissolves other than the strictly proteid precipitates. Still, from the *a priori* probability that non-proteid precipitable substances are present in minute amount, from the experiments with urine and with starch and HCl, it seems a warrantable deduction that the so-called peptone precipitate is not exaggerated by more than 5 per cent. (taking 10 c.c. of original filtrate as 100 per cent.), and this possible fallacy does not interfere materially with the practical value of the test.

Realizing, then, that we are employing a purely clinical and approximate method of comparing the proteolytic power of different stomachs or of the same stomach at different times, the question presents itself, What practical conclusions can be drawn from the results? In looking over my tables, it has not been possible to recognize a definite relation between the proteid precipitates and any other single object of the routine examination, such as acidity. This is by no means a condemnation of the method. If proteolysis were a mathematical function of some other measurable factor, it would not be necessary to attempt the former investigation at all.

A priori, it would seem that the albumose precipitate or this and the peptone precipitate should rise and fall with the amount of combined hydrochloric acid, but I cannot discover any such direct relationship. However, in a series of notes on gastric analysis, published in *American Medicine* in 1902–1903, I have shown the fallacies of the sodium-tungstate test for combined acidity, and that by alizarin is probably not much better. Incineration methods are not adapted to clinical study, but it is possible that a really accurate estimation of combined hydrochloric acid would show a correspondence to the proteolytic tests.

When the albumin precipitate is high and the peptone precipitate low, poor digestion is suggested. One of the reasons for abandoning the separate precipitation of albumose was that the intermediate position of this precipitate and its small amount prevented any positive deduction. It often happens, however, that there is an abundant precipitate in both or all three steps in the process. This suggests that there has been a recent acceleration in the acidifying or early stages of digestion, and certainly does not seem to indicate an impairment of digestion. On the whole, the most definite information seems to depend upon the amount of the final precipitate, which should amount to 20 per cent. to 30 per cent. Generally speaking, there is a fair correspondence between what has been alluded to as the optimum precipitates and a fairly normal acidity and ferment test. For instance, we may compare two tests made on the same case under similar conditions:

Total acidity.	Free HCl.	Combined HCl.	Albumin.	Albumose and peptone.	Rennet test.
48	22	19	trace.	8 per ct.	Weak.
90	45	29	1 per ct.	26 "	Strong.

When the investigandum is obtained late after a meal the digested proteids are low, usually about 10 per cent., whether the hydrochloric acidity is excessive or nil. Disturbances of the normal distribution of acidity in general seem to be inimical to digestion. While the alizarin test may not be reliable for the estimation of combined hydrochloric acidity, any great difference between the readings of acidity by dimethylamidoazobenzol and alizarin indicates fermentation acidity, and if the sum of free hydrochloric and so-called combined hydrochloric acidity does not nearly equal the total, the peptonization is usually low. For instance:

	Total.	Free HCl.	Combined HCl.	Fermentation.	Albumin.	Albumose.	Peptone.
F. G	85	15	27	85—(15+27)=43	1	trace.	10
J. B. B.	78	8	58	17	4	¼	22
G. L. S.	77	10	50	17	5	trace.	31
M.	80	34	37	9	2	......	23
E. A. S.	78	28	33	7	trace.	......	22
W. J. B.	70	22	23	25	½	......	14
J. P.	89	41	25	23	4	¾	17
C.	74	10	42	22	4½	1	16½

We cannot expect a very close correspondence in such examples, although I have selected several in which the total acidity is about equal. The phenolphthalein test for total acidity is fairly sharp and accurate. The alizarin reaction is sharp, but probably not very accurate. The dimethylamidoazobenzol test for free HCl is neither. As reported in the series of notes published in *American Medicine*, 1902–1903, the tedious method of titrating without an indicator and removing a drop of the investigandum from time to time and testing it with resorcin and sugar, has convinced me that an exaggerated reading for HCl is obtained, if we note the final but sharp end reaction with dimethyl. Instead, we must take the reading when the first slight but distinct change occurs from cherry to orange. This change occurs about fifteen degrees before the end reaction occurs, but I am unable to decide the point of change within an error of five degrees. As the alizarin method of estimating combined hydrochloric acidity is merely one of subtraction, it is immaterial for our present purposes whether this test is reliable or not, but the fact remains that when there is a considerable acid factor between the dimethyl reading and that by alizarin we may anticipate a low peptonization. This point may be illustrated by the diagram on opposite page. Unfortunately, we do not understand exactly how the acid salts and fermentation acids affect the various indicators. Apparently, a free organic acid acts precisely like a mineral acid, but much less energetically, and although I am convinced that the common practice of reading free hydrochloric acidity at the end reaction with dimethyl gives an exaggerated value and leads to the diagnosis of hyperchlorhydria in many instances in which there is really euchlorhydria—perhaps temporary—we must remember that all titration methods are purely approximate.

The method of proteolysis described, though approximately quantitative, must be thought of—like the acid estimations—as the measure of a rate of progress instead of a distance covered. There is no way of measuring the absolute amount of material digested by or in the stomach. We can, of course, weigh and analyze the entire test meal before ingestion and an hour or so afterward, resorting to thorough lavage. But we cannot be sure that some portion of the meal has not passed the pylorus undigested; on the contrary, we can be reasonably certain that considerable loss has occurred in this way.

The method described is more simple and easy and, *a priori*, more logical than those based on measuring the "left-over" digestive power. That it is crude and contains fallacies, is obvious, but all methods applied clinically to the very meagre amount of investigandum obtainable are subject to this limitation. I am rather preju-

TYPIC TITRATION OF CHYME.

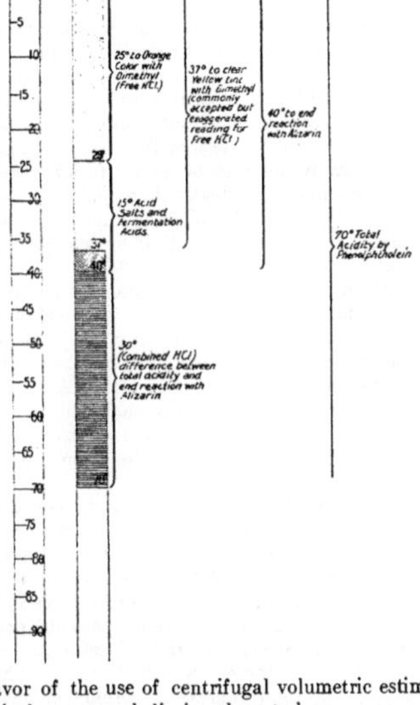

diced in favor of the use of centrifugal volumetric estimations for various clinical purposes, believing them to be more accurate on the whole than gravimetric methods employed under the unfavorable conditions common to most clinical investigations and than most clinical adaptations of elaborate methods, such as the Kjehlaahl nitrogen determinations. Meanwhile, assistance is desired in noting fallacies and in discovering more accurate means of separating the various proteids.

THROMBOSIS OF THE MIDCEREBRAL ARTERY CAUSING APHASIA AND HEMIPLEGIA.[1]

By Charles W. Burr, M.D.,

PROFESSOR OF MENTAL DISEASES IN THE UNIVERSITY OF PENNSYLVANIA.

REMARKS ON CEREBRAL SKIAGRAPHY.

By G. E. Pfahler, M.D.

The point to which we wish to direct attention in the following report is the usefulness of skiagraphy in diagnosing cerebral disease and in locating the lesion. The importance of the method in tumor of the brain is well established. It probably will become of great value in the differential diagnosis of so-called uræmic hemiplegia, in which there is no gross organic lesion, from hemorrhage and thrombosis. It may possibly prove to be an aid in differentiating between the two last conditions by means of the different location of the shadows, hemorrhage usually affecting the striate artery, thrombosis often of the main trunk as well as its branches. The patient's history is as follows:

R. C., a white woman, aged sixty-seven years, was admitted to the Philadelphia Hospital in February, 1901. She had a right-sided hemiplegia and was aphasic. We learned but little of her previous history. Thirty years before her admission she suddenly lost power on the right side and became speechless. After several months sufficient power returned in the leg to enable her to walk a little, but speech never returned. Ever since the onset of the palsy epileptiform convulsions have recurred at long and irregular intervals.

When examined, the day after her admission, she could stand alone and, with the aid of a cane, walk a little. The gait was very hemiplegic. The right arm was completely and absolutely paralyzed. There was very slight palsy of the lower part of the face and none of the tongue. The right leg was slightly rigid. The right shoulder was very stiff, the forearm rigidly flexed upon the arm, but the wrist and fingers were relaxed. Passive movement of the right arm caused pain in the elbow and shoulder. The left knee-jerk was normal, the right increased. Ankle clonus and Babinski's reflex were present on the right side. There was slight wasting of the right arm from disuse, but no neurotic atrophy. Tactile sensibility could not be determined on account of the inability of speech. Sensibility to pain was certainly preserved. Her only speech was the recurrent utterance "no, no, no—no, no." This was expletive, not intellectual. It was spoken on every

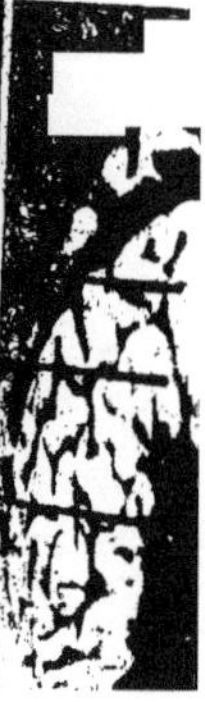

[1] Read at the Pennsylvania State Medical Society, June 24, 1908.

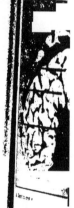

attempt to speak, and I am sure that sometimes it was uttered unconsciously in direct consequence of some external stimulus without any willed effort. It probably, therefore, was, in the latter case, not even emotional, but purely reflex. She showed by gestures indicating their uses that she recognized the nature of familiar objects by sight, but of course she could not name them. She did not recognize written or printed words at all. She certainly recognized letters to be such and seemed to know the specific meaning of four or five. She recognized the nature and uses of familiar objects put in her left hand, but with the right hand she recognized

FIG. 1.

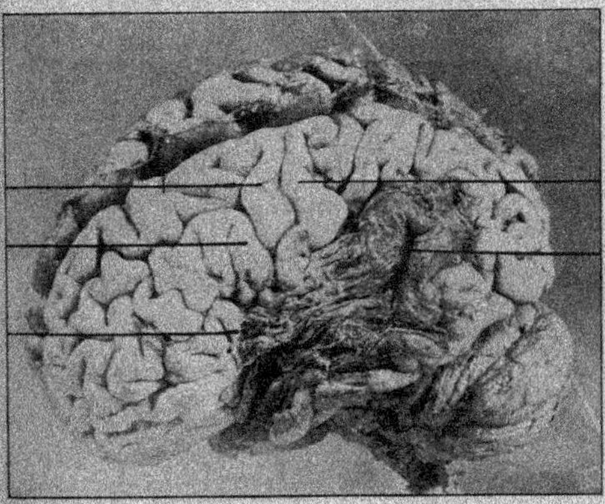

A

A. Dent in cyst wall. B. Ascending frontal convolution. C. Second frontal convolution. D. Third frontal convolution.

nothing. The significance of this could not be determined owing to the impossibility of discovering the condition of tactile, weight, thermal, and space sensibility. It may have been caused by a disturbance of sensibility or been the result of a true cortical tactile amnesia. She could not write at all either from dictation or copy. She was not completely word deaf. She obeyed all simple verbal commands even when great care was taken that she should not be able to guess the meaning of the order from my gestures. Complex commands requiring long sentences to give she did not understand and did not obey. She could not understand any conversation except the simplest phrases. There was however, as I have said, a remnant of word hearing left. She was not deaf to sound. While in the hospital she had several convulsions and several attacks of unconsciousness. She had chronic nephritis and died in a uræmic attack in April, 1902.

A necropsy was made the same day. Examination revealed extensive destruction in the region of distribution of the left midcerebral artery. The destroyed area was covered over by a pseudocystic pial membrane. Fig. 1 gives a false impression in one regard, namely, the depression marked "A" is not, as it appears to be, a fissure surrounded by a convolution (the angular gyre), but merely a dent made in the cyst wall at the time the photograph was taken. The lower halves of the ascending frontal and ascending

FIG. 2.

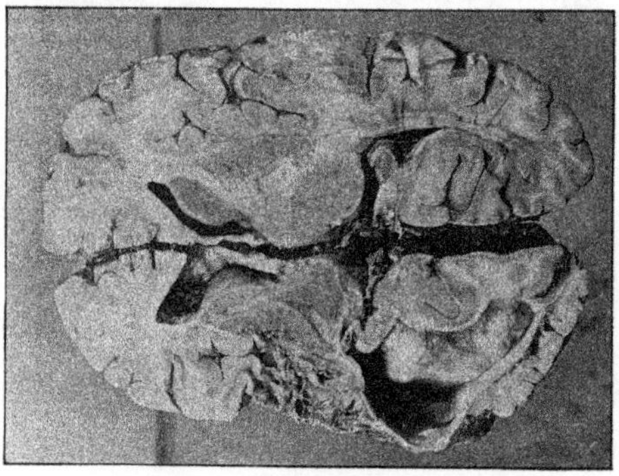

Horizontal section of brain, showing atrophy of left side.

parietal convolutions were completely destroyed; the upper halves were somewhat atrophied. Nothing remained of the island of Reil and only a small portion of Broca's convolution. The supramarginal, angular, and first temporal convolutions were absent. A part of the second temporal was also destroyed. The basal ganglia were quite a little smaller on the left than on the right, and the left internal capsule was atrophied. The anterior half of the posterior limb of the capsule was more affected than the posterior half. (Fig. 2.) The posterior horn and middle portion of the left ventricle were much enlarged and the outer wall was entirely lateral membranous, the cortex and underlying white matter being entirely destroyed. It is remarkable that the patient was not completely word deaf. The amount of speech hearing she possessed must have been due to the education and vicarious action of the right temporo-sphenoidal lobe.

The case is interesting in many ways, for example, as regards aphasia and differences in vascular distribution, for it is probable that there is quite a variation in the arterial distribution in different brains, but I wish to use it here simply as showing the possibilities of skiagraphy in the hands of an expert such as my friend Dr. Pfahler.

FIG. 3.

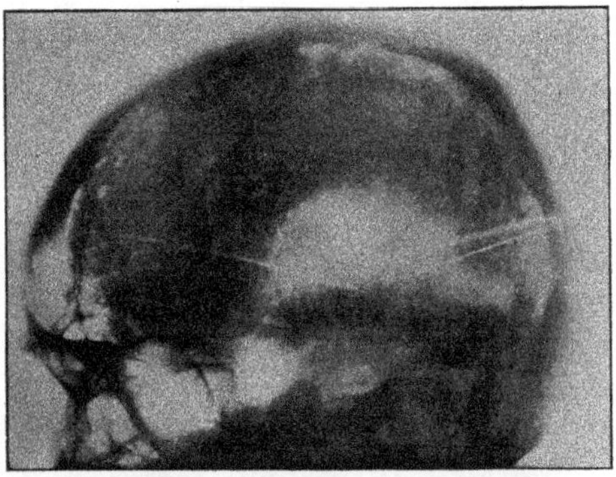

Skiagraph showing the outline of the skull, the frontal sinuses, the orbits, the base of the skull. The middle meningeal artery, the division between the cerebrum and the cerebellum, and the light area in the cerebrum corresponding exactly to the area of softening.

Remarks on Cerebral Skiagraphy. By G. E. Pfahler, M.D.

At the February meeting of the College of Physicians of Philadelphia,[1] I demonstrated, in connection with the case reported by Dr. Mills, that brain tumors can be skiagraphed. Some of these skiagraphs showed the absence of brain tissue, others a disturbance of brain tissue without any actual absence. Basing my opinion upon these facts I believed that an area of softening of the brain could be shown. My first opportunity to test this point developed at the autopsy in Dr. Burr's case just reported. The brain was replaced in the skull and an attempt made to photograph it by

[1] Philadelphia Medical Journal, February 8, 1902.

means of the Roentgen rays. I first made a negative of the affected and then one of the opposite side, because I believed that possibly the normal side could be used for comparison with the diseased. The present case demonstrates, however, that this cannot be relied upon, for the lesion was shown upon both negatives, but with much more definite outline on that of the affected side. In studying a skiagraph it is important to recognize the shadows of normal structures first. If these are not shown well, abnormal shadows must be accepted with doubt. If, however, normal shadows are clear and definite, I believe that abnormal shadows will be of great value in making a diagnosis.

FIG. 4.

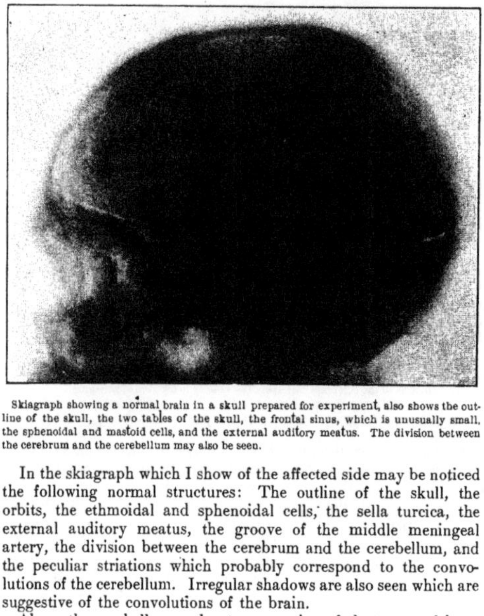

Skiagraph showing a normal brain in a skull prepared for experiment, also shows the outline of the skull, the two tables of the skull, the frontal sinus, which is unusually small, the sphenoidal and mastoid cells, and the external auditory meatus. The division between the cerebrum and the cerebellum may also be seen.

In the skiagraph which I show of the affected side may be noticed the following normal structures: The outline of the skull, the orbits, the ethmoidal and sphenoidal cells, the sella turcica, the external auditory meatus, the groove of the middle meningeal artery, the division between the cerebrum and the cerebellum, and the peculiar striations which probably correspond to the convolutions of the cerebellum. Irregular shadows are also seen which are suggestive of the convolutions of the brain.

Above the cerebellum and petrous portion of the temporal bone may be seen the light area which corresponds to the outline of the area of degeneration. A light space is seen above the sella turcica which shows where the brain tissue had not been properly replaced. The saw cuts may also be seen. (Normal brain, Fig. 4.)

From an experience in fifty-five brain examinations I am convinced that the Roentgen rays will be of considerable value in the diagnosis of cerebral lesions. I believe that we shall be able to diagnose most large lesions, such as new-growths, softening, hemorrhage, and abscess.

REPORT OF A CASE OF TUMOR OF THE BRAIN, AN ENDOTHELIOMA OF THE DURA; OPERATION; RECOVERY; DEATH IN 108 DAYS FROM RECURRENCE OF THE DISEASE.

By William J. Taylor, M.D.,

OF PHILADELPHIA,

ATTENDING SURGEON TO THE ORTHOPEDIC HOSPITAL AND INFIRMARY FOR NERVOUS DISEASES AND TO ST. AGNES' HOSPITAL; CONSULTING SURGEON TO THE WEST PHILADELPHIA HOSPITAL FOR WOMEN.

A boy, aged fifteen years, born in America, of Russian-Jewish parentage, was seen first with Dr. Theodore Sprissler on January 25, 1903.

He had been perfectly well until ten weeks before, when he misbehaved at school, and his teacher, becoming angry, seized him by the neck and bumped the right side of his head against a wall. He came home and immediately complained of headache. Shortly after this, still complaining of headache, he was taken to see Dr. Theodore Sprissler, who examined his head carefully and could find no evidence whatever upon the scalp of any violence, as there was no abrasion, no bruise, nor swelling. He did, however, have some slight fever—a little over 100° F.—and Dr. Sprissler sent him home and to bed, fearing that he might be contracting typhoid fever, but he did not think that the knock on the head had anything to do with his condition. This fever soon passed away.

He did not see him again for some little time, and then only for headache, which the boy always complained of as being localized in his right temporal region. Of late this headache had become more marked and there had been some vomiting, but there were periods of entire freedom from pain.

Thinking the headache might be due to some ocular defect, he was sent to Dr. F. M. Perkins on January 20, 1903, who made this record:

"*Examination.* No external variation from normal appearances. Vision normal. Pupils respond to light, convergence, and accommodation. Neither eye goes out under covering hand; has full vision with either eye and reads 0.5 type. Instilled homatropine for ophthalmoscopic examination with following results:

"Right eye: media clear, H. 2 D.; veins and arteries slightly tortuons, but vessel contours nowhere blurred. No retinal or choroidal changes. L. E.: the same conditions exist as in right eye.

"*January* 21. Atropine sulphate 0.01 gives in either eye H. 2 D. Headaches still persist. Ophthalmic examination gives same appearances as on January 20th.

"*27th.* Patient was seen at office January 22d and 25th, and no changes in eye-ground appearances of January 20th noted, but on this date, at an examination made at the patient's home, the following was noted:

"Right eye: pressure neuritis; full, tortuous veins; lymph spaces full and at places contours of vessels almost lost; edges of disk hazy. Left eye: same conditions as in other eye, except in less degree."

The boy would have periods of headache, at other times was perfectly free from it, and during the time of freedom from pain ran around and played like other children, and attended school for five or six successive days before Dr. Perkins' first examination. These paroxysms of headaches were of such a character that at times he was thought to be shamming, but soon vomiting occurred, and of a cerebral type.

In view of this condition, he suggested to Dr. Sprissler that I see the boy.

Now there was a very slight swelling over the squamous portion of the temporal bone, about the point of the insertion of the temporal muscle, and this was the spot at which he complained of his intensest pain, and it was somewhat tender on pressure.

When I saw him, on the 25th, the boy had been losing flesh, but there were no palsies. His station was perfectly good, but he complained of intense and increasing headaches, which were now almost constant, with occasional vomiting. I advised that he be seen by Dr. C. W. Burr, and also to increase the dose of potassium iodide, which he had been taking. The boy was evidently getting much worse, and on the 28th I saw him again, in consultation with Drs. Burr and Sprissler. We now were fully convinced that we had to do with a cerebral growth rapidly progressing. The symptoms had all increased; he had the most typical cerebral vomiting I have ever seen, and this occurred repeatedly while we were examining him. The slight enlargement on the right side of the skull had increased very materially and was extremely tender on pressure.

Medical Examination by Dr. Burr.

"I saw the boy for the first time on January 28th. On the right side of the head above the ear was a swelling about as large as a fifty-cent piece and circular in outline. It was painful and sensitive on pressure. There was no palsy of either arm or leg, or of the face. He used the left arm a little awkwardly. Sensibility to touch was normal on the face, arms, and legs, and there was no astereognosis. The left knee-jerk was a little diminished; the right normal. There was no muscular rigidity, nor ankle clonus. Stroking the sole on either side caused quick and rapid extension of the toes. He could walk a little, but staggered much, and attempts at walking caused vomiting. I was not sure whether the staggering was due to ataxia or to weakness and the violent head pain. Several times during the examination he had attacks of cerebral vomiting. Speech was normal. His mental state was good. He did not like to talk much on account of the violent headache, but there was no clouding of consciousness nor was he mentally dull or silly. He answered all questions intelligently."

We believed the condition to be due to a growth of the skull, most likely an osteosarcoma, and that it was growing downward and producing pressure upon the brain, and not likely to be a growth of the brain itself.

As he was growing so much worse and so rapidly, we all advised that he should be taken to St. Agnes' Hospital at once, and that his skull be opened the next day.

On Thursday, January 29th, four days after he was first seen, I operated. His condition was growing rapidly worse; evidence of pressure had distinctly increased, the pulse was 56, the temperature was normal, and he complained of intense pain in his head. His head was shaved, washed, and the scalp thoroughly disinfected, and, in the presence of Drs. Burr, Perkins, Sprissler, and a number of others connected with the hospital, I made a large flap over the temporal region and turned down the scalp. The flap, which was oval, was three and one-half inches across at its widest point. I found that a growth had eroded the skull and was attached to the temporal fascia and under portion of the scalp. This diseased portion I dissected away. I now with a chisel made a circular opening in the skull and lifted out a button of bone, two inches in diameter, the centre of which was the perforated portion of the skull. This was very vascular and evidently had undergone in almost its entire extent changes which, from macroscopic appearances, resembled sarcoma. In paring off the underlying growth I thought at first that I had opened into a large infiltrating growth of the brain. This was very dense and contained numerous fibrous bands. I next took a rongeur forceps and cut away the bone in front, at the back, and particularly toward the zygoma, and at last reached the limit of the growth. In working around the edges of the growth I found it was outside of the dura. The circumference of the dura was intact, but in the centre it had a base of about one inch, which was adherent. I now cut the dura completely around the growth and found a large tumor growing from the dura and projecting into the tissues of the brain, but entirely free from attachments in every direction. This I shelled out without much hemorrhage. I used hot water to control the bleeding in the scalp and in the bone, as well as Horsley's putty, then packed lightly with iodoform gauze and closed the scalp.

He reacted well from the shock of operation and loss of blood, and in forty-eight hours the packing was removed. His condition was now most satisfactory: headache had ceased almost at once, his temperature had been good, but at the end of seventy-two hours there was evidence of a fungus cerebri. There had been comparatively little bleeding, but tremendous weeping of cerebro-spinal fluid, necessitating frequent dressing.

I did not believe at the time of operation that all of the diseased bone and dura had been removed, but all was taken away which had the appearance of disease. His condition was alarming, and I feared that he would die on the table from hemorrhage. I believed there would be a speedy recurrence of the growth.

Every other case of dural tumor that I have seen, with one exception, has died from hemorrhage either at the time of operation or within the first twelve hours. The exception that I mention was a fibroma of the dura, removed by Dr. Keen in 1887. I have seen a number of other cases, and all have died from hemorrhage.

February 3d. Dr. Perkins made this note: "Ophthalmoscopic examination (in bed with candle-light) shows in each eye distinctly made out contours of all vessels; no neuritis present."

By February 13th, or in fifteen days, he was up and about the ward. The wound had healed throughout, except at one small place, where there had been packing, and from this there still was a discharge of cerebrospinal fluid, but this was gradually diminishing each day, and ceased on the 15th. He had absolutely no pain nor tenderness, nor any interference with his eyesight, nor any evidence whatever of trouble with his brain.

February 21st. Dr. Perkins made this note: "Examination with student lamp at St. Agnes, boy sitting in chair in the dark room, conditions for examination thoroughly satisfactory. Right eye: no vessel tortuosities or dilatation; macular region is the seat of fine, silvery bands; otherwise fundus normal. Left eye: same ophthalmoscopic appearances as in other eye."

On March 6th, after an absolutely uninterrupted recovery, he returned to his home with the wound completely healed, except, possibly at one place, where there was a line of granulation about one-half inch long by one-eighth of an inch wide. The eye-grounds were normal and he seemed to be perfectly well.

On March 12th he complained of a stiffness in the neck and inability to open the mouth wide, but this he had at the hospital, and was probably due to the irritation of the temporal muscles. He had no pain, headache, nor any symptoms of intracranial pressure, but there was certainly a greater amount of bulging at the site of the wound than before. The whole of the flap was pushed out and there seemed to be a rather hard, nodular swelling beneath the scalp.

I believed the growth returning and sent him to Dr. Burr for his examination and then to Dr. Perkins.

March 12th. Boy seen at his office by Dr. Perkins, who noted: "Pupils responsive to light, convergence, and accommodation. Neither eye out under cover; red Maddox rod, with rotary prism, with small electric light as object, gives at 20 cm.: exophoria, 0 to 2 degrees; hyperphoria, 0; and at six metres esophora, 1 degree; hyperphoria, 0. Right eye vision, 6/6; left eye, 6/6; no lenses used. Instilled homatropine for ophthalmoscopic examination, which gives the following findings: either eye media clear, and no pathological fundus appearances. The silvery macular bands noted on February 21st have entirely disappeared."

On March 16th, as there was distinct recurrence and no further operative measures could be undertaken, Dr. S. Mason McCollin began the use of the *x*-rays; but in two days there had been a rapid increase in the size of the growth, and he had slight headache, and his father noticed for the first time a slight discharge, which came from a small spot about one quarter of an inch in diameter at the upper anterior angle of the wound, and here and there at several spots over the surface of the projection were small points, which evidently would break down in the course of a few days.

I had never seen such a rapidly progressing growth.

By March 22d he had grown so much worse and his weakness had increased to such an extent that he was no longer able to go back and forth to Dr. McCollin's office, and he therefore entered St. Agnes' Hospital for further treatment by the *x*-rays. The growth had enlarged very much, and his general condition was weaker; he was pale, complained of pain in his head, and slept badly.

By March 31st the growth had increased somewhat in size, although this could only be estimated. He had had no headaches for a week, and this freedom must be attributed, I think, to the *x*-rays. He complained of a great deal of stiffness and pain in the neck, and of some numbness in the thumb and forefinger of the left hand, and stated that he could not move his thumb freely, although, when his attention was directed to it, it seemed to me that he could do so.

March 26th. Ophthalmoscopic examination made by Dr. Perkins showed in either eye slight vessel tortuosity, otherwise normal fundus. Red Maddox and rotary prism gave no muscle imbalance; and on April 2d: "In either eye the presence of undoubted neuritis, with swollen disks; the edges of the nerve entrance obscured, the vessel contour at places (even on general retinal level) being obscured for small areas. There was no evidence of enormous lymph extravasation or extensive hydraulic pressure, as was present at the commencement of the case—*i. e.*, before operation—but the eye-ground appearance was indicative of small encroachments on the calibres of the efferent vessels; presumably, therefore, commencing basilar interference. An examination made about four days before showed only vessel tortuosity, but no nerve head uplift above general retinal level. The Abney pellet test shows no central scotomata. There was no essential difference between the fundus appearances of either eye."

On April 13th he was taken to his home. He had now total paralysis of his left arm and hand, some paresis of his right hand; his speech was becoming impaired; he was very somnolent, sleeping almost all of the time, but he did not complain of much pain. Shortly after this he was placed under the care of another surgeon, who ligated the external carotid artery, evidently attempting to produce starvation of the growth by cutting off the blood supply. In this he was unsuccessful, as the boy died on May 17th, 108 days from the date of the removal of the tumor from the brain. No post-mortem examination was made by the physician then in attendance, and I did not learn of his death until some days after the funeral, and too late to make an attempt to procure one.

Remarks by Dr. Burr.

"I saw him again two days ofter operation. His condition was excellent. He was free from headache, bright and cheerful. There was neither anæsthesia nor palsy of either arm or leg. On March 12th he walked to my office and still was in excellent condition, except for a slight rheumatic wryneck, which passed away in a few days. The tumor had, however, already begun to grow again, and I advised against operating a second time. When I first saw him the diagnosis of tumor of the brain was not difficult, but I was in error as to its nature. I thought it was most probably an osteosarcoma; it was an endothelioma.

"There is not the slightest doubt that Dr. Taylor's operation not only prolonged the boy's life, but gave him a period of entire relief from very serious symptoms. Had he not been operated on I am sure he would have died a few days after my first examination.

"The tumor, of course, affected only the prefrontal lobe. It pushed aside but did not penetrate the brain mass; it was not an infiltrating growth. Whatever relation there may be between the prefrontal lobes and mental processes, this case proves that there may be serious and rapidly increasing pressure on the right prefrontal lobe without any mental symptoms whatever."

Pathological Report by Dr. D. J. McCarthy.

"Sections were cut from the tumor mass, the dura, and the bone. Sections of the dura and its free edges showed the connective-tissue nuclei larger than normal, but there was no evidence of tumor-cell infiltration. Sections of bone over the tumor showed a sclerated condition of the bone with absence of diploë, but there was no evidence of a malignant condition of the bone tissue. The sections from the tumor, and also sections cut through both the tumor and the dura, showed a tumor formation evidently starting from the meninges. The cells were arranged in rows following a racemose arrangement, and were in close contact with the interstitial tissue. Two types of cell were present: a large cell with small nucleus and relatively larger quantity of cell body, and a small round cell in the centre of the cell nests. The accumulations of cells in the dura between the bands of connective tissue gave somewhat the appearance of scirrhus, but the racemose type of infiltration following the lymph paths and the arrangement and type of cell lead us to make a diagnosis of endothelioma starting from the meninges."

A REPORT OF FIVE CASES OF TUMOR OF THE BRAIN, WITH OPERATION.[1]

By William G. Spiller, M.D.,

ASSOCIATE PROFESSOR OF NEUROLOGY AND PROFESSOR OF NEUROPATHOLOGY IN THE UNIVERSITY OF PENNSYLVANIA.

During my recent term of service at the University Hospital five cases of tumor, the growths being situated at different parts of the brain, were under my care, and in all operation was done by Dr. C. H. Frazier.

The first case was one of multiple sarcomatosis, and has been reported already in The American Journal of the Medical Sciences, July, 1903. A tumor was believed to be in the cerebellopontile angle, and it was found at this place. Multiple sarcomata of the central nervous system were not suspected before the operation, because they did not cause symptoms. I have already discussed this case and shown that symptoms of these numerous growths were absent because the tumors were so soft they caused no pressure and little or no destruction of tissue. This case is referred to here in connection with the other four, because all five cases occurred within a few months and in the same service.

Case II. *Tumor of the motor area, correctly localized and operated upon, with much improvement in the patient's condition during a period of seven weeks; return of the growth, with fatal termination.*— G. K. was referred to me by Dr. B. Kohn, April 21, 1903, with the following notes:

The patient denied having contracted syphilis, but said he had had gonorrhœa. He had used alcohol formerly to excess. He had had

[1] Read before the College of Physicians of Philadelphia, December 2, 1903.

headache for several years, but the pain had been growing worse since last summer, and had been especially severe during the previous two weeks. The pain was more or less over the whole head, but was more on the left side, especially in the forehead, and was more severe at night, and was not constant. He had noticed weakness in the right arm and hand for about two months. Since December, 1902, he had had convulsions—at first once a week, but lately not so often, and had had none during the previous two weeks. He always knew when they were coming on by a twitching in the right eye for about five minutes before the spasms developed. The attack began with a peculiar sound in the throat, the eyeballs then rolled about, and the right arm and hand became implicated in the convulsive movements. Sometimes the right lower limb was affected, but never the left side. Consciousness was not lost, and the man did not fall into sleep after the convulsions. The attacks occurred usually when the man was awake, but several times while he was asleep. The convulsions lasted about three minutes; sometimes longer. The patient had noticed for about a month that he had difficulty in speech, but his family had observed the indistinctness of speech only for about five to seven days. The disturbance of speech was purely motor in type.

The right eye had been weeping for three weeks. He had noticed dimness of vision, especially in the right eye, for some time. Mentality was sluggish and memory was poor. He had no delusions, no nausea, no vomiting, no incontinence of urine, no paræsthesia, and no pain except in the head.

A partial paralysis of the right side of the face had not been noticed by the family. The nasolabial groove was less distinct on the right side. He could not whistle well, and could not draw up the right corner of the mouth so well as the left. He was able to wrinkle the forehead and close the eyelids perfectly. The tongue when protruded deviated to the right. The pupils were equal, and the light response was preserved, but was slow on the right side. Local tenderness of the scalp to percussion was not obtained. The patellar reflexes were increased. Station was very poor, and the man was not able to stand without support. The right arm and hand were very weak and the grasp was poor.

Dr. Kohn said that he had noticed an appreciable increase in the aphasia and loss of power since he first saw the patient, one week previous. He could then stand and walk without support.

My notes, made April 25th, are as follows:

The patient is unable to give his history because of partial motor aphasia. He can speak some words and give his name. When asked his age he says fifty-two. He is unable to speak an entire sentence correctly, and has paraphasia. He understands all that is said to him. He says that he has severe headache, that it is constant, and places his hands over the forehead and over the occipital region. He seems to be unable to read at all. He wrinkles his forehead equally well on the two sides; shuts his eyes tightly and equally well on both sides. The right side of the face in the lower distribution of the seventh nerve is paretic. The tongue when protruded deviates a little to the right. No tenderness is felt on percussion of the scalp.

The right upper limb is very paretic. The grasp of the right hand is very feeble. The biceps tendon reflex on each side is about normal; the triceps tendon reflex is not obtained on either side. Sensation for touch and pain is preserved in the right upper limb. The muscles of the right forearm and hand are more wasted than those of the left.

The right lower limb is very paretic. He is able to flex the limb at the hip and knee. The patellar reflex is prompter on the left side than on the right, and yet it is a little below normal on the left side. Ankle clonus is not present on either side. The Achilles jerk also is weaker on the right side and about normal on the left side. The Babinski reflex is not obtained on either side, the toes being flexed on irritation of the sole of the foot. Sensation for touch and pain is normal in the lower limbs. In walking he drags the right lower limb and allows the right upper limb to hang at the side of his body.

April 27th. Percussion of the head does not give positive results. He has no loss of stereognostic perception. He denies positively a syphilitic infection and says he has not had dizziness.

The report of the ophthalmologic examination, April 25th, in Dr. de Schweinitz's service, by Dr. E. A. Shumway, is as follows: Vision, R. E., 6/150; L. E., 3/150. Pupils: reaction very prompt. Muscle balance: rotation of eyeballs seems unlimited in all directions. Eye-grounds: the left eye shows some fulness of central lymph sheaths; the lower inner margins of the nerve are slightly veiled, but there is no other lesion. The right eye has entirely normal eye-ground. Hypermetropia of about 5 D. in each eye. Impossible to obtain fields on account of mental condition. Visual acuity, for the same reason, very uncertain.

The report of the urinary examination, made April 29th, was cloudy; alkaline; specific gravity, 1024; albumin, a trace; sugar negative; phosphates; few epithelial cells and leukocytes.

My notes, made April 30th, are as follows: The man's account of himself is reliable, and he says positively that his convulsions have been confined to the right side of his face and right upper limb, and that the right lower limb has not been affected. The motor aphasia to-day is much greater than at any time since he has been in the hospital. The right patellar reflex is a little below normal, and the left is about normal. Bakinski's reflex is absent on each side, as on each side the toes are distinctly flexed.

On May 1st I noted that the motor aphasia seemed to be more pronounced. The right patellar reflex was about normal, and there seemed to be a slight indication of the Babinski reflex on the right side—*i. e.*, the smaller toes on the right side were extended two or three times in repeated attempts to obtain this reflex, but the big toe was not moved. When a board containing movable letters was shown to the patient he was able to pick out six or seven letters correctly on command, and he, therefore, was not letter-blind. He said he had had very little headache on the right side of the head and that his headache had been especially severe in the left frontal region.

Dr. de Schweinitz examined the eyes on this date, and reported that the condition in the left eye-ground could not be considered positively a beginning choked disk, but that it was suggestive, and within six months choked disk might be pronounced.

The patient was agraphic.

A diagnosis of tumor of the lower left motor area was made. It was supposed to affect Broca's area by pressure, or to invade it slightly, inasmuch as the motor aphasia was incomplete. The operation was done May 2, 1903, and a tumor was found in the opening of the skull, and was removed. Microscopic examination showed it to be a small spindle-cell sarcoma.

On May 5th, three days after the operation, my notes were as follows: The man can reply to questions, but still has much motor aphasia, and more than he had before the operation. The paresis in the lower distribution of the right seventh nerve and in the right upper and lower limbs is nearly the same as before the operation. He has no word-deafness. His general health is good, and he is very cheerful. The patellar reflex on each side is a little below normal. Ankle clonus is not present on either side. Achilles-tendon reflex is about normal on each side. Babinski's reflex is not present on either side, and the toes are distinctly flexed. The biceps tendon, triceps tendon, and wrist reflexes are much diminished on each side. Stereognostic perception in the right hand is much impaired; but this may be the result of motor weakness.

By the end of May the man was able to be out of bed, and walked about the ward without assistance. He improved steadily, the right hemiparesis almost disappeared, his speech improved, his headache ceased, his cheerfulness was very marked, and he seemed to be almost entirely well. On June 20th he had a severe convulsion, involving the whole right side of the body, and he became paralyzed on the right side, but he soon regained some power in the paralyzed limbs. About July 7th signs of right-sided pneumonia developed. By July 16th the right upper and lower limbs had become completely paralyzed and speech was much affected.

July 25th. He has great difficulty in swallowing, and is completely paralyzed in the right upper and lower limbs. He can say only a few words, and these indistinctly. The biceps and triceps tendon jerks on the right side are a little prompter than normal. The patellar reflex is about normal on the left side, but a little diminished on the right side. Ankle clonus and Babinski's reflex are not present on either side. Stereognostic perception and sense of position cannot be determined, because of the difficulty in getting the man to respond. Sensation for pain is present in all parts of the body. The face is very slightly affected on the right side, and the tongue is protruded straight.

The man's general condition did not permit a second operation. He died July 26th with signs of pneumonia; but as the lungs could not be examined at the necropsy, we were in doubt whether he had pneumonia or a tumor of the lung.

A necropsy was obtained, but permission was given for removal of only the brain and spinal cord. A tumor was found in the posterior part of the left second frontal convolution, extending into the middle of the precentral convolution and the upper part of Broca's area. The growth was infiltrating and at no part sharply defined from the surrounding tissue. It was, as already said, a small spindle-cell sarcoma. A small tumor about the size of a pea was found also on the right sixth cervical anterior root.

This case was seen in consultation by Dr. Mills, and he was also present at the operation.

CASE III. *Subcortical tumor, outer edge of tumor 1.5 cm. below the surface of the brain and within the white matter. Correctly localized as regards the portion of the brain affected, but not found at the operation because of its deep situation within the substance of the brain.*—T. S., a male, aged forty-seven years, was referred to me by Dr. L. J. Burns, April 27, 1903.

The man said he had contracted syphilis twenty-eight years previous. He had had a chancre, followed by sore throat and alopecia. He was married and had eight children living. His wife said that most of them were unhealthy and were anæmic. The wife had had four miscarriages. The man had had constant general headache during many years, but had had what he called "painful headache," confined to the left side of his face and head, during the last five years. He had paralysis of the right internal rectus; but this, he said, had been present for eight years. Since February 22, 1903, he had had convulsions, confined to the left side of the face and left upper limb. The convulsions always began in the lower part of the face, with a drawing sensation; then the jaws became locked, and the spasm extended to the upper distribution of the left seventh nerve. After the spasm in the face had reached its height, twitching of the left thumb was observed, and sometimes the left hand was forcibly rotated inward at the wrist. The left lower limb was never implicated in the convulsion. He had not lost consciousness more than once. The attacks lasted about three minutes. He had had as many as three or five in one day. When the attacks occurred he was unable to speak. He had attacks in which the speech became thick and convulsions did not occur. The warning was always a creeping sensation in the left lower jaw. He did not have nausea, vomiting, or dizziness. He complained of general weakness, but there was no objective weakness detectable except in the lower part of the left side of the face. The biceps tendon and triceps tendon and wrist reflexes of the upper limbs were about normal. The patellar reflex was almost normal on each side. The Achilles jerk was prompt on each side, but a little more so on the left side. Ankle clonus and the Babinski reflex were not obtained on either side. The stereognostic perception was good in each hand. He had complained of a sensation of itching for years. His speech had been getting thicker during the previous two weeks. He had no tenderness on percussion of the scalp.

An examination of the eyes by Dr. W. C. Posey, April 28, 1903, gave the following results:

O. D. inward motion abolished beyond the median line. Downward motion extremely limited, even down and out. External motion fully preserved. Upward motion lost. O. D. does not react to light or in accommodation. O. S. does react to light, but slowly in accommodation. Disks somewhat gray in their deeper layers. Vision: O. D. 5/12??; O. S. 5/5??

The man was admitted to the University Hospital, and while there a convulsive attack was seen by Dr. Willetts. It began with a creeping sensation in the left lower jaw; this was followed by twitching of the left platysma and of the left angle of the mouth. The entire left side of the face was drawn up, and the spasm was tonic. Flexion of the left thumb also was observed.

The report of the ophthalmic examination by Dr. E. A. Shumway, May 26, 1903, was as follows:

Ophthalmic diagnosis: Paralysis of third nerve O. D.; paresis of fourth nerve. Partial retention of motion of eyelid; gray degeneration of optic nerves; sheaths full.

Vision: R. E., 6/12??; L. E., 6/7.5? A. R. E. 2 D., p.p. 18 cm.; A. L. E. 0.75, p.p. 22 cm.

Pupils: O. D. pupil dilates to 7 mm. No response of iris to light or in accommodation. O. S. pupils responds sluggishly to both light and accommodation. O. D. lid droops slightly; movement inward entirely abolished; secondary contracture of external rectus, so that eye can hardly be brought to median line. Downward and upward motion lost, except slight down and out (fourth). O. S. movement good.

Eyegrounds: Media transparent; nerves show decided fulness of perivascular lymph sheaths; gray atrophy of nerve.

Dr. Harland reported that there was no involvement of the larynx, but the soft palate and pharyngeal constrictors (right side) seemed partially paralyzed.

On June 5, 1903, another examination was made. The tongue was protruded straight, and showed no tremor and no atrophy. The nasolabial fold on the right side was more distinct than on the left side. When the mouth was opened the teeth were not shown as distinctly on the left side as on the right. The patient could not draw up the left corner of the mouth alone at all, but could draw up the right corner.

Resistance to passive movements in the left upper limb was possibly not so good as in the right. The grip of the left hand was weaker than that of the right, and the left thumb was especially weak. The biceps tendon, triceps tendon, and wrist reflexes were about normal in each upper limb.

Resistance to passive movements in the lower limbs was about equal on the two sides. The patellar reflex was prompt on each side and equal on the two sides. The Achilles jerks were present and normal. Flexion of the toes occurred on irritation of the sole of the foot.

The left thumb felt numb, and the sense of position in the left thumb was much impaired, and the thumb was distinctly weak in resisting passive movements. Tactile and pain sensations were impaired in the left upper limb, and stereognostic perception was affected in the left hand. He called a dollar fifty cents, a twenty-five-cent piece a nickel. No impairment of stereognostic perception was detected in the right hand. Sensation for touch, pain, and temperature was not so distinct in the lower part of the left side of the face as in the right side. He called a pinprick sometimes a touch. The sensation of the upper part of the left side of the face was normal. He felt a pinprick less on the left side of the tongue, left side of the mouth and nose, and complained of a numb sensation in the lower part of the left side of the face like that in the left thumb.

Gait and station were normal, even with eyes shut.

A note was made that until the last two or three weeks his convulsions had always commenced in the lower left side of the face, and from here had extended to the neck, forehead, and eyeballs. Within the past two or three weeks, in five or six attacks, the convulsions had commenced in the thumb of the left hand, and had not extended farther than the wrist.

While under my care he had received mercurial inunctions and iodide of potassium until gastric symptoms developed.

A diagnosis of tumor of the right lower parietal and motor areas was made, because of the impairment of sensation in the lower left side of the face and in the left upper limb, and because of the impairment of stereognostic perception and sense of position in the left hand. The left lower limb was so little affected that the lesion was not believed to be high in the cerebral hemisphere nor to implicate the motor fibres of the lower limb in their passage to the internal capsule. Because of the convulsive movements of the left side of the face and of the left hand the tumor was believed to be cortical. An operation was performed by Dr. Frazier June 5, 1903; but, although a large opening was made, no lesion sufficiently intense to explain the symptoms was found.

An examination made June 23d, eighteen days after the operation, showed that the left upper limb was almost completely paralyzed. He could raise the left hand a little from the trunk while in bed. The grasp of this hand was very feeble. He could flex the left forearm slightly on the arm. The left upper limb was very flaccid. The biceps tendon and triceps tendon reflexes on the left side were a little exaggerated. The left lower limb was moved voluntarily and freely. The lower distribution of the left facial nerve was completely paralyzed, but the upper distribution was only slightly affected. The intelligence was good. The right side of the body was not affected.

The man had convulsions after the operation, and one of these was witnessed by Dr. C. K. Mills and myself, but the dictated notes were lost. My recollection is that they were typically Jacksonian in type and were on the left side.

Dr. de Schweinitz examined the eyes July 6th, and reported: O. D., oculomotor palsy; gray disk, with distention of the central lymph sheath, no neuritis. O. S., external muscles apparently normal; no neuritis.

He was examined on July 8th by Dr. Frazier and myself. The mental condition was bad. He did not recognize anyone. He did not reply intelligently to questions. The right pupil was much larger than the left. He had become emaciated since the operation. The left upper and lower limbs were completely paralyzed. When the left limbs were stuck with a pin they were not moved; but the movements of the right limbs when the left limbs were irritated showed that the pain sensation was preserved in the latter. The left side of the face was only partially paralyzed. We could not determine by sticking the face with a pin whether the upper distribution of the left seventh nerve was affected or not. The left limbs were flaccid. The patellar and Achilles tendon reflexes were diminished on each side equally, but were not lost. The biceps tendon and triceps tendon reflexes were also much impaired.

On July 9th Cheyne-Stokes breathing was observed, and the man was unconscious. He died on the afternoon of July 9th.

We had hoped to have a second operation. I felt sure that a lesion must be present in the area previously exposed, but the man's general condition was such that we could not feel justified in attempting another operation, especially as a very careful examination of the brain had been made at the first examination.

At the necropsy a tumor was found beneath the cortex, its central portion being below the right middle motor area. Its outer border was 1.5 cm. below the surface of the brain. The lower portion of the tumor was softened. The growth extended downward only as far as the upper level of the caudate nucleus, and at no place did it extend to the cortex. A line drawn across the brain from the fissure of Rolando would pass directly through the centre of the tumor. In transverse direction the tumor measured 4 cm., and from before backward 5 cm. Microscopic examination showed it to be a mixed sarcoma, consisting of round and small spindle cells.

CASE IV. *Multiple tuberculous tumors (méningite en plaque) of the parietal lobe, correctly localized and exposed at operation; removal of growths impossible.*—F. F. was referred to me May 26, 1903, by Dr. Theodore B. Appel, of Lancaster, Pa., with the following notes:

The patient, a white man, aged thirty-one years, had been married some years, and had no children. The family history was obscure. The mother was alive and well. F. was splendidly developed physically, and had never been sick before the summer of 1898, when he was taken ill in Florida while serving as a volunteer, and was sent North. He was confined for six weeks in a Philadelphia hospital with typhoid fever and malaria. He recovered completely, and became a barkeeper in Lancaster. He acquired the reputation of being able to drink more and mix his drinks more than any man of his age. About July 1, 1902, he was taken ill with what his physician diagnosed as typhoid fever. He had a low fever for twelve weeks, never reaching 101° F., not accompanied by headache, intestinal disturbance, nor a great amount of depression. He was never the same man after this attack, though he went back to his work and returned to his habits as regards alcohol. He had been free sexually, but denied having contracted any venereal disease. After working for four weeks he was confined to his bed for five days with an attack of influenza. This was followed by recurrent headaches, becoming more and more severe, and both frontal and occipital. These headaches occurred every two or three days and lasted about twelve hours. The day following he usually felt well. About December 1st, while asleep, he had a rather severe left-sided convulsion, lasting about ten minutes. He came out of it somewhat dazed, but after a few minutes dressed and went to work. The next evening he had another convulsion, involving the entire left side, and after this he remained in a stupor about three hours. These convulsions, as well as all he has had, came without warning. He was still able to attend to his work, and about January 3d, while coming out of a saloon, he slipped and fell, cutting his head over the external angle of the left eye. He was unconscious about two hours, and he may have had a third convulsion, as the next morning he had partial loss of power in the left arm. The following week he had a very severe convulsion of a similar character, lasting about half an hour, and followed by still more loss of power in the left arm. On March 2d he had a peculiar staring look and rather slow, monotonous speech. His patellar reflexes were very much exaggerated and the tonicity of the muscles on the left side was increased. After walking a short distance he had a tendency to bend backward, and he would prop himself against a convenient pole or wall until he had rested. He had decided loss of motion in the arm, but he could use it better than he had done a month previous. He showed no signs of syphilis.

On March 25th he had a fourth severe convulsion, limited to the left side, and followed by loss of power in the leg and left side of the face. Examination showed chronic inflammation of the optic nerves—more on the left side. He had some paralysis in the left side of the palate and throat muscles. He then was confined to bed. About April 10th he had another convulsion, which left him with the left side of his thorax absolutely paralyzed and an increased spasticity of arm and leg. His mental powers had steadily deteriorated, and occasionally he had visual hallucinations, and usually was like a child. His appetite was excessive. He had not had vomiting or fever. Occasionally he had involuntary evacuations of the bladder and he complained frequently of cramp-like pains in the spastic muscles of the leg and arm. The movement of the left thorax was very limited. Sensation for touch and pain was normal. The muscles of the left hand were slightly atrophied.

While under the charge of Dr. Appel he was treated with iodide and mercury until he developed coryza, sore throat, etc.

I first saw F. F. June 6, 1903. He had then just arrived from Lancaster. He had a staring expression, suggestive of brain tumor; his intellect was much clouded, but he understood simple questions, and replied to them correctly. $3+2$ he said $= 6$. $8-2 = 6$; $8-4 = 4$. His speech was thick and somewhat difficult to understand. His breath was offensive. He could move his head freely from side to side. The masseter muscle contracted firmly on each side. It was difficult to get him to draw up either corner of the mouth, and it was difficult to say whether or not the muscles about the corner of the mouth were weak, as he would not separate his lips. The tongue was protruded straight; it was not atrophied and showed no fibrillary tremor. The movements of the eyeballs were normal. Hearing was not determined, on account of the patient's stupor. He did not appear to be word-deaf.

The grasp of the left hand was fair, but not normal, and a little better than that of the right hand. Resistance to passive movement in both upper limbs was fair, but not normal. The muscles on the extensor surface of each forearm were somewhat atrophied. The biceps and triceps tendon reflexes and wrist reflexes were a little exaggerated on each side, but distinctly more so on the right side than on the left. His answers regarding sensation were not reliable, and yet when the upper limbs were stuck with a pin he made an effort to move them. The left upper limb was somewhat spastic; the right was not.

The left side of the thorax was flat and moved very little in respiration. Dulness on percussion was obtained over the upper part of the left thorax. A cardiac pulsation and thrill were felt in the left second intercostal space. A murmur also was heard at this place, and was presystolic in time. Pulse was rapid, 112, and regular.

The movements of the lower limbs were very weak; those of the left lower limb more so than those of the right. The lower limbs appeared to be weaker than the upper. He could draw up the right lower limb with difficulty, but could not draw up the left at all, and merely raised this limb from the bed. He was able to put both upper limbs above his head. The lower limbs were emaciated, and the left was very spastic and distinctly more so than the left upper limb. The right lower limb was a little spastic, but not nearly so much so as the left. The patellar reflex was exaggerated on each side. The Achilles jerk was exaggerated on the left side. The Babinski reflex was not obtained on the left side; the big toe did not move at all, and the other toes were flexed. The Babinski reflex was obtained on the right side, and the big toe was moved slowly and distinctly upward. The man was unable to stand even with support, as his legs were flexed on the thighs and the thighs on the abdomen. A bedsore was present over the sacrum.

I was informed by Dr. Appel that the man had lost power first in his left upper limb. Each convulsion began in the left upper limb; the eyes were turned to the left, and the face was contracted on the left side. The left lower limb was never involved in the spasm until after the upper limb.

June 9th. Dr. Shumway reported as follows: Beginning optic neuritis; more decided in the left eye, in which the nerve shows some swelling. Nerve edges are obscured. Moderate tortuosity of veins.

Stereognostic perception is lost in the left hand and is normal in the right hand. He is unable to recognize a knife, pencil, or key with the left hand, but does so easily with the right hand. Sense of position is also lost in the left hand, and is normal in the right hand. He is unable to place the first finger of the right hand on the end of the first finger of the left hand if the eyes are closed. Pinprick is felt in both hands and forearms.

The left lower limb, except the toes, is almost entirely paralyzed. Any movement of this limb causes pain in the knee, and the knee is swollen; this possibly may explain why the weakness is greater than it was a few days ago. The patient is able to say correctly and without hesitation whether the big toe of either side is bent up or down; therefore, the sense of position in these toes is preserved.

11th. The mental condition is much better; he replies promptly to questions and understands better what is said to him. He does not draw up either corner of the mouth very far, but he seems to draw up the left corner a little farther than the right. When he closes his eyelids he has a peculiar fluttering of the upper lids, so that he is unable to keep the lids closed. He hears a low-ticking watch in each ear at the distance of about four inches. The grasp of each hand is feeble and about equal in the two hands. The interossei muscles in each hand are somewhat atrophied and about equally so. The biceps and triceps tendon reflexes and wrist reflexes appear to be a little prompter in the right upper limb than in the left. Sensation for touch is much impaired, but not lost in the entire left upper limb, including a part of the left shoulder. Sensation for pain is almost normal in these parts, and both forms of sensation are normal in the right upper limb. The left upper limb is still somewhat spastic as compared with the right. He complains of tenderness on percussion in a spot about four inches directly above the external auditory meatus (probably the right side was meant). It is impossible to detect any change in the note in auscultation percussion of the head.

The left lower limb is very weak—much weaker than the left upper limb—and is very spastic. The right lower limb is apparently normal. The patellar reflex is much exaggerated on each side. The Achilles reflex is prompt on each side. The Babinski reflex is present on the right side, but feeble, and is not present on the left side. The lower limbs are emaciated and equally so. Stereognostic perception in the feet is uncertain. Sensation for touch and pain seems to be about normal in the lower limbs and feet. Ankle clonus is not obtained on either side. The patient is unable to stand even with assistance.

14th. Dr. de Schweinitz reported as follows: Double optic neuritis; 4 D.; right slight, and more extended in O. S. Paresis of right external rectus, with lateral diplopia in right field and nystagmic movement on right outer rotation. Visual fields normal with hand. Convergence near-point poor. O. D. diverges first.

15th. When he is told to place the first finger of the right hand upon the first finger of the left hand with eyes closed he seems to have no idea of the position of the left hand, and can touch his fingers only by feeling his way along the hand. If the hand of the examiner be placed near the patient's left hand he may touch the former and think it is his own hand. His mental condition has greatly improved. He has no hemianopsia. The left lower limb he can move with more power than he could a few days ago.

19th. The weakness of the left upper limb is greater to-day than it has been for several days, and the mental condition is not so good.

22d. The grasp of the left hand is more feeble than it has been since the first few days after he came to the hospital. The movements of the left fingers are awkward. The left lower and upper limbs are spastic. The right upper limb is a little spastic. The biceps and triceps tendon reflexes and wrist reflexes are exaggerated on both sides. Diarrhœa is severe to-day. Mercury and iodide are discontinued.

Because of the greater weakness in the left lower limb as compared with the left upper limb, the loss of stereognostic perception and of the sense of position in the left hand, the impairment of tactile sensation with preservation of pain sensation in the left upper limb, the ataxia of the left hand, and the convulsive movements of the left side, a diagnosis of tumor of the right parietal lobe, encroaching especially upon the centre for the lower limb, was made. An operation was done by Dr. Frazier on July 23, 1903, and numerous small plaques were found in the right parietal region, extending into the area for the lower limb. They were too numerous to permit of removal.

An examination made July 25th, two days after the operation, showed that the man's mental condition was poor. He did not move his left upper limb when asked to do so. The left side of the face and the left upper and lower limbs were paralyzed, but he could move the left lower limb a little. He was said to move the right limbs freely. The right lower limb was rigid.

He died a few days after the operation, and the necropsy showed that these plaques were almost confined to the parietal lobe, but extended onto the median side of the lobe and the upper part of the postcentral and precentral convolutions. One or two small plaques were found elsewhere. None were found within the white matter of the brain, except where they had grown inward from the pia. They varied in size, but some were about a half-inch in one diameter and were flat against the brain. The microscope showed that they were tuberculous.

Case V. *Tumor of the right cerebellar lobe at its union with the pons, correctly localized, and operation attempted but abandoned before the dura was opened, because of the patient's serious condition.*—W. C. B. was referred to me July 3, 1903, by Dr. W. F. Randall, of Dushore, Pa. The patient was a man past middle life. About Christmas, 1902, he began to complain of dull headache, not severe, and not occurring daily. During the past month or six weeks the headache had been severe. It had been frontal or occipital, and sometimes general; it came at any time, and usually lasted only a short time. The patient began to vomit about April, 1903; at first he vomited only in the morning, but now vomits at any time. Dizziness does not appear to have been present. He has not had convulsions. His sight has been poor for two months; his intelligence is good. He has been growing weak during the past three weeks, and the weakness is general—not greater on one side than on the other. The grasp of the hand is good on each side. The movement of the lower part of the right side of the face is not so good as that of the left side. The forehead is moved voluntarily and equally well on each side. He closes the eyes firmly on each side. The tongue is protruded straight, and not atrophied. Voluntary movements of the upper limbs are free, and the grasp of each hand is good. The biceps tendon and triceps tendon jerks and wrist reflexes are about normal on each side. Touch and pain sensations are normal in the face and upper and lower limbs. The patellar reflex is prompt on the right side but diminished on the left side. Ankle clonus and

Babinski's reflex are not present on either side. He has dizziness when he sits up, and in walking staggers and always toward the right. He is unable to stand erect with feet together, and his wife says that his tendency to fall is always toward the right. His memory has been failing during the past month.

July 16th. The patellar reflex is diminished on each side—a little more so on the left. Ankle clonus and Babinski's reflex are not present on either side. Achilles jerk is present but diminished, and more so on the left side. Hemiasynergy is very pronounced in the right lower limb, and is not present in the left. When the right leg is flexed on the thigh and the thigh on the abdomen as far as possible, and then an attempt is made to extend the right lower limb, he extends first the right thigh, and later, when the limb is almost ready to be placed upon the bed, he extends the leg on the thigh.

The patient's wife said that before he came to the hospital he yawned much in the daytime.

He has no tremor in movement of the upper limbs. He places the first finger of either hand on the end of the nose well.

The report of the ophthalmic examination by Dr. de Schweinitz is as follows: Double optic neuritis (choked disks); swelling about 5 D.; many hemorrhages; paresis apparently of right external rectus; pupils prompt; right halves of visual fields contracted, but line does not run quite to fixation point left and only half-way right. They seem somewhat uncertain.

The report from Dr. B. A. Randall is as follows: The right ear hears all tones less distinctly than the left, but distinguishes from 200–20,000 d. v. s. Bone-conduction preponderates over air, but is slightly subnormal where it should be exaggerated if trouble were tympanic only. Drumheads fair in appearance. No acoustic defect of left noted. There seems to be nerve lesion combined with tympanic on the right.

Examination of the blood showed: hæmoglobin, 75 per cent.; red blood cells, 5,312,000; white blood cells, 9840.

23d. During the past three days the patient has had very severe attacks of headache, usually frontal, but occasionally occipital, and during these attacks he has been very restless. He has had some morning vomiting. His wife says that his mental condition is worse, and he does not understand what is said to him. Stereognostic perception is normal in each hand. Right hemiasynergy is distinct. Resistance to passive movements is normal in the upper and lower limbs. Some nystagmoid movement is present on looking to the right or left. Sense of position is normal in the hands, but the tests for the toes give uncertain results.

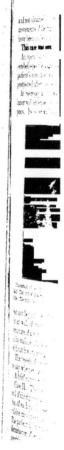

25th. The right side of the forehead is not wrinkled as well as the left, nor does he draw up the right corner of the mouth as well as the left. He yawns frequently. No tenderness of scalp is found on percussion. The patellar reflex is much diminished on the right side, and not obtained on the left side. The patient has had fine twitching movements of the right extremities, although at times the movements have been on both sides of the body.

This case was seen by Dr. C. K. Mills in consultation.

An operation for the removal of a tumor believed to be in the right cerebello-pontile angle was done by Dr. Frazier July 23, 1903. The patient's condition was so serious that further operation had to be postponed after the bone was cut through. He died July 24th.

At necropsy a cyst was found in the right cerebellar lobe. Its inner wall extended to the union of the right cerebellar lobe with the pons. Its outer wall extended to the surface of the cerebellar lobe,

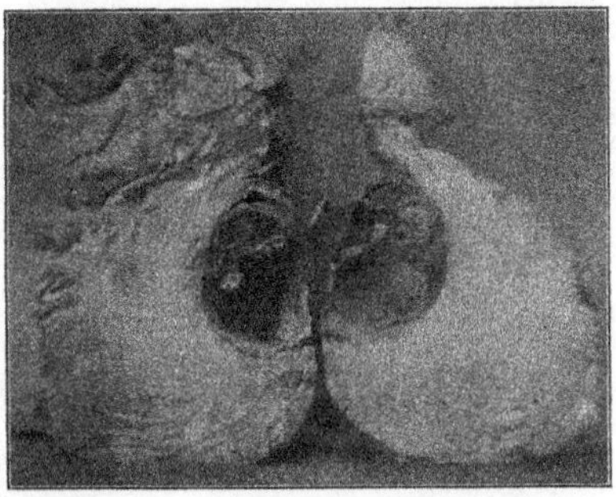

Photograph of the right lobe of the cerebellum from Case V. The lobe has been cut in half. The cyst, with a small tumor in its wall, is shown at the lower part of the cerebellar lobe. The upper part of the photograph represents the medulla oblongata.

but not beyond. Small tumor masses were found in the upper and inner wall of the cyst, and these, under the microscope, had the structure of a spindle-cell sarcoma. The cyst, with the tumor masses in its walls, could be easily enucleated. It measured 3.3 cm. from without inward and 2.4 cm. from above downward.

The vessels of the brain had been torn away, and it was impossible to say whether thrombosis had occurred or not.

A brief summary of the last four cases is as follows:

Case II. The symptoms were paresis of the right side of the face and of the right upper and lower limbs, some motor aphasia, diminution of each patellar reflex, frontal and occipital headache, and convulsive movements of the right upper limb, but not of the lower. The patient did not have nausea, vomiting, vertigo, Babinski's sign, disturbance of sensation, loss of stereognostic perception, nor optic neuritis.

An infiltrating spindle-cell sarcoma was found in the second left frontal convolution, extending into the middle of the precentral and postcentral convolutions and the upper part of Broca's area.

Case III. Syphilitic infection was acknowledged. The symptoms were severe headache on the right side during five years, convulsive movements of the left side of the face and of the left upper limb, but not of the left lower limb, a little weakness of the left side of the face, and nowhere else, gray degeneration of the optic nerves, paralysis of one third nerve and paresis of one fourth nerve, and loss of the iritic response to light and in accommodation. The patient did not have nausea, vomiting, dizziness, optic neuritis, alteration of tendon reflexes, Babinski's sign, nor loss of stereognostic perception. Later, some weakness of the left upper limb was noticed, and sensation became impaired in the left upper limb and in the left side of the face, and stereognostic perception and sense of position became impaired in the left hand. Still later, the left upper and lower limbs became completely paralyzed, and motion in the left side of the face became imperfect. A subcortical mixed sarcoma (round and small spindle cells) was found in the right cerebral hemisphere. Its central portion was beneath the middle part of the motor area. Its outer border was 1.5 cm. below the surface of the brain.

Case IV. The symptoms were frontal and occipital headache, convulsive movements of the left side of the body, impaired mentality, some weakness of upper and lower limbs, greater on the left side than on the right, spasticity of the lower limbs, exaggeration of tendon reflexes, Babinski's sign on the right side, but not on the left; optic neuritis greater in the left eye, loss of stereognosis and of the sense of position in the left hand, impairment of tactile sensation, but not of pain sensation, in the left upper limb, and awkwardness of the movements of the left fingers. Numerous tuberculous plaques were found, almost confined to the right parietal lobe, except where they extended into the upper part of the postcentral and precentral convolutions.

Case V. The symptoms were occipital, frontal, or general headache, vomiting, general weakness, paresis of the lower part of the right side of the face, dizziness, staggering toward the right, diminished patellar reflexes, right hemiasynergy, frequent yawning, double optic neuritis, paresis of right external rectus, central deafness on the right side, some nystagmus on lateral movement, and impaired mentality. A cyst with small sarcomatous masses in its walls was found in the right cerebellar lobe at its union with the pons.

In Case II. the convulsions in the right side of the face and in the right upper limb, the weakness of the right side of the face and of the right upper and lower limbs, the partial motor aphasia, were indicative of a focal lesion, probably a tumor, in the left side of the brain, and chiefly in or near the centre for the upper limb. As the convulsions probably had not implicated the right lower limb, it seemed more likely that the tumor had grown inward and involved the fibres coming from the centre for the lower limb in their course from this centre to the internal capsule. The absence of convulsions in the right lower limb seemed to indicate that the cortical centre for this limb was not irritated or else irritated after the fibres from this area had been cut. It was not surprising, therefore, to find a tumor within the brain in the area indicated. Especially noteworthy in this case was the absence of optic neuritis, nausea, vomiting, and dizziness.

The tumor was entirely removed, so far as we could determine, and was one of the smallest I have ever seen taken out at an operation. It was not very much larger than an English walnut. Our desire should always be to remove a tumor while it is still very small, but we are usually unable to accomplish this, as the symptoms are not sufficiently indicative of the position of the new-growth in its early development.

We felt very much pleased on account of the great improvement and, indeed, almost complete recovery following the operation for a period of about seven weeks. If the tumor had been well defined from the surrounding tissue a return might not have occurred. The necropsy showed a tumor that could at no point be outlined from the surrounding brain tissue.

We were very desirous of making another attempt to remove the growth, but the man's general condition was not such as to warrant this on account of signs of pneumonia.

Restoration to health for a period of seven weeks is by no means to be despised, and if, at the operation, we had removed more of what seemed to be healthy cerebral tissue surrounding the tumor the recurrence might have been prevented or delayed much longer. In every case in which a tumor is infiltrating and has the appearance of a sarcoma I would recommend that surrounding brain tissue should be removed, even though it appears to the naked eye to be healthy, and even though paralysis is likely to be increased by this removal.

In Case III. syphilis was acknowledged, and the headache existing many years, the paralysis of the right internal rectus extending over a period of eight years, and the loss of the iritic response to light and in accommodation made the case appear as one of syphilitic meningitis. Antisyphilitic treatment was thoroughly employed, without distinct benefit, but this did not prove that the case was not one of syphilitic meningitis. I have seen vigorous administration of mercury and iodides have little effect on advanced cerebral syphilis where many symptoms suggested the existence of brain tumor. These cases should be regarded, at least clinically, as cases of brain tumor, and so treated—*i. e.*, by operation, where operation is permissible.

The convulsions involving the left side of the face and the left upper limb were indicative of a lesion in the corresponding cortical centres for these parts. At first there was weakness only in the lower part of the left side of the face, but later the left hand-grasp became weak. The stereognostic perception became impaired in the left hand, the sense of position became impaired in the left thumb, and tactile and pain sensations became impaired in the left upper limb. Sensations of touch, pain, and temperature also became a little impaired in the left side of the face. The lesion seemed to be in the face and upper limb centres and the adjoining part of the parietal lobe, and it was believed to be cortical or very near the cortex, because of the typical Jacksonian epilepsy.

The area mentioned was exposed, but a distinct tumor could not be found. I regret that the brain was not punctured more freely in the exposed area. I have seen punctures made so often at operations for brain tumors without any effect, except possibly some increase in the paralysis after the operation, that I had grown a little lukewarm toward this procedure. In Case III. the tumor was softened and partly fluid in its lower portion, and repeated punctures might have caused the escape of some of the fluid and the detection of the tumor. It was so far below the cortex that its complete removal might have been uncertain, and, probably, would have been impossible.

In this case, as well as in Case II., optic neuritis did not exist, and this sign was, therefore, absent in two of the five cases, and yet in each of the two cases the diagnosis of tumor of the brain was made. One was a tumor of the middle motor area, and the other a subcortical tumor of the lower parietal and lower motor area. Choked disk is one of the most common signs of brain tumor, but is not always present. Oppenheim,[1] in his monograph on brain tumors, in regard to this subject says that he has found typical choked disk in fourteen and optic neuritis in five of twenty-three cases—*i. e.*, in 82 per cent.; that Gowers found it in four-fifths of his cases, and Knapp in two-thirds of his cases. Oppenheim expresses the opinion that, as in recent years the diagnosis of brain tumor has been made earlier and confirmed by operation, choked disk is not so frequently seen. Although papillitis does not depend entirely on the location of the tumor, he thinks it is almost a constant and early sign of tumor of the cerebellum. It is relatively often absent when the tumor grows from the meninges and presses against the brain, also in cases of cortical tumors that do not penetrate far into the white matter, and of tumors of the pons, medulla oblongata, and corpus callosum. Tumors of the occipital lobe, he thinks, cause optic neuritis late.

Mills,[2] in his text-book, remarks that optic neuritis is probably present on both sides in from 60 to 80 per cent. of all the cases of

[1] Die Geschwülste des Gehirns, second edition, p. 63.
[2] The Nervous System and Its Diseases, p. 510.

brain tumor, but that statistics on the subject are somewhat conflicting. It has been noted, he says, in only about 50 per cent. in tumors of the motor cortex.

Starr[1] says unhesitatingly that optic neuritis is present in 80 per cent. of the cases of brain tumor.

The occurrence of Jacksonian epilepsy in Case III., in which a tumor existed 1.5 cm. below the cortex, was somewhat misleading in making a diagnosis.

In the third edition of his text-book Oppenheim[2] says that unilateral convulsions may occur from lesions of the subcortical substance, especially when they implicate the fibres from the motor zone. The convulsions are not exactly like those of Jacksonian epilepsy, and when they resemble them more closely they are caused by lesions that affect the cortex by pressure, etc.

Dejerine,[3] in speaking on the same subject, remarks that typical attacks of Jacksonian epilepsy rarely may occur from limited subcortical lesions. He observed a case in which the convulsive movements began in the hand, and a tubercle was found in the white matter of the brain 1 cm. beneath the cortex.

In Case III. typical Jacksonian epilepsy was observed when the tumor was so far as 1.5 cm. below the cerebral cortex, and as the growth was 4 cm. in transverse diameter it must have been still further below the cortex when it first developed. This is possibly the first case in which a subcortical tumor so deeply situated caused typical Jacksonian epilepsy.

In Case IV. paralysis of the left side of the thorax was said to have occurred during a convulsion. The necropsy showed that the left lung was entirely atelectatic. It seemed to me impossible that the left side of the thorax could be completely paralyzed as a result of a unilateral cerebral lesion. I have never observed such a condition, and I am not aware that others have. Muscles on the two sides of the body that contract synchronously are not paralyzed by a unilateral cerebral lesion.

Especially interesting in this case, and of great diagnostic value, were the loss of stereognostic perception and of the sense of position in the left hand, the awkward movement of the left fingers, and the impairment of sensation for touch, but not for pain, in the left upper limb. These signs were indicative of a lesion of the parietal lobe. Absence of hemianopsia made an implication of the sensory fibres in the internal capsule and, therefore, a lesion near the visual fibres, improbable, and the typical Jacksonian epilepsy pointed to a cortical lesion.

The loss of the sense of position was so marked in this case that the patient was unable to find his left hand with his right hand when

[1] Organic Nervous Diseases, p. 600.
[2] Lehrbuch der Nervenkrankheiten, third edition, p. 605.
[3] Sémeiologie du Système Nerveux, p. 523.

his eyes were closed, and he frequently took hold of my hand believing it was his own.

Although I fully believe that a lesion of the parietal lobe may cause ataxia, loss of stereognostic perception, and loss of the sense of position and some disturbance of tactile and possibly of pain sensation in the limbs of the opposite side, I have not been convinced that a lesion of the motor area will give none of these symptoms.

In a recent paper Marinesco[1] remarks that Jonesco removed a part of the cortical centre for the left upper limb in a man. After the operation the patient could move his shoulder and elbow very well, but not his hand. Nine months later the movements of the left hand were very imperfect, and tactile sensation, the sense of position, and stereognostic perception were diminished in the left hand. In another case Jonesco removed the centres of the face and upper and lower limbs of the right cerebral cortex. A year after the operation there was much weakness of the left side of the body, and the sense of position, stereognostic perception, and tactile sensation were affected in the left upper limb. Thermal and painful sensations were preserved. These operations were done for epilepsy, and in one case, at least, and probably in both, the cortical motor areas were determined by the electric current.

I have observed loss of stereognostic perception caused by lesions much below the cortex of the brain, viz., in a case of tumor of the pons (Potts and Spiller) and in a case of tumor compressing the medulla oblongata (case of Dercum); but where the symptoms indicate a tumor of the cerebrum that probably is cortical, I believe the loss of stereognostic perception and of the sense of position and ataxia of the upper limb of the side opposite to that in which is the lesion indicate much implication of the parietal lobe.

In 1898, at a meeting of the Philadelphia Neurological Society, I[2] referred to a case that I had seen in the service of Dr. Lloyd, at the Philadelphia Hospital, which seemed to show that the cortical representation of the sense of position is in the parietal lobe. A man complained, during the night preceding his attack, of fatigue, headache, and inability to sleep. The following morning he fell on the floor on attempting to rise from his bed, but was not unconscious. When he was found he had paresis of the left limbs and of the left side of the face and tongue. Later the patient could raise his left upper limb above his head, but every movement of this limb was ataxic in an extreme degree, though the limb was not paralyzed. The mental condition of the patient prevented an examination of the condition of sensation. At the necropsy a hemorrhage was found in the right parietal lobe. The hemorrhagic area was about 2 cm. in diameter, and extended inward in the form of a cone to the lateral ventricle, having its base in the cortex. It

[1] Semaine médicale, October 7, 1903, p. 325.
[2] Journal of Nervous and Mental Disease, January, 1899, p. 43.

was situated about 4 cm. from the longitudinal fissure and about 2 cm. or 3 cm. behind the Rolandic fissure. The brain had been cut into frontal sections about 1 cm. apart, when we had an opportunity to examine it, and, although the injury to the cerebral tissue prevented an exact determination of the location of the hemorrhage, it was evidently in or very close to the supramarginal gyrus. The ataxia was probably caused by a loss of the sense of position.

This was probably one of the first cases reported in this country, showing that ataxia from a loss of the sense of position may be caused by a lesion of the parietal lobe. The case of Starr and McCosh preceded it.

A case that Dr. C. K. Mills and I saw together, June 3, 1901, in consultation, the case being under the charge of Dr. Ida Richardson, affords evidence also of the localization of the stereognostic perception and of the sense of position in the parietal lobe. The patient's left upper limb was decidedly ataxic, paretic, and astereognostic, and the head was retracted and rigid. The necropsy was made by Dr. W. F. Hendrickson. An area of depression, indefinite in outline, but about 6 cm. in diameter, was found in the parietal lobe of the right cerebral hemisphere just posterior to the fissure of Rolando. Palpation revealed less resistance at this point than over the surrounding tissue. On section this area was found to be the seat of extensive softening. The process implicated practically the entire right parietal lobe.

The case reported by C. K. Mills,[1] which was seen by me and others in consultation, was one of the first to establish the localization of the stereognostic perception in the parietal lobe. A diagnosis of tumor of this lobe was made because of the loss of the sense of position, the impaired cutaneous sensibility, astereognosis, and ataxia. The case has been so fully reported by Dr. Mills and is so well known that I need not refer to it further.

Oppenheim,[2] after giving a description of his case of parietal tumor with operation, remarks that lesions of the parietal lobe cause ataxia of one or both limbs of one side. Irritative or paralytic motor symptoms are absent, or when they occur they are the result of pressure. The sensory disturbance is always a partial hemianæsthesia, in that pain and temperature sensations are preserved, while tactile sensation and especially the sense of position and the stereognostic perception are impaired or lost. Such a symptom-complex occurs when the lesion does not extend far into the white matter of the parietal lobe. He says, also, that the cases in which tumor of the parietal lobe has been so accurately diagnosed that a radical operation was possible are very few.

This case of Oppenheim was reported by him February 12, 1900,

[1] Mills, Keen, and Spiller. Journal of Nervous and Mental Disease, May, 1900, p. 244.

[2] Mitteilungen aus den Granzgebieten der Medizin und Chirurgie, 1900, vol. vi. pp. 382, 383.

and published in the third number of the sixth volume (1900) of the *Mitteilungen.*

In his monograph[1] on tumors of the brain he says that in the majority of cases of tumor of the parietal lobe sensory irritative and paralytic phenomena were observed. He refers to Mills' case, but adds that the cases are not sufficient to permit us to regard the above-mentioned phenomena as positive evidence of lesions of the parietal lobe. The evidences of the localization value of these symptoms are, however, rapidly accumulating.

In March, 1901, C. W. Burr[2] reported a case in which there were slight hemiplegia, slight tactile anæsthesia, astereognosis, mind blindness, loss of the temperature sense on one side, sensory aphasia varying in intensity, and mental dulness. In this case a tumor was found in the parietal lobe, pressing against but not invading the ascending parietal convolution, partially destroying the angular gyrus, and involving almost the entire posterior parietal lobule.

The meningitis in plaques that occurred in Case IV. is of a very unusual character. The best paper on the subject that I know of is by Combe. He says that the meningitis in plaques (méningite en plaque of the French writers) is an unusual form of tuberculosis, and yet one that should be recognized. Tuberculosis of the central nervous system may appear as one or more tumors of different size, some small and some large; or it may appear as numerous minute tubercles scattered along the bloodvessels; or it may appear in plaques. Combe described the last form in 1898, although it was known to Landouzy, Dupré, and Chantemesse. The meningitis in plaques, as described by Combe, predominates on the convexity of the brain, and scarcely implicates the base at all. The inflammation is circumscribed and causes little exudation; it is almost always situated about and in front of the fissure of Rolando—*i. e.*, in the motor zone. It occurs as one or several plaques of different size and thickness, and consisting of agglomerated granulations and fibrinous deposits. The pia is thickened about the plaques and contains miliary tubercles. The pia is normal over the rest of the brain, or else hyperæmic and thickened. The base of the brain, the interpeduncular space, the bulb, and the cranial nerves are not affected.

This form of meningitis does not cause basal symptoms; usually there is no vomiting, no constipation, no slowness and no irregularity of the pulse, no strabismus, no intense headache, no choked disk. The localization in the motor area explains the Jacksonian epilepsy and paralysis of the opposite side of the body. It is not surprising, therefore, that most of the cases mentioned by Chantemesse had not been correctly diagnosed from the clinical symptoms.

The common form of tuberculous meningitis occurs more fre-

[1] Oppenheim. Die Geschwülste des Gehirns, second edition, p. 116.
[2] THE AMERICAN JOURNAL OF THE MEDICAL SCIENCES, March, 1901, p. 306.

quently in children, while the meningitis in plaques is found more frequently in adults.

Combe[1] says that in every case in which the meningitis in plaques appeared to be primary, miliary tuberculosis or local tuberculosis not causing any symptoms has been found.

The dura is usually normal, but sometimes adherences with the plaques are found. The paracentral lobule is the part usually affected.

According to F. Raymond[2] these plaques are really tubercles, and are caused by an infection conveyed by means of the cerebrospinal fluid.

E. F. Trevelyan[3] says that he has seen nine cases of the meningitis in plaques.

In my Case IV. the plaques were situated behind the fissure of Rolando in the parietal lobe, and not in front of the fissure, where Combe says they are more commonly found. The dura was adherent to a few of these plaques. The optic chiasm examined by microscopic sections showed no evidence of meningitis, and yet this part is usually a favorite location for meningitis.

In Case V. the movement of the lower part of the right side of the face was not so good as that of the left side. The patient always staggered toward the right in walking, and hemiasynergy of the right lower limb as described by Babinski was found on two or three occasions—*i. e.*, when the right leg was fully flexed on the thigh, and the thigh fully flexed on the abdomen, and the patient then attempted to extend the limb and place it on the bed, the movements of the lower limb were not synergic; the leg was not extended simultaneously with the thigh. Babinski thinks that this hemiasynergy is present on the side on which the cerebellar tumor exists. I have observed the sign in four cases of supposed cerebellar tumor, but only in this, Case V., have I been able to establish its reliability by necropsy. In Case V. the patellar reflexes were diminished on each side. Deafness of central origin in the right ear was reported by Dr. B. A. Randall. Nystagmoid movements were present when the patient looked to either side. These were the chief signs that led me to diagnose a tumor of the right cerebellopontile angle, and the diagnosis was correct.

Repeated yawning was observed in Case V. I have seen this when the symptoms indicated a lesion somewhere at the base of the brain, and I look upon it as a sign of a lesion at this part and not in the cerebral cortex. Oppenheim thinks it is not a rare sign of cerebellar tumor, but I believe it may be seen in cases of tumor elsewhere at the base.

I was unable to observe that the nystagmus was greater in devia-

[1] Revue médicale de la suisse romande, 1898.
[2] Leçons sur les maladies du système nerveux, 1900, fourth series, p. 24.
[3] Lancet, November 7, 1903, p. 1276.

tion of the eyes to the right, the side of the lesion, than in deviation toward the left. In a case of cerebellar abscess that I saw in consultation with Dr. B. A. Randall the nystagmus was much greater when the eyes were turned toward the side of the lesion than when they were turned away from it. I have not been able to make this observation in any other case, but I speak of it in the hope that it may prove to be of clinical value.

Oppenheim describes involuntary movements, tremor, occurring in cases of cerebellar tumor, and such movements were present in Case V.

A DISCUSSION OF THE SURGERY OF TUMORS OF THE BRAIN, WITH A RESUME OF THE OPERATIVE RECORDS OF FOUR CRANIOTOMIES.

By Charles H. Frazier, M.D.,

PROFESSOR OF SURGERY, UNIVERSITY OF PENNSYLVANIA; SURGEON TO THE UNIVERSITY HOSPITAL.

The statistics of the last five years give us every reason to take a more hopeful view of the surgery of cerebral tumors. It will be admitted without question that the greater attainments of more recent years are to be attributed to an earlier recognition of the tumor, to a correspondingly earlier resort to operation, to more accurate localization, and, finally, to certain distinct improvements in the technique. The latter may be said to include a speedier method of opening the skull, the exposure of a much larger area of the brain than was possible before the introduction of the osteoplastic flap, the adoption of the two-stage operation in those cases in which the blood pressure is materially depressed by the preliminary procedures. Many of the improvements or modifications of the technique in operations upon the brain have in view a common object, the prevention of shock. Operating as we are upon such a highly sensitive organ as the brain, and upon the organ which presides over functions so essential to the maintenance of life, additional precautions must be taken. The precautions which one ordinarily takes to prevent shock in operations upon other organs must be observed in brain operations the more stringently; the avoidance of unnecessary exposure, the avoidance of unnecessarily prolonged operation, the prevention of excessive hemorrhage, the avoidance of unnecessarily rough manipulations of the tissue, the administration of the anæsthetic by an experienced man; careful observation of the patient's condition, more particularly of the circulatory function, throughout the operation at frequent intervals; these are all points to which the greatest importance should be attached.

METHOD OF MAKING THE OSTEOPLASTIC OR WAGNER FLAP. The instrument which in our experience at the University Hospital seems to meet every indication is the so-called dental engine armed with a trephine and drill. Given an area of brain to expose, an osteoplastic flap of corresponding size can be made with much less traumatism and in a much shorter time with this instrument than with any other. Objections to other instruments may readily be found. In fashioning the flap with chisel and mallet a degree of traumatism must be inflicted upon the nervous structures within the skull, which is, to say the least, undesirable, and in the opinion of some surgeons the hammering increases the shock, and thereby adds to the risk of the operation. As compared with any of the other methods this is by all odds the crudest. The Gigli saw may be used, but a good deal of time is consumed in making the necessary number of trephine openings, and passage of the saw from one opening to another is neither an easy nor, in all cases, a safe procedure. The Stellwagen trephine, which was placed on the market a little over a year ago, is an ingenious instrument, but, from the mechanical point of view, is not to be compared with the dental engine. The efficacy of the Stellwagen trephine depends upon the ability to fix the central plate —this can only be accomplished by screwing the plate to the skull; but even after the central plate has been secured in place it requires a good deal of practice and force to be able to saw through the entire thickness of the skull in a reasonably short time. But there is still another and what I consider a very serious objection to this instrument, namely, the loss of a considerable amount of blood before the flap is reflected and the hemorrhage controllable. The greatest amount of bleeding comes from the venous channels in the diploë; with the Stellwagen trephine one begins to saw through the skull layer by layer from without inward until one reaches the diploë; upon reaching the inner table of the skull, one must proceed more slowly and with greater caution, because of the danger of penetrating the dura and injuring the brain. Meanwhile, hemorrhage from the diploic vessels is very free, and, of course, uncontrollable until the bone is entirely divided and the flap reflected. The drill of the dental engine divides the entire thickness of bone as it proceeds; furthermore, it seems to crush and occlude the openings of the diploic sinuses, and in that way spontaneously controls hemorrhage. Including the series of cases recorded in this paper, I have performed in the last six months some ten craniotomies with the dental engine, and I believe that with this instrument a given area of the brain can be exposed with the minimum degree of traumatism and in the minimum amount of time. The element of time plays a most important part in the outcome of operations for brain tumor. Mills,[1] in a paper presented to the College of Physicians in 1902, said: "I

[1] Philadelphia Medical Journal, September 27, 1902.

am satisfied that the present dangers to life in operations for brain tumor are from hemorrhage and prolonged operation.". Therefore, the addition to our armamentarium of an instrument which economizes time will tend toward lowering the mortality. In the absence of complications it is quite possible without undue haste to completely divide and reflect the bony flap in eight minutes. It requires but very little practice to become proficient in the use of this instrument. After the incision has been made in the scalp, corresponding to the size and shape of the flap, an opening in the skull at one extremity of the incision is made with a small trephine operated by the engine. This will consume but a fraction of a minute. A small dural separator is inserted in the opening in order to make sure that the dura is free from the bone before the bone-drill is introduced. This can be attached to the engine without any risk of the operator's hand coming in contact with any portion of the engine that may not be sterile. The drill is now introduced and the bone divided from one extremity of the incision to the other. To guard against the possibility of the wound becoming infected from particles of dust that may be cast off from the arm or pulleys of the electric motor, an assistant plays a stream of sterile water or normal salt solution over the field of operation while the machine is in motion. But two objections to this method of performing craniotomies suggest themselves: one, the possibility of infection; the other, the possibility of dividing the dura and lacerating the brain substance should the dura be adherent.

I have already referred to the manner in which infection may be guarded against. The danger of dividing the dura and lacerating the brain substance in those cases in which the dura is adherent is not incurred by this method more than by any other. No matter what the instrument selected for dividing the bone, if the dura be firmly adherent to the skull it will be exposed to the possibility of laceration. One of the advantages of making the flap of liberal dimensions is that there will be a margin of normal tissue between the lesion and the edges of the osseous opening. The possibility of the line of the bone-flap traversing the affected area is more remote.

McCosh, of New York, makes use of the electric engine in his craniotomies. A small bulb of the shape of a pear, about one-quarter of an inch in diameter, is attached to the engine, and with this bulb four or five holes are bored through the skull; the cone shape of the bulb allows the point to penetrate through the skull as it is revolved, and yet prevents the shaft from entering the skull or penetrating the dura. When the holes have been made the bulb is removed, and there is substituted a small circular saw, and the bone between the holes made by the burr sawed through. A small projecting and protecting flange is screwed to the side of the circular saw, so that the blade of the saw is exposed only for the depth of the skull as measured through the holes, and in this way the danger of sawing through the dura is wholly obviated.[1] This instrument would, it seems to me, require much more practice in order to enable one to operate it with safety. If one depends, in the adjustment of the flange, upon the depth of the skull measured at any one of the holes the danger of sawing through the dura cannot, as it is claimed, be wholly obviated. The depth or thickness of the skull varies, so that there would always be the possibility of the saw penetrating the dura if the skull were thicker at one of the holes than elsewhere, or what is also an objection, though not such a serious one, the saw would not penetrate the entire thickness of the skull if the skull were thinner at the point measured than it was at some other point along the projected incision.

Control of Hemorrhage. Exceptional precautions should be adopted to control hemorrhage from the very outstart. The amount of blood which will be lost from an extensive incision of the scalp might be considerable. The loss of blood will be reduced to a minimum by the application of a tourniquet around the head. I have been in the habit of using for this purpose rubber tubing. Dr. Cushing showed me recently an appliance for this purpose which seemed to me very superior. It consists of an inflatable tube, which fits snugly the head of the patient, and with a small bicycle pump can be distended sufficiently to exert the necessary degree of pressure. If no tourniquet is used, it is a good plan to make the incision section by section, stopping to control the hemorrhage from one section before proceeding to the next. Hemorrhage from the diploic sinuses is satisfactorily controlled by Horsley's wax. When we come to the question of the control of hemorrhage from the brain and tumor itself, we are confronted with a more difficult problem. But two courses are open: one to pack gauze firmly into the wound, the other to close one or both carotids temporarily. The latter course would seem to be the ideal course were the practice of it unattended with risk. Crile, to whom we are indebted for this suggestion, performed this preliminary operation in a series of cases without any serious after-effects. It seemed to me that, if as in Crile's hands this operation were free from danger, a very important contribution had been made to the technique of brain surgery. My personal experience, however, has not confirmed these views. In the first place, temporary closure of the carotids does not altogether control hemorrhage; it controls arterial hemorrhage, but upon the venous hemorrhage, which is the much more troublesome, it has little effect. But in addition to the control being ineffectual, it is not unattended by risk, at least it has not been in my hands. I have practised temporary closure of the carotid but five times in all, including two of the cases in this report, and from this limited experience I am firmly of the opinion that Crile's method should be reserved for the extreme cases, and in these should be confined to one side.

The posture of the patient during the operation should, of course,

[1] Starr. Journal of Nervous and Mental Disease, July, 1903.

not be overlooked. Hemorrhage will be less free if the patient's head and body are well elevated. Unless the patient is in a state of shock I am in the habit of continuing elevation of the head and shoulders after the patient is transferred from the operating-table to his bed.

Observations upon the Blood Pressure. One of the signs of increased intracranial tension of whatever origin is elevation of the blood pressure. It is present in depressed fractures of the skull, in intracranial hemorrhage, in cerebral contusion and concussion, as well as in brain tumor. In a very exhaustive work on concussion and cerebral compression by Kocher and his students, the effects of intracranial tension upon the circulation of the brain were studied. It was observed that when the compression was of a very moderate degree there developed primarily a venous stasis or disdiamyrrhosis. This was due to the obstruction of the venous circulation by the increased intracranial pressure. If this pressure continues or increases the circulation of the brain becomes re-established; this phenomenon is attributed to a stimulation of the vasomotor centre, which, acting through the peripheral vessels, causes such an increase in the arterial pressure as will compensate for the increased cranial tension. And so it is that in the presence of a brain tumor we often find the blood pressure elevated above normal. In all operations for the removal of brain tumors I have made it a practice to make an observation of the blood pressure before the operation and to have the observations upon the blood pressure continued throughout the operation. These observations are recorded on a chart designed for this especial purpose; on it are recorded by an assistant a tracing of the pulse and blood pressure in such a way that the operator can see at a glance what the pulse rate and degree of blood pressure may be. The sphygmograph,[1] which is used in my clinic, is very simple in its construction, and can be operated without any difficulty by an untrained assistant.

The object in having this record made throughout the operation is twofold. In the first place, generally speaking, the condition of the blood pressure is the most reliable index of the patient's condition; when the normal blood pressure is sustained throughout the operation we are assured that the operative procedures have not been of sufficient gravity to induce shock. This applies, of course, to operative procedures generally, and is not confined to those upon the brain; but in operations for the removal of tumors of the brain the blood pressure index is of much greater significance, in that it assists us in determining whether the operation should be performed in one or two stages.

Indications for Two-stage Operation. It has been said that 25 per cent. would be considered a conservative estimate of patients who died immediately from the effects of operation. In some cases death is attributed to shock, in some to concussion, and in some to

[1] It is a modification of the Riva-Rocci instrument that was worked out by Dr. Stanton, Instructor in Medicine at the University of Pennsylvania.

"unknown causes." In a discussion on the subject of brain tumors at the October meeting of the College of Physicians I said that I was inclined to believe that in the latter class of cases death was due to the sudden withdrawal of intracranial pressure. In the investigations of Kocher, that have already been referred to, it was demonstrated that the sudden withdrawal of intracranial pressure, after the blood pressure had been forced to a considerable height, may be followed by paralysis or break down of the vasomotor mechanism. If we are correct in assuming that this theory will explain many of the fatal terminations in a given number of cases, we should give more serious consideration to the advisability of dividing the operation into two stages. Horsley recommends the adoption of this procedure in every case without exception, and v. Bergmann, though not going so far as Horsley, recommended the two-stage operation in cases in which the patient's general condition was below par, or in which the tumor was a particularly large one. Horsley's recommendation seems to me unnecessarily radical, and that of v. Bergmann too indefinite. It seems to me a rule may be formulated which is based upon a much more scientific basis, namely, that when after the relief of pressure, such as would follow the removal of the osteoplastic flap and the reflection of the dura, there is a very decided fall in the blood pressure, an attempt should not be made at that sitting to remove the tumor. The completion of the operation should be postponed until the circulatory equilibrium has been restored, that is, until the circulation of the brain has become adjusted to the newly instituted physical conditions. This may mean the delay of a week or a delay of but forty-eight hours. [In order to determine in more exact terms the effect of the sudden removal from the brain of such pressure as would be exerted by a tumor, I am conducting a series of experiments upon dogs, in which an inflated rubber bag is introduced beneath the dura and distended so gradually as to simulate the growth of a tumor; when the bag is distended to a considerable size the fluid will be withdrawn suddenly, and the effect of the collapse of the bag upon the blood pressure will be recorded.]

In Case III. of this series such a course was adopted. The patient had a large subcortical tumor. Soon after the dural flap was reflected there was such a fall of blood pressure that I decided to postpone for the time being further operative intervention. The patient soon recovered from the effects of the preliminary step, but I feel quite sure that if I had continued with the operation and attempted to remove the tumor the circulatory disturbance would have been aggravated, and the patient would have died. In Case II. it will be noted in the chart that after the completion of the first stage of the operation the patient was not suffering from depression of the circulation. Accordingly, I proceeded and removed the tumor. The tumor proved to be a small one, so small that its presence had not caused enough increased tension to disturb the circulation, and the removal was effected, therefore, without affecting the blood pressure.

Sommer[1] reports his experience in an operation for sarcoma of the brain. Death ensued a few hours afterward for no demonstrable reason. The author says that in this as in many other cases death is due to sudden change in the circulation. His views coincide with mine. As a means of relieving pressure he recommends lumbar puncture in addition to the reflection of the osteoplastic flap as a preliminary measure, postponing for a few days any attempt to remove the growth. Lumbar puncture would no doubt relieve pressure temporarily, but whether its effects would be enduring enough to be of any practical value I am not prepared to say. Furthermore, lumbar puncture is in itself a dangerous procedure, and especially so in brain tumors. A number of sudden deaths have been reported as having been caused by this procedure.

As to the Question of Bulging of the Brain. If the most alarming feature of brain operation is hemorrhage, the most troublesome is the bulging of the brain that follows reflection of the dura. In the course of our operations Dr. Spiller and I have made certain observations bearing upon this subject. As a preface to these observations it should be stated that a distinction is made between the bulging which occurs immediately after the dura is reflected, which will for convenience sake be termed "initial" bulging, and that which manifests itself during the subsequent exploratory manœuvres, or "consecutive" bulging.

First, when a tumor is present there may be little or no initial bulging, but there is not likely to be any consecutive bulging. By this we mean that, given a case in which the tumor has been localized accurately and occupies the field bounded by the opening in the skull, there may be little or no bulging, even though the tumor be one of very considerable dimensions. In Cases II. and III. of this report there were present a small and a very large tumor respectively, and yet in neither case was there any initial or consecutive bulging. No doubt the character of the tumor would have some effect—thus a very vascular sarcoma would be more likely to bulge through the opening than a gumma. The release of pressure from a growth abounding in large vascular channels would result in a reactionary dilatation, more particularly of the venous channels, and this in turn might be followed by such circulatory disturbances as would readily lead to cerebral œdema. What we want to call particular attention to is this: that in the absence of bulging one must not be led to believe that there can be no tumor present.

Secondly, that when the tumor was not found, and if present was not situated at or beneath the area exposed, "consecutive" bulging was a very conspicuous feature, and the degree of bulging far exceeded the initial bulging observed when tumors were present. This at first thought seems as it were paradoxical, but upon further consideration is readily explained. It is due to the fact that normal brain tissue being the more sensitive reacts more rapidly to the insult of trauma-

[1] Beiträge zur Psychiatrie klinik, 1902, vol. i. p. 5.

tism. When the looked-for lesion does not present itself on the surface of the brain at the site of exposure certain exploratory measures are **instituted**: the brain is palpated to determine its consistency, exploratory incisions are made into the cortex to determine whether the growth is subcortical, and the exploratory needle is introduced in the search for deep-seated collections of fluid. Meantime the brain surface is subjected to the injurious influence of a comparatively low temperature. Each one of these exploratory measures inflicts a traumatism of greater or less degree, and, as a result of their combined effects, the brain swells with amazing rapidity, so that within a few moments it protrudes so beyond the dura that it becomes a physical impossibility to replace it sufficiently to unite the edges of the dural wound. The actual cause of the swelling is no doubt the development of œdema. As pointed out by Cannon, who conducted a series of experiments in order to explain the secondary increase of intracranial pressure in head injuries, the swelling and pressure are wholly independent of any increase of blood pressure whatever, and are the result of certain chemical changes in the brain substance itself, whereby the osmotic pressure is so increased that the brain rapidly becomes œdematous.

The practical lessons to be learned from these observations are easily foreseen. In the first place, have we not in this rapid and consecutive œdema a sign that the tissue presenting in the opening is chiefly normal brain tissue, and that if there be a tumor present in the region exposed it is in all likelihood a very small one? Secondly, these observations should teach us the importance of carrying out the exploratory measures in an expeditious manner. To be sure, we should not proceed with undue haste, but once the dura is exposed the various methods of exploration should be carried out in a methodical and unhesitating manner. A definite plan of procedure should be outlined before the operation begins, the instruments for exploration should be at hand, and once the dura is reflected the operator should, without a moment's delay, proceed with his investigation, and in the following order: 1. A careful inspection of the exposed cortex, noting whether pulsation is visible, whether the brain is of normal color, and noting the condition of the bloodvessels. Inspection should precede all the other forms of examination because soon after exposure of the brain to the traumatism inflicted by the examining finger the brain begins to bulge. The operator should palpate, gently of course, the cortex, both the part exposed and, if nothing abnormal be found there, the parts immediately surrounding. By palpation one can discover variations in consistency and in tension. V. Bergmann recommends in those cases in which the tumor cannot be felt that the patient be raised to a sitting posture, "whereupon the tumor may become visible or palpable, the area exposed sinking in somewhat from the atmospheric pressure in connection with the lessened blood pressure."[1] 2. If by palpation one discovers an in-

[1] Woolsey. The American Journal of the Medical Sciences, December, 1903.

crease in the consistency, and inspection fails to reveal a growth involving the cortex, an incision of from 1 to 3 cm. should be made in the direction of the suspected lesion. The importance of making more than a nick in the surface of the brain needs no explanation. In Case III., although the tumor would not have been removed at the first operation, it was not discovered, simply because the incision was not deep enough to expose it. 3. Failing to reveal the lesion, an exploratory needle, constructed especially for this purpose, should be introduced in two or three directions, but always through the same opening. The instrument best adapted to this purpose is a small cannula armed with a blunt obturator. The instrument should be introduced to the maximum depth, the obturator removed, and the instrument gradually withdrawn. The ordinary exploratory needle is useless, because upon its introduction the orifice becomes plugged with cerebral tissue, and the communication between a cyst or an abscess is thereby cut off.

Given a case in which the brain has bulged to a very considerable degree, how should this complication be treated? Three courses are open to the operator: the first to attempt to restore the brain to its normal confines and to close the dural wound; the second, to disregard absolutely the dura and to terminate the operation by closing the wound in the scalp; and the third, to make no attempt to replace the brain, but to repair the defect between the dural edges with a graft dissected from the pericranium. The adoption of one or the other of these three courses should depend upon existing conditions.

For purposes of illustration, imagine a case in which the tumor has not been found and in which there is an element of uncertainty in the diagnosis as to the existence of tumor. Under these conditions, if the dural edges cannot be approximated without such pressure upon the bulging brain as would lead inevitably to an undesirable amount of laceration of the brain substance, such a plan as that suggested by Keen should be carried out, namely, to dissect from the pericranium a graft large enough to fill the gap between the edges of the dura. This plan was adopted in Case IV. of this series. A diagnosis of tumor of the brain had been made, but instead of a tumor a tubercular meningitis almost confined to the parietal lobe was found. Shortly after the dura was reflected and the field explored the brain began to bulge in an amazingly and alarmingly rapid manner; to have attempted to suture the dura without removing a large section of the brain would have been a physical impossibility, and, inasmuch as there was no indication for the relief of pressure, the gap in the wound was closed in the manner as above described. As illustrating another phase of the question, picture a case in which a tumor was undoubtedly present, but had been localized inaccurately —a case in which headache was one of the conspicuous and most distressing symptoms. A radical operation in such a case is, for the time being at least, out of the question; but we have every reason to believe that in relieving pressure the patient will enjoy a temporary period of relief. If, then, the indication is clearly to relieve pressure, it would be the height of folly to attempt to sew up the dura, as by so doing the intracranial pressure would be as great as it was before the operation. Under these circumstances the dura should be disregarded absolutely, the bone of the flap should be removed, and the wound in the scalp closed with great precision.

Palliative Operation. In every operator's experience there will be a certain number of cases which for one reason or another are not suitable for the radical operation, either because the tumor is inaccessible, or because it may be too large, or because accurate localization is impossible. Under any of these circumstances when the patient is suffering, evidently from the effects of increased intracranial tension—*e. g.*, headache, or choked disk—the palliative operation should be performed. I say "should be" because I believe an operation under these circumstances is more than a question of propriety; it should be regarded as imperative. Were it not for the headache the patient might enjoy for the rest of his days freedom from pain, if pressure is relieved. I have under my care now a patient that was referred to me by Dr. Hermance and Dr. Spiller, a patient who has unquestionably a tumor, but no symptoms sufficiently pronounced to make localization possible. He suffered from attacks of such violent headache that his reason became impaired; his suffering was intense and only to be compared with that attending the paroxysms of tic douloureux. Opiates did not relieve him. A section of bone was removed from the skull, and with but two exceptions, when the attacks were not severe and of very short duration, he has enjoyed absolute relief from pain, and is as contented and placid as one could be under the circumstances. The same gratifying effects may be obtained in cases of choked disk. When this condition has not existed so long as to have caused atrophy of the optic nerve an early operation for the relief of pressure will be followed by marked subsidence of or disappearance of the choked disk and by a corresponding improvement of vision. We are thus enabled to restore to a greater or less degree the patient's vision for the remainder of his life. In a case recently operated upon the effect of craniotomy and consequent relief of pressure was very strikingly illustrated. The choked disk, which was present to a very marked degree, subsided at least one-half within three weeks of the date of the operation. Unfortunately in this case the operation was not performed soon enough to save the patient's vision, as very marked atrophy of the optic nerve had already occurred. For the relief of these two conditions, namely, headache and impairment of vision, I lay stress upon the importance of the palliative operation. In performing this operation a section of bone representing about three square inches should be removed and a dural flap fashioned and reflected, and the wound in the scalp closed. This will afford the desired relief of tension.

RESULTS. As to the more recent statistics upon the results of surgical intervention for cerebral tumor, Woolsey[1] has collected 101 cases of cerebral tumors which have been operated upon during the past five years. Of this series he says: "Twelve cases, 11.8 per cent., died within twenty-four hours, and twenty-six, or 25.7 per cent., within three weeks." Here at once we see a very marked reduction in the immediate mortality. Von Bergmann regards 25 per cent. as a very conservative estimate of the number dying as the direct result of the operation. Of the eighty-eight cases of Woolsey's series, of which an exact localization was made, the mortality was but 22.7 per cent., as against 46 per cent. among those not exactly localized. In Gussenbauer's series of twelve cases there was but one death, and that due to pneumonia. "As to the more remote results, six died within three weeks and three months; nine between three months and one year, and three between one year and two years. As almost all of these died from the effect of the tumor the mortality within two years is 43.5 per cent." This high mortality, both immediate and remote, Woolsey says is not greater than that following radical operations for malignant growths in some other situations, and that considering "the otherwise hopeless condition of these cases, the difficulties of exact diagnosis, the inaccessibility of the tumors, and the marked relief of symptoms in almost all cases not dying at once, we may take courage and feel some degree of satisfaction." Woolsey says "that we should feel still more encouraged when we consider the length of time during which some cases remain free of recurrences. Cases of sarcoma are reported four years, four years and one month, five and one-half years, and eleven years after operation. A case of fibroma was reported well eight years, cases of gummata two and one-half years, a case of glioma three and one-half years, and one case, in which the variety of tumor was not given, nine years after the operation. Seven cases of sarcomata are reported to have recurred at periods ranging from three months to eleven years, and averaging two years and four months, or, exclusive of the latter case, nine and one-third months."

It is needless to say that the prognosis in the case of benign tumors and cysts and in cases of well-encapsulated sarcomata is much better than in operations when the growths are of malignant and infiltrating type.

RESUME. 1. All measures recognized as prophylactic of shock should be observed stringently. In these we have the most effectual means of reducing the mortality. The most important of them are (*a*) the avoidance of prolonged operation; (*b*) the prevention of excessive hemorrhage, and (*c*) the avoidance of unnecessarily rough manipulation of the brain substance.

2. A given area of brain can be exposed with the least minimum degree of traumatism and greatest economy of time by the electric engine.

3. Temporary closure of the carotids in operations upon the brain is ineffectual and not unattended by danger. It should be reserved for extreme cases, and practised on one side only.

4. Observations should be made upon the blood pressure immediately before and at frequent intervals during the operation. Object of same twofold: (*a*) as the most reliable index of patient's condition; (*b*) as the only exact method of determining whether operation should or should not be carried out in two stages.

5. Two-stage operation is indicated when there has been a decided fall in blood pressure after the relief from intracranial tension, such as follows reflection of the Wagner flap and dura.

6. Lumbar puncture as a means of relieving pressure is a temporary, not to say dangerous, procedure.

7. Bulging of the brain is one of the most embarrassing features of cerebral operations. A distinction may be made between that which occurs immediately after reflecting the dura, "initial" bulging, and that which follows as a result of subsequent exploratory manipulation, "consecutive" bulging.

8. "Initial" bulging is due to the increased tension exerted by a tumor. It is not always present, is often not excessive, and is not likely to be followed by "consecutive" bulging.

9. "Consecutive" bulging is due to the cerebral œdema set up in normal brain tissue by trauma inflicted by the exploratory manipulations. "Consecutive" bulging far exceeds in magnitude initial bulging, and suggests the absence of a tumor of considerable size at the seat of operation.

10. In order to avoid this "consecutive" bulging, which is a most embarrassing feature of these operations, exploration should be carried out in the most expeditious manner.

11. When the edges of the dural wound cannot be approximated without undue tension or without great laceration of brain substance, the gap should be closed by a graft taken from the pericranium, providing the tumor has not been found and there is reason to question the accuracy of the diagnosis.

12. When there is every assurance of a tumor being present, but it proves to be inoperable or was imperfectly localized, no attempt should be made to close the dura, as in so doing the best possible palliative effects of the operation would be counteracted.

13. Palliative operations should be regarded not merely as operations of propriety, but should be considered imperative whenever the tumor cannot be found or cannot be removed.

14. A statistical study of the results of the last five years is encouraging. The mortality, both immediate and subsequent, has been reduced materially. Recurrence after operations for malignant growths of the brain is no greater than after operations for malignant growth of other structures.

Resume of the Operative Records.[1]

Case II.—*G. K.; operation May 2, 1903; osteoplastic resection of the skull; exposure and removal of cortical sarcoma; recovery from immediate effects of operation; marked improvement in patient's condition during a period of several weeks; return of the growth, with fatal termination.*

Upon reflection of the osteoplastic flap and dura an area was exposed to view which, to the touch and sight, was unquestionably pathological, and proved to be the tumor. Before proceeding to remove the tumor, consideration was taken of the patient's condition, and more particularly of his circulation. If from the effect of the preliminary procedures the patient's circulation had been depressed, further manipulation would have been postponed for twenty-four to forty-eight hours, or until the circulation was re-established. In the absence of any alarming evidence of depression, the operation was continued and the tumor removed. There were no technical difficulties nor hemorrhage attending this step of the operation.

The tumor was not situated in the centre of the area which was exposed, but quite near the margin of the opening, so that if the opening in the skull had been a small one it is quite possible that the tumor might have escaped the eye of the operator.

At the end of the operation the patient's temperature was 96° F., his pulse 92, and his respirations 28. The patient reacted quite promptly, and at no time did we entertain doubt as to his recovery from the immediate effects of the operation. On the evening of the operation there was complete paralysis of the right arm and leg, and aphasia; but the following morning the function of both limbs was partially restored and the patient could speak, but very indistinctly. On the fifth day a very decided improvement was observed, both in the size of his vocabulary and in the rapidity with which he could give expression to his thoughts. Generally speaking, there was a decided improvement over his condition before the operation. The headache of which he had complained so bitterly was almost entirely relieved. Occasionally he complained of a soreness in his head, but the constant distressing headache so characteristic of brain tumor had disappeared. Two weeks after the operation he left his bed, and would have been discharged from the hospital had it not been thought desirable to keep him under observation for a longer period.

Case III.—*Thomas S., aged forty-seven years; operation June 5, 1903; osteoplastic resection of the skull; subcortical tumor below the surface of the brain within the white matter; not found because of its deep situation within the substance of the brain; operative recovery; death thirty-four days after the operation.*

After preliminary closure of the carotids the osteoplastic flap and

[1] Editorial Note.—The clinical histories of these cases appear in full in the article by Dr. Spiller in this number of the Journal.

its dura were reflected and the brain exposed. When the dura was divided the brain did not protrude, as it so often does. Its surface was inspected and several gross lesions were noted in the field exposed. These lesions were quite superficial and were not sufficiently intense to explain the symptoms. Several incisions were made into the cortex of the brain about a centimetre in depth, with a view toward exposing a subcortical growth, but the incisions were not deep enough to have revealed the tumor which was discovered at the autopsy. The flaps were replaced and the wound closed. In this, as in the former case, the patient reacted promptly from the operation, and after a slight febrile reaction, running over a period of eight days, the temperature returned to normal. During the convalescent period the patient had some convulsions, Jacksonian in type, and his left upper limb became almost completely paralyzed. He was, however, almost entirely relieved of the headache from which he had been suffering. He was transferred to Dr. Spiller's ward three weeks after the operation.

CASE IV.—*F. F.; operation June* 23, 1903; *osteoplastic resection of the skull; exposure of multiple tubercular tumors (meningitis en plaque) of the parietal lobe; removal of growths impossible.*

Several observations upon the blood pressure were made prior to the operation, and, as is now my practice, these observations were continued at intervals of not less than five minutes throughout the operation. Anticipatory of hemorrhage, both common carotids were closed temporarily. A horseshoe-shaped flap composed of the scalp was fashioned with the knife of the Stellwagen instrument and the bony flap with the drill and dental engine. Upon attempting to reflect the dura numerous adhesions were discovered between it and the cortex, but these were separated without much difficulty. Upon reflection of the dura numerous lesions, some isolated, some confluent, were revealed distributed over the entire area of the cortex which had been exposed to view. Upon introducing my index finger between the dura and exploring the cortex in all directions, I discovered more adhesions. The discovery of the latter was sufficient to warrant the assumption that the process was too diffuse and of such a nature as to render it positively inoperable. Although the manipulations had up to this time been neither prolonged nor of such a character as to inflict serious traumatism upon the cerebral tissue, yet the brain had bulged to such an extent that it became quite evident that I would not be able to bring the edges of the dura into apposition. In order to guard against the development of a hernia or a fungus cerebri, a section of pericranium was removed of a size sufficient to fill in the gap in the dural wound. Within a few minutes of the time the brain was exposed, although nothing more than a careful inspection and exploration with the finger had been resorted to, the circulation began to fail, becoming more and more depressed until the termination of the operation, when the pulse was weak and the blood pressure alarmingly low (75). His condition for the first forty-eight hours was critical, but in the third day improved to such an extent that I began to feel more hopeful of his recovery from the operation. This reaction was only temporary, however, as œdema of the lungs rapidly developed, and on the fourth day after the operation the patient died.

CASE V.—*W. C. H.; tumor of right cerebellar lobe at its union with the pons; operation July 23, 1903; craniotomy of the cerebellar fossa; second stage of operation (opening of dura and exploration for tumor) postponed because of patient's serious condition.*

Realizing the difficulty with which all the surfaces of the cerebellum are exposed through a small unilateral opening and anticipating very free hemorrhage, not only from the scalp but from the diploic sinuses, I decided before the operation to secure a better opportunity to examine the suspected hemisphere by making a very liberal opening in the skull, one extending from one side to the other, and to control at least some of the hemorrhage by preliminary but temporary closure of the carotids. Proceeding along these lines, after the Crile clamps had been applied to the carotids I fashioned a horseshoe-shaped flap by making an incision from one mastoid process to another parallel to and 1 cm. above the superior curved line. After clamping the bleeding points in the flap, an opening in the skull was made with chisel and mallet 2 cm. below and 2 cm. from the median line. This opening was enlarged with the rongeur forceps equally in all directions until it extended above to the superior curved line and almost to the median line. A similar opening was made in the opposite side. By means of a Gigli saw the intervening bridge of bone was divided above and below and removed. With this the first stage of the operation was completed. The patient's condition at this time was such as to make it unwise to proceed to search for the tumor. From the beginning of the operation there was some evidence of impairment of the respiratory or circulatory function, perhaps both. This may or may not have been due to the anæsthesia (ether), to the loss of blood, to the fact that the position of the patient may have embarrassed respiration. At all events, he was more or less cyanosed throughout, and when the first stage of the operation was completed his pulse was very rapid (170 to 180), although his blood pressure was high (158). Immediately after his recovery from ether it was noted that he was hemiplegic. During the night his respirations were of the Cheyne-Stokes type, and there were some twitchings of the left side of the face. On the following morning, at 9 o'clock, his pulse reached its lowest rate (120), but from that time on until the patient's death, thirteen hours later, the pulse and temperature began to rise. The last registration was: pulse, 180; respiration, 24; temperature, 103.8° F.; blood pressure, 90.

REVIEWS.

Diseases of the Skin: Their Description, Pathology, Diagnosis, and Treatment, with Special Reference to the Skin Eruptions of Children, and an Analysis of Fifteen Thousand Cases of Skin Disease. By H. Radcliffe-Crocker, M.D. (Lond.), F.R.C.P., Physician for Diseases of the Skin in University College Hospital; Honorary Member of the American Dermatological Society; Membre Correspondant Etranger de la Société Francaise de Dermatologie, etc. Third Edition, revised and enlarged, with 4 plates and 112 illustrations. Philadelphia: P. Blakiston's Son & Co., 1903.

This new edition of Dr. Crocker's well-known work on *Diseases of the Skin* is a ponderous volume of almost 1500 pages, one-half larger than the previous one, convincing evidence of the author's industry and of the great activity prevailing in this particular field of medical research. Marks of careful and judicious revision are visible in every part of the book, which has been thoroughly brought up to date. Many new articles have been added, among the most important of which are those upon *x*-ray Dermatitis, Toxin Serum Eruptions, Porokeratosis, Sarcoid, Leukæmia and Pseudoleukæmia Cutis, Endothelioma Capitis, Hydrocystoma, Acne Necrotisans, Folliculitis Decalvans, and Blastomycosis Hominis. The excellent plan of putting in small type matters of minor importance has been followed in this, as in former editions.

After giving a definition of eczema, the author proceeds to make clear what forms of inflammation of the skin he includes under this term, a quite necessary step, owing to the increasing confusion among recent writers as to just what is meant by eczema. He excludes all forms of seborrhœic dermatitis as well as those due to strong irritants, but he also calls attention to the fact that certain substances which are commonly innocuous may, in certain individuals, produce a dermatitis indistinguishable from eczema, and for this and other reasons it is best to consider such inflammations among the forms of eczema. In the treatment of this oftentimes very obstinate disease turpentine internally, in 10-minim doses, is recommended as very beneficial in uncomplicated cases, care being taken to accompany it with large quantities of some diluent to avoid irritation of the genito-urinary tract. In those cases characterized by frequent exacerbations counterirritation over the nape of the neck or in the lumbar region, in the shape of dry heat or mustard plasters, has been found extremely serviceable by the author in promptly relieving the itching.

In recent years the view that lupus erythematosus should be ranged among the diseases due, directly or indirectly, to tuberculosis has been gaining ground; but Crocker is not at all inclined to accept this view. He believes the affection is "primarily a vasomotor disturbance leading to an inflammation of the skin, perhaps of toxic but not of tuberculotoxic origin, especially predisposed to by a feeble blood current," with secondary microbic invasion.

Unna's view that psoriasis is but a part of the seborrhœic process obtains no support from the author, who believes it is most probably due to a microparasite which finds a suitable soil only in certain individuals. This organism probably at first attacks the skin; but its rapid spread and wide distribution are best explained by supposing that it penetrates the circulation later, and is distributed by the blood current.

The colored plates representing the principal syphilides which have been added to this edition will afford but indifferent aid in diagnosis, since they are anything but accurate representations of the lesions they are supposed to depict.

The enviable position which this treatise at once assumed upon its first appearance is easily maintained by this edition, and the student, the general practitioner, and the specialist will find it an accurate and complete presentation of the subject of dermatology, useful alike as a text-book and as a work of reference. M. B. H.

Nurses' Guide to Surgical Bandaging and Dressings. By William Johnson Smith, F.R.C.S., Principal Medical Officer, Seaman's Hospital, Greenwich. Philadelphia: J. B. Lippincott Co. London: The Scientific Press, Limited.

This is a good book badly named—one that any nurse can read with advantage. It is an excellent, handy pocket manual on surgical nursing with a title in part too modest, yet otherwise misleading. It is not with bandaging that the greater number of these pages deal, but, adapted to the needs of nurses, they contain a concise, plain, and sufficient statement of the pathology and treatment of wounds, ulcers, burns, infection, and sepsis; also of the principles and comprehensively of the practice of asepsis, antisepsis, and of special surgical nursing, and a useful chapter on splints. Of all this the cover fails to hint.

A subordinate part of the book, a couple of chapters on bandaging, through being alone honored in the title, unjustly forces comparison with works devoted solely to this topic, notably an ideal one by an American author and from the press of the same publisher. Judged by this standard, it cannot escape harsh criticism on the score not only of incompleteness, but of insufficient illustration of the bandages described.

Had the title of this attractive little book indicated that it was a manual on surgical nursing and dressings with hints on bandaging, it would not challenge criticism, but invite praise and more than honor the promise of its back. J. M. S.

HYPERÆMIA AS A THERAPEUTIC MEASURE (HYPERAMIE ALS HEILMITTEL). By PROF. AUGUST BIER, of Greifswald. Leipzig: F. W. C. Vogel, 1903.

PROFESSOR BIER has been animated by two facts in his endeavors to gain for hyperæmia a permanent place in therapeutics—that hyperæmia is one of nature's great remedial agents, for it is a well-established observation that every diseased process which the body itself attempts to cure immediately becomes surrounded by an area of hyperæmia; and that physicians should be under obligations to imitate those natural processes by which the organism is constantly combating the inroads of disease.

He divides his book into two parts. In the first he discusses active or arterial hyperæmia, and passive or venous hyperæmia, and also the methods for the practical application of these. Hot air and vacuum apparatus, the constricting bandage, and dry cupping are described, and in a separate chapter the physiological action of dermal irritants is fully discussed. Another chapter is devoted to the description of the analgesic, bactericidal, absorbent, dissolving, and nutrient actions of hyperæmia. The second division of the book is taken up with the consideration of the methods and results of the treatment of various diseases by means of induced hyperæmia. Tuberculosis of the joints is first discussed. Here passive hyperæmia only can be employed, as the more pronounced active form can effect great harm. Bier recommends the procedure perfected by Tillmann, which consists of applying a constricting bandage for one hour daily sufficiently tight to induce a well-marked passive hyperæmia. There should be no pain from this, and the appearance of red blotches on the skin must be avoided. It is not necessary to bandage the parts on the peripheral side of the elastic bandage, nor is it essential to apply the constricting band immediately above the diseased joint. Thus in tuberculosis of the joints of the hands or feet the elastic bandage may be readily applied on the upper arm or the thigh. Cold abscesses should be evacuated through a small incision and the compression commenced two or three days later. If abscess formation comes on during treatment, an incision is likewise made and the treatment interrupted for a few days. The fistulous tracts close quite readily and Bier has also observed the expulsion of bone sequestra during the time of treatment. Permanent fixation as a routine is not recommended, but, on the contrary, active and passive movements are begun as soon as possible. In this way Bier was able to cure cases of joint tuberculosis which experienced surgeons had designated for primary amputation.

The author of the book believes that this is the most conservative method in the treatment of joint tuberculosis, which is followed by good results without the slightest danger, and with which the function of diseased joints can be restored in a manner superior to all other conservative procedures. The method is, however, not infallible, and the condition of the patient's blood undoubtedly plays an important rôle in the success of the process.

The acute gonorrhœal inflammations have also been most favorably influenced by passive hyperæmia. Here it is necessary to apply the elastic bandage for somewhat longer periods, at least ten to twelve hours daily. The analgesic effects are particularly well marked; it is possible to move joints both actively and passively after the bandage has been in place for a short time, in which motion had previously caused most acute pain, and the wished-for sleep soon follows. In some cases the method failed, but fortunately the best results were secured in the worst cases. Bier also treated with excellent outcome instances of acute articular rheumatism and also certain inflammations of the soft parts, such as erysipelas and some varieties of phlegmonous processes, but in the latter case the author advises caution and abandons the method unless an immediate result is achieved.

Active and passive hyperæmia are both of undoubted value in the treatment of chronic articular inflammations and their consequences. In these cases the vacuum apparatus accomplishes good results. The general procedure is as follows: application of hot air daily for one hour, use of the vacuum apparatus once or twice daily for twenty to thirty minutes at a time, compression with the elastic bandage for eight to twelve hours a day, and massage and elevation of the limb during the interim.

Treatment with hot air, because of the absorption induced by the hyperæmia, has a favorable effect in removing the œdema which often results after the healing of fractures. It was also used with gratifying results in a case of elephantiasis of the leg. Mention must also be made of the fact that neuralgic pains are benefited by active hyperæmia, and headaches, especially those accompanying an anæmia, by passive hyperæmia produced by the application of a rubber bandage around the neck.

The book is the result of most careful observation and is based on the author's personal experiences in over one thousand cases of various diseases where positive and favorable effects were obtained by this method of treatment. In this country but few physicians have made such extensive trials of these measures, and the good results obtained by Professor Bier with this method should animate others to make further experiments and to add their knowledge gained to this interesting department of therapeutics. S. E. J.

HIGH-FREQUENCY CURRENTS IN THE TREATMENT OF SOME DISEASES. By CHISHOLM WILLIAMS, F.R.C.S. EDIN., etc. London: Rebman, Limited, 1903.

IN this work the author offers "a short account of the treatment of some diseases by means of electric currents of high frequency and high potential." The main source of the account is given as from the author's own practice, supplemented by selections from "diverse journals not readily accessible to the busy practitioner." His experience with the therapeutic use of these currents dates from 1898, and in his introduction he at once arouses interest by stating that high-frequency currents "have been proved to produce extraordinary and peculiar results in the alleviation of some diseased conditions."

Certainly the uniformly excellent results secured by him in "atonic dilatation of the stomach—results far in advance of those obtainable in the same length of time by any other therapeutic agent—stir up hope that here is a form of treatment worthy of extended trial. The scope of the work includes a discussion of the different "sources of energy," of various apparatus, of the properties of the currents from physical and physiological standpoints, and lastly a consideration of therapeutic methods.

While we agree with the statement that a "certain amount of elementary electric knowledge is necessary," we cannot recommend the "elementary electrophysics" which the author gives as being either accurate or useful. The following archaic view of what takes place in a primary battery when the external circuit is closed will serve as an illustration: After describing a cell in which plates of copper and zinc are immersed in dilute sulphuric acid, he goes on to state, "When the electricity generated is allowed to circulate externally by joining the plates one notices that on each plate gas bubbles are formed from the electrolytic decomposition of the water, hydrogen and oxygen being liberated, and these bubbles interfere more or less with the chemical activity between the liquid and the metals, so that the E. M. F. and with it the tension tend to rapidly decrease; this action is termed polarization."

Now, the oxygen and hydrogen gases set free at the electrodes are obtained as the result of a secondary action in the dilute sulphuric acid (the electrolyte): in this, while the hydrogen is set free at the kathode, the negative ions of SO_4 decompose the water at the anode and combine with its hydrogen to form hydrogen sulphate and set the oxygen free; the term polarization refers to the production in the cell of an electromotive force counter to the normal one.

Under the head of Sources of Energy are discussed primary and secondary batteries, commercial electric mains, and static machines. The author's description of a static machine is not applicable to the associated cut on page 42, which is directly referred to. The machine is stated to "produce electricity by friction," whereas it is really generated by induction, the difference of potential existing between the disks at rest being increased by rotation.

In the chapter devoted to the description of apparatus the "elementary electrophysics" is of a nature to arouse interest. We quote as a sample from page 105: "Most of us have seen the experiment of two tuning forks tuned to the same pitch giving the same harmonic. If one be vibrated by a blow or by the fingers the second fork will start vibrating by itself and give off the same harmonic; because it is syntonous or vibrating in unison with the former, it will reinforce the sound given by the first vibrator." Now, the tone of the tuning fork is a practically simple one—*i. e.*, a fundamental one—the overtones being inappreciable, and therefore the term harmonic is inaccurate; the second tuning fork *responds* to the tone of the first; it does not reinforce. This is based on the well-known principle of sympathetic vibrations.

The book will prove of interest to electrotherapeutists for the reason that it gives the opinions of a man of considerable practical experience as to the selection and use of the apparatus essential in the production of high-frequency currents. H. M. W.

A Text-book of Diseases of Women. By Barton Cooke Hirst, M.D., Professor of Obstetrics in the University of Pennsylvania; Gynecologist to the Howard, the Orthopedic, and the Philadelphia Hospitals. Pp. 683, with 655 illustrations, many of them in colors. Philadelphia, New York, and London: W. B. Saunders & Co., 1903.

Dr. Hirst has been a consistent advocate of the opinion entertained in Germany that obstetric and gynecic surgery should always be combined. The present work, he announces in the preface, is "a companion volume to the author's *Text-book of Obstetrics*; the two volumes covering the whole subject of gynecology." Knowing as we do his unusual experience in both branches, as well as his high reputation as a teacher and indefatigable worker, we are prepared to find his latest work a valuable addition to the literature.

The section on diseases and injuries of the vagina, includes nearly seventy pages, with no less than sixty cuts, nearly all original. We note several pages on the treatment of gonorrhœa and an excellent description of the manner in which the pelvic floor is lacerated during labor. The author rightly believes that only by understanding how the injury occurs can one recognize afterward the exact nature of the lesion and the indications for operation. The detailed description of complete laceration, admirably illustrated, deserves careful study. The writer's conservatism is indicated by his adherence to the use of pessaries for cystocele. His operation for the cure of this condition is certainly an advance on the usual oval and circular methods of denudations. As he rightly says, Martin's operation "does not unite the torn muscles which should support the lower anterior vaginal wall and the urethra, and therefore it is not always permanently successful."

The writer prefers Emmet's operation for the repair of laceration of the pelvic floor, which is thoroughly described and fairly well figured. He uses silkworm-gut in all his plastic work, his experience with chromicized catgut being less satisfactory than that of most operators. We must take exception to some of the illustrations (especially Figs. 196–198), which are more intelligible to the expert than to the tyro.

Injuries of the cervix are profusely illustrated, unnecessarily so, the critical reader may think. We are thoroughly in accord with the statement that "whenever one is in doubt as to the suitable form of operation, it is better to decide on an amputation." Figs. 228 and 229 do not bring out with sufficient clearness the depth and extent of the denudation. Silkworm-gut is preferred for trachelorrhaphy, a conservative practice which is opposed to that of most gynecologists, who obtain equally good results with chromic gut, while the patient is spared the pain and annoyance consequent upon the removal of sutures while the perineal wound is still weak and sensitive.

The section on carcinoma is excellent. There seems to be no good reason for confusing the student by adding "malignant adenoma" as a separate variety. The paragraphs on symptomatology and diagnosis are clear and concise. Some of the illustrations, though excellent in themselves, might be dispensed with.

In common with recent views, the author prefers abdominal to vaginal extirpation, or rather the combined method, although from his description it is not clear what advantages he gains, since he does not advocate routine removal of the lymph-nodes. His lucid descriptions of surgical operations are well exemplified in the pages devoted to the technique of hysterectomy.

His conclusions with regard to prognosis after operations are fair and conservative, his immediate mortality after vaginal and combined hysterectomies being 7 per cent., while four of his patients were known to be alive at the end of five years.

We are glad to note that the author still believes in the non-surgical treatment of uncomplicated retrodisplacement, and does not reject the use of tampons in adherent retroflexion. In this he is, as ever, a safe guide to the student, who is only too apt to infer that so-called medical gynecology is a thing of the past. The descriptions of the use of pessaries and of Alexander's operation (he prefers Edebohls' method) are especially good. He seems to have had better results from plastic operations alone, with accompanying ventrosuspension, than have most of his confrères. He does not favor the recent vaginal operations of Wertheim, Freund, and others.

The section on fibromyomata and operations for their removal is ample and is beautifully illustrated. The same applies to the sections on endometritis and malignant disease of the endometrium. One is rather surprised to miss any reference to deciduoma malignum. The Fallopian tubes form the subject of Part VIII. Here, again, some of the cuts are superfluous. One characteristic illustration of each of the diseased conditions would be sufficient. The paragraph on the preventive treatment of tubal disease (pages 415–416) ought to be read by every layman, as well as physician. The author rightly believes that the palliative treatment of salpingitis should receive a fair trial before resort is had to an operation.

The section on extrauterine pregnancy is, as will be inferred from the writer's wide experience, up to date. The criticism might be offered that too little stress is laid upon the difficulties of diagnosis in many cases, as every gynecologist has experienced in his own practice. Explorative vaginal section deserves mention. The author is apparently one of the few operators who still use the old-fashioned glass drainage-tube. He states that he now rarely irrigates the abdominal cavity except to remove blood-clots after operations for ectopic gestation. The description of the operation for intraperitoneal rupture (page 441) is a model of terse writing.

Part IX., on diseases of the ovaries, leaves little to be desired. The cuts are many and original and the technique of ovariotomy most satisfactory.

Upward of fifty pages are assigned to diseases of the urinary tract, cystoscopy and catheterization of the ureters being carefully described. Ten are devoted to floating kidney, an innovation in a work on diseases of women, doubtless in deference to the especial interest which gynecologists have taken in this subject, much to the distaste of the general surgeon. We are pleased to note that the author does not subscribe to the indiscriminate practice of performing nephropexy on slight indications, since he found it necessary to operate in only 5 out of 200 cases.

The excellent concluding chapter on the technique of gynecic surgery in quite a model in its way, the lucid descriptions being illustrated by over 100 figures. Nothing has been omitted to furnish a safe and trustworthy guide to the beginner. It serves as a true index of the careful, conscientious work which distinguishes the author.

We have been unable in this brief review to do justice to this the latest work on gynecology. Our object has been rather to stimulate the reader to make a careful study of it for himself. While a critical reviewer might take exception to some minor defects, we are so impressed with the honest conservative tone maintained throughout, and with the fact that it is based entirely upon the personal experience and convictions of the writer, that we have only commendation for this fresh product of his wonderful industry. We have already called attention to the number and beauty of the illustrations, and to the clear, common-sense manner in which each subject is treated. While we are not prepared to admit that the present book is equal to the companion *Text-book of Obstetrics*, the fourth edition of which appears simultaneously with it, we have no doubt that it will achieve the same widespread popularity, which is all that the most ambitious author could desire. H. C. C.

GYNECOLOGY. A TEXT-BOOK FOR STUDENTS AND A GUIDE FOR PRACTITIONERS. By WILLIAM R. PRYOR, M.D., Professor of Gynecology in the New York Polyclinic Medical School; Attending Gynecologist to the New York Polyclinic Hospital; Consulting Gynecologist to St. Vincent's Hospital, New York City Hospital. Pp. xvi., 380, with one hundred and sixty-three illustrations. New York and London: D. Appleton & Co., 1903.

THE preface of this excellent book indicates clearly its purpose, which is to present the subject in such a practical, dogmatic way as "a professor of gynecology in any of the colleges has to lecture." Rare diseases, bacteriology and minute anatomy, and "matters which strictly belong to other branches of medicine" are accordingly omitted.

We have not been disappointed in our favorable anticipations. Dr. Pryor has not only succeeded in writing a readable book, but one which in many respects is in a class by itself. At the outset we note with approval its division into two parts, the first, including nine chapters, being devoted to diseases and non-surgical treatment; the second to descriptions of the various gynecological operations.

In the introductory chapter on examination of the patient there are several useful practical hints with regard to the proper practice of the bimanual, important points being emphasized in large type. The illustrations are few, but satisfactory, unless we except the cut showing Trendelenburg's position, in which the elevation is extreme, at least for most American operators. The writer still prefers Sims' position for examination and minor operations.

With Chapter II. (pages 14 to 68) we are introduced at once to the subject of inflammation, beginning with vulvitis and concluding with oöphoritis. The important subject of gonorrhœal infection receives especial attention, in quite sharp contrast to the superficial way in which it is treated in most text-books. If space permitted we would like to quote several of the italicized sentences. The pages on gonorrhœal and septic endometritis deserve careful study, since they contain an unusual amount of information condensed within a small compass.

The much-vexed subject of metritis is disposed of with less verbiage and clearer insight than is the case with most writers, for which students will feel devoutly thankful, however one may differ from the author's radical views. Peritonitis receives careful attention, twelve pages being devoted to it. With the conclusion that "peritonitis is an exponent of an infectious process rather than a disease *per se*," few, if any, will dissent.

Salpingitis (another subject which has been rendered unnecessarily complicated to the student) is happily elucidated. We note in passing one of the many dogmatic statements in large type which often arrest the reader's attention and present in a few words the gist of the treatment of pyosalpinx, viz., "Suppuration in a preformed sac is cured either by removal of the sac or by its obliteration."

The concluding section on inflammations of the ovaries is another example of the process of condensation, which may not always suit the pathologist, but certainly will relieve the student's perplexity. Here again the writer shows that he holds decided views and is not afraid to express them. Referring to ovarian sclerosis (a better term, by the way, than the common "cirrhosis"), he affirms that "as the symptoms produced by such a condition are so little understood, sclerosed ovaries should never be removed unless the uterus also needs to be sacrificed."

We agree heartily with the statements that "there is no standard of gross appearance to guide the surgeon in his operations upon the ovaries," and that "few symptoms are produced by ovarian inflammations which are not easily referable to associated diseases."

Chapter III., on "Distortions and Displacements," is on the whole quite satisfactory, although some of the statements may be questioned, notably this, that "the ligaments play no part in maintaining the uterus in position until their uterine attachments are rendered tense by displacement of the uterus." The author's views with regard to the treatment of anteflexion are well known. Those on retrodisplacement are sound. Believing, as he does, that "not so much the displacement as the accompanying or causative lesions produce the symptoms," he would naturally emphasize his opinion that "there is too great a tendency in the profession to perform operations for retrodisplacement without employing less severe methods first." This is sound teaching for the modern medical student, who is in danger of forgetting that gynecology is not synonymous with surgery.

Sections on laceration of the cervix and perineum seem rather out of place in this chapter. The writer assigns less importance to cervical tears than other authors, not regarding this lesion as the cause of sterility, abortion, or reflex nervous symptoms, while he admits that it is a direct etiological factor in the production of cancer. In common with most gynecological surgeons, he finds that amputation is indicated much more frequently than trachelorrhaphy.

Under Chapter IV., on Diseases of the Vulva, are included diseases of the vagina and cervix, a confusing arrangement, especially as the concluding subject under cervical conditions deals with vaginismus (?). Doubtless the author will see the propriety of a rearrangement of the subject-matter in a subsequent edition, or at least a change in the heading. The important subject of pruritus deserves a place here instead of the brief mention which it receives on page 17 under the section on Bartholinitis.

Genital fistulæ are well treated in Chapter V., though here again we note with surprise the appearance of a sub-heading on "Diseases of the Urethra and Bladder," with no less than eight pages on the ureters, a disproportionate amount of space, it would appear, in a work intended for students and practitioners, for whom the subject presents rather a scientific than a practical interest. The whole subject of diseases of the urinary tract is handled in a satisfactory manner, and we note with approval the author's original work in this field, with which the profession is already familiar.

Chapter VIII., on Cancer, is one of the best, especially the paragraphs on symptoms, which are expressed in a terse, dogmatic way well calculated to impress them upon the mind of the student. The writer thinks that the first symptom is "an increase in that leucorrhœa which the woman habitually has," bleeding being a subsequent indication. Contrary to usual observations, he does not find that menorrhagia is present. In referring to the examination of scrapings in suspected cancer of the body of the uterus he emphasizes the fact too often lost sight of, that "the positive evidence furnished by the curette and microscope is infallible, but the negative by no means shows that cancer does not exist."

With Chapter IX. we enter upon the second part of the book, where the author is entirely at home. Operations on the cervix are first considered, beginning with dilatation and curettage, and concluding with amputation. Perineorrhaphy receives careful attention. We note with some surprise that the author still uses silver wire, and does not move the bowels until the seventh day, which accounts for the statement that it may be necessary to break up hard fecal masses with a dull curette (!).

Contrary to the general opinion with regard to Pryor's radical methods, he is an advocate of conservative operations on the adnexa, while recognizing justly their limitations. The introductory paragraph under Chapter XV. represents a common-sense view of this much-discussed question. An interesting presentation of his opinions on vaginal section and drainage in acute salpingo-oöphoritis and acute pelvic peritonitis will be found on pages 279 and 280. The operation may strike the ordinary reader as revolutionary, but if the writer is right, "it is not only conservative, but is curative."

In Chapter XVII. there is a clear description of the author's radical operation for pelvic suppuration, with the details and remarkable results of which gynecologists are already familiar. The accompanying cuts are excellent. In the chapter on removal of the cancerous uterus the writer begins with the propositions that "no radical operation should be attempted unless the section of the tissues can pass outside the cancerous field," and that "the merits of an operation for the relief of this condition are determined by the ultimate results rather than by the immediate." He prefers the abdominal method of extirpation, since after vaginal extirpation 60 per cent. recur within the first year.

Chapter XIX. deals with various subjects, viz.: hernia, cystotomy operations during pregnancy, and a short section on the results of castration; Chapter XX. with hæmostasis, and the concluding chapter with the operative treatment of anomalies of the genitals. Following these is a "song without words," headed Chapter XXII., which includes five pages filled with cuts of instruments, without accompanying text.

We have reviewed in a most superficial way a work which deserves careful perusal if for no other reason than it is an honest book, written by an honest man. We may dissent from some of his views and may think that his tone is often too positive and dogmatic, but we cannot deny the virility and originality which characterize his exposition of them. Looked at from a critical standpoint we cannot regard the arrangement of the book as free from faults, since the sequence is often interrupted, and there is not that natural coherence which one looks for in a scientific work. But the book must obtain prompt and widespread recognition by reason of its intrinsic excellence. The style is condensed, but never to the point of obscurity. There is no padding and no borrowing from mediæval sources, but it is essentially an exponent of personal observation. There is no doubt that the circle of readers will be larger than the author modestly hopes, for he may be sure that it will "interest even those of large experience."

When we add that the drawings are mostly original and that they are reproduced with that beauty for which the well-known firm of publishers is famous, that the text, paper, and binding are of an equally high class order, we have added enough to convince the reader that he will find the volume a distinct addition to the already formidable list of gynecological text-books. H. C. C.

PROGRESS

OF

MEDICAL SCIENCE.

MEDICINE.

UNDER THE CHARGE OF

WILLIAM OSLER, M.D.,

PROFESSOR OF MEDICINE IN THE JOHNS HOPKINS UNIVERSITY, BALTIMORE, MARYLAND,

AND

W. S. THAYER, M.D.,

ASSOCIATE PROFESSOR OF MEDICINE IN JOHNS HOPKINS UNIVERSITY, BALTIMORE, MARYLAND.

A Case of Pentosuria.—ERNST BENDIX (*Münchener med. Wochenschrift*, September 8, 1903, No. 36) states that although almost a decade has passed since Salkowski first taught that pentosuria is a nutritional anomaly, *sui generis*, very few cases of this condition have hitherto been described. This probably proceeds from the fact that many cases are overlooked on account of lack of symptoms, while others, as a result of insufficient urine examination, are called diabetes mellitus. In preparing his monograph upon this subject Bendix found only about one dozen cases in the literature: three cases by Salkowski and Jastrowitz and Salkowski and Blumenthal, two cases from Bial, one from F. Meyer, two from Brat, one from F. Blumenthal, and three cases from the Italian literature by Luzzato Reale and Colombini, the two last-mentioned cases being doubtful. In addition, three cases of Caporalis are probably not true pentosuria, but cases of glycuronic acid, leaving in all twelve cases in the whole literature. The case reported was from the practice of Dr. Auerbach, in Cologne. The patient was a merchant, aged fifty-two years. Family history good. Neither disturbances of nutrition nor nervous disease among his relatives. His parents died at about the age of eighty years. He himself, from his eighteenth or nineteenth year, suffered with his stomach. Otherwise had never been very strong. Alcoholic and venereal history were negative. About one and a half years ago he suffered severely from influenza, with subsequent stomatitis. Convalescence was very tedious, and the patient lost much weight. At this time it was first ascertained that there was albumin in the urine and that Fehling's solution was also reduced. Since the fermentation test was negative and the urine optically inactive, the reduction of

Fehling's solution was not attributed to the presence of grape-sugar. Bendix was fortunate enough at this time to find that the reducing substance was pentose. The patient was living on a mixed diet. His general nutrition was excellent. The organs of the chest were essentially normal. There was no polyphagia nor polyuria. The patient had never used alkaloids, such as morphine and cocaine. The urine had been repeatedly examined by Bendix and always showed an acid reaction, the specific gravity varying from 1016 to 1028. The albumin test was always positive, the amount varying from ½ to 1½ grams *pro mille.*

Microscopically the cellular elements were scarce; a few leukocytes and epithelial cells were present; casts had never been found. In many of the specimens were uric acid crystals, often calcium oxalate crystals; acetone and acetoacetic acid test negative. Test for indican and diazo negative. Trommer and Fehling tests were positive and perfectly typical in the manner which Salkowski first described for pentose urine. The color change and the separation of oxydul did not occur immediately upon boiling, but only after cooling, and then very suddenly throughout the whole column of fluid. Fermentation was negative. The plane of polarized light was not turned. The phloroglucin reaction and the orcin reaction (the latter also with Bial's modification) were strongly positive. The golden yellow osazone, according to Salkowski's directions, gave the characteristic peculiarities for pentosazone (melting point,155; solubility in hot water and nitrogen content of about 17 per cent.). The amount of pentose in the urine varied from 0.4 per cent. to 0.6. per cent. In this case, then, it is certainly demonstrated that there was an optically inactive pentose in the urine. Probably by analogy with Nenberg's findings it may be an arabinose.

The Influence of the Concentration of the Urine upon the Outcome of the Reactions for Albumin.—DR. BENNO HALLAUER (*Münchener med. Wochenschrift,* September 8, 1903, No. 36, p. 1539) found that if normal human urine of ordinary concentration is evaporated on the water bath or *in vacuo* to one-half of its volume and then has added to it 4 per cent. of a serum containing 32 per cent. of albumin, that albumin tests performed upon this urine differ in their results from those given by ordinary albuminous urine. The boiling test gave a stronger reaction than in the case of non-concentrated urine. The Heller's reaction and the acetic-acid-potassium-ferrocyanide reaction are negative, however, with the concentrated urine. But in these cases a precipitation occurs as soon as the urine is diluted with water. The boiling test also fails with the concentrated urine if nitric acid is first added to the specimen. In this case, also, addition of water completes the reaction. He found that if the urine is still further concentrated to about one-quarter of its volume or less, even the boiling test fails to show albumin; but the addition of water restores the normal reactions. The author has tried these experiments with a great number of specimens, using serum from the horse and ox, urine from cases of nephritis, and crystallized serum albumin. The results were always essentially the same. The potassium-ferrocyanide-acetic-acid test, which has hitherto been considered a most delicate clinical test, is the first to disappear. The Heller's test often requires slightly greater concentration.

As to the cause of these phenomena, it appears that urea blocks the

Heller test, while boiling reaction is stopped by urea and neutral salts and the ferrocyanide reaction by certain salts, especially the phosphates.

Concerning the Diagnosis of Chronic Nephritis.—SCHWARZKOPF (*Münchener med. Wochenschrift*, September, 1903, No. 35, 50th Jahrg., pp. 1493, 1494) states that Nothnagel was the first to call attention to the occurrence of casts in the urine without simultaneous albuminuria. Nothnagel observed this in patients with icterus. Since attention has been turned to this subject a number of cases of "cylindruria" have been reported. Most of these were cases of drug-poisoning rather than of nephritis proper, there being a transitory injury to the kidney. The best known cases are those of Lüthje (*Arch. f. klin. Med.*, vol. lxxiv., S. 163), who found in all of his cases, after administering salicylic acid, casts, for the most part, not accompanied with albumin. Trük's dissertation (Tübingen, 1902) gives a résumé of the literature. Schwarzkopf reports five cases considered to be chronic nephritis, in which casts occurred without albumin either for part of the time or for the whole time the patient was under observation. The author agrees with Stewart (THE AMERICAN JOURNAL OF THE MEDICAL SCIENCES, 1893) in dwelling upon the importance of remembering this in making a diagnosis in the early stage of chronic nephritis, especially in those cases which are free from cardiac and vascular signs.

Concerning the Absence of Casts from the Urine of Patients with Nephritis.—ADOLF TREUTLEIN (*Münchener med. Wochenschrift*, September, 1903, 50th Jahrg., No. 35, pp. 1494–1496) concludes from his work that casts may be absent from a certain number of cases which otherwise are typical cases of nephritis. He concludes that in these cases the casts are destroyed by lysis resulting from the action of the bacillus coli, the bacillus coli in such cases being an inhabitant of the bladder or of the pelvis of the kidney.

Is Sugar Destruction Completely Stopped after Extirpation of the Pancreas?—LUTHJE (*Münchener med. Wochenschrift*, September, 1903, 50th Jahrg., No. 36, pp. 1537–1539) points out the experimental difficulty of removing all trace of the pancreas. He calls attention to the difference between sugar formation and sugar destruction. The pancreas certainly is concerned in the latter process. There is no ground to believe that the pancreas is the only organ concerned in sugar formation. Minkowski and others have noted that if a dog has its pancreas removed and is kept in a fasting condition the sugar disappears from the urine sooner or later. Lüthje considers this strong evidence that the sugár formed in the body by other organs is being converted. The author reports an extensive experiment in which the duodenum and pancreas were removed, gastroenterostomy between the posterior wall of the stomach and a loop of intestine was performed, and the gall-bladder was tied off. The experimental animal (a dog) was starved from the fifth day before operation. On the sixth day of hunger, that is, the first after operation, the percentage of sugar in the urine was 1.35, with a total of 13.5 grams of sugar. On the second day after operation, 2.25 per cent., a total of 9 grams of sugar. On the third day, 1.8 per cent., a total of 18 grams. On the fourth day after operation, 0.4 per cent., a total of 4 grams of sugar, after which from the fifth to the tenth day sugar disappeared. The specimen of blood drawn from the femoral vein on the seventh day after operation gave strong reaction with Trommer's test and showed quantitatively 0.312 per cent. of sugar in the blood. The dog died on the tenth day. At autopsy there was a small abscess in the region of the union between the stomach and gut. Lüthje concludes from this that it is definitely proven that even complete extirpation of the pancreas in a dog does not entirely destroy the dog's ability to consume sugar. He discusses the possible factors in sugar metabolism other than the pancreas. (1) The possibility of one or more organs partially taking the place of the pancreas and (2) the possibility that sugar formed in the body after pancreas extirpation has a different chemical origin. He notes the striking fact that the sugar first disappears from the urine of dogs after removal of the pancreas when the dogs have established a constant starvation nitrogen value. It is to be supposed that at this time the animals are beginning to consume their own "organized" albumin and that the "reserve" albumin has been used up. Possibly sugar thus arising from albumin of cells has a different mode of breaking down. This possible hypothesis throws light on the varying amounts of sugar shown by extirpated dogs of differing degrees of nutrition and by well-nourished and cachectic human beings. It explains the fact noted in one of his experiments that after sugar had disappeared from the urine of an operated dog a small feeding of nutrose at once brought about a return of glycosuria.

Leukæmia and Tuberculosis.—SUSSMANN (*The Practitioner*, October, 1903, p. 536) finds that there are only 25 undoubted cases of tuberculosis complicating leukæmia in the literature. He is inclined to the view that it is a rare complication of either the splenomedullary or the lymphatic form. He finds that, whereas tuberculosis is found to be present in from 11 per cent. to 12 per cent. of the necropsies in a series of over 7000, it occurs in only 2.4 per cent. of the autopsies in leukæmia. When the combination does occur, it is two and one-half times more frequent in the lymphatic than in the splenomedullary form. It is six times as common in the male as in the female. The tuberculosis may be found latent and obsolete or it may supervene as a terminal infection. It may be latent and be lighted up as a result of the leukæmic infection. This is the condition most commonly found. When the two diseases occur together the leukocytes are liable to diminish in number and the spleen and glands tend to decrease in size. The writer thinks that this antagonism is possibly due to the excess of nucleo-albumin and the increased phagocytic power of the blood, both of which conditions, he claims, are present in the leukæmic patient.

Arterial Thrombosis of Gonorrhœal Origin.—NORMAN MOORE (*Lancet*, December 16, 1903, p. 1714) reports a case of arterial thrombosis due to the gonococcus, and held to be the first case of the kind reported. A young man, aged twenty years, was admitted to the Manchester Royal Infirmary with gonorrhœa and with early dry gangrene of the left leg. Four days previous to admission he became chilly and feverish. The day before entrance he complained of coldness and pain in the left leg. On admission the left leg was cold, waxy, pulseless, and anæsthetic below the tubercle of the tibia. The three outer toes showed mummification, and there was discoloration about the ankle. The left common iliac was found not to pulsate. The patient died four days after admission. The evening before death he complained of pain in the right leg, and the pulsation in the right femoral was inappreciable. The limb below the knee was cold, pulseless, and anæsthetic.

The autopsy revealed a thrombus occluding the aorta from the renal arteries to its bifurcation. Both common iliacs and the external and internal iliacs were also filled by the thrombus. The rest of the arterial system was normal. There were no vegetations on the cardiac valves, nor were there any thrombi in the cavities of the heart. Histological examination of the thrombosed arteries showed that there was a definite acute endarteritis. Gonococci were demonstrated by Gram's method in the thrombus. No blood cultures, however, were made before or after death. Moore, nevertheless, concludes that the patient had a gonorrhœal septicæmia; that an acute endarteritis was consequently set up, and that this inflammatory process caused the local development of the thrombus.

SURGERY.

UNDER THE CHARGE OF

J. WILLIAM WHITE, M.D.,

JOHN RHEA BARTON PROFESSOR OF SURGERY IN THE UNIVERSITY OF PENNSYLVANIA; SURGEON TO THE UNIVERSITY HOSPITAL,

AND

F. D. PATTERSON, M.D.,

SURGEON TO THE X-RAY DEPARTMENT OF THE HOWARD HOSPITAL; CLINICAL ASSISTANT TO THE OUT-PATIENT SURGICAL DEPARTMENT OF THE JEFFERSON HOSPITAL.

The Operation of Gastroenterostomy, with Indications for its Performance.—Mayo Robson (*Archives international de chirurgie*, 1903, vol. i., No. 1) states that the operation of gastroenterostomy is imperative in the following conditions as soon as the diagnosis is established: 1. In cases of pyloric stenosis leading to dilatation of the stomach; here gastroenterostomy provides a new outlet for the passage of the stomach contents, and thus saves the patient from starvation and death. The advantage of this operation over pyloroplasty is that in the latter operation contraction of the new orifice occasionally occurs, and this is especially apt to take place if there be active ulceration going on at the time of the operation. 2. In malignant stenosis of the pylorus; the operation has been followed by brilliant results in this class of cases and the author's experience has shown the immediate results to be almost equal to those of simple stenosis. 3. A degree of congenital stenosis is doubtless a frequent though often an unrecognized cause of dilatation of the stomach in young adults. A number of such cases have been reported and gastroenterostomy has been followed by brilliant results. 4. Congenital atresia of the pylorus, in which no passage exists between the stomach and intestine, is a defect which in all recorded cases has run a rapidly fatal course. If diagnosed early it should be treated by gastroenterostomy. 5. In chronic ulcer, with tumor of doubtful character, too extensive or adherent for effectual removal, this operation has in some cases, where merely temporary relief only was anticipated, been followed by a complete and permanent cure. 6. In cancer or tumor of the duodenum producing obstruction to the onward passage of the stomach contents, gastroenterostomy acts in exactly the same manner as in cancer of the pylorus. As a rule, this form of disease in the second part of the duodenum is removable only with the greatest difficulty, in consequence of the important structures in the border of the lesser omentum being involved. 7. Hour-glass contraction of the stomach may be due to chronic ulcer or to cancer. If the contraction be due to simple ulceration, gastroplasty is the operation of choice, and in a number of cases the results have been excellent; but if the stricture be a long one and the thickening be very extensive, then gastroenterostomy, in which the proximal cavity is united to the jejunum, is the better operation; but great care must be observed that the junction is not made between the bowel and the distal cavity, otherwise no benefit will ensue. It should be the operation of choice when pyloric stenosis is associated with hour-glass contraction. 8. In perigastritis with adhesions the operation of gastroenterostomy may be entirely curative; at least, it has been so in many cases; but there are some cases where the adhesions are so extensive and the secondary dilatation of the stomach is so well marked that to rest content with simply detaching adhesions would be to court failure. If the pylorus is patent, yet embarrassed by adhesions, one should always separate them, and try to avoid their recurrence by interposing the right free border of the omentum between the raw surfaces left by the gastrolysis, thus substituting a long, freely movable attachment for short binding ligaments should adhesions re-form. If, however, adhesions are very extensive and very short, dense, and firm, the operation of posterior gastroenterostomy had better be done, and this especially if at the same time there is stenosis of the pylorus or hour-glass stomach. 9. In tumor outside the pylorus, but pressing on it and causing obstruction to the passage onward of the stomach contents, gastroenterostomy may be required at the same time that the tumor is treated. The following indications apply only after the failure of systematic medical treatment: 10. In ulcer of the stomach, whether acute or chronic, not yielding to medical treatment, surgical treatment is in the greater number of cases the only satisfactory method of dealing with these refractory cases, and operation should be resorted to at a much earlier period than has hitherto been the custom, and always before the patient is so far reduced by pain and starvation or the supervention of serious complications that weakness and anæmia render any operative procedure hazardous. Before the abdomen is opened it is quite impossible to say what operation or operations will be required, and the surgeon must be prepared to adapt himself to circumstances on discovering the position of the ulcer and the conditions associated with it, especially as to the presence or absence of adhesions and other complications. Gastroenterostomy acts by securing physiological rest of the stomach and, at the same time, curing the hyperchlorhydria which is usually present. 11. Duodenal ulcer very frequently fails to yield to general treatment, and the author believes it is much more frequently the cause of fatal symptoms than is generally recognized. 12. In hemorrhage from the stomach or duodenum, as shown by hæmatemesis or melæna, where general treatment has been tried or failed and where the bleeding is persisting or recurring after brief intervals, operation is advisable, with a view to find and to secure, if possible, the bleeding point or points, or of performing gastroenterostomy in order to obtain physiological rest and thus to favor natural hæmostasis. 13. In persistent spasm of the pylorus, or Reichmann's disease, leading to dilatation of the stomach, pylorodiosis or stretching the sphincter may be effectual in relieving spasm and in producing immediate relief to the obstruction, but as it is apt to be followed by relapse, gastroenterostomy would seem to be the better operation. 14. Hyperchlorhydria is a concomitant of ulcer of the stomach, though it may occur apart from ulceration. As a rule, it yields to medical and general treatment, but where this fails to relieve and the life of the patient is being made miserable by constant indigestion with acid eructation, the operation of gastroenterostomy is well worth consideration, especially when in such a case it can be performed with almost no risk, for in the absence of complications such as occur in ulcer or cancer, the operations, when properly performed by an expert, ought to have no mortality. 15. Persistent gastralgia: Cases must have occurred in the practice of every physician where, although the positive signs of ulcer were absent, gastralgia of such intensity had persisted and in case of temporary relief had recurred so regularly that the patient is brought to the last stage of exhaustion by an utter inability to take food because of the pain induced by even a mouthful of solid food. Some of these cases are doubtless due to simple ulcer, but in others the absence of tenderness in the epigastrium, of rigidity of the recti, of regular vomiting, and of hæmatemesis, makes the diagnosis extremely doubtful. Even rectal feeding and absolute rest in bed do not always cure the condition, and the patient gradually loses weight and strength and lapses into a state of chronic invalidism without any positive sign of organic disease. After all ordinary means have failed, gastroenterostomy is well worthy of consideration, and in one case in the author's experience it led to an excellent result. 16. In tetany of gastric origin. The prognosis of tetany occurring in gastric dilatation is undoubtedly very serious, and, according to some authorities, death occurs in 75 per cent. of the cases. The largest mortality occurs in cases where the cramps in the extremities are associated with tonic spasms in the head and trunk muscles or with clonic spasm. The author's experience would tend to show that the early surgical treatment of these cases may be followed by most beneficial results. 17. Acute gastric dilatation is one of the most serious diseases that can be encountered. But that the condition is not hopeless has been well shown by one case where lavage was followed by a cure. As yet gastroenterostomy has not been tried as a means of relieving this condition. 18. In an exceptional case of ulcer of the stomach eroding the pancreas and producing pancreatitis, with abscess draining into the stomach, a gastroenterostomy apparently saved the life of the patient by draining the very foul contents directly into the intestine. 19. Cholelithiasis may lead to perigastritis, and the contraction of bands of lymph around the pylorus may produce obstruction or kinking, thus leading to dilatation of the stomach, at the same time that the concretions lead to obstruction of the bile ducts. As a rule, the condition can be relieved by gastrolysis, but where the adhesions are extensive or the thickening of the pylorus is very pronounced, the operation of gastroenterostomy may have to be performed at the same time as the cholecystotomy. Gallstones may also lead to fistula between the gall-bladder and pylorus and the thickening of the pyloric canal may lead to obstruction, for which gastroenterostomy may be the most suitable operation, though in the cases that have come under the care of the author the repair of the fistula in one case and pyloroplasty in another were sufficient, when combined with cholecystotomy, to remedy the disease. 20. In atonic dilatation of the stomach, general and medical treatment, supplemented, if need be, by electrical treatment and lavage, if carried out systematically and for a sufficient length of time, usually yield good results; but in some cases, despite regular lavage of the dilated organ, well-regulated diet and general medical treatment, the dilatation persists and the nutrition of the patient and the general health become seriously impaired. In such cases the operation of gastrorrhaphy or gastroplication may be worth considering, though in certain cases gastroenterostomy may possibly be performed with advantage. The indication for operation in these cases is not so distinct as in the case of dilatation due to pyloric obstruction, seeing that the cause is a general one; nor is the recovery after operation so rapid and satisfactory. The general health requires considerable attention at the same time that the stomach is being dealt with.

Splenectomy for Banti's Disease.—QUEEN and DUVAL (*Revue de chirurgie*, October 10, 1903) state that the principal characteristics of this affection are: 1. Obscure etiology; neither alcohol, syphilis, nor tuberculosis apparently being a factor. 2. The enlargement of the spleen in all directions is the initial symptom. 3. As a result of this enlargement there develops an anæmia, which is fatally progressive, but whose duration is variable, but always long, varying from three to twelve years. 4. During this anæmia the urine contains urobilin, the skin and the conjunctiva become jaundiced, and a diarrhœa appears and usually lasts for some months. 5. The ascitic phase then appears. The liver is sclerosed and the cirrhosis of Laennec, which makes rapid progress, appears. 6. During the disease there is no leukocytosis, but there is a diminution of hæmoglobin and corpuscles. 7. The morbid pathology consists in an enormous enlargement of the spleen, of from one to two kilograms in weight. Histologically there is an atrophy of the pulp and a sclerosis, with hypertrophy of the capsule and the reticulum and a partial sclerosis of the Malpighian corpuscles. The liver is small, hard, granular, with a cirrhosis, presenting all the characteristics of Laennec's atrophy. 8. The bacteriological examination of the blood and the spleen is always negative. 9. The extirpation of the spleen is followed by a radical cure of the disease. If there exists a beginning hepatic cirrhosis, the splenectomy arrests its development. The authors report one case in their own experience and six others collected from the literature in which splenectomy was followed by a complete recovery.

Adrenalin in Local Anæsthesia.—BRAUN (*Centralblatt für Chirurgie*, 1903, No. 38) states that the two most important points to be considered in the use of adrenalin for this purpose are the dose and the danger of secondary hemorrhage. As regards the dose, such a very powerful drug as it is should only be used with great care. A dose of 1 milligram is entirely too big to be subcutaneously injected. In one case an injection of 20 c.c. of a 0.5 per cent. solution of eucaine "B." with 10 drops of the 1:1000 adrenalin solution, caused vomiting and prostration, which lasted for an hour; in several other cases this dose caused some cardiac palpitation. Hartwig and others have had some very unfavorable symptoms from this dose, and Enderlen has reported a case where the injection of 8 cg. of cocaine, with 8 drops of adrenalin solution, was followed by a fatal result. The best solution would seem to be one composed of hydrochloric acid, 0.2; sodium chloride, 0.8; and distilled water, 100 parts. Then 10 c.c. of this mixture should be placed in a test-tube and heated to the boiling point, and then 1 cg. of adrenalin added, and the solution again boiled. This will give a colorless solution, in which the greater part of the salt is neutralized by the adrenalin. 2 drops of carbolic acid should be added and then the fluid should be kept in bottles holding from 3 c.c. to 5 c.c.; this solution will keep indefinitely. As regards hemorrhage, it is apparent that the anæmia resulting from the use of adrenalin is not followed by hyperæmia nor tissue paralysis, and it is not possible to secure accurate hæmostasis in the presence of adrenalin. So care should be taken to use a very small dose of adrenalin; this markedly intensifies the duration and degree of the anæsthesia, but will not contract the arteries so as to interfere with the proper control of any bleeding that may occur.

Retroduodenal Choledochotomy.—QUERVAIN (*Centralblatt für Chirurgie*, 1903, No. 40), after mentioning the work of Berg, Lane, Kocher, etc., states that though this operation is but rarely performed, still it may not be considered as a new method. After noting in detail a case operated upon by this method with a perfect recovery, the author states that, as regards technique, the incision of the duodenum must be done very carefully and most accurate hæmostasis secured, and so any drainage to the intestinal wall will be avoided, as well as serious hemorrhage. Should the duodenum be turned over inward, then one should incise the choledochus at the point where it is not covered by the pancreas. The best indication of the point to cut is usually the easily felt stones. As to the choice between the retroduodenal and transduodenal methods, the former method is to be recommended in all cases where the duodenum may be easily removed. If, however, it and the pancreas are closely matted together with adhesions and further progress by the retroduodenal route is distinctly dangerous, then one should abandon all attempts at further separation and at once proceed with the transduodenal operation.

Ogston's Operation for Clubfoot.—LAUENSTEIN (*Centralblatt für Chirurgie*, 1903, No. 39), after considering the question in detail, reaches the following conclusions: 1. Experience has shown that this operation is not a difficult one. 2. A careful examination with *x*-rays should be made in every case, and whenever possible a radiograph should be taken. 3. The amount of bone removed must be gauged by the circumstances present in each individual case. 4. When sufficient bone has been removed, then the abnormal position can be easily and thoroughly corrected, and retention in good position can be easily obtained. 5. The after-treatment is shorter; at the end of eight weeks the child may safely be allowed to walk with a properly fitting shoe. 6. Radiographs taken subsequent to the operation show that there is absolutely no danger of any failure of development of the foot. 7. To just what age this operation should be limited has as yet not been determined.

A New Modification of Maydl's Operation for Congenital Ectopy of the Bladder.—BORELIUS (*Centralblatt für Chirurgie*, 1903, No. 29), after noting in detail two cases in which he used the modified method, states that the essential points in the technique are: 1. A careful separation of the bladder and the forming of an elliptical piece, which includes the ureters. 2. The opening of the abdominal cavity so that the sigmoid flexure may be pulled well forward. 3. A lateral anastomosis between the upper and lower portions of the sigmoid. 4. A longitudinal incision at the top of the flexure and the implantation of the ureters. 5. The wound should then be closed with sutures.

Wound of the Epigastric Vessels as the Result of Puncture for Ascites.—BAUM (*Deutsche Zeitschrift für Chirurgie*, August, 1903) reports the case of a man, aged fifty-five years, who presented himself for treatment with cirrhosis of the liver with marked ascites. Puncture being decided upon, it was done in the usual manner in the median line and a large quantity of fluid withdrawn. As the fluid rapidly accumulated, another puncture was made 1 cm. to the left of the linea alba and 8.5 cm. above the symphysis, and then 4300 c.c. of fluid was withdrawn. The patient was not uncomfortable until three hours later, when he complained of much pain in the abdomen and a sense of distention as from tympanites. Examination showed the abdomen markedly distended, more especially so on the left side, more or less rigidity, an increase of pain on pressure, and dulness on percussion over the distended area. The skin was apparently unaltered, and fluctuation could not be elicited. A diagnosis of laceration of the epigastric artery having been made, the abdomen was opened at once under local anæsthesia at the point where the puncture was made. The fatty tissue was found to be infiltrated with blood, and as soon as the peritoneum was opened there was a rush of blood from the wound. Many blood clots were found and these were removed after the torn epigastric vessels had been ligated. The wound was drained at each end and then the intervening portion closed with sutures. The further course was in every way normal, the patient making an uninterrupted recovery. In view of this case, it would seem important to remember that when this accident does occur an immediate laparotomy is indicated, and that it is much less likely to occur if the puncture be made in the median line.

Adenoma of the Umbilicus.—KOSLOWSKI (*Deutsche Zeitschrift für Chirurgie*, August, 1903) states that in the embryo the middle intestine is a straight tube, which communicates with the yolk sac. About the fourth week the intestine is twisted toward the umbilicus and becomes joined with it, and about the eighth week the ductus omphaloentericus becomes obliterated into a thin cord, which is still present at the third month. Seldom is this obliteration of the ductus omphalomesentericus complete; it retains its connection with the intestine and causes an inversion of the intestinal canal (Meckel's diverticulum), which is connected to the umbilicus by this obliterated cord. This may give rise to various pathological conditions; among the most interesting is the following case of fibroid adenoma. The patient states that five weeks ago he noticed in the median line, between the symphysis and the umbilicus, a small and somewhat painful swelling, which had increased in size until it was about as large as a walnut. The area of pain seemed to be enlarging and involved all the abdomen. The patient, though fifty-five years of age, looked to be over seventy years, with marked arteriosclerosis, emphysema, and an unusually poor general appearance. On examination there is a small tumor in the median line, about midway between the symphysis and the umbilicus, very painful on pressure; the skin over it is freely movable, but the tumor itself is hard and more or less adherent to the surrounding structures. Toward the umbilicus a cord can be made out. The abdominal walls are rather thin and the urogenital and intestinal tracts present nothing abnormal. The median position of this tumor with the presence of this cord induced the diagnosis of epithelioma and an operation for its relief was performed. An incision in the median line was made over the tumor; this incision was continued on either side of the tumor until the peritoneal cavity was opened. The tumor was then pushed upward and it was found to be a fibroma of the ductus omphalomesentericus. Extirpation of the tumor and the cord was then done and the wound closed. The patient made an uninterrupted recovery. Wyssokowitsch, who made the pathological examination, reports that the tumor is a submalignant fibroadenoma. It is of interest to note that but four other analogous cases have been reported.

THERAPEUTICS.

UNDER THE CHARGE OF

REYNOLD WEBB WILCOX, M.D., LL.D.,

PROFESSOR OF MEDICINE AND THERAPEUTICS AT THE NEW YORK POST-GRADUATE MEDICAL SCHOOL AND HOSPITAL; VISITING PHYSICIAN TO ST. MARK'S HOSPITAL.

Colloidal Silver.—Dr. H. S. Loebl has treated various forms of sepsis, erysipelas, and puerperal processes by intravenous injections of this substance. When the intravenous method is impossible he makes use of rectal injections, 1:500 or even 250 parts of distilled water, the amount of menstruum employed being 3½ ounces, twice daily. The injection is preceded by a cleansing enema. The advantages of this method are obvious, while the results are usually satisfactory.—*Wiener klinische Wochenschrift*, 1903, No. 44, p. 1230.

The Abortive Treatment of Gonorrhœa.—Dr. Ferdinand Fuchs recommends the use of albargin in this connection. This preparation contains 23.6 per cent. of silver nitrate, while protargol contains only 8.3 per cent., and is easily soluble in water. The treatment must be instituted not longer than seventy-two hours after the suspected coitus, and is still more successful if forty-eight hours or less have intervened. Thus early in the infection microscopic examination of the urethral secretion shows squamous epithelial cells, leukocytes, and a few gonococci, sometimes free, sometimes in the epithelial cells, but seldom within the leukocytes. The technique of the treatment is as follows: A 2 per cent. albargin solution is injected by means of an olive-tipped hand syringe into the anterior urethra until the patient complains of a sensation of distention. This injection is retained for five minutes and is then allowed to escape. A second injection is now given and the solution retained for three minutes. This is followed by a third, which is retained for two minutes. It is seldom that pain is complained of, but on the following night the patient may be troubled with frequency of urination. After the injection examination shows fewer leukocytes and no gonococci, and in about fourteen days the secretion entirely disappears. No complications have followed in six cases reported by the author, and in all of them equally good results have been attained. —*Therapeutische Monatshefte*, 1903, No. 10, p. 508.

Hedonal.—DR. JOHANN FRACZKIEWICZ reports that this new hypnotic, the chemical formula of which is $CONH_2OCHCH_3C_3H_7$, which physically is a white cr stalline powder easily soluble in alcohol, ether, and boiling water, and less so in tepid water. Its taste resembles that of menthol. He uses the drug in doses of 20 grains for women and 30 grains for men. In these doses it produces in from fifteen minutes to one hour a moderately deep dreamless sleep, lasting from five to eight hours, and not followed by unpleasant after-effects, such as headache, dizziness, or ringing in the ears. During the slumber the heart action and respiration are not affected. In persons with normal kidneys the drug has a slight diuretic action, but is not so active in this regard as to disturb the rest of the patient. When there is kidney disease the diuretic effect seems to be *nil*. In cardiac disease the drug seems to do no harm. In conclusion, the author asserts that hedonal appears to be useful in the insomnia of hysteria, neurasthenia, marasmus senilis, and in psychoses of the milder grades. In these conditions it does no harm, even when continued for a considerable period; its diuretic effect is not cumulative. In insomnia due to pain it is useless.—*Therapeutische Monatshefte*, 1903, No. 11, p. 572.

Phosphorus in Psychasthenia.—DR. ALFRED MARTINET asserts, as a result of his clinical observations upon phosphoric medication in psychasthenia, that in the accidental forms of the condition when taken early the treatment is quickly followed by a return of the mental processes to a normal state. In habitual psychasthenia of long standing the treatment when continued for considerable periods of time results in a progressive amelioration of the condition. In psychataxia with agitation the phosphoric medication produces a rapid aggravation of the pathological state. The phosphorus is prescribed as follows: Official phosphoric acid, 10; acid sodium phosphate, 20; distilled water, 200. Of this the patient takes at first 30 drops in a glass of water with each meal, progressively increasing the number of drops taken to 100. If there are dyspeptic or other symptoms, these are treated at the same time according to ordinary methods.—*La presse médicale*, 1903, No. 93, p. 805.

Lecithin.—DR. HENRI LABBE believes that this drug fulfils all the indications of phosphorus and the glycerophosphates. In rickets with cod-liver oil (lecithin, 1; cod-liver oil, 250) it seems to cause a cessation of the disease in from four to six months. In cases of defective growth it has also given favorable results. It is indicated in dyspepsia with phosphaturia, unless this latter is due to overfeeding, in which case, however, it may be given in small doses ($\frac{3}{4}$ to $1\frac{1}{2}$ grains) in connection with a properly regulated diet. In neurasthenia and anæmia it relieves the symptoms, increases the patient's strength and the hæmoglobin and the number of red blood cells. In tuberculosis and senile debility it betters the general condition, but in the former disease the lesions do not seem to be modified. In diabetes, especially of the pancreatic variety, it increases the strength and weight, but does not alter the amount of sugar in the urine. In cachectic and convalescent states, except those following malaria, it is a valuable aid in the regeneration of the blood. In certain cases it acts as a heart stimulant when digitalis is useless. The continued administration of the drug is entirely harmless.—*Revue de thérapeutique*, 1903, No. 21, p. 721.

The Treatment of the Cardiac Complications of Rheumatism.—DR. F. COMBEMALE believes that if murmurs appear the cardiac condition should be closely watched for at least four weeks, during which period treatment by means of sodium salicylate should be continued; the patient should remain absolutely at rest in bed, and all excitement must be avoided. When acceleration of the pulse is noted sparteina in the following formula is prescribed: sparteina sulphate, 1; syrup of tulu, 10,000; distilled water of linden, 20,000. Of this two tablespoonfuls are given daily. Precordial pain calls for counterirritation by means of cupping or vesicants, which measures should be continued if the pain persists. If the pulse becomes irregular, as well as rapid, digitalis in the following formula: powdered digitalis leaves, 50; water, 120; fluid extract of convallaria, 30. The daily dose of this mixture is 7 to 8 drachms. Caffeine should not be employed unless myocarditis is present. —*Annales de la Polyclinique de Paris*, 1903, No. 11, p. 261.

Arsenous Acid in Cancerous Ulcerations.—DR. ROUX DE BRIGNOLLES is inclined to the theory that the topical application of arsenous acid exerts a specific action in certain forms of epitheliomatous ulcerations. In two types of cancerous lesion he has found its use followed by most happy results. These are ulcerations recurrent in the cicatrix after operation for carcinoma of the breast and cutaneous epitheliomata. Such lesions taken early and before gland involvement may be readily cured. He believes that the curative effect of the arsenic is due to a dehydration of the cancerous tissue in the presence of fresh blood and alcohol and the combination of the drug with the cancerous elements to form an albuminate and to lessen the degeneration of the connective tissue. He uses the arsenous acid in the following formula: powdered arsenous acid, 1; ethyl alcohol and distilled water, of each, 50. With this mixture the cancerous surface is painted after having been cleansed, during which process a few drops of blood, not more, must have been caused to flow. The application is allowed to evaporate and no dressing need be applied. On the next day the surface which has been treated will be covered by an eschar, which is not removed, but upon which daily applications like the first are made until the crust becomes completely black and easily movable upon the tissues beneath. The crust may now be removed and another application made; if on the next day the resulting crust is easily movable one may be sure that the treatment is successful. If the crust is firmly fixed the treatment must be continued as before until the entire disappearance of the cancerous elements.—*Gazette médicale de Paris*, 1903, No. 47, p. 389.

Empyroform.—DR. ALFRED KRAUS reports upon this new tar preparation, which is a condensation product of birch tar and formalin. It is used as a 1 per cent. solution with chloroform and acetone, as a paint with chloroform and traumaticin, or as a 5 per cent. ointment with equal parts of lanolin and vaselin. It is most useful in chronic eczema, relieving the itching in a decided manner, and it is even useful if there be acute symptoms. In psoriasis, lichen urticatus, prurigo, pityriasis rosea and versicolor it has given good results.—*Prager medicinische Wochenschrift*, 1903, No. 33, p. 419.

The Action and Therapeutic Application of Radium.—DR. JUMON reports encouraging results from the therapeutic use of this substance in lupus. After the radium rays have been applied for five or six days the surfaces to which they have had access become reddened, and after prolonged application an appearance like that of a second-degree burn or an ulceration of the surface may be produced. The ulcers are whitish or yellowish, shallow, not indurated, painless, and slow to heal. This latter process may be facilitated by the use of dressings wet with boric acid solution. If pus germs gain access to the abraded surface suppuration may ensue. When the healing is complete, white, soft, superficial cicatrices usually result. If the application of the rays has been too short the ulceration produced is too superficial, and recurrence of the original lesion is likely to take place. On the other hand, permanent cure follows the application of "plaques" of radium of an intensity of from 5000 to 19,000 for from twenty-four to thirty-six hours. Such a treatment results in a white, pearly cicatrix, sometimes surrounded by a zone of brown pigmentation. The scar is flexible, not indurated, and unlike that produced by ordinary measures. So far as immediate result is concerned, the curative effects seem excellent; what the ultimate result will prove to be only time will tell. The advantages of the treatment are its simplicity, its freedom from pain, and the comparatively short time needed for its completion. Undoubtedly study of the subject will be followed by modifications of the technique of the use of the substance.—*Revue de thérapeutique*, 1903, No. 20, p. 692.

Ascites Treated by a Diet Free from Chlorides.—M. ACHARD reports two cases of ascites, one due to hepatic cirrhosis, the other to mitral insufficiency, where a diet in which the chlorides were reduced was followed by good results after a milk diet had failed to benefit the patients. The diet prescribed was as follows: sixteen ounces each of meat and potatoes, two ounces of rice, five ounces of sugar, and forty-five grains of salt. The first patient's weight fell in twenty-five days from 138 to 119 pounds, and so remained after an ordinary diet had been resumed; the diet prescribed was but slightly poorer in salt than the milk diet, but the diuresis due to the sugar and starches aided the organism in the excretion of the chlorides. The ascites of the second patient increased under ordinary diet, but being put upon a diet lacking in salt her weight remained stationary for twelve days, after which the daily ingestion of 5 drachms of salt resulted in an increase of the ascites and an increase of eight pounds in weight in six days. Examination of the ascitic fluid showed a diminution in its chlorides when the patient was upon the diet lacking in salt and a rapid increase in these elements when ordinary regimen was resumed.—*La semaine médicale*, 1903, No. 45, p. 369.

PEDIATRICS.

UNDER THE CHARGE OF

LOUIS STARR, M.D.,

OF PHILADELPHIA,

AND

THOMPSON S. WESTCOTT, M.D.,

OF PHILADELPHIA.

Infections of the Newborn.—S. McC. Hamill and W. R. Nicholson (*Archives of Pediatrics*, September, 1903, p. 641) report a series of cases of infections of the newborn, and present the conclusions from their study. They do not incline to accept as pathological entities such conditions as melæna neonatorum, hemorrhagic disease of the newborn, Buhl's disease, Winckel's disease, etc. According to their observations, and in accordance with the literature, all the clinical symptoms described under these various titles may exist as manifestations of a number of different infections, the nature and severity of the symptoms depending upon the character of the infecting organism. Any classification, therefore, must depend upon a bacteriological basis.

In the six cases recorded six different micro-organisms were isolated, viz., the bacillus pyocyaneus, the bacillus lactis aërogenes, the colon bacillus, the staphylococcus aureus, the bacillus coli immobilis, and a streptococcus. In their complete list of cases, amounting to about fifteen, only one other micro-organism, an unclassified micrococcus, has been encountered. Various other organisms have been found in similar infections, but those most commonly encountered are the streptococcus, the bacillus coli communis, and the staphylococcus. Délestre, for instance, in thirty-seven positive cultures from infected infants, found the streptococcus fourteen times, the colon bacillus ten times, and the staphylococcus six times.

The post-mortem findings may be summed up in the words "congestion" and "hemorrhage," varying in degree in different cases. There is usually a considerable degree of congestion of the spleen, the mesenteric lymph nodes, the kidneys, suprarenals, liver, stomach, or intestines. Ulceration in various portions of the gastrointestinal tract has been recorded. The liver, kidneys, and the suprarenal glands may be the seat of hemorrhages. Hemorrhages into the serous cavities are common.

The bladder may contain bloody urine, and sometimes ecchymosis of its mucous membrane is present.

The principal changes in the thoracic organs are: enlargement and congestion of the mediastinal glands, congestion in the lungs, areas of atelectasis or pneumonia. The heart muscle is sometimes soft and frequently its vessels are enormously distended.

Histological studies are incomplete. The changes are those commouly found in infectious conditions, namely, cloudy swelling, fatty degeneration and infiltration of the liver and kidneys, in addition to the changes resulting from hemorrhage.

Most of these infections occur in maternity hospitals, where the opportunities for the spread of disease germs are great. It is possible that the origin of these infections depends upon the presence of the various micro-organisms which bacteriological investigations have demonstrated in the air and dust of wards.

The mother's milk also has been held accountable, and not only in the presence of suppurative lesions of the breast, but also in milk from apparently normal breasts, have pathogenic organisms been isolated. The use of the same bath for several infants and the bedding together of the infected and the non-infected has resulted in conveying the infection.

Admitting the possibility of these sources of infection, the authors, nevertheless, incline to the belief that the most common medium is the poorly trained or careless nurse. In the institutions in which they have observed these cases they have noted that they were not confined to one ward; that they have been handled by the same nurse, and that the bacteriological studies have shown the presence of different organisms in the different cases. The literature shows few examples of any one organism being held accountable for all the cases in an epidemic. These facts, they think, are against the greater frequency of air infections.

The authors believe that the cord has been given too much prominence as the point of entrance, and that the most common ports of entry are the buccal cavity, the tonsils, and the remainder of the alimentary tract, and next in order the lungs.

As very little can be done in the way of treatment when infection is once established, the necessity for prophylactic measures by improving the general aseptic technique of maternity wards is of great importance.

Absolute cleanliness on the part of the attendants, careful handling of the napkins, bed-pan, etc., separate wards and special nurses for the infants are some of the measures which would prevent, to a certain extent, these infections. The advisability of the routine practice of cleansing the infant's mouth is questioned. The recognition of any pathological condition of the breasts, such as erosions or fissures, should be a signal for the immediate withdrawal of the infant.

The Overlying of Infants—WESTCOTT (*British Medical Journal*, November 7, 1903) gives some statistics upon this too frequent cause of death among infants in England.

During the last decade there were 15,009 overlain infants in England and Wales, and for the year 1902 London alone presented the shameful mortality of 588 deaths from this cause.

The danger diminishes with the age of the infant, until at a year old the risk of suffocation by the mother is trifling.

The dead infants presented the well-known signs of death by suffocation: bluish lips, flexion of the legs and arms, clenched hands, and froth, often blood-stained, in the nostrils and mouth. Many showed undoubted marks of pressure—for example, a flattened nose. The common post-mortem findings in an infant that has died from suffocation are: engorged lungs, sometimes œdematous; congestion of the brain and meninges, the right heart containing soft clot and the left heart empty; the pleura and pericardium showing minute ecchymoses.

Westcott deplores the fact that this habit of mothers taking infants to their own beds is so common in England, and, as it is impossible to punish parents under the existing laws, even when drunkenness is proven, he thinks it should be declared an obligation on every parent to provide a cot or cradle for the infant's use.

GYNECOLOGY.

UNDER THE CHARGE OF

HENRY C. COE, M.D.,

OF NEW YORK.

ASSISTED BY

WILLIAM E. STUDDIFORD, M.D.

Examination of the Blood in Cases of Ovarian Cyst.—POZZI and BENDER (*Annales de Gynécologie et d'Obstétrique*, October, 1903) conclude a paper on this subject with the following deductions: 1. In the majority of the cases the benign or malignant character of an ovarian cystoma may be inferred from examinations of the patient's blood. 2. If the red cells are normal and the white are in the proportion of from 6000 to 8000, the tumor is benign. 3. A moderate leukocytosis with a normal number of red cells may indicate suppuration, though an increase in the white cells is noted in the case of large cysts; no positive inference can be drawn with reference to malignity. 4. With a diminution of the red cells and a leukocytosis from 12,000 to 20,000 malignant degeneration may be suspected.

The presence of anæmia is a more important indication than the increase in the white cells. The percentage of hæmoglobin is of course an important aid. The writers add that blood examinations are of especial value from the standpoint of prognosis, citing two cases in which patients with marked diminution of red cells and leukocytosis succumbed quickly after operation, without infection

Cystitis in the Female.—VEDELER (*Norsk Mag. for Laegerid.; Zentralblatt für Gynäkologie*, 1902, No. 42) found only 380 patients with cystitis among 10,000 gynecological cases. He regards coitus as an etiological factor. Only 1.5 per cent. of the cases occurred in virgins, 2.5 per cent. in widows, but over 5 per cent. in married women. Of the 3 cases in little girls 2 were due to gonorrhœa following attempted coitus. Four cases resulted from the use of catheters, and in 22 cystitis was referred to syphilis, typhoid, tuberculosis and lithiasis. In only 45 was there no accompanying disease of the urethra and genital organs. Menstruation, the climacteric, and early pregnancy seemed to have no influence upon the condition, though menstruation apparently caused an exacerbation of existing cystitis.

[We are surprised to note that so few cases were traced to the use of the catheter, which, according to our observation, is the commonest cause of post-operative cystitis.—H. C. C.]

Plastic Operation for Hydronephrosis.—PETERSEN (*Münchener med. Wochenschrift*, 1903, No. 11) describes an ingenious operation for the relief of obstruction to the ureter following incision and drainage of a hydronephrotic kidney. The obstruction proved to be a valvular fold of mucous membrane at the entrance of the ureter. This was removed by making a longitudinal incision as in pyloroplasty and closing it transversely with catgut sutures. The renal sac was then folded on itself at several points and the folds were sutured, so as to reduce the size of the pelvis as much as possible. The drainage of urine through the wound rapidly diminished, and at the end of six weeks the patient was discharged cured.

Paraffin Injections in Incontinence of Urine.—HOCK (*Prager med. Wochenschrift*, 1903, No. 6) reports the case of a girl, aged twenty-three years, who six years before had had a calculus removed per urethram, with resulting incontinence which resisted all treatment. After two operations for narrowing the urethra, and one in which torsion was performed, her condition was worse than before. A second torsion gave only slight relief. Two injections of paraffin (75 grains each time) were made at the neck of the bladder, when the incontinence was speedily cured. Three months later the patient again began to have dribbling of urine, and the injections were twice repeated, with permanent relief. The paraffin remained unchanged at the point of injection.

Operations for Uterine Fibroid.—CZEMPIN (*Zentralblatt für Gynäkologie*, 1903, No. 42) reports 140 cases in which the principal indication for operation was obstinate menorrhagia. He prefers the vaginal route, saving the uterus if possible. Of the 58 vaginal operations hysterectomy was performed 17 times with no deaths. In 82 of the abdominal operations supravaginal amputation was performed 19 times with 4 deaths, and hysterectomy 44 times with 6 deaths. Two deaths were due to embolus, 5 to shock, and 3 to sepsis. There was no mortality in 19 conservative abdominal operations.

Myoperithelioma.—GOTTSCHALK (*Zentralblatt für Gynäkologie*, 1903, No. 42) reports the following case, which he regards as unique: The patient, aged fifty-one years, had multiple uterine nodules, which grew rapidly and were accompanied by a constant bloody discharge. The diagnosis of fibroids with malignant degeneration was made, and the uterus was removed successfully. Numerous fibroid nodules were found, especially sessile submucous. The latter were covered with papillary excrescences, as well as the surrounding endometrium.

Microscopic examination showed that the growths had developed from the perithelia of the adventitia and from the deeper, rather than from the superficial vessels. In the sections of the myomata the ordinary alveolar structure of cancer was found, while in the superficial portion the pure perithelial type prevailed. The conclusion drawn by the writer was that the malignant change began in those vessels of the myoma just beneath the mucosa.

Retroflexion.—KOVWER (*Zentralblatt für Gynäkologie*, 1903, No. 42) found 239 cases of retroflexion in 2800 gynecological cases (8.5 per cent.), of which 210 were treated. In 135 the uterus was movable, and in 75 adherent. Of the latter only 7 were operated upon, the remainder being treated with tampons. Thirty-one patients were subsequently able to wear pessaries; 25 per cent. were cured. One hundred and twenty cases of movable retrodisplacement were treated with pessaries; in 6 no treatment was necessary, and of 9 patients operated upon, 10 per cent. were cured. Only 16 out of the 239 patients (6 per cent.) were operated upon. Alexander's operation was preferred in movable retroflexion, 9 operations being recorded with 6 cures.

The writer notes that in the 5 abdominal operations for adherent retrodisplacement not a single patient was permanently relieved. He is entirely opposed to the surgical treatment of retroflexion, since by no method can the uterus be restored to its normal position. This is possible in some cases by the use of pessaries. Young girls should be treated as little as possible.

[The frank pessimism of this writer is in striking contrast with the enthusiastic reports of most surgeons. In fact his skepticism is so avowed as to awaken the suspicion that he is an extremist. Between the views of those who denounce the use of pessaries and the opinions above expressed there is certainly a middle course which is safer than either extreme.—H. C. C.]

Treatment of Inoperable Cancer of the Uterus.—BLAU (*Zentralblatt für Gynäkologie*, 1903, No. 45) reports the result of palliative treatment in 408 cases of inoperable cancer in Chrobak's clinic. The routine method consisted in removing as much of the diseased tissue as possible with the sharp spoon and cauterizing the new surface with fuming nitric acid or the Paquelin. The cavity is then tamponed with iodoform gauze, which is removed in four days. To promote granulation and cicatrization applications of tincture of iodine are made every two or three days. At intervals of three or four months the surface is touched with nitric acid or a 20 per cent. alcoholic solution of bromine. Iodoform is used freely for foul discharges, with injections of permanganate of potash or creolin. Only two patients succumbed to the operation.

342 patients were kept under observation. In three cases which presented all the clinical appearances of cancer of the cervix (though the specimens were not examined microscopically) one patient lived for eleven years before succumbing to the disease, one was alive at the end of nine years, and one at the end of six years.

The average duration of life after the operation was 252.3 days. Two patients now under observation were living after two to three years, four after three to four years, and one after eleven years. 109 patients (31.8 per cent.) lived over a year after operation, and thirty-three (9.6 per cent.) over two years.

Epidural Injection in Enuresis.—KAPSAMMER (*Wiener klin. Wochenschrift*, 1903, Nos. 29 and 30) made 300 injections without a single accident. He used at first 5 cm. of cocaine solution (one-half of 1 per cent.), but subsequently found that normal saline solution produced the same result. The needle is inserted at the junction of the coccyx and sacrum, so that the solution reached the roots of the cauda equina without entering the dural sac. Usually one injection is sufficient. The result of the trauma is to stimulate the *nervus erigentes* and to restore the tone of the vesical sphincter.

Streptococci in the Normal Urethra.—ASAKURA (*Zentralblatt für die Krankheiten der Hern. med. Sexualorgane*, Band xiv., Heft 3) examined the secretions found in the fossa muscularis in 112 apparently healthy men and found the streptococci pyogenes present in fourteen (12.5 per cent.). This fact the writer regards as of especial interest to gynecologists, since it proves that streptococci may be introduced into the vagina during the sexual act.

The Operative Treatment of Cancer of the Uterus.—KLEIN (*Münchener med. Wochenschrift*, 1903, Nos. 11 and 12), after a careful study of the statistics, concludes that the percentage of cases (now 13.4 per cent.) can be still further increased by the earlier recognition of the disease by the general practitioner. To this end he should learn to diagnose the condition in its incipient stage. At the same time, the opposition of patients and their friends to early radical operation must be overcome. The laity should understand that cancer of the uterus is curable if attacked under the most favorable conditions.

OPHTHALMOLOGY.

UNDER THE CHARGE OF

EDWARD JACKSON, A.M., M.D.,
OF DENVER, COLORADO,

AND

T. B. SCHNEIDEMAN, A.M., M.D.,
PROFESSOR OF DISEASES OF THE EYE IN THE PHILADELPHIA POLYCLINIC.

The Use of a Mydriatic after the Age of Forty-five.—STARKEY, of Chicago (*Journal of the American Medical Association*, April 25, 1903), concludes that: "No age can be arbitrarily fixed beyond which cycloplegics must not be used, and while they are as necessary in certain cases after forty-five years as they are before, they are required in fewer and fewer cases as life advances. But since there is more danger of glaucoma in the elderly, and as mydriatics tend to increase intraocular tension, these drugs should be used with caution after the age of forty years, and in certain cases should not be used at all."

Of a number of ophthalmologists to whom questions bearing upon this point had been sent by the author, the majority agree in the main with the above conclusion.

Periscopic Lenses.—Percival, Newcastle-on-Tyne (*Arch. of Oph.*, July, 1903), gives the following table for the requisite curvatures of the two surfaces of periscopic lenses. These lenses will be accurately periscopic for all eccentric vision within a solid angle of 50 degrees between — 8 D. and — 14 D. For powers beyond this range extreme eccentric vision will not be so good as centric vision—*e. g.*, with a + 12 D. lens the vision will be distinct within a solid angle of 40 degrees—that is, 20 degrees on either side of the middle line. The index of refraction of the glass is assumed to be 1.54.

Power.	Anterior surface.	Posterior surface.
— 1 D	+ 5.5 D	— 6.5 D
— 2 D	+ 5 D	— 7 D
— 3 D	+ 4.5 D	— 7.5 D
— 4 D	+ 4 D	— 8 D
— 5 D	+ 3.5 D	— 8.5 D
— 6 D	+ 3 D	— 9 D
— 7 D	+ 2.5 D	— 9.5 D
— 8 D	+ 2 D	— 10 D
— 9 D	+ 1 D	— 10 D
— 10 D	Plane	— 10 D
— 12 D	Plane	— 12 D
— 14 D	Plane	— 14 D
— 16 D	— 0.5 D	— 15.5 D
+ 1 D	+ 6 D	— 5 D
+ 2 D	+ 8 D	— 6 D
+ 3 D	+ 10 D	— 7 D
+ 4 D	+ 12 D	— 8 D
+ 5 D	+ 13 D	— 8 D
+ 6 D	+ 15 D	— 9 D
+ 7 D	+ 16.5 D	— 9.5 D
+ 8 D	+ 17.75 D	— 9.75 D
+ 9 D	+ 19.5 D	— 10.5 D
+ 10 D	+ 21 D	— 11 D
+ 12 D	+ 23 D	— 11 D
+ 15 D	+ 27 D	— 12 D

Intraocular Lipæma.—White, of London (*Lancet*, October 10, 1903), reports a case of pronounced diabetes, in which the retinal vessels, both arteries and veins, contained blood of a deep cream color, passing into pale salmon in the larger vessels. The vessels appeared a little larger than usual. The whole retina was pale.

Examination of the blood taken during life showed that, in addition to a precipitated proteid, a substance was present which, although allied to fats, was not a true fat, so that the term "lipæmia" is not strictly correct. As the diabetes improved the color in both sets of vessels became more healthy, and, finally, quite natural.

Similar cases had been previously recorded by Heyl, *Transactions of the American Ophthalmic Society*, 1880; Fraser, *British Medical Journal*, May 23, 1903; and Reis, abstracted in the *Ophthalmoscope*, August, 1903.

Examination of 4608 Railroad Employes for Acuity of Vision, Hearing, and Color Perception.—Murray, of Scranton (*Annals of Ophthalmology*, January, 1903), found that of the above number 3.01 per cent. were color blind, 2.58 per cent. had weak chromatic sense, and 9.44 per cent. were in need of glasses or other means to improve their vision for distance.

OTOLOGY

UNDER THE CHARGE OF

CLARENCE J. BLAKE, M.D.,

OF BOSTON, MASS.,
PROFESSOR OF OTOLOGY, HARVARD UNIVERSITY.

ASSISTED BY

E. A. CROCKETT, M.D., PHILIP HAMMOND, M.D., E. DE WOLF WALES, M.D., AND WALTER A. LE COMPTE, M.D.

Ueber Horubungen Mittlest des Phonographen.—HERMANN GUTZMANN (*Monatsschrift für Ohrenheilkunde*, September, 1902) appreciates the strain upon the voice of the practitioner who undertakes exercises for the improvement of hearing. For this purpose he uses the phonograph. Tubes from the phonograph are placed in the patient's ears and all external sounds and influences excluded. The same exercise at different speeds and intensities are repeated as often as necessary.

The writer reports a case of a child, aged thirteen years, with catarrh of the middle ear as a result of scarlet fever at the age of five years. Since that time the child has developed slowly, is small for her age, head small and elongated, and nose narrow and palate high. A few adenoids present in the vault, she drags her feet when walking, and is slow to learn and is easily tired. The hearing in the left ear is absent. In the right ear tones above B are heard, and perception of the voice impossible, except upon shouting. The mechanical control of the tongue is poor, and in the production of the vowels *u*, *e*, *i*, they are often changed to *a*, *o*, etc. A phonograph was obtained and six cylinders, with letters in different sequences and intensities of tone, were used. In the beginning the vowel *a* was heard correctly; the other vowels and most of the consonants were heard incorrectly. After fifteen days all of the vowels were heard correctly, and a marked improvement in the voice production was evident.

The writer believes that the phonograph can be a great aid in vocal exercises and saves time and also strain upon the voice.—H. D. W.

The Pathological Anatomy of the Temporal Bone.—A. SONNTAG (*Monatsschrift für Ohrenheilkunde*, November, 1902) describes an interesting anomaly of the jugular fossa. The fossa usually extends to the level of the tympanic cavity. In this case he noticed that pressure upon the jugular vein caused a movement of the drum membrane. Investigating further he found that the bulb of the jugular was almost in apposition with the drum membrane and was covered only by mucous membrane. A large defect in the bone occupying part of the posterior half of the internal wall of the tympanum and part of the posterior wall as well was seen. The defect was kidney-shaped and about 9 mm. by 5 mm. in size. The sigmoid sinus was very far anterior. This coincides with Zuckerkandl's view that the deeper the jugular fossa the farther forward is the sinus.

Such a location of the jugular vein is extremely important in case of paracentesis, the danger of injury and infection is evident. The blue color of some membranes has been described, but it would be difficult to recognize such a case in an acute otitis media.

A second interesting specimen was one of complete ankylosis of the malleus and incus, so that the line of the joint could not be seen. Bridges of bone passed to the inner and anterior walls of the tympanic cavity. The promontory, stapes, etc., could not be identified. The mucous membrane was thickened and in the place of the drum membrane a thin layer of bone was found occupying its position. The process was evidently one of osteosclerosis.—H. D. W.

Ueber den Einfluss des Telephonierens auf das Gehoerorgan.—In an exhaustive review of this subject, BRAUNSTEIN (*Archiv f. Ohrenheilkunde*, B. lix., H. 3 und 4) not only collects the conclusions of other writers, but gives the results of his own observations, which were made to include the objective and subjective examination and the reported experience of a large number of telephone operators doing from six to eight hours continuous daily service in the telephone offices in Munich. The conclusion reached is in accord with that of the majority of the writers upon this subject, whom he quotes, and is to the effect that, aside from the mechanical effect of the constant wearing of a telephone headpiece and the influence upon the general nervous system of protracted strained attention, no deleterious effects were produced; on the other hand, there were instances in which, evidenced both by the experience of the telephone operators and by subjective examinations, the hearing, for sounds of moderate intensity, was improved. Of 450 operators examined, 150 had left the service; in no instance was this on account of the prejudicial influence of the telephone upon the hearing, and of those remaining in the service no one was liable to discharge because of increasing disability referable to continuance in the service.—C. J. B.

Recent Theories on Sound Conduction.—TREITEL (*Archives of Otology*, vol. xxxii., No. 5) summarizes the recent contributions to the vexed question of sound transmission through the middle ear, in contradistinction to the theory of Helmholtz of the resonance value of the drumhead and the major transmission through the ossicular chain, and shows that both from a physical and a physiological basis molecule vibrations must be admitted as possible to explain both the limit of sound-perception in the human subject and the transmission through different media to the labyrinthine capsule.

Among the first to doubt the Helmholtz theory of the function of the drumhead and ossicles was Beckman, who sees in this so-called sound-transmitting apparatus only a dampening mechanism for the very unstable labyrinthine fluid, the equlibrium of which he claims is preserved through both the fenestral membranes; in the case of the round window by its elasticity, and in the oval window by adjustment of the complicated control apparatus, the drumhead, muscles of accommodation, and ossicular chain, of which the stapes forms the terminal member. The possibility of sound transmission through the round window as a direct route, Beckman does not admit, and the improvement in hearing by use of an artificial drum-membrane he explains, not by the transmission to the stapes of a larger segment of the sound wave, but by the weighting, artificial control effect, upon the stapes itself. In support of this idea, Beckman further cites the considerable increase in hearing by bone-conduction, with slightly decreased hearing by air-conduction, in cases of acute otitis media with intact drumhead when the drumhead and malleo-incudal movements are partially inhibited and the stapes left, supposedly, free to act.

Zimmerman is of the same opinion as Beckman as to the dampening value of the drumhead and ossicular chain, but for sounds of major intensity only, not for ordinary sound-conduction, which he claims is direct through the promontory wall for all tones, because bone is the best conductor. This proposition leaves out of view the law governing the loss of force in the translation of sound waves from one medium to another, a loss which would variously affect the partials of any compound sound wave. As an offset to this is the claim that the equilibrium of the labyrinthine fluid is maintained only through the membrane of the round window, which, because of its structure and surroundings, can only be displaced outward and cannot be regarded as a medium for the transmission of sound waves in the opposite direction.

Zimmerman further questions the conclusions arrived at by Helmholtz and Politzer in their tests of the sympathetic movements of the individual ossicles by means of an organ-pipe tone, on the ground that the sounding body was hermetically attached to the external auditory canal and that the effects produced were those under increased air pressure; he denies, on both physical and physiological grounds, the capacity of the drumhead to react to sound of great amplitude of vibration, and regards the sympathetic vibration of the drumhead as a resonator membrane to all tones as impossible, and endeavors to explain, upon the basis of his theory of bone-conduction solely, the phenomena of lengthened bone-conduction in cases where the drumhead is absent, of improvement in hearing in such cases by application of an artificial drumhead and of paracusis.

Lucae, among others who seek to maintain the theory of sound-transmission through a middle-ear conducting mechanism, is directly opposed to the exclusive bone-conduction theory of Zimmerman, holding that while the sound waves pass directly to the labyrinth wall they are so dampened by the drumhead as to be inoperative, and that the round-window membrane is capable of responding to and transmitting sound waves, as demonstrated in the investigations of Johannes Müller.

Kleinschmidt regards the middle ear, including the mastoid cells, as an air chamber for the transmission of sound waves, the resonating effect of that cavity when filled with air under the normal condition of a patent Eustachian tube being a matter of little importance. He doubts the transmission of all notes through the ossicular chain, on account of the minimum amplitude of many of the appreciated tones, and also the ability of the accommodative muscles to act with a rapidity equivalent to the rapid succession of sounds, provided that the transmitting apparatus act as a whole. Accepting the proposition that the membrane of the round window can be set in vibration only by waves conveyed to it through the medium of the air in the middle ear, and that the stapes, with the drumhead, is actuated by low tones, this action coming later than the movement in the labyrinthine fluid due to movement of the membrane of the round window, he considers the ossicular chain to have a dampening effect, the intrinsic muscles having no other office than that of protection of the labyrinth from excessive impulses.

Dennert, by experiments with tuning-forks vibrating in air and fluids, and Kaiser, by experiments with immersed telephones, seek to support the theory of Helmholtz, the former concluding that in air-conduction an external auxiliary apparatus especially adapted for the transmission of sound-vibration to the labyrinthine fluid is necessary, and the latter that while molecular vibration plays a part in the sound-transmission, the Helmholtz theory of mass-vibration is capable of normal acceptance.

The latest contribution to this discussion is the work of Secchi, who maintained more than ten years ago that the only access of sound waves to the labyrinth from the air in the middle ear was through the membrane of the round window, and who further maintains, as the result of clinical observations, supplementing laboratory experiments, that the drumhead serves only as a sound check or as a passive regulator of pressure, the ossicles, under action of the intrinsic muscles, regulating the intratympanic pressure during attentive hearing and serving as a protective apparatus against the effect of major excursions upon the labyrinth.—C. J. B.

PATHOLOGY AND BACTERIOLOGY.

UNDER THE CHARGE OF

SIMON FLEXNER, M.D.,

DIRECTOR OF THE ROCKEFELLER INSTITUTE FOR MEDICAL RESEARCH, NEW YORK.

ASSISTED BY

WARFIELD T. LONGCOPE, M.D.,

RESIDENT PATHOLOGIST, PENNSYLVANIA HOSPITAL.

The Dwarf Tapeworm (Hymenolipsis Nana), a Newly Recognized and Probably Rather Common American Parasite.—STILES (*New York Medical Journal*, 1903, vol. lxxviii. p. 877). The dwarf tapeworm was first described in France by Dujardin, in 1845, as a parasite of the brown rat, but the term mus decumanus, which Dujardin gave to the parasite, cannot stand, since, in 1789, Gmelin used it for a different parasite. The correct name is hymenolipsis nana. About 100 cases have thus far been recorded in man, the greatest majority of them being reported from Sicily, where it is estimated that 10 per cent. of the children are infected. Before 1902 only two or three cases had been recognized in this country, but within the year the author has diagnosed the parasite in 18 infected individuals, living principally in the Southern States. Since September, 1902, the Hygienic Laboratory has examined about 3500 patients for intestinal parasites, and while "tænia solium" was not found in a single instance, and "tænia saginata" but twice, the dwarf tapeworm was discovered sixteen times. The dwarf tapeworm measures from one-fifth to slightly less than two inches in length; it has four suckers on the head and a crown of hooks. The presence of three testicles in each segment is characteristic for the genus hymenolipsis. The eggs are quite characteristic and have two distinct membranes. It has been shown by Grassi and others that in rats the life cycle of this tapeworm takes place in the intestinal villi, and it is probable that in man autoinfection occurs, either per os and anum or by reverse peristalsis, development of the eggs through an intermediary host being unnecessary. The method of primary infection is not definitely known, but it is assumed that it occurs through the droppings of infected rats or mice in pantries and kitchens, where bread and other food may become contaminated. The dwarf tapeworm inhabits the ileum and may be present in thousands or only in very small numbers.

The symptoms produced by its presence are usually slight and may be absent altogether. Severe symptoms, however, such as persistent diarrhœa, epileptiform attacks, etc., occasionally are seen. Perhaps 10 to 12 per cent. of the cases exhibit severe nervous symptoms. The diagnosis is readily made by finding the characteristic eggs in the stools. Male fern is the only drug which has met with any degree of success in the treatment of the affection. Prevention of infection is secured by cleanly personal habits and by keeping mice and rats away from food supplies.

Localization of the Pneumococcus.—WANDEL (*Deut. Arch. f. klin. Med.*, 1903, vol. lxxviii. p. 1) reviews the literature concerning the localization of purulent infections secondary to pneumonia, and reports in detail four cases of acute pneumococcic endocarditis and three cases of pneumococcic pyæmia, with joint or heart lesions following chronic pneumococcic pneumonia. An attempt was made to trace the passage of the bacteria from the lung into the general blood stream. The fact that in pneumonia the bronchial glands are frequently swollen, and often hemorrhagic suggested that the pigmented lymph glands might act as a locus minoris resistentia for the development of the pneumococcus. In the above cases the lymph glands at the root of the lungs showed more or less coal pigmentation, with swelling and softening, and in one or two instances presented small abscesses. Pneumococci were found in great numbers in cultures and cover-slips from the pus of these abscesses, although they could only be grown in extremely small numbers from the lungs themselves. Under such conditions the normal filtration apparatus of the glands is materially interfered with, and bacteria are allowed to pass freely either into the thoracic duct or into the small bloodvessels of the lymph gland, thereby gaining entrance into the general circulation. This opinion was confirmed by microscopic examination, and the author believes that the origin of general systemic infections and purulent inflammations complicating pneumonia at a distance from the lungs is thus adequately explained.

A Delicate Test for the Demonstration of Bile Pigments in Urine.—JOLLES (*Deut. Arch. f. klin. Med.*, 1903, Bd. lxxviii. p. 135) has made certain modifications in the method which he formerly used to detect the presence of bile pigments in urine, and has found that this modification increases the reliability and delicacy of the reaction.

About 10 c.c. of urine are shaken in a test-tube with 2 to 3 c.c. of chloroform and 1 c.c. of a 10 per cent. solution of barium chloride. The mixture is then centrifugalized and the fluid above the sediment and chloroform drawn off with a pipette. Water is now added and the chloroform and sediment washed, the whole centrifugalized, and the water removed by a pipette. Next 5 c.c. of alcohol are added and shaken well with the chloroform, after which 2 to 3 drops of an iodine solution are put into the mixture, and the whole filtered. If even the slightest trace of bile is present the fluid, after a few moments' standing, assumes a characteristic greenish color. If the urine is highly concentrated the reaction is best obtained by heating the mixture at 70° C. over a water bath before filtering. The reaction is not interfered with, either by indican or hæmoglobin. The iodine solution is prepared in the following manner: 0.63 gr. of iodine and 0.75 gr. of bichloride of mercury are dissolved separately in 125 c.c. of alcohol, the two solutions brought together, and the volume made up to 250 c.c. with concentrated hydrochloric acid. If the iodine solution is protected from the light in dark bottles it keeps indefinitely.

The Role of the Omentum in the Course of General Infections.—SIMON (*Presse Méd.*, 1903, T. ii. p. 726). It is already known that the omentum plays a very significant part in the cicatrization of abdominal wounds, in protecting torn or sutured peritoneal surfaces, and in walling off local infections of the peritoneum from the general cavity, but the changes in the omentum during a general infection have received but little attention. Simon found, after subcutaneous injections of lethal doses of diphtheria toxin, followed by injections of antitoxic serum, that the omentum reacted much as the spleen does under such conditions. Diapedesis of red blood corpuscles, migration of the polymorphonuclear leukocytes from the bloodvessels, and production of large phagocytic cells were noted, while, later, accumulations of plasma cells were seen about the bloodvessels. After four or five days the reaction subsides and the omentum gradually assumes its normal appearance.

The omentum in man was found to undergo much the same series of changes in diphtheria and in variola, although the intensity of the reaction varied somewhat in the individual cases. The author concludes that the omentum does not remain inert, even in general infections, and believes that it plays a definite part in the defence of the organism and probably in the development of immunity.

An Experimental Study of Nephrotoxins.—PEARCE (*Univ. of Penna. Med. Bull.*, 1903, vol. xvi. p. 217) says the subject of nephrotoxins has been studied in a somewhat superficial manner, particularly by the French and Italian observers, and the author in his work has repeated many of the experiments of Nefidieef, Castaign and Rathery, Ascoli and Figari, and others, frequently arriving at results which warranted conclusions quite different from those of the authors just cited. It was found impossible to produce an autonephrotoxin in rabbits or rats by several methods employed. Ligation of the ureter or of the entire pedicle of one kidney brought about only such lesions in the opposite kidney as occurred after unilateral nephrectomy, namely, a compensatory hypertrophy. It was equally impossible to produce an isonephrotoxin either by injections of serum from animals treated in the manner just described into other animals of the same species or by injecting serum produced by inoculating one animal's kidney into another animal of the same species. With heteronephrotoxins the conditions were found to be quite different. When the serum from a rabbit, which had been treated with successive doses of dog's kidney, was injected into dogs, these animals developed a pronounced acute nephritis, evidenced by the appearance of albumin and numerous casts in the urine, together with a marked hæmoglobinuria. Control experiments made by injecting dogs with the serum of normal rabbits produced no such effect. Since the heteronephrotoxic serum was hæmolytic *in vitro* for dog's erythrocytes it was thought that possibly a part of the renal disturbance might be dependent upon this factor; and to exclude this possibility the dog's kidneys were thoroughly washed before the immunizing doses were given to rabbits. By this means a serum was produced in rabbits which set up an intense albuminuria with numerous casts, both conditions persisting for many days, but did not give rise to hæmoglobinuria. The histological lesions in the kidneys resulting from the injections of this toxic serum consisted in an extensive granular degeneration of the convoluted tubules and a fatty metamorphosis limited almost exclusively to the loops of Henle. Granular and hyaline casts were found in the tubules of the kidney, and minor changes occurred in the glomeruli. The heteronephrotoxic serum was found to be active after heating for half an hour at 56° C. Serum prepared from the cortex of the kidney proved to be much more toxic than that obtained by injections of the medullary portions. If the liver of dogs, instead of the kidney, was used for immunizing purposes a serum was obtained which gave rise to symptoms and lesions; when injected into dogs, similar to those called forth by inoculations of heteronephrotoxic serum. In the course of the experiments several dogs were found which were the subjects of a spontaneous nephritis; and it was discovered that their blood serum was capable of giving rise to an acute nephritis when injected into healthy dogs. This effect could be produced even to the second remove. All attempts to produce chronic renal lesions by successive inoculations of heteronephrotoxic sera were unsuccessful. No immediate effect was noted upon the blood pressure following injections of heteronephrotoxic sera into dogs or of isonephrotoxic sera into rabbits. From the foregoing experiments the author believes that the correlative action of different kinds of serum upon different body cells is demonstrable and that specificity is a function of receptors and not of cells in their entirety.

HYGIENE AND PUBLIC HEALTH.

UNDER THE CHARGE OF

CHARLES HARRINGTON, M.D.,

ASSISTANT PROFESSOR OF HYGIENE, HARVARD MEDICAL SCHOOL.

Effects of Compressed Air on the System.—Drs. Leonard Hill and J. J. R. Macleod (*Journal of Hygiene*, October, 1903, p. 401) have made an experimental study of the action of compressed air, which leads them to the conclusion that with proper choice of men and regulation of the shift and decompression period work can be carried on without loss of life at a depth as great as 200 feet, at which depth the pressure will exceed 100 pounds per square inch, or about 7 atmospheres. Their experiments with animals show that compressed air above 5 atmospheres lessens the output of carbon dioxide and lowers the body temperature, and that oxygen at and above 1 atmosphere has the same effect. It is a sign of oxygen poisoning. Compressed air at 10 atmospheres is more damaging, at least to small animals, than oxygen at 2 atmospheres. It increases the loss of body heat, because it is a better condnetor and because it is saturated with moisture. The saturation of the air in caissons with moisture does not prevent evaporation from the body, because the skin temperature is higher than that of the air, and the wet air increases the heat loss by dampening the clothes or fur. Highly compressed air may possibly interfere with the diffusion of carbon dioxide from the alveolar air, and may, owing to increased friction, hinder the passage of air in and out of the air-tubes. The nitrogen output in dogs is not altered in any noteworthy degree by exposure to 8 atmospheres for six hours. Inflammation and consolidation of the lungs are produced by exposure to 8 atmospheres for twenty-four hours, or to 1.5 atmospheres of pure oxygen; and the higher the oxygen tension the more rapidly the inflammation ensues. It does not seem likely that inflammation of the lungs is produced with the pressures and length of exposure usual in caissons. The cause of caisson sickness is the escape of gas bubbles in the bloodvessels and tissue fluids during decompression, but recompression causes them to go into solution again, and if it is applied quickly enough the circulation rebegins. After death following rapid decompression, the bubbles can be seen in the bloodvessels, heart, retinæ, aqueous humor, connective-tissue spaces, and elsewhere, and the alimentary canal is blown out with gas. The varying symptoms of caisson sickness are due to the varying seat of the air emboli. Owing to the elasticity of their tissues and to the greater facility for collateral pathways of circulation, young men escape the sickness, so that by choosing suitable men and regulating carefully the periods of compression and decompression, caisson and divers' sickness can be avoided. Gradual decompression is most important, and, provided two hours are spent in decompression, animals can safely be exposed to 8 atmospheres for four hours.

Factors which Determine the Local Incidence of Fatal Infantile Diarrhœa.—DR. H. MEREDITH RICHARDS (*Journal of Hygiene*, July, 1903, p. 325) calls attention to the fact that the various problems of infantile mortality are, with the continued fall in the birth rate, calculated to assume even greater practical importance in the near future, and that of these problems none is more in need of solution than the exact etiology of infantile diarrhœal diseases. He discusses the influence of methods of feeding, seasonal incidence and meteorological relations, influence of social status, physiography, pollntion of the soil and its effects, and concludes that fatal infantile diarrhœa is usually a form of food-poisoning; that infection usually takes place at the home; that urban conditions are chiefly hazardous from the amount of polluted soil found in the roads and yards of urban districts; that infinite care is needed if babies are to be hand-fed in towns; and that practical preventive measures should include (*a*) impermeable roads with efficient channelling, (*b*) copious swilling of roads, (*c*) education of mothers as to the necessity of scrupulous cleanliness, (*d*) the co-operative or municipal provision of specially prepared modified milk, which should be sterilized during the diarrhœal season, (*e*) a more efficient control of the milk trade, with special reference to the provision of cooled, approximately sterile milk from healthy cows, and (*f*) the provision of houses which shall be sufficiently convenient to allow of their being cleansed with the least possible expenditure of energy.

Dr. Arthur Newsholme (*Public Health*, August, 1903, p. 654) asserts that much of the relative immunity from diarrhœa at Brighton, England, in 1902, was due to the rainfall, for frequent rains during the summer weeks, even though the total fall be not great, is one of the most effectual means of keeping down the diarrhœa death rate. The obvious course to pursue is, then, in time of drought, to replace the natural scavenging of rain by municipal scavenging; that is to say, by wetting the dusty streets, thus converting the dust into mud, and gathering and removing the mud, rather than merely sprinkling water to lay the dust. With regard to soil temperatures at a depth of four feet, which are regarded as an important index of the possibility of prevalence of epidemic diarrhœa, he shows that Ballard's rule that diarrhœa must be expected when the soil temperature at a depth of four feet reaches 56° F. is fallacious, for on June 24th the temperature was 56° F.; on June 30th it was 58.4° F.; during the second half of July it was between 60° F. and 61° F.; in August it reached 61.8° F.; on September 10th it reached the maximum, 62.6° F., and then, slowly falling, it kept above 56° F. until October 19th, when it dropped to 55.8° F.; but no deaths occurred from diarrhœa, and, contrary to the rule, the highest number of deaths from diarrhœa occurred three weeks later than the week in which the soil temperature attained its mean weekly maximum. "The temperature conditions were favorable to diarrhœa; the rainfall prevented it. The facts for the present year justify the conclusion that rainfall is more important than temperature in relation to epidemic diarrhœa."

Dr. Herbert Peck, M. O. H. for Chesterfield (*Ibid.*, p. 655) is also of the same mind, for he ascribes the low death rate from diarrhœa in his district in 1902 in great part to the frequent showers. The amount of rain is of less importance than the number of showers, as is shown by a table of the rainfall for eight years. He concludes that frequent watering of the streets and roads in the more populous parts of the district would do much to prevent deaths from this cause.

[The first to call attention to the influence of rainfall on the death rate from diarrhœal diseases was Dr. E. W. Hope, who, in 1899, made known that at Liverpool during a period of twenty years the highest death rate occurred in the driest summer and the lowest in the wettest. The fourteen years in which the mean summer rainfall was 10.9 inches showed an average rate of about 50 per cent. higher mortality than the six wet years, with a mean rainfall of 13.8 inches for the corresponding months.—C. H.]

The Relation of Sulphur in Illuminating Gas to Air Vitiation.—The oppressive quality of air which is much vitiated by combustion of illuminating gas is the subject of an interesting contribution by Dr. J. S. Haldane (*Journal of Hygiene*, July, 1903, p. 382), who excludes the carbon dioxide produced by combustion and the attendant decrease in oxygen and increase in temperature as the causes thereof. The quantity of sulphur in ordinary gas is so small that his hypothesis that this substance is the cause of the unpleasantness may, he says, at first sight seem improbable. English gas contains, as a rule, less than 20 grains of sulphur per 100 cubic feet, and hence, as gas forms about half its volume of carbon dioxide in burning, the products of combustion would contain less than ½ gram of sulphur per 500 litres of carbon dioxide, and this would yield about 1 gram, or ⅓ of a litre, of sulphur dioxide to 500 litres of carbon dioxide, or 1 volume in 1500. Hence, air vitiated by gas combustion to the extent of 30 parts of carbon dioxide per 10,000 would contain less than 0.02 sulphur dioxide, or 1 part in 500,000, which proportion is not very much smaller than Lehmann found would produce perceptible irritation of the nose and throat. Part of the sulphur is, however, in Haldane's opinion, present as sulphuric acid and in a particulate form, in which condition it has not the same specific taste as sulphurous acid, but is extremely irritating and unpleasant. In order to investigate the relation between the proportion of sulphur in gas and the unpleasantness of air vitiated by the products of combustion, he made a series of experiments, which proved that the degree of unpleasantness varies directly with the amount of sulphur, and that gas which is purified of its carbon disulphide is greatly superior, from the hygienic standpoint, to that which is purified only of its hydrogen sulphide. Unfortunately, no process is known which will remove all of the sulphur from gas; but were it possible to do this, there would be no objection to the free use of gas for both heating and lighting and to the escape of the products of combustion into the room. He found that the air of a room in which good oil was burned in a lamp was not noticeably unpleasant, apart from the heat, even where the carbon dioxide rose to 75 parts per 10,000; but that when gas was burned the air was distinctly unpleasant when vitiated to the extent of 30 to 40 parts of carbon dioxide per 10,000, and very unpleasant when this impurity rose to 60 parts.

The Relationship of Human and Bovine Tuberculosis.—MESSRS. D. J. HAMILTON and J. MCLAUCHLAN YOUNG (*Transactions of the Highland and Agricultural Society of Scotland*, 1903, and *Public Health*, September, 1903, p. 689) undertook a series of twenty experiments designed to test the validity of the assertion that human tuberculosis differs so much from bovine that it cannot be transmitted to calves, and arrived at the following conclusions: 1. Although human tuberculosis is probably not so virulent for the calf as that derived from bovines, yet it can readily be inoculated upon that animal. 2. This holds good whether the tubercle inoculated be derived from tubercular lymph glands, tubercular lung, tubercular sputum, or tubercular urine. 3. It produces this positive result irrespective of whether it be introduced by feeding the animal with the tubercular material, by subcutaneous inoculation upon a peripheral part, by respiring a spray containing the bacillus, or by injection into the venous system. 4. The organs most affected are those in immediate connection with the part operated upon. 5. The lymphatic system is constantly involved in the resulting tuberculosis. 6. When administered by the mouth, tubercular sputum induces an abdominal lymph-gland tuberculosis without necessarily involving the intestine in any way. 7. When tuberculosis from a human source has been ingrafted upon a calf, it grows enormously in virulence by being reinoculated upon a second calf. 8. The morphological characters of the bacillus may vary according to circumstances, and are no guide to the source of the organism under observation. 9. The above facts go to favor the view that the human bacillus and that of bovines are identical, but modified somewhat by their environment, and directly contradict the results alleged to have been obtained by Koch and Schütz.

Prophylaxis of Malaria.—At the Eleventh International Congress of Hygiene and Demography, at Brussels, September 2–8, 1903, PROFESSOR A. CELLI recommended as prophylactic measures against malaria the production of artificial immunity by means of quinine, disinfection of the blood of malarial persons with quinine, mechanical protection of dwellings and of exposed parts of the body, isolation of patients, destruction of anopheles, and drainage for the destruction of their breeding places. For the production of artificial immunity, he recommended either daily doses of 5 or 6 grains of quinine (children half as much) or weekly doses of 15 grains on Saturday and Sunday evenings. The daily dose is more efficient and less unpleasant, and its action is cumulative and produces an almost complete mithridatism. The specific disinfection of the blood requires long treatment and especial care in pre-epidemic times. The Italian Government prepares quinine salts and sells them throughout the kingdom at lowest prices to apothecaries, tobacconists, and salt dealers. The peasants who work in malarial districts are supplied free of cost to themselves, the landowners being charged for it. Laborers on public works can have all they need, and the contractors for whom they work are held accountable for all deaths due to lack of supply.

The Use of Chemical Preservatives in Foods.—In a communication before the International Congress of Medicine, at Madrid, PROFESSOR BROUARDEL (*Annales d'hygiène publique et de médecine légale*, 1903, vol. xlix. p. 420) maintained that the claim made by those interested in the addition of chemical preservatives to foods, that the amounts employed are too small to produce harmful results, and that the substances used cannot be classed as harmful, because they are employed extensively as drugs in medical practice with good results, should be quite ignored and disregarded. He relates that Dubrisay has reported the finding of as much as 2 grams of salicylic acid per litre of wine, 1.25 grams per litre of beer, and 1.6 grams per kilo of butter. He regards the establishment of a maximum permissible amount of antiseptics as not worthy of consideration, since prolonged use of them may act injuriously and escape detection as the real offender. That acute poisoning has not been observed is no argument in their favor, for obviously any substance which could cause acute symptoms in the amounts used would be avoided.

THE

AMERICAN JOURNAL

OF THE MEDICAL SCIENCES.

MARCH, 1904.

PERINEAL ZOSTER, WITH NOTES UPON CUTANEOUS SEGMENTATION POSTAXIAL TO THE LOWER LIMB.

BY HARVEY CUSHING, M.D.,
ASSOCIATE PROFESSOR OF SURGERY IN JOHNS HOPKINS UNIVERSITY, BALTIMORE, MD.

THE infrequency of herpes zoster in the cutaneous areas supplied by the sacral nerves may be gathered from Henry Head's comparatively recent tabulation in Allbutt's *System of Medicine*.[1] Of the 378 cases which his exceptional opportunities have enabled him personally to observe, in seven instances only did the lesion occur in the sacral areas: once in the first, once in the second, and five times in the third segmental distribution.

If I am not at fault, the eruption which occurred in the first of the cases to be described corresponded to a lesion of the fourth (possibly of the fourth and fifth) posterior root ganglion. It is not unusual in zoster for an outlying area of hyperæsthesia to give evidence of some disturbance with the adjoining ganglia: so here there were indications that the third and second sacral were involved, the lesion, however, not being sufficient to occasion an herpetic rash. I had originally thought that the fifth sacral alone was represented by the outcrop of vesicles in this case, believing from a study of segmental cord lesions that had the fourth been involved the area would have included the posterior and lower part of the scrotum. Dr. Bardeen, however, assured me, from his reconstruction studies of the plexus in the embryo, that only in case the fifth sacral was here of the prefixed type could it have supplied this region in the perineum.

[1] System of Medicine, 1899, vol. viii. p. 616.

I am unaware that a case of zoster limited to this particular territory has been described. The clinical history follows:

The patient, Mr. J. P. B., aged fifty-three years, consulted me in July, 1903, for a right-sided trigeminal neuralgia of ten years' standing. The paroxysms, having originated in the area of the N. infraorbitalis, had finally involved the other two divisions of the fifth nerve. He presented the usual pitiable appearance of those who suffer from this fearful malady in its major form.

On July 27th, under chloroform anæsthesia, the right ganglion was removed *in toto*. The case proving to be an exceptionally bloodless one, the extirpation was more rapid and easy than usual. During the final steps, in elevating the superior dural envelope from the ganglion, in order to expose the sensory root, the customary escape of a small amount of cerebrospinal fluid took place. No other events seem particularly deserving of mention here. A small rubber protective drain was left in the posterior inferior angle of the incision, a provisional suture having been taken at its site.

On the following day, July 28th, the drain was removed and the provisional suture tied. There had been an abundant escape of cerebrospinal fluid. Patient comfortable, except for persisting nausea. Highest temperature 100° F. It was presumed that he would have the usual rapid and uneventful recovery so characteristic of these cases.

July 29th (second day). Patient complains of some frontal headache, confined to the unoperated side;[1] this was accredited to the escape of cerebrospinal fluid of the preceding day. Temperature 98.6° F.

30th. As usual on the third day the fine interrupted sutures were removed from the incision and a collodion dressing applied. There was no reaction about the wound. Complaint of some discomfort in back.

August 1st (fourth day). Severe backache, with pain running down back of legs to calf. Cannot be comfortable.

3d. Left frontal headache continues. Severe backache, with great soreness of muscles. Paquelin cautery brushed over lumbar region without giving relief. Patient can hardly move himself in bed, body or legs, without great pain. Sedatives. A few herpetic blisters forming on upper lip and ala of nose of left (sound) side (Fig. 1).

4th (seventh day). Attention called for first time by orderly to a "rash," which has appeared on the patient's perineum. Examination disclosed in the areas indicated by the accompanying diagram

[1] It is a point in favor of the dural origin of headache that should they occur from one cause or another after ganglion operations, provided the extirpation is complete or the trigeminal root has been divided, they are, according to my experience, invariably hemicranial and referred to the sound side. The dura, as well as the face, receives its sensory supply from the N. trigeminus, and, except for the region about the foramen magnum (pneumogastric supply), becomes anæsthetic on the side of operation.

(Fig 2) a crop of newly formed and forming vesicles confined to the right side and most numerous about the margin of the anus. Thence they spread anteriorly as far forward as the posterior edge of the scrotum, and externally as far as the tuber ischii, the most external vesicle being about 6 cm. from the median raphe, with the legs in the position of the photograph. There were no vesicles on the scrotum; none on the penis; none within a radius of 3 cm. from the tip of the coccyx. Two very suspicious small red spots, which might have been broken vesicles, were present on the skin over the sacrum, just below the level of the right posterior inferior iliac spines. I could not be certain of their nature, for this was the area of the patient's maximal pain and "soreness," and it had been brushed over the day before with the Paquelin cautery.[1]

FIG. 1.

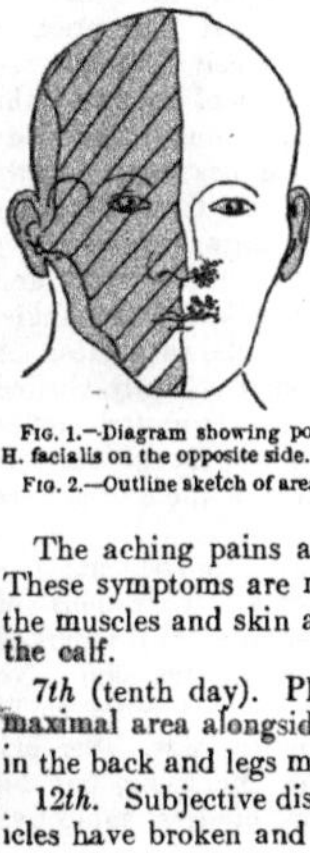

FIG. 2.

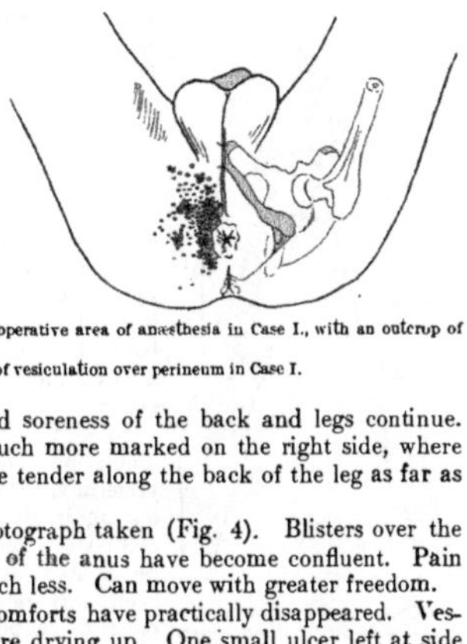

FIG. 1.—Diagram showing postoperative area of anæsthesia in Case I., with an outcrop of H. facialis on the opposite side.

FIG. 2.—Outline sketch of area of vesiculation over perineum in Case I.

The aching pains and soreness of the back and legs continue. These symptoms are much more marked on the right side, where the muscles and skin are tender along the back of the leg as far as the calf.

7th (tenth day). Photograph taken (Fig. 4). Blisters over the maximal area alongside of the anus have become confluent. Pain in the back and legs much less. Can move with greater freedom.

12th. Subjective discomforts have practically disappeared. Vesicles have broken and are drying up. One small ulcer left at side and slightly anterior to the anal margin. Patient sitting up with some degree of comfort for the first time, with "no pain, just soreness." There is still some tenderness present on the supporting surface while sitting; the area of eruption, however, hardly overlaps onto this area, the vesicles barely reaching the tuberosity of the ischium in the sitting posture. When the patient stands the eruption

[1] If, as is presumed, these were true herpetic vesicles they may be taken to represent the posterior primary division.

is hardly visible, being concealed in this position between the mesial surfaces of the buttocks (Fig. 3).

It is quite possible to delineate the cutaneous areas of disturbed sensation over the buttock and back of the right leg (Fig. 3) by gently pinching the skin; similarly the muscular areas of soreness by pressure. The cutaneous areas, although tests with the hair æsthesiometer and graded thermic tests show that there is considerable actual tactile and thermic hypæsthesia, nevertheless are hyperæsthetic to painful stimuli, pressure, pinching, pricking or scratching with pin, etc. This area of "painful hypæsthesia" includes the lower portion of the right half of the scrotum, as well as the territory shown in Fig. 3 over the gluteofemoral region. The area of maximal tenderness, both surface and deep, lies over the sacrum, just below the level of the posterior iliac spine. The muscles underlying the entire territory are tender ("sore") on pressure well down on to the calf. No evidence of disturbed sensation of the sole of the foot could be made out. The body temperature, which has been slightly subnormal since the third day, has again reached the normal point.

FIG. 3.

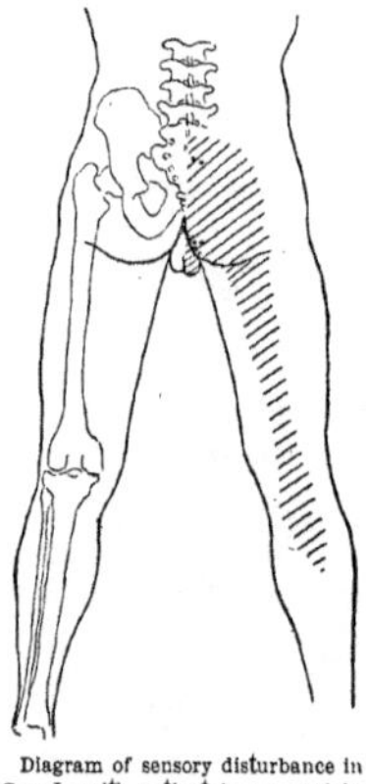

Diagram of sensory disturbance in Case I., with patient in an upright posture, showing the few vesicles at the edge of the buttock, which were visible in this attitude. Shaded area indicates the hyperæsthetic zone, presumably S. II. and S. III.

The deep reflexes are present and active both at the knee and ankle. They are equal on the two sides. A normal plantar reflex is easily elicited on either side. No cremasteric reflex could be brought out, though the vermicular movements of the dartos were active.

13th. Continued improvement. Examination confirms observations of yesterday. Hyperæsthetic area marked out again by pinching the skin. No cremasteric and no anal reflex could be elicited on either side. Sensory symptoms remain the same, but the patient complains of less subjective discomfort.

24th (twenty-eighth day). For the past week the patient has been absolutely free from subjective sensations. There is no trace at present of the hyperæsthetic zone corresponding to the second and third sacral areas. The scars of the eruption are not tender. Some diminution of thermic sense alone persists in patches over the area occupied by these scars. The anal and cremasteric reflexes have returned.

The patient has gained seventeen and one-half pounds in weight since August 10th (fourteen days).

In my personal series of twenty cases of Gasserian ganglion extirpation, this is the second time in which an herpetic eruption has occurred as an evident sequel of the operative procedure. The earlier case consequently may be deserving of mention here, for, although the eruption of vesicles was entirely confined to the areas of the trigeminal and cervical nerves, a bilateral hyperæsthesia of the fourth and fifth sacral territories accompanied it. In the light of the more recent observation, I cannot believe otherwise than that the process was occasioned by some disturbance with the lower sacral posterior root ganglia, which stopped short of causing an herpetic eruption.

The case in brief is as follows:

Case II.—The patient, Alexander D., aged thirty-eight years, entered the Johns Hopkins Hospital in January, 1900. He was suffering with a severe right-sided trigeminal neuralgia, which had thrice recurred after peripheral operations, and had finally involved all three divisions of the nerve. A suboccipital extension was also present.

On January 15th the right ganglion was removed *in toto*. The extirpation presented no great difficulties, although the case was a bloody one. The wound was closed without drainage, as the oozing ceased after removing the ganglion.

His convalescence promised to be without incident. The temperature registered 100° F. the day ofter the operation, its highest point. The sutures were removed from the wound on the third day. It apparently was healing without reaction. He was allowed to be up and about the following day. Temperature normal.

Five days later—that is, on the ninth day after operation, he exposed himself in a chilly bath-room during his morning ablutions and sneezed violently three times. He immediately cried out with severe pain in the head, spine, and down the back of his legs. He had a chill, during which his temperature rose to 104.8° F., but fell again after a few hours to normal, where it remained.

In forty-eight hours an extensive crop of herpes had developed, with a distribution as follows (Fig. 5): On the left side of the face, chiefly on the nose, upper lip, and cheek (second division of the N. trigeminus), and also on the neck overlapping the angle of the jaw (N. auricularis magnus, third or second cervical) were large areas of closely placed vesicles, many of which subsequently became confluent. On the right side also was a symmetrically placed patch (cervical distribution) near the angle of the jaw, entirely outside of the postoperative area of anæsthesia (Fig. 5). Of course, no eruption of the nature of true zoster could occur in the right trigeminal area. In addition to this extensive bilateral outcrop of vesicles, with its attendant discomforts about the head, pain and paræsthesia were complained of at the opposite pole of the body, and on examination it was found that a symmetrical area (Fig. 6), including the margin

FIG. 4.

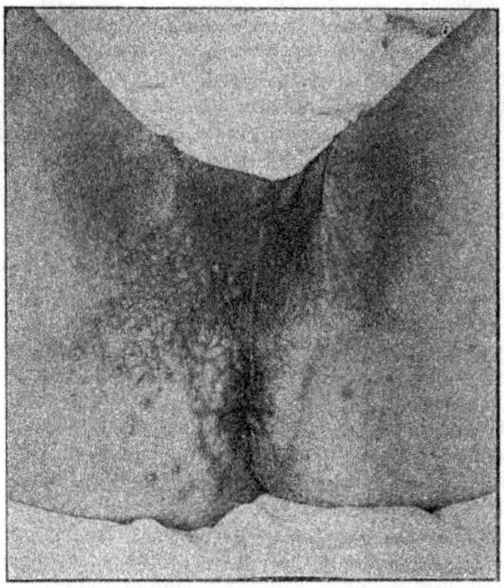

Photograph of perineal zoster in Case I., showing condition of eruption on the third day after its appearance.

FIG. 5.

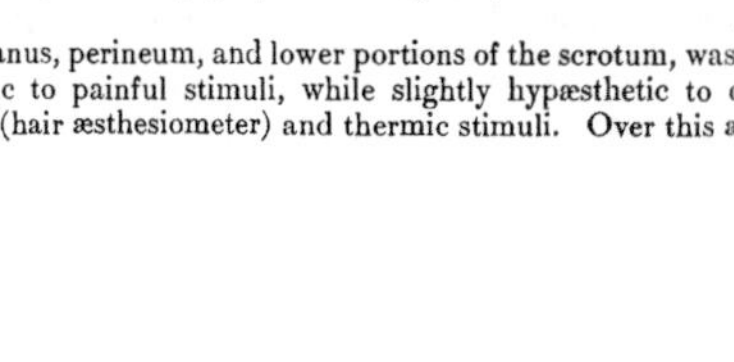

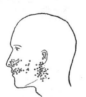

CASE II.—Distribution of facial and bilateral cervical herpes. Note that the postoperative anæsthetic area remains free, indicating that the other eruptions presumably originated from lesions in the posterior root ganglia (cervical and trigeminal).

of the anus, perineum, and lower portions of the scrotum, was hyperæsthetic to painful stimuli, while slightly hypæsthetic to delicate tactile (hair æsthesiometer) and thermic stimuli. Over this area the patient experienced a most disagreeable sensation of formication. An herpetic rash was anticipated, and though it did not materialize, I nevertheless considered that the condition was resultant to a lesion of the corresponding posterior root ganglion (herpes zoster, without the eruption).[1]

Some tenderness of skin and muscles on pressure existed over the buttocks and down the back of the legs, extending on one side as far as the sole of the foot. These symptoms all cleared up in the course of a few days, together with the disappearance of the herpetic eruption on the face. It was necessary, however, to catheterize the patient for some time after the onset of the attack.

FIG. 6.

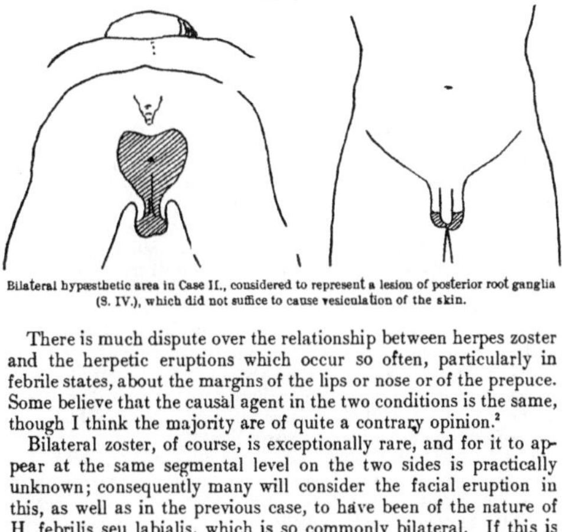

Bilateral hypæsthetic area in Case II., considered to represent a lesion of posterior root ganglia (S. IV.), which did not suffice to cause vesiculation of the skin.

There is much dispute over the relationship between herpes zoster and the herpetic eruptions which occur so often, particularly in febrile states, about the margins of the lips or nose or of the prepuce. Some believe that the causal agent in the two conditions is the same, though I think the majority are of quite a contrary opinion.[2]

Bilateral zoster, of course, is exceptionally rare, and for it to appear at the same segmental level on the two sides is practically unknown; consequently many will consider the facial eruption in this, as well as in the previous case, to have been of the nature of H. febrilis seu labialis, which is so commonly bilateral. If this is so, there can be little doubt, from these observations, but that the

[1] Although "herpes zoster" would be an absurd misnomer for such conditions, there being neither a rash nor a girdle-like distribution, James Mackenzie (Some Points Bearing on the Association of Sensory Disorders and Visceral Disease, Brain, 1893, vol. xvi. p. 344) nevertheless contends that essentially the same disease of the posterior ganglia may be present without producing vesiculation of the skin, the pain and sensory disorders alone indicating the nature of the lesion and its site.

[2] Those inclining to one or the other view are cited in Spitzer's recent Sammel-Referate, Neuere Erfahrungen über den Herpes Zoster, Centralblatt f. d. Grenzgebiete d. Med. u. Chir., 1901, Bd. iv. p. 548.

presence of the Ganglion semilunare, which is the cranial homologue of the spinal posterior root ganglia, is essential for the production of herpetic eruptions of this nature, since in both cases the cutaneous area rendered anæsthetic by the extirpation remained free from vesiculation.

It is curious that these two cases should both have presented symptoms not only of disturbance in the intact and remaining Ganglion semilunare (mild in the case first reported and severe in the latter one), but also of disturbance with the posterior ganglia of the most remote sacral segments (severe in the first case and mild in the latter one). It would almost seem that gravitation must have played a part in bringing about a deposition of the infective agent, whatever it may have been,[1] in the caudal portion of the meningeal sac, and the anatomical position of the terminal sacral ganglia (Fig. 7) at the very lowermost part of the sac would perhaps favor such a view. It seems unlikely that there should have been a different etiological factor at work in bringing about the trigeminal and the sacral processes.

On Sensory Segmentation Postaxial to the Lower Limb.

As is well known, several methods may be utilized for the approximate determination of the cutaneous areas presided over by the individual units of the spinal cord.

ANATOMICAL. In the first place, by dissection the nerves may be traced from the cord to their finer cutaneous ramifications. For those parts of the body in which the successive trunks retain the semblance of their primitive segmental character, this anatomical method presents no great difficulties. It is quite otherwise, however, with the nerves destined to supply the limbs, since by their fusion into a plexus they become complicated to a most puzzling degree. This is true, even in the early embryo, for, as Dr. Bardeen's morphological studies have demonstrated, the plexuses have begun to form long before the nerves have reached their destination in the skin covering the budding extremity.

Careful anatomical dissections, such as those of Paterson,[2] Eisler,[3] and others, serve to show the great variations as regards their spinal roots which exist for the lumbosacral nerves, and how difficult it is by the dissection method to obtain any clear conception of cutaneons segmentation such as would be of use for clinical purposes.

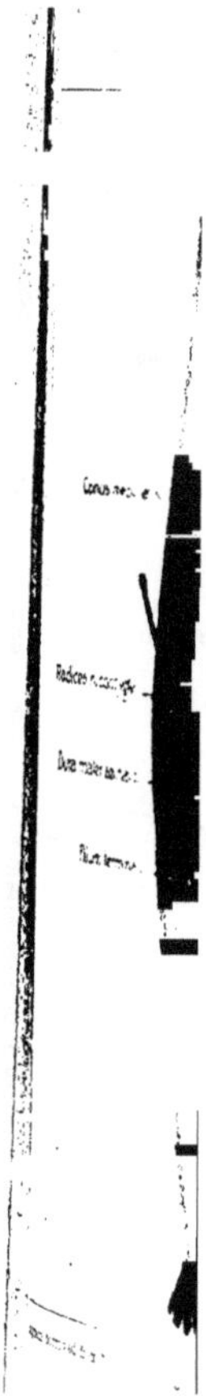

[1] From an etiological standpoint I am unable to account for the eruption in these cases Presumably there was an infective agency of some kind. In the first case, however, the temperature remained normal or slightly subnormal during the entire period of eruption. In the second case an alteration in the temperature curve like that of a malarial paroxysm took place. Unlike the malarial chill, however, there was an associated rise in leukocytes, from 4800 to 22,000. Both the leukocytosis and pyrexia quickly returned in a few hours to their normal points.

[2] The Origin and Distribution of the Nerves to the Lower Limbs, Journal of Anatomy and Physiology, 1893-1894, vol. xxviii. pp. 84 and 169.

[3] Der Plexus lumbosacralis des Menschen, Halle, 1892.

FIG. 7.

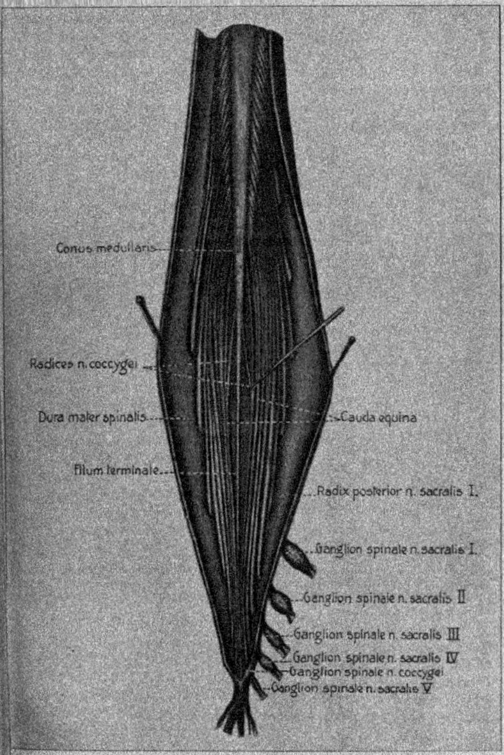

Diagram borrowed from Toldt's Anatomisches Atlas, 1903, showing the situation of the lowermost posterior root ganglia at the extremity of the meningeal sac.

In the region caudal to the extremity with which we are dealing, there is, to be sure, a return again to a somewhat more simple type of root distribution. In the average individual, that is one in whom the plexus is neither placed higher nor lower in relation to the limb (prefixed or postfixed, according to Sherrington's terminology) than the normal type, it may be said that the second sacral is the lowest of the roots to enter completely into a leg distribution. The segments below this level (third sacral to coccygeal) supply the terminal or caudal end of the body, where, uncomplicated by the growing ex-

FIG. 8.

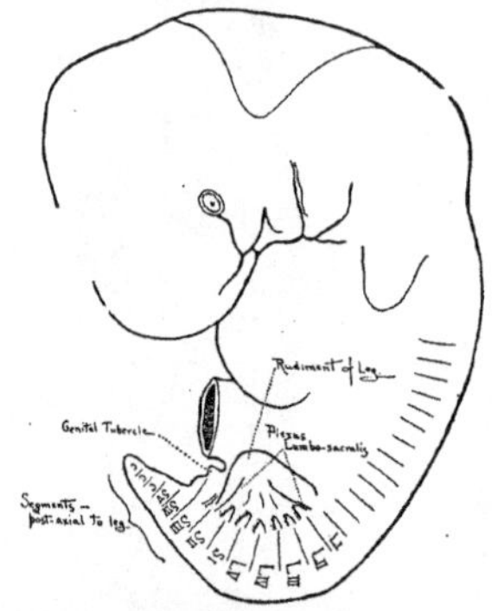

Diagrammatic outline of a four and one-half weeks' embryo, showing the segments (S. III.—coccygeal) postaxial to the rudimentary hind limb. The nerve roots (LI. to S. II.) form the lumbosacral plexus, destined for the most part for distribution in the leg. The sensory elements of the four lower miatomes (S. III.—coccygeal) are destined for the parts about the cloaca, penis, scrotum, perineum, anal region, and buttock. For comparison with adult distribution see Fig. 10. (Sketch adapted from Bardeen and Lewis, American Journal of Anatomy, vol. i., No. 1, Plate III.)

tremity, their cutaneous areas present a zonal distribution running clearly from mid-dorsum to mid-venter. The anatomical arrangement is not quite so simple, however, as in the trunk above the limb, for these lower nerves do enter into a certain plexiform arrangement, the so-called plexus pudendus (anat. nomen.) or plexus finalis trunci (Renz), and beyond the stated fact that the skin over the genitalia, perineum, buttock, and ischioanal region is supplied usually by segments below the second sacral, there is but little attempt anatomically to indicate any clear zonal distribution.

In the upright attitude of the adult, all evidence that the original situation of these parts was postaxial to the limb is lost, and only by a morphological comparison with their primitive simple arrangement is it possible to obtain a clear idea of their subsequent configuration. In very schematic fashion I have endeavored to indicate by the accompanying sketch of a four weeks' embryo, kindly supplied by Dr. Mall, the position of these lower cutaneous zones before the growth of the leg led to their distortion (Fig. 8).

PHYSIOLOGICAL. Secondly, the experimental method, although exact in many ways, nevertheless presents serious drawbacks, chiefly owing to the difficulty of interpretation of sensations in their transference from animals to man. Were it not for this factor, the physiologist would be able accurately to delineate the cutaneous strips of each segment by a procedure which Head has appropriately called "the method of remaining æsthesia." This method, first practised by Sherrington, consists in the division of the posterior roots of two or more segments, both above and below the particular zone which is to be studied. Thus, there should remain an æsthetic zone of skin with intact nerve supply in the midst of an anæsthetic field, and with no confusion from overlapping. Owing to this functional overlap of neighboring segments, as Sherrington first demonstrated, the division of a single posterior root does not suffice to produce a strip of "resultant anæsthesia." The subject could not, therefore, be studied in any such simple way. Charts, furthermore, based upon observations from lower animals, are not easily transferable to the cutaneous fields of man, and there is considerable evidence, as Head and Thorburn have pointed out, that the sensory fields of the spinal segments are more sharply defined than are the root areas with which experimental physiologists and anatomists have chiefly concerned themselves.

CLINICAL. 1. *Traumatic Paralyses.* A third and possibly the most satisfactory method of delineating at least the upper margins of the several segmental areas occurs in association with cases of spinal injury, in which a clean-cut, total, transverse lesion of the cord has occurred. By the combination of a sufficient number of such cases, especially when the level of the lesion has been determined by a post-mortem study, the sensory zones for the individual segments may be accurately mapped out. The areas thus determined and figured by Allen Starr, 1892; Thorburn, 1893; Kocher, 1898; and Wichmann, 1900, furnish data for the best-known and most carefully represented charts of this kind (Fig. 9).

It is, however, very unusual for traumatic injuries to pick out the tip of the conus medullaris, enclosed and protected as it is by the powerful lumbar vertebra, without injuring at the same time the neighboring strands of the cauda equina, thus giving a picture a segment or two higher than the level of the actual cord lesion. It is very rare, on the other hand, for cases of injury limited to the cauda equina and occasioned by sacral injuries to occur low enough to involve the roots below the third sacral and to leave those above unaffected.[1] Thus Thorburn[2] gives in his diagram no segmentation below the third sacral, remarking that "the fourth sacral and sub-

FIG. 9.

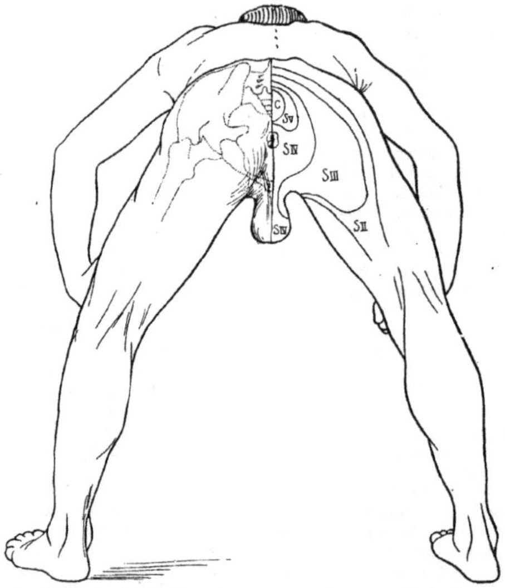

A representation of the sacral areas as indicated by the diagrams of Starr, Thorburn, Head, Kocher, and Wichmann. The corresponding zones in each figure have, for ease of comparison, been shaded in a similar way. It will be noted that there is considerable unanimity in the configuration at the area accredited to the third sacral (S. III.). Wichmann's figure alone fails to indicate the "saddle-shaped" form, though his context mentions it as characteristic of this zone.

jacent roots are not indicated, being placed too low down in the perineum for representation in these sketches" (Fig. 9).

[1] Cases of pelvic operation by the sacral route (Kraske), in which by resection of the coccyx and oblique division of the lower part of the sacrum including, at least on one side, the foramina of exit of S. V. or IV., or even in some cases S. III., seemingly would offer favorable opportunities for the study of the sensory areas of the corresponding roots. I have as yet been unable to make any satisfactory observations on patients with such surgical lesions.

[2] The Sensory Distribution of the Spinal Nerves, Brain, 1893, vol. xvi. p. 355, and elsewhere.

The lowest area represented in Kocher's[1] otherwise remarkably perfect series is the third sacral and one, according to my interpretation, in which this territory possibly is indicated only in part, together with the fourth and lower areas, so that its representation is somewhat larger than the actual distribution of the fourth sacral as usually indicated.

Wichmann[2] has adopted in his diagram a spectral color scheme, which, when familiarized, is in many respects useful for purposes of orientation. In the extremities, however, he has allowed for variation and overlapping to such an extent that the separate segmental units are not as clearly outlined as his individual cases seemingly would justify; consequently, in these areas (second lumbar and second sacral, inclusive) the diagram is confusing. This is not the case, however, with the zonal arrangement of those segments of the trunk which have not been distorted by the outgrowth of the limb. Following Renz, he includes, under the heading *Plexus finalis trunci*, the third, fourth, and fifth sacral and the coccygeal segments, whose areas all lie caudad to the lower extremities. The third sacral alone overlaps slightly on the extremities, so that its area of representation is no longer circular like those which lie below it, but has become distorted into the familiar figure ("saddle-shaped") noted by many observers as resembling the imprint which the buttock makes upon a chair. This configuration, though alluded to in his context and apparent in the sketches of his individual cases, he has failed to indicate in his combined diagram (Fig. 9).

Starr's[3] figure, although antedating those of Kocher and Wichmann by several years, and in spite of its deficiencies to which many have called attention, nevertheless, seems to me, so far as the scheme of representation of the three lower areas goes, to be much the more satisfactory. In it each of the sacral segments on the buttock, starting below at the fifth, successively encircles the area caudad to its own representation, and thus the principle of segmentation posteriorly on the trunk is more or less graphically indicated, and the effect which the growth of the limb has had in distorting the original circular strips becomes intelligible. Whether or not a successive diminution in the diametrical width of these areas on the buttock, from the first sacral tailward, is clearly demonstrable, I cannot from personal observations take a positive stand, but my impression, in accord with Thorburn and Starr, is that the diameters do so diminish.

2. *Referred Pain and Zoster*. In addition to those mentioned above a final method remains.

The demonstration by Mehlis (1818), that a herpetic eruption

[1] Die Verletzungen der Wirbelsäule zugleich, also Beitrag zur Physiologie des menslichen Rückenmarkes. Mitteil. a. d. Grenzgebieten d. Medizin u. d. Chirurgie, 1898, Bd. i. xxv. p. 415

[2] Die Rückenmarksnerven und ihre Segmentbezüge, Berlin, 1900, Tafel i.

[3] Local Anæsthesia as a Guide in the Diagnosis of Lesions of the Lower Spinal Cord. The American Journal of the Medical Sciences, 1892, vol. civ. p. 15.

follows the distribution of peripheral nerves, and later by v. Bärensprung (1863), that it was a manifestation of lesions of the posterior root ganglia, paved the way for subsequent observations, which have culminated in the valuable studies of Henry Head on the cutaneous distribution of zoster. Head, by tabulating and plotting a large number (412) of these cases, was enabled to make a diagram of segmental cutaneous areas for almost the entire body, which in many ways proved corroborative of the facts determined by a study of cord lesions. His demonstration, furthermore, that the eruption in zoster corresponded with the areas of referred cutaneous pain and tenderness, associated with visceral disease, led him to the important conclusion that the fields which were delineated by zoster represented segmental cord areas rather than the less definitely outlined fields presided over by the individual roots. In the region, however, with which this paper deals, his chart is very incomplete from insufficiency in the number of the rarer cases of zoster which occur in the lower sacral segments. This may, in part, account for the obscure topography which his well-known figures give for the lowermost zones, where, to the uninitiated, all semblance of any segmental characteristic has been lost. This was especially true for this earlier diagram (1893), which is the one most widely copied, and, although the later one (1900)[1] is more satisfactory, it still remains somewhat confusing. The scheme of the sacral areas in this latter diagram is reproduced here (Fig. 9), and it will be seen that his third and fourth sacrals more nearly correspond with these territories as figured by others than they did in his original scheme.

Unless I have overlooked it, there is no mention in his classical papers in *Brain* of zoster occurring in or limited to the fourth and fifth sacrals and coccygeal areas. In his first communication[2] there is cited as a great rarity a case from the original article of v. Bärensprung,[3] which would appear to indicate an involvement of the lower sacral areas. There, unfortunately, is some confusion in the context, for, in describing this case, it reads "the eruption almost exactly corresponds with the *two upper*[4] sacral areas." This may possibly have been a slip for the "two middle," for, although v. Bärensprung does not especially state his opinion, nor at the time of this, his first paper, had there been definite proof of the relationship of zoster to lesions of the posterior root ganglia, nevertheless, he leads one to believe, from his description of the course of the N. pudendus, which supplies this area in large part, that it arises from the three middle sacral nerves. Also, the third and fourth sacral

[1] Head and Campbell. The Pathology of Herpes Zoster and its Bearing on Sensory Localization, Brain, 1900, part iii., p. 353, plate 17.

[2] Henry Head. On Distribution of Sensation, with Especial Reference to the Pain of Visceral Disease, Brain, 1893, part i., vol. xlvi. p. 1.

[3] Die Gurtelkrankheit. Armalen des Charite-Krankenhauses zu Berlin, 1861, Bd. ix. p. 100. Vierundfumfzigster Fall.

[4] Italics mine.

would more nearly correspond with the territories which Head himself figures in his last diagram. Mackenzie[1] regards this, as well as another of v. Bärensprung's[2] cases, as probably indicating the distribution of the fourth sacral. Personally, inasmuch as the eruption included the præputium clitoridis, vulva, perineum, and buttock, extending slightly on to the leg, I would think that the third sacral was also included, for if there is one segmental area regarding whose representation most writers are in accord, it is the third sacral, which closely corresponds with the herpetic field in this oft-quoted case. (See the area of the third sacral in Fig. 10.)

It is, of course, to be borne in mind that a herpetic eruption may only appear in patches, or maximal points, over the skin in the cutaneous zone corresponding to the involved posterior root ganglia, and, indeed, only a very small crop may be present, whereas the segment may have a broad area of representation. Furthermore, more than one segment in this situation is apt to be affected at a time which adds greatly to the difficulty of accurate demarcation of the individual ones. In the first of the cases above reported, as I have already stated, there was presumably an involvement of the ganglia from the second to the fourth sacral, inclusive, although the lesion in the latter alone sufficed to call out a herpetic rash over its own cutaneous territory.

By the "referred pain" method, Head was unable to give illustrations which would show the separate sacral areas. He calls attention to the fact, saying "that the areas making up the tract of skin over the perineum, scrotum, and penis, a portion of the buttocks, and posterior aspect of the thigh, calf and sole of the foot appear with decreasing frequency from above downward, and that if one of the lower ones is involved, it is practically always accompanied by one of the areas above it." The referred tenderness of painful bladder lesions is apt to be localized in this territory under discussion, and one of the cases which he records presented an area of cutaneous hyperæsthesia, which involved the zones probably represented by the third, fourth, and fifth sacral together. It is not at all improbable that areas of referred tenderness, or even of zoster in the sacral regions lower than the third, may, for obvious reasons, have been overlooked or unrecorded.

According to the theory originally promulgated by Ross, the limbs in their outgrowth from the trunk carry with them and distort the simple, ring-like, cutaneous units corresponding to those miatomes which enter into the limb construction. The lower four segments, lying caudalward from the hind limbs, build, just as do the dorsal nerves, more or less complete circular and concentric zones. These serially diminish in size until they reach the tip of the coccyx, which,

[1] Herpes Zoster and the Limb Plexuses of Nerves, Journal of Pathology and Bacteriology. 1893, vol. i. p. 332.

[2] Loc. cit., p. 99. Dreiundfunfzigster Fall.

FIG. 10.

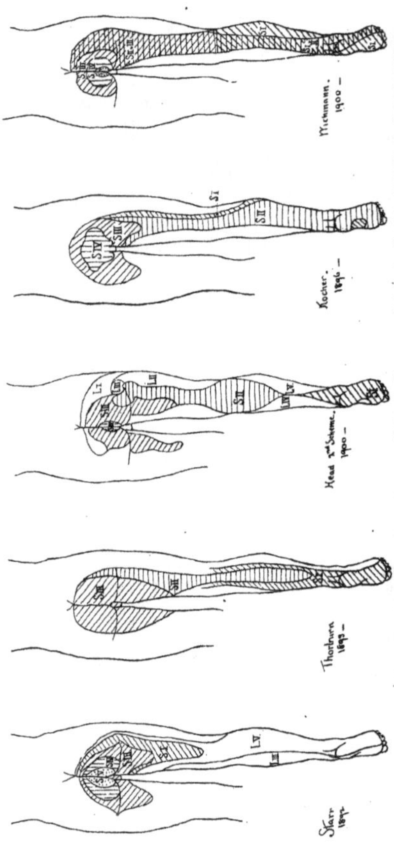

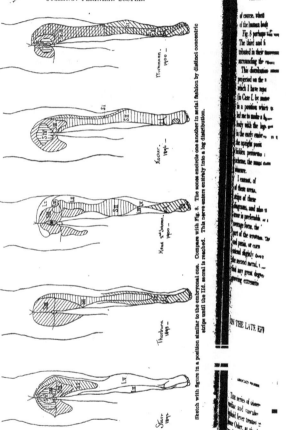

Sketch with figure in a position similar to the embryonal one. Compare with Fig. 8. The zones encircle one another in serial fashion by distinct concentric stripe until the IId. sacral is reached. This nerve enters entirely into a leg distribution.

of course, whether in embryo or adult, represents the terminal point of the human body.

Fig. 8 perhaps will elucidate this more clearly than a description. The third and fourth sacral, as indicated in the figure, are distributed in their midventral portion to the rudiments of the genitalia surrounding the cloaca.

This distribution presumably holds true when the segments are projected on the rounded end of the adult body. In the two cases which I have reported, the fact that most of the territory involved (in Case I. by zoster, in Case II. by an area of hyperæsthesia) was in a position which in the customary diagrams is concealed, has led me to make a figure (Fig. 10) which shows the nether pole of the body with the legs somewhat in the position which they occupied in the early embryo. In the diagrams, such as are shown in Fig. 9, the upright position, causing, as it does, a deep gluteal fold, with a hidden perineum and scrotum, makes, even in Starr's excellent scheme, the zonal distribution for these lower sacral areas somewhat obscure.

I cannot, of course, pretend to any great accuracy in the outline of these areas, believing only that the figure makes the cutaneous strips of these lower segments more intelligible than do the older diagrams, and also that for purposes of clinical utility a margin of error is preferable to a certainty of confusion. I have taken, as the average form, the fourth sacral as supplying the perineum and lower part of the scrotum, the third sacral the upper part of the scrotum and penis, or corresponding organs in the female, and beginning to extend slightly down the back of the leg. It is not until we reach the second sacral, which has a leg distribution in its entirety, that we find any great degree of distortion to have resulted from the outgrowing extremities.

ON THE LATE EFFECTS OF TYPHOID FEVER ON THE HEART AND VESSELS.

A CLINICAL STUDY.

By W. S. Thayer, M.D.,

ASSOCIATE PROFESSOR OF MEDICINE IN THE JOHNS HOPKINS UNIVERSITY.

The series of observations here recorded is part of a study of the cardiac and vascular complications and sequels of the cases of typhoid fever treated in the last fourteen years in the clinic of Professor Osler, at the Johns Hopkins Hospital. Though not yet as complete as might be desired, the material already gathered seemed to me to be sufficient to justify an analysis of the results so far obtained.[1]

* * *

The infrequency of endocarditis as a complication of typhoid fever is generally recognized. Only 11 cases were noted among the 2000 Munich necropsies, while but 3 have been observed in nearly 100 necropsies at the Johns Hopkins Hospital.

The grave myocardial changes which may occur during the disease are well known, thanks to the studies of a large number of observers, from Laennec,[2] Louis,[3] and Stokes,[4] whose observations relate only to the gross appearances, down to the more minute histological investigations of Stein,[5] Zenker,[6] Hayem,[7] Déjerine,[8] Romberg,[9] Landouzy and Siredey,[10] Renaut,[11] Mollard and Regaud,[12] Giacomelli,[13] and many others. The extent of their clinical significance and their relation to the cardio-vascular manifestations of typhoid fever are still, however, questions of dispute. That the cardiac lesions as such may account for sudden collapse and death is scarcely to be doubted, but the clinical discrimination between the collapse due to disease of the heart muscle and that in which the condition is rather one of vaso-motor paralysis is often a difficult and uncertain matter. The interesting studies of Pässler and Rolly[14] would tend to support the idea that the latter mechanism may ac-

[1] Read before the New York Academy of Medicine, October 20, 1903.

[2] Traité de l'auscultation, etc., Paris, 1819, 8°, vol. ii. pp. 286 et seq.

[3] Anatomical, Pathological, and Therapeutic Researches upon the Disease known under the Name of Gastroentérite, etc. Translated from the original French by H. I. Bowditch, Boston, 1836, 8°, vol. 1. pp. 282 et seq.

[4] Diseases of the Heart and the Aorta, Philadelphia, 1854, pp. 366 et seq.

[5] Untersuchungen über die Myocarditis, Munchen, 1861, 8°, J. J. Lentner, p. 115.

[6] Ueber die Veranderungen der willkürlichen Muskeln in Typhus abdominalis; fol. Leipzig, Vogel, 1864, pp. 29 et seq.

[7] Recherches sur les rapports existant entre la mort subite et les altérations vasculäires du coeur dans la fièvre typhoïde, Arch. de phys, 1869, vol. ii. p. 698. Des complications cardiaques de la fièvre typhoïde, Gaz. hebd. de méd., Paris, 1874, 25, vol. xi. pp. 796, 815.

[8] Sur les alérations du myocarde (désintegration granuleuse) comme cause de la mort subite dans la fièvre typhoïde, Compt. rend. de la Soc. de biol., 1885. 8s., vol. ii. p. 769

[9] Ueber die Erkrankungen des Herzmuskels bei Typhus abdominalis, Scharlach und Diphtherie, Deutsch. Arch. f. klin. Med., 1891, vol. xlviii. p. 369; 1892, vol. xlix. 413

[10] Contribution à l'histoire de l'artérite typhoïdique; de ses conséquences hâtives (mort-subite) et tardives (myocardite scléreuse) du coeur, Rev. de méd., Paris, 1885, vol. v. p. 843. LANDOUZY, La fièvre typhoïde dans ses rapports avec l'appareil vasculaire et cardiaque, Gaz. d. hôp., Paris, 1886, vol. lix. p. 323. LANDOUZY et SIREDEY, Étude sur les localizations angio-cardiaques typhoïdiques, leurs conséquences immediates, prochaines et éloignées, Rev. de méd., Paris, 1887, vol. vii. pp. 804, 919,

[11] Les myocardites aigues, Congrès Français de médecine—V. session, Lille, 1899; Paris, 1899, t. ii. pp. 1-83.

[12] État des artères du coeur dans les myocardites aiguës, Congrès Français de méd., 1899, vol. v. p. 280. MOLLARD, Les troubles cardiaques dans la convalescence de la fièvre typhoïde, Presse méd., Paris, 1900, vol. i. pp. 19-22.

[13] Il miocardio nelle infezioni, intossicazioni, avvelenamenti. Ricerche anatomo-patologiche e sperimentali, Policlinico, Roma, 1901, viii., M., pp. 145-155.

[14] Experimentelle Untersuchungen über Kreislaufstörungen bei acuten Infectionskrankheiten, Deutsch. Arch. f. klin. Med., 1903, vol. lxxvii. p. 1.

count for more instances of collapse in acute disease than has generally been supposed.

The part played by infectious processes in the ætiology of acute and chronic changes in the vessels is also a point toward which considerable attention has been directed in recent years.

The relative frequency of venous thrombosis in typhoid fever is familiar enough, and the probability that this is, in many instances, associated with a phlebitis depending upon local infection would seem to result from various studies of recent years.

The not infrequent arterial thromboses and acute arteritides, notably of the vessels of the extremities and of the brain, which have been studied particularly by French observers, need not be recalled. Potain[1] has called attention to the occurrence of acute aortitis.

The influence of infectious diseases in general on the production of the more insidious endarteritic changes in the aorta and other vessels—in other words, the relation of acute infections to the development of atheroma of the aorta and arterio-sclerosis in general—is a question of great importance, to which, it seems to me, we have scarcely directed sufficient attention. Numerous observers have noted the frequency of fresh gelatinous and fatty sclerotic plaques in the aorta and larger vessels in individuals dead of various acute infectious diseases, while Gilbert and Lion,[2] Crocq,[3] and others have produced sclero-calcareous and fatty sclerotic changes in the aorta of rabbits by the injection of pathogenic bacteria after previously inflicting slight mechanical injury to the walls. Indeed, Gilbert and Lion have, in several instances, succeeded in producing changes which they believe to be closely analogous to those observed in human arterio-sclerosis by the intravascular injection of pathogenic organisms without the previous production of a point of least resistance by injury. On the other hand, Thoma[4] mentions typhoid fever among the ætiological elements in the production of that angiomalacia which he believes to be the primary lesion in the development of arterio-sclerosis.

In brief, there is much which goes to suggest that acute infections, and typhoid fever among them, play an important part in the ætiology of arterio-sclerosis. Some observers who have especially studied this question believe that after acute rheumatism typhoid fever is the infectious disease most frequently resulting in changes in the heart and vessels.

[1] De l'aortite typhique, Semaine méd., Paris, 1894, vol. xiv. p. 460.

[2] Artérites infectieuses expérimentales, Comptes rend. de la Soc. de biol., Paris, 1889, 9s., vol. i. p. 583.

[3] Contribution à l'étude expérimentale des artérites infectieuses (abstr.), Arch. de méd. exp. et d'anat. path., Paris, 1894, vol. vi. pp. 583-600.

[4] Ueber das elastiche Gewebe der Arterienwand und die Angiomalacie, Verhandlungen des XIII. Cong. f. inn. Med., Wiesbaden, 1895, p. 465.

The observations of Landouzy and Siredey[1] are especially striking. These authors report the case of a man, aged twenty-three years, who died suddenly on the fifteenth day of typhoid fever. Two years before he had passed through a serious typhoid infection of six weeks' duration. The heart muscle showed extensive acute inflammatory and degenerative changes in association with grave older sclerotic alterations. There was nothing in the history of the patient, beyond his previous typhoid fever, to which these alterations could be ascribed. Out of 15 typhoid patients between five and forty-eight years of age, followed by Landouzy for a period of nine years, there were 3 in whom marked cardiac disturbance had persisted after recovery from the acute disease. These 3 patients, five, three, and two years after the disease, all showed a certain degree of hypertrophy, with cardiac irritability. As a result of their study, Landouzy and Siredey maintain among their conclusions that: "The secondary angio-cardiac complications of typhoid fever are more frequent than is generally believed and than has been generally acknowledged up to the present time.

"After acute articular rheumatism, typhoid fever appears to give rise to more angio-cardiac complications than any of the other infectious diseases.

"Among the most important and commonest of these complications are those which arise insidiously during the course or decline of the disease. The angio-cardiac lesions are important to recognize, less because of the prognostic reserve which they demand during the course of the disease itself (collapse, sudden death) than for that which they impose upon us for the future."

And Lacombe,[2] among the conclusions of his thesis, maintains that: "The disorders of the heart appearing some years after recovery from typhoid fever may be legitimately ascribed to this disease, if no other malady capable of compromising the integrity of the heart, either before or after the typhoid, has occurred."

* * *

The communications of Landouzy and Siredey especially suggested to me that it might be of interest to make a series of observations as to the condition of the heart and vessels in a number of individuals who had had typhoid fever in the wards of the Johns Hopkins Hospital during the past fourteen years, comparing these results with the previous hospital records, which, in many instances, are fairly complete. This proceeding appealed to me the more because, so far as I know, it has never been previously attempted. With this end in view, I sent out letters to all patients who had had typhoid fever in the wards of the hospital since its opening in 1889—over 1400 in all. In the majority of instances, as might have been expected, the letters failed to reach their destination and were returned, but 183 patients presented themselves for examination.

[1] Op. cit., 1885. [2] Localizations angiocardiaques de la fièvre typhoïde, Paris, 1890, 4°.

The majority of these patients were examined at the hospital between 3 and 5 o'clock on Sunday afternoons. About 30 per cent. of the cases were studied in the Out-patient Department between the hours of 10 and 12 in the morning. The measurements of the heart, the record of the pulse, and the estimations of the blood pressure were made in the recumbent posture for comparison with the hospital records.

AGE AND DATE OF ATTACK.

The ages of the patients varied between three and sixty-nine years, while the periods which had elapsed between the discharge from the hospital and the subsequent examination ranged from one month to thirteen years. In all cases the patient was questioned as to the maladies from which he might have suffered since his discharge from the hospital. The following table will show the period of time which had elapsed between the discharge from the hospital and the subsequent examination of the patients:

TABLE I.

Showing the length of time which had elapsed between the discharge of the patient from the hospital and his subsequent examination.

Months.		Years.												
1-6[1]	6-12	1	2	3	4	5	6	7	8	9	10	11	12	13
22	26	18	20	23	21	11	13	11	8	6	2	0	1	1 = 182

PULSE.

(*a*) *Rate.* Most of the patients at the time of their examination had already rested for some little period of time after their arrival at the hospital. In a large proportion of the cases, however, there was a manifest nervousness; no more, probably, than is common on the examination of any one under similar circumstances; perhaps a trifle less, inasmuch as the patients were for the most part old friends.

The following table shows the rate of the pulse in 182 cases:

TABLE II.

Rate of the pulse per minute.

50-60	60-70	70-80	80-90	90-100	100-110	110-120	120-130	Not noted.	Total.
1	17	42	50	26	23	8	8	17	182

In this table it will be seen that in 110 instances, or 60.4 per cent. of the cases, the pulse ranged between 60 and 90. In 16 instances, or 8.7 per cent., it was above 110.

(*b*) *Regularity.* In 30 instances irregularity of the pulse was noted; four of these were cases in which the rate was not recorded.

Of the cases in which the pulse was over 90, irregularity was noted in 18.3 per cent.

Of the cases in which the pulse was under 90, irregularity was observed in 12.7 per cent.

(*c*) *Intermittence.* In only 3 instances was the pulse distinctly intermittent. One of these was a well-marked case of hypertrophy

[1] There were but three cases seen under three months from the time of discharge.

with mitral insufficiency. There were 2 cases in which a strikingly collapsing character of the pulse was noted. In each of these instances an aortic diastolic murmur was present.

BLOOD PRESSURE.

In 165 of these cases the systolic blood pressure was taken by means of the Riva-Rocci apparatus. This proceeding was made the last step in the examination, in order that the patient might be in as placid a condition as possible. The estimations were repeated several times until constant readings were obtained. The band was always placed around the middle of the upper arm, right or left.

The results of these estimations are indicated in the following table :

TABLE III.

Showing the averages of the systolic blood pressure in 165 old typhoids arranged by age according to decades.

1–10	10–20	20–30	30–40	40–50	50–60	60–70
112.4 mm.	135.2 mm.	153.5 mm.	161.5 mm.	170.2 mm.	179.6 mm.	215 mm.
(5 cases)	(39 cases)	(58 cases)	(44 cases.)	(15 cases.)	(3 cases.)	(1 case.)

Struck by the high averages of the systolic blood pressure in this group of cases, I sought for statistics with which these figures might be compared, but soon found that it would be necessary, in order to reach a fair conclusion, to make myself a series of observations upon normal individuals under conditions as similar as might be. I have, therefore, in the last several months made 276 estimations of the blood pressure in presumably healthy individuals. These observations were made upon physicians, nurses, and employés of the hospitals, friends of patients, healthy children in several different asylums and schools, and upon various of my own friends. I did not allow myself to record the blood pressure of any patient, surgical or medical, no matter what his complaint. The records were taken between the hours of 3 and 5 in the afternoon or between 10 A.M. and 1 P.M.; in other words, several hours after a meal. They were all taken in the recumbent posture, sufficient time being taken to allow the individual to recover from the preliminary nervousness; that is, under conditions similar to those employed in making the observations upon the previous group of patients. The averages of this table, which may be seen upon Chart I., show a distinctly and uniformly lower blood pressure than in the old typhoids.

TABLE IV.

Showing the averages of the systolic blood pressure in 276 healthy individuals and 165 old typhoids arranged according to age by decades.

			Old typhoids.			
1–10	10–20	20–30	30–40	40–50	50–60	60–70
112.4 mm.	135.2 mm.	153.5 mm.	161.5 mm.	170.2 mm.	179.6 mm.	215 mm.
(5 cases.)	(39 cases.)	(58 cases.)	(44 cases)	(15 cases.)	(3 cases.)	(1 case.)
			Healthy individuals.			
104.6 mm.	128.7 mm.	136.9 mm.	140.8 mm.	142.2 mm.	154 8 mm.	180 mm
(37 cases.)	(87 cases.)	(89 cases.)	(37 cases.)	(20 cases.)	(5 cases.)	(1 case.)

Inasmuch as all observers agree that the average blood pressure is slightly lower in women than in men, it may be well to note that the proportion of women was higher among the old typhoids than among the cases from which the control table was constructed, the exact figures being 38.7 per cent. for the old typhoids and 33.3 per cent. for the normal cases.

CHART I.

SHOWING AVERAGES OF THE SYSTOLIC BLOOD PRESSURE IN 165 OLD TYPHOIDS AND IN 276 HEALTHY INDIVIDUALS ARRANGED ACCORDING TO AGE BY DECADES.

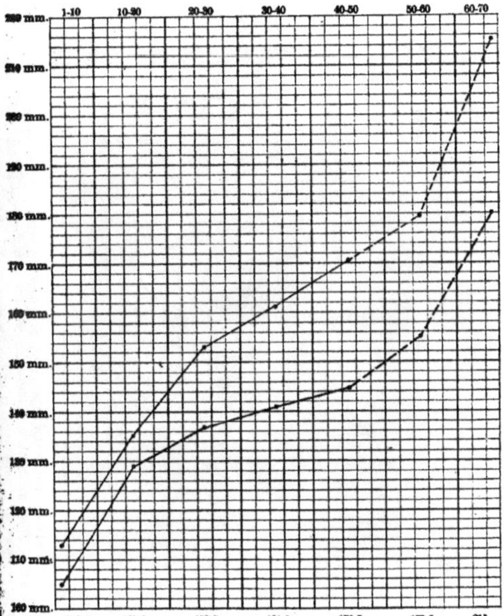

OLD TYPHOIDS	112.4 ([illegible] cases)	135.2 ([illegible] cases)	153.5 ([illegible] cases)	161.5 (44 cases)	170.2 (15 cases)	179.6 ([illegible] cases)	215 (1 case)
HEALTHY INDIVIDUALS	104.6 ([illegible] cases)	128.7 ([illegible] cases)	136.9 ([illegible] cases)	140.8 ([illegible] cases)	142.2 ([illegible] cases)	154.8 ([illegible] cases)	180 (1 case)

On the other hand, more of the normal cases were examined during the morning hours than of the old typhoids, the percentage being 40.5 per cent. to 30.3 per cent.

A closer analysis of the figures upon which these tables are based reveals the fact that among the old typhoids there were 54 cases in which the blood pressure was above 160; this group comprises over 50 per cent. of the cases over thirty years of age.

In the much larger number of observations upon healthy individuals there were but 10 such cases, 6 of which gave a history of preceding serious infectious disease, while in 1 there was a good suspicion of alcoholism. Of the 54 old typhoids, in but 17 was a similar history obtainable.

CHART II.

SHOWING THE AVERAGES OF THE SYSTOLIC BLOOD PRESSURE IN OLD TYPHOIDS AND IN NORMAL INDIVIDUALS FROM WHOM ALL CASES WITH A HISTORY OF SERIOUS INFECTIOUS DISEASE OR ALCOHOLIC HABITS HAVE BEEN EXCLUDED.

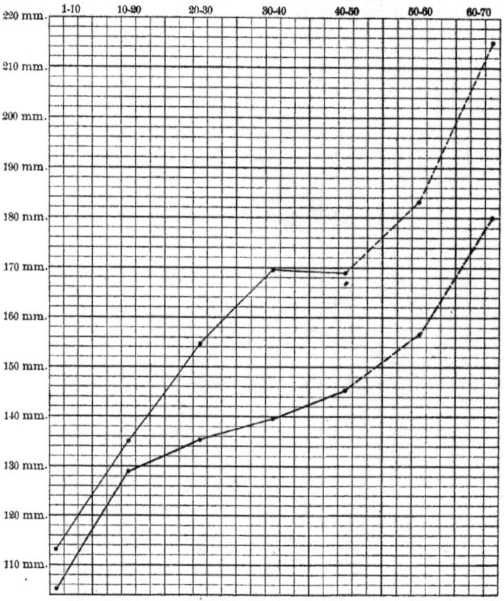

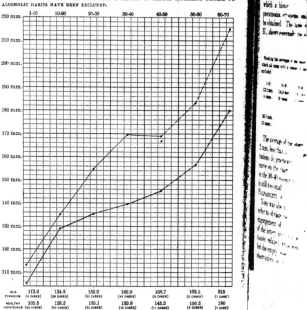

	1-10	10-20	20-30	30-40	40-50	50-60	60-70
OLD TYPHOIDS	113.2 (4 CASES)	134.9 (28 CASES)	152.2 (32 CASES)	169.9 (24 CASES)	168.7 (6 CASES)	183.5 (2 CASES)	215 (1 CASE)
HEALTHY INDIVIDUALS	105.5 (32 CASES)	128.3 (67 CASES)	135.1 (52 CASES)	139.8 (19 CASES)	145.2 (11 CASES)	156.2 (4 CASES)	180 (1 CASE)

The highest record of blood pressure among the cases in healthy individuals was 180, and that in a woman aged sixty years, while among the old typhoids there were 27 cases in which the pressure was above 180, a number of which were striking examples of hypertension, 10 showing a record of 200 or above.

It might be objected that to ascribe this difference between the two curves to changes dependent upon the preceding typhoid fever would be a rash conclusion, inasmuch as a great number of other influences must have come into play, while the number of cases studied is too small to justify positive conclusions. In order to rule out some of these disturbing influences, I have prepared a table in which I have eliminated from each list all those cases in which a history of scarlet fever, diphtheria, acute rheumatism, pneumonia, erysipelas, smallpox, syphilis or alcoholic habits could be obtained. This table, which is represented graphically on Chart II., shows essentially the same relation between the two curves:

TABLE V.

Showing the averages of the blood pressure in old typhoids and normal individuals, from which all cases with a history of serious infectious disease or alcoholic habits have been excluded.

	1-10	10-20	20-30	30-40	40-50	50-60	60-70
Old typhoids.	113 2 mm. (4 cases.)	134.9 mm. (28 cases.)	152.2 mm (32 cases.)	169.9 mm. (24 cases)	168.7 mm. (8 cases.)	183.5 mm. (2 cases.)	215 mm. (1 case.)
Healthy individuals.	105.5 mm. (32 cases.)	128 3 mm. (62 cases)	135.1 mm. (52 cases.)	139.8 mm. (19 cases.)	145.2 mm. (11 cases.)	156.4 mm. (4 cases.)	180 mm. (1 case.)

The average of the observations upon healthy individuals is about 2 mm. less than in the uncorrected list. That of the typhoid observations is practically unchanged. The alteration in the typhoid curve on the chart arranged by decades, due to the higher figures in the 30–40 column, emphasizes the fact that the number of cases is still too small to allow of the construction of final charts.

PALPABILITY OF THE RADIAL ARTERIES.

Note was also made of the palpability of the radial arteries. In order to obviate the common confusion arising from a full vessel or engorgement of the venæ comitantes, the blood was milked out of the artery and veins with the fingers of both hands, the tense tissues relaxed, while with a third finger an attempt was made to feel the empty vessel. The following table will show the results of observations on 181 old typhoids:

TABLE VI.

Showing the palpability of the radial arteries in 181 cases arranged by age according to decades.

Age.	Cases.	Not palpable.	Palpable.	Per cent. of palpable vessels.
1–10	5	5	0	0
10–20	42	30	12	28.5
20–30	62	29	33	53.2
30–40	54	25	29	53.7
40–50	14	7	7	50
50–60	3	0	3	100
60–70	1	1	0	0

A glance at these figures reveals the striking fact that over 50 per cent. of our cases above twenty years of age showed palpable radial arteries. In 2 instances in which the radials were not palpable, 1 the

CHART III.

SHOWING THE PERCENTAGES OF PALPABILITY OF THE RADIAL ARTERIES IN OLD TYPHOIDS AND IN HEALTHY INDIVIDUALS ARRANGED ACCORDING TO AGE BY DECADES.

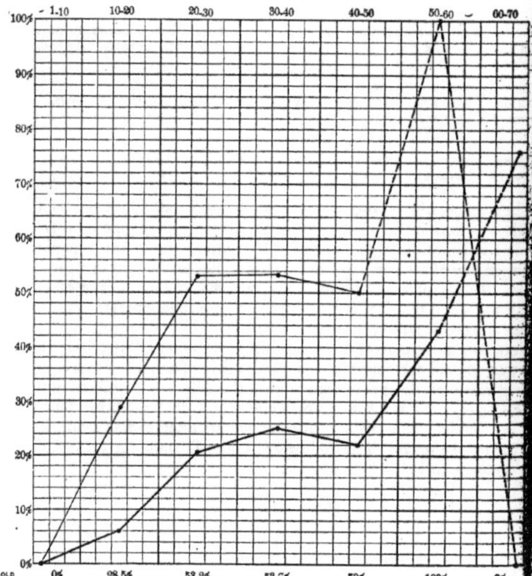

	1-10	10-20	20-30	30-40	40-50	50-60	60-70
OLD TYPHOIDS	0% (5 CASES)	28.5% (42 CASES)	53.2% (62 CASES)	53.7% (54 CASES)	50% (14 CASES)	100% (3 CASES)	0% (1 CASE)
HEALTHY INDIVIDUALS	0% (37 CASES)	6.1% (98 CASES)	20.4% (185 CASES)	25% (61 CASES)	22% (97 CASES)	42.8% (7 CASES)	80% (5 CASES)

case of a man aged twenty-five years, and 1 that of a woman aged forty-seven years, one or the other of the temporal arteries was distinctly thickened. In general, I have in these studies been impressed with the irregularity in the distribution of the sclerotic processes in peripheral vessels. It is by no means uncommon to find one radial or temporal distinctly thickened or tortuous, while the other is apparently unaffected.

A comparison of the observations recorded in this table with those made upon the patients while in the hospital is of little value, in view of the fact that a definite note as to the palpability of the radials was made in but 48 cases. These figures, which were even more striking than the high averages of blood pressure, could, it seemed to me, be fairly compared only with a similar series of observations made by myself upon supposedly healthy individuals who had not suffered from typhoid fever. Within the last several months, accordingly, I have examined the radials and temporals of 421 individuals who have never had typhoid fever. The accompanying table, illustrated on Chart III., shows a comparison of the percentages of palpable radials arranged by decades in our old typhoids and in healthy individuals:

TABLE VII.

Showing the percentages of palpability of the radial arteries in old typhoids and in healthy individuals arranged according to age by decades.

Old typhoids.

1–10	10–20	20–30	30–40	40–50	50–60	60–70
0 %	28.5 %	53.2 %	53.7 %	50 %	100 %	0 %
(5 cases.)	(42 cases.)	(62 cases.)	(54 cases.)	(14 cases.)	(3 cases.)	(1 case.)

Healthy individuals.

1–10	10–20	20–30	30–40	40–50	50–60	60–70
0 %	6.1 %	20.4 %	25 %	22 %	42.8 %	80 %
(37 cases.)	(98 cases.)	(86 cases.)	(61 cases.)	(27 cases.)	(7 cases.)	(5 cases.)

By these figures it appears that between the ages of ten and fifty years 46.8 per cent. of the old typhoids showed palpable vessels as compared with 17.6 per cent. of the normal cases.

I have also prepared comparative tables, as in the case of the records of blood pressure, based upon an analysis of those cases only in which a history of serious infections or of habits which might induce arterio-sclerosis was wanting. This table is illustrated by Chart IV.

TABLE VIII.

Showing the percentages of palpability of the radial arteries in old typhoids and in healthy individuals from which all cases giving a history of serious infections or alcoholism have been excluded.

Old typhoids.

1–10	10–20	20–30	30–40	40–50	50–60	60–70
0 %	22.5 %	54.2 %	62.9 %	57.1 %	100 %	0 %
(4 cases.)	(31 cases.)	(35 cases.)	(27 cases.)	(7 cases.)	(2 cases.)	(1 case.)

Healthy individuals.

1–10	10–20	20–30	30–40	40–50	50–60	60–70
0 %	4.2 %	21.3 %	22.2 %	18.7 %	33.3 %	75 %
(32 cases.)	(70 cases.)	(103 cases.)	(27 cases.)	(16 cases.)	(6 cases.)	(4 cases.)

As in the case of the observations upon the blood pressure, the total average is slightly lower among the healthy individuals—15.1 per cent. : 17.5 per cent. Among the typhoids the average palpability of the vessels in this list varies but little from that in the previous table—45.7 per cent. : 46.1 per cent.

HEART.

Position of the Apex. Measurements of the distance of the apex of the heart from the median line were made in 180 of the old typhoids. The average distance of the apex from the median line as determined by palpation, percussion, and auscultation in individuals between the ages of twenty and fifty years was 9.12 cm.

Similar measurements made in 102 of these cases on admission to the hospital showed an average of 8.7 per cent.

CHART IV.

SHOWING THE PERCENTAGES OF PALPABILITY OF THE RADIAL ARTERIES IN OLD TYPHOIDS AND IN HEALTHY INDIVIDUALS AFTER THE REMOVAL FROM EACH LIST ALL CASES IN WHICH THERE IS A HISTORY OF SEVERE INFECTIOUS DISEASE OR OF ALCOHOLIC HABITS.

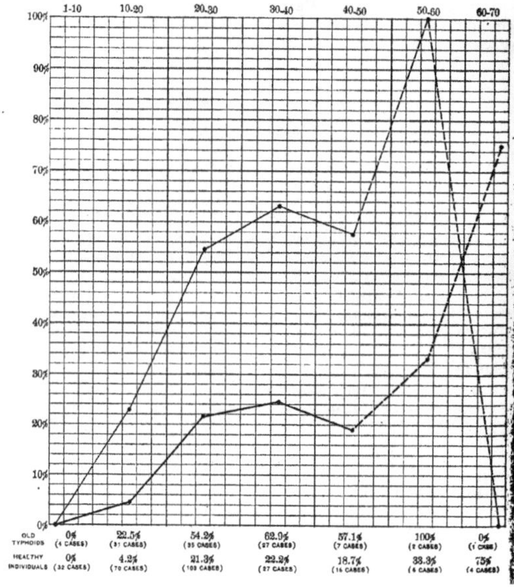

The following table shows the averages, arranged according to age by decades, of 102 cases which were examined on admission to the hospital, side by side with the records of those examined later:

TABLE IX.

Showing the average distance of the cardiac apex from the median line in 102 cases of typhoid fever on admission to the hospital, and of 180 cases examined later.

Old typhoids.

1-10	10-20	20-30	30-40	40-50	50-60	60-70
6.3 cm.	7.7 cm.	8 9 cm.	9.1 cm.	9.8 cm.	9.5 cm.	12 cm.
(5 cases.)	(41 cases.)	(63 cases.)	(52 cases.)	(15 cases.)	(3 cases.)	(1 case.)
During attack.						
5.7 cm.	6.6 cm.	8.5 cm.	8.5 cm.	9.6 cm.		
(5 cases.)	(36 cases.)	(38 cases.)	(14 cases.)	(9 cases.)		

It will be noted that the average measurements in the old typhoids are slightly but constantly larger than in the cases examined on admission to the hospital. Though this difference, as shown by the table, is trivial, it should, perhaps, be borne in mind that there is not infrequently in typhoid fever a slight dilatation of the heart, and that most of these examinations were made when the fever was well under way.

Inasmuch as 46 of these cases entered the hospital when they were under twenty years of age, that is, at a time when, in many instances, they had not attained full development, it seemed wise to investigate the position of the apex in individuals over twenty years at the time of their admission, where notes had been made both in the hospital and subsequently. There were 59 such cases. At the time of admission the average distance of the apex from the median line was 8.82 cm.; subsequently it was 9.14 per cent., a slight difference, but one which corresponds closely with the larger averages.

Extent of the Cardiac Dulness to the Right. In 158 cases examined by myself a note was made as to the extent of the cardiac dulness to the right of the midsternal line. The average distance for each decade is shown in the following table:

TABLE X.

Showing the average extent of the cardiac dulness to the right of the midsternal line in 158 old typhoids arranged according to age by decades.

1-10	10-20	20-30	30-40	40-50	50-60	60-70
2.4 cm.	3.12 cm.	3.45 cm.	3.39 cm.	3.47 cm.	3.4 cm.	5 cm.
(3 cases.)	(36 cases.)	(54 cases.)	(47 cases.)	(14 cases.)	(3 cases.)	(1 case.)

The greatest extent of dulness to the right of the median line among these cases was 5 cm., in a man with dilated heart and mitral insufficiency.

In but 1 case, that of a man aged thirty years, was no dulness to the right to be made out. This case accounts in great part for the slightly lower average in the fourth decade.

There is nothing remarkable about these figures, which are, indeed, a trifle smaller than those given by Riess.[1]

Heart Sounds, In the Hospital. In 170 of these cases in which notes with regard to the condition of the heart sounds were made in the hospital, murmurs were noted in 39 instances, or 29 per cent. In 31 cases the murmur was a soft systolic blow heard at the apex, and only once was the sound transmitted to the axilla. In a number of cases this murmur was heard only on admission or at the height of the disease, disappearing with convalescence. In 5 of these 31 cases the pulse in the hospital was above 140, one case, however, being under fifteen years of age.

On Later Examination. Notes on the heart sounds were made in all but 2 of the 183 old typhoids. 88, or 48.6 per cent., of these cases showed murmurs. In all of these the murmurs were systolic, although in 2 instances an aortic diastolic murmur was heard in addition, and in one case a doubtful mitral presystolic.

In only 38 cases was the systolic murmur audible at the apex. In the majority the murmur was a soft blow, with its maximum intensity at the base of the heart, in the pulmonic or aortic area.

In 11 cases an apex systolic murmur was transmitted to the axilla, and in 7 was audible also in the back. In 7 cases the symptoms justified the diagnosis of mitral insufficiency (Nos. 9921, 10,704, 10,714, 31,173, 17,636, 28,249, 36,210). One further case (20,507), an instance of aortic insufficiency, showed also evidences of mitral incompetency. In one case (32,037) there were signs suggesting mitral stenosis.

In 2 instances aortic diastolic murmurs were heard in cases which had previously shown no evidence of cardiac trouble (39,371, 26,507). One of these individuals, who was examined nearly four months after discharge from the hospital, was seen again five months later, at which time the diastolic murmur had entirely disappeared and the size of the heart had slightly diminished. This case must probably be regarded as one of functional insufficiency, due to relaxation of the aortic ring.

Reduplication of the First Sound. In 14 of the old typhoids a reduplication of the first sound at the apex or tricuspid area was observed. One of these was a case of well marked hypertrophy, with mitral insufficiency; another was a case of Graves' disease, with high arterial tension. In general, it was noted that the arterial tension in cases showing reduplication of the first sound was high, the average pressure being 164.9. In 3 cases the pressure was above 200. In only one of these reduplications did it seem possible to determine the cause of the split in the first sound. In this case it was clearly due to delay in the closure of the tricuspid valve.

[1] Sahli. Lehrbuch der klinischen Untersuchungsmethoden, Leipzig u. Wien, 8 Auflage, 1901, 8°, p. 165.

Reduplication of the Second Sound. In 82 of the old typhoids there was a reduplication of the second sound. This, in every instance but one, was audible at the base and usually limited to the pulmonic area. In 73 cases the reduplication was clearly dependent upon delay in the closure of the pulmonic valves. The reduplications were usually slight and heard only at the end of inspiration—cases such as would fall into Galli's[1] class of "reduplications of the first grade." In 10 cases, however, the reduplication was heard throughout the entire cycle.

The proportion of reduplications is not far from that observed by Galli, who, in his 120 carbineers, found 19 per cent. of such reduplications in the morning, 40 per cent. at noon, 56 per cent. in the afternoon.

The blood pressure of these cases was slightly below the general average for the old typhoids of the same decades—148.3 : 152.

Accentuation of the Second Sound. Out of 161 cases in which the relative accentuation of the aortic or pulmonic second sounds was noted, the pulmonic second was accentuated in 82, or 50.9 per cent. The following table will show the relative percentages of accentuation of the second aortic sound, arranged according to decade:

TABLE XI.

Showing the percentage of cases in each decade in which the aortic second sound was accentuated.

1–10	10–20	20–30	30–40	40–50	50–60	60–70
20 %	30.3 %	48.2 %	44.6 %	46.6 %	100 %	100 %
(5 cases.)	(33 cases.)	(58 cases.)	(47 cases.)	(15 cases.)	(2 cases.)	(1 case.)

Compared with the figures of Cabot,[2] the percentages in the lower decades are high, while those above the third decade are low. I do not, however, attach any great importance to these figures. In using the term "accentuated" I have intended to indicate that sound which was actually the louder of the two. In a number of instances, however, the second aortic sound, while not apparently as loud as the second pulmonic, was ringing, liquid, musical and suggestive of high tension. Again, the study of reduplications of the second sound, among other things, proves, I think, clearly that in many instances the closure of the aortic valve plays the greater part in the production of the loud sound which one hears in the pulmonic area.

SUMMARY OF THE GENERAL ANALYSES.

To summarize the results of these general analyses we have found:

1. That our old typhoids show an average blood pressure higher than that observed in control tables of normal subjects of the same age and under the same conditions, while the individual

[1] Münch. med. Wochenschr., 1902, vol. xlix. pp. 95, 1005, 1049.
[2] Physical Diagnosis of Diseases of the Chest, 2d ed., 1903, 8°, p. 124.

records in a considerable proportion of cases exceed the figures usually regarded as normal.

2. That in these same cases the radial arteries are palpable with much greater frequency than was observed in a series of control observations in individuals who had never had the disease.

3. That there is some evidence of cardiac enlargement, as indicated by the results of measurements of the distance of the apex from the median line when compared with figures for the same decade resulting from observations made at the time of admission to the hospital.

4. That there were among these 182 old typhoids 10 instances of cardio-vascular lesions, which had developed following typhoid fever in the absence of the ordinarily recognized ætiological elements; 7 cases of hypertrophy with mitral insufficiency (10,704, 10,714, 31,173, 17,636, 24,675, 28,249, 36,210);[1] two of aortic insufficiency (39,371, 20,507); one of marked arterio-sclerosis with hyper-tension in a young man (17,632).

In addition to these cases there was one instance of possible mitral stenosis (32,037).

* * *

Are the more serious cardio-vascular manifestations during typhoid fever common precursors of permanent lesions? Is it in cases presenting such symptoms that the grave, later changes develop? Is it possible to recognize at the time of their origin the development of those processes which subsequently exert a permanent effect upon the organism?

In order to obtain some light upon these questions, it was determined to examine separately into the subsequent condition of:

1. Those cases in which, during the attack, extreme rapidity of the pulse was noted.
2. Those cases where irregularity of the pulse was observed.
3. Those cases in which an apical systolic murmur was heard.

1. The Subsequent Condition of Those Cases of Typhoid Fever in Which Extreme Rapidity of the Pulse was Noted during the Attack.

Rate of the Pulse: In 19 cases a pulse of 140 or above was recorded during the attack. 9 of these patients were under twenty years of age at the time of admission. The rate of the pulse in the remaining 10 cases on subsequent examination shows no great variations from the general average. In 2 instances the rate was not noted. In one, a case of Graves' disease, it was 120; in one, 104; in one, 92; and in the other 5 instances, or 50 per cent., the pulse was between 68 and 84.

Systolic Blood Pressure. Of the 19 cases in which an extremely rapid pulse was observed in the hospital, 9 who were under twenty

[1] In one other case (9921) it is well possible that the typhoid fever may have been the exciting cause of the condition.

years of age have been omitted from the list; it is easily conceivable that in individuals under twenty years a pulse of 140 may not represent the same conditions as a pulse of that rate at a later age. Of the remaining 10 cases, varying in age from twenty-two years to fifty-three years, the average systolic pressure was 166.8. The general average of the old typhoids for these decades was 159.2. There were among these 10 cases, 2 with a blood pressure above 200, and 5, or 50 per cent., with a pressure above 160.

Palpability of the Radial Arteries. In 4, or 40 per cent. of these 10 cases, the radial artery was palpable. The general average for these decades among the old typhoids was 53.7 per cent.

Position of the Apex of the Heart. In only 4 of the 10 cases were measurements made during the disease. The average distance of the apex from the median line in these cases was 7.37 cm. In 10 cases examined subsequently the average distance was 8.48 cm. In the 4 cases in which a hospital record was made the average distance of the apex from the median line in the later examinations was 8.5 cm. If we compare these figures with the average of the measurements on admission to the hospital—8.82—and the average for the old typhoids—9.14—we find that they are lower in both instances. The difference, however, between the measurements during the disease and later is greater in the smaller group.

Extent of the Cardiac Dulness to the Right. In none of these 10 cases were measurements of the cardiac dulness to the right made during the fever. The average extent of dulness to the right of the median line on subsequent examination was 3.61, or slightly more than the total average for the same decades—3.44.

In review, then, we have found that in 10 cases over twenty years of age who, during their typhoid fever, showed extreme rapidity of the pulse, there was on subsequent examination, an average blood pressure somewhat higher than that observed in the mean of the whole 165 cases; the percentage of palpability of the radial arteries was less; the distance of the apex of the heart from the median line was somewhat less; while the extent of the dulness of the heart to the right of the median line was a trifle above the general average. The increase in the size of the heart during the period subsequent to the illness was somewhat above the general mean. Two cases showed distinct hypertrophy, with hyper-tension (11,331 and 14,675); in one of these there was evidence of mitral insufficiency.

2. SUBSEQUENT CONDITION OF THOSE CASES IN WHICH IRREGULARITY OF THE PULSE WAS NOTED DURING THE ATTACK.

Rate and Rhythm of the Pulse. Irregularity of the heart's action was noted in 12 cases during the attack. In 1 of these the irregularity occurred in association with the bradycardia (46) of convalescence. In 2 cases irregularity was observed on the subsequent examination. In the remaining 10 nothing remarkable was noted as to rate or rhythm of the pulse.

The Systolic Blood Pressure. In 11 of these 12 cases the average blood pressure on the later examination was 152.2 mm., as compared with the general average of 152 mm. 3 cases were under fifteen years of age. If we put aside these 3 cases in which the average pressure was 113.3 mm., there are left 8 cases, aged between twenty years and forty-two years, in whom the average pressure was 166.8 mm. The average pressure among the old typhoids for these decades was 158.6 mm. In 2 instances the pressure was above 200.

Palpability of the Radial Arteries. The radial arteries were palpable in but 3, or 27.2 per cent., of these cases.

Position of the Apex. The position of the apex was noted in the hospital in 9 of these cases. In 4, under twenty years of age, the average distance of the apex from the median line was 7.12 cm. In 5, over twenty years, the average distance was 8.2 cm. Of the 12 cases on the later examination, in 3, under twenty years of age, the average distance of the apex from the median line was 6.6 cm. In 9, over twenty years, it was 8.18 cm. In the 4 cases in which a hospital note was made the average distance of the apex from the median line on subsequent examination was 8 cm., or 0.2 cm. less than the average in the hospital.

Extent of Dulness to the Right. In none of these cases was a measurement made in the hospital of the extent of the cardiac dulness to the right. In 11 instances a record was made on the later examination. In 3 cases, under twenty years of age, the average was 3 cm. In 8 cases, over twenty years, the average was 3.35 cm.

Review. In the 12 cases which in the hospital showed irregularity of the pulse, as in the cases with rapid pulse, the blood pressure, on later examination, was found to be distinctly higher than the general mean of the 165 old typhoids. On the other hand, there was no evidence of cardiac enlargement; the distance of the apex from the median line was, indeed, less than in the general mean, or in the same cases on admission to the hospital. The percentage of palpability of radial arteries was also lower than the general average.

3. The Subsequent Condition of Those Cases in Which an Apical Systolic Murmur was Noted during the Attack.

The Rate of the Pulse. Of the 31 patients in whom during their fever a systolic murmur was observed, in 29 the rate of the pulse was noted in the subsequent examination. Twenty-one, or 72.4 per cent. of these cases, showed a pulse between 76 and 88. In 2 instances the pulse was between 90 and 100; in 5, between 100 and 110; and once only 120, a case of Graves' disease. When these figures are compared with the foregoing records for the total number of cases, it becomes evident that there is no apparent tendency in this group of cases to an increased rapidity of the pulse.

Palpability of the Radial Arteries. In 30 of these cases in which a note as to the palpability of the radial arteries was made, the vessel was to be felt in 11, or 36.6 per cent., as compared with the general average of 46.1 per cent.

The Systolic Blood Pressure. In 28 of these 31 cases the systolic blood pressure was taken in the later examination. The average of these 28 cases was 158.5 mm., against the general average for the total number of cases of 152.4. This higher average was observed in every decade excepting the first, in which there was but 1 case, and the third, in which there were but 4. In 18 cases, over the age of twenty years, the average pressure was 169.2, as compared with the general average of 159.6 for the same decades. In 5 cases the pressure was 200 mm. or above.

Position of the Apex. In 22 of these cases the position of the apex was determined in the hospital, the average distance from the median line being 7.1 cm. In 30 cases a subsequent note was made, the average being 8.9 cm. The former figures are slightly lower than the general average, the latter slightly higher. If we subtract from this list of cases those who were under twenty years at the time of admission, the average becomes 8.54 cm. in 11 hospital cases, against 9.4 cm. in 19 cases examined later. If we further compare only the 11 cases in which notes were made both in the hospital and later, the averages are, respectively, 8.54 cm. and 9.25 cm. Comparing these figures with the general hospital averages for the same decades, 8.70 and 9.22, it is evident that this small group of cases in which systolic murmurs were heard at the apex during their attacks showed, on later examination, measurements essentially the same as in the general average, despite the fact that at the onset of the disease the average for these same cases was slightly below the general mean.

Extent of Cardiac Dulness to the Right. In none of these cases was the dulness to the right measured while the patient was in the hospital. In the subsequent examinations a record was made in 29 cases, the average extent of dulness being 3.39 cm., as compared with the total average for all decades of 3.35. 9 of these patients who were under twenty years of age showed an average measurement of 3.3 cm., as against the general average of 3.08, while the 20 cases over twenty years of age showed an average measurement of 3.43, as compared with the general average of 3.44.

Heart Sounds. In but 2 of the 31 cases in which a systolic apical murmur was heard in the hospital was the sound transmitted to the axilla, and in neither of these instances were the signs such as might have justified a diagnosis of organic cardiac disease.

On the later examination:

In 11 instances the heart sounds were clear.

In 1 case there was a slight cardio-respiratory murmur at the apex.

In 6 cases there was a soft systolic murmur at the base, in some instances heard also over the right ventricle.

In 13 cases there was a systolic murmur at the apex of the heart. Of these 13 cases:

In 5 the murmur was a soft systolic blow heard at the apex, and in 3 instances also over the rest of the cardiac area. In the 2 cases where the murmur was limited to the apex it disappeared in the erect posture.

In 5 the signs justified the diagnosis of mitral insufficiency.

In 1 there were signs suggestive of mitral stenosis.

In 1 there was marked arterio-sclerosis, with hyper-tension, and a slight systolic murmur at the apex, tricuspid, and pulmonic areas.

In 1 there was Graves' disease, with a systolic murmur all over the cardiac area. This condition was present also at the time of the fever.

Review. On considering these figures, we find that the 31 cases in which systolic murmurs were observed during the fever showed, on later examination, nothing remarkable with regard to the pulse, while the palpability of the peripheral arteries was below the general average for the old typhoids.

On the other hand, the blood pressure was strikingly higher than the general average, one-half of the cases of extreme hyper-tension (200 mm. or above) being observed in this small group. The size of the heart was also increased, as compared to the mean of our observations upon the old typhoids, while the actual increase in those cases in which measurements were made in the hospital and later was also greater than the general average.

Seven or nearly one-quarter of these cases, showed, on subsequent examination, evidence of organic cardiac lesions, while another case was a striking example of general arterio-sclerosis, with hyper-tension, in a young individual.

* * *

Among these 183 cases there are several which deserve special attention.

CASE I. *Hypertrophied heart; mitral insufficiency.*—Mrs. H. B. (Hospital No. 9921), aged forty years, was admitted to the hospital on April 19, 1894, where she passed through a typhoid fever of thirty days' duration, complicated with neuritis of the left ulnar nerve. The urine was free from albumin. Previously she had been a healthy woman, excepting for an attack of acute articular rheumatism at six years, and three attacks since then. In the hospital records it was noted that there was no increase in the area of cardiac dulness; that the sounds were clear at the apex. The highest recorded pulse was 116.

On January 5, 1903, the patient reported for examination in answer to my letter. She had had no illness since leaving the hospital. She had, however, complained of late of being somewhat short of breath on exertion. The pulse was 22 to the quarter, regular, of good size, rather long duration. The radial artery was just palpable; temporals not prominent. Systolic blood pressure, 200 mm.

Heart. Point of maximum impulse in the fifth space 10 cm. from the midsternal line. Dulness extends 4 cm. to the right of the midsternal line. At the apex the first sound is replaced by a well-marked blowing systolic murmur; the second is clear. The murmur is heard distinctly throughout the axilla and in the back. It is audible also in the tricuspid, pulmonic, and aortic areas, over the manubrium, and in the carotids. The aortic second sound is sharp, though scarcely as sharp as the second pulmonic, which is accentuated. There are one or two reduplications of the second sound in the pulmonic area at the end of each inspiration, the second part of the split sound being accentuated. This reduplication is occasionally heard in the aortic area, where the accented part is clearly the first.

In this case it is possible that a valvular lesion, though not evident at the period when she was in the hospital, may have dated from her preceding attacks of rheumatism.

Case II. *Moderate hypertrophy of the heart; mitral insufficiency.*—E. T. E. (Hospital No. 10,704), aged twenty-five years, entered the hospital on August 23, 1894, where he passed through a typhoid fever of very moderate intensity and without complications beyond albuminuria, with granular casts, and some epithelium. He had had measles, scarlet fever, and mumps as a child; no venereal history; used alcohol in moderation. The note on the heart states that: "The point of maximum impulse is in the fourth space, a little inside the mammillary line. Relative dulness not increased to the right. Pulse slow, of good volume and tension. Sounds clear, of normal relative intensity." No further note was made on the heart.

On January 18, 1903, the patient returned for examination. He had been well since discharge. He was rather flushed and excited; pulse, 24 to the quarter, of good size, duration fair; vessel wall just palpable. Brachial pulse visible at the bend of the elbow, and temporals visible, but not especially thickened. Blood pressure, 180 mm.

Heart. Impulse marked in the third and fourth interspaces; of maximum intensity in the fifth interspace in the mammillary line 10.5 cm. from the midsternal line. Dulness extends 3.2 cm. to the right of the midsternal line.

At the apex the first sound is prolonged and followed by a soft systolic murmur, which is heard throughout the axilla; second clear. In the tricuspid area the sounds are clear and sharp. In the pulmonic area the first sound is prolonged and continued into a slight systolic murmur; the second, loud and sharp. The murmur is also heard in the aortic area, over the manubrium and in the carotids.

Occasionally a very slight reduplication of the pulmonic second sound is to be heard at the end of inspiration. In the erect posture a soft systolic souffle is well heard in the left back, though audible at the apex.

There may be some question as to the existence of mitral insufficiency in this case, but the high tension, the rather large size of the heart, and the audibility of the murmur in the left back are suggestive.

CASE III. *Hypertrophy and dilatation of the heart; mitral insufficiency.*—J. H. (Hospital No. 10,714), aged sixty-one years, was admitted to the hospital on August 24, 1894, where he passed through a typhoid fever of seventeen days' duration, of moderate severity. The urine during the attack showed a trace of albumin, hyaline and granular casts. He had had previously no serious illnesses; had used alcohol in moderation. The pulse was full, soft, regular in force and rhythm, 92. Tension not increased. Vessel wall not thickened.

Heart. Apex-beat in the fifth space, 3 cm. inside the nipple line. The first sound at the apex was occasionally followed by a soft systolic puff, not transmitted (cardio-respiratory?). Sounds at the base clear, of normal relative intensity.

On January 18, 1903, the patient returned to the hospital in answer to my letter. Up to a week before he had been fairly well. For a week he had been complaining of shortness of breath on exertion. He was somewhat cyanotic, the respirations labored and rather wheezing. The pulse was 22 to the quarter, of good size; duration fairly good; vessel wall not palpable. Blood pressure, 215 mm.

Heart. Point of maximum impulse neither visible nor palpable. By percussion and auscultation it was localized in the fifth interspace, 12 cm. from the midsternal line. Dulness 5 cm. to the right. Sounds: first, reduplicated at the apex; second, clear. The reduplication was not clearly heard in the tricuspid area. At the base the sounds were clear in both the pulmonic and aortic areas, the aortic second sharply ringing, greatly accentuated. Fine râles were heard at both bases.

The patient was admitted to the hospital on the following day, at which time the apex was found 1 cm. farther out, and a systolic murmur was audible at the apex, transmitted but a short distance outward. The sounds were feeble over the precordium. The second sounds were clear. After rest in bed the patient improved greatly. The fine râles cleared up, and eleven days later the patient was discharged. The apical murmur, however, persisted. The blood pressure in bed was 165 mm. The urine at first showed a trace of albumin, which disappeared later; specific gravity normal.

This was a well-marked case of dilatation, with mitral insufficiency.

CASE IV. *Hypertrophy of the heart; mitral insufficiency.*—A. B. (Hospital No. 31,173), a young woman aged twenty-four years, was admitted to the hospital on July 9, 1900, where she passed through an attack of typhoid fever of forty-six days' duration without serious complications. The urine was at all times free from albumin. As a child she had had measles, mumps, and scarlet fever, the latter followed by nephritis; the radial arteries were not palpable.

Heart. Point of maximum impulse not palpable. Sounds best heard in the fourth space, 9 cm. from the median line. First sound rather feeble. The aortic second louder than the second pulmonic. There was no further note on the heart.

On December 22, 1902, the patient returned for examination. She had been married and had had one child since discharge. Since the birth of the child she had not felt well.

Pulse, slightly irregular in rhythm, 27 to the quarter, occasionally intermittent, of moderate size, and good duration. The vessel wall was not palpable. Blood pressure 170 mm.

Heart. Apex impulse in the fourth space, 10 cm. from the median line. Dulness extended 3 cm. to the right of the median line. The impulse was strong, rather snapping, associated with and apparently preceded by a very slight thrill. "The first sound at the apex is rather sharp, followed by a slight systolic murmur. This murmur is heard in the axilla and faintly in the back; it is a little louder in the tricuspid area. In the pulmonic area there is a loud systolic murmur. The second sound is sharp and clear, relatively accentuated, as compared with the second aortic; no reduplication. In the aortic area there is a well-marked systolic murmur transmitted upward over the manubrium and into the carotids. The second sound is clear."

In this instance the enlargement of the ventricle and the slight irregularity of the pulse, as well as the transmission of the systolic murmur, all tend to suggest that a true mitral insufficiency exists. The snapping character of the first sound and the slight suggestion of a palpable thrill, although no corresponding murmur was to be heard, are in favor of the existence of an actual valvular lesion.

CASE V. *Mitral stenosis and insufficiency (?).*—A. S. (Hospital No. 32,037), a girl aged ten years, was admitted to the hospital on September 3, 1900, where she passed through a typhoid fever of thirty-four days' duration, complicated by cystitis. The case was of moderate severity, the pulse not particularly rapid at any time. As a child she had had measles, tonsillitis, and bronchitis at three years, and again the winter before entry.

In the hospital record it was noted:

"*Heart.* Point of maximum impulse in the fourth space, 6 cm. from the midsternal line. Both sounds well heard at the apex. Loud systolic murmur at the base. At the apex the first is accompanied by a very faint systolic murmur; the second pulmonic, not accentuated."

Later on it was again noted that there was a faint systolic murmur all over the precordium, loudest in the pulmonic area. No note was made on the heart at the time of discharge. The patient was not, however, supposed to have a cardiac lesion.

On December 22, 1902, the patient returned for examination. She had been perfectly well since discharge. The pulse was regular, 25 to the quarter, of moderate size, and rather long duration. The vessel wall was not palpable. Blood pressure 135 mm.

Heart. Apex visible and palpable in the fourth space, 7 cm. from the midsternal line, just inside the mammillary line. Dulness 2.25 cm. to the right of the median line. The impulse was strong, rather prolonged, preceded by a suggestion of a thrill. The first sound at the apex was prolonged and booming. There was a distinct echo in the latter part of diastole, which was almost loud enough to be called a true presystolic murmur, having all the characteristics of a presystolic murmur of slight degree. The first sound was succeeded by a very soft, slight systolic murmur, which was heard in the axilla, but not in the back. Second sound well heard at the apex. In the tricuspid area there was a soft systolic murmur which became louder as one reached the pulmonic area. The second sound in the pulmonic area was sharp and clear. The same murmur was heard at the aortic orifice feebly, but better than in the pulmonic area; also over the manubrium and in the carotids. At the time of the examination it was noted: "It would seem that the apex murmur (presystolic) was doubtless produced at the time of entrance of blood into the ventricle from the left auricle, and, in all probability, at the mitral valve. The case may be one of mitral stenosis, though it is not impossible that the heart may be quite normal."

CASE VI. *Hypertrophy and dilatation of the heart; mitral insufficiency; hyper-tension.*—M. Z. (Hospital No. 17,636), a woman aged forty-three years, was admitted to the hospital on October 19, 1896, where she passed through a typhoid fever of sixty-four days' duration, without complications. The urine showed a trace of albumin, and once a hyaline cast. She had been previously a perfectly healthy woman, excepting for an attack of typhoid fever seven years before and for occasional pains in her joints, unassociated with fever or swelling. She had had twelve children and two miscarriages.

When in the hospital it was noted that at the apex the first sound was replaced by a soft systolic whiff, faintly transmitted to the axilla.

The second sounds were clear. The heart's action was rather irregular. The murmur could be heard all over the base of the heart. The highest recorded pulse in the hospital was 120. No further note was made upon the circulatory apparatus. On discharge the patient was considered to have a normal heart.

The patient returned to the hospital on February 16, 1903, in answer to my letter. For two months she had suffered from shortness of breath, especially on excitement and exertion. This was also worse at night, so that at times she had to sit up in bed. On physical examination the pulse was 26 to the quarter, of fairly good size; duration long; vessel wall not palpable. The blood pressure was 200 mm. The urine was free from albumin.

"*Heart.* Point of maximum impulse palpable in the fifth interspace, 9.50 cm. from the median line. Dulness extends 2.75 cm. to the right of the median line. Sounds: The first at the apex is followed by a well-marked blowing systolic murmur heard faintly throughout the axilla; second clear. In the tricuspid area the murmur is less marked; the second sound clear. In the pulmonic area the first sound is represented by a slight systolic murmur; the second sharp and loud. In the aortic area the first is followed by a very soft systolic murmur heard over the manubrium, not in the carotids. The second pulmonic is sharper than the second aortic. No reduplication of the second sound. In the erect posture the murmur persists at the apex, but is not heard in the back." Two months later the patient returned to the Out-patient Department again, complaining of shortness of breath. At this time the apex had moved outward 2 cm., while in other respects the signs were about the same.

CASE VII. *Hypertrophy; mitral insufficiency.*—B. W. (Hospital No. 24,675), a woman aged twenty-six years, was admitted to the hospital on September 11, 1898, where she passed through a long typhoid fever, with two relapses, complicated with arthritis of the ankles. The urine was free from albumin. The patient had always been healthy and had had previously no serious illnesses. In the hospital the following note was made on the heart

"*Heart.* Point of maximum impulse, fifth space, 3 cm. inside the mammillary line. At the point of maximum impulse there is a soft, blowing systolic murmur, not traceable into the axilla. Sounds at base clear; of normal relative intensity. Pulse regular; good volume; 36 to the quarter." In several notes there is no mention of palpable radials. Later it was stated that the second pulmonic was accentuated, and that the murmur was traced to the anterior axillary line.

The patient was examined on March 6, 1903, five and a half years later. After leaving the hospital there was another relapse, with left-sided femoral phlebitis. For some time afterward there was œdema of the feet. Otherwise she has been quite well. The pulse was 80, regular, of fairly good size; long duration. Artery just palpable. Blood pressure 210 mm.

"*Heart.* Apex impulse in the fifth space, 10.5 cm. from the median line. Dulness extends 3.5 cm. to the right of the midsternum. At the apex the first sound is followed by a systolic murmur, which is heard all over the cardiac area, though best at the point of maximum impulse; it is transmitted as far as the mid-axilla. In the erect posture it is still heard at the apex, though with much diminished intensity. In the back as the patient sits up, it is a question whether at times a faint suggestion of a murmur may not be heard. The second sounds are both strong; the second pulmonic is distinctly accentuated."

CASE VIII. *Mitral insufficiency; hypertrophy of the heart;*—E. R. (Hospital No. 28,249), a colored woman aged thirty-eight years, was admitted to the hospital on October 24, 1899, where she passed through a mild attack of typhoid fever of seventeen days' duration. The urine contained a trace of albumin, and hyaline and granular casts. As a child she had had measles, mumps, and chickenpox. No other serious illnesses.

In the hospital it was noted that "the point of maximum impulse is in the fifth space, 8.5 cm. from the median line. Impulse punctate, rather heaving; slight suggestion of a thrill running up to the impulse. At the point of maximum impulse the first sound is replaced by a short blow, which is preceded by a very short, indistinct rumbling. This latter is to be heard above and outside the point of maximum impulse. The systolic murmur is heard over the base. The second pulmonic is slightly accentuated and clear. The aortic second sound is clear." No note as to the palpability of the radial arteries. About two weeks before discharge it was noted that there was a systolic murmur at the apex and pulmonic areas, but on discharge it was stated that the heart sounds were clear.

On August 12, 1903, the patient returned in answer to my letter. She had had one child since leaving the hospital. For three months she has felt rather poorly, the catamenia having been profuse and of late rather irregular—possibly menopause. The pulse was regular, excepting for occasional intercurrent beats, 17 to the quarter; of moderate size, long duration. The vessel wall was just palpable on the right side; not on the left. Temporals not sclerotic. Blood pressure 165.

Heart. Point of maximum impulse visible and palpable in the fifth space, 11.5 cm. from the median line, 1 to 2 cm. outside the mammillary line. The dulness extended 3.7 cm. to the right. Impulse, heaving, stronger than usual. " The first sound at the apex is prolonged and followed by a distinct systolic murmur heard throughout the left axilla and faintly in the back. The second sounds are sharp. In the tricuspid area the murmur is not distinctly audible. The second pulmonic is fairly sharp, and is reduplicated with about two beats on inspiration. The second aortic is not as loud as the second pulmonic. The reduplication of the second sound is not heard in the aortic area, and is clearly due to pulmonic delay. In both pulmonic and aortic areas there is a slight suggestion of a systolic murmur, which is not heard in the carotids."

CASE IX. *Hypertrophy and dilatation of the heart; mitral insufficiency.*—J. F. (Hospital No. 36,210), aged eighteen years, was admitted to the hospital on September 9, 1901. He passed through a typhoid fever of very moderate intensity, the probable length of fever being only about thirteen or fourteen days. The urine showed a slight trace of albumin on entrance and a few coarsely granular casts, but both albumin and casts disappeared later. There were no complications. He had had chickenpox when young, but knew of no other serious illnesses. Is a farmer, and exposed to a good deal of bad weather. Does not drink nor use tobacco.

In the hospital the pulse was 21 to the quarter; marked sclerosis of radials. "Heart sounds loud and booming. Systolic murmur in pulmonic area. Second sound clear." No further note was made on the heart. The highest recorded pulse was 112. During convalescence the pulse was as low as 48.

In September, 1903, he reported in answer to my letter, and, in my absence, was examined by Dr. Briggs. He had been perfectly well since leaving the hospital. "Radials much sclerosed. Brachials thickened and visibly pulsating at the elbow. Pulse 24 to the quarter, slightly irregular in force and rhythm, with rare intermissions of rather short duration; large volume; not collapsing. Blood pressure 182."

Heart. Point of maximum impulse in the fourth interspace, 8 cm. from the midsternal line, though the impulse was to be felt as far out as 14 cm. from the median line in the fifth interspace, with which dulness was practically coexistent. Relative dulness extended 5 cm. to the right of the midsternal line. The systolic impulse was forcible; the shock of both sounds well felt; no thrill. At the apex both sounds were well heard, the first booming, and followed by a rather intense, blowing, systolic murmur, transmitted to the axilla, but not to the back. "In a small area upward and inward from the apex in the fourth space the second sound has at the beginning of examination a faintly rumbling echo, not running through diastole; this disappears on resting, reappearing after examination. In the tricuspid area and over the precordial region the systolic is well heard; the second sound is clear. In the pulmonic area the systolic is louder than over the right ventricle; not so loud as at the apex. The second pulmonic is louder than the second aortic and is reduplicated, the accent being on the second part of the reduplication, and the length of the interval being more marked during deep inspiration, though present throughout the respiratory phases. The aortic sound is clear, ringing, bell-like, and, though not so loud, is more intense than the second pulmonic. The first sound is fainter. No systolic murmur audible. There is no diastolic murmur to be heard at the base nor along the border of the sternum."

CASE X. *Four months after discharge, aortic insufficiency which had disappeared five months later.*—J. C. (Hospital No. 39,371), a man aged twenty-two years, entered the hospital on June 26, 1902. Here he passed through a typhoid fever of moderate severity, without complications, leaving the hospital on August 9, 1902. The urine showed a trace of albumin at the height of the disease. He had had measles as a child; denied venereal disease; habits good. In the hospital it was noted that the radial artery was palpable. On two occasions during the disease the blood pressure was 128.

Heart. Dr. McCrae noted that the point of maximum impulse was very feeble, visible (?) in the fifth space, 10.5 cm. from the midsternal line. The first sound was everywhere of rather an indefinite quality, but there was no actual murmur.

On November 30th, about sixteen weeks after discharge from the hospital, he reported in answer to my letter. The pulse was 27 to the quarter (the patient was rather nervous), collapsing, but of clearly high systolic pressure. Vessel wall not palpable. Blood pressure 174 mm.

Heart. Apex in the fourth interspace, 10.5 cm. from the midsternal line. Sounds clear and strong at the apex. A soft systolic murmur was heard at the tricuspid area and at the aortic area transmitted upward over the manubrium. The second aortic sound was very loud; no murmur. Both sounds were heard in the carotids, the first prolonged as a roughened murmur. No murmur was heard in the pulmonic area. The systolic murmur was distinctly loudest at the aortic area, and was transmitted upward. *There was a very soft diastolic murmur, heard along the left sternal border.* This murmur was extremely slight, but was heard by Dr. Briggs, as well as by myself.

Five months later, on April 21st, the patient reported at the dispensary. He had been complaining of a slight cough, the last stage of a cold which he had had for about a week. He was still hoarse, with a teasing cough. Had not been working regularly on account of nervousness. The lungs were clear. The pulse was regular, of good size; nothing remarkable about its quality.

"*Heart.* Apex impulse not seen nor felt. By stethoscope and percussion it was localized 9.5 cm. from the median line, in the fifth space. Dulness extends 3.5 cm. to the right of the median line. At the apex and all over the cardiac area, most marked in the aortic area, there is a soft systolic murmur, which wholly disappears in the erect posture. The sounds are otherwise clear, excepting that in the pulmonic area there is a reduplication of the second sound, which occurs several times during ordinary inspiration, the delayed part being clearly the second pulmonic. This reduplication is heard at times in the aortic area. There is no diastolic murmur either in the erect or recumbent posture."

The case is one of much interest. May it have been an instance of transient dilatation of the aortic ring?

CASE XI. *Aortic insufficiency.*—L. R. (Hospital No. 20,507), a man aged thirty-nine years, was admitted to the hospital on September 4, 1897, and passed through a typhoid fever of fifty days' duration, followed by a relapse, associated with bronchitis and a pemphigoid eruption on the hands. The urine contained no albumin, but an occasional hyaline and granular cast was found. As a child he had had scarlet fever, and almost every fall had had malarial fever. Four years before entry he had had another attack of typhoid fever; four years before, urethritis. The pulse was not remarkably rapid at any time during the course, and the only note with regard to the circulatory apparatus was "heart negative."

On February 15, 1903, the patient reported in answer to my letter, and, in my absence, was examined by Dr. Briggs. The patient had been well since discharge, but had lived a life of hard work and exposure. "Pulse 82; slightly irregular in force and rhythm; distinctly collapsing; vessel wall moderately thickened; marked visible pulsation in brachials and carotids; none in the temporals. Marked capillary pulsation. Systolic blood pressure, 185 mm.

"*Heart.* Point of maximum impulse just visible and palpable in the fourth space, 12 cm. from the median line, in the left mammillary line. Impulse faint; no thrill. The relative dulness begins at the second left interspace and extends to the right sternal margin at the level of the fourth rib. No absolute cardiac dulness. At the apex both sounds are heard; the first rather muffled, followed by a soft systolic puff, carried to the mid-axilla, and faintly heard at the xiphoid. The second sound is sharp and clear. Just above the nipple, in a small area, there is a short, faint rumble in diastole, ending before the first sound, which is not snapping. Both sounds are heard over the right ventricle, with a systolic murmur, which becomes more marked in the second, third, and fourth left spaces, and is heard at the base, though not over the manubrium, and in the neck. The pulmonic second is louder, accentuated; occasionally a faint reduplication with inspiration. The aortic second is soft, but clear. In the second and third left interspaces close to the sternum there is a very short, faint diastolic murmur following the second sound."

CASE XII. *Marked arterio-sclerosis.* C. Z. (Hospital No. 17,632), a boy aged thirteen years, was admitted to the hospital on October 19, 1896, where he passed through a typhoid fever of seventeen days' duration, without complications, being discharged on November 19, 1896. There was a trace of albumin, with hyaline and granular casts, during the height of the fever. He had suffered from no previous serious infections, and, so far as could be determined, was a boy of good habits. The highest recorded pulse in the hospital was 112. A full note on the heart was made by Dr. McCrae. Pulse 21 to the quarter, soft, and easily compressible; synchronous in radials and femorals.

Heart. Point of maximum impulse in fourth space, 7 cm. from the median line; wavy; no thrill. Area of cardiac dulness not increased. Sounds: A soft, systolic murmur was heard at the apex, not especially carried around to the axilla; best heard over the second and third left spaces. The second sound was very loud at the apex and much accentuated in the second left space. No further note as to the heart.

On January 4, 1903, he returned in response to my letter. Three years ago he had had an attack of tonsillitis, after which his tonsils were removed. Beyond this he had considered himself quite well. The pulse was 25 to the quarter, showing rather marked irregularities in rhythm; of good size and long duration. The vessel wall was much thickened; readily rolled under the finger. The temporals were tortuous, prominent and somewhat thickened. The systolic pressure was 200 mm.

Heart. The apex impulse was visible and palpable in the fifth space just inside the mammillary line, 8.7 cm. from the median line. The dulness extended 3.2 cm. to the right of the midsternal line. Sounds. The first at the apex was prolonged and booming, followed by a very slight systolic murmur, which was lost before one reached the mid-axilla. "A much more distinct, high-pitched, blowing systolic follows the first sound in the tricuspid area and over the right ventricle in the third and fourth spaces. It is, however, barely audible in the pulmonic area, and is not heard in the aortic area or over the manubrium. It is not affected by change of position. Sounds at the base clear. The second aortic is accentuated." At the time that this note was made the following remarks were added: "In this instance there is a distinctly hypertrophied heart, with marked sclerosis of the radials and temporals. The murmur heard in the tricuspid area is not of the ordinary character of a functional murmur, being higher pitched and having a very blowing sound."

This case, it seems to me, is one of particular interest, in view of the fact that beyond the tonsillitis the only element to which one could reasonably ascribe the cardio-vascular abnormalities was the preceding typhoid fever.

* * *

Summary.

A study of the condition of the heart and vessels in 183 individuals who have passed through typhoid fever at the Johns Hopkins

Hospital within the last thirteen years has revealed the following facts:

1. The average systolic blood pressure in these old typhoids was appreciably higher than in control observations upon healthy individuals.

2. The higher average of the blood pressure was constant in every decade.

3. In many instances among the old typhoids the blood pressure exceeded appreciably the limits of what is usually regarded as normal.

4. The radial arteries in the old typhoids were palpable in a proportion nearly three times as great as that found in control observations upon supposedly healthy individuals who had never had the disease.

5. The average size of the heart was greater among the old typhoids than in the same cases at the time of admission to the hospital. The difference held good also when the cases were classed according to age by decades.

6. Cardiac murmurs were heard with considerably greater frequency among the old typhoids and in the same cases during the attacks.

7. In 8 cases where, on discharge from the hospital, the heart was considered normal, subsequent examination revealed hypertrophy, with mitral insufficiency. One case showed a possible mitral stenosis; one an aortic insufficiency; one a striking general arteriosclerosis, with hyper-tension.

8. In one case an aortic diastolic murmur was present four months after discharge, but had disappeared five months later.

9. Those patients whose pulse during the disease was remarkably rapid or irregular, showed, in general, on later examination, a blood pressure above the common average for the old typhoids. In other respects, however, their condition differed but little from the general run of cases.

10. Those cases in which a systolic murmur at the apex of the heart was observed during the attack showed later an increase in the blood pressure and in the size of the heart, as compared both with the mean of the observations made upon the same cases on admission to the hospital and with the general average for the old typhoids. Nearly one quarter of those cases in which during the attack, systolic apical murmurs were detected, showed, on later examination, evidences of organic heart disease. Indeed, the majority of all the cases of organic cardiac lesions among the 183 old typhoids came from this small group of 31 cases.

It is recognized that these results are based upon the analysis of a number of cases too small to justify final conclusions; the next 200 cases may considerably modify the figures. Yet the fact that these 183 old typhoids are materially older, from a point of view of their hearts and arteries, than the average individual who has not had typhoid fever, would tend to support the views of those who regard this disease as an active element in the ætiology of a considerable number of cases of cardiac hypertrophy and dilatation coming on sometimes in early life, as well as an important factor in the production of those vascular changes which Cazalis has happily called "*la rouille de la vie.*"

MULTIPLE SARCOMA.[1]

By Thomas A. Claytor, M.D.,

PROFESSOR OF THERAPEUTICS, COLUMBIA UNIVERSITY; PHYSICIAN TO THE GARFIELD AND TO THE UNIVERSITY HOSPITALS, WASHINGTON, D. C.

This subject is one so broad that it becomes of interest alike to the internist, the surgeon, and the dermatologist.

The particular class of cases which I propose to consider is that in which there are multiple sarcomatous growths in the skin and subcutaneous tissue, excluding that class of tumors characterized by lymphoid cells, in which are included leukæmia, pseudoleukæmia, and malignant lymphoma, and also the so-called sarcoid group, comprising idiopathic hemorrhagic sarcoma, sarcoma cutis, and multiple benign sarcoid. Cases have been reported in which the tumors seemed to have been multiple from the beginning, but it seems more probable that there was a primary growth which may have escaped notice, so rapidly was it followed by an outburst of metastatic tumors. The secondary growths may be pigmented or non-pigmented, or may be mixed—*i. e.*, some may show melanotic material, while others are entirely white, which was observed in one of my cases to be reported later. They may belong to the round, spindle, or myeloid form of sarcoma, or the cells may change from one form to another during the progress of the disease. The tumors usually appear as small, round nodules, the size of a shot, which rapidly develop into oval or round plates, which may be somewhat depressed in the centre. The size to which they may grow is indefinite; as a rule, however, few reach a greater diameter than one inch. They are situated either in the skin proper, or in the deep fascia, hence may move with the skin or the skin may move freely over them. Ulceration may occur either from pressure or from apparently spontaneous breaking down of the new tissue. They may or may not be encapsulated. The latter condition is said to improve the outlook. The appearance of the cutaneous or subcutaneous nodules is either preceded or rapidly followed by involvement more or less

[1] Read before the Medical Society of Washington, D. C., October 7, 1903.

general of internal organs and tissues, which in a longer or shorter time, usually the latter, causes death.

After a careful study of a number of reported cases, I find it unprofitable to attempt any statistical classification of the seats of primary growth, there being apparently no special points of predilection

The primary growth may be a pigmented mole situated anywhere upon the skin; it may be in the subcutaneous tissue, or may spring apparently from the bone, skull, vertebræ, etc., or from an internal organ.

The following reports of cases, two of which I have observed myself and the others selected from the literature, will give a clearer idea of this most fatal affection:

CASE I.—R. C., white, male, married, aged thirty years, butcher, was admitted to Garfield Hospital December 4, 1902. His father died of pneumonia; his mother is living and in good health. C. had the usual diseases of childhood, including measles, mumps, whooping-cough, etc., from which he made good recoveries; had enteric fever when fifteen. He went to school until he was twelve, and then worked for ten years in a factory. Since then he has been a butcher. Three years ago he had erysipelas extending over the scalp, face, and neck. The attack resulted from a scalp wound. Immediately after this a swelling was noticed on the right side of the head in the occipital region, which increased in size very slowly until the present time, when it is about the size of a large walnut. For the past eighteen months the stomach has been irritable, the meals being frequently vomited. These periods have been intermittent, however, and at times his stomach gives him no trouble. The vomitus has never contained blood. Had gonorrhœa eight years ago, but has never had syphilis. Uses no alcohol. He was married six years ago, but his wife has borne no children.

The present attack may be dated from the first appearance of the tumor on the back of his head, which was three years ago. The growth of the tumor has been intermittent, there being periods when it did not seem to enlarge for some time. No other enlargement was noted until last May, seven months ago, when a nodule began to develop on the right side of the neck about two inches below the mastoid process. This gradually increased in size until two months ago, when it seemed to diminish a little. In July another nodule appeared under the skin near the umbilicus. The tumor on the neck caused pain and stiffness until it stopped growing. About this time, because of his general debility and anæmic appearance, he was advised to take a trip to California. About September 1st nodules began to appear on the chest and a few on the abdomen. None of them gave any pain and moved freely under the skin. Nodules then appeared on the right arm and in the right axilla. Those in the axilla gave pain, with a feeling of contraction. Later the growths appeared on the left arm. About October 15th slight swelling of the abdomen was for the first time noted, which has gradually increased. Complains of pain across the shoulders and chest, which keeps him from sleeping. There is no cough, but considerable dyspnœa on slight exertion.

Physical Examination. Emaciated and anæmic. In the right posterior occipital region is a tumor about the size of a walnut, which is just beneath the scalp, very slightly movable on the skull, and of almost bony hardness. This is probably the primary growth which was first noticed three years ago. Numerous smaller nodules may be felt in or under the scalp. On the right side of the neck, rather toward the posterior aspect, is a firm, nodular tumor, three and five-tenths inches long by three inches in the anteroposterior diameter. About the periphery are numerous smaller nodules. The large tumor is quite firmly fixed, though it is not absolutely so, the smaller ones being freely movable. There are nodules in the left postcervical region; there is a small nodule situated over the inner third of each clavicle. Numerous small nodules are seen upon the anterior aspect of the right arm, one upon the right forearm. The right epitrochlear gland is slightly enlarged. There are numerous small nodules extending from the right axilla down to the ilium; also in the right interscapular, right lumbar, and sacral areas posteriorly and on the right side of the chest anteriorly. One tumor, larger than the rest, about half an inch in diameter, two inches to the right of the umbilicus. One situated about midway between the umbilicus and ensiform cartilage, about a quarter of an inch in diameter, is red, and is said to discharge pus from time to time. This is the only tumor which seems to be attached to the skin, all the others apparently growing from the deep fascia, being alike freely movable upon the muscles and under the skin. Growths are also seen in and about the left axilla, upon the left arm, left side of the chest and back, but are not so numerous as upon the right side. A few nodules are upon the right thigh and in the right inguinal region.

The growths vary in size from a shot to a large marble, except the primary growth on the head and the first secondary on the neck; some are plate-like, others round. They are firm, elastic, and not painful. There is no discoloration of the skin, except over the one situated on the abdomen, near the umbilicus, which has broken down.

The pulse is weak and compressible. No abnormality is to be discovered in the heart or lungs; the liver and spleen cannot be satisfactorily examined because of a large ascitic collection. (These organs were found at the autopsy not to be enlarged.)

Between the date of the first examination and that of the patient's death numerous hard masses, about the size of a fist, were detected in the abdominal cavity. They seemed to be quite freely movable in the ascitic fluid and were proven at the autopsy to be sarcomatous masses in the omentum.

The patient said that the nodules first appeared about the size of a pinhead and gradually increased without pain, except when they were subjected to pressure against a bony surface.

One of the smaller growths was removed on December 11th. It was encapsulated. The following is the report by Dr. J. B. Nichols:

Alveolar, large, round-celled sarcoma. Areas of beginning necrosis scattered irregularly throughout. Blood examination showed 3,710,000 reds, 6300 whites, hæmoglobin 65 per cent.; no abnormality in size or shape of red cells. A differential count of the white cells showed: small mononuclears, 13.8 per cent.; large mononuclears and transitional, 8 per cent.; polynuclear neutrophiles, 78 per cent.; eosinophiles, 0.4 per cent.; mast-cells, 0.8 per cent.

The urine showed no abnormality, except a rather high specific gravity.

Examination of the stomach contents after an Ewald test breakfast showed: total acidity, 31; acidity due to HCl, 11; free HCl, 0.04 per cent.; lactic acid, 0; pepsin deficient, etc.

The most distressing symptoms were due to the rapid and persistent accumulation of ascitic fluid. For twenty-four to forty-eight hours after a tapping there would be comparative comfort, only to be followed by intrathoracic pain, nausea, vomiting, dyspnœa, etc., as the fluid accumulated. The temperature was irregular, ranging from subnormal to 100° F.; the pulse and respirations were never frequent.

Death occurred on January 29, 1903, about three years after the appearance of the primary growth beneath the scalp, and about nine months after the appearance of the first secondary growth, which was on the right side of the neck, and about four months after general subcutaneous involvement.

Necropsy. Multiple, hard, subcutaneous nodules (for size and situation see case history). Emaciation extreme. Heart: weight, 265 grams; small; fat diminished, muscle dark red. Myocardium of every chamber contains deeply pigmented nodules situated subendo- and subpericardially and intramurally, varying in size from a pea to a hazelnut. Valves normal, coronaries patulous, aorta slightly atheromatous. Pericardium contains a few cubic centimetres of straw-colored fluid. Lymph glands frequently sarcomatous. Spleen: weight, 171 grams. One nodule at the hilum, two of larger size deep in the splenic substance. Right lung: weight, 285 grams. Moderately pigmented; a small, caseous, firmly encapsulated area in the apex; interlobular adhesions; two subpleural sarcomata over middle lobe; a few small sarcomata in the lower lobe, one large tumor at the root. Left lung: weight, 250 grams. A few nodules in the lower lobe, otherwise negative. Stomach: mucosa congested. Small intestine: sarcomatous nodules generally distributed over serous coat. Large intestine: a large nodule situated at the ileocæcal valve. Subperitoneal sarcomata everywhere; a nodular mass at the splenic flexuræ.

Peritoneum: moderate amount of straw-colored fluid. The omentum solid, firm, dark red; a mass of sarcomatous nodules 4.7 cm. at the thickest portion. Liver: weight, 1550 grams; two small nodules on the peritoneal aspect of right lobe; in the substance of the lobe are four nodules. Kidneys: the only point worthy of note is the difference in size and weight of these organs; the right weighs 170 grams, the left 57 grams.

Unfortunately, there could be no examination of the brain or cord.

Treatment consisted of hypodermic injections of Fowler's solution twice daily, beginning with three drops. The X-ray was also tried, but neither had any beneficial effect, though there was an increase in the number of red cells and in the hæmoglobin until a short time before his death. The subcutaneous nodules continued to appear, and the internal growths increased in size. That the primary growth was that of the right occipital region I see no reason to doubt, and whether or not its prompt and complete removal would have changed the outcome is the important question.

CASE II.—A. S., male, white, aged twenty-eight years, brakeman, was admitted to the University Hospital July 7, 1903 (on the service of Dr. W. P. Carr, by whose courtesy I have been allowed to observe and report the course of the disease). One grandfather died of tuberculosis, otherwise the family history is good. He was a healthy child; had measles at three and typhoid fever at twelve, from which he made good recoveries. Uses tobacco freely and drinks a great deal of coffee, but no alcohol. He has had no venereal disease. Went to school until he was sixteen and since has worked. Has always been strong and healthy until the beginning of the present illness. Last February he began to feel languid and at about the same time noticed for the first time a nodule behind the left ear on the mastoid process. The growth increased in size and was removed in the middle of April.

Two other nodules had already appeared on the chest when the growth over the mastoid was removed, and these were rapidly followed by others. On June 2d one of the nodules was excised for diagnostic purposes. It was found to be a large round-celled sarcoma, the picture being very similar to that in the previous case. On July 8th Dr. Carr removed the recurrent growth, which had extended well down on the lateral aspect of the neck, had broken down, and was giving considerable trouble. At the same time he removed a number of the subcutaneous growths from the chest and upper abdomen.

July 21st the red cells numbered 4,312,000, whites 18,000; the hæmoglobin was 60 per cent. A differential count showed: large mononuclears, 11 per cent.; small mononuclears, 5 per cent.; polynuclears, 72 per cent.; eosinophiles, 11.5 per cent.; myelocytes, 0.5 per cent. I am unable to account for the eosinophilia. The urine was negative.

Symptoms. The chief trouble from the beginning in February was weakness. There was abnormal pain and occasional nausea and vomiting.

Physical examination July 28th showed marked paleness and emaciation. Over the chest, back, and abdomen were numerous nodules, varying in size from a shot to a small marble. There was no discoloration of the skin over these nodes, which were not painful to the touch, except those which had been subjected to the X-ray. They were freely movable, being for the most part subcutaneous, moving on the muscle and under the skin. Some, however, were attached to the skin. There were a few growths on the arms, thighs, and legs. The heart was in its normal position, but there was a systolic murmur, heard with greatest intensity at the apex and transmitted into the axilla. The lungs were apparently normal, though there was an area of dulness at the base of the right lung, which may have been due to an upward enlargement of the liver. The latter organ extended two inches below the costal border. A large, hard mass, the size of the double fist, was felt in the median line of the abdomen, just above the pubes. Between this and the umbilicus another smaller mass was felt. Neither was painful. The spleen could not be felt. As to which was the primary growth, it may be said that the one over the mastoid was first noticed, but the abdominal pain began at about the same time, and the abdominal mass was of large size. The small nodules continued to multiply, and the patient left the hospital in September, and has since died. His illness lasted about seven months from the appearance of the primary growth.

The X-ray was also used in this case without curative effect.*

J. Sabrazès and L. Muratet[1] report a case, in a man aged sixty-six years, of very general involvement, which was fatal in eight months. The previous history showed nothing worthy of note. Following a supposed attack of grip, there appeared a small growth below the right clavicle, which was rapidly followed by a multiplicity of tumors over the body. At the same time tumors developed in the abdominal cavity. The growths under the skin varied in size from a shot to large nodules, raising the skin, and readily made out by palpation. The principal parts involved were the trunk, upper portion of the arms, and face, while the forearms, legs, and feet were free. Death occurred after eight months, during which time the tumors continued to increase. The autopsy showed the growths to have developed in the subcutaneous connective tissue. The skin was movable over them. There were also tumors on the long bones of the upper extremities or adherent to the periosteum, in the kidneys, and in the pericardium and myocardium. The blood count showed only 8060 leukocytes.

Levi[2] reports a case of melanotic sarcoma in a man aged fifty

[1] Arch. de méd. expér. et d'anat. path., 1902, vol. xiv.
[2] Bull. soc. anat. de Paris, 1899, lxxiv.

years. The primary growth was situated on the inner surface of the fourth toe on the left foot. It was first noticed when about the size of a pea. As the man was a baker and went without his shoes a great part of the time, it was thought that some traumatism was probably the cause. The disease, which had begun six months previously, extended rapidly to the neighboring toes, thence to the groin, where a hard tumor, the size of a fist, formed. The primary growth broke down and ulcerated. Small black nodules like the primary one appeared on the leg and in the popliteal space. During the later stages small melanotic subcutaneous nodules appeared on the outer surface of the right thigh, the edge of the right upper eyelid, the scalp, etc. Signs of pulmonary involvement then were noted, and a vague delirium, with prostration, preceded death.

Autopsy showed melanotic nodules involving the subcutaneous cellular tissue. Numerous sarcomatous nodules, both melanotic and non-melanotic, were found in the lungs, kidneys, and brain.

J. H. Musser[1] reports an interesting and frequently quoted case of universal melanotic sarcoma in an old woman, who, on January 19, 1878, had had the right eye removed for supposed glaucoma (probably sarcoma). She was readmitted in September, 1887, with a small tumor on the left side of the neck, which was painless, slightly elastic, about the size of a walnut, adherent to the skin, the surface of which was bright red and puckered. One week later another tumor was found on the right arm, it was subcutaneous, not so red or as prominent as the former. Other tumors rapidly developed, most of them on the trunk and upper extremities, a few on the thighs. They were more abundant on the right half of the body. A great number were movable under the skin, some adherent to it, and presented a reddish hue. They were abundant in the scalp. She died March 4, 1888, about six or seven months after the appearance of the tumor on the neck.

The autopsy showed involvement of nearly all the internal organs, including the heart, lungs, liver, adrenals, ovaries, uterus, etc. There was no examination of the brain or cord.

D. Grant[2] gives a partial report of the following interesting case: A man, aged twenty-seven years, gave a history of having had a black mole on the deltoid of his right arm since birth. Three years previously it had been wounded by the horn of a sheep, but soon healed; some time afterward it was hurt again, and then spread to the size of a finger-tip. Eighteen months after receiving the first injury it was bruised again, and this time did not heal readily. A few additional small patches appeared in close proximity. The whole area was then excised. This was the end of June, 1896. In November a lump appeared in the right axilla, which was excised, but since a large number of growths in the skin have appeared over

[1] Philadelphia Hospital Reports, 1893.
[2] Intercolonial Medical Journal, Melbourne, Australia, 1897, ii.

the trunk, both front and back. The general health was excellent, but the condition was considered so grave that he was sent to the Pasteur Institute to receive the Coley treatment. This is a striking example of the serious results which may follow injuries to congenital moles

Charles F. Withington[1] reports, among others, a case of multiple sarcoma, in which the primary growth had existed twenty or thirty years without giving any signs of malignancy. It occurred in a man aged seventy years, of good personal and family history. Six months before admission he noticed a number of small black tumors on the surface of the body, which had increased since then. About the same time he began to lose weight and strength. It was then learned that he had had for twenty or thirty years a tumor on the posterior aspect of his shoulder, non-pigmented and painless. Death occurred only six or seven months after the secondary tumors appeared. Autopsy showed extensive metastasis in the brain and internal organs, especially the heart.

F. C. Shattuck[2] reports a wonderfully rapid case, in which death occurred in less than four weeks after the appearance of the subentaneous nodules. There was extensive involvement of the internal organs. The primary growth was thought to have been in the dorsal vertebræ.

ETIOLOGY. Concerning the cause of sarcoma, whether single or multiple, practically nothing is known. It may follow an injury or may take its origin from old scar-tissue, or there may be no discoverable cause. The parent tumor in the variety of multiple sarcoma now under consideration is not infrequently a pigmented mole, which suddenly takes on the characteristics of a malignant growth. The usual cause for this change is an injury accidentally sustained or friction from the clothing. It may be as well to state here that it has been shown by several authorities, notably Chambard, J. Hutchinson (Jr.), Unna, and Gilchrist (Crocker), that all melanotic growths are not sarcomata, and Unna states that all growths with metastasis which start from pigmented moles are really melanotic carcinomata rather than sarcomata. The clinical behavior, however, is the same.

Concerning the pathology, I shall say nothing.

SYMPTOMATOLOGY. The symptoms are not distinctive. Besides wasting, there are likely to be those which arise from the presence of tumors, such as pain, ascites, etc.

The blood, so far as I know, shows nothing except the conditions found in any severe secondary anæmia. My case (II.) had a lenkocytosis of 18,000, but at the time the examination was made there was a suppurating wound.

DIAGNOSIS. In a fully developed case, with more or less widely scattered subcutaneous nodules, the diagnosis is simple, especially after once having had one's attention called to the condition. In the

[1] Medical and Surgical Reports, Boston City Hospital, 1897.
[2] Boston Medical and Surgical Journal, 1894.

early stages, however, when, as is often the case, there appears an irregularly nodular bunch on the side of the neck, with, perhaps, a few small nodules in the neighboring lymphatic areas, there are several possibilities which suggest themselves, namely, leukæmia, pseudoleukæmia, lymphosarcoma, tuberculosis, or syphilis. The fact that all of these conditions involve the lymphatic glands, and hence are found in lymphatic areas only, is of diagnostic importance, for the sarcomatous growths are not confined to these localities. In fact, they are usually in greatest abundance on the outer surfaces of the arms, on the chest, etc., localities where lymphatic glands are not found. Lymphatic leukæmia may be excluded by a blood examination, the other possibilities only after observation of the case for a longer or shorter time, depending on the rapidity of the appearance of metastatic growths. The most satisfactory method is to remove one of the smaller nodules for microscopic examination. This very simple procedure is, however, not without danger, since operations upon sarcomata are often followed by rapid and more malignant recurrence. If the skin has been involved the growth is almost sure to recur at the original site, but if subcutaneous the danger is much less.

TREATMENT. The rational course would seem to be that of prompt and complete removal of all suspicious growths, especially if they show the slightest signs of activity. It is a fact, however, that in many of these cases the extirpation of the primary growth is so quickly followed by an outburst of secondary tumors that we are forced to ask ourselves if the operation did not act as a stimulant to a more or less quiescent condition, and in that way only hasten the inevitable result. The question of operation, then, is one which requires careful consideration.

So far as drugs are concerned, arsenic is the only remedy which has proven of any value. Köbner's[1] case is frequently referred to as an example. He gave Fowler's solution hypodermically, at first from $2\frac{1}{4}$ to 4 drops daily, diluted with an equal volume of water, to an eight-year-old girl, who suffered from multiple sarcoma. The treatment was begun September 12, 1881, and was continued with increasing doses (up to 9 drops) until January 5, 1882. The nodules decreased greatly in number and size and the enlargement of the liver and spleen decreased. The treatment was continued until March, 1882, and in January, 1883, the condition was much improved; the body weight had increased; there were only a few nodules in the skin, and these were much less pigmented.

Sherwell's[2] case showed improvement, but the patient was unable to continue the use of the arsenic, and died.

Other cases of great improvement or of apparent cure have been reported from time to time from the use of arsenic, but the outlook under any circumstances is very dark.

[1] Berliner klin. Wochensch., 1883.

[2] THE AMERICAN JOURNAL OF THE MEDICAL SCIENCES, vol. civ.

TUBERCULOUS STRICTURE OF THE ASCENDING COLON, WITH SUDDEN TOTAL OBSTRUCTION OF THE BOWEL; PERFORATION OF THE INTESTINE; REMOVAL OF THE CÆCUM AND HALF THE ASCENDING COLON; RECOVERY.

By Thomas S. Cullen, M.B.,

ASSOCIATE PROFESSOR OF GYNECOLOGY, JOHNS HOPKINS UNIVERSITY, BALTIMORE, MD.

The careful and exhaustive articles bearing on lesions of this character that have already appeared render it superfluous for me to enter into a detailed consideration of the subject. Before describing the present case, therefore, I shall merely enumerate briefly the salient pathological and clinical features of the disease. Those wishing to study the subject fully are referred to the interesting articles of Henri Hartmann and Pilliet,[1] and Reclus,[2] in the French; of Hofmeister,[3] Adolf Hartmann,[4] and Gross,[5] in the German, and of Lartigau,[6] in this country. Hofmeister has tabulated all the cases he could find in the literature, and his consideration of the subject is most thorough, while Baumgarten, through his students, Hartmann and Gross, has contributed not a little to the pathological aspect of this disease. The works of Lartigau and Hofmeister should be carefully read by all particularly interested in this class of cases.

Tuberculous ulceration of the intestine is relatively frequent, as evidenced by the findings at autopsy, but stricture of the lumen of the bowel following as a result of this condition is somewhat rare. Hofmeister says that Eisenhardt, in 1000 autopsies on tuberculous patients, found intestinal lesions 566 times. In only 9, however, was there a more or less definite stricture of the bowel.

Tuberculous strictures of the bowel are usually single and situated at the ileocæcal valve. The cæcum is converted into a sausage-shaped mass, which is adherent, as a rule, posteriorly and occasionally laterally. The omentum, although at times adherent to the growth, is not as prone to engraft itself on the tumor as in cases in which appendicitis exists. The outer surface, while relatively smooth, may be studded by a few tubercles. At one point the gut shows a constriction, and usually around this the adipose tissue is very dense. Where the cæcum is cut into the mucosa frequently shows considerable alteration. It is sometimes studded with irreg-

[1] Note sur une variété de typhlite tuberculeuse simulant les cancers de la région, Bull. de la Soc. anat. de Paris, 1891, vol. lxvi. p, 471.

[2] Typhlite et appendicite tuberculeuses, Cliniques Chirurgicales de la Pitié, 1894, p. 317.

[3] Ueber multiple Darmstenosen tuberkulösen Ursprungs, Beiträge zur klinischen Chirurgie, 1896, Bd. xvii. S. 577.

[4] Ein Fall von tuberkulöser Darmstenose, Inaug. Diss., Tübingen, 1897.

[5] Ueber Stricturirende Darmtuberkulose, Inaug. Diss., Tübingen, 1901.

[6] Journal of Experimental Medicine, 1901, vol. vi. p. 23.

ular or serpiginous tuberculous ulcers, while the intervening mucous membrane is the seat of a chronic inflammatory process. At the point of stricture the lumen of the gut is so narrow that the tip of the finger can hardly be introduced. In some cases so small is the calibre of the bowel that a sound is passed with difficulty, and in our case a small bird-shot was sufficient to completely occlude the canal. The degree of alteration in the cæcum varies with the individual case, and it is only necessary for the reader to picture the tuberculous process advancing until the cæcum becomes matted and densely adherent to all the neighboring structures, and, in rare instances, the process gradually involves the abdominal wall until finally there is a fistulous opening on the surface. Even in the early stages the mesenteric glands are enlarged and already involved in the tuberculous process, and where the cæcal invasion is apparently in its incipiency there may be caseation of these glands.

Tuberculous stenoses of the gut, when multiple, are almost invariably situated in the ileum. Anywhere from one to twelve strictures have been noted in the same patient. In one case Hofmeister found twelve strictures scattered over a distance of about seven feet of gut. The bowel between the strictures is frequently distended, and in rare cases has been known to reach 17 cm. in circumference. Lartigau draws especial attention to a group of these cases, in which, associated with the tuberculous process, there is a marked diffuse thickening of the bowel wall, which occasionally reaches 1 cm. or more in thickness.

The appendix is usually adherent, but, except where the tuberculosis of the cæcum is far advanced, shows no implication in the specific process. Our case proved no exception to the rule. Although bound down by adhesions, the appendix was otherwise normal.

Histological Picture. In sections from the cæcum the edges of the ulcers may show tuberculous tissue, but, as a rule, epithelioid cells or typical tubercles are wanting, and nothing but granulation tissue can be made out. In the vicinity of the muscle, however, groups of epithelioid cells, and now and then tubercles, are seen. The peritoneal surface is usually free from tuberculous nodules until the disease is far advanced or unless the cæcal lesion has been associated with tuberculous peritonitis. Sections from the stricture are composed entirely of connective tissue; sometimes with, at other times without areas even slightly suggestive of tuberculosis. The adipose tissue surrounding the gut at the point of stricture is much infiltrated with small round cells, rendering the fat exceedingly hard and firm. Sections from the lymph glands in the region of the cæcum almost invariably yield typical tubercles.

Naturally the tuberculosis gradually extends to the muscle and outer coats of the bowel. The farther away the process extends from the lumen of the bowel, the more characteristic will be the specific lesions, since the inflammatory changes produced by the intestinal bacteria have less opportunity of masking the tubercles. The diffuse thickening or "chronic hyperplastic tuberculosis" of the intestine yields a very different picture to that of simple tuberculosis, as has been clearly pointed out by Henri Hartmann, Lartigau, and others. In these cases the tuberculous process has been relegated entirely to the background, while the mucosa and muscle have been overrun with round cells. Intestinal bacteria have doubtless gained entrance to the walls through the tuberculous lesions and have continually kept up a chronic inflammation of the bowel wall so widespread in character that the tuberculosis is entirely overshadowed. At a few points, however, it will still be demonstrable, and can be detected with certainty in the mesenteric lymph glands. Even in the cæcal wall, when the typical lesions are totally wanting, tubercle bacilli can still be readily demonstrated.

Clinical History. Patients presenting tuberculosis of the cæcum are usually between twenty and thirty years of age. The condition, however, may be found in the very young, and has been noted in persons fairly advanced in years. Quite commonly the patient has suffered from an old tuberculous process in the lungs or has a suspicious family history. In many of the cases which have come to autopsy healed lesions in the lungs have been demonstrated, while in a few instances there has been swelling of the cervical, axillary, or other lymph glands coincident with the cæcal lesion. One of the first symptoms is constipation. After a time dull or sharp pain is felt in the appendiceal region. As the constriction develops there may be an intermittent diarrhœa, with the gradual narrowing of the bowel, and fulness may be noted over the cæcum. Where there is much infiltration of the intestinal wall the gut becomes very firm and feels like a sausage-shaped tumor. With the gradual growth of tuberculous tissue and narrowing of the bowel symptoms of obstruction manifest themselves, as evidenced by abdominal distention, colicky pain, marked peristalsis, vomiting, and rapid loss in weight.

But although these symptoms may be present, in some instances definite indications of the presence of the lesions may be entirely absent. In our case the patient felt well until the day before operation, complaining only of slight discomfort near the appendix.

Diagnosis. With the increased attention paid to cæcal tuberculosis the possibilities of overlooking these lesions will be lessened. It was only a few days after our case was operated upon that Dr. Finney saw a patient giving symptoms sufficiently suggestive of a tuberculous lesion in the cæcum to render such a diagnosis justifiable. At operation the cæcum was found to be the seat of a most extensive tuberculous ulceration. Fortunately, it was found possible to excise the whole of the diseased area.

Given a tumor in the right iliac fossa of slow growth, a clinical history pointing to a previous pulmonary tuberculosis, and a comparative absence of temperature, it is highly probable that tuberculosis is present. If a patient be fairly well advanced in years, of course, the possibility of a malignant growth must be considered. As pointed out by Hartmann, Lartigau, and other authorities, tuberculosis of the cæcum, especially of the hyperplastic form, has often been taken for sarcoma. This has been due to the massive infiltration with small round cells. But provided that we remember that they form a definite infiltration, instead of one or more large foci, and further, that the cells are uniform in size instead of being large and small and actively dividing, confusion is not likely to occur.

The gross diagnosis between tuberculosis and carcinoma of the cæcum may offer numerous difficulties, but on microscopic examination no confusion can exist, as in the tuberculous process the epithelial elements play an entirely passive rôle or have disappeared. Moreover, the demonstration of the tubercle bacilli is generally easy.

The diagnosis between cæcal tuberculosis and appendicitis is usually dependent on the tuberculous history and the slow growth of the tumor, together with the absence of a temperature suggestive of a pus accumulation. Of course, in a case similar to the present one, a differential diagnosis would be absolutely impossible.

TREATMENT. If tuberculosis of the cæcum be diagnosed early operation is indicated. Resection of the entire diseased area is, of course, necessary for an absolute cure. Lateral anastomosis between the ileum and ascending colon is the ideal operation. If after resecting the diseased portion of the gut very little mobility be obtainable, in order to avoid tension an end-to-end anastomosis is the only alternative. Where there are numerous strictures scattered over an area of several feet of gut, the question arises as to whether the entire diseased area be excised or several anastomoses be made, removing only the diseased segments and leaving the intervening normal gut. If the span of gut involved by the tuberculous process be not over three or four feet, it is wiser to remove this portion in its entirety. In one of the cases reported between six and seven feet were removed, and the patient recovered. With the diseased cæcum it is always necessary to carefully examine the glands of the mesentery, and if they be involved, they too should be excised. The results from resection have been very gratifying, Hofmeister in his table of 83 operative cases showing a recovery of 62 per cent.

Tuberculous stricture of the ascending colon, with sudden total obstruction of the bowel; perforation of the intestine; removal of the cæcum and half the ascending colon. Recovery.—The following is taken from my case-book, November 29, 1902: At 11 P.M. I saw, in consultation with Dr. Charles E. Simon, Miss K. G., aged twenty-four years. The day before she had indefinite pains in the region of the appendix. They were, however, not very severe and lasted but a short time. To-day she did her work as usual and prepared supper, but shortly afterward was taken with severe pain in the right side and was forced to go to bed. At 9 P.M. Dr. Simon saw her.

There was marked rigidity of the right rectus over the appendiceal region. There was little temperature. On examination of the blood Dr. Simon noted that all eosinophiles had disappeared and that there was an evident leukocytosis.[1] When I saw her two hours later the rigidity of the right side had in part disappeared, probably as she was slightly under the influence of morphine. The general condition was good; pulse full and regular. Nevertheless, I advised immediate operation.

At 1.30 A.M. the abdomen was opened and a thin, watery pus immediately escaped from the peritoneal cavity, and the pelvis was found to be completely filled with pus. The intestinal loops, however, on the whole, presented a fairly normal appearance. Here and there they were covered by a few flakes of fibrin. The appendix was easily recognized and was bound down by adhesions. It was tied off from tip to base. As the distal extremity appeared to be normal, we expected to find a perforation near the cæcum, but on complete removal of the appendix it was found that, apart from adhesions, no alteration was present. After removing the pus from the abdomen a sponge was passed into the right renal pocket to see if any pus was there, and, to our surprise, some dark fluid escaped. This was entirely different from that found in the pelvis. The abdominal incision was continued upward to the ribs, and we immediately saw a perforation, about 4 mm. in diameter, in the ascending colon. As there was a good deal of fluid escaping, I temporarily closed this fistulous opening with a purse-string suture. I then drew the ascending colon out and made a longitudinal incision, and on introducing the finger into the colon found total obstruction a short distance above the ileocæcal valve. The lower third of the ascending colon, the cæcum, and a small portion of the ileum were tied off and removed, together with some enlarged glands in the mesocolon. The ascending colon and ileum were then united by end-to-end anastomosis. Lateral union would have been preferable, but we had no choice, as the tissues would have been on too great a tension. A Connell suture was employed for two-thirds the circumference of the gut, the remaining third being turned in with rectangular mattress sutures. The entire line of suture was reinforced by running mattress sutures. The pelvis was carefully sponged out, the intestinal loops brought up into the abdomen, and the entire pelvis loosely packed with iodoform gauze.[2]

[1] Simon lays much stress on the frequent absence of eosinophiles where pus is accumulating, and thinks that this sign is of more practical value than the degree of leukocytosis.

[2] For several years, where the pelvis has been filled with free pus, I have made it a practice, after having wiped the pelvis and intestines off, to place the patient for a moment in the Trendelenburg posture. The pelvis has then been loosely but fully packed with gauze, the ends of which are brought out through the appendix incision. My object has been to prevent the intestinal loops from dropping down and becoming adherent or kinked in the pelvis. In my hands this procedure has yielded very gratifying results. The loops, although still liable to become adherent, are on a level and are not nearly so prone to become obstructed.

A gauze drain was also left at the site of the anastomosis. The patient stood the operation well. Her pulse did not rise above 100. The outlook, however, was not particularly flattering, considering the fact that there was a commencing peritonitis and also considerable œdema of the intestinal wall. Eight days after operation, on removing the last of the gauze, some fecal matter was found on the dressing. The fistula gradually closed, and the patient made an excellent recovery.

February 12, 1904. The patient has been at work for several months, performing general household duties without the slightest inconvenience. Her general condition is excellent. From her I learned that she had had typhoid (?) fever six years previously and was in bed for two weeks. For the last year she has had cramp-like pains throughout the abdomen two or three times a month, and recently the bowels have been more constipated than usual. She gives no history whatever of injury or bruising of the abdomen. For about a week before her admission to the hospital she had had intermittent abdominal pain. From the family history we were unable to get any data suggestive of hereditary tuberculosis.

Pathological Report. (Gynecological Pathological No. 6316.) The specimen consists of a small portion of the ileum, of the cæcum, and of about one-half of the ascending colon. The mucosa of the ileum is unaltered, that of the cæcum in most places is normal, but at a point directly opposite the ileocæcal valve is a perforation 5 mm. in diameter (Fig. 1). The walls of the perforation are rather smooth and the surrounding mucosa, over an area 1 cm. in diameter, is somewhat thickened. The ascending colon, about 5 cm. above the perforation, shows a marked constriction. At this point the lumen narrows down until it is not more than 2 mm. in diameter. Indeed, so small is it that a fine bird-shot would lodge and completely plug the canal at this point (Fig. 2). The intestinal wall at the point of constriction varies from 5 mm. to 8 mm. in thickness and is exceedingly firm in consistence. The constriction is 1 cm. in length and the ascending colon above this point is unaltered.

Histological Examination. The appendix, beyond showing a few adhesions on its outer surface, is normal. The cæcum in the vicinity of the perforation has entirely lost its glandular elements, the specimen consisting almost entirely of granulation tissue. The underlying muscle shows a varying amount of small round-celled infiltration. This is especially abundant in the vicinity of the peritoneal covering.

Along the margin of the perforation there is also much granulation tissue, and the underlying muscle is everywhere infiltrated by small round cells. The ulceration is evidently an old process, as nowhere is a very acute inflammatory reaction present. The walls of the stricture are, to a great extent, composed of fibrous tissue. Here and there we have some light areas somewhat suggestive of tuberculosis. No giant cells are, however, demonstrable. Several mesenteric glands were removed with the intestine. Some of these reached 1.5 cm. in diameter. On histological examination

FIG. 1.

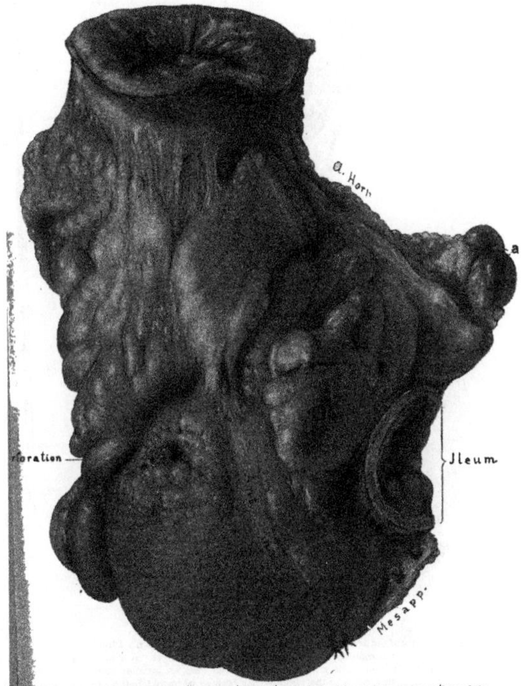

Tuberculosis of the cæcum with perforation (natural size). Above is a cross-section of the ascending colon. Below and to the right the ileum. At a point directly opposite the ileum is a perforation of the cæcum, and just above the perforation the adipose tissue is thickened and there is a constriction of the gut. At *a* are two enlarged and tuberculous lymph glands. For the interior view of the specimen, see Fig. 2.

these show typical tubercles, some sections of which contain four or five giant cells. The tuberculous process in the lymph glands has here and there advanced to caseation.

Fig. 2.

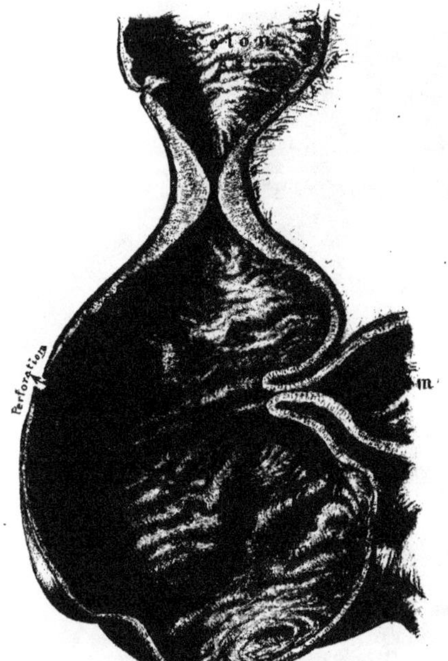

Tuberculous stricture of the ascending colon with perforation of the cæcum. Directly opposite the ileocæcal valve is a small perforation with slightly ragged edges. A short distance above this point the intestinal walls grow thicker and then form an annular constriction. The lumen of the ascending colon at the stricture has been so narrowed that a small bird-shot, when introduced, lodged therein and completely plugged the gut.

The following points merit attention in this case:

1. The total absence of definite symptoms until a few hours before operation.

2. The presence of symptoms identical with those of acute appendicitis.

3. Marked contraction of the stricture.

4. The advisability of always exploring the right renal pocket in all cases in which there is free purulent fluid in the pelvis.

As seen from the history, the patient had practically no symptoms until about five hours before operation, and then there was moderate pain over the appendix, accompanied by rigidity of the right rectus.

Examination of the blood showed a total absence of eosinophiles. The only way in which we can account for the lack of symptoms is that for some reason there occurred an acute contraction of the stricture, which, up to this time, had permitted the free passage of feces. The possible existence of such a condition supplies another indication for early operation whenever trouble exists in the appendiceal region. Already peritonitis had developed, although the symptoms had existed for so short a time; and had we delayed until morning there would have been little chance of saving the patient.

After having removed the appendix and wiped the pus from the pelvis, the abdominal cavity appeared normal, and I probably should not have explored the right renal pocket had I not been familiar with the renal work of Max Broedel, who has shown clearly that where there is a free accumulation of fluid in the region of the appendix that by gravity it will travel down into the right renal fossa.

I should have preferred lateral anastomosis, but we were forced to make an end-to-end union on account of tension.

A STUDY OF NORMAL AND PATHOLOGICAL CONDITIONS OF THE BURSÆ OF THE NECK, WITH SPECIAL REFERENCE TO THE SUBHYOID BURSA.*

By Willis S. Anderson, M.D.,

ASSISTANT TO THE CHAIR OF LARYNGOLOGY, DETROIT COLLEGE OF MEDICINE; LARYNGOLOGIST TO THE HARPER HOSPITAL POLYCLINIC, ETC., DETROIT, MICHIGAN.

We find on searching the literature of the older writers references to cystic tumors of the neck, some of them, no doubt, of bursal origin; but from the descriptions given it is impossible to know their exact nature. Commencing with Celsus, who mentions tumors of the neck,

* Thesis presented to the Council of the American Laryngological, Rhinological, and Otological Society, April, 1903.

down to the latter half of the eighteenth century, we find occasional references to these conditions; but not until the beginning of the nineteenth century can we find any definite literature on the subject.

Boyer,[1] in his treatise published in 1831, describes cysts of the neck as follows: "There is sometimes found between the hyoid bone and the thyroid cartilage, upon the membrane uniting them and behind the thyroid muscle, an encysted tumor, containing a viscous, yellowish fluid." He further states that they usually cause no trouble except that the deformity may be annoying, especially to women. While Boyer's cysts are undoubtedly hygroma of the subhyoid bursa, he did not recognize them as such, nor did he seem to have any knowledge of the existence of a bursa normal to this region. Voillemier and Vidal appear to have had a vague knowledge of its existence, but Malgaigne,[2] in 1838, was the first to describe accurately this bursa. Verneuil,[3] in 1853, published a careful study of the bursæ of the neck and their affections under the title "Recherches anatomiques pour servis a l'histoire des Kystes de la partie supérieure et médiene du cou." In this monograph he gives the location of the different bursæ found in this region. The most complete study of the subject the writer has found is a thesis by Batut,[4] published in 1886.

Besides the above-mentioned, a few scattered articles in German, French, and English have been found, and an occasional brief reference in some of the more complete works of surgery.

The fairly constant serous bursæ of the neck, according to Verneuil, are three in number: 1. Subcutaneous antethyroid, also called præthyroid. 2. Deep subhyoid (Boyer's bursa). 3. The superficial or sushyoid.

The subcutaneous antethyroid bursa, described by Beclard,[5] lies in the loose areolar tissue over the Adam's apple. This bursa is not always present, and when existent it varies in size from a mere space to a well-defined sac easily demonstrated. It is difficult to differentiate any bursa in the loose tissue in women and children; in men it is usually present and tends in both sexes to grow larger as age advances. It develops as the result of friction between the subcutaneous tissue and the prominence of the thyroid cartilage.

The subhyoid bursa, described by Malgaigne, is the one more directly to be considered. It is situated between the hyoid bone and the thyrohyoid membrane. Superiorly, it is limited by the insertion of the thyrohyoid membrane to the lower lip of the upper border of the body of the hyoid bone; anteriorly, its wall is formed by the posterior surface of the hyoid bone at its upper portion and the cervical aponeurosis below; posteriorly, it is limited by the thyrohyoid membrane; inferiorly, it reaches to the upper portion of the thyroid cartilage by an infundibuliform prolongation; laterally, it may extend under the thyrohyoid muscle, but its usual limit is the inner border of the muscle. It is about 2 cm. long by 1 cm. broad, and larger in men than in women and children. Verneuil found it rudimentary in a fetus, and constantly present in fifteen adult subjects. The subhyoid bursa is rarely absent. Malgaigne describes it as a single sac, with two lateral prolongations, while the more accurate dissections of Verneuil show it to be a double bursa, with a partition in the median line. The latter observer explains the development of this double bursa as the result of friction between the upper border of the thyroid cartilage and the hyoid bone, and, because of the thyroid notch in the median line, less friction is experienced at this point, a fact which accounts for the median wall of connective tissue separating the two bursæ. There is sometimes a connection between the antethyroid bursa and the subhyoid bursa.

The superficial or sushyoid bursa described by Verneuil lies between the geniohyoid and the geniohyoglossal muscles. Besides the three above-mentioned bursæ, which are fairly constant, others have been found and described by various observers. Among these may be mentioned a second bursa lying in the concavity of the hyoid bone, described by H. Luschka.[5] Fleichman described a bursa on the geniohyoglossi next to the frænum of the tongue as the bursa sublingualis. Rosenmüller, quoted by Luschka,[6] described the bursa sternohyoidea between the sternohyoid muscle and the hyoid bone. Others have been described as the thyroidea lateralis (Gruber),[7] stylohyoidea, cricothyrothyroidea (Calori), and thyrotrachealis (Calori).

While considering the location and structure of this bursa, mention ought to be made of the remains of the thyreoglossal duct. There is in the embryo (His)[8] a prolongation of the thyroid gland upward, forming a duct or tract. This tract runs (Butlin)[9] from the foramen cæcum at the base of the tongue downward in the raphé between the geniohyoglossi muscles to the hyoid bone. It is intimately connected with the body of the hyoid bone, with its periosteum, and with the subhyoid bursa behind. Below the mylohyoid muscle the tract can be traced from its close connection with the lower and posterior edge of the hyoid bone downward in front of the thyrohyoid ligament to the pyramidal lobe of the thyroid gland beneath the raphé uniting the sternohyoid muscles. This tract may remain open in a portion of its extent, which accounts for the cysts of this duct. There is found frequently in its course small masses of thyroid gland tissue, which are known as the accessory or parathyroids. This duct is lined by ciliated epithelium, and is in close relation with several bursæ of the neck, especially the subhyoid bursa.

The gross anatomy of the bursæ of the neck has been studied by a number of observers, but there does not seem to have been any attention given to their histological structure. The writer has made a number of dissections of subhyoid bursæ, with the object, first, to confirm the work of other observers; and, second, to demonstrate the histological structure of these sacs. Several dissections of embryos and children at term show the bursa in a very rudimentary state. On gross inspection all that is evident are the small spaces in the very loose areolar tissue lying between the body of the hyoid bone and the thyrohyoid membrane. Dissections from one subject, examined histologically with a low power, revealed a fair-sized space in the loose areolar tissue. There was no distinct limiting membrane lining the whole of the cavity, but in places with a high power there was a suggestion of such a limiting membrane lined by flattened endothelial cells. It would seem that in early life this bursa was nothing more than a mere space in the areolar tissue without a distinct lining membrane. The bursa in adult subjects was regularly found larger in men than in women. It occupied considerable space in the loose tissue behind the hyoid bone. The interior of the sac was smooth, and had the appearance of a serous lining. In some cases trabeculæ could be seen running across the cavity. Histologically, no continuous lining could be demonstrated, but in places a limiting membrane lined by flattened cells was observed. The lining membrane was much more distinct in the specimens taken from the children at term. In no instance were columnar ciliated cells found.

The results obtained from this limited study are in harmony with what we should expect from our knowledge of subcutaneous bursæ in general. Since these bursæ develop as the result of friction between the adjacent parts, we should expect them to vary considerably in size and structure, and also to be more developed in advanced age. Schafer[10] says: "It must, however, be observed that among the subcutaneous bursæ some are reckoned which do not always present the characters of true synovial sacs, but look more like mere recesses in the subcutaneous areolar tissue, larger and more defined than in the neighboring areolæ, but still not bounded by an evident synovial membrane. These may be looked upon as examples of less developed structure, forming a transition between the areolar tissue spaces and the perfect synovial cavities; indeed, it may happen that what is a well-developed synovial bursa in one subject is merely an enlarged areola in another. Many of the bursæ do not appear until after birth, and they are said to increase in number as age advances. The synovial membranes are composed entirely of connective tissue with the usual cells and fibres of that tissue. There exist on the synovial membranes no complete lining, although patches of cells may, it is true, here and there be met with which present an epithelioid appearance."

No definite etiology of cysts of the subhyoid bursa has been found. It is thought that trivial traumatisms, so slight as to escape the memory, may be the cause. Tight collars, especially when the edges press at that point, may be the exciting factor. The latter cause is the one given by a patient who consulted the writer. They are never congenital.

Symptoms. As a rule, these cysts cause but few subjective symptoms. The symptoms are proportionate to the size of the tumor, and are caused naturally by the mechanical presence of the growth. If the cyst is small no inconvenience is felt; the larger ones sometimes interfere with deglutition or respiration and give rise occasionally to a sense of stiffness of the muscles of deglutition. In rare instances cysts have attained such a size as to give rise to serious symptoms. One author claims that these swellings may be visible on the floor of the mouth, but it would seem that this was an error in diagnosis, as the thyrohyoid membrane, which limits the upper border of the bursa, is a firm resisting membrane. The cysts develop slowly and are not painful or tender to the touch. They vary in size from a slight swelling to a tumor the size of an orange. Usually they are the size of a hazelnut. They are found just below the hyoid bone, in the median or just to one side of the median line, and they are firmly attached to the underlying tissue. The tumor is usually globular and tense; the skin over it freely movable, and shows no sign of inflammation. They are usually smooth, but in long-standing cases a roughened surface has been detected. Fluctuation may be present, depending on the size of the growth, the contents, and the possibility of fixing the tumor while the sign is being elicited. They are said to be more common in men. The cases seen by the author were in females, but the sensitiveness of women to any deformity may account for it apparently being more common in them. In the few cases reported where the cysts have attained a larger size, there are, in addition, pressure symptoms, which may give rise to interference with circulation in the neck, to dyspnœa, or to dysphagia.

The clinical history of these cases varies. They may remain for years, causing but little inconvenience and not increasing appreciably in size; they may disappear under treatment so simple that one feels that the treatment was not the cause of their disappearance. Such was the fact in one of the writer's cases, although it has been claimed by some that they never disappear spontaneously. They may vary in size from month to month, as in one case now under observation. They may spontaneously open, or open as the result of local treatment, and leave a chronically discharging sinus. They may become infected and form an abscess.

The differential diagnosis between the hygroma of the subhyoid bursa and other tumors of the neck ought not to be difficult in the majority of cases. It can be distinguished from a cold abscess by the absence of induration at the base and by the freedom from evidences of inflammation and constitutional symptoms. Its situation above the thyroid cartilage will easily differentiate it from ordinary enlargement of the thyroid gland. An enlarged lymphatic gland would be unusual in the median line, although a single lymphatic gland has been demonstrated in this region. As a rule, enlarged glands are situated at the side of the neck, and are dependent upon tuberculosis, syphilis, or some point of infection in the nose and throat. Aneurysms of the neck give rise to pulsating tumors, which easily distinguishes them from cysts, although the possibility of the pulsation from a vessel transmitted through a tumor must be remembered. If the tumor can be moved toward the median line and drawn away from the vessel the pulsation will cease. If the possibility of lipoma must be eliminated, this can be done by an exploratory puncture. Sebaceous cysts are indolent, inflammatory swellings, with a black point at the summit of the swelling, and the integument is closely adherent. Cystic swellings of other bursæ must be differentiated by their situation. The diagnosis between median branchial cysts, thyroglossal cysts, and cysts of the subhyoid bursa is more difficult, and much confusion exists. A study of the literature and reported cases of cysts in this region shows that a clear distinction between the various cysts has not been made. The important diagnostic point is the histological structure of the sac. If the wall of the sac is lined by ciliated epithelium, the cyst is a branchial or thyroglossal duct cyst; if lined by flattened endothelium, it is of bursal origin. Such examination ought to be made in every case. Branchial cysts in this region have a pedicle adherent to the hyoid bone.

The two cases seen by the writer were probably hygroma of the subhyoid bursa. It is to be regretted that no histological examination of the wall of the sac could be made. The diagnosis was made by the location, the character, and appearance of the swelling.

CASE I.—Girl, aged twelve years. Family and personal history has no bearing on the case. Five or six months previous, before she came under observation, her mother noticed a lump on the child's throat in the region of the hyoid bone. At first it was small, but it grew gradually larger. No history of traumatism or other etiological cause was obtained. The tumor at no time gave rise to any symptoms referable to the interior of the throat, except, perhaps, a little stiffness on swallowing. The general health of the child was excellent. Examination showed a tumor about the size of a marble, which lay in the median line, on a level with or just below the body of the hyoid bone. The tumor moved with the hyoid bone, but it did not seem to be attached to the body of this bone, as it could be moved independently of the bone. The growth was circumscribed, and to the touch was of a cystic nature. The skin was not adherent, and there was no evidence of inflammation. The parents declined operative treatment. About a year later the patient was seen, and the tumor was found to have completely disappeared. The father reported that the tumor had remained stationary for several months and then, without treatment, had gradually grown smaller. The possibility of this being a cyst of the thyroglossal duct or a parathyroid, which developed about the time of puberty, cannot be excluded.

CASE II.—Woman, aged forty-three years. Referred to the writer by Dr. W. R. Parker. General health good. About five years before consulting the writer she noticed a swelling just to the right of the median line of the neck, about on a level with the hyoid bone. There was no enlargement of the thyroid gland. The patient thinks the pressure of a high collar may have caused the swelling. There was observed no relation between the growth and her menstrual function. Examination showed a cystic tumor about the size of a large marble, situated just below the hyoid bone, as if it came out from under the body of that bone. The skin was freely movable over the growth, and there was no induration at its base, nor signs of inflammation. There were no constitutional symptoms, nor any subjective symptoms, except possibly a little stiffness on swallowing. As the patient did not wish any operative interference, she was advised to use tincture of iodine locally. The tumor decreased in size and remained so for about a year, then increased again, and later again diminished. It has never entirely disappeared. She does not think the variation in size has been the result of treatment.

A careful study of the literature on this subject shows that comparatively few cases of undoubted bursal cysts have been reported, and in still fewer cases has a microscopic examination of the sac proven beyond doubt their bursal nature. Any attempt to tabulate the cases reported would be unprofitable, because so much uncertainty exists as to the exact nature of many of the cysts of the hyoid region. These cysts are probably not so rare as the meagre number of cases reported would indicate. The following, cited by various writers, compose the bulk of cases found after careful search. It is evident that some of the cases are not of bursal origin.

Three cases are quoted by Batut:[4]

Case I.—Male, aged twenty-three years, had a seromucous cyst of subhyoid bursa, about the size of a pigeon's egg, situated a little to the right in the thyrohyoid region. It contained a viscid, stringy, serous fluid. It was unsuccessfully treated by an injection of tincture of iodine and alcohol, but was finally cured by a single injection of chloride of zinc.

Case II.—Male, aged twenty-four years; tumor, the size of a hazelnut, situated above the thyroid cartilage, in the median line of the neck. Various methods of treatment were used, but a chronic discharging fistula resulted.

Case III.—Male, aged twenty-nine years; tumor, the size of a walnut, situated to the right of the median line. The contents of sac was a mucous fluid, which contained no pus or epithelial cells. The tumor was completely extirpated, but later the patient died of œdema of the glottis.

Dressel[11] describes at length a case in a girl aged eighteen years. Preceding the fistula there was a cystic tumor, the size of a hazelnut, above the thyroid cartilage. As a result of local applications the cyst opened and a chronic fistulous tract resulted. A study of the lining of the membrane of this tract proved that it was lined by ciliated epithelium, and he rightly concluded that the case was a fistula following a cyst of the remains of the thyroglossal duct, and not a subhyoid bursa. This author quotes thirteen cases gathered from various sources, but on studying their histories it is not easy to tell definitely the nature of the cysts. In none of the cases was the cyst wall examined microscopically. Cholesterin crystals were noted in the contents of the three cases.

Dr. A. Friedlowsky[12] describes a case of cystic degeneration of the subhyoid bursa. It was more prominent posteriorly and pushed the epiglottis backward. It was a small, firm, round tumor, filled with a viscid, amber fluid. The walls were tolerably thick. It was found to be a degeneration of the subhyoid bursa. No microscopic examination was made of the sac.

Dr. R. F. Weir[13] reports a case of the extirpation of the subhyoid bursa. It returned after being tapped and injected with iodine. He emptied the cyst with a trocar, injected melted paraffin, allowed it to solidify, and then dissected out the whole cyst. He speaks of the value of this method, which enables one to dissect out the entire cyst wall, and thus prevent a persistent fistula.

In the London *Lancet*[14] a case is reported as a subhyoid dermoid cyst in a girl aged twelve years. The tumor was noticed for five or six years; it gradually increased in size, and it was situated in the median line. On opening the cyst it was found to pass backward and behind the hyoid bone. The contents consisted of oily matter and crystals of fatty acids. No microscopic examination of the sac was made, but it was described as resembling mucous membrane. The author assumed that it was lined by columnar, ciliated epithelium and that it was a dermoid. It is to be regretted that a microscopic examination of the wall of the sac could not have been made, as this may have been a case of a cyst of the subhyoid bursa.

Ingalls[15] reports a case, in a male aged thirty years, of a hemispherical growth, about one inch in diameter, situated just above the thyroid cartilage, and causing no inconvenience. History of syphilis several months before. The growth was movable and slightly fluctuating. An exploring-needle proved it contained pus. The diagnosis of a suppurating bursa was made, the fluid was withdrawn, and a 5 per cent. to 10 per cent. carbolic solution was injected. Result not given.

Dr. Hamilton,[16] in a paper on "Supralaryngeal Encysted Tumors of Bursal Origin," reports ten cases. No examination of the walls reported. They contained a thin yellow serum. Dr. Elsberg, in the discussion of the above paper, reported three cases. He also referred to the dissections he made of the bursæ. He found the bursal space either with or without distinctly developed membranous walls. The cysts contained a watery serum, varying in consistency and color, more or less viscid, synovial or mucoid. They usually contained cholesterin crystals, a large quantity of albumin, and the soluble salts of the blood. Besides the above-mentioned, cases have been reported by Malgaigne, Boyer, Rognette, Hyrtl, and others.

It is the general experience that these cysts do not spontaneously disappear of their own accord, but, on the contrary, have a tendency to become inflamed and to open by ulceration. This gives rise to a chronically discharging fistula, which may persist indefinitely, causing much annoyance to the patient.

The different methods of treatment may be divided into:

1. General and local absorbents.
2. Simple incision and drainage.
3. Drainage and the use of a local irritant to produce adhesive inflammation.
4. Partial excision of the cyst wall.
5. Complete extirpation.

1. There is no reason to believe that the internal use of diuretics, iodides, mercurials, or other absorbents have any beneficial effect in bursal affections. The local use of absorbents, irritants, or vesicants seldom does any good, although an occasional report favorable to their use can be found. In a case which the writer reported above the cyst disappeared entirely without treatment. No local application should be used that will cause inflammation or vesication, as a chronic fistula has followed too active local treatment.

2. Simple incision with drainage is of no avail. If the incision closes, recurrence is the rule; if it remains open a chronic fistula is the result.

3. Drainage of the sac and the use of local irritants to produce closure has been tried successfully in a number of cases, but failures are also reported. In some cases a chronic suppurating fistula, with all its annoyances, has resulted. The method is a familiar one in surgery and depends on the ability to obliterate the entire sac by adhesive inflammation. The cause of the failure seems to be that the local irritant cannot be brought into contact with all parts of the sac or that a too strong application is followed by suppuration, which persists with the development of the fistula. When it is recalled that the sac normally extends up behind the hyoid bone, narrowing as it ascends, and is usually prolonged downward to an infundibuliform prolongation, we can understand why it is not easy to obliterate the whole sac. Incision and cauterization of the wall with nitrate of silver, chloride of zinc, or caustic potash, have been tried and good results reported. Solutions of iodine, carbolic acid, alcohol, chloride of zinc have been used as injections, with varying results. Panus cured a case by injecting a solution of chloride of zinc into the sac without evacuating it. This lessens the danger of severe inflammatory reaction.

4. Partial extirpation of the cyst is unsatisfactory and not to be advised.

5. Complete extirpation of the cyst is by far the most satisfactory method of treatment, although in Boyer's time he considered it impossible. Difficulty has often been experienced in dissecting out the entire sac. Weir's method is an excellent one. He injected the sac with melted paraffin, and allowed it to harden before attempting to dissect out the sac. This method allows the cyst to be shelled out entire.

The writer wishes to acknowledge his indebtedness to E. H. Hayward, who prepared the histological sections at the Detroit Clinical Laboratory.

BIBLIOGRAPHY.

1. Boyer. Traité des Maladies chirurgicales, 1831.
2. Malgaigne. Anat. Chir., 1838, t. ii p. 40.
3. Verneuil. Archives générales de médecine, 1853, vol. i, pp. 185 and 450.
4. Batut. Étude sur l'hygroma de la bourse thyrohyoidieme et sou traitément. Bordeaux, 1886.
5. Beclard. Emmert's Lehrbuch der Chirurgie, Stuttgart, 1854.
6. Luschka. Die Anatomie des Menschen, Tübingen, 1862.
7. Grüber. Archiv f. Anat. u. Physiol., Leipzig, 1875, p. 590.
8. His. Anatomie menschlicher Embryonen.
9. Butlin and Spencer. Diseases of the Tongue, 1900, p. 4.
10. Schäfer. Quain's Anatomy, 1891, part ii., vol. i p. 393.
11. Dressel. Beitrag zur Geschichte der Fistula Bursae Subbyoideae, 1888.
12. Friedlowsky. Allgemeine Wiener med. Zeitung, 1868, No. 22.
13. Wier. New York Medical Journal, vol. lv. p. 285.
14. London Lancet, November 23, 1889, p 1058.
15. Ingalls. Medical News, February 13, 1897.
16. Hamilton. Medical Record, 1869–70, p. 545.

HÆMOLYMPH NODES.[1]

BY HUGHES DAYTON, M.D.,

ALUMNI FELLOW IN PATHOLOGY, COLLEGE OF PHYSICIANS AND SURGEONS, COLUMBIA UNIVERSITY.

THE earliest mention of the occurrence of nodes macroscopically resembling the spleen was that of Leydig, in 1857, who described their occurrence along the abdominal aorta. Since 1875 the presence of lymph nodes of a red color or containing red blood cells has been noted by a number of observers, and various explanations have been offered to interpret these findings. To Warthin, of the University of Michigan, we are indebted for the most systematic and extensive study of these structures, and in his recent articles are contained the most convincing proof of the existence of the so-called hæmolymph node as an organ *sui generis*.

It is not the purpose of the writer to review exhaustively the work of others in this field, or to describe in detail the histology of these nodes, but rather to present the results of a personal study of their

[1] A study from the Department of Pathology of the College of Physicians and Surgeons, Columbia University, New York.

individuality and functions. A summary of the work of others in this field had been prepared, but the literature has since been so satisfactorily abstracted by Warthin in his most recent publication that this and the complete bibliography are omitted. The histology is well presented in his other articles.

These so-called hæmolymph nodes have been found by various observers in man, monkey, ox, sheep, goat, horse, pig, dog, cat, weasel, ferret, stoat, rabbit, squirrel, rat, mouse, bat, water-vole, mole, fowl, and turkey.

The structures denominated hæmolymph nodes vary in size from that of a pinhead to that of a lymph node, though averaging smaller than the latter. They are dark red, brown, or mottled red and white, usually smooth, soft, and elastic, but easily ruptured. Few or many bloodvessels surround or enter the nodes, in some cases at a hilum. Lymphatics are apparently absent in some cases. When ruptured the nodes resemble a blood clot. Each node possesses a delicate capsule of connective tissue with some non-striated muscle fibre. Just within the capsule is a peripheral blood sinus from which irregular prolongations run throughout the node. Between the sinuses are cords of lymphoid tissue, and usually cell collections resembling lymph follicles toward the periphery of the node. In some cases the division into cortical and medullary portions is very indistinct, and the relative amount of lymphoid tissue is generally smaller than in a lymph node. The sinuses are traversed by an irregular reticulum, usually finer than that of a lymph node, this and the sinus walls apparently being lined with endothelium. Proliferation of the endothelium appears to furnish the large phagocytes lying in the sinuses and in some cases nearly filling them. An artery enters at and a vein emerges from the hilum. The artery divides into branches which run in trabeculæ extending from the capsule through the sinuses. The finer branches sometimes appear to terminate in the sinuses; others break up into capillaries in the lymph cords, some of these capillaries apparently emptying into the sinuses. The sinuses terminate in veins which unite into one, emerging at the hilum. In some nodes small arteries enter at various points in the capsule, and in the transition forms afferent lymphatics may be seen entering the peripheral sinus. In some transition cases the blood and lymph sinuses seem to be separate systems; in others bloodvessels and lymphatics appear to mingle their contents in common sinuses. The sinuses contain varying numbers of red cells, either free or in various stages of disintegration within the phagocytic cells already mentioned, and leukocytes. The characteristic feature is said to be the occurrence normally, in the sinuses of a node, of destruction of red cells which have been brought to the node by bloodvessels.

The various interpretations which have been placed upon the presence of red blood cells within the sinuses of structures resembling lymph nodes, or the occurrence of bodies macroscopically suggesting accessory spleens or red or mottled lymph nodes, are that they are: (1) neoplasms; (2) masses of newly formed splenic tissue; (3) lymph nodes engaged in the formation of new red cells; (4) lymph nodes whose sinuses contain blood as the result of congestion, hemorrhage, diapedesis, absorption of extravasated blood, etc.; (5) hæmolymph nodes.

The interpretation as neoplasms was advanced by but one observer, Mosler, who described the dark-red nodules found in the greater and lesser omenta of a splenectomized dog and termed them "hemorrhagic telangiectatic lymphomata." Their microscopic structure was the same as that described by others as hæmolymph nodes. Tizzoni and others have interpreted them as newly formed splenic tissue, basing their view upon their occurrence in animals the spleens of which they had removed. The investigations of Morandi and Sisto, and of Warthin appear to have conclusively disproved the splenic nature of these nodules. The idea that the lymphoid nodules with sinuses containing red cells were structures engaged in the formation of red blood corpuscles has been supported by a number of the earlier observers, but recently by Retterer only. Some were led to this belief by finding in the sinuses large cells containing what appeared to be red blood cells, some of which they described as being extruded. These are now generally regarded as endothelial cells displaying phagocytic activity and ingesting the red cells. Retterer believes that lymph nodes produce blood plasma, leukocytes, and red cells, the last derived from lymphocytes by a hæmoglobin change of the nucleus. The evidence of all other investigators appears to disprove this construction of the presence of red cells. The view that the appearance of red cells in the sinuses is due to hyperæmia, hemorrhage, diapedesis, or the absorption of extravasated blood by normal lymph nodes has been advocated by several writers, of whom Saltykow is the most decided representative at present. His study of the subject has been careful and systematic. Examination of sixty autopsy cases has convinced him that the red nodes are merely lymph nodes whose sinuses contain blood brought by lymph vessels from regions in which hemorrhage has occurred, or entering them by diapedesis from capillaries in the node, or by hemorrhage from them into the lymphoid tissue or sinuses, the presence of red cells in the sinuses exciting the endothelial cells of the latter to intense phagocytic activity. His reasons for assuming that the nodes are merely lymph nodes are: in a large proportion of the cases an extravasation of blood is found in the node itself or the surrounding cellular tissue; in many nodes the vasa efferentia and subcapsular sinus are the only or chief containers of red cells, giving the impression that they are filled from without; the red nodes are found in the situations of normal nodes, and all transition forms to the ordinary type exist.

The interpretation as organs *sui generis*, variously denominated hæmolymph, hæmal, and hæmolytic nodes, dates from the time of Gibbes' preliminary report in 1884. Since the present writer began his investigations the ground has been covered with remarkable unanimity by Morandi and Sisto, Weidenreich, Lewis, and Warthin, to whose articles he would refer those desiring the bibliography, review of the literature, and full description of the histology. They agree that the hæmolymph nodes are a distinct set of organs whose functions are the production of leukocytes, and especially the destruction of red cells and to a less degree of leukocytes. Morandi and Sisto give as their reasons for ascribing to these organs a hæmolytic function the constant occurrence in their sinuses of cells containing red cells in various stages of disintegration, and the increase of those phagocytic cells after splenectomy, and still more after subsequent administration of hæmolytic substances. The writers mentioned agree also that there is a complete series of transition forms from the structure of the spleen to that of an ordinary lymph node. Warthin regards them as a set of structures subject to variation, one form passing into another as the needs of the body require. He describes the formation of new hæmolymph nodes as beginning with angiectatic dilatation of the capillaries of a fat lobule, the fat cells becoming enlarged, the capsule of the lobule thickened. Lymphocytes are infiltrated along the walls of the capillaries; fat cells are absorbed, and some are converted into reticular cells; proliferation of endothelium in the dilated capillaries divides them into blood sinuses. Continued lymphoid formation, development of sinuses, and absorption of fat complete the transition into a hæmolymph node. Progressive hyperplasia of lymphoid tissue encroaching upon the sinuses may transform this or a previously existing hæmolymph into a lymph node.

In the writer's own investigations hæmolymph nodes have been observed and studied in the adult, infant, dog, cat, red deer, rabbit, and guinea-pig. Failure to discover them in the gray squirrel was probably due to incomplete examination of a single subject.

In all experimental cases the nodes were removed immediately after death and fixed in Orth's or Zenker's fluid, alcohol, or formaldehyde solution. Celloidin was usually employed for embedding, occasionally paraffin. Hæmatoxylin and eosin were ordinarily used in staining. The experimental work was confined to the dog and rabbit, the normal condition of these animals being verified by autopsy and microscopic examination.

I. Evidence in Favor of Other Interpretations than Organs Sui Generis.

In support of the view that red cells in the sinuses are brought by afferent lymphatics from regions in which there is extravasation of blood is the fact that in a number of cases in which the sinuses of nodes contained red cells large numbers were seen in surrounding lymph spaces. This is not at all conclusive, as similar collections of red cells were found in the lymph spaces surrounding nodes whose sinuses showed no characteristics of hæmolymph nodes. In several cases nodes containing red cells were observed in which afferent lymphatics were filled more or less completely with red cells. In these the appearances of a hæmolymph node were present, yet there was distinct proof that red cells were being brought by lymph vessels. An example is shown in the accompanying figure.

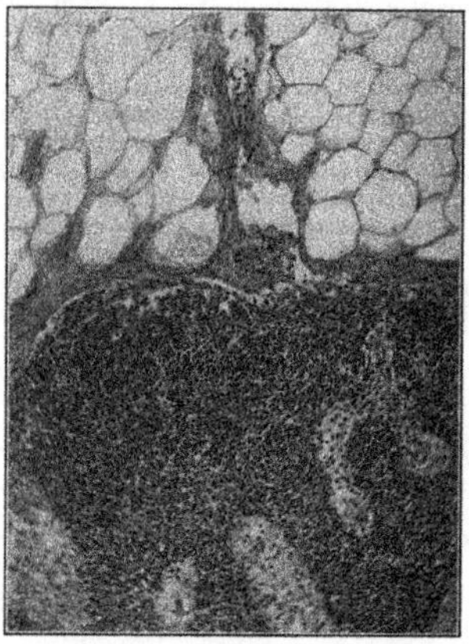

Lymph node, showing red blood cells in sinuses and in afferent lymphatic.

This is reproduced from a photomicrograph of an axillary node removed during an amputation of the breast for carcinoma. In this case there was obviously extravasation of blood in the region whose lymphatics were tributary to the node. Several other such instances were found. The fact that in some instances red cells are brought to a node by afferent lymphatics does not prove that this is the invariable explanation of their presence. In a red deer examined a few minutes after death, immediately following a wound with comminution of the pelvic bones and extensive laceration of the adjacent soft parts, large numbers of small dark-red nodes were found in the prevertebral region of the abdomen and thorax and along the renal vessels. The peripheral and central sinuses of these nodes contained many red cells but no evidence of recent or former phagocytosis, while in places where the sinuses were completely filled with red cells the adjacent lymphoid tissue was also so densely packed with red cells as to suggest a local hemorrhage. The blood-vessels of the nodes were greatly congested. There were no hemorrhages in the neighboring tissues. While these nodes were so extensively distributed as to suggest that local extravasation of blood could not have been responsible for their appearance, the complete absence of phagocytosis in all examined would suggest that the red cells had entered the sinuses only shortly before fixation of the tissues. The presence of hemorrhages in the lymphoid tissue would also favor the view that these were ordinary lymph nodes with recent hemorrhages into the lymphoid tissue and thence into the sinuses, caused probably by great disturbance of the circulatory system incident to the traumatism and shock.

With a view to determining the possible influence of circulatory disturbances in producing appearances which might be described as hæmolymph nodes, the following experiment was carried out: A rabbit was anæsthetized with ether and the inferior vena cava ligated in two places, just above and below the left renal vein. The animal was found dead in the morning, about twenty hours later. Viscera normal, except great congestion of the left kidney and spleen. In contrast to the negative results obtained in previous examinations for nodes containing red cells in normal rabbits, red corpuscles were discovered in six of the nodes studied.

That circulatory disturbances will not, however, always cause the presence of red cells in lymph nodes was demonstrated by two other experiments upon rabbits. In one, ether anæsthesia, ligation of aorta, inferior vena cava, and right ureter *en masse*. Rabbit found dead next morning. Viscera normal, except congestion of kidney and desquamation of cells of its tubules. In spite of the intense circulatory disturbances, red cells were found in the sinuses of only three of eleven nodes, and of the positive specimens one showed hemorrhages into the lymphoid tissue and blood in adjacent lymph spaces. In another rabbit: ligation of the right femoral vessels after bleeding from the artery, under ether anæsthesia, repeating this eighteen days later with the left femoral vessels, and killing a day later by severing the medulla. General anæmia; cheesy area surrounded by consolidation in lung; other viscera practically normal. Nodes from the immediate vicinity of the former and recent operations showed no red cells in their sinuses. In one mesenteric node they were found enclosed in phagocytes; in two others pigment masses were observed in such cells.

Hæmolymph nodes were found in cases in which there was no hyperæmia.

These observations would seem to show that circulatory disturbances may cause the pressure of red cells in sinuses of nodes, but are not sufficient to account for their appearance in most cases.

That the presence of red cells in the sinuses may be caused by toxic substances within the body was shown by subcutaneous injection of ricin into a normal dog. In all of twenty-one nodes from the cervical, axillary, bronchial, retrosternal, gastric, mesenteric, retroperitoneal, and pelvic regions many red cells were found in the sinuses and in adjacent lymph spaces, with marked congestion of bloodvessels. Similar results, with marked endothelial hyperplasia in the sinuses, were obtained by ricin injection into a rabbit. While these experiments demonstrate that a poison in the circulation may induce the presence of red cells in the sinuses of lymph nodes the toxic action was too severe to draw strict inferences in regard to the behavior of nodes under comparatively normal circumstances.

In three dogs examined, into the peritoneal cavities of which 1 per cent. solution of zinc chloride had been injected for experimental purposes, the abdominal cavities were found post-mortem to contain bloody exudate. In one animal red cells were found in the sinuses of eleven out of fifteen mesenteric and prevertebral nodes; in a second dog, red cells in sinuses of six out of eight nodes from the anterior mediastinum; in the third, red cells or their remains free or in phagocytes in all but two of twenty-seven nodes from the prevertebral, renal, mesenteric and anterior mediastinal regions. In some cases the adjacent lymph spaces contained red cells. The red corpuscles in these nodes were evidently brought by afferent lymphatics, although none of the sections studied showed their entrance, since at various points in their circumference the peripheral sinuses were closely packed with red cells, and communicating portions of the sinuses contained phagocytes filled with red cells and some red cells free, while toward the centre of the node phagocytosis was just beginning, and since adjacent lymph spaces were filled with red cells. It is unlikely that all of the nodes containing red cells were hæmolymph nodes. Probably many were lymph nodes whose endothelium was exerting phagocytic powers in response to stimulation by the toxic substance, zinc chloride, or by some substance produced by its action, perhaps by damaged red cells from the peritoneal cavity. The occurrence of red cells in many of the nodes in these cases may, therefore, have been due to absorption of extravasated blood or to the presence of a toxic substance in the blood. That the presence of toxins does not necessarily cause phagocytic destruction of red cells in the sinuses was shown by negative findings in two rabbits. One of these had been injected with the toxin of the bacillus of rabbit septicæmia (Lartigau); the other had been subjected to the influence of the toxin of tubercle bacilli.

To summarize: absorption of extravasated blood, circulatory disturbances, and toxic substances in the circulation may cause the appearance of red cells in the sinuses of lymph nodes, but there are many nodes in which this explanation is unsatisfactory.

II. Evidence in Favor of Interpretation of "Hæmolymph Nodes" as Organs Sui Generis.

1. *Constant Occurrence.* The constant occurrence of hæmolymph nodes in the dog was shown by the following experiments: Four dogs were instantly killed by dividing the medulla, two of these subsequently being found to have microscopically normal viscera, two chronic diffuse nephritis and associated cardiac lesions; one by bleeding while chloroformed, viscera microscopically normal; one by chloroform alone; three by intravenous injections of staining fluid or pigment in suspension, viscera normal, except congestion. In each of three cases a number of hæmolymph nodes were found. The occurrence of all stages of phagocytic destruction of red cells in the sinuses in normal animals killed without unnecessary traumatism, and the nodes of which were hardened within a few minutes after death, shows that this presence of red cells in the sinuses and this blood destruction were not the result of the manipulations or a pathological condition but evidence of the performance of a normal function of the nodes. In one guinea-pig killed by chloroform a hæmolymph node was found, showing red cell destruction by phagocytes. In two of three cats examined after killing with chloroform nodes were obtained, the sinuses of which contained red cells free and in phagocytes. Although red cells were found in lymph spaces in fat surrounding the nodes, there was no reason for attributing the presence of red cells in the sinuses to pathological conditions caused by killing with chloroform, or by rupture of bloodvessels while struggling, since some of these cells were already within phagocytes. In three normal rabbits, two with cholecystitis from bacterial injection, two injected with bacterial toxines, and one splenectomized and subsequently immunized to bullock's blood, red cells were not found in the sinuses, though others have detected them in rabbits, but pigment masses were observed in some phagocytes in sinuses. In human subjects nodes containing red cells were discovered in such varied cases as infants dying from asphyxia neonatorum, gastroenteritis, status lymphaticus, and cerebral hemorrhage after forceps delivery; adults, from pneumonia, pulmonary and laryngeal tuberculosis and splenic anæmia. In a number of autopsy cases in which but few nodes were studied hæmolymph nodes were not found.

2. *Intimate Association with Ordinary Lymph Nodes.* The nodes whose sinuses contain red cells are often closely connected with ordinary lymph nodes. In one normal dog examined two nodes

were found so closely approximated as to be separated by only a few connective-tissue fibres, except at the point where blood and lymph vessels were situated. The circulatory relations could not be exactly determined. One was a typical lymph node with fine reticulum and no red cells in its sinuses; the other possessed a coarser reticulum and its sinuses contained many red cells. The two nodes were so closely connected that if the presence in the blood of some substance stimulating lymph nodes to accomplish the destruction of red blood cells was the cause of the one assuming the appearance described as that of a hæmolymph node, it would seem certain that the same influence would have acted upon the other node. On the contrary, the general appearance of the two nodes was so different and the distribution of red cells in one so distinctly marked that it would appear there was a fundamental difference in their structure and circulatory connections.

3. *Circulatory Relations.* The most direct evidence of the existence of hæmolyph nodes as organs *sui generis* would seem to be the demonstration of bloodvessels directly entering the sinuses, though it is possible that diapedesis may be responsible in some cases for the presence of red cells in them. In both dog and man I have been able to discover what appeared to be direct termination of a capillary in a sinus, but the possibility of artefacts in so delicate a tissue as a capillary wall or the lining of a sinus makes such ocular evidence unreliable. Many hæmolymph nodes appear to be more vascular than lymph nodes. The interstitial injections which have been employed by others seem unreliable, as the needle may pass into either a lymph or a blood sinus, or both, so that both systems may be injected, rendering differentiation uncertain. Two attempts to make a physiological injection of dogs through the femoral vein failed, one because the insoluble substance suspended caused embolism, the other because of the diffusibility of the material employed. In a third case insoluble Berlin blue suspended in normal salt solution warmed to body temperature was slowly injected into the proximal stump of a divided femoral vein of an anæsthetized dog, while bleeding was permitted from the distal stump in order to prevent undue increase of blood pressure. After ten or fifteen minutes of such injection the animal died. The pericardial, thoracic, and abdominal cavities were at once injected with 5 per cent. formaldehyde solution to fix the tissue cells, and the body placed in cold storage for thirty-six hours. All organs normal. In twelve of twenty-five nodes examined red cells were discovered in the sinuses. In only three was the Berlin blue found in the sinuses with the red cells, but in these three at least the coincident presence in sinuses of the recently injected pigment, together with fresh red cells not in phagocytes, would strongly point to a direct communication between the circulatory system and the sinuses of the nodes.

4. *Histological Differentiation.* The greater coarseness of the reticulum of hæmolymph nodes as compared with that of lymph nodes has been confirmed by the present study, as has the lack of differentiation between cortical and medullary regions in typical hæmolymph nodes. The frequent presence of mast cells and also of eosinophiles has been noted. The eosinophiles seem most frequent in hæmolymph nodes and in lymph nodes in cases with extreme hæmolysis such as splenic anæmia. This suggests an association between the eosinophilic granules and the destroyed red cells. Warthin's statement that phagocytes containing red and white cells are found in all sinuses of hæmolymph nodes, while in lymph nodes they are usually confined to the medullary portion, appears to be borne out.

While having no positive evidence to present in favor of the belief that transformation of fat lobules into hæmolymph or lymph nodes, or of the latter into each other, occurs, the writer has observed, in several instances, appearances which favor this view.

5. *Functions.* No evidence of red cell formation could be found. The chief function is obviously destruction of red blood cells; others are formation of leukocytes, their destruction by phagocytes, and probably formation of blood plasma. They may also be concerned in the production of eosinophiles and of phagocytes for the general circulation.

That destruction of red blood cells is an intermittently exercised function and often a purely local process, not due to hæmolytic substances in the general circulation, is shown by the occurrence simultaneously in different nodes or in different parts of the same node of its various stages. These stages are: red cells free in sinuses; apparently adherent to the periphery of the phagocytes; unchanged but contained in enlarged phagocytes; red cells disintegrating within phagocytes which are now stained more deeply red by eosin; red cells not seen, phagocytes deep reddish-yellow; phagocytes smaller, staining normally, containing granules or globules of brownish-yellow pigment; phagocytes of normal size, pigment free in sinuses.

In a node physiologically injected with Berlin blue, for example, one portion of the sinuses contained red cells which had entered long enough before to have been nearly destroyed by phagocytes, while in another portion were fresh red cells which had entered with the injected pigment immediately before death. In explanation of this intermittent action it seems most logical to believe that in some cases the bloodvessels bringing the red cells become blocked temporarily by the mass of red cells and enlarged and proliferated phagocytes in the sinuses. Blood pressure in the node is probably an important factor. In other cases the intermittent action is difficult to explain, but it may be due in some to the presence of hæmolytic substances in the blood plasma. These might cause changes in either blood cells or vessel walls which would lead to diapedesis into the sinuses.

CONCLUSIONS. Both histological and experimental evidence is strongly indicative of the existence of the hæmolymph node as an organ *sui generis*. In the light of our present knowledge the chief practical point, however, is to recognize the capability for phagocytic destruction of red blood cells which is possessed to a high degree by certain lymphoid structures, rather than to dwell upon the individuality of the hæmolymph node. The occurrence of transition forms from the node containing blood sinuses only to that with sinuses containing lymph alone renders a strict classification impossible. For practical purposes Warthin's grouping of all varieties under the heading of *hæmolymph nodes* appears eminently satisfactory.

To Dr. George C. Freeborn I am indebted for many valuable suggestions in connection with this investigation; to Dr. A. J. Lartigau for aid in the operative work, and to Dr. Edward Leaming for the accompanying photomicrograph.

BIBLIOGRAPHY.

Lewis. Journal of Physiology, 1902, vol. xxviii., Nos. 1 and 2.
Morandi and Sisto. Archiv. per le Sci. Med. 1901, vol. xxv., No. 13.
Retterer. Comptes Rendus de la Soc. de Biol. 1902, T. liv., p. 33.
Saltykow. Zeit. für Heilkunde. Abtheil für Path. Anat, 1900, S. 301.
Warthin. Journal of the Boston Society of the Medical Sciences, vol. v. p. 415.
Warthin. Journal of Medical Research, 1902, vol. ii. p. 435.
Warthin. THE AMERICAN JOURNAL OF THE MEDICAL SCIENCES, October, 1902.
Warthin. Transactions of the Chicago Pathological Society, November, 1902, vol. v., No. 8.
Weidenreich. Anatom. Anzeiger, 1902, Ergänzungsheft, Bd. xxi., S. 47.

SYPHILITIC AFFECTIONS OF THE SKIN AND OSSEOUS SYSTEM IN THE NEWBORN.

BY W. REYNOLDS WILSON, M.D.,
OF PHILADELPHIA.

SYPHILITIC infection may be transmitted in varying degrees of intensity. Its manifestations follow certain definite rules. Every newborn infant, the victim of transmitted syphilis, may not necessarily exhibit the taint; on the other hand, in the largest number of conceptions occurring in the earlier stages of syphilis transmissible from one or both parents, abortion or premature expulsion of the fetus is liable to result.

The opportunity of infection occurs:

1. In the presence of a coexistent infection in both parents. This usually results in abortion (Baginsky), although Neumann has recorded the birth of healthy infants under such conditions.

2. In the presence of infection of the male parent alone at the time of conception. In this case the infection is transmitted directly to the fetus, and is in reality the result of direct contagion. Although the pregnancy may not be interrupted, the infant mortality is great, the children succumbing in proportion to the primariness of the infection in the parent.

3. In the presence, at the time of conception, of maternal infection alone. As in the case of paternal infection, the infant may escape transmission if the paternal disease has reached its tertiary form.

4. In the presence of maternal infection during gestation. The intensity of the infection in such instances depends upon the degree of postponement of the postconceptional infection in the mother.

According to Fournier, syphilis in the newborn may present direct congenital manifestations or indirect evidences of infection. In the latter case it is spoken of as hereditary syphilis. The lesions in hereditary syphilis may be either precocious or deferred as to the date of their appearance.

Congenital syphilis in the newborn is marked by signs of an infection the evolution of which has been completed in utero. Should the infant be born alive, it presents localized areas of separation of the epidermis in the form of blebs, accompanied by excoriation. The skin resembles the condition of maceration in stillborn infants. There is also present retrograde bony development (imperfectly expanded thorax, craniotabes, etc.), enlargement of the liver and spleen. Such infants are usually premature.

Hereditary syphilis in its precocious form affects especially the newborn infant. It is marked by snuffles, hoarse cry, pendulous abdomen, splenic and hepatic enlargement, and the characteristic syphilides.

The subject of hereditary syphilis with deferred manifestations may present at the time of birth a perfectly healthy appearance. More frequently, however, the infants are emaciated, the skin being of a dull yellowish color and the face presenting a characteristic senile expression.

Syphilis in the newborn may be considered in reference to the skin localization as follows:

1. The pathognomonic form of eruption in early syphilis is that of a pemphigus (Gastou). The lesion may either exist as a congenital manifestation or may make its appearance at the end of the first week of life. The character of the eruption is twofold. It may appear, first, in the form of violet or reddish patches protruding slightly beyond the surface of the skin and surrounded by a zone of moderate hyperæmia. The elevation of the surface affected is due to the displacement of the epidermis by the accumulation of a sanguinolent fluid, which may rapidly change in color to a greenish-yellow. The size of a fully-formed vesicle usually equals that of a small pea. The diameter, however, may reach 1 cm. or more in

extent. The border may be circular or polygonal. Rupture of the bleb leaves an ulcerated, uneven base. Recovery takes place by the formation of a brownish crust, the neighboring skin remaining reddened and squamous. Secondly, the syphiloderm may begin as a pustular eruption the lesions of which proceed rapidly to maturation and take on a varioloform appearance. If the pustules coalesce, the resulting exfoliation may assume the character of a squamous dermatitis, producing a condition resembling ichthyosis. Syphilitic pemphigus usually attacks the palmar and plantar surfaces, especially in its vesicular form. The pustular form is found most frequently in the region of the buttocks and genitalia. It may, however, show no elective tendency as to location, appearing on any part of the body or face.

Jacquet regards the pemphigus of hereditary syphilis in the newborn in the light of a developed form of a papulomacular syphilide, corresponding to that observed usually as a later manifestation. The exuberance of the lesions resulting in the bleb-like development, according to his view, is due to the normal congestion of the skin and the delicacy of the epithelial layer in the newborn.

2. A further manifestation often met with is the papuloerosive syphiloderm, which makes its appearance in the crevices of the skin, where moisture is apt to be present, as, for instance, in the genitocrural folds, the axilla, the region of the umbilicus, and the interdigital spaces. The efflorescence occurs in the form of small papules of a yellowish-gray color and a diphtheritic surface, accompanied by a local erythema. This usually results in erosion, which attacks the summit of the papules and permits the escape of a thinnish exudation. The erosion extends peripherally rather than in depth.

3. Probably the most frequently observed syphiloderm in hereditary syphilis is that of erythema. The rash begins very much as a simple erythema, attacking the region of the genitalia and nates. It, however, may not be confined to these points of election, as it frequently makes its appearance on the face, especially on the forehead and body. The eruption may even extend to the scalp. The eruption is apt to spread rapidly, showing a tendency to infiltration, and resulting in the development of small papules, which show, as the result of erosion, a moistened surface. The efflorescence remaining after the disappearance of the acute erythema presents a copper-colored, papular syphilide characteristic of secondary manifestations. Frequently the papules are disposed at the verge of the anus and the commissure of the lips (Van Harlingen). There may be active desquamation resulting in the formation of thick, yellowish crusts, which, in separating, leave a moist, infiltrated base. Syphilitic erythema, when attacking the region of the umbilicus, very often results in an impetiginous rash, which terminates in local desquamation. Complicating the erythema, there is frequently observed a macular and squamous eruption of the palmar and plantar surfaces.

4. Furunculoid lesions attacking the corium, as well as tuberculous eruptions, are not uncommonly found coincidently with the more typical skin manifestations. Gastou calls attention to the existence of a gummatous condition, which exists in the form of deep tumefactions, in the region surrounding the articulations. This condition must not be mistaken for the infiltration due to periarthritic abscess. It is not uncommonly seen in instances of fatal congenital syphilis.

As in acquired syphilis, the lesions are apt to be symmetrical and are characterized by polymorphism. Owing to the latter characteristic, it is sometimes difficult to differentiate the varieties in syphilitic erythema, the simple form frequently merging into the squamous and impetiginous forms.

Paronychia may be mentioned among the syphilides appearing in the newborn. Although the infiltration surrounding the matrix may be extensive, it is not likely to result in ulceration. Fissures occurring at the borders of the mucous membrane are commonly seen, situated in the region of the anus and lips. Fissures in the epidermis of the scrotum, and, in the female, in the region of the fourchette, may be observed.

Mucous Membranes. Syphilis of the mucosæ may appear frequently as the primary manifestation in hereditary transmission. In this way the coryza may appear as the initial manifestation. The nasal secretion is at first sanious, becoming afterward greenish and purulent. It is frequently mixed with blood. It is irritating to the adjacent skin and often fetid. The crusts which form from the drying secretions may give rise, through their detachment, to epistaxis. The mucous membrane becomes swollen and the submucosa infiltrated, often to such extent as to interfere with the nasal respiration. The buccal mucous membrane, the tongue, the hard palate may become individually the seat of mucous patches, the sites of which offer local areas of ulceration in the process of cicatrization. The pharynx is usually swollen and reddened. The laryngeal mucous membrane may also partake of the hyperæmia and swelling, causing characteristic hoarseness, and leading often to extinction of the voice. Dyspnœa may sometimes occur, simulating laryngismus stridulus and resulting rapidly in death by asphyxia. Inflammation of the middle ear, accompanied by otorrhœa, is of infrequent occurrence.

The Osseous System. The changes in the osseous system affect the long bones as a rule, less frequently the phalanges. The pathological changes in the cranial bones are usually associated with the evolution of infantile syphilis in its later stages. The bones of the head may present, however, a condition of craniotabes. Undue protrusion of the parietal eminences with deeply-marked sutures (natiform cranium) may rarely be observed. Microcephalus or hydrocephalus may be present in cachectic infants.

The abnormalities occurring in the long bones affect usually the juncture of the diaphysis and epiphysis. In an undeveloped state the lesion may exist as an osteochondritis, which may offer no external evidence. In acute or progressive form it is marked clinically by an indifferent swelling, which may not be detected beneath the soft tissue; occasionally by a palpable enlargement. The condition may make its appearance soon after birth. If the lesions be multiple and pronounced in development they may present the appearance of pseudosyphilitic infantile paralysis. The clinical picture of this disease is described by Parrot. When the infant in a pronounced case is suspended by the axillæ the extremities hang flaccid. If the skin is pinched the muscles move, but the position of the member is not changed. On the other hand, the infant will suffer without resistance such displacement of its extremities. If the legs are extended while the child is in the dorsal decubitus they will resume their flexed position, but the movement is accompanied by pain. The joints may be tumefied. Crepitation and fluctuation may be present. Such extensive involvement usually results in a fatal outcome. The inflammation and loss of continuity producing the symptoms just described are due, according to Gastou, to a justo-epiphyseal osteitis. The suppuration which is present usually invades the joint and leads uniformly to the destruction of the cartilage and the separation of the epiphysis. The apparent muscular relaxation present in such cases may be confused with paralysis of central origin, due to such causes as intracranial hemorrhage and obstetrical traumatism. It may likewise simulate the muscular immotility present in fractures and luxations. The condition is not to be confused with epiphyseal separation due to the destruction of the cartilage, found in the putrefactive invasion of the tissues in macerated infants. In instances of the purulent destruction of the epiphyseal attachment, the presence of streptococcus denotes the possibility of the septic process occurring secondarily to the specific inflammation. The lesion may be found at either end of the femur, at the distal end of the tibia, and the bones of the forearm (Ziegler).

As to the pathology, the site of the lesion is the so-called zone of proliferation—*i. e.*, the transitional cartilaginous area that separates the epiphysis from the shaft of the bone. According to Kassowitz and Heubner, the progress of the condition may be divided into three stages: 1. A premature deposit of the primary calcareous infiltration in the original cartilaginous substance. 2. An irregular invasion by this calcifying process of the area of intermediary cartilage (the area in which the cartilage cells begin to arrange themselves to form the primary cartilaginous trabeculæ), with an overgrowth of the cartilaginous trabeculæ and with the premature deposit of bone. 3. The development of a granulation zone between the epiphysis and apophysis, followed in some instances with the actual secretion of pus.

Macroscopically the yellowish line of demarcation at the apophyso-epiphyseal juncture corresponding to the zone of proliferation, found post-mortem in newborn infants, represents the early stage of the process just described.

The digital phalanges may be the seat of the bony involvement in congenital and hereditary syphilis. The periosteum and fibrous structure surrounding the bone are usually affected. Secondarily, the skin and subintegumentary tissues become involved. Suppurative changes resulting in ulcerations are usually not to be observed, on account of the readiness with which the specific infiltration yields to treatment. The proximal phalanx is more frequently involved than the distal phalanx. The finger is apt to be swollen at its base, presenting a pyriform appearance with the characteristic discoloration of the skin. Baginsky has observed a bony deformation of the fingers, resulting in syndactylism in a syphilitic child.

A STUDY OF THE CALORIC NEEDS OF PREMATURE INFANTS.

By John Lovett Morse, A.M., M.D.,

INSTRUCTOR IN DISEASES OF CHILDREN, HARVARD MEDICAL SCHOOL; ASSISTANT PHYSICIAN AT THE CHILDREN'S HOSPITAL AND AT THE INFANTS' HOSPITAL, BOSTON.

Vierordt and Rubner were the first to investigate the metabolism of the infant. Camerer, in 1889, collected a large amount of material and endeavored to determine in heat units the nutritive needs of infants of various ages. He calculated the caloric contents of breast milk on the basis of Pfeiffer's analyses. A considerable number of observations have been made by different men since that time. Each one has, as a rule, made but one or two. Most of them have been made on breast-fed infants; a few on artificially fed. Some of them have extended over the first year, but most of them only over short periods of time. Czerny and Keller, in their hand-book published in 1902, have reviewed the work of previous observers in detail and added a considerable amount of material of their own. Since then Beuthner has studied three cases, one of which was fed entirely on breast milk, the others partly on breast milk and partly on artificial food. In 1902 he summed up the cases fed on breast milk hitherto studied in private practice. He included the cases of Ahlfeldt (2), Camerer (4), Feer (3), Hähner (4), Laure (1), Pfeiffer (2), Weigelin (1), Oppenheimer (1), and his own (3). The average number of calories per kilo taken daily was as follows:

1 week	59 calories.	10 weeks	104 calories.
2 weeks	100 "	14 "	96 "
4 "	106 "	17 "	91 "
7 "	114 "	30 "	85 "

In all these experiments the caloric worth of the nourishment was reckoned on the usual basis that 1 gram of albumin equals 4.1 calories, 1 gram of carbohydrates 4.1 calories, and 1 gram of fat 9.3 calories. There must be some doubt, of course, whether these figures, which were calculated expressly for the mixed food of a man, can be used in estimating the nutritive value of milk for an infant. In the mixed diet of the adult about 8 per cent. of the total worth is lost in the feces. Czerny and Keller have shown that this loss is much less in healthy children fed on milk. All these observers estimated the caloric value of human milk at 650 calories per litre, and of cow's milk at 670 calories per litre. This standard for the caloric contents of woman's milk is based on an estimated composition. Everyone knows that the milk of different women varies, especially in its fat contents, and that the milk of the same woman varies from day to day and from nursing to nursing. These physiological variations in the composition of woman's milk make an average caloric worth elusory. This average figure is still more elusory when we realize that the accepted caloric value of 650 calories per litre is based on the average of the analyses of the milk of two women, one of whom had a milk poor in fat, the other a milk rich in fat. Schlossmann, moreover, obtained as the result of 218 analyses of woman's milk an average value of 782 calories per litre. He used this figure as the basis of his investigations. It is evident that the figures of previous observers will be materially altered if this caloric value is accepted. It is evident, therefore, that figures based on such an average caloric value per litre of milk cannot be of great value.

Heubner draws the following conclusions from the cases of Feer, Finkelstein, Camerer, and others: An alimentation whose quotient of energy does not exceed 70 calories is insufficient for an infant, even if breast-fed, to prosper on, at least during the first six months. In order to get a normal gain a quotient of energy of at least 100 calories with natural alimentation and of 120 with artificial alimentation is necessary. After the sixth month a given quotient of energy gives better results as regards gain in weight than in the first six months ; that is to say, in the second half of the first year the organism works more economically than at the beginning of life. In order to obtain the same results a larger quotient of energy is required in artificial alimentation than in natural alimentation. He believes that the less favorable results of artificial food are due to the greater work which cow's milk imposes on the digestive organs. This work absorbs a certain number of calories which normally are made use of by the organism. Other writers have attributed the difference in the results to the difference in the casein of woman's and cow's milk.

In attempting to determine how much nourishment a healthy suckling needs it is of the greatest importance to determine by what standard the amount of this need is to be measured. In adults under physiological conditions enough nourishment must be taken to keep up the weight. This is not sufficient for infants in the first year, who must take enough nourishment to make possible a gain in body substance. This gain must also be of a certain definite kind. A gain in weight alone is not sufficient and cannot be accepted as a reliable guide to the worth of the food. At present we are not in a position to say what substances and what quantities of these substances are necessary to meet the loss of the body and to make possible a normal gain in development. We do know that the infant must have albumin, but that it can thrive on a comparatively small amount. Whether fat or carbohydrates can be omitted without causing harm to the organism has not yet been determined in the healthy infant. Single observations on sick children point to an affirmative answer.

The number of experiments which have thus far been made in the metabolism of infancy are too small to justify any general and sweeping conclusions. It must be remembered, moreover, that figures based on an average caloric contents of milk show nothing more than does the quantity of the nourishment. A study of the curve of nourishment in healthy infants shows in the beginning for a longer or shorter time a daily increase in the amount of milk taken, which increase, nevertheless, steadily diminishes as the infant becomes older. In the first weeks of life, in breast-fed children, the amount of nourishment taken is about one-fifth of the body weight. It gradually diminishes and from the middle of the first to the middle of the second quarter-year remains between one-sixth and one-seventh, and at the end of the first half-year is about one-eighth of the body weight.

The variations in the rate of development of children who take the same quantity of woman's milk may be largely explained by the differences in the chemical composition of the milk which they receive. Moreover, as the result of the variations in the area of the surface of the body different percentages of the energy taken in are given off in the form of heat. Finally, it is possible that the differences in the composition of the body substance in different children may play a part.

Czerny and Keller think that the figures which have been obtained by averaging the number of calories taken by the various infants which have been studied are larger than the nutritive need of a healthy infant. One of the infants studied in their clinic shows that Heubner's assumption that an intake of less than 70 calories per kilo, even in breast-fed infants, is not consistent with a normal increase in weight for the first half-year is erroneous. In this case less than 70 calories per kilo were taken for six weeks. The increase in weight was, nevertheless, 15 grams daily. They also give various observations which show that in breast-fed infants less than 100 calories per kilo is completely sufficient for a satisfactory development.

They do not agree with Heubner's assertion that with an artificial food satisfactory development is impossible on less than 120 calories per kilo daily. Heubner based his opinion on Finkelstein's study of a healthy infant. Another case of Finkelstein's which was also on an artificial food did well and gained regularly on much less than 120 calories per kilo, taking an average of 103.6 calories per kilo in the first quarter-year, 102.5 in the second quarter, and 99 in the third quarter. They consider that the quantity of milk necessary to give 120 calories per kilo of body weight is overfeeding.

They do not agree with Heubner that a larger caloric worth of cow's milk is necessary than of breast milk. They state that metabolism experiments have thrown but little light on the comparative nutritive worth of woman's and cow's milk for healthy infants. (They quote Rubner and Heubner's experiments.) These show no important differences as regards the utilization of the constituents of cow's and woman's milk, the physiological results being almost the same in both cases. They assert that the caloric need of a healthy infant is no greater when nourished on cow's milk than on human milk, and that the assumption that when cow's milk is taken more of the energy ingested is used up by the digestive tract than when breast milk is taken is therefore unwarranted.

It is a well-known fact that small bodies have a greater surface area in proportion to their mass than have large bodies. The loss of heat is therefore relatively greater in proportion to the weight in small than in large bodies. Rubner first recognized the importance of this fact in relation to tissue changes in living animals, and demonstrated that the tissue changes are proportional at every age to the size of the surface of the body. Young individuals, therefore, show a relatively greater destruction of material than older, and hence require relatively larger amounts of nourishment. This difference in size explains to a certain extent, but not entirely, the far greater number of calories per kilo required by infants than by adults in order to thrive. The rest of the infant's greater requirement is accounted for by the fact that the infant uses up a considerable amount of energy in growth.

Reasoning on the same lines, premature infants, being so small, should require even more calories per kilo than full-term infants in order to thrive. Heubner compared an artificially-fed premature infant studied by Finkelstein with a breast-fed full-term infant studied by Feer and another artificially-fed full-term infant studied by Finkelstein, and found that it did not do so well as the others. Its gain was only one-half as rapid as that of the artificially-fed infant, although after the sixth week it took as many or more calories per kilo of weight. During the first three weeks it took an average of 25 calories per kilo and made no gain, while in the two weeks following it took between 50 and 90 calories per kilo and made a slight gain. During the next four weeks it took an average of 104 calories per kilo, and from the tenth to the seventeenth weeks inclusive 135 calories per kilo. It averaged 120 calories per kilo from the eighteenth to the thirty-ninth week inclusive, and 107 calories per kilo from the fortieth to the fifty-second week. During the first quarter of the year it made an average daily gain of 12 grams, in the second one of 18 grams, in the third one of 15 grams, and in the last one of 2 grams. Its initial weight was 1350 grams, while at the end of the year its weight was 5750 grams. It was fed on peptonized milk.

Heubner explains the smaller gain on a relatively equal or greater intake of energy on the principles detailed above. Another possible reason why premature infants might be expected to require a relatively greater intake of energy lies in the comparatively undeveloped condition of the digestive power which results in a less complete utilization of the food ingested. No proof of this latter assumption is, however, at hand.

Beuthner studied an infant six or seven weeks premature for twenty-five weeks. It was entirely breast-fed for seven weeks, and was then given in addition cow's milk diluted with a cereal decoction to the end of the twenty-fifth week, at which time the observation was discontinued. It weighed 2400 grams at birth and 6800 grams at the end of the twenty-fifth week, having made an average daily gain of 25 grams. During the first quarter it took a daily average of 113.1 calories per kilo, and during the second quarter one of 92.2 calories per kilo.

Schlossmann studied an infant four or five weeks premature from the twelfth to the eightieth day. It was breast-fed. It weighed 2230 grams on the twelfth day and 3310 grams on the eightieth day, having made an average daily gain of 16 grams. It took an average of 119 calories per kilo daily and made an average daily gain of 5.5 grams per kilo.

These cases, as far as they go, confirm Heubner's assumption that premature infants require a relatively greater amount of nourishment than full-term infants, and that a larger number of calories is necessary in a substitute food than in breast milk. The differences are so slight, however, that but little importance can be attached to them.

During the past winter I have studied from the point of view of the quotient of energy the feeding of six premature infants, five of them at the Infants' Hospital and one in private practice. All were fed on modified cow's milk of definite percentages prepared at the Walker-Gordon Laboratory. The composition of the food being known, it was easy to calculate its caloric contents. It is possible that the composition of the food may not always have been exactly what it was supposed to be. Edsall's recent analyses of milk prepared at the Walker-Gordon Laboratory show, however, that these variations must have been very small, certainly not large enough to have vitiated to any extent the value of the results. They certainly must be more accurate than those obtained on the basis of the average analyses of woman's and cow's milk. The amount of food taken at each feeding was carefully measured. The caloric value was calculated on the basis that 1 gram of sugar or proteids equals 4.1 calories, and 1 gram of fat 9.3 calories.

Unfortunately all the babies did not do uninterruptedly well. One died when twenty-seven days old, of a congenital cardiac lesion complicated by atelectasis of the lungs. Its digestion had been good from the first, however, and it had shown no signs of its cardiac or pulmonary lesions until its sudden collapse and death. One left the hospital when three weeks old, not gaining, but doing very well in other ways. Two did very well and gained steadily. One gained steadily for ten weeks and another for eight weeks, after which both had more or less disturbance of digestion and did not gain regularly, sometimes gaining and sometimes losing. Most of them showed a tendency to have too many dejections. These were, as a rule, of good color and odor, but were rather loose and contained fine curds. They did not seem to interfere with the gain in weight, but suggested that a portion of the food was not properly utilized. The histories with charts are given in more detail below:

Ruth C. was brought to the Infants' Hospital February 1, 1903, when six hours old. She was thought to be two months premature. The physical examination showed nothing abnormal. Her cry was strong. Her weight was 2500 grams. Her temperature was about normal during the whole of her stay in the hospital. She always took her food well and never vomited. She had from one to four movements daily, usually one or two, which were generally a little green and contained a few curds. The movements were not as good on February 12th. She was given calomel and her food was cut down for forty-eight hours. She was discharged February 22d at her parents' request. She had been taken out of the incubator and was doing well. Her weight was 2440 grams.

James McL. was admitted to the Infants' Hospital April 24, 1903, when twenty-four hours old. He was supposed to be two months premature. He was feeble and had a feeble cry. His extremities were cool. The heart sounds were normal, the rate slow. No further examination was made. His weight was 1170 grams. He was at once put in the incubator. His temperature remained subnormal until May 9th, after which it was irregular, but usually elevated. He took his food well from a Breck feeder, but was not able to take an ordinary nipple. He regurgitated a little during the last two or three days. During the first nine days he had one movement daily which, after the meconium was passed, was well digested. After that time he had from two to six movements daily, usually well digested. They were well digested on the day of his death. He seemed to be doing finely until the weather suddenly became hot. He immediately began to fail and died May 20th. His weight on the day of his death was 1040 grams. The autopsy showed that both the foramen ovale and the ductus arteriosus were open and that portions of both lungs had never expanded.

CHART I.

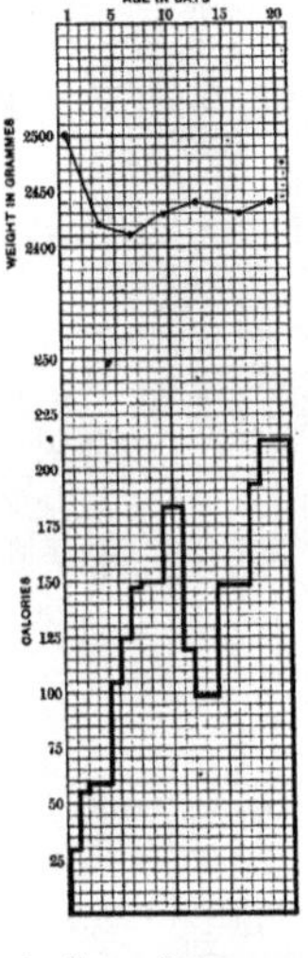

CHART II.

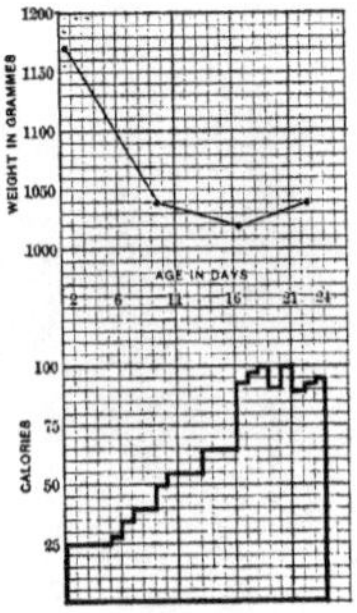

Charles S. was first seen on February 3, 1903 when twelve hours old. He was at least four weeks premature. Physical examination showed nothing abnormal. He acted fairly vigorously and had a strong cry. His weight was 1530 grams. He was put in a padded crib. When five days old he suddenly collapsed and almost died. After this he was feeble for a considerable time. At first he had to be fed with a Breck feeder and sometimes with a dropper. He usually took his food fairly well, but showed a tendency to spit it up if he were at all overfed. The food supply had to be cut down several times temporarily on this account. There was a slight tendency to constipation, but the movements were, as a rule, well digested. He had a good deal of colic. The observation was stopped on May 19th, when he was fifteen weeks old, because the family were going into the country for the summer, where they had to use a home modification of milk. His weight at that time was 2620

CHART III.

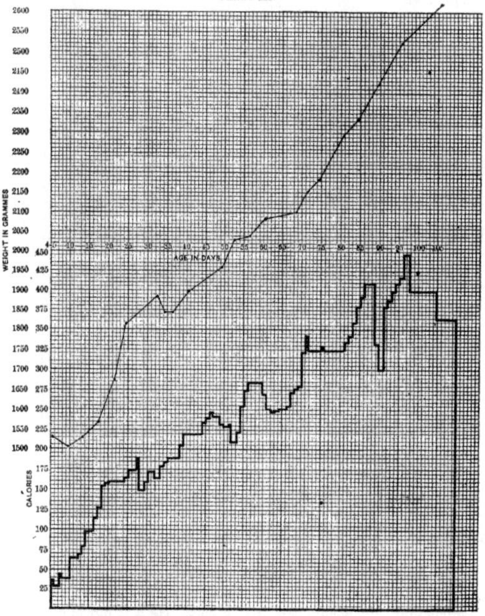

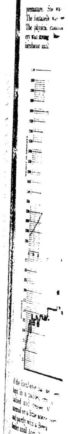

grams, making an average daily gain of a little over 10 grams. He was doing well at that time and has continued to do so.

Pauline J. was admitted to the Infants' Hospital March 20, 1903, when two weeks old. She was born at the Lying-in Hospital and had been in an incubator there before she came to the Infants' Hospital. She was supposed to have been about two months premature. She was small, emaciated, and markedly jaundiced. The fontanelle was depressed, and the cranial bones overlapped. The physical examination showed nothing else abnormal. Her cry was strong. Her weight was 1180 grams. She was kept in an incubator until April 25th, and would have been kept there longer

CHART IV.

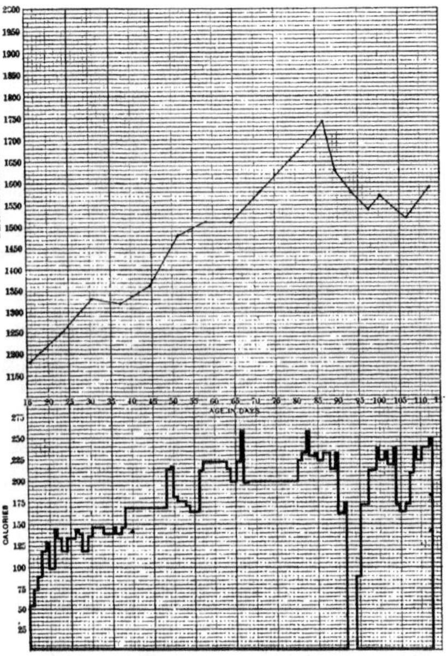

if the incubator had not been needed for another baby. She was kept in a padded crib until the middle of June. She was first bathed and dressed May 18th. Her temperature was usually normal or a little above normal. She was fed partly with a dropper and partly with a Breck feeder until March 24th, then with a Breck feeder until April 23d, after which she took the nipple. She usually took her food fairly well. She did not vomit at all until about the second week in May, after which she at times vomited a good deal and at others not at all. On this account the food supply had to be cut down on several occasions and at one time milk was omitted entirely. After May 1st there was a slight tendency to looseness of the bowels. At times she had as many as seven or eight in twenty-four hours. These were either yellowish or yellowish-green, with fine curds and occasionally a little mucus. The movements, however, on the whole, were not bad. They certainly did not interfere with her general condition or prevent her from gaining until June 1st, when she was twelve weeks old. She then weighed 1720 grams, having made an average daily gain of 8 grams. She did not do as well after the hot weather began in June, although she developed no new symptoms, did not vomit any more or have a greater number of movements. She was discharged June 29th, when sixteen and one-half weeks old, because the hospital was closing for the summer. At that time she was not doing very well, was having many movements and vomiting a little. Her weight was 1600 grams. She was evidently sick after June 1st, and hence her records from this date on can hardly be properly used in estimating the caloric need of a normal infant.

Emanuel B. was admitted to the Infants' Hospital January 17, 1903, when two weeks old. He was supposed to be about two months premature. He had spent the first two weeks in an incubator at the Lying-in Hospital. While there he vomited every few days and was constipated. The physical examination showed nothing abnormal. His weight was 1370 grams. He was put in a padded crib, dressed March 5th, bathed March 23d and taken out of the padded crib April 26th. His temperature was subnormal during the first two weeks, but after that was normal. He always took his food well and very seldom vomited, at one time not for ten weeks. He had from two to five movements daily, which were usually yellow but sometimes green, and often contained small curds and sometimes a little mucus. On the whole the movements were mostly satisfactory except that they were increased in number. He was doing fairly well when he left the hospital, May 19th. He was then nineteen weeks old and weighed 2640 grams. He had had a little fever, had not taken his food quite as well, and had not gained during his last ten days in the hospital. Nothing definitely wrong was made out, however. It is hardly fair, nevertheless, to consider him a well baby after May 9th. The last ten days should not be counted in drawing conclusions. From the fifteenth to the one hundred and twenty-fifth day he made an average daily gain of a little over 12 grams.

James J. was admitted to the Infants' Hospital January 22, 1903, when fourteen days old. He was supposed to have been one month premature. He spent the first two weeks in the Lying-in

Hospital. He was thin and the anterior fontanelle was somewhat depressed. The physical examination was otherwise negative. His weight was 1820 grams. He was put in a padded crib. He had to be fed with a Breck feeder until March 10th. He was bathed March 13th and taken out of the padded crib April 26th. His temperature was subnormal for nearly a month, after which it

CHART V.

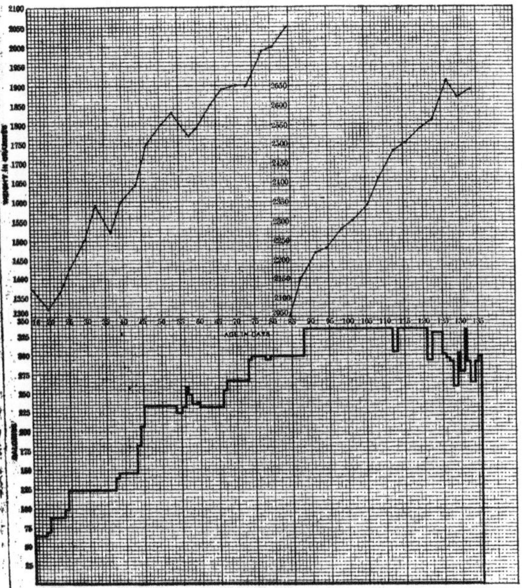

was usually about normal. He was never vigorous and never took his food very well. He did not vomit until the middle of May, after which he vomited occasionally. He had from two to four movements daily up to about the middle of March, after which he had too many movements, often as many as six or eight in twenty-four hours. After April 1st, when he weighed 2430 grams, any attempt to increase the amount or strength of the food caused an increase in the number of movements. These movements were yellowish, or yellowish-green, and contained fine curds. On several occasions the food had to be cut down decidedly, and once milk was entirely omitted. During the last five weeks he had a sore mouth and tongue from time to time. He was much depressed by the first hot weather, which occurred in the middle of May. It was at that time that the milk had to be stopped. He never did as well afterward. He was discharged June 18th in fair condition and gained

CHART VI.

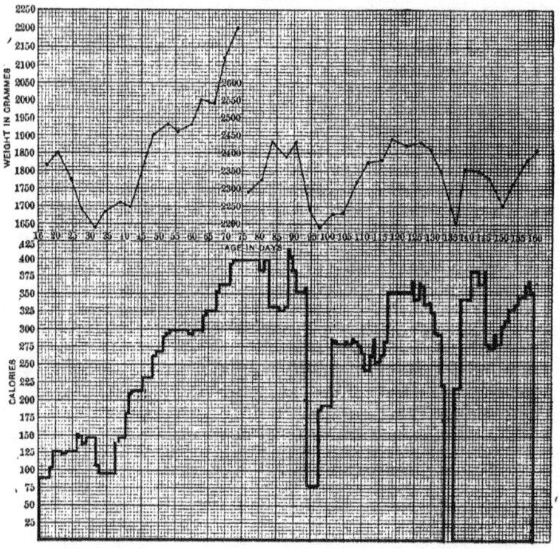

in weight. His mouth was well. He was taking his food rather better, was vomiting about once a day and having from three to four movements daily, some of which were normal and some of were green and contained curds. His weight was 2410 grams. The only period in which he did almost uninterruptedly well was from the thirty-second to the eighty-third day. During this time he made an average daily gain of more than 15 grams. His subsequent record is of chief interest in showing the rapid fall in weight when the nourishment was cut down, with a correspondingly rapid rise when it was again increased. It is worthy of study in this connection.

Age in days.	Average calories per kilo ingested daily.						Average daily gain. Grams per kilo.						Number of cases	Daily average calories per kilo.
	Grossman.	McLeod.	Stone.	Jeffrey.	Blaikie.	Joyce.	Grossman.	McLeod.	Stone.	Jeffrey.	Blaikie.	Joyce.		
1-5	24.8	20.5	...	...	...	...	lost	lost	...	...	...	...	2	22.6
5-10	61.7	34.5	33.6	...	...	...	even	lost	lost	...	...	...	3	43.3
10-15	53.5	56.7	59.0	...	...	...	even	even	6.5	...	...	...	3	56.4
15-20	75.4	85.4	94.4	77.7	52.7	55.2	even	even	14.8	6.6	lost	2.2	6	73.5
20-25	...	72.1	95.1	100.8	72.5	70.3	...	even	17.0	8.0	13.1	lost	5	82.2
25-30	...	...	90.8	103.8	87.2	83.3	...	...	4.3	9.3	12.3	lost	4	91.3
30-35	...	...	98.5	109.0	82.8	72.4	...	...	lost	even	6.5	2.4	4	90.7
35-40	...	...	114.9	116.5	86.9	75.2	...	...	7.6	1.5	6.3	2.3	4	98.5
40-45	...	...	121.0	126.4	101.5	120.0	...	...	3.1	4.5	10.9	11.4	4	117.2
45-50	...	...	119.4	134.5	135.0	132.0	...	...	7.0	12.8	11.4	11.8	4	130.2
50-55	...	...	123.4	119.7	129.0	152.3	...	...	2.9	5.4	2.2	even	4	131.1
55-60	...	...	133.9	138.6	137.2	156.2	...	...	3.8	2.6	lost	2.0	4	141.5
60-65	...	...	120.3	143.0	122.7	158.6	...	...	even	even	6.1	6.1	4	136.1
65-70	...	...	147.9	141.5	137.2	170.3	...	...	6.6	7.7	4.2	12.6	4	149.2
70-75	...	...	151.0	126.1	145.5	180.6	...	...	6.4	6.3	2.0	9.2	4	150.8
75-80	...	...	145.9	122.3	152.4	176.2	...	...	8.0	6.0	7.1	8.8	4	149.2
80-85	...	...	161.3	121.8	157.2	156.5	...	...	5.1	6.5	6.2	8.4	4	149.2
85-90	...	...	152.6	134.3	148.1	149.5	...	...	7.4	lost	13.4	even	2	150.3
90-95	...	...	165.0	...	158.7	131.7	...	...	6.4	...	3.7	lost	2	161.8
95-100	...	...	160.4	129.3	148.5	64.8	...	...	3.9	even	4.4	lost	2	154.4
100-105	...	...	148.4	141.2	149.9	117.1	...	...	3.0	lost	4.3	1.8	2	146.6
105-110	...	...	...	130.3	140.7	124.0	...	...	...	2.5	8.4	8.7	1	140.7
110-115	...	...	...	...	133.7	112.1	...	...	...	...	4.8	4.2	1	133.7
115-120	...	...	...	...	138.7	135.5	...	...	...	...	4.1	4.1	1	138.7
120-125	...	...	...	...	121.4	146.0	...	...	...	...	6.2	even	1	124.4
125-130	...	...	...	...	110.6	145.5	...	...	...	...	even	lost		
130-135	...	...	...	...	111.4	...	...	...	...	...	1.5			
135-140	...	...	...	...	...	...	...	...	...	...	...	.		
140-145	...	...	...	...	...	158.7	...	...	...	...	...	even		
145-150	...	...	...	...	...	132.0	...	...	...	...	...	lost		
150-155	...	...	...	...	...	141.4	...	...	...	...	...	7.0		
155-160	...	...	...	...	...	150.9	...	...	...	...	...	5.9		

Further analysis of this table shows that these cases took from the fifteenth to the ninetieth day, that is, during the first quarter after the first two weeks, a daily average of 122.7 calories per kilo of weight, and that from the ninetieth to the one hundred and twenty-fifth day, that is, during the early part of the second quarter, a daily average of 142.9 calories per kilo of weight.

In the first few weeks these infants took less than the average given in Beuthner's table. As they did not gain at first it is probable, however, that in order to avoid upsetting the digestion they were somewhat underfed. These figures justify Heubner's assertions that not less than 70 calories per kilo are necessary during the first six months, and that with artificial alimentation at least 120 calories per kilo are necessary to get a normal gain. They correspond fairly closely with the results obtained by other observers in premature infants during the first three months, Beuthner's infant having averaged 113.1 calories per kilo, Schlossmann's 119 calories per kilo, and Finkelstein's 120 to 135 calories per kilo. In contradistinction to other figures they show a progressive increase in the quotient of energy toward the end of the first quarter and at the beginning of the second quarter. In spite of the high quotient of energy these infants did not gain as rapidly as the average normal full-term infant, thus confirming Heubner's assumption that premature infants require a relatively greater amount of nourishment than do full-term infants.

It is very difficult to draw any very satisfactory conclusions from these figures. In some instances when two babies of the same age were taking almost exactly the same relative amount of nourishment one gained and the other lost. In other instances the baby taking the smaller amount of nourishment gained while the other lost. For example, between the fifteenth and twentieth days baby J. gained on 55.2 calories per kilo, while baby B. lost on 52.7 calories per kilo. Between the twentieth and twenty-fifth days baby B. made a large gain on 72.5 calories per kilo, while baby McL. just held his weight on 72.1 calories per kilo and baby J. lost on 70.3 calories. Between the thirtieth and thirty-fifth days baby J. gained on 72.4 calories, while baby S. lost on 98.5 calories. Between the fifty-fifth and sixtieth days babies S. and J. gained on 133.9 calories and 138.6 calories respectively, while baby B. lost on 137.2 calories.

In some cases in which two babies of the same age were taking practically the same relative amounts of nourishment, one gained two or three times as much as the other; for example, between the fortieth and forty-fifth days baby J. took a daily average of 120 calories per kilo and made a daily gain of 11.4 grams per kilo, while baby S. took 121 calories and gained only 3.1 grams per kilo.

Again, babies of the same age gained essentially the same amounts on widely differing amounts of nourishment; for example, between the seventieth and seventy-fifth days baby S. made an average daily gain of 6.4 grams per kilo on 151 calories per kilo, while baby J. gained 6.3 grams on 126.1 calories.

In other instances one baby did better than another for a time, and then a little later the second baby did better than the first; for example, between the twentieth and twenty-fifth days baby B. took 72.5 calories per kilo and gained 13.1 grams per kilo daily, while baby J. lost weight on 70.3 calories. Between the forty-fifth and fiftieth days baby B. took 135 calories per kilo and made a daily gain of 11.4 grams per kilo, while baby J. took 132 calories and gained 11.8 grams. Between the eightieth and eighty-fifth days baby B. took 157.2 calories and gained 6.2 grams, while baby J. took 156.5 calories and gained 8.4 grams.

Again, the same baby did not gain in proportion to the amount of food taken; for example, baby J., between the fortieth and forty-fifth days, took an average of 120 calories per kilo and made an average daily gain of 11.4 grams per kilo; between the forty-fifth and fiftieth days he took 132 calories and gained 11.8 grams; between the fiftieth and fifty-fifth days, 152.3 calories with no gain; between the fifty-fifth and sixtieth days, 156.2 calories with a gain of 2 grams; between the sixtieth and sixty-fifth days, 158.6 calories with a gain of 6.1 grams; between the sixty-fifth and seventieth days, 170.3 calories with a gain of 12.6 grams, and between the seventieth and seventy-fifth days, 180.6 calories with a gain of 9.2 grams.

The only conclusion which it seems possible to draw from these contradictory figures is that the gain seemed to depend as much, or more, on the digestion and metabolism of the given baby at the given age as on the amount of the food, the age of the baby, or any inherent differences in the individual babies.

CONCLUSION. The conclusion seems justified from these figures that the caloric need of premature infants is relatively greater than that of full-term infants. This greater need is due in part to the small size and comparatively large surface area of premature infants, which cause them to lose heat faster than do larger, full-term infants, and partly to the incomplete development of their digestive powers, on account of which they utilize a relatively smaller proportion of the caloric value of the food ingested. This conclusion emphasizes the importance of protecting premature infants against loss of heat and of providing for them a food which will throw the least work on the partially developed digestive powers.

BIBLIOGRAPHY.

Beuthner. Jahrb. f. Kinderheilk., 1902, vol. lvi. 446.
Czerny and Keller. Des Kindes Ernährung, Ernährungsstörungen u. Ernährungstherapie, 1902, Abth. iii. u. iv.
Heubner. Zeitschr, f. Diätet. u. physik. Therap., 1901, vol. v. 13.
Schlossmann. Archiv f. Kinderheilk., 1902, vol xxxv. 339.

AN EXPERIMENTAL STUDY OF THE RELATION OF CELLS WITH EOSINOPHILE GRANULATION TO INFECTION WITH AN ANIMAL PARASITE (TRICHINA SPIRALIS).[1]

BY EUGENE L. OPIE, M.D.,

ASSOCIATE IN PATHOLOGY, JOHNS HOPKINS UNIVERSITY; FELLOW OF THE ROCKEFELLER INSTITUTE FOR MEDICAL RESEARCH.

THE present study has been undertaken in order to determine how the eosinophile leukocytes react when subjected to influenees which increase their number in the blood or elsewhere. The leukocytosis which follows infection with bacteria on the one hand has been carefully investigated. Leukocytosis caused by infection with a variety of parasites belonging to the animal kingdom, it is well known, is characterized by an increase of the eosinophile leukocytes; the conditions which influence this phenomenon, on the contrary, are incompletely understood.

[1] The present investigation has been conducted with the aid of a grant from the Rockefeller Institute for Medical Research.

Müller and Reider,[1] studying the blood of patients suffering with a variety of diseases, found in an individual infected with uncinaria duodenalis that the eosinophile leukocytes constituted 9.6 per cent. of the total number of leukocytes. In a similar case Zappert[2] noted a proportion of 17 per cent., and, at the same time, observed Charcot-Leyden crystals in the feces. Bucklers[3] directed his attention to a variety of parasitic infections and found a considerable increase of the eosinophile cells in association with uncinaria duodenalis, strongyloides intestinalis, and even with such relatively harmless forms as ascaris lumbricoides, tænia solium, and tænia saginata. In one case of uncinariasis or ankylostomiasis eosinophile cells formed 53.6 per cent. of the white corpuscles, while the total number of leukocytes was 20,600 in one cubic millimetre of blood; infection with ascaris lumbricoides caused eosinophilia of 10 per cent.; infection with both ascaris lumbricoides and oxyuris vermicularis 19.3 per cent. In a fatal case of infection with uncinaria duodenalis Strong[4] found the mucosa, the muscularis mucosæ, and the submucosa of the small intestine infiltrated with eosinophile cells. In a similar case described by Yates[5] the same local accumulation was noted, and in the basal part of the mucosa eosinophile cells were so numerous that seventy-five were counted in one field of the oil immersion lens (obj. 1-12th).

To the list of animal parasites causing eosinophilia may be added trichina spiralis (Brown[6]), filaria bancrofti (Calvert,[7] Gulland[8]), and bilharzia hæmatobia (Coles[9]). The studies of T. R. Brown and of others who have confirmed his observations have shown that eosinophilia is so constantly associated with trichinosis that its presence may serve as an important factor in the diagnosis of the disease. In the blood of a patient in whose muscles Brown subsequently demonstrated trichinæ eosinophile cells constituted, on admission to the Johns Hopkins Hospital, 37 per cent. of the total number of leukocytes. The proportion was somewhat diminished for a time, but subsequently rose and on the fiftieth day after admission reached 68.2 per cent. The total number of leukocytes varied during the greater part of the illness from 15,000 to 30,000 per cubic millimetre. In specimens of muscle removed at a period preceding the maximum eosinophilia extensive degenerative changes had resulted from the presence of embryonic trichinæ, and in the altered tissue eosinophile cells with polymorphous nuclei had accumulated in large numbers. Similar phenomena were exhibited by subsequent cases.

[1] Deutsches Arch. f. klin. Med., 1891, vol. xlviii. p. 96.
[2] Zeitsch. f. klin. Med., 1893, vol. xxiii. p. 227. [3] Münch. med. Woch., 1894, vol. xli. p. 23.
[4] Circulars on Tropical Diseases, No. 1, Chief Surgeon's Office, Manila, 1901.
[5] Bulletin of the Johns Hopkins Hospital, 1901, vol. xii. p. 366.
[6] Journal of Experimental Medicine, 1898, vol. iii. p. 315.
[7] Bulletin of the Johns Hopkins Hospital, 1902, vol. xiii. p. 133.
[8] British Medical Journal, 1902, vol. i. p. 831. [9] Ibid., p. 1137.

H. U. Williams and Bentz[1] have digested trichinous pork for forty-eight hours at 36° C., with artificial gastric juice containing pepsin and 0.2 per cent. of hydrochloric acid, and have introduced the dried residue into dogs, cats, and frogs. In a considerable proportion of these experiments eosinophile leukocytes in large numbers have collected about it. The phenomenon, as Williams and Bentz state, is probably due to some substance derived from the bodies of the worms, but the experiments, they think, do not entirely exclude the possibility that the result may be due to the action of hydrochloric acid and pepsin or to the agency of bacteria.

The foregoing has shown that a considerable number of diverse animal parasites cause an increase of the eosinophile cells in the general circulation and in several instances a local accumulation in the neighborhood of the parasite. It is not improbable that the parasite secretes some product which has a specific influence upon the eosinophile cells, causing their multiplication. Should it be possible to produce a similar condition experimentally, we would have a ready means of studying the somewhat obscure activities of these cells. It is, moreover, of considerable importance to determine if the eosinophile cells of man and of the lower mammals bear a similar relation to entozoan infection. Study of conditions under which the eosinophile leukocytes are increased in number offers the readiest means of determining their much disputed origin and seat of multiplication.

Calamida[2] has prepared from the tapeworms of the dog, tænia cucumerina and tænia coenurus, an extract which he claims exerts a chemotactic influence upon the eosinophile cells.

The parasites, previously washed in sterile salt solution, are rubbed with ground glass in a mortar and at the same time treated with salt solution. By means of a Berkefeld filter is obtained a filtrate which, concentrated by evaporation, produces death when injected into rabbits and guinea-pigs. This material is hæmolytic for the red blood corpuscles of the rabbit and of the guinea-pig and, injected into the circulation, rapidly causes fatty degeneration of the liver. If a capillary tube containing the fluid is placed in the subcutaneous tissue of the rabbit, at the end of twenty-four hours it will be found to contain leukocytes, of which the greater number are eosinophile cells. Injected into the circulation, Calamida states, leukocytosis results in six to eight hours, eosinophile cells being increased in greater degree than other forms.

METHODS. Hoping to obtain a substance by which the eosinophile leukocytes might be increased at will, I have employed an extract prepared by grinding in a mortar with sand and normal salt solution the body of tænia saginata, first washed with sterile salt solution. By passing the extract through a Pasteur filter a clear yellow fluid

[1] Transactions of the Association of American Physicians, 1903, vol. xviii. p. 152.
[2] Cent. f. Bakt. und Par., 1901, vol. xxx. p. 374.

is obtained. This filtrate injected into the subcutaneous tissue of guinea-pigs, as much as 10 c.c. being used, failed to produce a noteworthy increase of the eosinophile cells. In one instance their number rose from 1 per cent. to 5 per cent. on the fourth day; in another, from 1.3 per cent. to 5.8 per cent. on the fifth day. The results were somewhat inconstant and, fresh tæniæ being difficult to obtain, this method of increasing the eosinophile cells was discarded.

Since many lower mammals are readily infected with trichinæ, the observations of T. R. Brown upon human infection suggests the possibility of increasing the eosinophile leukocytes experimentally by this means. H. U. Williams and Bentz, however, found no noteworthy increase of the eosinophile cells in the blood of rats and cats artificially infected with trichinæ.

For the purpose of the experiments to follow, the guinea-pig has proved convenient. The methods of obtaining the blood and of counting the leukocytes have been described in a previous paper.[1] In any experimental study of the eosinophile cells in the guinea-pig variations in the normal proportion of these cells must obviously be taken into consideration. These variations have been described in the article just cited. A slight increase of eosinophile leukocytes might give uncertain evidence of the results of infection, yet when examinations, continued from day to day, show that their number exhibits characteristic changes, little opportunity for doubt remains. The charts to follow will show that trichinosis in these animals has an effect upon the eosinophile cells which is similar to that observed in man, even though the details of the process are not always the same.

It soon became evident that the severity of the infection exerts an important influence upon the reaction exhibited by the blood, and hence it has been essential to adopt some means by which this factor may be estimated. By the following method the number of trichinæ fed to a given animal is determined with approximate accuracy. A small piece of trichinous pork measuring hardly more than 4 cm. in length and half as much across the fibres is freed as far as possible from fat and fascia. The infected pork used in these experiments was obtained from the United States Bureau of Animal Industry through the courtesy of Dr. D. E. Salmon, to whom I desire to express my obligation. From various parts of the meat selected small masses are removed and adjusted to a weight of 0.05 gram. When this particle is teased in glycerin containing 5 per cent. of acetic acid and pressed between two glass slides the number of encapsulated trichinæ can be conveniently counted with low magnification. From an average of five such counts it is possible to determine how much meat contains a given number of trichinæ, and though the cysts are not evenly distributed, the following figures will show that an approxi-

[1] The American Journal of the Medical Sciences, February, 1904, p. 217.

mate estimate of their number can be made if a small piece of muscle is used:

Specimen of pork No. 1.	Number of trichinæ in 0.05 grm.	124
"	"	91
"	"	113
"	"	100
"	"	128
	Mean	111.2
Specimen of pork No. 2.	Number of trichinæ in 0.05 grm.	40
"	"	63
"	"	71
"	"	54
"	"	74
	Mean	60.4
Specimen of pork No. 3.	Number of trichinæ in 0.05 grm.	121
"	"	155
"	"	120
"	"	117
"	"	103
	Mean	123.2

Increase of Eosinophile Leukocytes with Mild Trichinosis. Pork containing 2000 to 3000 trichinæ fails to cause death or does so only after several weeks. A larger dose is usually fatal within a week or ten days. The milder infection, which will be first considered, is accompanied by characteristic changes in the number and distribution of the eosinophile cells. The reaction exhibited by the blood is best described by the following experiments, of which the results have been repeatedly confirmed by observations to be cited later.

Experiment 1. A guinea-pig weighing 481 grams received pork containing 2000 trichinæ. The proportion of eosinophile cells in the blood and the weight underwent the changes indicated below:

Day.	Eosinophile leukocytes.	Weight.	Day.	Eosinophile leukocytes.	Weight.
1st	1.3 per ct.	481 grm.	34th	5.0 per ct.	
9th	2.5 "	496 "	43d	4.0 "	
18th	7.5 "		49th	8.5 "	462 grm.
21st	15.5 "	477 "	51st	3.0	
25th	6 "		57th	1.8 "	429 "
32d	10.5 "	509 "	65th	1.3 "	430 "

The animal finally recovered and regained its former weight.

Experiment 2. A guinea-pig weighing 695 grams received 3000 trichinæ. The changes in the proportion of the eosinophile cells and their number in 1 c.mm. of blood are well shown by Chart I.

The record of the total number of leukocytes in 1 c.mm. of blood was as follows: First day, 13,900; ninth, 17,200; twelfth, 24,600; fifteenth, 25,300; eighteenth, 18,700; twenty-second, 25,900; twenty-sixth, 15,100. The proportion of eosinophile cells being known, their absolute number is readily estimated, and has been indicated in the chart.

During the first ten or twelve days after ingestion of trichinous meat there is no noteworthy alteration in the number of eosinophile cells; a gradual increase follows and reaches a maximum during the latter part of the third or the beginning of the fourth week. The number of eosinophile leukocytes may remain elevated several weeks, but should death ensue a more or less rapid decrease precedes the fatal termination. In one animal the blood contained 1.3 per cent. of eosinophile leukocytes at the onset of the experiment; in a second, 15.3 per cent., yet in the two experiments the number of eosinophile cells underwent similar changes.

CHART I.

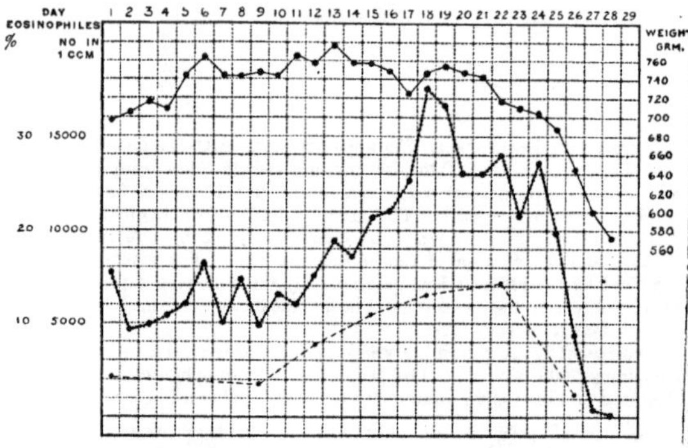

Showing changes in the number of eosinophile leukocytes and of polynuclear leukocytes with fine granulation after infection with 10,000 trichinæ. The percentage of eosinophile leukocytes is indicated by a dotted line; their number in 1 c.c. of blood by a broken line; the number of polynuclear leukocytes with fine granulation in 1 c.c. of blood by a broken and dotted line; the weight of the animal by a continuous black line.

According to the observations recorded by Leuckart[1] the encapsulated parasite in the muscle of the hog or other animal is set free by the action of the gastric juice within three or four hours after it is taken into the stomach and, passing to the small intestine, attains sexual maturity within from thirty to forty hours. Before the end of the second day copulation has taken place, and on the sixth or seventh day ripe embryos are first observed in the uterus of the female worm. At this time all of the female parasites have not

[1] Die menschlichen Parasiten, Leipzig und Heidelberg, 1876, vol. ii.

its maximum distention. On the ninth or tenth day after infection embryos have begun to reach the muscles. The foregoing experiments show that the eosinophile cells of the blood increase and reach a maximum at a time when embryonic trichinæ are passing in great numbers from the intestine to the muscles. The adult parasites in the intestine gradually diminish in number and have disappeared at the end of five or six weeks. In the guinea-pig the disease is apparently of shorter duration, for I have never found adult trichinæ in the small intestine after the fourth week of infection.

In Experiment 2, in which the total number of leukocytes have been repeatedly determined, leukocytosis has been found associated with increase in the proportion of eosinophile cells. When from the total number of leukocytes and the percentage of eosinophile leukocytes the number of the latter in 1 c.mm. of blood is estimated, the absolute and relative numbers are found to undergo corresponding changes: until the middle of the second week there is no increase, but subsequently the chart shows a gradual rise, which reaches a maximum on the twenty-second day. The maximum percentage of eosinophile leukocytes noted on the eighteenth day is apparently due to a diminution of the other leukocytes rather than to an actual increase of the eosinophile cells.

In the experiments to follow, guinea-pigs were infected with trichinæ in large number. Though death followed more rapidly than in the preceding experiments, the eosinophile cells exhibited changes similar to those already noted.

Experiment 3. A guinea-pig weighing 667 grams ingested pork containing 7500 trichinæ. Following is a record of the changes in weight and proportion of eosinophile leukocytes:

Day.	Eosinophile leukocytes.	Weight.	Day.	Eosinophile leukocytes.	Weight.
1st . . .	2.3 per ct.	667 grm.	11th . . .	4.5 per ct.	
2d . . .	6.5 "		12th . . .	2.0 "	610 grm.
3d . . .	8.8 "		13th . . .	2.5 "	604 "
4th . . .	3.0 "		14th . . .	....	
5th . . .	1.7 "	646 "	15th . . .	9.2 "	606 "
6th . . .	0.5 "		16th . . .	....	
7th . . .	0.8 "	601 "	17th . . .	12.0 "	
8th . . .	1.3 "	582 "	18th . . .	....	
9th . . .	0.3 "	576 "	19th . . .	7.7 "	473 "
10th . . .	0.5 "	585 "			

The animal died on the twentieth day after infection, and adult male and female trichinæ were present in immense number in the small intestine. Loosely coiled embryos were very numerous in the voluntary muscles.

Experiment 4. An animal weighing 718 grams received 10,000 trichinæ. The weight and percentage of eosinophile leukocytes are recorded in the accompanying chart. At the onset of the experiment the number of leukocytes per cubic millimetre was 10,800; on the ninth day the leukocytes numbered 10,200, but subsequently increased and were as follows: Fifteenth day, 21,300; seventeenth, 20,400; twenty-first, 20,800. Shortly before death, which occurred on the twenty-fifth day, the number of leukocytes was 17,400. From the figures just given, together with percentages determined by differential count, the number of eosinophile lenkocytes and of polymorphous leukocytes with fine granulation has been estimated.

By frequently repeated examination of the blood of his first patient infected with trichinæ, Brown demonstrated a remarkable relationship between the neutrophile and eosinophile leukocytes.

CHART II.

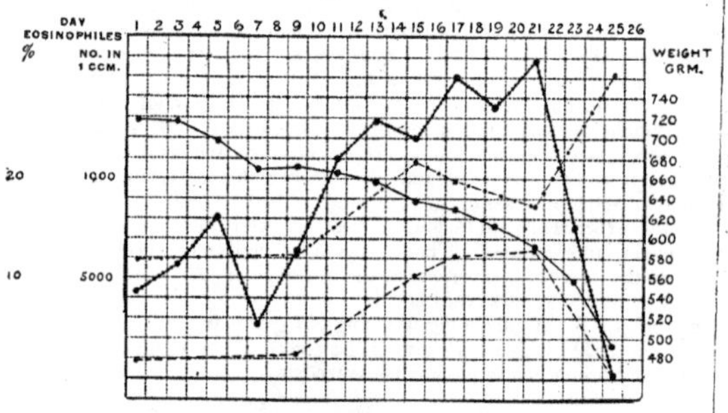

Showing changes in the number of eosinophile leukocytes and of polynuclear leukocytes with fine granulation after infection with 10,000 trichinæ. The percentage of eosinophile leukocytes is indicated by a dotted line; their number in 1 c.c. of blood by a broken line; the number of polynuclear leukocytes with fine granulation in 1 c.c. of blood by a broken and dotted line; the weight of the animal by a continuous black line.

Daily estimation of the number of these cells in one cubic millimetre of blood showed that when the eosinophile cells increased the neutrophile leukocytes exhibited a corresponding diminution in number, so that when the eosinophiles had reached a maximum percentage of 68.2 the number of neutrophiles in one cubic millimetre of blood was less than normal, even though there was at the time a marked leukocytosis.

In Experiment 4 the total number of leukocytes was markedly increased after the second week of infection with trichinæ.

In Chart II. both eosinophiles and finely granular polynuclear leukocytes undergo a parallel rise, but with further increase of the absolute number of eosinophile cells the finely granular leukocytes exhibit the inverse relation noted by Brown. With the terminal decrease of eosinophile cells there is a very great increase of finely granular forms. It will be subsequently shown that increase of the eosinophile leukocytes in the blood is often associated with such great multiplication of eosinophile cells in the bone-marrow that other cells are in part replaced. It is not improbable that this great accumulation of eosinophile cells retards the multiplication of polymorphous cells with fine granulation, so that their number in the blood diminishes. It is, then, unnecessary to assume that diminution of finely granular leukocytes, accompanying increase of eosinophile leukocytes, is due to transformation of the former into the latter.

DECREASE OF EOSINOPHILE LEUKOCYTES WITH SEVERE TRICHINOSIS. Charts I. and II. exhibit certain peculiarities which other experiments have shown are not accidental. With the less severe infection caused by 3000 trichinæ (Chart I.), the weight of the animal was maintained, indeed with a slight increase, during almost three weeks. The more severe effect of 10,000 trichinæ is shown by Chart II., where the weight of the animal gradually diminished from the onset of the infection. In this case the animal, which at first was large and healthy, survived twenty-five days, and the eosinophile cells, which rose more quickly than in the former experiment, reached approximately the same number. In other experiments, where trichinæ were administered in very large number, little resistance to the infection was shown, the weight of the animal diminished with great rapidity, and death followed within two weeks. The following experiments illustrate the condition:

Experiment 5. To a guinea-pig weighing 604 grams was fed pork containing 6500 trichinæ. The changes in weight and percentage of eosinophile cells were as follows:

Day.	Eosinophile leukocytes.	Weight.
1st	10.3 per ct.	604 grm.
5th	5.7 "	590 "
9th	6.3 "	490 "
12th	0.3 "	448 "

The animal died on the twelfth day after infection. In the small intestine adult trichinæ were present in great number.

Experiment 6. A guinea-pig weighing 609 grams received 10,000 trichinæ. The animal had been infected seven months before with 2000 trichinæ, but had completely recovered and had gained 100 grams in weight. Death occurred on the seventh day of the second infection.

Day.	Eosinophile leukocytes.	Weight.
1st	22.3 per ct.	609 grm.
5th	0	532 "
7th	0	483 "

The small intestine contained adult trichinæ in immense number, while in the muscles were encapsulated trichinæ in abundance.

Experiment 7. A guinea-pig weighing 607 grams received 20,000 trichinæ:

Day.	Eosinophile leukocytes.	Weight.
1st	7.7 per ct.	607 grm.
4th	0.3 "	547 "

Death occurred on the fourth day after infection, and adult trichinæ in great number were present in the small intestine.

In the experiments which precede those just described eosinophile cells of the blood have diminished with greater or less rapidity just before death. The weight of the animal doubtless gives the best indication of the effect of the infection upon its nutrition, and changes in weight can serve as an index of the power of resistance. The diminution in weight which precedes death is accompanied by a corresponding diminution in the number of eosinophile cells. This is well seen in Chart I., where the weight, after increasing during the first two weeks, subsequently falls, gradually at first, but later more rapidly. In Chart II., even though the weight gradually diminishes from the onset of infection, decrease of eosinophiles corresponds with a more sudden fall in weight. In Experiments 5, 6, and 7 the rapidity with which the resistance of the organism has been overcome is shown by the sudden fall in weight; the eosinophile cells rapidly diminish in number, and subsequent anatomical studies will demonstrate how injurious is the effect of the infectious agent upon these cells.

Local Accumulation of Eosinophile Cells. Several experimental studies have sought to determine the pathological changes produced in lower animals by trichina spiralis, and especial attention has been given to the muscle fibres invaded by the parasite. The purpose of the present investigation has been to study the relation of the leukocytes and notably of the eosinophile cells to the parasite or to poisons produced by it. Since the eosinophile cells are increased in the blood the attempt has been made to determine how they multiply, where they accumulate, and what alterations they undergo. The final object of such study is to determine, so far as possible, what part the eosinophiles play in resisting invasion of an animal parasite.

According to Leuckart, whose view has long been accepted by pathologists, the embryos of trichina spiralis set free by the female worm within the lumen of the intestine make their way by aid of their own activity through the intestinal wall into the peritoneal cavity, and hence, following the loose connective tissue, reach the various voluntary muscles. Leuckart had rarely, if indeed ever, seen embryos free within the intestinal lumen. Cerfontaine[1] and, later, Askanazy[2] have shown that the mature female worm penetrates the mucosa and there expels her young. Transmission by

[1] Arch. de biol., 1893, xiii., i., 125.

[2] Virchow's Arch., 1895, cxli., 42.

way of the lymphatic vessels through the mesenteric lymphatic glands and thoracic duct to the vascular system affords a simple explanation of the rapidity with which trichinæ are carried to the muscles throughout the body.

The observations of Askanazy are of especial interest. Many female trichinæ pierce the villi, and in part, or with their entire body, enter the central chyle vessel, within which free embryos can be found; female worms also penetrate the mucosa, where they usually enter a lymphatic vessel. A few parasites apparently fail to find a lymphatic vessel and deposit their young within the mucosa, whence not improbably they migrate by their own activity through the intestinal wall into the peritoneal cavity. Repeated observations have, however, shown that the embryonic trichinæ, an insignificant number excepted, enter the lymphatic vessels and are carried to the mesenteric lymph glands, where, in rabbits, according to Askanazy, embryos are readily found during the latter part of the second week after infection. From the lymph glands by way of the lymph stream, trichinæ enter the thoracic duct and hence are carried through the heart and lungs to the systemic circulation, thus reaching, ten to fourteen days after infection, the voluntary muscles, which alone afford a suitable site for further development. In the lungs of infected rabbits Askanazy has rarely failed to find small red areas where the bloodvessels are dilated and hemorrhage has occurred into the alveoli; at a later stage fibrin and some leukocytes are present. Within such areas he has repeatedly found embryonic trichinæ, which acting, he believes, as emboli, cause the lesion and afford further evidence in favor of a hæmal distribution of the parasite.

I have studied the relation of the eosinophile cells to the lesions of experimental trichinosis in a considerable number of animals, some dead as the result of infection, others killed at varying intervals after infection. In the four experiments to follow, a uniform dose of 2500 trichinæ was administered; the blood was examined at intervals of four days, and the animals were allowed to live periods varying from approximately one to four weeks. Subsequent observations made for the most part upon animals spontaneously dead after infection have shown that these experiments fairly represent the course of infection.

Experiment 8. The animal was killed on the ninth day after receiving 2500 trichinæ.

Day.	Eosinophile leukocytes.	Weight.
1st	5.7 per ct.	487 grm.
5th	11.7 "	482 "
9th	11.7 "	484 "

Experiment 9. The animal was killed on the fifteenth day after infection with 2500 trichinæ.

Day.	Eosinophile leukocytes.	Weight.	Day.	Eosinophile leukocytes.	Weight.
1st . . .	1.7 per ct.	336 grm.	13th . .	10.7 per ct.	432 grm.
5th . . .	4.3 "	396 "	15th . .	9.3 "	432 "
9th . . .	5.7 "	397 "			

Experiment 10. The animal was killed on the twenty-second day after infection with 2500 trichinæ.

Day.	Eosinophile leukocytes.	Weight.	Day.	Eosinophile leukocytes.	Weight.
1st . . .	5.7 per ct.	567 grm.	17th . .	15.3 per ct.	572 grm.
5th . . .	6.3 "	584 "	21st . .	19.7 "	570 "
9th . . .	2.0 "	566 "	22d . .	17.3 "	566 "
13th . . .	6.7 "	579 "			

Experiment 11. An animal which had received 2500 trichinæ was killed on the twenty-ninth day after infection.

Day.	Eosinophile leukocytes.	Weight.	Day.	Eosinophile leukocytes.	Weight.
1st . . .	6.7 per ct.	586 grm.	17th . .	15.7 per ct.	680 grm.
5th . . .	6.7 "	635 "	21st . .	18.8 "	690 "
9th . . .	4.3 "	630 "	25th . .	21.7 "	692 "
13th . . .	9.7 "	668 "	29th . .	17.7 "	674 "

In accord with the observations of Cerfontaine and Askanazy upon the hæmal dissemination of the parasite, increase of the eosinophile leukocytes, previously described, is associated with local accumulation in the mesenteric lymph glands and in the lung. No noteworthy increase of these cells in the intestinal mucosa was noted, though in no instance was I so fortunate as to obtain a section through a worm which had penetrated into the mucous membrane. During the third week (Experiments 3 and 9), at a stage when trichinæ are entering in large number the lymphatic vessels of the intestine, eosinophile cells accumulate in the lymphatic glands at the base of the mesentery, and may be collected in such numbers that they give the appearance of a small abscess in which ordinary polynuclear cells are replaced by eosinophile leukocytes. There is, however, no evidence of necrosis or of liquefaction of tissue in such a focus. The occasional presence of numerous epithelioid cells, commingled with eosinophiles in the centre of the lesion, gives evidence that proliferation of the fixed cells may occur. At a later stage eosinophile cells disappear from the gland, in part at least, and in one instance (Experiment 12), in an animal which died during the sixth week after infection, eosinophile cells had almost completely disappeared, but small nodules of newly formed tissue, containing many epithelioid cells, apparently represented the lesion which at an earlier stage had been found infiltrated with leukocytes.

In one instance (Experiment 3) there was inconclusive evidence that accumulation of eosinophile cells was caused by the presence of an embryo of trichinæ. In the centre of a focus, where proliferating cells of epithelioid type were commingled with eosinophile leukocytes, was a small amount of hyaline material. Indefinitely defined structure suggested the presence of a much altered parasite. In one instance an embryo was found within the mesenteric gland. but eosinophiles were not numerous about it

Only in the lung does one find accumulations of eosinophile cells approaching in extent those of the mesenteric lymphatic glands. Embryonic trichinæ, or toxic products associated with their presence, after leaving the lymphatic glands would first reach this organ. Askanazy has directed attention to small hemorrhagic foci in the lung of rabbits infected with trichinæ and has been able to demonstrate the parasite within the lesion. Similar ecchymoses occur in the lungs of infected guinea-pigs after the beginning of the fourth week. At times the interalveolar capillaries are much dilated and red blood corpuscles have escaped into the alveoli. In one instance (Experiment 4) fibrin was also present and leukocytes, with eosinophile granulations, had accumulated in the periphery of the focus. In Experiments 10 and 11 the lungs contained small nodules of consolidated tissue in which eosinophile cells were massed in immense numbers. The alveolar walls were thickened and the alveoli were either filled by large desquamated epithelial cells or replaced by fibrous tissue. In the centre of the nodule eosinophile cells were so closely packed together that in sections stained with eosin the tissue had an almost homogeneously red color. In the walls of the adjacent alveoli eosinophile cells were scattered in countless number. In none of these lesions have I found trichinæ.

During the third week after infection trichinæ are readily found in the voluntary muscles. The changes that follow their penetration into the muscle fibres have been carefully described in recent years by Ehrhardt[1] and others. Degeneration of the fibre is associated with proliferation of its nuclei. At no stage of the disease have I found eosinophile cells even in small number in the neighborhood of the degenerate fibres. In this respect trichinosis of guinea-pigs differs from that of the human subject.

Multiplication of Eosinophile Cells. Examination of the blood has shown that the eosinophile leukocytes, which begin to increase during the second week of trichinosis, reach a maximum during the latter part of the third week. These cells, which do not differ from those ordinarily present in the blood, are a little larger than the finely granular leukocytes and possess polymorphous nuclei. The eosinophile cells which accumulate in the lymphatic glands of the mesentery and in the lungs are identical in structure. Their nuclei are polymorphous and never give evidence of mitotic division. In the bone-marrow, however, eosinophile cells can be shown to proliferate actively.

During the first two weeks after infection the number of eosinophile cells in the bone-marrow is not notably altered, but at a later

[1] Ziegler's Beiträge, 1896, xx., 1, 43.

period the cellular elements are increased at the expense of the fat and the number both of eosinophile myelocytes and of forms with polymorphous nuclei is very greatly increased, while mitotic division is encountered much more frequently than in the normal marrow.

In a preceding article I have shown that the proportion of eosinophile leukocytes in the blood of apparently healthy guinea-pigs is subject to great variation, the percentage count ranging from less than one to more than thirty. Corresponding to this varying proportion of eosinophile cells the bone-marrow exhibits noteworthy peculiarities. In animals of which the blood contains approximately 1 per cent. of eosinophiles fat is abundant and the cells of the marrow occupy the space between the fat cells. Cells with eosinophile granulation are fairly numerous and are in part myelocytes with eosinophile granulation, large cells with large, round, oval, or slightly irregular nuclei; in part smaller cells with polymorphous nuclei, resembling the eosinophile leukocytes of the circulating blood. In animals containing a higher proportion of eosinophile leukocytes, for example, 5 or 10 per cent., fat is somewhat less abundant and eosinophile cells form a much greater proportion of the marrow cells. Where, however, eosinophile leukocytes form from 15 to 30 per cent. of the white blood corpuscles the bone-marrow presents a characteristic appearance. Fat is largely replaced by myeloid cells, of which those with eosinophile granulation form a large proportion. Particularly numerous are myelocytes with eosinophile granulation. Similar cells in process of mitotic division, though never very abundant, are more numerous than is usual.

A brief description of the bone-marrow from Experiments 8 to 11, in which animals were killed at the end of one, two, three, and four weeks after infection with trichinæ, will show that the eosinophilia of trichinosis is accompanied by changes in the marrow similar to those just described. In none of these experiments did the proportion of eosinophile leukocytes equal 10 per cent. at the time when infection occurred. At the end of the first and of the second week after infection eosinophile cells are present in moderate number and mitotic figures are found only after continued search At the end of the third week (Experiment 10), when, as has been shown, the eosinophile leukocytes of the blood attain a maximum, the fat of the marrow is largely replaced and eosinophile cells are present in very great number. Eosinophile myelocytes are particularly numerous, and dividing forms are abundant. Mitotic figures are readily recognized by the hyperchromatic condition of the nuclei. The diaster stage of division is not infrequently encountered, while at times complete division of the cell body has occurred. At the end of the fourth week (Experiment 11) the appearance of the marrow is similar to that just described, but mitotic division is somewhat less frequent in the sections. When an animal dies during the fourth week of infection the bone-marrow resembles that of animals killed at the height of eosinophile leukocytosis, even though the number of eosinophile leukocytes has diminished shortly before death. This fact is well illustrated by the bone-marrow from Experiments 2 and 4, where death has occurred on the twenty-eighth and twenty-fifth day after infection. Fat is largely replaced and eosinophile cells are present in very great number; eosinophile cells with polymorphous nucleus are, however, much more numerous than myelocytes, and only in the marrow from Experiment 4 has one mitotic figure been found.

The changes observed in the bone-marrow of guinea-pigs in which the eosinophile cells of the blood have been increased by trichinosis are comparable to those which have been found associated with the ordinary form of leukocytosis, in which the polymorphonuclear leukocytes with fine granulation (neutrophile in man, amphophile in rabbit) are increased. Ribbert[1] first showed that the injection of micro-organisms causes an increase of the finely granular myelocytes and a diminution of fat in the bone-marrow. Roger and Josué[2] studied the changes in the marrow accompanying suppuration and noted that an increase of the finely granular myelocytes, together with a diminution of fat, is caused by the injection of various toxic and infectious agents. Muir[3] has studied the changes in the bone-marrow consequent upon the repeated injection of staphylococcus pyogenes aureus into rabbits. Cellular elements increase at the expense of fat, and finely granular myelocytes, which divide by mitosis, are present in greatly increased number. Both Muir and Roger and Josué distinguished two types of cellular proliferation in the bone-marrow. When, as the result of hemorrhage or of abnormal destruction of red blood corpuscles, the nucleated red corpuscles proliferate by mitosis, the marrow assumes an appearance which is distinguishable from that associated with prolonged leukocytosis; an erythroblastic type can be distinguished from a leukoblastic type of marrow.

The experimental study of trichinosis has shown that the eosinophile leukocytosis of this disease is associated with changes in the bone-marrow which are analogous to those accompanying the more common leukocytosis caused by bacterial infection and by other means. The eosinophile leukocytes of the blood are derived by mitotic division from eosinophile myelocytes, which are analogous to the finely granular myelocytes. With continued proliferation of these cells their number in the bone-marrow so increases that, replacing the fat, they give a characteristic appearance to the tissue. A coarsely granular or eosinophile variety of the leukoblastic type

[1] Virchow's Arch., 1897, cl., 391.
[2] Compt.-rend. Soc. de biol., 1896, p. 1038; and 1897, p. 322.
[3] Journal of Pathology and Bacteriology, 1901, vol. vii. p. 161.

of marrow is then distinguishable from the more common finely granular variety.

DEGENERATIVE CHANGES IN EOSINOPHILE CELLS WITH SEVERE TRICHINOSIS. Infection with trichinæ in such number that the animal survives or dies only after several weeks causes active multiplication of the eosinophile cells. Infection with a very large number of trichinæ, fatal within one or two weeks, is followed by rapid diminution of the number of these cells in the blood, and study of the internal organs from guinea-pigs used for Experiments 5, 6, and 7 have shown that the eosinophile cells under such conditions undergo degenerative changes which further indicate that the toxic products of the parasite exert a specific action on them. The organs obtained from animals used in the two following experiments, in which trichinæ in great number were administered, have been studied in order to confirm these observations.

Experiment 13. A guinea-pig weighing 648 grams was fed with pork containing 5300 trichinæ and died on the eighth day after infection. Adult trichinæ were found in immense number in the small intestine.

Experiment 14. A guinea-pig weighing 679 grams received 7500 trichinæ. Two months before, the animal had been infected with 2000 trichinæ and had completely recovered, the weight increasing almost 150 grams. Following the second infection the weight rapidly decreased and death occurred on the ninth day.

Day.	Eosinophile leukocytes.	Weight.
1st	0.7 per ct.	679 grm.
5th	0.7 "	623 "
9th	....	523 "

Of much interest are the changes in the bone-marrow caused by rapidly fatal trichinosis. Here the number of eosinophile cells undergoes no noteworthy alteration, and both myelocytes and forms with polymorphous nuclei are present in moderate number. The nuclei of the myelocytes exhibit greater irregularity of outline than is usual, so that they not infrequently assume an irregularly lobed form, the size of the cell distinguishing it as a myelocyte. Mitotic figures are occasionally seen. The nuclei of the smaller eosinophile cells frequently stain deeply, are very irregular in outline and often have a shrivelled appearance. Particularly noteworthy is the presence of eosinophile cells in which the nuclei have undergone fragmentation. The number of such cells is variable, and those affected appear to be both myelocytes and polymorphonuclear forms. Throughout such a cell are scattered spherical globules of chromatin, varying in size and staining deeply and homogeneously. The body of the cell appears to be unchanged, and the eosinophile granules take their usual brilliant stain.

Eosinophile cells, with similarly shattered nuclei, have been found in other organs. In Experiments 5 and 13 many eosinophile cells in the mucosa of the small intestine had undergone nuclear fragmentation, and the same process was observed in the mesenteric lymph glands. In one instance (Experiment 5) eosinophile cells were numerous in the mesenteric lymph gland, and at one point had accumulated to form an abscess-like focus similar to those already described; here nuclear fragmentation was particularly frequent.

CONCLUSIONS.—The administration of trichina spiralis to the guinea-pig causes an increase of the eosinophile leukocytes in the blood, comparable to that which accompanies human infection. There is no constant alteration of the number of these cells until the end of the second week after infection, when their relative and absolute number rapidly increases and reaches a maximum at the end of the third week. At this time embryonic trichinæ are in process of transmission from the intestinal mucosa by way of the lymphatic vessels and the blood through the lungs to the muscular system.

Eosinophile cells accumulate in the mesenteric lymphatic glands and in the lungs and form foci which resemble small abscesses in which polynuclear leukocytes are replaced by eosinophile cells. These cells are provided with polymorphous nuclei and do not differ from the eosinophile leukocytes of the circulating blood. Accumulation of eosinophile cells in the mesenteric lymphatic glands and in the lungs is explained by the transmisson of the embryonic parasite through these organs.

Increase of eosinophile cells in the blood and in other organs is accompanied by characteristic changes in the bone-marrow. The fat is diminished in amount, and cellular elements replace it. Cells with eosinophile granulation are present in immense number, and particularly numerous are the eosinophile myelocytes, cells peculiar to the bone-marrow, while such cells, undergoing mitotic division, are more numerous than usual. The bone-marrow is the seat of multiplication of the eosinophile leukocytes.

The number of eosinophile leukocytes in the blood always diminishes before death, so that the proportion usually becomes less than 1 per cent.

Infection with a very large number of trichinæ causes a rapid diminution of the number of eosinophile leukocytes and is quickly fatal. The eosinophile cells of the bone-marrow exhibit degenerative changes, of which nuclear fragmentation is most characteristic. Similar changes may affect the eosinophile cells of the intestinal mucosa and of the mesenteric lymph glands. Mild infection stimulates the eosinophile cells to active multiplication, but severe infection causes their destruction.

A BRAIN TUMOR INVOLVING THE SUPERIOR PARIETAL CONVOLUTION; TWO OPERATIONS FOR ITS REMOVAL; PARTIAL SUCCESS, WITH SOME RELIEF OF SYMPTOMS; DEATH TWO YEARS LATER; AUTOPSY.[1]

By Theodore Diller, M.D.,
(of Pittsburg)
NEUROLOGIST TO THE ALLEGHENY GENERAL HOSPITAL; PHYSICIAN TO THE INSANE DEPARTMENT OF ST. FRANCIS' HOSPITAL.

Clinical Summary. *Man of good habits, aged fifty-six years; neurasthenic symptoms for one year; then during four years frequent attacks of Jacksonian epilepsy, initial convulsive movements beginning in the left great toe; general symptoms of brain tumor appear only after these attacks had been present for two years; two operations; tumor only partly removed because of hemorrhage; partial relief; death five years after onset and two years after the operation. Autopsy: A large spindle-celled sarcoma in the right superior parietal convolutions and adjacent mesial convolutions.*—J. H., a man, aged fifty-six years, a druggist, had always enjoyed good health until the spring of 1898. His family and personal history were negative; he denied specific disease. No history of traumatism.

In the spring of 1898 he felt tired and often complained of weariness. Slumber refreshed him much less than formerly, being often disturbed by dreams. He often sung in his sleep. The patient frequently remarked that he "could not keep up with the procession." These neurasthenic symptoms continued until February, 1899 (*i. e.*, about one year), when, without the slightest warning, he was seized with an attack as follows:

His left great toe felt as though in a "cramp." This sensation continued for five minutes, when he sat down. By this time the foot began to twitch. This also continued five minutes. Then convulsive movements began to ascend the body, involving, in the order named, the muscles of the left side of the trunk, the neck, causing here a sense of choking, and, finally, the muscles of the chest and neck, especially those of the right side, the head moving forward and backward, striking with force against the floor. These convulsive movements were maintained without intermission from 1.30 to 5 P.M., when they ceased for a time. Soon there was a resumption of the movements in the left trunk, which, with intermissions, were kept up until 2 A.M. the next day. He was conscious throughout the attack, at times engaging in conversation. The arm and face were at no time involved in convulsive movements. During the

[1] A paper read before the Allegheny County (Pa.) Medical Society, November 17, 1903.

attack he experienced a peculiar sensation in the left leg "like electricity going through it."

Following this seizure, moderate but distinct loss of power in the left arm and leg were noted by the patient. He stayed in bed more or less for a period of three weeks, when he felt as well as ever, except for a certain loss of control of the left arm and some "clumsiness" of the left leg. Four weeks after this attack he was in better health than at any subsequent period.

Five weeks after the attack just described a second occurred; and this was followed by a third, fourth, and fifth seizure, the intervals between them being from ten to fifteen days. These attacks lasted from ten to twenty minutes each, and always began by twitchings in the left great toe, which marched up the leg, thigh, and trunk, as in the first attack. In no seizure was the face or arm involved in convulsive movements; but the latter felt numb and weak during the attack.

Now several attacks occurred in which the entire left leg was at once involved in convulsive movements. In a few attacks the muscles of the calf or thigh seemed to be first involved

Since the first dozen attacks they have occurred at irregular intervals of from ten days to six weeks up to the time of the operation. The great majority of all these seizures began by convulsive movements in the left great toe; although others occurred in which the muscles of the entire left leg were apparently simultaneously involved.

Usually (not always) the patient could predict an attack from a few minutes to twenty-four hours in advance by a peculiar sensation in the leg. After each attack the left arm and leg were weak for a time; but usually recovered within the ensuing five or six days. Convulsive movements ceased in all muscles simultaneously.

His consciousness was entirely preserved throughout all the seizures. The left arm and face were never involved in the convulsive movements. The eyes never turned to one or the other side during a seizure.

The patient had never had headache, vomiting, vertigo, loss of vision, diplopia, or disturbance of hearing.

The last attack before the operation occurred in the latter part of April, 1901, and about twenty-six months after the initial seizure.

He went to bed complaining of a great sense of weariness and fell into an unusually heavy sleep. The next day he complained of severe headache located in the occiput. The next night he was taken with a severe seizure of the usual type while on the street. For thirty-six hours following he was dull, stupid, restless, delirious. The second evening after this attack, when he was examined by Drs. Montgomery, Stieren, and myself, he was still somewhat dull and clouded mentally; but when aroused he recognized members of his family and conversed a little. Palsy of the right third nerve was apparent, as evidenced by a dilated pupil, external squint, and ptosis in the right eye. Dr. Stieren discovered optic neuritis of the right eye and an appearance suggestive of this condition in the left eye.

Close questioning of members of the family developed the fact that the patient was believed to have undergone moderate but progressive mental deterioration since the first convulsion, as evidenced chiefly by a growing lack of interest in affairs, dulling of perception, a lessened sense of responsibility, and a considerable loss of self-reliance. It also developed that the patient had suffered a progressive loss of power in the left arm and leg, aside from the temporary losses following the seizures.

Examination, May 16, 1901. There is in the median line of the skull posteriorly, about four or five inches anterior to the inion, two inches posterior to the Rolando fissure, a bony protuberance, which his wife believes has grown during the last few years.

The mental condition is one of mild, moderate dementia. Memory is fairly good. He is somewhat careless in his habits. His interest in affairs has diminished. He does not read, go to church, etc., as formerly.

Muscular Sense and Stereognostic Appreciation. He recognizes objects placed within either hand readily. Stereognostic appreciation by his feet seems equal. Fingers of left hand, placed in various positions, are not correctly reproduced in right hand.

Special Senses. Hearing and eyesight normal. Taste normal.

Eyes. No apparent extraocular palsy. He moves his eyes in all directions readily. Pupils equal; they react moderately but promptly to light and also to accommodation.

Sensation. Temperature sense, normal; tactile, normal; pain, normal.

Motion. Grasp of left arm distinctly less than that of the right, probably about one-third less. There is about the same degree of loss of power in the left leg.

Reflexes. Knee-jerks: right is normal; left is greatly increased. Ankle clonus absent on both sides. Plantar reflexes on both sides are very active. Babinski sign absent on both sides. Cremaster reflex present on both sides. Abdominal reflex absent on both sides. Biceps-jerk: absent on right side; present on left side. Triceps-jerk: left, absent; right, absent also. Scapular reflex not obtainable.

Percussion. No difference in percussion note over the skull. More pain is produced over the protuberance on the skull previously mentioned than elsewhere.

Viscera. Heart, lungs, and liver normal. Pulse 100.

Diagnosis. A tumor of unknown character in the superior Rolandic region of the right side involving the leg centre.

Operation, May 20, 1901, by Dr. R. W. Stewart, at the Mercy Hospital.

It was proposed to make an opening, the centre of which should be over the right superior parietal convolution, just behind the Rolandic fissure and as near to the median line as possible; but when the flap of scalp was turned back, the long protuberance already referred to became very striking; and here the bone was found to be very thin, soft, and evidently diseased; so it was hastily concluded to make the opening at this point—*i. e.*, about one inch directly posterior to the point at first intended. This bony protuberance proved to be soft, spongy, thin, eroded skull, very dark in color, which was readily removed. The healthy dura beneath was incised when a tumorous mass was readily made out. But with beginning attempts to remove it the patient fell into a condition of collapse, due largely or wholly probably to a continuous and persistent oozing hemorrhage from the seat of the operation. The wound was, therefore, packed, and the operation hastily concluded. The patient recovered fairly well and seemed to be in good condition on the next day. A microscopic section of a portion of the tumor removed proved to be a spindle-celled sarcoma (Dr. Singley).

A second operation was undertaken by Dr. Stewart six days later, Drs. McKennan, Werder, Buchanan, Mayer, and others being present. As soon as the packing was removed a steady and persistent hemorrhage at once began, which repeated packings failed to control. An enlargement of the opening in the skull failed to reveal cerebral convolutions at any point. Dr. Stewart was, however, able to get his finger between the tumor and the brain structure and thought the growth extended in a forward direction. After the removal of a number of small pieces of the tumorous mass, the operation was again hastily terminated, since the patient was again going rapidly into a condition of collapse. He made an uneventful recovery from the second operation.

I examined the patient on July 25, 1901, when I found the wound well healed. He expressed himself as feeling brighter and happier than for several months past. He had resumed smoking, a habit he had given up some months before the operation because of a lack of desire for tobacco. Members of his family, too, regarded his mental condition as much improved. In the two months since the operation he had had two convulsive seizures of the usual type.

The patient lived a little longer than two years after this examination; but during this time he was not again examined by me. His family report, however, that for the most part he was fairly comfortable; that the convulsive seizures occurred with somewhat less frequency and severity than during the two years preceding the operation; that he was troubled with headache but seldom; and that he never vomited; that his eyesight seemed good; that he was hopeful, cheerful, and on the whole happy; that, although much improved mentally, a certain psychic reduction was noticeable; and that a certain degree of weakness of the left arm and leg was observable (more at some times than at others). In short, both the patient and his family felt that he had been much benefited by the operation.

Last January he developed an attack of pneumonia, and following convalescence from this illness considerable increase of his mental reduction was noticed; and from this time on loss of power in his right arm and leg, especially the latter, steadily increased and became very marked. However, only a few days before his death he walked about the neighborhood with the aid of a cane and visited some friends. With the aid of his glasses he was still able to read a newspaper. Although he seldom complained of headache, he often spoke of a fulness about the head.

Fig. 1.

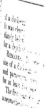

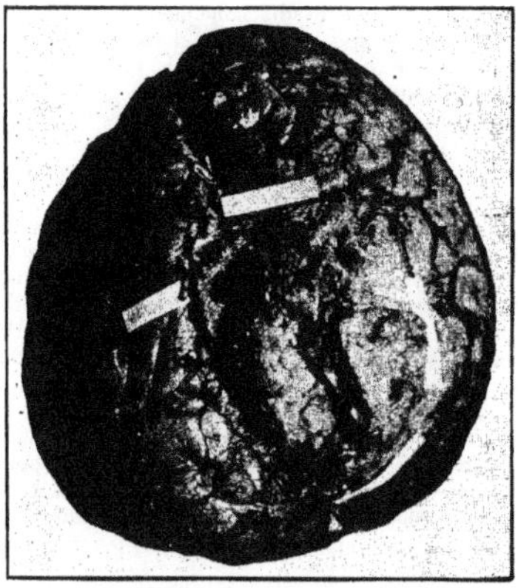

On July 31, 1903, he was seized with two general convulsions. Following the second attack coma developed, and death occurred on August 2d.

An *autopsy* was performed by Drs. Daggett, Litchfield, and myself sixteen hours after death. The scalp over the opening in the skull was found much depressed and united by thin cicatricial bands to the underlying structure, and these in turn to the tumor mass. Part of the tumor adhered to the skull-cap upon its removal.

The tumor was found to extend from the upper extremity of the Rolandic fissure to the parieto-occipital fissure, posteriorly. On the convexity of the brain it extended downward to the upper portion of the inferior parietal convolution. On the mesial aspect of the brain it extended down to the upper third of the gyrus fornicatus. It bulged beyond the median line, producing a large concavity on the mesial aspect of the opposite lobe, at one point, over the paracentral convolution, giving off two tit-like projections, which produced deep indentures in the corresponding convolutions of the left side. The tumor, therefore, involved the superior parietal, the paracentral, and quadrate convolutions chiefly and the inferior parietal convolution and the gyrus fornicatus also partially. No other tumor was discovered.

The tumor was dense in structure and easily palpable in the fresh specimen from the surrounding cerebral tissue, and about the size

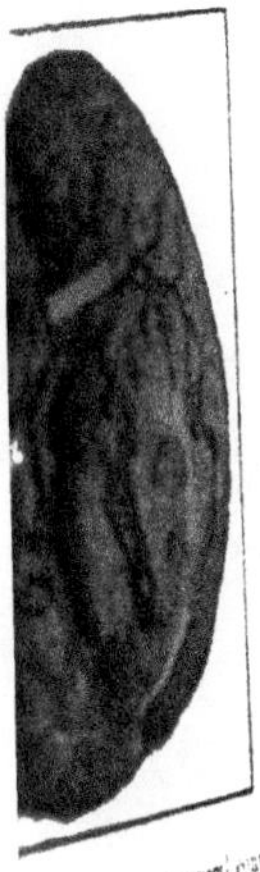

FIG. 2.

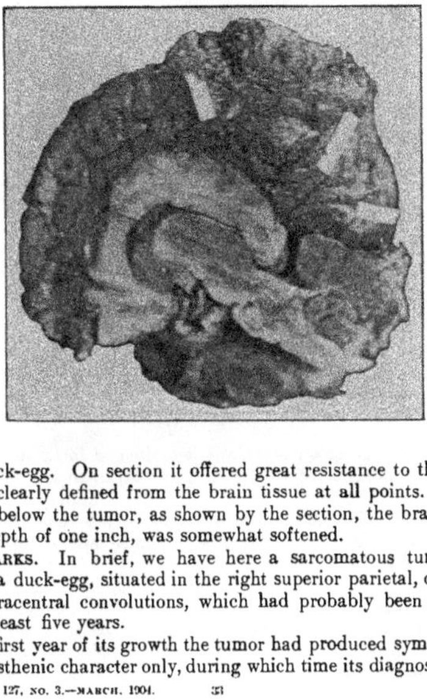

of a duck-egg. On section it offered great resistance to the knife. It was clearly defined from the brain tissue at all points. Immediately below the tumor, as shown by the section, the brain mass, for a depth of one inch, was somewhat softened.

Remarks. In brief, we have here a sarcomatous tumor, the size of a duck-egg, situated in the right superior parietal, quadrate and paracentral convolutions, which had probably been growing for at least five years.

The first year of its growth the tumor had produced symptoms of a neurasthenic character only, during which time its diagnosis would have been impossible. Fourteen months later Jacksonian epileptic attacks, with the signal symptom in the left great toe, began, and were maintained at intervals until death. Only three years later, or two years after the first of these attacks, did any other symptoms of the growth manifest themselves, the patient during this time being free from optic neuritis, headache, vomiting, vertigo, and cranial nerve palsies, the common symptoms of brain tumor; and so during this period a positive diagnosis of the growth was impossible. Nevertheless, even during this period the tumor had been strongly suspected. I saw the patient for the first time on November 14, 1899, with Dr. Litchfield, at that time the attending physician (*i. e.*, about nine months after the initial seizure). Dr. Litchfield had already reached the conclusion that the attacks of Jacksonian

FIG. 3.

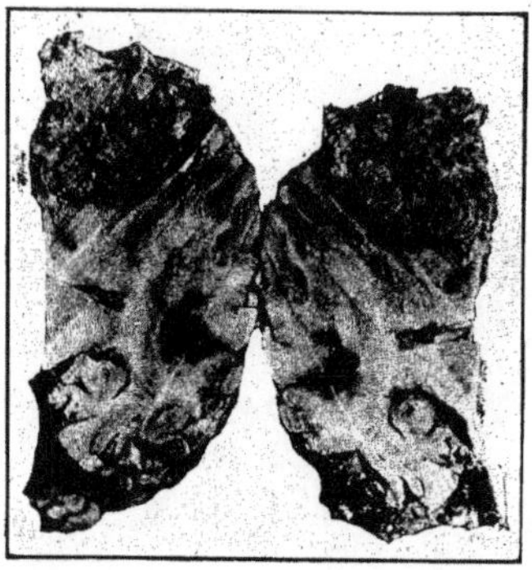

epilepsy were due to an organic lesion, situated in the motor cortical region for the left great toe, and had urged an operation, with a view of exploring this region, having proven antisyphilitic treatment useless. I concurred in this view. Had Dr. Litchfield's advice been acted upon at this time or shortly afterward, it seems to me not unlikely, if not, indeed, probable, that the growth would have been successfully removed, since we must suppose it was then much smaller than it was at the time of the operation, eighteen months later, and since the point at which it was then proposed to trephine would have discovered the growth. Indeed, nearly all the favorable features for a successful operation were then present, viz.,

FIG. 4.

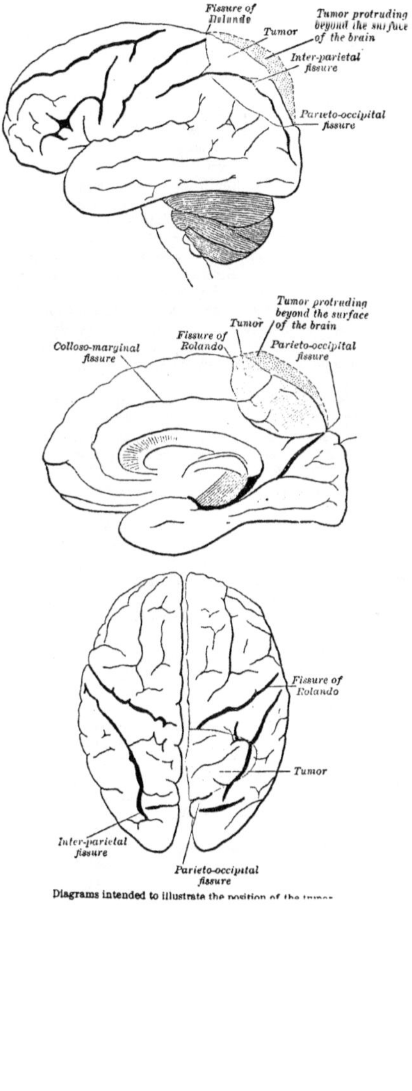

Diagrams intended to illustrate the position of the tumor

a single hard, circumscribed sarcoma, moderate in size, non-infiltrating and situated in one of the most accessible areas for surgical intervention, and in an area which permitted the maximum of certainty in localization by the clinician.

These same favorable features were present at the time the operation was undertaken, eighteen months later, except that the tumor was then doubtless larger. But, on the other hand, with the appearance of headache, optic neuritis, and stupor the probability that the organic lesion was a tumor had grown to a practical certainty.

Even as it was, one cannot escape a feeling of disappointment that the growth was not entirely removed at the operations, since even then it was still an unusually favorable one for surgical intervention. But I will say no more of the surgical aspect of the case, since Dr. Stewart has kindly consented to offer some discussion of this phase of the subject; his remarks are appended to this paper.

Although the character of the tumor was not diagnosed, yet consideration of two features pointed to sarcoma, viz., the slow growth of the tumor and the fact that sarcoma occurs more frequently than any other brain tumor in adults.[1] In a negative way the absence of carcinoma or tubercle in other parts of the body also lent support to this view.

As to the light this case sheds on cerebral localization, not a great deal can be said, because of the considerable size of the tumor, and since its exact starting-point cannot be known. In general, however, it conforms to the commonly accepted view that the cortical motor representation for the left great toe is situated in the opposite superior parietal convolution. It argues against the location of stereognostic appreciation taking place in this convolution. It also argues against the views of those who would place the motor cortical representation for the great toe in the superior precentral convolution—*i. e.*, anterior to the Rolandic fissure; and, on the contrary, it affords support to the views of those who localize this function in the superior parietal convolution, well back of the Rolandic fissure. It will be remembered that the tumor extended anteriorly only to the Rolandic fissure.

If we may judge by the bony protuberance on the skull, the growth began midway between the Rolandic and parieto-occipital fissure, next to the longitudinal fissure.

A noteworthy feature of the case was the absence of some and the late appearance and temporary character of other of the general symptoms of brain tumor. Headache was severe once only, in the attack just before the operation. Vomiting and vertigo were never symptoms. The optic neuritis probably subsided, since no appreciable defect of vision was present at any time after it was discovered. The third nerve palsy was, I believe, correctly interpreted

[1] Starr. Organic Nervous Diseases, p. 585.

at the time as a "distant symptom," and not due to direct involvement of this nerve or its nucleus.

One more point seems worthy of comment, viz., protrusion and erosion of the bone over the growth. The question arises in my mind, Was this due to the hard and unyielding character of the neoplasm which, by pressure, had shut off the blood supply to the superimposed cranial bone? It would seem so.

I am indebted to Dr. Litchfield for his notes on the earlier history of this case; to Dr. A. Lévété for the excellent photographs which illustrate this paper; and to Dr. R. W. Stewart for consenting to offer some discussion of the surgical aspects of the case. To each of these gentlemen I desire to express my thanks.

Remarks by R. W. Stewart, M.D.

The improvement, both in the mental and physical condition of this patient which followed partial removal of the tumor, makes it all the more regrettable that the whole growth was not enucleated. Had this been done, it is quite probable that there would have been a permanent recovery, as these growths are, as a rule, only semi-malignant in character and with but little tendency to infiltration.

The difficulty which I experienced with this case was the alarming hemorrhage following the attempt at removal of the growth, which apparently had opened the longitudinal sinus. The hemorrhage was so severe that the patient immediately went into collapse, and a fatal issue was only prevented by packing the cerebral cavity and the resort to hypodermic stimulation.

After the lapse of a week I was in hopes that the packing could be safely removed and the operation completed; but the attempt to do so was followed by exactly the same experience as in the former trial, and only a small portion of the tumor was removed at this time.

As the microscopic examination showed the tumor to be a sarcoma, and as no definite idea was obtained as to the limits of the growth, no further attempt was made to remove it.

The light shed on the case by the post-mortem evidence showed that the tumor was not inoperable, and I feel that I erred in two things. First, in not doing the operation in two steps as follows: First: removal of the skull over an area sufficiently extensive to expose the dura over the entire underlying tumor. The flap is then stitched back in position, and in the course of a week the second operation should be undertaken.

This consists in reopening the wound, incision of the dura over the entire extent of the tumor, and the control of all hemorrhages as the operation progresses. In this case it would probably have been necessary to ligate the longitudinal sinus at each side of the tumor. The tumor is then dissected out very much in the manner in which it is done in the post-mortem room, hemorrhage being controlled by ligation of the vessels as the operation progresses.

The chief advantage in doing the operation in two steps is that it minimizes the shock, which is the greatest danger confronting the patient. Had this been done and a sufficiently extensive area of the skull removed, it is probable that there would have been no opportunity for post-mortem findings in this case.

CONGENITAL CYSTS OF THE FOURTH VENTRICLE.[1]

A REPORT OF TWO CASES ASSOCIATED WITH TUMOR OF THE OPTIC THALAMUS AND CRUS CEREBRI.

By J. Ramsay Hunt, M.D.,
(OF NEW YORK)
ASSISTANT INSTRUCTOR IN NERVOUS DISEASES IN THE CORNELL UNIVERSITY MEDICAL COLLEGE, NEW YORK; NEUROLOGIST TO THE CITY HOSPITAL; ASSISTANT PHYSICIAN TO THE MONTEFIORE HOME.

(From the Pathological Laboratory of the Cornell University Medical College.)

Introduction. The pathological conditions resulting in the formation of cysts within the fourth ventricle or a cystic dilatation of the ventricle are as follows:

1. Parasitic: Cysticercus or echinococcus cysts.
2. Cystic degeneration of a tumor.
3. Cystic degeneration of the choroid plexus.
4. Cystic dilatation of the fourth ventricle from occlusion of its communications.
5. Congenital cysts.

These are of pathological rather than clinical importance because of their rarity and the atypical character of the symptoms produced.

Both cases forming the subject of the present study are examples of brain tumor in young subjects with *congenital* cysts of the brain stem projecting into the fourth ventricle.

In both the intimate structural relation of cyst and tumor was demonstrable.

Summary.

Case I.—A boy, aged seven years, previously healthy, developed symptoms of brain tumor referable to the left optic thalamus. The important objective symptoms were: hemiparesis and hemiataxia of the right arm and leg; paralysis of the emotional innervation of the right side of the face; paresis of the left external rectus; nystagmus; hearing impaired on the right, both to aerial and bone conduction; no hemianopsia; no objective sensory disturbances.

Autopsy. Large tumor (mixed-cell sarcoma) situated in the left

[1] Read in abstract at a meeting of the New York Neurological Society, January 5, 1904.

optic thalamus, infiltrating the subjacent structures and appearing on the basilar surface of the pons.

The fourth ventricle is dilated by a large cyst, which is firmly attached to the floor, penetrates the substance of the pons Varolii, terminating in the midst of the neoplasm. Serial sections show the presence of glia and nerve fibres in all parts of the cyst wall continuous with the nerve structures of the pons.[1]

History. A boy, aged seven and a half years, previous history negative, was admitted to the Montefiore Home September 12, 1896. Complains of headaches, vomiting, defective vision, uncertainty of gait, and an awkwardness of the right side; mentally clear, but apathetic and lacks energy; speech stammering; awkwardness and weakness of the whole right side; tongue deviates to the right. Station uncertain; gait ataxic; hemiplegic. Pupils medium size, the right larger than the left; all reactions prompt. Lateral nystagmus; slight convergent squint; vision $\frac{3}{46}$ on both sides. Optic neuritis greater on the right side. Hearing both to bone and aerial conduction is impaired on the right. Percussion of skull negative. Smell and taste normal.

Note November 26, 1897. Is dull and forgetful; explosive laughter; hearing on right defective; skin reflexes active; tendon reflexes active and greater in the right side; right ankle clonus. The active innervation of the face is alike on the two sides. In repose and when responding to psychical and emotional stimuli, paralysis of the right side of the face is evident. Inco-ordination of the right arm and leg, which are flabby and thinner than in the left; no disturbance of sensation; left parietal region, slight tenderness on percussion. (Under antisyphilitic treatment the general symptoms subsided, including the optic neuritis, and the objective symptoms showed great improvement.) Discharged.

Readmitted April 9, 1900 (Dr. Abrahamson). Ataxia, atony, and weakness of the right side. The volume of the extremities is diminished on the right side. Asymmetry of the face; in repose the right side drooping; this inequality is reversed on emotional innervation, and disappears on voluntary innervation. Paresis of left external rectus with internal strabismus; lateral nystagmus; no hemianopsia; no limitation of visual fields. Vision: O. S., $\frac{20}{20}$; O. D., $\frac{20}{30}$. No objective sensory disturbance; knee-jerks elicited by reinforcement, left $>$ right; Achilles jerks lively; abdominal reflexes present, more active on the left side. Right ear defective to bone and aerial conduction.

Note September 10, 1900. Apathetic and somnolent; vertigo, headache, and vomiting; pupils equal and rather small. The direct and consensual reactions to light on the left side are sluggish and

[1] Patient was presented at the January meeting of the New York Neurological Society, and subsequently was reported clinically by Dr. Joseph Fraenkel in the Journal of Nervous and Mental Disease, 1899, p. 427.

at times absent; accommodation sluggish on both sides. Paresis of left external rectus; nystagmus; knee jerks are variable, diminished, sometimes absent; Babinsky phenomenon on the right; Achilles jerks lively on both sides; no objective sensory disturbances; abdominal reflex is absent on the right, feeble on the left.

Grew rapidly worse; progressive increase of the general cerebral symptoms. Died September 30, 1900.

Autopsy. Only the brain was removed. The skull, meninges, and vessels of Willis were normal. The pons contains a tumor within its substance on the left side throwing its noımal contour into irregular nodulations. The left fifth nerve at its exit from the pons is compressed and flattened, while the left third, fourth, and sixth nerves stand in dangerous proximity to the growth.

Section through the hemispheres on a plane with the corpus callosum exposes a large tumor situated in the left optic thalamus and continuous with the infiltration in the pons. (Fig. 1.) It measures three inches in the longitudinal and two and one-half inches in the transverse diameter, and is rather sharply circumscribed from the surrounding brain substance by a lamellated periphery. It is of firm consistency and of a deep-red color (hemorrhagic). Some portions, chiefly on the periphery, are of a pinkish hue; others of a translucent appearance.

Hemorrhagic dots and minute areas of necrosis are scattered over the surface of section. The growth bulges into the third ventricle, the middle commissure of which is flattened out into a thin membrane, and encroaches posteriorly on the corpora quadrigemina.

The pineal gland is enclosed in a dense accumulation of connective tissue, but is otherwise normal. The hypophysis cerebri was normal.

On separating the medulla and the cerebellum at the foramen of Magendi a firm epiglottis-like prolongation appears. This on removal of the right lobe of the cerebellum is found to be the posterior tip of a large cyst, filling up and distending the fourth ventricle. (Fig. 1.) This cyst is one and three-quarter inches long and one and one-half inches wide. Its walls are thick, wrinkled posteriorly, smooth, and distended anteriorly and laterally. The outer layer of the wall strips readily, as in a fibrinous exudation, exposing a smooth surface with prominent and injected vessels beneath. It is accurately moulded to the interior of the fourth ventricle and on its basilar surface is firmly attached to the floor. The attachments of its upper surface to the cerebellum are slight and easily separated. The width of the vermis of the cerebellum is reduced by pressure to five-eighths of an inch and the lateral recesses appear as deep excavations.

The medulla is broader and flatter than normal. The posterior orifice of the aqueduct of Sylvius is free. The whole ventricular system of the brain is distended, more so on the left side. Numerous ependyma granulations. A small portion of the cyst wall was cut away, exposing the interior, which was smooth, containing only a small quantity of clear fluid.

Microscopic Examination. The medulla, pons, left hemisphere of the cerebellum, and the enclosed cyst were hardened and embedded in bulk and cut serially. Approximately every tenth section was prepared and mounted by the Weigert-Pal method; half of these were subjected to a contrast stain (acid-rubrin).

Cyst. The cyst begins on a level with the tip of the calamus scriptorius, gradually increasing in size to the plane of the striæ acusticæ. From this level it becomes smaller and the walls thicker, dipping down into and becoming an integral part of the left side of the pons. On a level with the posterior corpora quadrigemina it terminates as a small triangular cleft, in the neighborhood of the left pyramidal tract.

From the tip of the thalamus to the striæ acusticæ the cyst wall has no connections with the floor of the ventricle, save to the ala pontis (ponticulus) on either side. From the striæ acusticæ to its termination the cyst wall is intimately associated with the neural structures of the pons.

The nerve tracts form a decussation on its under surface, which pass upward into the cyst wall on either side. (Figs. 2, 3, and 4.) The cyst wall may be divided into three layers. An inner one is composed of glia; a thick middle layer of medullated nerve fibres which encircle the wall as a heavy band; and an outer layer in which the network of medullated nerve fibres is sparse, resembling gray matter. No ganglion cells could be demonstrated in the cyst wall, which possessed a rich supply of bloodvessels. No ependyma cells could be demonstrated lining the cyst wall. Here and there flat cells were seen, apparently of epithelial origin.

Cerebellum. The vermis and hemispheres of the cerebellum were compressed, and as a result showed changes in their configuration but without atrophy.

Medulla and Pons. The left pyramidal tract is small and pale. The lemniscus and fasciculus long. posticus are normal on both sides. The columns of Goll and Burdach are paler than normal, probably due to ascending intramedullary posterior root degenerations. (As the cord was not removed this cannot be definitely stated.)

The medulla, except for a moderate flattening and lateral elongation, maintains its normal configuration to a level with the acoustic nuclei. Here the cyst becomes incorporated with the floor of the ventricle on the left side, nerve fibres decussating on its under surface and passing up into the cyst wall. This decussation is largely formed of the coarse fibres composing the middle peduncles of the pons, and increases considerably as the level of the superior olive is approached. Tegmental fibres, as well as a few fibres from

FIG. 1.

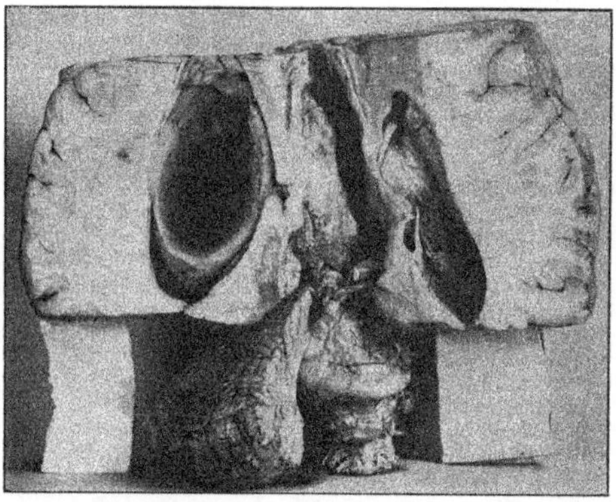

CASE I.—Tumor of left optic thalamus and congenital cyst distending the fourth ventricle.

FIG. 2.

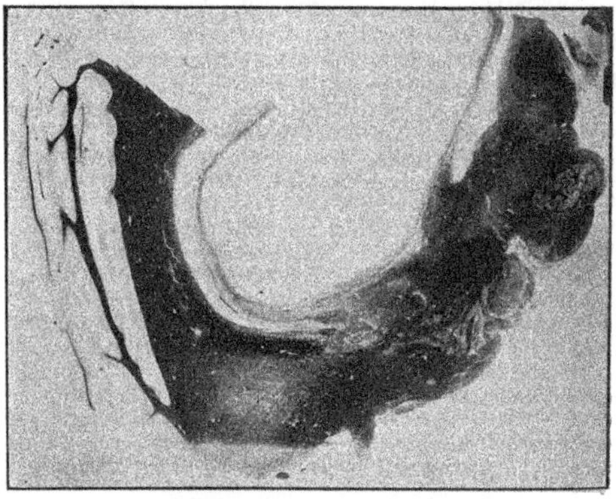

CASE I.—Weigert-Pal method. Level of striæ acusticæ. Showing intimate relation of cyst wall to floor of ventricle.

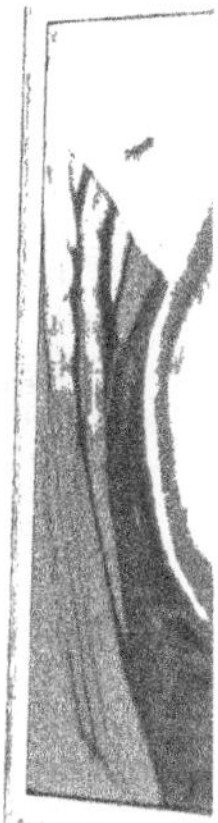

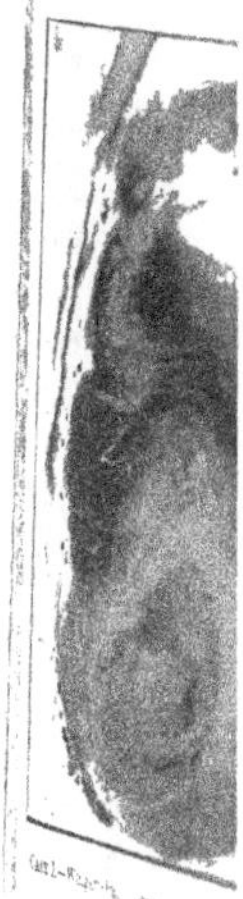

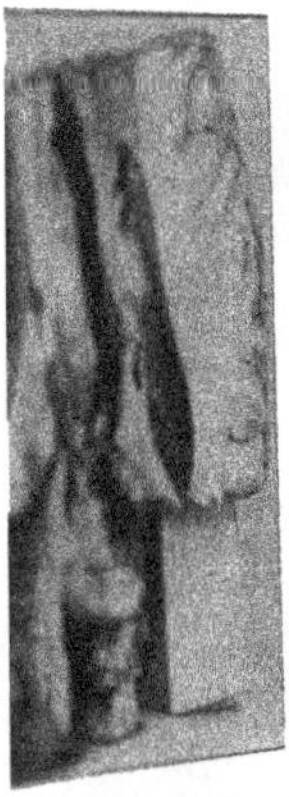

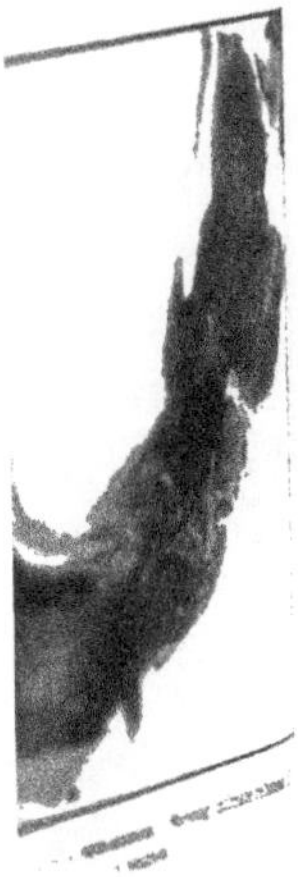

FIG. 3.

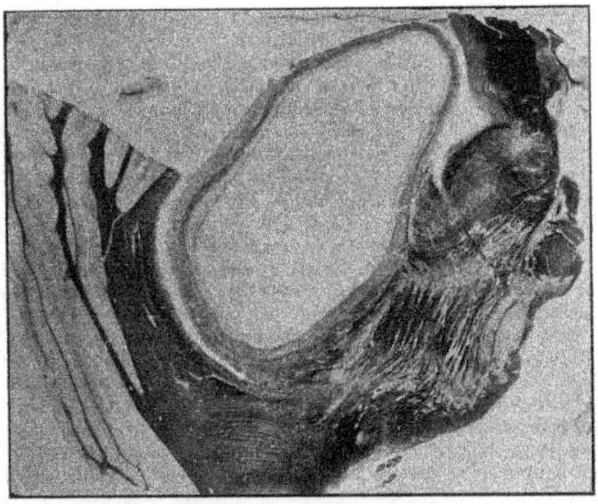

CASE I.—Weigert-Pal method. Level of the superior olive. Showing thick band of medullated nerve fibres in wall of cyst, continuous with the neural structures of the pons.

FIG. 4.

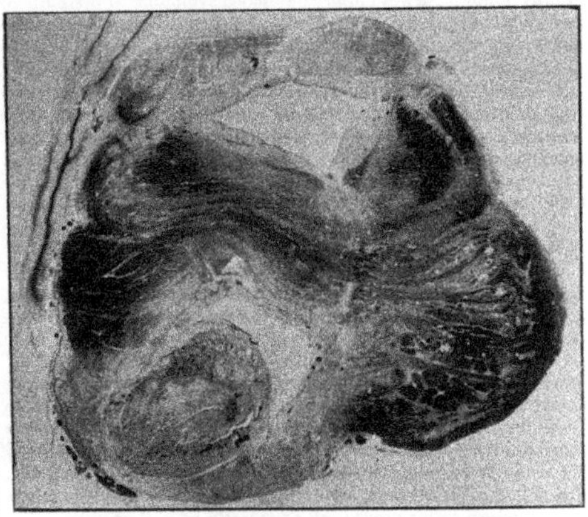

CASE I.—Weigert-Pal. Level of the posterior corpora quadrigemina. Cyst terminating in tumor as a narrow cleft.

the left median fillet and fasciculus long. posticus may be traced upward into the wall of the cyst.

At a level with the superior olivary body, where the cyst begins to sink gradually into the pons, the number of nerve fibres decussating on its under surface and passing up into its walls is very large. Most of these are derived from the pontine peduncle, so that these fibres on the right side of the pons are comparatively sparse.

Notwithstanding the distortions and changes in the configuration of this area, the important structures may all be discerned—*i. e.*, the superior olive, the ascending root of the fifth, lemniscus, and the fasciculus long. posticus.

On a level with the posterior corpora quadrigemina the cyst has tapered off to a small triangular slit in the region of the left pyramidal tract, and is here completely encircled by the tumor, which projects ventrally as a nodular swelling. (Fig. 4.)

Tumor. The pontine tumor and the large thalamus tumor are continuous and have the same histological peculiarities—*i. e.*, a polymorphous cell sarcoma, composed of round cells, spindle cells, and giant cells. The growth is extremely vascular, with numerous hemorrhages.

CASE II. *Summary.* A boy, aged seventeen years, previously healthy, following a head injury developed symptoms of brain tumor referable to the right crus cerebri. Weber's syndrome; left hemiplegia with extreme spasticity; complete right and partial left oculomotor paralysis; explosive laughter.

Autopsy. Glioma of the right crus cerebri extending posteriorly and infiltrating adjacent structures in the pons. A cyst of the fourth ventricle penetrating its floor, perforating the substance of the pons beneath and distinct from the aqueduct of Sylvius and appearing on the under surface of the right crus, terminating in the tumor mass.

Microscopically the cyst wall is composed of medullated nerve fibres and glia continuous with the nerve structures of the pons.

History. M. H., admitted to the Montefiore Home November 8, 1901; cash boy, aged seventeen years; family history negative. Previous history: was always a healthy boy, not subject to headaches or vertigo. (*Would frequently become nauseated while riding in street cars.*)

On June 7, 1901, he was hit in the back of the head by a swinging door, falling down a short flight of stairs. He received a scalp wound in the occipital region, but was not unconscious and in a short time was able to return home. In the street car, as had happened frequently before, he became nauseated and vomited. For a day or so he had moderate headache and in three days was able to return to his occupation apparently as well as ever.

One month later internal strabismus of right eye with ptosis developed and was soon followed by a weakness and stiffness in the left arm. The weakness in the arm increased and became apparent in the left leg as well. He was inclined to somnolence and got very dizzy, but no headaches or vomiting. About the same time it was noticed that he laughed inordinately on slight provocation and sometimes spontaneously.

The patient was examined in the neurological department of the German Hospital and was referred to the surgical ward for operation, under the supposition that a post-traumatic cyst had developed at the base of the brain in the region of the right crus cerebri.

Operation August 28, 1901. An osteoplastic flap five inches in diameter was thrown back; the middle meningeal artery was resected and, after retraction of the temporal lobe, four exploratory punctures were made in the direction of the right crus, with negative results. Discharged November 7, 1901, unimproved.

Status præsens, November 9, 1901. Head dolichocephalic; face asymmetrical; teeth viciously implanted; torus palatinus; complete ptosis of right eye, partial of left; divergent strabismus on both sides; paralysis of the upward, downward, and inward movements of the right eye. The inward and downward movements of the left eye are limited in their excursion and accompanied by nystagmus. Nystagmoid twitchings were present in the right eye on attempted movement. The right pupil is widely dilated and fixed. The left pupil is normal in size and all reactions are present but sluggish. Paralysis of the left face, arm, and leg, with spasticity; clonus; Babinsky phenomenon; no objective sensory disturbances. Skin reflexes were absent on the left side; hearing, smell, and taste normal; no limitation of visual fields. Station; body is bent toward the left side with a tendency to fall in the same direction. There was uncontrollable and involuntary laughter from time to time, especially when starting to speak. Mentally, he was bright and clear; speech normal.

Optic Nerves. The vessels of the disks were congested and the upper margin was hazy; urine negative.

Note, March 12, 1902 (Dr. Abrahamson). General condition is much worse. His speech is indistinct. Any question or command induced uncontrollable laughter; no weeping. The right arm and leg are the seat of slow co-ordinated movements, which may be controlled on command. The cessation is only temporary, however. There is contraction of the left upper extremity, the clenched hand resting in contact with the shoulder; extensor contraction of the left lower extremity. The tongue deviates toward the left. There is complete ptosis of the right eyelid and partial of the left. The right eye is turned upward and slightly outward, the only movement preserved being feeble external rotation. The left eye is turned outward and downward, with preservation of the excursions downward and inward. Right pupil is large, with

FIG. 5.

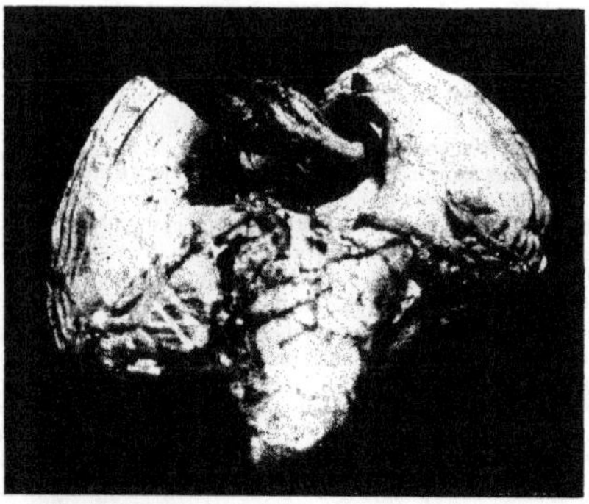

CASE II.—Vermis of cerebellum removed, exposing cyst in fifth ventricle.

FIG. 6

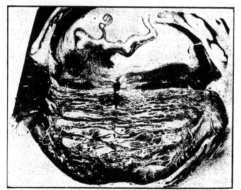

CASE II.—Weigert-Pal. Level of the fifth nuclei. Showing relation of cyst to floor of ventricle and thick layer of medullated nerve fibres in cyst wall.

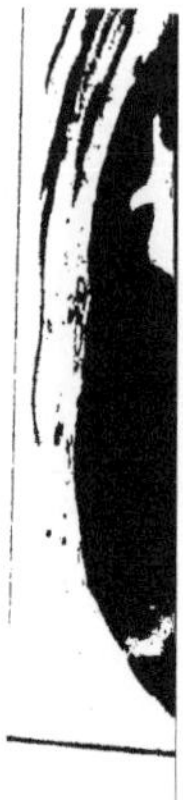

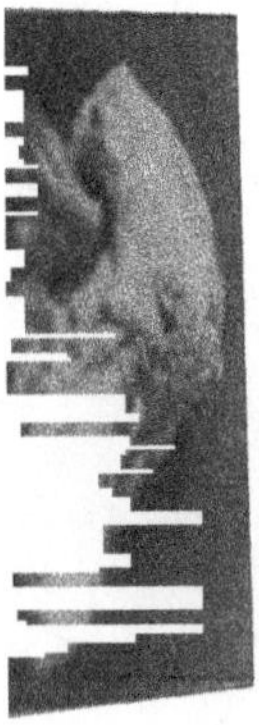

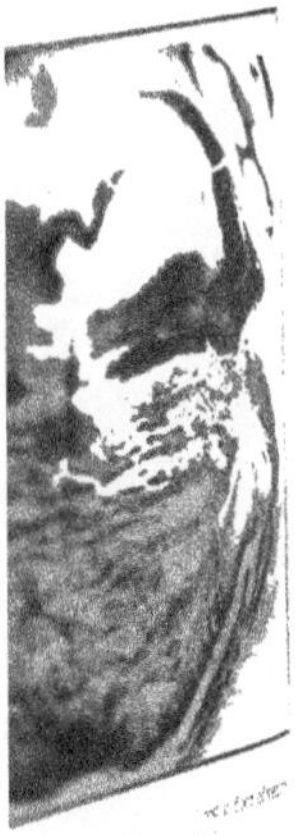

Fig. 7.

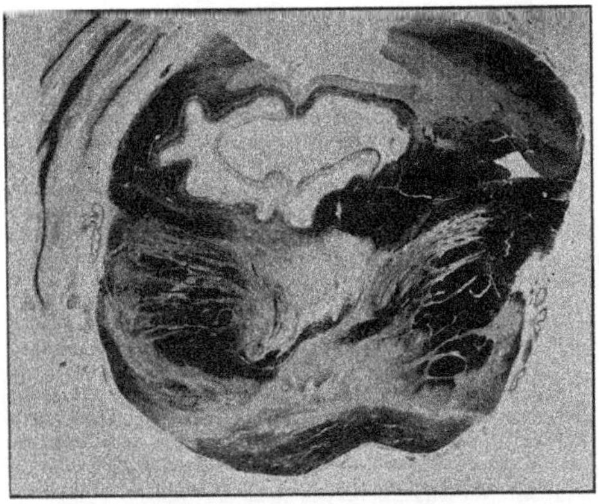

Case II.—Level of the posterior corpora quadrigemina. The cyst is beneath and distinct from the aqueduct of Sylvius, the roof of which is torn across. Cyst wall has collapsed on one side. Gliomatous infiltration of pons.

Fig. 8.

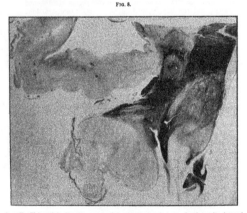

Case II.—Weigert-Pal. Showing crus cerebri, optic tract and chasm: basal ganglia, internal

irregular outline, and fixed. Left pupil is normal in size, with sluggish reactions. Other cranial nerves are negative.

Note, July 12, 1902. Emaciation is most extreme. The left hand and arm are in extreme flexion contracture, the hand resting on the acromion; left leg shows extension contracture. The left side of the body is cooler than the right. He hears and attempts to respond to some questions, but the response is inarticulate and indistinguishable. During the past four months there have been no paroxysms of forced laughter. He can tell the number of fingers held before either eye. The patient leads a purely vegetative existence; never speaks; sleeps most of the time; points to the mouth to indicate desire for food or drink. He recognizes members of the family and calls them by name. He drinks large quantities of water, and for three months has passed urine and feces in the bed, and if not watched will carry excrement to his mouth. The movements of the tongue and palate are slow and feeble, but there are no evidences of cranial nerve palsies other than those mentioned, with the exception of the motor portion of the right trigeminus nerve, the jaw deviating toward the right side. Pain impressions are equally keen on both sides of the body; no albumin or sugar in the urine.

Autopsy Cadaver is in a state of extreme emaciation; sacral and trochanteric decubitus; tubercular focus in left apex; central pneumonic area in the left lower lobe. Chronic cystitis; otherwise the examination of the thoracic and abdominal contents was negative. There was incomplete union of the osteoplastic flap at the site of the operation. The dura mater over this region is thickened and adherent and the inferior surface of the right temporal lobe shows old superficial foci of softening, with pial thickening. The sinuses of the dura and the vessels of Willis are normal; moderate internal hydrocephalus.

Description of Crural Tumor and Cyst. Springing from the right crus cerebri is a firm, nodular, grayish-white mass filling up the interval between the cerebral peduncles. The outer side of the growth is in close relation with the right optic tract; the inner side encroaches on the third nerve. The right third nerve is compressed and atrophic. The basilar surface of the pons and medulla oblongata with their respective cranial nerves are normal in appearance.

On splitting the cerebellum to afford inspection of the interior of the fourth ventricle, a cyst is disclosed springing from the anterior portion of its floor, to which it is firmly attached. (Fig. 5.) The posterior orifice of the aqueduct of Sylvius is free. The cyst is flattened and measures one and a quarter inches in its long and about five-eighths of an inch in its short diameter. The cyst wall is tough and dense and the surface is wrinkled. The interior is smooth and the only contents a clear fluid. The ependyma of the ventricle is dotted with numerous granulations. The cyst wall, at its attachment to the ventricular wall, dips down into the substance of the pons, through which it passes beneath the aqueduct and appears on the inferior aspect of the right crus cerebri, where it stands in immediate relation to the tumor. The growth is firmly adherent to the superior wall of the cyst, which is collapsed in this region.

Microscopic Examination. A series of sections was prepared from various levels of the medulla, pons, and crus cerebri, including the cyst, according to the Weigert-Pal method with contrast stain. The medulla shows atrophy of the right pyramidal tract; the right spinal trigeminus root is normal. The central canal in the lower portion is obliterated and Helweg's tracts are degenerated. In the pons at the level of the fifth nucleus the cyst wall becomes firmly attached to it, forming an integral part of the floor of the ventricle. Numerous bundles of nerve fibres pass into and encircle the cyst wall, which contains a rich supply of medullated nerve fibres and glia cells. (Fig. 6.) The fasciculi long. postici are contained in the left wall of the cyst at its junction with the floor. The right fifth nerve root is atrophic. At this level no evidence of tumor infiltration is seen.

On a plane with the trochlearis nucleus the cyst is enclosed within the substance of the pons below the aqueduct, with which it has no communication, and a little to the right of the median line. (Fig. 7.) The configuration of the surrounding parts has been somewhat distorted; the important structures are, however, easily discernible—*i. e.*, the median and lateral fillet, the roots of the cerebral trigeminus and the trochlearis, and the trochlearis conjunctivum. The latter is displaced toward the left side. The dense bundles of the fasciculi long. postici are distributed over the superior portion of the cyst wall. At this level, below the lemnisci, infiltrating gliomatous tissue is already apparent.

Sections through the right crus cerebri include the thalamus, the lenticular nucleus, optic tract, and chiasm, and the inferior convolutions of the temporal lobe. (Fig. 8.) The normal outline of the crus is obliterated and is replaced by a tumor mass. On the under surface of and attached to the growth is the collapsed cyst wall. In the wall of the cyst medullated nerve fibres are still demonstrable. The wall is composed of a coarse, wavy glia tissue in which the fibrillar elements preponderate, and containing a sparse network of medullated nerve fibres. At several points lining the interior distinct areas of columnar epithelial cells are seen resembling the ependymal lining of the ventricles.

The tumor proliferation begins in the outer layers of the cyst wall and is here firm in texture, the spindle type predominating, forming interlacing waves and bands; numerous giant cells. In the periphery of the growth the proliferation is more typically gliomatous, merging gradually into normal areas. The vascular supply is rich.

The *cyst wall* may be roughly divided into two layers, the inner composed of coarse glia and an external rich in medullary nerve fibres. The interior lacks a continuous epithelial lining, but a few remnants still persist. These consist of columnar cells, flat cells, and stratified layers of cells, the latter suggesting an epithelial metaplasia. No ganglion cells were observed.

Remarks. The occurrence in the brain of congenital cysts, while rare, is recognized in all classifications of the subject. They originate in offshoots of the primary cerebral vesicles. Bruns mentions, in connection with gliomata of the pons, the occurrence in the brain stem of minute cysts lined by ependyma and evidently separations from the primary neural tube. Stroebe demonstrated in gliomata of the brain minute cysts lined by columnar epithelium, probably sprouts of the primary cerebral vesicles.

In spinal cord pathology the relation of central gliosis, gliomata, and syringomyelia to developmental defects and embryonal rests of the central canal is fairly well established. In brief, abnormal offshoots and diverticula of the primary neural tube in any portion of its course may furnish the incentive to morbid proliferation.

Cysts of the size, location, and nature just described are unique in my pathological experience. A parasitic origin could be definitely excluded by the nature of the histological findings.

In favor of a congenital origin are:

1. The cyst wall throughout was composed of medullated nerve fibres and glia.
2. The intimate relations of the cyst wall with the adjacent nerve structures as it traverses the brain stem; the cyst is not intercalâted, but forms an integral part of the pons.
3. Remnants of an epithelial lining.
4. The associated neoplasms.
5. The absence of cerebral symptoms preceding the development of tumor.

The gross anatomical relations of the cysts in my cases suggest an origin from that portion of the medullary tube engaged in the formation of the second and third primary cerebral vesicles.

The developmental changes in these vesicles, which form the mid-brain and hind-brain, are especially conspicuous and complicated. This portion of the fetal brain is wedged in between the head and neck bend, flaring out laterally to form the expansions of the floor of the fourth ventricle, corresponding to the lateral recesses.

The evaginations of the *Rauten lippen*, which develop subsequently, enfolding and covering in the ventral and dorsal zones of His, further complicate matters and would favor the occurrence of developmental defect. The frequency of gliomata in this region is well known.

In conclusion, I would emphasize the importance of subjecting the so-called old, sterile, *parasitic* cysts in the neighborhood of the ventricular cavity, to serial study and the Weigert method before excluding a congenital origin.

A CASE OF ACCIDENTAL POISONING BY AN UNKNOWN QUANTITY OF ATROPINE SULPHATE; RECOVERY.

By Samuel Stalberg, M.D.,
(of Philadelphia)
CLINICAL ASSISTANT, OUT-PATIENT SURGICAL DEPARTMENT, POLYCLINIC HOSPITAL; ASSISTANT PHYSICIAN, CHILDREN'S DISPENSARY, JEWISH MATERNITY HOSPITAL; EXAMINING PHYSICIAN, ST. VINCENT'S HOSPITAL.

The great majority of the cases of belladonna poisoning are accidental in origin. Thus, of 466 recorded cases of poisoning by belladonna and its alkaloid, collected from medical literature by Witthaus,[1] the drug in 344 cases was taken by accident, either in mistake for some other preparation or in overdose through some error of the druggist. In 35 cases it was administered with either homicidal or suicidal intent, while in 87 cases the cause was uncertain.

Following is a history of my case:

D. L., Hebrew, aged fifty years, has been suffering for several years with a chronic bronchial cough, accompanied by profuse expectoration. For this he was given, in a local dispensary, a pill, to be taken t. i. d., and containing, as I subsequently learned, strychnine, $\frac{1}{60}$ grain; codeine, $\frac{1}{2}$ grain, and atropine sulphate, $\frac{1}{240}$ grain.

He had taken thirty of these pills during two weeks, when, being improved, he was advised to have his prescription renewed. This he did, taking the first pill of the second instalment on the evening of December 30, 1902, after having intermitted their use for two days. He took the second pill of this lot—the pill that no doubt contained the overdose—at about noon of the next day, and the toxic effects of the atropine began to manifest themselves about an hour later, when I was hastily summoned by the patient's daughter, who declared that her "father lost his voice."

Upon arrival I found the patient on his feet; at times attempting to stagger across the room; at others, stooping and supporting himself on the bed-post. His eyes were wild, brilliant, and staring, and the pupils dilated to their utmost. I do not remember, however, having noticed diplopia, amblyopia, or other disturbances of vision often seen after an overdose of atropine. Face was flushed, and somewhat expressive of terror. Fingers were restless, continually buttoning and unbuttoning the vest, suspenders, etc. He several times bent under the bed, as if in search of something. He was semidelirious, and chatted continually and incoherently. Several times he exclaimed: "Let me bark! I want to bark!" His voice was husky, and his mouth, tongue, and pharynx parched. He had a constant desire to micturate, and passed a quantity of urine every few seconds.

Temperature was normal; pulse 120; respiratory rate not observed. Patellar reflexes exaggerated.

At first puzzled as to the cause of the man's behavior, the thought of some drug intoxication soon suggested itself, and, upon inquiry, I found that he had been taking the above-mentioned pills. I immediately thought of atropine, and, telephoning to the drug-store, learned of their contents.

The diagnosis established, the indications for treatment were clear. Obviously, it was too late for the exhibition of chemical antidotes, and stomach-washing was impracticable. Pilocarpine hydrochlorate and morphine sulphate, somewhat antagonistic physiologically to atropine, were therefore immediately administered. One-sixth of a grain of the former and one-eighth of a grain of the latter were given in solution, *per orem*.

The morphine was repeated in about twenty minutes, and the pilocarpine hourly for three or four hours. The drugs were exhibited in this manner rather than by the more prompt hypodermic method, for the simple reason that the soluble hypodermic tablets were unobtainable—an argument for the necessity of every physician to be equipped and ready for any emergency. The difference in the rapidity of action, however, could not have been great, since both pilocarpine and morphine, especially the latter, are rapidly absorbed from the stomach.

According to Kerr,[2] the physiological effects of morphine may manifest themselves in from two to three minutes when the drug has been taken hypodermically, and in four to five minutes after it has been swallowed in solution. I also catheterized the patient, with a view to prevent reabsorption of the poison from the urine, but without success. Of course, he was ordered to bed, but there was trouble in keeping him there.

Probably as a result of the morphine he slept a while, but his sleep was interrupted and restless. By 6 P.M. of the same day most of the alarming symptoms had either entirely disappeared or were greatly improved. He was no longer delirious, and spoke rationally, but his voice was still rough, mouth dry, and pupils dilated. The latter did not come down to normal for about seven days, and his pulse rate kept above normal for the same period. During, and for a few days succeeding the attack, the heart action was weak, so that, partly at the suggestion of Dr. A. A. Eshner, who was called in consultation, varying quantities of strychnine and digitalis were administered after the subsidence of the acute attack. The test for sugar in the urine of the patient, taken during the attack, was negative; but this may have been due to the fact that the urine had been standing for a few months —owing to the illness of the writer—before the test was made. F. Raphäel[3] reports the excretion of 0.4 per cent. sugar in the urine of a man moderately poisoned by atropine.

This case, as is seen, is a fairly typical one; but there are a few features which deserve comment. In my case the temperature was normal. This is contrary to what usually obtains. In 19 reported cases[4] in which the temperature was recorded, there was in every instance an increase in temperature of from 1° to 6° F. Others, like Boehm, Schaunstien, Kobert, and Schroff,[5] hold that there is always a constant diminution in the body temperature in atropine poisoning. In a case of atropine poisoning recently reported by Cortright,[6] the temperature was supernormal for about sixteen hours from the time of poisoning, the highest temperature being 103.03° F. Looking at this question from the point of view of the physiological action of atropine, we find that moderate doses cause a pronounced rise in temperature, while large toxic doses lessen animal heat.

According to H. C. Wood,[7] this increase is due to paralysis of thermogenetic inhibition. According to Ott and Collmar,[8] this increase is due to increased heat production, the result of stimulation of the thermogenetic centres in the spinal cord. The final fall in temperature is probably due, according to H. C. Wood, to vasomotor paralysis. The rise in temperature in atropine poisoning would seem to be a perfectly logical outcome, however, of the chief, characteristic, ultimate effect of the drug, viz., that of a paralyzant of inhibition. Another unusual feature of this case is the frequent and free micturition during the attack. Usually, as a result of the depressant action of the drug on non-striated muscle fibres, there is retention. A few cases, however, have been reported[9] in which this frequent urination was present.

The present status of opinion regarding the place of morphine in the treatment of atropine poisoning is important. Among others, Reichert,[10] as a result of experimental work, holds that morphine and atropine, far from being antagonists, are synergists, atropine therefore being of very limited utility in morphine poisoning.

In regard to atropine poisoning itself, he[11] believes that death in that case results from paralysis of the respiratory centre, but that the centre has great recuperative power, so that if artificial respiration is properly practised the centre recovers its activity, when there is in consequence a marked improvement of other depressed states.

Pilocarpine is considered a most efficient antagonist to the poisonous action of belladonna, the action of the two drugs upon the heart having been demonstrated[12] to be directly opposite, pilocarpine restoring the inhibitory action of the vagus after it has been destroyed by atropine. Pilocarpine also promotes the action of the sudoriparous and salivary glands, and is supposed to favor the excretion of the poison by its action on the emunctories. Symptomatic treatment is also of great importance in atropine poisoning.

REFERENCES.

1. Witthaus and Becker. Text-book of Medical Jurisprudence, vol. iv. p. 662.
2. Norman Kerr. Twentieth Century Practice, vol. iii. p. 71.
3. Quoted in American Year Book of Medicine and Surgery, 1901.
4. Witthaus, loc. cit.
5. Quoted by Witthaus, loc. cit.
6. Cortright, C. B. A Case of Atropine Poisoning. New York Medical Journal, Sept. 5, 1903.
7. Wood, H. C. Text-book of Therapeutics, 11th ed., p. 175.
8. Quoted by Wood, loc. cit.
9. Bond. British Medical Journal, 1881, p. 639. Quoted by Witthaus.
10. Therapeutic Monthly, May, 1901. Quoted by American Year Book of Medicine and Surgery, 1902.
11. Philadelphia Medical Journal, January, 1901.
12. Small. Twentieth Century Practice, vol. iii. p. 513.

THREE CASES OF PERNICIOUS ANÆMIA, WITH A DESCRIPTION OF THE PATHOLOGICAL CHANGES FOUND IN THE SPINAL CORD.

BY ROBERT REULING, M.D.,
OF BALTIMORE, MD.

CASE I.—W. H., male, aged forty-six years; white, born in the United States; widower. Was seen by me in consultation during December, 1901. His occupation has been variable. For several years he was clerk in the Baltimore & Ohio Railroad office. For six years he travelled as salesman for a commercial house, and at thirty-five years he settled in South Carolina, where he started a small general store in one of the small towns in the northeastern part of the State. His family history is negative. No history of tuberculosis, anæmia, or neuroses. He has always lived fairly well, but in his occupation as salesman his food was frequently not of the best, and he had frequent attacks of gastric discomforts. His stomach became so deranged that his general health was much affected, so that he gave up his position as salesman and went into business for himself. As a child when six years old he had scarlet fever. Pneumonia when seventeen years old. No sequelæ. From his nineteenth to his twenty-third year he was very nervous, apparently suffering from sexual neurasthenia. Gonorrhœa at twenty-two years, without complications. No history of syphilis or its secondary manifestations.

The patient dates his present illness from an attack of fever and marked malaise, associated with severe muscular pains, which was pronounced influenza by the attending physician. This was in November, 1899. He remembers several people that were similarly affected in the town; he was living in South Carolina at the time. He remained in bed for almost three weeks, and from his description the myalgia must have been unusually severe; the pains were especially marked along the spine and in the muscles of the legs. The fever was high and lasted about six days. There was gastric disturbance, marked nausea, but no vomiting. Bowels constipated. On leaving his bed he felt extremely weak, very depressed, and had lost much flesh. After two months he began to feel somewhat better, but he was still not the same man, and anorexia, with mental depression, was still present. About six months after this illness he was taken suddenly ill with severe pains in the abdomen coming on during the night, almost constant vomiting for forty-eight hours, and marked diarrhœa, with tenesmus. The prostration must have been pronounced. This disturbance was apparently due to eating ice-cream and drinking considerable beer later. He now began to have frequent attacks of gastric disturbance, and he says "his stomach has not been right since." As a rule, anorexia, rarely vomiting, but considerable gastralgia have been persistent symptoms during the last year or more. The extreme pallor was first noted one year ago and has been gradually increasing. The patient was treated six months ago in Greensborough, North Carolina, and thinks he was given quinine, arsenic, and iron. He thinks he has had some little fever at intervals. He improved for a time, but six weeks ago he decided to visit relatives in Baltimore, as he realized his disease was taking a serious course. The journey north tired him a great deal, and he almost fainted in the station here, and in Washington he was obliged to take whiskey at short intervals. His friends here were shocked at his appearance. He was treated by a physician, who pronounced the case cancer of the stomach, and advised operation. As a medical student was living in the house in whose ability the people had confidence, they asked his opinion about the case, and, as he differed from the former diagnosis, I saw the case as a third party.

Notes at Bedside. A man of large frame, looks older than forty-six years. Extremely anæmic tongue, lips and finger-nails show extreme pallor. He is still fairly nourished, but signs of loss of flesh apparent. The skin in general has a dirty, very light lemon color; this is more marked over lower abdomen and the face. Hair is gray and very dry. Breath bad. Several decayed teeth, especially the left first molar. No pus apparent about the teeth. Tongue coated slightly, thickened, but not tender. No subcutaneous hemorrhages. Lungs clear on auscultation and percussion. Heart impulse just in nipple line; soft blowing systolic murmur over body of heart, not transmitted to right or left. Liver not enlarged, not tender. Abdomen in general looks natural. Stomach area about normal on percussion. Deep pressure in epigastrium gives rise to some pain, and the patient is immediately nauseated. Slight œdema over dorsum of the feet and over ankles. Both patellar reflexes are abolished; the plantar reflexes are still present. No apparent atrophy of any group of muscles. No sensory disturbance elicited; feels heat and cold everywhere. When asked to walk there is no difficulty apparent. There is, however, considerable Romberg symptom present. When the patient attempts with eyes closed to touch the knees with the heel of the opposite foot he comes rather wide from the mark, and there is a slight ataxic swaying of the extremity. It is difficult to say if this is a true ataxia, as the extreme muscular weakness might account for it. No bladder or rectal disturbance. Vision good.

Ophthalmoscopic examination shows two punctiform hemorrhages in the right eye in the lower quadrant of the fundus and a small hemorrhage just at the edge of the disk in the left eye. No nystagmus. Pupils react to light and accommodation.

Fig. 1.

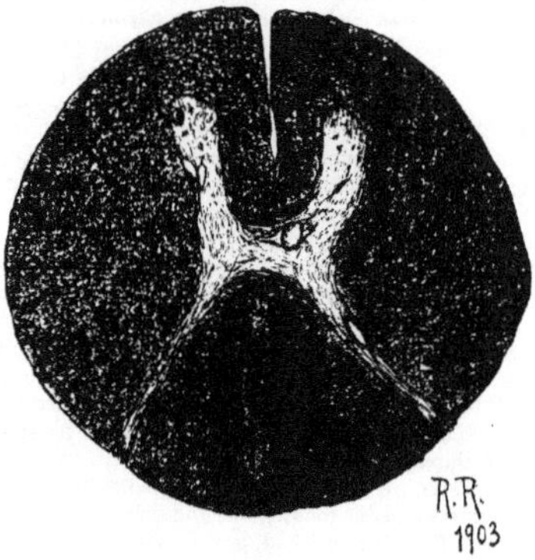

Case I.

Blood Examination. 1,800,000 erythrocytes, 7000 leukocytes, and 22 per cent. hæmoglobin. Specimens were stained after drying on copper plate and also after fixing in absolute alcohol and ether. Specimens show a marked poikilocytosis; almost every corpuscle is distorted. Many microcytes and a few macrocytes and about forty nucleated red blood cells were found in a blood smear. The first specimen showed no megaloblasts; the second, which was examined with the sliding stage, showed six. They were typical. Urine contains a trace of albumin; specific gravity, 1016. No casts; no diazo.

The patient was seen four or five times, but I made only two personal blood examinations, and, as my student friend had little opportunity to carry these out, my report is rather incomplete.

When last seen the blood count had improved slightly, 2,000,000, but there are several megalocytes now seen in the stained specimen, February 11, 1902. The patient died on March 2, 1902, from bronchopneumonia.

A complete autopsy was not granted, and I was only allowed to remove the cord, and this was not an easy matter in a private home.

Description of Cord. No macroscopic changes evident; meninges normal.

Description of Microscopic Changes Found in the Spinal Cord in Case I. Small pieces from every portion of the cord and medulla were placed in formalin and in a mixture of Müller's fluid and formalin. After hardening they were stained by the Weigert, Weigert-Pal, Van Gieson, and eosin and hæmatoxylin methods. In this case the Marchi stain was not employed. In every specimen examined, no matter what the staining method was, it was quite evident that a narrow strip of degeneration was present in both the column of Goll and that of Burdach, most marked in the former in most sections. The degeneration was most apparent in the lower cervical and upper dorsal regions. The drawings from this case were made from specimens stained by the Weigert-Pal staining method, and the blanched area in the posterior tracts of the cord represents the degenerated fibres. In the Van Gieson specimens it was clearly shown that these degenerated fibres had lost their myelin sheaths, and very few axis-cylinders could be made out in the degenerated areas. The remainder of the cord was absolutely normal. There were no hemorrhages found; the bloodvessels were normal, as were also the meninges. In all sections examined the same degeneration was apparent as far down as the upper sacral cord.

CASE II.—This case is of special interest, I think, in that the spinal symptoms seemed to precede the onset of the anæmia. Mrs. M., seen in November, 1902, aged thirty-four years; mother of two children, and who has had two stillbirths; the last child was born when seven months old, in 1900. Family history negative, except that one maternal uncle died of phthisis. She has had scarlet fever and measles. Typhoid fever at twenty years. No sequelæ. Has been of a neurotic disposition, and for several weeks during her first pregnancy was quite hysterical. No history of syphilis or its secondary manifestations.

She dates her present trouble to her last pregnancy, which resulted in a miscarriage at the seventh month of gestation, in 1900. She had fever for three weeks after this, and was a very sick woman. No marked rigor, but chilly feelings. Some muscular pains, but these were not marked. No swelling of the joints. After spending seven weeks in bed she was allowed to sit up, but was too weak to walk, even about the room. She has always had a rather sallow complexion, but has generally weighed between 130 and 135 pounds. In the early part of 1901 the patient was still run down, but was able to attend to light household duties. About this time she noticed a peculiar feeling and sensation of cold in the right thigh; this was especially marked when fatigued. Later a very similar sensation was noticed in the left thigh, but more over the buttocks. At times she had a feeling as though hot water was being poured over her lower extremities. This was nothing that troubled her. In August, 1901, she was in a driving accident, which left her very nervous, and she was subject to crying spells and suffered with pain down the back, and she seemed to have slight difficulty in walking, especially in the dark. No lancinating pains, but she still felt the sensations described above. She began to suffer with her stomach, and had constant feelings of weight in the epigastrium, and the pressure

FIG. 2.

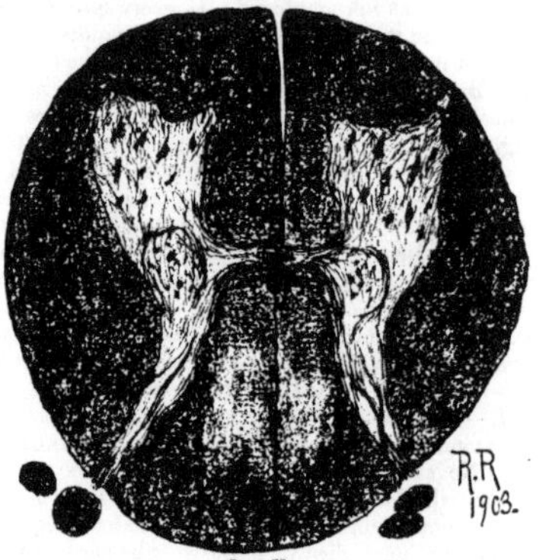

CASE II.

of clothing was very annoying. She did not vomit, but was frequently nauseated, especially in the morning. At this time she began to get pale. She took iron and quinine, probably arsenic, but her anæmia, except with periods of improvement, has steadily increased.

Notes at Bedside. A moderately well-nourished woman; subentaneous fat well preserved. She is extremely pale, and the skin has a faint suggestion of a yellow tinge. Tongue coated and rather sensitive to pressure and feels hard and is somewhat thickened, especially the anterior two-thirds. Teeth in fairly good condition. No glandular enlargement. Hair very dry and without lustre; not gray. Lungs clear throughout, except a few moist râles at the left base. Heart: A very loud hæmic murmur over the base, which is transmitted to the vessels of the neck. Apex-beat about the nipple line. Liver slightly below the costal border, 3 cm. Stomach is also displaced downward. The right kidney is readily palpable and slightly movable; in fact, a moderate degree of Glénard's enteroptosis exists. Test meal shows trace of hydrochloric acid. No lactic acid. Motor function of stomach evidently sluggish and some hypersecretion present.

Blood Count. 2,000,000 erythrocytes, 9000 leukocytes, and 32 per cent. hæmoglobin. Stained specimen with Ehrlich's triple stain shows marked poikilocytosis. Microcytes numerous; also macrocytes in several fields; and in about every fourth or fifth field an atypical megaloblast is visible, with very dark nucleus. Beautiful karyokinetic figures are seen in some of the nucleated corpuscles, and several erythrocytes show the polychromatophilic degeneration.

Examination of Nervous System. Gait is rather stiff, but no typical ataxia when the eyes are open. She watches the floor very intently. With closed eyes there is evidently a slight ataxia. Well-marked Romberg symptom. Both patellar reflexes absent. Plantar reflex present. No Babinsky reflex. No atrophy of any muscles. Apparently a slight dulling to the differentiation of heat and cold over the right thigh, but this is slight. Touch normal. No other sensory disturbance; patient says she is rarely free lately of the paræsthetic sensations in the lower extremities. No lancinating pains present. Has never noticed any bladder or rectal symptoms. Patient seen on one more occasion, and this was two weeks before her death, which occurred in January, 1903. Post-mortem limited to removal of cord and brain and inspection of abdominal viscera, which could not, however, be removed.

Cord. Macroscopic appearance normal.

Description of Microscopic Examination of Cord from Case II.— The entire cord was removed and sections from all regions placed in formalin, Müller's fluid with formalin added, also a few sections stained by the Marchi method, besides Van Gieson and eosin and hæmatoxylin staining. In all sections from whatever regions of the cord, except the very lower dorsal, ninth to the twelfth segments, and the sacral portion, a well-marked degeneration, involving almost the entire posterior tract of fibres, including the columns of Goll and Burdach. In this, as in the former case, the change was most pronounced in the upper dorsal and lower cervical regions. With the Weigert-Pal method a slight blanching of both right and left lateral columns was evident, but it was only after using the Marchi stain that it became evident that a considerable number of nerve fibres had degenerated in these lateral areas, this degeneration being probably of recent date. The anterior portion of the cord was normal. No hemorrhage found. The bloodvessels, nerve cells, and meninges were apparently normal. Nissl's stain was not employed, so one can say nothing in regard to the nerve cells, except that they showed no marked shrinkage.

In this case the reader will remember that there was evidence of spinal disease preceding the onset of anæmia for several months; in fact, the pronounced paræsthesias rather diminished toward the end of the disease. Several cases of this description are now found in the literature. It is most probable that more than one toxin exists in pernicious anæmia, one having a predilection for causing degenerative changes in the red blood cells, while the other seems to have a special affinity to the spinal cord fibres.

The theory that these degenerations start from hemorrhagic foci is rather losing ground lately, and it seems much more likely they are due to diffuse degeneration affecting certain fibre columns, for in just the cases where hemorrhages occur no such degenerations are usually found.

CASE III.—A male aged forty-eight years; married; born in Bohemia, but came to the United States when ten years old. The cord from this case was kindly given me by Dr. Flexner. The patient was admitted to the Johns Hopkins Hospital in 1901; the autopsy was performed at the hospital. Unfortunately, I can only present a few clinical facts in connection with the case, as I have not obtained the history in full; these notes were taken from the history when the cord was obtained. The patient complained of extreme weakness, breathlessness, and vertigo. His occupation has been a coal-miner, and he has been in Pennsylvania about the mines since his boyhood. His previous health has been fairly good. Remembers no serious illness whatever. No pneumonia or typhoid. He has had occasioual severe attacks of tonsillitis, which would make him quite ill; he has had about four of these; during one pus was discharged from the tonsil. He has always drunk considerable whiskey. No history of lues or gonorrhœa.

The patient attributes his present illness to stomach trouble, he being fully convinced he has cancer of the stomach, which he believes was caused by a wooden beam striking him across the belly. This was two years before his admission to the hospital. This accident happened after an explosion in the mine, and he, being one of the rescuing party, was exposed to many dangers and to the action of the gases formed by the explosion. He is quite positive that from this day his general health has not been the same. He was very excited at the time and was laid up for about two weeks. The gastric symptoms have been heavy, painful feeling in the epigastrium; occasional attacks of more acute pain. Vomits at times, more in the morning; this has occurred since entering the hospital. No history of jaundice. None of rheumatism. Bowels frequently loose, with intermittent constipation. Notes on physical examination lost.

Description of the Pathological Changes in Case III. The same staining methods were employed in the cord from this case as in Case I., the Marchi method not being used. The only change from the normal are several small circumscribed areas of degeneration, which are readily seen under the lowest power of the microscope; these were limited to the anterior parts of the cord. On closer examination it is evident that these degenerated fibres were caused by small hemorrhages into the cord substance. Several were found in the upper sacral region, as shown in the illustration, and two well-marked hemorrhages in the dorsal region between the third and fifth segments. In these the presence of blood pigment is clearly seen, and it easily explains why they should occur in the anterior portion of the cord, this being the most vascular portion. In this case the posterior and lateral columns are absolutely normal. As to the cause of these hemorrhages, they are no doubt due to some changes in the coats of the smaller vessels, very likely a form of hyaline degeneration; no doubt the effect of the unknown toxin, which seems to be the etiological factor in this most perplexing dis-

FIG. 3

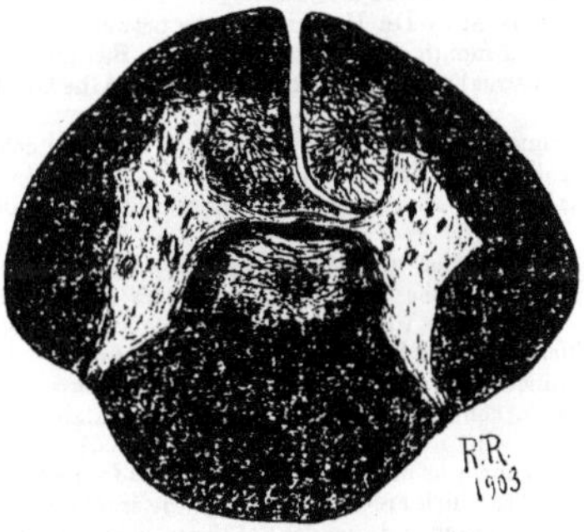

CASE III.

ease. That such degenerations are not found in the ordinary secondary anæmias, even the most severe cases, as those seen after infection with the bothriocephalus, etc., this is well shown in the cases and pathological report of Minnich and Nome on cases of pernicious and secondary anæmias. Lichtheim was the first to call attention to the tabetic-like changes in the spinal cord in pernicious anæmia. In this country the most important article on the spinal changes in this disease is that of Putnam, who also reports several cases in which well-marked spinal symptoms, mostly of a tabetic character, with paræsthetic sensations, preceded the onset of the pernicious anæmia. The reader is also referred to articles of Gold-scheider, Nome, Marie, Turner, Minor, and Grasset.

A HUMAN EMBRYONIC VESICLE SHOWING EARLY PLACENTA FORMATION.

By John M. Swan, M.D.,
PATHOLOGIST TO ST. MARY'S HOSPITAL, PHILADELPHIA.

(From the Pathological Laboratory of St. Mary's Hospital.)

The specimen from which the sections exhibited were taken was given to me in the laboratory of St. Mary's Hospital in June, 1903, by Dr. D. F. Harbridge. It had been passed from the vagina of one of his patients about June 16th. After the passage of the specimen the patient had profuse hemorrhage for a week, and had fainted on account of the loss of blood.

On November 17, 1902, the woman had been in a trolley accident, and six days later she had a miscarriage. The product of conception was estimated by Dr. Harbridge to be between the sixth week and the second month of development. Since this miscarriage the patient's menstrual periods had been irregular and the flow had been profuse.

The specimen was a spherical, fleshy mass, brown in color, about 0.5 cm. in diameter. On section it was found to contain a cavity, which was lined by a membrane that resembled amnion in appearance.

Microscopically this membrane proved to be chorion, with its villi projecting into the maternal blood spaces and bathed in the maternal blood. The villi are seen to be composed of fetal mesoderm, which is limited by two layers of tissue: first, a layer of distinctly outlined columnar cells, each containing an oval nucleus; and second, a continuous layer of cytoplasm containing irregular nuclei, but showing no demarcation into cell areas. The former of these layers, known as the layer of Langhans, is formed of the fetal ectoblastic cells, which are the remains of the trophoblast; and the latter is the syncytium, a descendant of the trophoblast.

The tissue at the periphery of the section is the decidua placentalis, and shows the dilated vessels which ramify in it.

The earliest recorded human placenta that has been examined is that described by H. Peters, of Vienna, in 1899. The following is a brief résumé of Peters' conclusions, after studying the appearances of the developing embryonic vesicle, which he estimated to be four days' old:

By the time the impregnated ovum reaches the uterine cavity it is surrounded by a chorion, which is covered on its free surface by epithelial cells of ectoblastic origin. The embryonic vesicle is lodged in a fold of the decidua, and, by a process of erosion, eats its way into the stroma of that membrane, the point of entrance of the embryonic vesicle into the stroma of the decidua being marked by a blood clot. In this way the decidua placentalis is produced between the muscular wall of the uterus and the embryonic vesicle, and the decidua capsularis is produced between the embryonic vesicle and the cavity of the uterus.

The epithelium of the chorion proliferates and forms a dense mass of cells known as the trophoblast, which presents villous projections, with intervillous spaces. The villi grow into the decidua placentalis and become attached to the deeper layers of that tissue or to the

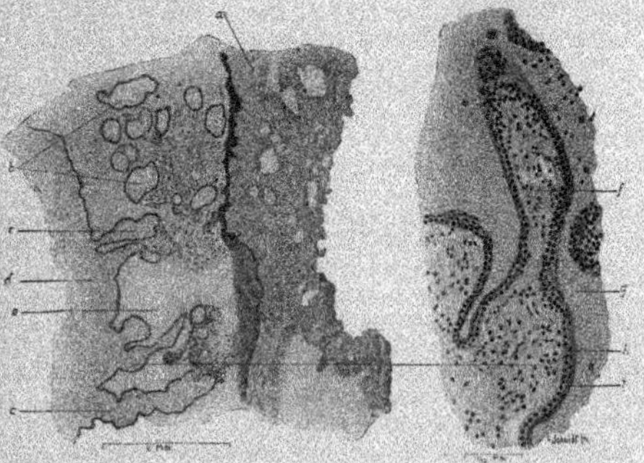

Section of young human placenta. *a.* Decidua placentalis. *b.* Chorionic villi in cross-section. *c.* Chorionic villi in longitudinal section. *d.* Chorion. *e.* Maternal blood space. *f.* Mesodermic core of chorionic villus. *g.* Red blood corpuscles in maternal blood spaces. *h.* Layer of Langhans. *i.* Syncytium.

muscular wall of the uterus, coming in relation as they grow with the dilated decidual capillaries. By phagocytic action the cells of the trophoblast absorb the endothelial lining of these capillaries, allowing their contained blood to lie between the projecting villi. The villi, at first simple, subsequently become branched, the branches lying free in the decidual blood spaces. Coincidently with these changes, the chorionic mesoderm becomes vascularized by the ingrowth and extension of the allantoic bloodvessels, by which means the fetal blood is carried into the chorionic villi in close relation with the maternal blood spaces. The maternal blood on the one side and the fetal blood on the other side absorb the cells of the trophoblast until only two layers are left, the layer of Langhans and the syncytium. In the future development the former layer is absorbed so that in the placenta at term the syncytium is all that remains of the original ectoblastic covering of the chorion. Then the fetal blood is separated from the maternal blood by the syncytium, the interposed mesoderm of the villus, and the endothelium of the fetal capillaries.

REVIEWS.

INTRODUCTION TO THE STUDY OF MALARIAL DISEASES. By REINHOLD RUGE. Translated by P. EDGAR and M. EDEN PAUL. London: Rebman, Limited, 1903.

IN spite of its modest title this book represents a fairly comprehensive exposition of the subject and strikingly shows the direct application of scientific research work to practical questions of hygiene and practice. This is brought out very clearly in the chapters on Epidemiology, on Therapeutics, and on Prophylaxis, which ought to be carefully read and assimilated by everyone engaged in medical education, whether in the narrower sense of lecture-hall and clinic-room instruction, or in the sense of education of the public. In the first—the choice of chapter headings is not altogether a happy one—which deals with the origin of malaria, there is brought forward such an array of convincing arguments in support of the theory of the dissemination of malaria by mosquitoes and a refutation of the objections that have been urged against it as to sweep the last vestige of doubt from the most skeptical mind.

The treatment of malaria obviously resolves itself into the proper method of administering the sovereign drug, quinine, and on this subject the author's ideas are quite definite, if somewhat radical. Briefly stated, his directions for the administration of quinine in benign (tertian and quartan) intermittent fever are to give "one gram or fifteen grains of quinine four or five hours before the impending paroxysm, and repeat this dose at the same hour every day for six successive days." He believes that fifteen grains is the minimum dose for an adult if the blood is to contain a quantity of quinine sufficient to be effective against the parasite. The same large dose is therefore required when quinine is given to control the fever permanently or as a prophylactic measure, for both of which objects it is to be prescribed on two successive days at intervals of ten days, for he has ascertained that two successive doses of quinine have a more powerful effect than one isolated dose. This periodic administration of quinine, corresponding to our "tonic" dosing, is to be kept up for three months after the disappearance of the paroxysms and of the fever, even when the patient has removed to a region where he is no longer exposed to fresh infection. With regard to the method of administration Ruge arbitrarily condemns all but the drug in solution or in wafers; "tabloids" especially are treated with utter contempt. The reader will bear in mind, however, that the book is written by a naval surgeon and primarily for the use of naval and military surgeons, who are less bound by prejudices and traditions than any other class of practitioners. Incidentally it is also written by a German, and the writer's national pride asserts itself in the liberal references to Koch, who, it would appear, according to the author, has done most, if not all, the recent important work on malaria. The latter's method of prophylaxis, consisting in the hunting down and curing with quinine of every individual case of malaria, especially the slight cases which are ordinarily overlooked, and the cases of relapse which keep up the disease during the off season, is the one that seems to the author to be the most effective, supplemented by personal prophylaxis. Methylene blue is the only drug that is capable of taking the place of quinine and, accordingly, finds its chief use in the treatment of black-water fever.

The author, with an implied apology, devotes a great deal of space in the chapter on Diagnosis to a description of the technique of making blood preparations, as "good preparations are, above all, needed for the successful demonstration of malaria parasites." His methods differ in a number of points from those usually employed; thus he obtains the blood neither from the tip of the finger nor from the lobe of the ear, but prefers "the back of one of the ungual phalanges," where the prick is less painful and the skin is thinner, so that the drop appears almost immediately. For spreading the film the ingenious method of Jancso and Rosenberger is advised, by which an even film of the desired thinness is obtained and the blood is spread without the least pressure, thus preserving the morphological integrity of the corpuscles. R. M. G.

ATLAS OF THE EXTERNAL DISEASES OF THE EYE. INCLUDING A BRIEF TREATISE ON THE PATHOLOGY AND TREATMENT. By PROF. DR. O. HAAB, of Zurich. Authorized Translation from the German. Second edition, revised. Edited by G. E. DE SCHWEINITZ, A.M., M.D., Professor of Ophthalmology in the University of Pennsylvania; Consulting Ophthalmic Surgeon to the Philadelphia Polyclinic; Ophthalmic Surgeon to the Philadelphia Hospital; Ophthalmologist to the Orthopedic Hospital and Infirmary for Nervous Diseases. With 98 colored lithographic illustrations on 48 plates. Philadelphia, New York and London: W. B. Saunders & Co., 1903.

THESE plates and descriptions with the companion volume upon the fundus are of inestimable value in the study and practice of ophthalmology. They replace, as far as may be, the clinic and instructor. Their low price and convenient form must cause them to supplant the larger plates. Practically all disease forms of the external and internal affections of the eye are portrayed in colors with full and clear descriptions in the text, including symptomatology, etiology, and treatment. Quite naturally all the plates are not of the same excellence, but no serious objection can be brought against any, and some are superb.

From considerable familiarity with the German edition, we have no hesitation in saying that the present descriptions in English (the plates are the same) are superior to the original in clearness, terseness, and ease of style. In this case it is not true that *traditore* is *tradutore.*

Of the comments added by the editor, Prof. de Schweinitz, we can only say that we wish there were more. They are valuable addenda, and occasionally rectify certain special views somewhat peculiar to the author.

The two volumes form a companion set which can with advantage be in the hands of every practitioner, even though he be not a specialist.

T. B. S.

INTERNATIONAL CLINICS. Edited by A. O. J. KELLY, A.M., M.D., Philadelphia, Pa. Vol. III., pp. 305. Thirteenth series. Philadelphia: J. B. Lippincott Co., 1903.

THE present volume opens with an excellent series of papers on "Diseases of the Gall-bladder and Gall-ducts." Musser discusses the medical aspects—some medical aspects, as he terms it—first presenting a skeleton, which he subsequently clothes with very substantial flesh, while Rudolph presents the "Causation, Symptoms, and Diagnosis of Gallstones." Stockton broadens the subject with his "Diagnosis and Medical Treatment of Cholelithiasis and Cholecystitis," while the surgical aspect of the case, so far as regards the indications and value of intervention, falls to Lejars. Deaver, on the "Surgical and Postoperative Treatment of Chronic Gallstone Disease," extends the subject. The symposium is completed by Weber, on "Biliary Cirrhosis of the Liver with and without Cholelithiasis." In the first place, it is apparent that in gallstones we have neither the beginning nor yet the end of the gallstone disease; further, that pathology and particular pathological findings, as shown by surgery, teach us that there is a medical aspect which is not to be ignored; and, finally, a careful diagnosis is essential and a working diagnosis possible in the great majority of cases. To one who wishes to know the present status of the gallstone question we can refer this volume, wherein a most satisfactory presentation is found. The one hundred and twenty pages constitute a veritable monograph.

Treatment is well represented by Finlay on "Pneumonia," Robin on "Gastric Cancer," Rose on "Carbonic Acid in Rectal Disease"—presumably meaning carbon dioxide gas—and Chantemesse on "Typhoid Fever Serum;" all good. Medicine is not far in the rear with Craig on "Malarial Infections," which clears the atmosphere; Leslie on "Clinical Types of Pneumonia," suggestive even to one whose experience has been so ample that he is alert for surprises; Mays on "Sudden Death Due to Respiratory Disorder" invoked the nervous system as an explanation, a paper for thought; Fowler writes on an "Intermediate Type of Leukæmia," as though we had not enough unsettled questions without the addition of another, and finally Poynton on the "Clinical Evidence of Myocardial Damage in Rheumatic Fever." With this valuable series of important papers surgery seems accorded hardly enough space. Bodine on "Cocaine Anæsthesia in Operation for Varicocele," Lewis on "General Anæsthesia," Lucas-Championnière on "Asepsis and Antisepsis," Rodman on "Gastrostomy; Concussion of the Brain," and Belfield, with a practical paper on "Intrascrotal Tumors," gives in small compass much valuable information, and Schwartz closes with the "Modern Treatment of Varicose Veins."

We have had in the past, at times, some misgivings as to the scope of this series. It seems to be intermediate between the journal and the monograph. In the past there have been volumes whose contents properly belonged to ephemeral journalism and the papers were tardy. At others an effort has apparently been made to cover too much ground. Again we have found articles which were almost monographs in their completeness. We believe the present volume meets our ideas. What has been selected has been thoroughly and ably done. The gallstone question in this volume, taken by itself, is notable and there is plenty more for good measure. May the editor continue to have the energy to draw out brilliant papers and the discrimination to properly group them! R. W. W.

The Decennial Publications. The Distribution of Blood-vessels in the Labyrinth of the Ear of Sus Scrofa Domesticus. By George E. Shambaugh, M.D. Chicago: The University of Chicago Press, 1903.

Dr. Shambaugh's monograph is a model of its kind. The work was undertaken for the purpose of studying the vascular supply in the labyrinth of the ear. A satisfactory study of the vessels in the adult is almost impossible, owing to their complexity, therefore the author was led to take up the study in the embryo. The difficulty of such a study may be realized from the fact that out of five hundred embryos injected only about one hundred of the specimens were found suitable for the study. The author describes carefully the methods which he employed, chiefly that of Eichler, which consists in making celloidin casts of the labyrinth, from preparations in which the bloodvessels had been previously injected. The methods used are described in full. A special feature of the monograph, however, will be found in the excellently colored plates. These are drawn with such evident accuracy that even if accompanied by a very slight text, they elucidate perfectly the points which the author brings out. On the whole, Dr. Shambaugh's study does not contain any startling anatomical find, but it does establish the anatomy of the circulation of the labyrinth on a definite basis, and therefore possesses the greatest value. F. R. P.

THE MEDICAL NEWS VISITING LIST, 1904. Philadelphia and New York: Lea Brothers & Co.

THE PHYSICIANS' VISITING LIST FOR 1904. Philadelphia: P. Blakiston's Son & Co.

BOOKS of this kind are an invaluable adjunct to the physician and his work, and the two under consideration are so well known to the medical profession that their characteristics need hardly be described. Some systematic form of record of visits, vaccinations, births, etc., is absolutely necessary to those engaged in practice. Both the *Medical News* and the *Physicians' List* have enjoyed continuous popularity with the profession for many years. Their general get-up and plan is the outgrowth of an intimate need of what is necessary in such volumes, and it is not likely that, having maintained their popular favor all these years, there can be found any plan to improve upon their scheme. J. H. G.

A TREATISE ON ORGANIC NERVOUS DISEASES. By M. ALLEN STARR, M.D., PH.D., LL.D., Professor of Diseases of the Mind and Nervous System in the College of Physicians and Surgeons. New York and Philadelphia: Lea Brothers & Co., 1903.

THE specialty of diseases of the nervous system has not, in late years at least, suffered from any lack of exposition of the subject through text-books and extensive monographs. There is, however, and always will be, a demand by the profession for text-books which embody the advance of knowledge in any particular line of work, with the basic and established principles. The text-book under discussion will be accepted by the profession in general, and neurologists in particular, as an example of a concise, clear-cut, complete presentation of an especially difficult and intricate subject. There has undoubtedly been a remarkable advance in our knowledge of the central nervous system and its diseases in recent years. The increase in the literature is out of all proportion to this advance. This is due in the main to single case reports and the tendency to individualize cases of a particular disease group, both from a clinical and pathological standpoint, has not only overburdened the literature of the subject, but has blurred the sharp outlines of the disease types to which we are accustomed in other branches of medicine. The result of all this is that the exposition of such a subject in order to be complete, and at the same time within convenient bounds, implies an ability for condensation, systematization, and digestion on the part of the author far beyond that called for in any other specialty. What Oppenheim has done for the German student Starr has succeeded in doing for the English, and much after the same method. The condensation and digestion is well carried out by means of footnotes, with references to the original articles, a distinct advantage over that of other works, where only the names of the investigators are given.

The personal element is strongly marked throughout the book. The author has drawn freely from his long and extensive practice in illustrating the different types of disease by the addition of case records, photographs, etc. Many of the sections illustrating diseased conditions are from his own cases and others from other American investigators, although a large number of these illustrations—*i. e.*, of the pathology—are drawn from the standard foreign works. In treatment the book is especially good, and here again, as in prognosis, long years of experience has lent that proper perspective to the value of methods and drugs and their results. Many of the chapters—Tabes, Anterior Poliomyelitis, Peripheral Neuritis—might be considered as monographs rather than chapters of a text-book.

The pathology of the different diseases is carefully considered and well illustrated by drawings and photomicrographs, as noted above. Sufficient attention, however, is not given at times to accuracy in the use of technical terms. The term neuron, quite needlessly, is used in a confused way to express the whole or part of the neuron. The posterolateral scleroses, both in the clinical and pathological descriptions, are insufficiently treated. The term sclerosis is used for the diffuse degenerations and no differentiation attempted. Putnam is given the credit of being the sole observer as to the different stages, etc., of the disease—*i. e.*, distinguishing between symptoms of long and short standing in the same case. That tumors of the pituitary are usually fibroma or myxoma will not be accepted by those who have studied the pathology of this gland carefully. These, however, are minor errors, which one may pick out of such a work easily enough, but have little influence in the estimation of its real value.

There is considerable room for improvement in the indexing,

reference of some authorities, and correction of typographical errors. The book itself is of 750 pages; the 275 engravings in the text and the 26 plates are very well executed and add greatly to its value. The paper is good and the printing and binding all that one might wish for. Altogether the book is a credit to American neurology, and will compare favorably with the standard text-books of other languages. D. J. McC.

RECHERCHES CLINIQUES ET THERAPEUTIQUES SUR L'EPILEPSIE, L'HYSTERIE, ET L'IDIOTIE. Volume XXI. Compte-rendu du service des enfants idiots, épileptiques, et arriérés de Bicêtre pendant l'année 1901. Par BOURNEVILLE. Paris: Félix Alcon, 1902.

THIS volume is more of an annual report of the department for epilepsy and idiocy of the Bicêtre than a volume of research, as its title would indicate. Over half the volume is concerned with a statistical study of the number of patients, movement of population, history of the service, etc. Then follow ten contributions to the study of idiocy and epilepsy by Bourneville and his assistants. The effect of bromide of camphor in epilepsy is studied with apparently favorable results, and is quite up to the standard of the clinical studies of the best French clinicians. The other articles, all original investigations, are as follows: "A Study of Puberty," by Bourneville; "A Contribution to the Study of Moral Idiocy, with Especial Reference to Lying as a Symptom," by Bourneville and Boyer; "A Study of the Relation of 'Muscular Impotence' and Bony Deformities in Infantile Hemiplegia," by Bourneville and Bangour; "Hemorrhages of the Skin and Mucous Membranes after Epileptic Attacks," by Bourneville; "Symptomatic Idiocy Due to an Atrophic Sclerosis of the Right Cerebral Hemisphere," by Bourneville and Crouzon; "Idiocy of the Mongolian Type," by Bourneville, and also another article on the same subject by Phillipe and Oberthur; "True Porencephaly and Pseudoporencephaly," by Bourneville and Morel. The titles indicate the substance of the articles given. They constitute a valuable addition to the pathology of idiocy.

A study of the schools for backward children will be of interest to those laboring with this difficult problem. D. J. McC.

NOSE AND THROAT WORK FOR THE GENERAL PRACTITIONER. By GEORGE L. RICHARDS, M.D. NewYork: International Journal of Surgery Company, 1903.

THIS little work is really a novelty in its own particular line, and its author is to be congratulated upon the most excellent way in which he has fulfilled the object which he intended to accomplish.

It is based throughout on his own extensive personal experience, and it is this which gives the keynote to the volume.

While giving the diagnosis and treatment of morbid conditions in the nose and throat, as they fall within the province of the general practitioner, Dr. Richards is careful to indicate the difficulties which confront those who are not especially skilled in rhinology and laryngology, and thus not lead them into attempts to do that which does not lie within their province. The book is not only adapted to the general practitioner, but will prove an especially useful guide to those who desire to take up laryngology and rhinology as special pursuits. It is in no sense of the word a compend, nor does it pretend to furnish a complete text-book. Dr. Richards writes in a clear style, admirably suited to his subject-matter. This book is a pioneer in its line and deserves the professional favor with which it is sure to be received. F. R. P.

A Narrative of Medicine in America. By James Gregory Mumford, M.D. Philadelphia and London: J. B. Lippincott Co., 1903.

This work covers the entire field of the history of medicine in America from the earliest time down to the present date. Its title has been well chosen by the author, who has given us what is truly a story or narrative of the medical profession rather than a dry series of historical facts. Within recent years there has been a great impetus given to the study of medical history, and much has been written upon it. Dr. Mumford has not only availed himself of the work which has been done in this field of investigation by others, but has gone to original sources and has authenticated or disproved many disputed statements.

In a book of this character it is most difficult to observe a proper proportion in dealing with various epochs or individuals, and its author is to be congratulated upon the skilfulness which he has shown in weaving the network of his narrative. Beginning with the early days of settlement, when the sick and injured depended for relief upon the amateur medical attentions of pastors or deacons, like Samuel Fuller, Dr. Mumford goes on to the real beginnings of medical history in this country, when bright young men who determined to practise medicine sought their knowledge at the feet of the best teachers in England and on the Continent, and brought back to this country the lessons which they had learned from the Hunters, Haller, Boerhaave, or Morgagni. Most interesting are his accounts of the careers of the founders of American medicine: Morgan, Shippen, Rush, and John Jones—each skilfully delineated, with the estimates of their characters and accounts of their mutual relations given. Coming to a later date, when medical science had extended from Philadelphia, Boston, and New York, penetrating other sections of the country, Dr. Mumford describes most sympathetically and graphically the great services rendered by pioneers, such as Drake and Dudley. In fact, among the most interesting portions of the book will be found those devoted to the careers of these men, many of whom figure to the present generation as names and naught else.

Although Dr. Mumford pays due attention to the founding of hospitals and medical schools, and describes the services of men like those above mentioned and the Warrens of Boston in this connection, we doubt if the histories of institutions will ever thrill us as do the life-histories of men who struggled through almost insuperable difficulties to the achievement of such tremendous benefits to humanity.

Dr. Mumford's book should not only be read but owned by every American physician, and we could think of no more stimulating gift to be put in the hands of the graduate than this narrative, in which are embodied the wonderful achievements of his predecessors in the healing art.

F. R. P.

PRACTICAL POINTS IN NURSING. For Nurses in Private Practice. By EMILY A. M. STONEY. Third edition. Philadelphia, New York and London: W. B. Saunders & Co., 1903.

THE third edition of this valuable book on nursing has been revised and brought up to date by a physician owing to the death of the able author.

The work itself, except for the revision made necessary by advance in knowledge, retains much of its originality. The authoress was peculiarly qualified by experience and position to write authoritatively, and she is to be doubly commended for omitting much that a nurse need not know, as well as for the good selection of what she should know.

The matter has been divided into seven chapters and an appendix: I. The Nurse; II. The Sick-room; III. The Patient; IV. Nursing in Accidents and Emergencies; V. Nursing in Special Medical Cases; VI. Nursing of Sick Children; VII. Physiology and Descriptive Anatomy. The appendix contains various kinds of useful knowledge, such as tables of weights and measures, recipes, dose list, glossary, etc. The difficulty in instructing nurses lies in knowing just how much to teach and how much to withhold. It is necessary for the modern trained nurse to have an intelligent knowledge of the reason for pursuing a particular course or abandoning another. It is not necessary, on the other hand, for a nurse to take a complete medical course. Miss Stoney's work contains many things of interest to physicians as well as to nurses, and should prove a valuable aid for nurses in their private work. The book has its need also, as private nursing is somewhat different from hospital work, and often a nurse is at a loss for many kinds of information not picked up at the hospital. J. N. H.

A MANUAL OF PLAGUE. By WILLIAM ERNEST JENNINGS, M.B., C.M., Major in the Indian Medical Service; Chief Medical Officer for Plague Operations in the Bombay Presidency, etc. With an Introduction by Surgeon-General G. BAINBRIDGE, M.D., M.R.C.P., I.M.S. London: Rebman, 1903.

THE extensive and really alarming outbreak of plague which but a few years ago threatened to spread from the East to Occidental nations has drawn particular attention to the study of this disease; and so important and numerous have been the discoveries concerning its etiology, treatment, and prophylaxis that a thorough exposition of the present knowledge concerning the subject can scarcely be gained from the ordinary text-book of medicine. In certain countries where plague is likely to occur it is absolutely necessary that the practitioner should be thoroughly conversant with every aspect of the disease. To this end the present manual is excellently adapted, for it treats of the subject from a practical standpoint, and is besides essentially up to date. The book opens with an introductory chapter upon the interesting history of plague epidemics, after which follow chapters on the bacteriology, pathology, treatment, epidemiology, symptomatology, etiology, etc. The diagnosis and prognosis are appropriately treated and many important pages deal with measures for the suppression and prevention of the spread of plague. The author's personal knowledge and extensive experience with the disease certainly give the book a practical value.

There are a number of illustrations, most of which are fairly good. The book is well printed and nicely bound. W. T. L.

A MANUAL OF HYGIENE AND SANITATION. By SENECA EGBERT, A.M., M.D. Third edition, enlarged and thoroughly revised. Philadelphia and New York: Lea Brothers & Co.

THE third edition of Dr. Egbert's very useful manual shows evidence of very careful and thorough revision of every chapter. New material and numerous additional illustrations have been introduced where needed. Disinfection has been divorced from Quarantine and placed in a chapter by itself, and the chapter on Laboratory Tests has been much improved. The first edition was a valuable addition to the literature of Hygiene, the second was an improvement over the first, and the third is better than the second. As the author keeps his work abreast of the times, each revision causes an increase in size; and it seems probable that before long he will have to determine where a cut can be made with least injury to the book as a whole. It is the opinion of the reviewer that the chapter on Bacteriology could well be spared even now, for it is slight and sketchy; it can be of no assistance to those who have had an elementary course in the subject, and is not full enough for those who have not. Moreover, a work on Hygiene should no more include elementary bacteriology than elementary physics, chemistry, or mathematics. C. H.

MODERN SURGERY: GENERAL AND OPERATIVE. By JOHN CHALMERS DA COSTA, M.D., Professor of Principles of Surgery and of Clinical Surgery, Jefferson Medical College, Philadelphia; Surgeon to the Philadelphia Hospital and to St. Joseph's Hospital, Philadelphia. Fourth edition, rewritten and enlarged, with 707 illustrations, some of them in colors. Philadelphia, New York and London: W. B. Saunders & Co., 1903.

ALTHOUGH the whole science of medicine is constantly and steadily progressing, perhaps the most noted advances are in the realm of surgery, where new methods, improved technique, and more modern patterns of instruments are ever pressing the old ones into the background. For this reason a text-book on surgery very soon becomes out of date unless continually revised and rewritten, for, though many of the procedures have come to be regarded as standard ones, student and practitioner alike will not be satisfied with a work containing these only, but demand methods of the day and hour, such as the Lorenz treatment and others of a kindred nature. In this aspect Da Costa's *Surgery* is excellent. This fourth edition has continued the many good points of the previous editions, but has been entirely rewritten, many procedures now obsolete having been dropped and their places taken by modern methods. It is not a large work, the general divisions corresponding to the generally accepted classification of subjects in all standard works on surgery. The discussions, both in regard to Symptomatology and Treatment, are brief but clear and concise and well adapted to teach what the author wishes. A chapter on Bacteriology precedes the surgical matter proper, as the author believes, and justly so, that without a clear idea of the causes of infection in its various forms the surgeon is but poorly equipped to guard against it. Fractures and Dislocations, on account of their great practical importance, receive a large amount of space and are treated in a rational manner, while for all but the more common operations on the Eye, Nose, Throat, and Ear, in common with most gynecological procedures, the reader is referred to special works on these subjects. The different operations on the intestines with their many advocates are carefully considered and clearly set forth with their various advantages and disadvantages, and the chapters devoted to these are both interesting and instructive. There are over seven hundred illustrations, many of them good half-tones, but, on the other hand, there are a number of old cuts which are hardly in keeping with a work in every other respect so up to date. The reproductions of *x*-ray photographs, of which there are a number, are excellent.

G. M. C.

A DICTIONARY OF MEDICAL SCIENCE. Containing a full explanation of the Various Subjects and Terms of Anatomy, Physiology, Medical Chemistry, Pharmacy, Pharmacology, Therapeutics, Medicine, Hygiene, Dietetics, Pathology, Bacteriology, Surgery, Ophthalmology, Otology, Laryngology, Dermatology, Gynecology, Obstetrics, Pediatrics, Medical Jurisprudence, Dentistry, Veterinary Science, etc. By ROBLEY DUNGLISON, M.D., LL.D. Twenty-third edition, thoroughly revised, with the Pronunciation, Accentuation, and Derivation of the Terms. By THOMAS L. STEDMAN, A.M., M.D. Philadelphia and New York: Lea Brothers & Co., 1903.

THE name of Robley Dunglison stands forth as that of the greatest medical lexicographer of the English language. For seventy-five years his work has been the standard dictionary used by the English-speaking medical world, and now in its twenty-third edition it is a pleasure to realize that it remains fully up to the standard of the most modern requirements. One thing which is particularly noticeable in the work is the great economy of space which its editor has succeeded in accomplishing by the elimination of obsolete terms and all matter which was not of distinct value in subserving the purpose of the dictionary. In the accomplishment of this object nothing has been omitted which could prove of any real service to the searcher after information, and room has been made to accommodate a wonderful line of new subject-matter. Space has also been obtained by cutting out the figured pronunciation, which is so often absolutely unnecessary. A number of most excellent cuts have been introduced. They have evidently been chosen for their real value, and not to catch the eye of a casual peruser of the work. Although the type is small, as is always necessary in a work of this nature, nevertheless it is so clear that it is easy to read. The publishers of this classical work are to be congratulated in having procured the services of an editor who, having preserved all the traditions which have given the book its pre-eminence, has at the same time brought it most thoroughly up to date. F. R. P.

THE AMERICAN ILLUSTRATED MEDICAL DICTIONARY. A New and Complete Dictionary of the Terms Used in Medicine, Surgery, Dentistry, Pharmacy, Chemistry, and the Kindred Branches, with their Pronunciation, Derivation, and Definition, Including Much Collateral Information of an Encyclopædic Character. By W. A. NEWMAN DORLAND, A.M., M.D. Third edition, revised and enlarged. Philadelphia, New York and London: W. B. Saunders & Co., 1903.

AMERICAN POCKET MEDICAL DICTIONARY. Edited by W. A. NEWMAN DORLAND, A.M., M.D. Containing the Pronunciation and Definition of all the Principal Terms Used in Medicine and the Kindred Sciences, along with over Sixty Extensive Tables. Fourth edition, revised and enlarged. Philadelphia, New York and London: W. B. Saunders & Co., 1903.

BOTH these dictionaries have gone through a number of editions, and have achieved a most enviable degree of favor from the medical profession. The large one indeed may be considered as an authoritative work of reference of the greatest value to the literature of the medical profession. Its definitions, though concise, are very lucid. The method of indicating the pronunciation of the terms is exceedingly simple. A feature of special value in the work is the excellent tables of muscles, nerves, bacteria, etc., with which it abounds. Although the illustrations are not very numerous, they are all such as possess real value to the reader.

The *American Pocket Medical Dictionary* will prove of special use to medical stenographers, nurses, and other persons who are required to be familiar with the definition and spelling of medical terms. Within its small bulk it practically comprises all the information of its nature with which, under ordinary circumstances, it would be necessary for them to be familiar.

Both of these dictionaries are most excellent in their typography and their arrangement. J. H. G.

PROGRESS

OF

MEDICAL SCIENCE.

MEDICINE.

UNDER THE CHARGE OF

WILLIAM OSLER, M.D.,

PROFESSOR OF MEDICINE, JOHNS HOPKINS UNIVERSITY, BALTIMORE, MARYLAND.

AND

W. S. THAYER, M.D.,

ASSOCIATE PROFESSOR OF MEDICINE, JOHNS HOPKINS UNIVERSITY, BALTIMORE, MARYLAND.

On the Tuberculous Serum Reaction.—MARCHETTI and STEFANELLI (*Riv. Crit. d. Clin. Med. Firenze*, 1903, vol. iv. pp. 657, 673, 689), in the clinic of Professor Grocco, of Florence, have made an interesting study of the value of the tuberculous serum reaction. As is well known, the possible diagnostic importance of this reaction was first suggested in 1898 by Arloing, whose later studies with Courmont have been followed by numerous observations with conflicting results; one party maintaining that the reaction when carried out under rigid rules and interpreted with proper reserve is of material value in the early diagnosis of tuberculosis; the other, among whom is Koch, denying absolutely its value. The Italian authors have studied seventy-three cases of varying characters. They emphasize the necessity of using cultures of carefully determined age and of following minutely, in every detail, the method of Arloing and Courmont. The results of their studies have been as follows:

They believe that the reaction is of no material value unless positive within the first six hours.

In grave tuberculosis, pulmonary or abdominal, the reaction was positive in 42 per cent. of the cases.

In early cases, mild or improving, the reaction was positive in 88 per cent.

In cases which were probably tuberculosis, but which clinically could not be positively determined, the reaction was positive in one out of four of the grave cases and in two-thirds of the milder forms of disease.

In three cases of lupus the reaction was negative.

In five cases which were proven by autopsy not to have been tuberculosis the reaction was always negative.

In cases in which clinically there was no evidence of tuberculosis and which did not come to autopsy, the reaction was negative nine times out of ten; it was positive in one instance of multiple sclerosis.

In general, the milder the lesion the more positive was the reaction, while in one case where the reaction was primarily positive it disappeared as death approached (tuberculous meningitis).

For six hours the reaction may be positive in clearly non-tuberculous cases.

They conclude that the Arloing-Courmont reaction, "studied accurately in all its most minute particulars and weighed with due restrictions, is a useful and not to be neglected diagnostic aid, especially in early and mild cases, the very instances in which the percentage of positive results is larger and more striking." But these cases are the very instances in which, from the point of view of prophylaxis and treatment, the early recognition of the process is of especial value. While they believe that there is a relation between the degree of specific agglutinative power in the tuberculous blood serum and the gravity of the infection, yet, in the present state of our knowledge, the results of the test do not justify prognostic conclusion.

Pneumothorax: An Historical, Clinical, and Experimental Study.—Emerson (*Johns Hopkins Hospital Reports,* vol. xi. pp. 1–450) has reviewed the literature of pneumothorax from the time of Hippocrates down to the present date. There are 358 very full abstracts of the most important contributions to the subject during this period. Hippocrates interpreted the splashing sound as a sign of empyema and not of pneumothorax, which he did not recognize. The writer emphasizes the fact that "succussion" is not the splashing sound heard, but the act of shaking which produces it, a distinction which clinicians do not sufficiently realize. Our knowledge of pneumothorax is usually stated to date from the thesis of Itard, published in 1803. He reported 5 cases of pulmonary tuberculosis with pneumothorax, but did not recognize the condition during life. Laennec, who published his observations in 1819, in his work on *Mediate Auscultation,* was the first to recognize the disease *intra vitam.* Owing to Hippocrates' belief that the succussion splash was a sign of empyema, it had fallen into disfavor and had been practically disregarded up to Laennec's time. The latter was the first to recognize its true significance and to add it to the symptom-complex. Comparatively speaking, little of importance has been added to our knowledge of the disease since the days of Itard and Laennec. They discussed the clinical symptoms very fully, and it is Itard's classification, with slight modifications, that is now in use. Since their day the cases of so-called idiopathie pneumothorax, that is, pneumothorax arising within the chest and in which the gas was not air, have been the cause of considerable dispute. In the last twenty years the therapeutics of the disease has been mainly under discussion.

Emerson reports at length the cases of pneumothorax that have occurred in Professor Osler's and Professor Halsted's wards at the Johns Hopkins Hospital. There were 48 in all. The largest number, 22, were due to pulmonary tuberculosis. Of these, 18 were men and 4 women. In 11 the pneumothorax was right sided and in 11 it was left sided. Statistics in general have shown the disease to be about twice as frequent on the left as on the right side. Of the 22 cases, 19 came to autopsy, and in 16 the perforation was found. It was in the upper lobe in 7, in the lower in 6, and in the middle in 3. The autopsies on cases of tuberculous pneumothorax represented just 4 per cent. of all the cases of pulmonary tuberculosis that came to autopsy.

There were 2 cases following bronchiectasis. There had been only 11 cases previously reported in the literature. Rupture of a metastatic abscess in the lung was the cause in 2 cases. One instance followed gangrene of the lung. Rupture of emphysematous blebs was the cause in 2 cases. Next to pulmonary tuberculosis, the largest number followed tapping of the chest for fluid. There were 10 due to this cause. In 1 the air was pumped into the chest; in a second it was allowed to enter through the unguarded needle; and in a third the lung was pricked by a hypodermic needle. The writer speculates as to the cause in the other cases. 5 of these 10 cases died. In 2 cases the pneumothorax resulted from rupture of an empyema into the lung. Traumatism was the cause in 6 cases. It is of interest that there were 14 other cases in Professor Halsted's wards in which the lung was known to have been injured by various forms of traumatism, but in which pneumothorax did not occur. There was 1 case in which the disease was a sequel to a hepatopulmonary amœbic abscess.

The writer discusses very fully the mechanics, symptoms, physical signs, course, prognosis, diagnosis, and treatment of pneumothorax. Emerson's original investigations in connection with the disease have been chiefly in a study of its mechanics and also in an endeavor to determine whether the pneumothorax be a valvular, open, or closed one from careful analyses of the gas contained in the pleural cavity. To both of these considerations he has made valuable contributions.

In regard to treatment, the concensus of opinion seems to be that the air in the chest may be usually disregarded. In other words, it is not necessary to aspirate it. If any considerable amount of fluid be present it should be aspirated, but with great caution. Too much fluid must not be removed and too great a negative pressure in the aspirator must be avoided, otherwise a closed pneumothorax may be converted into an open one.

The Results of Organotherapy in Addison's Disease.—E. W. ADAMS (*The Practitioner*, October, 1903, p. 473) has analyzed 97 cases of this disease reported in the literature and in which adrenal preparations in one form or other were used medicinally, with the object of determining the efficacy of this line of treatment. He classified the cases, with the results as follows: 1. Cases made distinctly worse, 7. 2. Cases deriving no real benefit, 43. 3. Cases showing marked improvement, 31. 4. Cases permanently relieved, 16. There has been a great diversity of preparations of the gland used. The successful results seemed to occur only in those cases where adrenal gland preparations were given solely by mouth. The subcutaneous and intramuscular injection of the adrenal preparation is useless, as it has been shown that the active principle is oxidized and rendered inert when injected into the tissues. Adams says that epinephrin and adrenalin, the newly discovered active principles, do not appear to have been given a trial. He does not state what preparation of the gland given by mouth seems to have proved most beneficial. From the post-mortem records he concludes that the cases most likely to derive benefit are those in which the tuberculous process is a chronic sclerosing one, and where the other organs are fairly sound.

The writer states, in drawing his conclusions, that there would appear to be a certain class of cases of Addison's disease which derives indubitable benefit from the exhibition of some form of suprarenal substance, although in any given case it remains up to now impossible to determine its probable response to the treatment. In any given case, selected haphazard, the probability is that disappointment will follow on the institution of organotherapy; but that probability is very distinctly less than that attaching to any alternative method of treatment at present known. He believes that the last word upon the preparation to be used and its method of administration remains to be said. The problem seems to be to get a sufficient and continuous dose of the pure and active principle unchanged into the blood stream. Intravenous injection is held to be impracticable.

SURGERY.

UNDER THE CHARGE OF

J. WILLIAM WHITE, M.D.,

JOHN RHEA BARTON PROFESSOR OF SURGERY IN THE UNIVERSITY OF PENNSYLVANIA; SURGEON TO THE UNIVERSITY HOSPITAL,

AND

F. D. PATTERSON, M.D.,

SURGEON TO THE X-RAY DEPARTMENT OF THE HOWARD HOSPITAL; CLINICAL ASSISTANT TO THE OUT-PATIENT SURGICAL DEPARTMENT OF THE JEFFERSON HOSPITAL.

The Treatment of the Appendix Stump after Extirpation.—RIEDEL (*Centralblatt f. Chir.*, 1903, No. 51) states that he differs most widely from the remarks of Zellar (an abstract appears in this number), and that the best method is as follows: the mesentery should be freely separated from the appendix and then the appendix should be ligated with catgut close to the gut. Catgut is preferable to silk, as it can be tied tighter, and it does not tend to injure the bowel. The appendix should again be ligated, this time with silk, 1 cm. away from the first ligature and then divided between them. The mucous membrane of this stump should then be excised with scissors and the remaining coats should then be closely approximated with three silk interrupted sutures; the temporary catgut ligature which was first applied should then be cut. In aseptic cases no drainage is necessary, but if indicated one should not hesitate to use it.

Extirpation of the Appendix.—ZELLER (*Centralblatt f. Chir.*, 1903, No. 45) states that one method of treatment of the stump of the appendix after extirpation is to leave a "cuff," which is then sewed over the stump; still another consists in the turning in or invagination of the stump into the cæcum, and then the area is closed by Lembert sutures. This method, however, may produce dangerous sequelæ, such as abscess, as in the case reported by Horman (*Centralblatt f. Chir.*, 1901, p. 1028), where the patient succumbed five days after operation from this cause. The author recommends as the best procedure to separate the appendix from its mesentery and then, taking care to prevent the escape of any of the intestinal contents, to cut it absolutely flush with the bowel, and then to close the resulting hole in the gut by two rows of Lembert sutures. This method has uniformly been followed by a good result and would seem to be the safest method of avoiding the formation of a fecal fistula.

The Treatment of Granulating Wounds.—WAGNER (*Centralblatt f. Chir.*, No. 50, 1903), after discussing in detail the treatment of these wounds by means of different ointments and aseptic dressings, states that his efforts have been directed toward lessening the period of granulation. In the large superficial wounds skin grafting has proved most efficacious on many occasions, but it is a useless procedure in the presence of active suppuration. In those cases where the granulations have a tendency to be œdematous and as a result the dressings are kept constantly moist by the discharge, ointments will prove to be useless, as they only tend to increase heat and moisture and at the same time absolutely prevent the contact of the air with the wound. If such cases have their wounds exposed to the air during the daytime one will soon see the whole aspect change; the secretion becomes much less and healing follows. At night they should be covered by a suitable dressing to prevent infection from the bed-clothes. The author notes having selected two practically similar cases and treated one by the "open" and the other by the "closed" method, and the one treated by the former method healed in much the shorter space of time. In no case did any infection result from the exposure of the wounds to the air.

A New Operation for Hemorrhoids.—LANDSTRÖM (*Centralblatt f. Chir.*, 1903, No. 47) states that extirpation and cauterization are well-known methods and that the treatment by ligature has also many advocates, but that lately he has used the following method in his hospital work, with excellent results. The principle of the operation is to exert strong pressure by means of forceps on the hemorrhoidal mass, which is thus excised. The blade of these forceps is about 7 cm. long by 5 cm. wide; they should be applied in a similar manner to the Langenbeck forceps. The patient is prepared in the usual manner, then placed in the side position, the sphincter dilated, the forceps applied, the hemorrhoidal mass removed, and the operation completed by the introduction of some iodoform gauze, which, however, should be removed on the second day. The operation requires but very few moments for its performance and the hæmostasis is nearly absolute, and so the operation is an admirable one for weak patients. The author notes the successful use of this method in 25 cases, and has found it to be a most satisfactory method of procedure.

The Radical Cure of Inguinal Hernia, with Especial Reference to the Anatomy.—HOFMAN (*Centralblatt f. Chir.*, 1903, No. 41) bases his observations upon an experience of 45 cases during the past year upon whom the radical cure was attempted. The most perfect asepsis is an absolute essential, for upon it depends the success of the operation.

Too much importance cannot be laid upon the absolute closure of the sac in the region of the parietal peritoneum and the restoration or re-establishment of a support for the same at the internal ring by one or more wire-thread sutures, but care should be taken at this time not to disturb the normal relation of the spermatic cord. This presents no extraordinary difficulty if proper care be taken in the insertion of a purse-string suture into the sac and in the subsequent sutures. The author's series of 45 cases made an uninterrupted recovery, and when examined a year later showed no evidence of recurrence.

THERAPEUTICS.

UNDER THE CHARGE OF

REYNOLD WEBB WILCOX, M.D., LL.D.,

PROFESSOR OF MEDICINE AND THERAPEUTICS AT THE NEW YORK POST-GRADUATE MEDICAL SCHOOL AND HOSPITAL; VISITING PHYSICIAN TO ST. MARK'S HOSPITAL.

Treatment of Mucomembranous Enterocolitis.—DR. PEROCHAUD asserts that the three principal indications in this affection are these: to modify the general state of the nervous system, to modify the local nervous conditiou, and to excite the trophic action of the abdominal nerves. If the disease is of long standing absolute quiet and milk diet must be enjoined. In the cases of short duration, in addition to milk, cereals, soft-boiled eggs, small quantities of the various meats—cut very fine—fish and the green vegetables are allowable. Fruit, if eaten at all, must be cooked, and bread should be eaten in small quantity. No fat soups may be taken. Water is the preferable beverage, but beer and wine together with the mildly alkaline mineral waters may be drunk in small amounts. Beverages are useful to combat the tendency to constipation, and milk drunk during meals often renders service in this connection. Highly seasoned food should be interdicted. In severe forms of the disease where absolute milk diet is intolerable, cereals and finely chopped meat may be given. It is very necessary that a daily movement of the bowels should be secured, but this must be done without irritating the intestine. The author recommends for this purpose injections of olive oil and castor oil by the mouth, but other laxatives may be employed; most important is the acquirement of the habit of going to stool every day at the same hour. Abdominal pain may be relieved by hot applications, cannabis indica, belladonna, and, as a last resort, morphine. Abdominal massage is useful in this connection as well as in combating the constipation. Intestinal lavage is to be employed for the removal of the products of the disease from the intestine. It should be given through a tube passed high into the rectum, and in atonic conditions of the intestine should be at a temperature of 103° F., while, if the opposite state obtains, at 98° F.; the quantity should be about two quarts and the procedure should take at least twenty minutes. Various solutions may be used. Naphthol, 1:300; ichthyol, 1:64; or solutions of sodium bicarbonate, sodium chloride, sodium borate, silver nitrate, etc. The author highly recommends beer yeast to be taken in doses of about one-half a drachm slightly diluted three times a day between meals, and asserts that his results from its use have been most excellent. General tonic treatment should also be prescribed, but the greatest care should be observed lest the digestive tract be disturbed by it. Massage, hydrotherapy, and electrotherapy, especially the latter, are important adjuncts to the other treatment.—*Gazette médicale de Nantes*, 1903, No. 51, p. 1021.

Wine and Alcoholic Beverages in Dyspepsia.—DR. ALBERT MATHIEU considers that the routine use of alcohol in gastric disorders is not to be tolerated, though Boas has shown that in small quantities it stimulates stomach digestion. Alcohol, when injected directly into the organ, has a direct action upon its lining and a chemical action upon its contents. Linossier has shown that alcohol diminishes the peptonizing power of the gastric juice and has the same action upon the trypsin. Alcohol also retards the inversion of saccharose in the presence of beer yeast. Dastre has proven as well that it also interferes with pancreatic digestion. It is therefore evident that in marked gastric lesions, such as ulcer, cancer, gastritis, with congestion of the peptic glands or atrophy of the same, alcohol is contra-indicated not only because it retards digestion and increases the pain, but also since it aggravates the lesion. The patients who appear to be benefited by the use of alcohol are those whose stomachs lack motor power and who have a sensation of weight or inflation after eating. Such find relief from a small glass of cognac or liqueur at the end of a meal. It is probable, however, that even in these cases the habit increases their disease in the end. They may better take a glass of hot, well diluted, red or white wine during or after the meal from time to time. The author believes that patients troubled by acid regurgitation may be relieved by taking white wine, preferably sparkling, well diluted. Wine, especially red wine, increases the discomfort of those with a tendency to gastric stasis and distress. In all cases the use of wine should be left off and renewed from time to time if it is to produce its best effect.—*Revue de thérapeutique*, 1903, No. 23, p. 798.

Renal Opotherapy.—M. RENAULT has administered the macerated kidney of the pig in various forms of renal disease with striking results. He states that this form of medication rapidly induces diuresis, and when continued brings the quantity of urinary secretion to normal and maintains it. It reduces the quantity of albumin excreted by the insufficient kidney and often causes its entire disappearance for considerable periods, consequently it favors the restoration of the epithelium of the organ to a histologically normal condition. The macerated kidney also exercises an antitoxic action and the antitoxin which it contains is not changed by the digestive processes. In some patients mild toxic symptoms may be produced, such as pruritis, urticaria, sudorific crises, slight gastric disturbance, etc., but aside from these its action is entirely beneficial. Arterial hypertension, excitability of the heart, and tendency to dilatation always lessen under its influence if it is administered for a sufficiently long time. It is a therapeutic agent that should be in general use, not as a substitute for other medication, but as an adjunct to it. The chief disadvantage of the treatment is that the kidney must be prepared freshly every day.—*Gazette médicale de Paris*, 1903, No. 52, p. 454.

The Prophylaxis of Gonorrhœa.—Dr. Jules Janet, after considering the use of most of the means recommended for the prevention of gonorrhœal infection, such as the condom, the application of vaseline to the meatus before coitus, and the injection of various antiseptics (mercury bichloride 1 : 1000 to 1 : 10,000; silver nitrate, 2 per cent.; protargol, 4 to 20 per cent.), concludes with the statement that, while he recommends to his patients the instillation into the fossa navicularis of several drops of a solution of silver nitrate 2 per cent., or of protargol 20 per cent., he believes the only true prophylaxis of the disease is not to lay one's self liable to infection.—*Revue de thérapeutique*, 1903, No. 24, p. 829.

The Internal Treatment of Gonorrhœa.—Dr. Edmund Saalfeld reports excellent results in a considerable number of cases from the internal administration of capsules of gonosan, which is a preparation of the resin of kava-kava and sandal oil. Under this agent the purulent discharge in a short time becomes mucoid, the pain is diminished, painful erections are rendered less frequent and distressing, and complications, such as epididymitis, prostatitis, cystitis, and adenitis are unlikely to occur. The author believes that gonosan is of especial value in patients in whom local treatment for any reason cannot be frequently applied.—*Therapeutische Monatshefte*, 1903, No. 12, p. 626.

Extract of Thymus in Chloroanæmia.—Dr. G. Marcolongo has experimented with the extract of the thymus gland in the chloroses of childhood and adolescence and has found that in five patients, varying in age from eight to twenty-one years, the hæmoglobin percentage and the number and resistance of the red cells rapidly increased. At the same time a considerable amelioration of the general condition and an increase in weight was noted. The preparation employed contained one part of the juice of the gland suspended in two parts of neutral glycerin. Of this, two and one-half drachms were given each morning and night.—*La semaine médicale*, 1903, No. 50, p. 412.

Potassium Iodide in Ophthalmology.—Dr. A. Leprince has had occasion to use this drug in various ophthalmic lesions, infantile cataract, episcleritis, scleritis, and iridocyclitis. In all the cases considerable improvement was shown after the first day and cure followed after varying periods of time, depending upon the severity of the disease. In rheumatic and arthritic lesions the treatment is especially applicable. The iodide is employed in strengths of from 1 to 2.5 per cent., depending upon the nature of the affection. Of this solution, from two to three drops are instilled into the eye from one to three times a day. The procedure is painless and provokes no reaction. In the author's opinion severe cases might be benefited by subconjunctival injections of the solution.—*Revue française de médecine et de chirurgie*, 1903, No. 57, p. 1361.

Sodium Salicylate in Lupus.—Dr. A. Plique calls attention to the use of sodium salicylate in two cases of lupus under his observation. Villemin the younger has experimented upon cultures of the bacillus tuberculosis and has found that only six agents produced complete sterilization; of these, four were salicylic acid derivatives, of which sodium salicylate seemed most applicable to the purpose in hand. The drug was used in the following solution: sodium salicylate, 1; distilled water, 8. Applications of this were made morning and evening to the involved areas. The only untoward effect produced was a slightly disfiguring white pellicle. The addition to the solution of a little fuchsin produced a rose color and greatly lessened the disfigurement. This latter should be added in as small quantity as possible, so as not to diminish the tolerance of the tissues and not to increase the irritation. The two cases treated were of long standing and obstinate facial lupus; in one six weeks and in the other one month of treatment produced a considerable amelioration. The cures are not complete, since certain small hard nodules remain. The author suggests that it would be interesting to inject the solution into these, but before doing this it would be well to further observe the results of topical application.—*Journal de médecine et chirurgie pratique*, 1903, No. 24, p. 929.

OBSTETRICS.

UNDER THE CHARGE OF

EDWARD P. DAVIS, A.M., M.D.,

PROFESSOR OF OBSTETRICS IN THE JEFFERSON MEDICAL COLLEGE; PROFESSOR OF OBSTETRICS AND DISEASES OF INFANCY IN THE PHILADELPHIA POLYCLINIC; CLINICAL PROFESSOR OF DISEASES OF CHILDREN IN THE WOMAN'S MEDICAL COLLEGE; VISITING OBSTETRICIAN TO THE PHILADELPHIA HOSPITAL, ETC.

Distention of the Lower Uterine Segment Before the Rupture of the Membranes.— GOLDNER (*Monatsschrift für Geburtshülfe und Gynäkologie*, Band xviii., Heft 4, 1903) contributes an interesting and practically important paper upon this subject.

He calls attention to reported cases of rupture of the uterus in which the ovum has been expelled into the abdominal cavity with unruptured membranes. His own observations cover a period of about three years with 9000 cases of labor, among whom there were 321 cases in which the lower uterine segment became abnormally distended, and of these in 19 this distention occurred before the rupture of the membranes. From these cases he concludes that this distention arises from the great predominance of the muscular tissues in the contractile segment of the uterus. He finds that a long continuance of labor pains, repeated labor, and early rupture of the membranes all tend to produce this condition. In his 19 cases, 17 were primiparæ of the average age of childbearing. No disease which might affect the muscular tissue of the uterus was present in these cases. The children were not abuormally large, nor were there pelvic conditions which obstructed birth. In 7 of the 17 cases the cranium remained high and movable above the entrance to the pelvis. Oligohydramnios was present in 9 of the 19 cases, five times with normal pelvis and four times with contracted pelvis. Some pelvic contraction was present in 8 cases, although but 3 of these had contraction sufficiently great to influence the course of labor. In 6 cases there was absolutely no abnormality to which could be ascribed the condition. Toughness and resistance of the membranes with oligohydramnios and a rigid and undilatable external os were the conditions which seemed to predispose to abnormal distention of the lower uterine segment with unruptured membranes. In 15 of these cases the contraction ring was as high as the umbilicus. In 10 cases the contraction could be plainly discerned immediately after the birth of the child.

In 13 of these patients it was necessary to interfere to expedite labor. It was in all these cases possible to examine the patient before active pai s came on and to be sure that the membranes had not ruptured through a laceration in the membranes high above the presenting part.

Tubal Gestation in Which the Ovum Continued to Grow about Four Weeks after Rupture, Becoming Implanted on the Omentum.—LOCKYER (*Journal of Obstetrics and Gynecology of the British Empire*, November, 1903) publishes the case of a patient who had attacks of irregular abdominal pain accompanied by collapse. A critical examination of the history revealed the fact that the patient had had four distinct attacks of internal hemorrhage. The left side of the abdomen was tender and considerably swollen, and upon opening the abdomen the omentum was pushed upward by extravasated blood. The fetus appeared in the wound and the placenta had been attached to the omentum near the left broad ligament. The placenta had also been attached to part of the rectum and the side of the p vi brim. The general oozing was stopped by gauze packing and stimulation was freely employed. The patient died in collapse twenty-four hours after operation.

Upon examination the fetus was four months advanced. There was no attempt at the formation of an hæmatocele, but the pregnancy had been secondary abdominal pregnancy, the tube having ruptured in the early weeks of gestation followed by the temporary recovery of the mother. The villi, penetrating the wall of the tube, had gained attachments upon the omentum, to the rectum, and to the peritoneum forming the posterior layer of the broad ligament. The fetus remained alive until it passed through a large tear in the secondary gestation sac.

A Statistical Study of Eclampsia.—In the *Archiv für Gynäkologie*, Band lxx., Heft 2, 1903, BUTTNER contributes the results of an extensive statistical study in eclampsia. The number of confinements available for study was 143,304. Among these occurred 321 cases of eclampsia, or 1 in 446.4. The frequency of eclampsia was considerably increased since the former statistics taken from 1885 to 1891. Among these patients, 73.7 per cent. were primiparæ, 26.3 per cent. multiparæ; 18 per cent. of the primiparæ were older than twenty-eight years and 5 per cent. were seventeen years and younger. Twin pregnancy was present in cases of eclampsia in 6 per cent. Although the frequency of eclampsia was increased in those portions of Germany from which these statistics were taken, the mortality was somewhat diminished. In the series of cases reported the mortality was 21.12 per cent., in contrast with a previous mortality of 34.8 per cent. The results of treatment are shown in the fact that in districts where physicians could be obtained with difficulty the mortality rose to 27.4 per cent. In three cases diagnosis was not made during life and the patients perished undelivered. The mortality of eclampsia occurring during labor was

20.5 per cent. Where eclampsia developed after labor the mortality was 24.07 per cent. The longer after delivery the eclampsia occurred, the better the prognosis for the mother. If, however, eclampsia develops during the latter portion of the first day after labor, the mortality rises cousiderably.

The mortality for the fetus was 29.7 per cent. Here again among cases in the country and in small hamlets the mortality among children was greatly increased, rising to 32.4 per cent. About 50 per cent. of the mothers required artificial delivery. It is shown that prompt interference during labor, resulting in the rapid delivery of the child, improves the mother's chances in those cases where eclampsia develops during parturition. When the mother dies of eclampsia during labor, fetal mortality is enormously increased. In cases where the mother dies after the delivery of the child the chances of the fetus for survival seemed to be fairly good.

Regarding the repetition of eclampsia in the same patient, it was found that 2.40 per cent. of the patients had eclampsia more than once. The effort was made to determine the influence of the weather upon the occurrence of eclampsia, and it was found that the colder months showed an increase in the percentage of cases. The percentage of moisture in the atmosphere seemed to influence the occurrence of eclampsia, as the drier the air the better the conditions for the patient. Extremes of heat or cold were both marked by an increase in eclampsia.

Regarding the question as to the relationship existing between eclampsia and labor pains or contractions of the uterus, it was determined that eclampsia is not caused by labor pains, but that eclampsia first occurs and then uterine contractions. Both contractions of the uterus and eclamptic convulsions result from irritation of the same poison.

As regards the occurrence of eclampsia in epileptic women, upon close examination of the history of cases, but two could be found in which it seemed probable that epilepsy and eclampsia occurred in the same person.

GYNECOLOGY.

UNDER THE CHARGE OF

HENRY C. COE, M.D.,

OF NEW YORK.

ASSISTED BY

WILLIAM E. STUDDIFORD, M.D.

Epithelial Spaces in Lymph Nodes—FALKNER (*Zentralblatt für Gynäkologie*, No. 50, 1903) found in 13 per cent. of Wertheim's cases of radical operation for cancer of the uterus peculiar spaces within the lymph glands lined with columnar epithelium. Eighty cadavers were examined (not cases of cancer) and the pelvic glands were studied microscopically without showing any of these spaces. Hence the inference that they are not related to the Wolffian bodies (as thought by various observers), but to the uterine carcinoma. Observations by

Meyer have subsequently shown that these may be due to some other irritation. The inference that these spaces always represent beginning cancerous degeneration is not correct, though in some instances Wertheim demonstrated the presence of epitheliomatous invasion of the spaces.

Exfoliative Endometritis.—GOTTSCHALK (*Zentralblatt für Gynäkologie*, No. 49, 1903) describes a specimen in which it was shown that the exfoliation was due to hemorrhage into the submucous layer. Numerous venous thrombi were present, indicating obstruction and resulting rupture of the vessels, doubtless due to diminished cardiac action. This was also indicated by the presence of slight œdema of the lower limbs. Although repeated curettement and intrauterine applications had failed to relieve the membranous dysmenorrhœa, it was cured by remedies indicated by the cardiac weakness.

Drainage.—MARTIN (Chrobak's *Festschrift; Zentralblatt für Gynäkologie*, No. 49, 1903) believes that it is impossible to predict before operation in a given case whether pus is infectious or not, although examinations of the blood are undoubtedly of value. It has been the writer's practise not to drain after laparotomy unless marked leukocytosis is present, and especially if a pus-sac is removed without rupture. If the intestine is injured or there are large raw surfaces which cannot be covered with peritoneum, the gauze tamponade is used and the ends are carried through both the abdominal and vaginal openings.

Modern Gynecological Operations.—FRITSCH (*Ibid.*) criticises the tendency of surgeons to adopt routine methods of procedure. While the vaginal route is preferable when a tumor is readily accessible, he believes that in the majority of cases abdominal section will be attended with the best results, whether the case is one of uterine fibroid, adnexal disease, or extrauterine pregnancy. He thinks that, while Alexander's operation is safer, ventrofixation gives the best results, and both are superior to vaginofixation.

Preservation of the Ovaries after Total Extirpation of the Uterus.—LEOPOLD AND EHRENFREUND (*Ibid.*) reports the results in 151 cases of vaginal hysterectomy for fibroids. The operation was limited to the removal of tumors not larger than a child's head. Ligatures were used, the mortality being only 3.9 per cent. Out of 102 patients who were kept under observation, all but four made a perfect recovery and were able to attend to their usual occupations. Although one or both ovaries was preserved, climacteric disturbances were frequently noted, though never so severe as to affect the patient's general health.

Fibromyoma of the Vagina.—POTEL (*Revue de Gynécologie*, Band vii., Heft 2–4) adds 2 cases to 160 in the literature. Eighty-four per cent. occurred in young women. The pedunculated form is most common, and 50 per cent. occur in the anterior vaginal wall. They grow slowly their growth being accelerated by pregnancy. In all but 6 cases the neoplasm was a fibromyoma. The only treatment is extirpation, which may require careful dissection from the rectum and bladder and ligation of the nutrient vessels, especially in the case of sessile growths.

Leukocytosis in Inflammatory Disease of the Adnexa.—KIRCHMAYR (*Wiener klin. Rundschau*, No. 11, 1903) found marked leukocytosis in all his cases of parametric and perimetric abscesses, 17,190 being the highest count noted. In several instances in which no pus was found the number of leukocytes was doubled after operation, probably due to fresh lymphatic infection. The writer infers that a leukocytosis of 30,000 points with great probability to the presence of pus, but that a moderate increase in the number of white cells is of little diagnostic value. The fact that there is no increase is not evidence that pus is absent.

Drainage in Laparotomy—DODERLEIN (*Zentralblatt für Gynäkologie*, 1903, No. 471) drained the pelvic cavity per vaginam in 161 out of 754 abdominal sections (21.3 per cent.), with a mortality of 8.7 per cent., losing only 2.3 per cent. of the patients where no drainage was employed, though in the former series the cases were more serious.

FEHLING (*Ibid.*) prefers drainage through the abdominal wound with a Mikulicz tampon. He drained only thirty-six times in 327 laparotomies, his general death rate being 4.5 per cent. In 55 pus cases (with a mortality of 1.8 per cent.) the Mikulicz tampon was used in 28, with 1 death; in 27 cases without drainage there was no mortality.

OPHTHALMOLOGY.

UNDER THE CHARGE OF

EDWARD JACKSON, A.M., M.D.,
OF DENVER, COLORADO,

AND

T. B. SCHNEIDEMAN, A.M., M.D.,
PROFESSOR OF DISEASES OF THE EYE IN THE PHILADELPHIA POLYCLINIC.

Possibility of Radium Rays in Blindness.—TRACY (*Journal of Advanced Therapeutics*, December, 1903) refers to the use of radium in optic atrophy and reports a case. Giesel's observation that when a tube of radium touched the eyelids of the closed eyes a sensation of light was produced, has suggested the attempt to employ this property to stimulate the optic nerve in cases of blindness from nerve disease with retention of light perception. Lunden, of Berlin, affirms that he obtained good results from radium in the case of two boys who were almost totally blind.

Tracy reports improvement in the case of a man fifty-two years of age who had been affected with optic atrophy for four years.

Cataract Extraction, with a Small Peripheral Buttonhole in the Iris; Report of 312 Cases.—CHANDLER (*Archives of Ophthalmology*, January, 1904) removes a piece of iris 1 mm. in diameter as near to its root as possible to prevent prolapse; the opening permits drainage of the aqueous and expression of the cortex. He usually makes it after extraction of the lens. It is necessary to use a forceps the teeth of which are at the tip end, and scissors with very thin blades.

Three hundred and twelve senile cataracts operated on by this method with one or two exceptions gave the following satisfactory results: vision above $\frac{1}{10}$, 91.2 per cent.; $\frac{1}{20}$, 3.5 per cent.; $\frac{1}{30}$, 2.6 per cent.; fingers and projection, 1.2 per cent.; lost 1.5 per cent. There were 4 cases of prolapsed iris, 2 the direct result of accidental violence after re-establishment of the anterior chamber. Iritis occurred in varying degrees in 32 eyes, with blocked pupil in 3 cases; 4 eyes were lost, 3 from corneal suppuration and 1 from panophthalmitis. Secondary operation was performed in 67 cases without any inflammatory reaction.

The average stay in the hospital was eighteen and two-third days.

Sympathetic Ophthalmia.—Ramsay (*Annals of Ophthalmology*, January, 1904) details the morbid changes in the exciting eye which are likely to give rise to sympathetic inflammation, such as penetrating wounds of the ciliary region, foreign bodies lodged within the eyeball, degenerative changes in an eye previously injured, corneal ulcers which have perforated. Sarcoma of the choroid or dislocation of the lens accompanied by plastic iridocyclitis may also induce sympathetic inflammation; but these are probably the only instances in which the disease arises apart from a perforating lesion of the exciter. The disease probably never occurs earlier than three weeks; after that there is no limit. On an average it develops most frequently five or six weeks after the accident. If the second eye escape until the one injured has healed, it will probably not occur at all unless fresh inflammation or degenerative changes occur in the exciting eye. It is more frequent in the young than in the old. Its onset is most insidious. Serious results are frequently not anticipated until the disease is thoroughly established. The prognosis is always grave.

Sympathetic inflammation must be distinguished from irritation; the latter is simply a neurosis and passes off without leaving any organic changes.

Mackenzie was the first to demonstrate the causal connection between the exciter and the sympathizing eye. He considered that the disease was transmitted by the optic nerve across the chiasm. Leber and Deutschmann have advanced the theory that sympathetic inflammation was the result of a septic infectious process in the injured eye and that the micro-organisms travelled along the optic nerves to the sound eye. Unfortunately subsequent investigations have failed to verify these conclusions and they are now generally discredited. All clinical experiences, however, go to support the theory that infection of the injured eye is necessary to cause inflammation in the other, but there seems no reason for supposing that a specific micro-organism is necessary. Injury of one eye is itself capable of producing nutritional disturbances in the other, but in addition to such vasomotor changes another factor must be present before true inflammation is excited; this other factor is no doubt microbic infection. The difficulty lies in demonstrating the channels of communication between the two eyes along which the microbiotic factor finds its way. There are three such passages: the bloodvessels, the ciliary nerves, and the optic nerves. The latter can be excluded from the clinical phenomena. It would appear that the infecting influence, microbe or toxin, reaches the sound eye through the blood stream and that its virulence is concentrated upon the anterior uveal tract, whose nutrition has already been lowered by the irritation of the ciliary nerves of the injured eye.

Enucleation of a severely injured eye is advised except under two circumstances, first, when there is still sight in the injured eye and no sign of sympathetic disturbance in its fellow; and, second, when sympathetic inflammation is in progress and there is still sight in the exciting eye.

The usual antiphlogistic regimen and treatment for iridocyclitis are recommended, special stress being laid upon mercury.

No operation ought to be attempted until some time after all acute symptoms have subsided.

DERMATOLOGY.

UNDER THE CHARGE OF

LOUIS A. DUHRING, M.D.,

PROFESSOR OF DERMATOLOGY IN THE UNIVERSITY OF PENNSYLVANIA,

AND

MILTON B. HARTZELL, M.D.,

INSTRUCTOR IN DERMATOLOGY IN THE UNIVERSITY OF PENNSYLVANIA.

Erythrodermia Exfoliativa Universalis Tuberculosa.—BRUUSGAARD, (*Archiv für Dermatologie und Syphilis*, Bd. lxvii., Heft 2), as a contribution to the study of tuberculous affections of the skin, reports the case of a woman, sixty-three years old, who developed an inflammation of the skin which, at first limited to the calves, in the course of some months became universal. The inflammation was accompanied by marked redness, infiltration, and exfoliation, without moisture. Upon the entrance of the patient into the hospital there was marked swelling of all the palpable lymph glands. The hair and nails were implicated early in the disease, and were gradually cast off. The severity of the inflammation increased, and a marked tendency to acute exacerbations appeared with increased exfoliation. The exacerbations were often accompanied by increased fever, dyspnœa, and intolerable itching. As the patient's general condition grew worse the exacerbations diminished in intensity and frequency. The final stages of the disease were characterized by increasing cachexia, a peculiar pigmentation associated with the follicles, and universal swelling of the lymph glands. The patient finally died of bronchopneumonia. At the autopsy the lymph glands were found to be markedly swollen and to contain large and small broken-down foci in which numerous tubercle bacilli were demonstrable. The liver and spleen also contained isolated miliary tubercles with giant cells, and the ileum contained a tuberculous ulcer. Sections of skin taken from various parts of the body showed typical tubercles with giant cells and bacilli. The tubercles were situated in the papillary and subpapillary layers of the skin, and in a single section were found plainly localized about a hair follicle.

A Year's Trial of the Light Treatment for Lupus.—C. M .O'Brien (*Dublin Journal of Medical Science*, August, 1903) used the French Lorbet-Genoud lamp, usually fifteen minutes being allowed for each sitting, and the current 12 ampères, but where it was tolerated by the patient, longer sittings were made use of (twenty to sixty minutes), with from 12 to 18 ampères. The author thinks that some of the failures attributed to the French lamp compared with the results from the Danish lamp. Lengthening may be overcome by the sittings. In cases attended with ulceration, where the pressure of the Danish method could not be tolerated, the Roentgen rays were used until sufficient healing had occurred to permit of further treatment by the ultra-violet rays. The results of the author upon the whole were highly satisfactory, and he thinks, as to permanency of cure, that the Danish light cannot be excelled. In circumscribed superficial lupus the Danish (Finsen) light, properly used, takes a conspicuous position among the most notable discoveries in modern medicine.

A Case of Erythema Induratum (Bazin) Combined with Lichen Scrofulosorum.—JULIUS SOLLNER (*Monatshefte für prakt. Derm.*, December 15, 1903) gives full notes of the case, with microscopic examination of the lesions. No tubercle bacilli were found. After consideration of the various relations of the two diseases, he concludes that the manifestation of erythema induratum is either tuberculosis or is related to that disease in a manner like that of lichen scrofulosorum to tuberculosis.

Protozoa in a Case of Tropical Ulcer ("Aleppo Boil").—J. H. WRIGHT (*Journal of Cutaneous Diseases*, January, 1904) states that this disease, which is generally believed to be of an infectious nature and capable of transmission from one individual to another by inoculation, but apparently not contagious in the usual meaning of that term, has considerable resemblance to tuberculosis and syphilis of the skin. A case was observed in Boston in the person of an Armenian child, aged nine years. In thin stained smears peculiar bodies having the following characters were discovered. They were round, sharply defined, and 2 to 4 micromillimetres in diameter. In each of the bodies there was a larger and a smaller lilac-colored mass. These bodies were present in very large numbers in the smears, and there is good reason for believing them to be micro-organisms and the infectious cause of the disease, and further that they are protozoa. Reference is made to the studies of other observers in the same disease. Photographs accompany the article.

Pyæmic Dermatitis.—LEBET (*Annales de Dermatologie et de Syphiligraphie*, No. 12, 1903), after a brief résumé of the literature concerning some of the dermatoses which occur as a complication of or, in some instances, as the chief symptom in general infectious diseases, reports a case of eruption consisting of pustules, macules, deep-seated nodules, and abscesses in a boy, aged seven years, as a sequel of an infected wound of the heel. The author's conclusions concerning pyæmic inflammations of the skin are as follows: In pyosepticæmic infections there are dermatoses produced by microbes (staphylococci and streptococci) brought to the skin through the bloodvessels—metastatic pyæmic dermatoses. These dermatoses may be multiform (purpuric, pustular, varioliform, and nodose). There is no reason for placing these affections in the group of angioneuroses; they are not erythemata, but inflammations. Bacteria may form superficial metastases in the capillaries of the papillæ, in the derma, or in the subcutaneous connective tissue, in the last case affecting the veins by preference. The virulence of the microbes brought to the skin by the blood seems to be at times attenuated by this transportation, as suppuration may be absent even in the presence of pyogenic micro-organisms.

A Rare Form of Xanthoma.—W. Moser (*New York Medical Journal*, October 10, 1903) records the case of an Italian boy with multiple, mushroom-like growths, varying in size from a pea to a hen's egg, of a bright yellow or yellowish-pink color, neither sensitive to pressure nor painful, smooth and not nodulated, tuberculated, nor fissured. They had existed for a long period and gave rise to no symptoms beyond the discomfort of their presence. The microscope showed them to be made up of a yellow fibrous tissue, the cellular elements being scanty, polymorphic, and pigmented.

HYGIENE AND PUBLIC HEALTH.

UNDER THE CHARGE OF

CHARLES HARRINGTON, M.D.,

ASSISTANT PROFESSOR OF HYGIENE, HARVARD MEDICAL SCHOOL.

Malaria in Places Usually Free from Anopheles.—Several cases are communicated by Dr. John Cropper (*Journal of Hygiene*, October, 1903, p. 515) illustrative of a difficulty which often occurs to those who study the agency of anopheles in the causation of malaria and which has led sometimes to disbelief in such agency. In a former paper on the "Geographical Distribution of Malaria in Upper Palestine" (*Ibid.*, 1902, p. 47) he had said that, although resident for some years in the town of Acre, he had never been able to find a single specimen of anopheles. This year his successor had two patients ill with malaria, and in their room the anopheles were found. The disease is rare in Acre, but common enough a mile away. The preceding winter was exceptionally wet, and the water covered the plain to within less than a half-mile from the town, near the wall of which the house of the patients was situate. At Shefa Amr, three hours from Acre, within reach of no running water except after heavy rains, two English ladies had malaria. Imagines of anopheles were not found, but the water of an open cistern contained the larvæ. At Nablous, where, in 1901, anopheles larvæ were found in a shallow cistern, an examination of several open cisterns in houses where the disease occurred gave negative results. Visitors come often from notoriously malarial districts within easy reach and introduce the parasite. "So it is, probably, with many if not all places in the Tropics not essentially malarious—*i. e.*, not furnished with an abundant supply of anopheles."

Formaldehyde Disinfection.—In disinfection of rooms with formaldehyde, the gas tends toward the ceiling, in spite of the fact that its specific gravity is slightly greater than that of air, and so the upper parts are more thoroughly disinfected than the lower. To overcome this irregularity, MAYER and WOLPERT (*Archiv für Hygiene,* vol. xliii. p. 171) introduced a rotary fan, which brought about a better result. The influence of temperature is shown by the fact that at temperatures below freezing the gas has no influence whatever on anthrax spores. Each degree increase beyond 50° F. to 60° F. shows a distinct increase in efficiency, and at 86° F. the action is very marked. (*Ibid.*, p. 222.)

Toxicity of Coal-tar Colors.—In Russia the use of coal-tar colors in articles of food and drink was prohibited in January, 1898, but nevertheless they are largely employed. For example, fourteen of fifteen confections examined at Dorpat were found to be so colored, and about the same results have been obtained at the public laboratories at Moscow, St. Petersburg, Odessa, Kiew, and Warsaw. In order to determine their toxicity, PROFESSOR G. W. CLOPIN (*Hygienische Rundschau,* August 1, 1903) examined 50 colors, which he gave to dogs in 1-gram to 3-gram doses daily for eight to fourteen days, and also applied to human skin, the subjects wearing woolen or cotton gloves or stockings which had been dyed with the various colors without the use of poisonous mordants. Of the 50 examined, 15, or 30 per cent., proved to be decidedly poisonous, either causing death of the dogs or such severe symptoms of poisoning that they would have died had the experiments continued, and 20, or 40 per cent., were found to cause disturbances of limited extent. Of the distinctly poisonous colors, only 2, ursol D and auramin O, proved to be skin poisons. Ursol D caused severe dermatitis and auramin O irritated the skin only feebly. Like other investigators, he found no red color to be poisonous.

PATHOLOGY AND BACTERIOLOGY.

UNDER THE CHARGE OF

SIMON FLEXNER, M.D.,

DIRECTOR OF THE ROCKEFELLER INSTITUTE FOR MEDICAL RESEARCH, NEW YORK.

ASSISTED BY

WARFIELD T. LONGCOPE, M.D.,

RESIDENT PATHOLOGIST, PENNSYLVANIA HOSPITAL.

A Note on Autolysis in Lobar and Unresolved Pneumonia.—FLEXNER (*Univ. of Penna. Med. Bull.*, 1903, vol. xvi. p. 185) concludes from a long series of experiments made with specimens of typical lobar pneumonia in various stages of the disease, and with ten or twelve examples of unresolved pneumonia, that the process of resolution is in main part accomplished by the self-digestion of the exudate in the pneumonic lung. When protected from the action of bacteria lungs in the stage of grey hepatization were found to undergo autolysis outside the body with great rapidity, while the specimens of red hepatization took much longer to autolyze and those of unresolved pneumonia showed scarcely any change, even after a considerable length of time. The process of autolysis is mainly dependent upon the number of leukocytes in the exudate, and it is this fact which explains the slow and incomplete liquefaction of the exudate in red hepatization and unresolved pneumonia. The exudate in a pneumonic lung which has not undergone resolution is exceedingly poor in cells, and many of the alveoli are plugged with dense hyaline, fibrinous masses. Unresolved pneumonia is, therefore, considered as an acute lobar pneumonia, in which the inflammatory exudate, either because of some disproportion between the leukocytes and other constituents, or because of other causes as yet unknown, failing to autolyze perfectly, cannot be absorbed and hence undergoes organization.

Etiology of the Sleeping Sickness of the Negro.—ALDO CASTELLANI (*Cent. f. Bakt. u. Parasit.*, 1903, Bd. xxxv. p. 62) describes a trypanosoma which he has found in the cerebrospinal fluid of twenty out of thirty-four cases of sleeping sickness investigated in Uganda. In order to demonstrate the parasite, it is necessary to collect about 10 c.c. of spinal fluid, centrifugalize and examine the sediment, when the trypanosoma, at first actively motile, are readily seen. The parasite was not found in the blood, but was discovered in the fluid removed from the lateral ventricles of the brain in two autopsy cases. The cerebrospinal fluid of twelve healthy individuals living in the Uganda district did not contain parasites. The author concludes that the sleeping sickness is in all probability caused by this particular species of trypanosoma.

The Effects of Lymphotoxins and Myelotoxins on the Leukocytes of the Blood and on the Blood-forming Organs.—BUNTING (*Univ. of Penna. Med. Bull.*, 1903, vol. xvi. p. 200) finds that the serum of the normal goose is, to a certain extent, toxic for rabbits when injected intraperitoneally or subcutaneously. This toxicity consists in a moderate depletion in the bone-marrow and lymph glands of preformed cells, and to an early and slightly excessive restoration of these elements after withdrawal. The depletion is in large part due to migration of the cells into the peritoneal cavity, during which process the circulating blood shows at first a scarcity and later an excess of these elements. Only slight signs of toxic action are found in the blood-building organs at a distance from the injections. Serum from a goose which had received successive injections of the bone-marrow of rabbits when inoculated into the rabbit gave rise to changes in the white cells of the circulating blood, and to lesions in the hæmopoietic organs in a measure similar to those produced by injections of normal goose serum. The characteristic action of the myelotoxic serum, however, was its marked effect upon the bone-marrow and the cells derived from the bone-marrow. Following injections of this serum in rabbits the circulating blood showed a sharp and marked rise in the total number of amphophile leukocytes, and a less pronounced increase in the lymphocytes, but still an increase above that called forth by injections of normal serum. The blood picture and the histological alterations in the bone-marrow suggested, therefore, that there had been a sudden and excessive demand upon the bone-marrow for the amphophile leukocytes. Large doses of the myelotoxic serum produced extensive destruction of the bone-marrow elements "in loco."

Serum obtained by treating geese with the lymph glands of rabbits gave rise to changes in rabbits which differed from those produced by normal goose serum chiefly in the fact that the toxic action of the serum was directed toward the lymphoblastic tissues. The circulating blood showed a primary lymphopænia, followed by a definite and often marked absolute lymphocytosis, while the effect upon the amphophile leucocytes was practically the same as that following injections of normal goose serum. A study of the lymph glands especially made it evident that there was an extensive primary injury to these tissues with a later excessive repair of cellular elements. It was found, moreover, that by increasing the hæmolytic power of goose serum for the erythrocytes of the rabbit, the toxic power of the serum for both amphophile leukocytes and lymphocytes of the rabbit was also increased; but these effects were of much less intensity than the characteristic specific changes called forth by injections of the myelotoxic and lymphotoxic sera. Bunting in his conclusions regards leukocytosis as the excessive reaction of leukoblastic tissue to a leukopenia of the circulating blood, due either to a withdrawal of leukocytes from the circulation or to their destruction within the circulation. The amphophile, eosinophile, and basophile leukocytes are derived from the bone-marrow, while the lymphoid cells are chiefly derived from the lymph glands and spleen, although the marrow is a lymphoid tissue and contains typical lymphocytes. Amphophile and eosinophile myelocytes may multiply by mitosis, and their number may be increased by the development of specific granules in the protoplasm of large mononuclear elements with scant basophilic protoplasm, a cell identical in appearance with the cells of the germinal centres of the lymph glands. Megaloblasts are a constituent of normal marrow and form the proliferating centre of erythroblastic tissue.

Further Observations on the Agglutination of Staphylococci.—Otto (*Cent. f. Bakt. u. Parasitten*, 1903, Bd. xxxiv. p. 44) concludes that of the many varieties of staphylococci there is only one which is really pathogenic for man. This variety may be easily diagnosed by its strictly specific agglutinability with the serum from an animal immunized against the pathogenic variety. The true pathogenic form, furthermore, is alone capable of producing hæmolytic staphylotoxin.

Notice to Contributors.—All communications intended for insertion in the Original Department of this Journal are received only *with the distinct understanding that they are contributed exclusively to this Journal.*

Contributions from abroad written in a foreign language, if on examination they are found desirable for this Journal, will be translated at its expense.

A limited number of reprints in pamphlet form will, if desired, be furnished to authors, *provided the request for them be written on the manuscript.*

All communications should be addressed to—

Dr. Francis R. Packard, 1831 Chestnut Street, Philadelphia, U. S. A.

THE

AMERICAN JOURNAL

OF THE MEDICAL SCIENCES.

APRIL, 1904.

THE INFLUENCE OF COMPLICATING DISEASES UPON LEUKÆMIA.*

By George Dock, A.M., M.D.,

PROFESSOR OF MEDICINE IN THE UNIVERSITY OF MICHIGAN, ANN ARBOR, MICHIGAN.

Investigations in leukæmia during the last decade have led to a great increase in our knowledge of the phenomena of that disease, especially of the minute changes in the blood and tissues. But the gains hitherto have added complexity to the subject by suggesting new problems, instead of clearing up the old ones. Failing the discovery of some microscopic germ as the cause from which the various changes can be traced, the elucidation of many details is likely to be brought about only by patient labor in piling up and analyzing observations.

With this idea I have examined one interesting feature, perhaps I should say one set of features in the disease, viz., the changes following or associated with intercurrent disease. Cases of this kind are rapidly multiplying in the literature, and, having had some instructive cases of my own, it seemed to me that a study of these and others might be useful. I soon found that the outcome would not be as rich as I hoped, but the subject seemed worthy of presentation on account of the nature of the material now available.

I will cite my most important case, leaving out many details of the history:

Case I. *Myelogenous (mixed-celled) leukæmia; influenza; reduction of leukocytes to 5000 and below; gradual rise of leukocytes six weeks after the complication, reaching 157,000 in another month;*

* Read before the Academy of Medicine of Cleveland, September 18, 1903.

death seventeen months after the complication.—Mrs. C. D. A., aged forty-two years, housewife, was first seen December 29, 1896. From the notes made then I quote: Patient complains of swelling in the left side, shortness of breath, and weakness. The family history is negative as regards ancestors. The husband, who seemed well during the patient's lifetime, developed splenic anæmia a year after her death. (See *Transactions of Association of American Physicians*, 1903.) The daughter, after the mother's death, had lymphoid hyperplasia in the pharynx and tongue and in the appendix. The latter was the seat of frequent and severe pain; it could be felt as a hard body, as thick as a lead-pencil, through the strong and well-nourished abdominal wall, and was removed at my advice and found to be free from evidences of inflammation, but with lymphoid tissue unusually developed.

Besides the usual acute infectious diseases, the patient had ague twice in childhood, but does not think she had enlarged spleen, "ague-cake" being a familiar sign in that vicinity at the time.

Menstruation began at thirteen years, and was always regular, except during pregnancy, up to two years ago. Since then the flow has been greater, but pale, and accompanied by bearing-down pains.

At nineteen years she had "dysentery," passing blood with the stools for one month. A series of furuncles on the arms and back followed this. She was then fairly well for ten years, was married, and, except for an abortion after the first pregnancy, remained well until her second and last pregnancy, eight years ago. About the fifth month she had a pain in the abdomen, back, and right shoulder, which closely resembled biliary colic. The patient ascribes all her trouble, however, to the confinement, which was difficult, but the exact results of which do not appear. Three months after it she became intensely jaundiced, and remained so for two weeks. The abdominal pain mentioned above returned then, and at intervals, but without jaundice, up to two years ago.

Two years ago the patient thinks the present disease began, with chilly feelings in the back and hands. In two days there was pain in the splenic region, sore throat, pain in the extremities, and slight fever. The chills lasted for two months, occurring sometimes twice a day, followed by fever and sweating. The pain in the left side continued up to six weeks ago. It was thought to be pleuritic. Three months ago the swelling on the left side was discovered by the patient. It was then about the size of an apple. Soon after the swelling was discovered the chills and fever returned, with paroxysms, usually about 11 A.M. and 2 or 3 P.M., but any exertion was likely to be followed by a chill. The tumor gradually became larger. About two months ago a throbbing pain began in the posterior part of it, and lasted about a month. Then severe and unexplained vomiting came on, and in a paroxysm of vomiting it seemed as if something had fallen in the splenic region. Since then the pain has been less severe. Shortness of breath on exertion has increased gradually in the last year. There have been no hemorrhages. Headache has been troublesome for some months.

Status præsens, December 29, 1896. Patient is of small size, medium frame, muscles and panniculus well nourished. The superficial lymphatic glands are not enlarged. The face and visible mucous membranes are of good color, but the hands are pale.

The thorax is symmetrical in the upper part. Examination of the lungs negative.

The heart is in the normal position; dulness not enlarged. There is a soft systolic murmur all over the heart area; the first sound is loud. Radial pulse small, quick, regular.

The abdomen is large, especially in the left upper part, where the thorax is also fuller. The recti are separated. The lower edge of the liver is almost at the navel line, but deep in the abdomen. The edge is thin and tender on pressure.

The splenic dulness begins in the seventh interspace and extends down into the mass below the ribs, evidently the spleen, which can be easily felt as a flattened body reaching to the level of the anterior superior spine of the ilium and to the median line. The edge is thick; there is a shallow notch on the inner side. There is palpable and audible friction over the surface. The patient says the mass is sometimes lower than at present. It is not unusually movable by pressure or position.

There is pain on pressure over the sternum and tibiæ.

The blood is pale, not very thin; fresh preparations show enormous increase of the leukocytes, among which large cells with fine or coarse granules are conspicuous. The blood count shows: red corpuscles, 2,500,000; leukocytes, 367,070; hæmoglobin (Fleischl), 50. Stained preparations show moderate poikilocytosis, many nucleated reds—1: 40 leukocytes, or 9074 per c.mm. About one-fourth have the size and appearance of megaloblasts, but the two forms run into each other by variations impossible to classify precisely. Differential count of the leukocytes shows: lymphocytes, 0.3; mononuclear neutrophiles, 48.8; polynuclear neutrophiles, 41.6; polynuclear eosinophiles, 0.7; mononuclear eosinophiles, 1.4; basophiles, 2; degenerated, 5. The lymphocytes are often smaller than red corpuscles, but do not show as intense staining of the nucleus as do typical small lymphocytes, and have usually a distinct rim of protoplasm. Many of the myelocytes have deeply indented nuclei, but the looser, skein-like structure of the nucleus distinguishes most of them from those denominated polynuclear. The eosinophiles, especially the mononuclears, vary much in size from that of a small lymphocyte to that of the largest mononuclears. The basophile cells are large or small in about equal proportions. The degenerated leukocytes are hard to classify, but seem to represent all the larger forms.

The diagnosis of myelogenous, mixed-celled leukæmia was given, the usual prognosis stated to the husband, and Fowler's solution recommended to the family physician.

February 1, 1897. The patient entered the medical clinic of the University Hospital. She says that two weeks ago she had influenza, with tonsillitis and coryza. The discharge was bloody, especially in the morning, and a week ago there was moderate nose-bleed. She complains now of great weakness, dyspnœa, pain in the left side, and general itching. She "feels as if walking on sticks."

Status præsens. The patient looks somewhat more anxious than before. The skin is not very pale. The hands feel numb when the arms are fully extended. There is no distinct tenderness over the nerve trunks of the extremities. The tongue is clean. There are no stomach symptoms. The pharynx shows moderate redness and swelling, with scanty mucopurulent exudate. The thoracic organs are negative, aside from a few small rales in both bases on deep inspiration, and a soft systolic murmur over the base of the heart. The abdomen is above the level of the ribs. The edge of the liver is within an inch of the navel line. The spleen extends three fingers' breadth below the margin of the ribs. The lower end is rounded, a shallow notch can be felt just above the point. The spleen is very tender on pressure, freely movable. There is distinct friction over it. The superficial lymphatic glands are not enlarged. There is no œdema of the ankles. The blood count: red corpuscles, 2,540,050; leukocytes, 7500; Fleischl, 50 per cent. Red corpuscles show marked vacuole formation; many polychromatophiles; some red corpuscles show mitotic figures. The arsenic had been increased up to 12 drops t. i. d.; it was continued, with extract of red bone-marrow (4 c.c. t. i. d.).

February 2d. Red corpuscles, 2,500,000; leukocytes, 8125; Fleischl, 50 per cent. Differential counts given in table.

7th. Patient complains of more numbness and also of itching. Arsenic stopped. Temperature has been up to 101° to 101.6° F.; pulse, 110; respiration, 22.

9th. Red corpuscles, 2,192,000; leukocytes, 4775; hæmoglobin, 50 per cent. Temperature has not been higher than 99.4° F.; pulse, 80 to 100; respiration, 22. Patient still complains of itching, also of weakness, headache, and slight dizziness.

12th. Red corpuscles, 2,863,000; leukocytes, 5000. The condition remained about the same. The temperature was rarely above normal; there was slight gain in weight. Itching was the most troublesome symptom.

March 3d. The leukocytes number 35,156; red corpuscles, 3,733,333; hæmoglobin, 60. The spleen can barely be felt on quiet breathing. On deep inspiration it extends three fingers' breadth below the ribs. Splenic dulness begins on the ninth rib and is 9 cm. long. On the right side there is dulness from the sixth intercostal space to an inch above the margin of the ribs and to the tip of the ensiform. The abdomen is slightly distended; no enlarged glands can be felt in it. The inguinal glands are slightly enlarged.

10th. Red corpuscles, 3,125,000; leukocytes, 40,170; hæmoglobin, 55. The systolic murmur over the base is still present. There is no œdema.

21st. Red corpuscles, 3,100,000; leukocytes, 90,000; hæmoglobin, 70. The patient feels better than before. Has no subjective symptoms. The spleen can barely be felt on quiet breathing; liver not enlarged. Patient has gained eight pounds in all since admission.

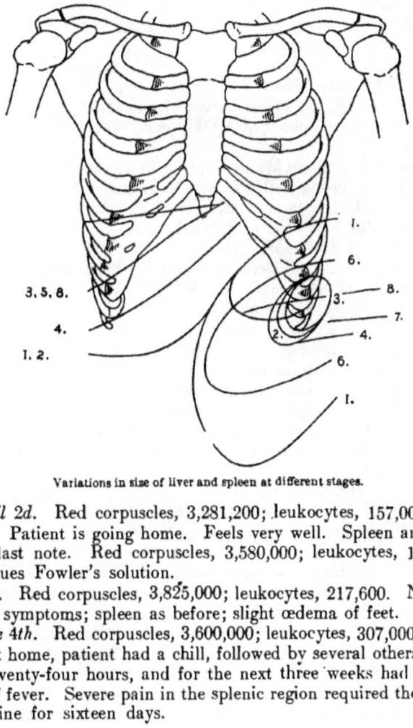

Variations in size of liver and spleen at different stages.

April 2d. Red corpuscles, 3,281,200; leukocytes, 157,000.

5th. Patient is going home. Feels very well. Spleen and liver as at last note. Red corpuscles, 3,580,000; leukocytes, 189,000. Continues Fowler's solution.

15th. Red corpuscles, 3,825,000; leukocytes, 217,600. No subjective symptoms; spleen as before; slight œdema of feet.

June 4th. Red corpuscles, 3,600,000; leukocytes, 307,000. Next day, at home, patient had a chill, followed by several others in the next twenty-four hours, and for the next three weeks had a good deal of fever. Severe pain in the splenic region required the use of morphine for sixteen days.

July 1st. Red corpuscles, 3,600,000; leukocytes, 307,000. The patient feels as well as before the febrile attack. She has tingling in the toes and fingers; otherwise well. She has gained eight pounds since leaving the hospital. The spleen is three fingers' breadth below the margin of the ribs on quiet breathing; it is hard and thicker than before. The liver is three fingers' breadth below the ribs, the edge thin and of normal consistency. Fowler's solution, stopped during the fever, renewed.

22d. Feels better. Took Fowler's solution up to 10 drops. The hands are better; the feet tingle slightly. Red corpuscles, 3,600,000; leukocytes, 178,000. The spleen is slightly smaller. Is now taking bone-marrow.

August 19th. Pain in the legs returned about ten days ago. Began Fowler's solution again, and pain ceased. Looks well; does housework, but tires easily. The liver is not palpable; the spleen is much larger than before, reaching two finger-breadths below the level of the navel; the upper border of dulness in the eighth interspace. Red corpuscles, 4,000,000; leukocytes, 165,000; hæmoglobin, 70.

October 21st. Patient has been taking Fowler's solution and bone-marrow and is feeling well, and now looks better than she has for a long time. The spleen is smaller, reaching only two and one-half fingers' breadth below the ribs. Red corpuscles, 4,000,000; leukocytes, 57,000; hæmoglobin, 70.

January 27, 1898. General condition has been fairly good. Red corpuscles, 3,095,000; leukocytes, 461,666. The spleen is a handbreadth below the margin of the ribs, 3 cm. from the middle line. The liver cannot be felt, except on deep breathing; there is dulness to the margin of the ribs. The superficial glands are not enlarged. Fowler's solution continued.

February 26th. General condition is good. Red corpuscles, 3,533,333; leukocytes, 279,260. Spleen as at last note. This was the last time the patient was seen. April 17th she wrote to say that she was not able to travel, on account of pain in the abdomen and enlargement of the spleen.

June 8th. Reported that patient, who had been trying to come to the hospital, had fever, chills, nausea, and vomiting, and was very weak. "The spleen fills the entire abdomen."

17th. "Patient is able to sit up, but still very weak. Is entirely deaf and complains of roaring in the ears." Soon after this she died, while I was away from home. An autopsy was made, but no tissues preserved.

Summary of the case: A woman with mixed-celled leukæmia, with greatly enlarged spleen. Two weeks after an attack of what was probably influenza, the leukocytes were found reduced from 367,070 to 7500, falling to 4775 in two weeks more, with reduction, but not disappearance, of the abnormal white and red cells. The spleen was much smaller; the liver became smaller later. In two months from the complication the leukocytes reached 40,000, in ten weeks 157,000, and in a year 461,666, having once been as low as 57,000 in the mean time. The liver and spleen remained small for many months, though the spleen was usually easily palpable. For the next six months the patient grew worse in every respect, and died a year and a half after the first observation. The most important stages in the blood are shown in the following table:

Date.	Red cells.	White cells.	Hæmoglobin.	Nucleated red cells.	Small lymphocytes.	Large lymphocytes.	Transition and large mononuclear.	Polynuclear neutrophiles.	Polynuclear eosinophiles.	Mononuclear eosinophiles.	Myelocytes (Ehrlich).	Basophile.	Degenerated.
Dec. 29	2,500,000	367,070	50	9074	0.00	0.30	00.0	41.6	0.7	1.4	48.8	2.0	5.0
Feb. 1	2,541,050	7,500	50										
" 2	2,500,000	8,125	50	2358	4.2	5.7	4.9	70.6	......	......	12.3	......	6.0
" 9	2,192,000	4,775	50	1224	2.5	11.8	10.1	56.0	......	1.4	11.1	1.0	6.0
" 12	2,863,000	5,000	...	416	1.6	13.3	3.3	63.8	0.3	0.6	9.6	1.0	6.6
March 3	3,733,333	35,156	60	524	0.4	7.6	7.1	66.2	0.2	......	15.5	......	2.7
" 10	3,125,000	40,170	55	362	0.15	5.2	2.4	54.4	......	......	20.9	......	16.4
" 14	3,125,000	40,170	50	500	0.8	2.4	1.4	62.0	......	0.2	29.9	......	3.3
" 21	3,100,000	90,000	50	few	0.1	2.3	3.2	63.7	0.4	0.2	22.3	......	6.4
Oct. 21	4,000,000	57,000	70	1760	1.3	3.5	7.7	62.0	1.2	1.3	20.8	0.9	2.3
Jan. 27	3,095,000	461,666	65	7387	2.3	1.3	4.4	63.2	0.4	0.7	27.0	......	0.7
Feb. 26	3,533,333	279,000	70	6700	8.8	6.0	3.0	41.0	1.0	0.3	34 0	1.0	5.0

Such a change, more marked than one usually sees in leukæmia under treatment, forces one to try to learn something from it, not only as regards pathology, but, even more imperatively, something of therapeutic value. The most important objective symptom, the excess of leukocytes, disappears. It would seem that by examining such cases one might discover something regarding the production of leukocytes and their appearance in the circulation, as well as their ultimate destruction; also something of the life of the red corpuscles, and of other details of the pathology of leukæmia. It might seem that the process could be imitated, and a symptomatic, if not a causal, treatment be discovered. Medical literature contains a number of such cases, though not so many as one might expect, remembering the vulnerability of the leukæmic to infection. Not only single cases have been reported, but studies have been made, and in the present article I am merely going over ground that has already been traversed by others, my only advantage being due to the fact that I am at present the latest inquirer.

The literature of the complications is unusually confused. Some of the cases have been reported two or even three times by the same or different authors. Besides unavoidable errors, such as those in ages, dates, and other minor details, author's names have been changed. H. Strangways Hounsell, one of the earliest authors, becomes Honsell, Hantell, Strongways, Srangways, and even, by an unnecessary comma, two authors, contributing a case each. Thorsch reported a case in his own name, from the clinic of von Limbeck, and at least two writers ascribe it to "Zeissl," whose name does not appear in the original article.

The subject is complicated by other things. A frequent cause is the lack of exact classification of the leukæmia. In many cases I have been obliged to follow the author's terminology and classify cases that should, perhaps, be otherwise arranged. With future cases this difficulty will become less frequent, and also another regarding the diagnosis of the complication. But owing to the chronic and obscure course of many cases and the tendency of patients to wander from one to another physician, incomplete observations will multiply, and will, nevertheless, often deserve publication.

I shall discuss the cases according to the nature of the complicating disease in the first place, and the variety of leukæmia in the second, and, without trying to follow a scientific order, will speak first of tuberculosis.*

Cases of Tuberculosis and Leukæmia.

The combination of tuberculosis and leukæmia was noted very early. Virchow[1] described a case in 1849, and his rival, Bennett,[2] noted 2 out of 23 cases collected in 1852. Virchow also made the anatomical examination in a case observed clinically by Bamberger[3] in 1857. According to Mosler,[4] there were 12 examples of tuberculosis in the 100 cases of leukæmia analyzed in Martin Ehrlich's thesis in 1872. Yet in the recent literature the combination is rarely mentioned. Many authors admit that they have never seen such a case. It was encountered only twice in the 37 cases observed in the Göttingen clinic,[17] with 10 autopsies. Among my own cases, 25 in number, there were no clinical evidences, but in 2 out of 6 autopsies miliary tuberculosis was found, once in a marked degree. I think that more extensive observations will show that the exclusion is not so absolute as has been thought. In my own clinical material leukæmia occurs most frequently in the early part of the fifth decade, when tuberculosis is relatively infrequent. Cornet, Moorehouse, and others have pointed out that this age period is one very prone

* Three articles were received too late to use in this paper. Tommaso Prodi, La Riforma Medica, July 22, 1903, A Case of Lymphatic Leukæmia, with Tuberculosis of the Larynx, Lungs, and Lymphatic Glands. W. J. Susmann, The Practitioner, October, 1903, Tuberculosis in One out of Forty-one Cases of Leukæmia Observed in Various London Hospitals. Wilhelm Neutra, Zeitschrift f. Heilkunde, Band xxiv., 1903, Two Cases of Lymphocythæmia; in one Pleurisy, with Leukocytes Dropping from 160,000 to 8800; in the other, Suppurative Pleurisy and Peritonitis; Blood Not Thoroughly Examined.

to tuberculous manifestations, but I think the whole subject is one that requires further investigation. This is one of many aspects of leukæmia that can be studied with advantage by the physician in private practice, where the whole course of the disease can be followed. Owing to the nature of the disease patients with leukæmia do not remain in hospitals as long as is desirable for extensive study.

Another fact requires some consideration. Small leukæmic growths closely resemble tubercles. The early literature has occasioual mention of leukæmic growths, sometimes of large masses that, especially in the lungs, break down and simulate ulcerative tuberculosis. At an early period Virchow, Boettcher, and Ollivier and Ranvier studied the peculiarities of the two growths, but it was not until the structure of tubercle had been more minutely described by Wagner, Schüppel, and Langhans, and especially after the discovery of the tubercle bacillus, that the differentiation was made certain. It would be interesting to re-examine some of the old museum preparations with reference to the breaking down of such growths. The analysis of cases published before 1882 is very unsatisfactory. The only cases necessary or profitable to examine now are those in which an effect on the blood or organs has been noted.

There are in the literature about 27 cases that either are cited in this connection or might be referred to. To these I add two imperfect observations not previously reported. The cases of Virchow and Bamberger, mentioned above, throw no light on the question now under consideration. That of Hounsell,[5] fairly well described, is of value also only in showing the association of diseases. Besides tuberculosis the patient had scarlet fever, tonsillitis, and secondary pneumonia. The leukæmia was probably acute lymphocythæmia. Ollivier and Ranvier[6] reported the case of a man, aged forty years, with miliary tuberculosis of the abdominal organs, old pulmonary tuberculosis, and leukæmia. The case cannot be analyzed for lack of details regarding the blood. The same difficulty exists in the report by Robin[7] of a case of extensive lymphatic tuberculosis with leukæmia. Still less available is a case mentioned by de Roth,[8] of miliary tuberculosis and leukæmia, observed by Knoepfelmacher, but not published. Brueckmann[9] has reported a case of splenic-myelogenous and lymphatic leukæmia with old and recent tubercles that has some incidental interest, because it appears that the examination of the blood made in a famous German clinic, in 1892, consisted in estimating the proportion of red and white cells in blood, "mit Wasser stark verdünnt." Two cases reported by Volpe[10] are even more imperfectly described, and do not add anything to the material, while several of 6 cases he quotes from the literature are cases of pseudoleukæmia. In a case of Musser and Sailer[11] there were "evidences of old tubercle" in the apex of one lung. This and a similar case reported briefly by Saundby[12] show that leukæmia can develop in bodies with old tuberculous foci, as is proved by some of the cases cited below. Sabrazès[13] has briefly mentioned a case of myelogenous leukæmia and tuberculosis of the lymph glands, with diminution of eosinophiles and mast-cells, and increased polynuclears. The patient reported by Strattmann[68] had a history of apical catarrh and pulmonary hemorrhages before the spleen became large, and may also have been tuberculous. The patient treated with tuberculin by H. Heuck,[64] mentioned below, also had slight signs of pulmonary tuberculosis.

Finally, in Kraus'[32] case, discussed below, there was miliary tuberculosis besides the streptococcus and diplococcus infections.

Of the other 15 cases 7 are examples of medullary leukæmia, with acute miliary tuberculosis. Of these, the cases of Quincke [14] [15] (2 cases), Lichtheim,[16] Schmidt,[17] Bezançon and Weil,[18] and Hirschfeld and Tobias[19] showed diminution of leukocytes as follows:

Quincke, Case 1	1 : 3	to	1 : 50
Quincke, Case 2	1 : 4	to	1 : 90
Lichtheim*	1 : 8	to	1 : 370 (250,000 to 8,900)
Schmidt	1 : 2.9	to	1 : 135 (962,000 to 28,000)
Bezançon and Weil	135,000	to	19,871, rising to 45,000
Hirschfeld and Tobias	331,000	to	110,937

In Schmidt's case there were small cavities in the lungs. In Hirschfeld and Tobias' case there were old lesions in the apices, but not cavities, and no clinical symptoms of tuberculosis. The miliary tuberculosis does not seem to have been very severe. No bacilli were found in sections. The leukocytes were as high as 434,000 nine months before the low count, 228,000 four months before, rising to 331,000 two weeks before the low count. Six months later, after a recurring pneumonia, they numbered 283,333, and death occurred five weeks later. In the case of de Roth[8] there was a rise toward the end.

Four cases of myelogenous leukæmia are recorded in which chronic tuberculosis existed, sometimes ending in miliary tuberculosis. These are reported by Elsner and Groat,[20] Sturmdorf,[21] Parker,[22] and Murrell,[23] though the tuberculosis in the latter case may not have been very chronic. In all there was a fall in the number of leukocytes toward the end. In some the lowest count was still so high as to leave little room for doubt as to the diagnosis, viz., in Elsner and Groat's case, 121,000; Sturmdorf's 116,000; Parker's, 100,000, later 130,000; but in Murrell's it was 16,200, from 220,000. Arsenic was freely used in this case.

The other cases show variations in the leukæmic condition and other features that make it necessary to consider them separately.

In the case of Stintzing[24] there was enlargement of the spleen and lymphatic glands, with old tuberculous lesions (cavities) in the

* Elsner and Groat and Hirschfeld and Tobias classify Lichtheim's case among lymphatic leukæmias, but as the author says the polynuclear and mononuclear cells were about equal, I agree with Baldwin and Wilder and Quincke in placing it with the splenomedullary cases, though the lymph glands were also enlarged.

lungs. The leukocytes decreased slightly, 1:100 to 1:150; the glands became smaller, but the spleen remained about the same size. It is difficult to understand the author's statement that the "leukæmia improved while the phthisis made great progress," particularly as the patient died, unless we take a very partial view of the case.

Juenger's[25] patient had enlarged lymphatic glands, and probably acute leukæmia, though the description of the blood leaves some doubt as to its precise character. Miliary tuberculosis of the glands and peritoneum, with early caseation, was found post-mortem. The leukocytes rose from 40,000 to 125,000 in two weeks, two and a half months before death, and fell to 68,800 six weeks before the end, following an attack of diarrhœa. Arsenical pigmentation was then present. The glands became smaller. An abscess in one of them was incised. The blood was not examined again until two days before death, and then showed no excess of leukocytes.

In Francksen's[26] case, probably also lymphatic leukæmia, there was tuberculosis of the lymph glands, spleen, and liver, with final bronchopneumonia. The leukocytes fell from 240,000 to 128,000 between observations four months apart, and did not fall lower in the next three days, or two days before death. The spleen became smaller toward the end.

Baldwin and Wilder[27] reported a case of probable chronic lymphocythæmia. In this lymphatic enlargement had lasted more than two years, chronic pulmonary tuberculosis, finally developing cavities, as long or perhaps longer. The leukæmia was observed for about two months. There were no recent miliary tubercles. The leukocytes numbered 695,000 at the beginning of the period, reached 1,113,000 nine days before the last count, and then fell to 943,500 and 959,500, without qualitative changes. The lymph glands and spleen grew smaller four days before the end.

From the available material it appears that chronic tuberculosis does not distinctly influence the course of leukæmia, or, as we shall see later, materially influence the leukocyte formula. Acute miliary tuberculosis, on the other hand, is followed by or associated with reduction of the leukocytes in the majority of cases. The exceptional cases may be due to the slight development of the miliary tuberculosis in extent, or to the fact that death occurs before the change has time to take place, though it may be, as de Roth has suggested, that in some cases the body becomes accustomed to the infection and the leukocytes are not affected, as in more acute cases.

Two of my cases, though imperfectly observed, add weight to both of the first two suppositions.

Case II.—M. T., domestic, aged twenty-five years, first seen June 2, 1896. "She was well until July, 1895, when swellings and red spots appeared on the right leg, and similar lesions appeared on various parts of the body up to the time of examination. The abdomen has been large for nearly a year. It was supposed to be due to uterine or ovarian tumor, for which an operation was advised by two physicians she consulted. Weakness present for three months." I found a mixed-celled leukæmia, with red corpuscles, 3,587,500; leukocytes, 598,000; hæmoglobin, 60. There were ecchymoses, up to the size of the palms, on the arms and legs. The spleen extended one inch beyond the middle line, and to the level of the anterior superior spine of the ilium. The liver was not enlarged; the axillary and cervical lymph glands were slightly enlarged, but not the inguinal glands. No pain or tenderness in the bones.

The patient was observed by Dr. Cowie and myself for two years, taking Fowler's solution as steadily as is usually possible. Within three weeks the ecchymosis ceased, menstruation reappeared after an absence of several months, but there was no marked fall in the leukocytes and no noteworthy change in the leukocyte formula. Myelocytes varied from 25 per cent. to 44 per cent.; polynuclears, 30 per cent. to 50 per cent.; lymphocytes, 1 per cent. to 6 per cent.; polynuclear eosinophiles, 1 per cent. to 3.2 per cent.; mononuclear eosinophiles, 1.2 per cent. to 1.8 per cent.

Becoming anxious for more radical treatment, the patient disappeared from our observation. A year later, three years after the first observation, Dr. Cowie and Dr. Warthin were given an opportunity of making an autopsy by the courtesy of Dr. J. A. Wessinger, who had been called upon in the last illness. The spleen was enlarged; the chief picture was that of a severe tuberculosis of the serous membranes. The blood showed no increase of leukocytes, and microscopic examination of the tissues revealed a complete absence of leukæmic changes, except in the bone-marrow, which was lymphoid.

In this case it is impossible to know when the change occurred. The tuberculosis was more severe than it seems to have been in many of the reported cases.

In Case III., to be reported more fully on account of other features, a man, aged twenty-nine years, died with so-called leukæmic apoplexy, without any decrease of leukocytes up to the moment of death. At the autopsy a slight recent miliary tuberculosis was found. Striking as the differences are in these two cases, I think we should await the publication of others before drawing conclusions from them.

Miscellaneous Infections.

There are 23 reported cases of intercurrent infection other than tuberculosis, including my own Case I. The infections represented are: In medullary or splenomedullary leukæmia: typhoid-like disease (Eisenlohr[28]), afebrile typhoid (Pal[29]), erysipelas (Richter[30]), also reported by Freudenstein;[31] erysipelas, streptococcus, and diplococcus infection with miliary tuberculosis (Kraus[32]), sepsis (H. F.

Mueller,[33] Koermoczi[34]), empyema (G. Heuck[35]), influenza (Kovacs,[36] Dock), peritonitis (Da Costa[37]).

In lymphatic leukæmia, acute in most cases: sepsis, angina (H. F. Mueller[38]), angina, streptococcus (Weil[39]), streptococcus infection (Wende[40]), sepsis (Cabot[41]), staphylococcus (Fraenkel[42]), colon baeillus (Fraenkel, *ibid.*), staphylococcus and colon (E. Mueller[43]), pneumonia (Oette,[44] Froelich,[45] Thorsch[46]).

Chronic lymphocythæmia was observed complicated by pneumonia by Grawitz[47] and Hart,[48] and bronchitis by Petit and Weil.[49] In some of the cases more than one complication was observed, and these I shall utilize as far as the data will permit.

The following may also be mentioned: Heusner, in discussing Strattmann's case,[63] mentioned a patient with leukæmia in which diminution in the size of the glands and spleen and improvement of the blood followed pneumonia, but relapsed. Rieder[50] (p. 38) has reported a case of medullary leukæmia with sepsis, and one of lymphatic leukæmia and sepsis, with increase of the leukocytes. The details are too scanty to use. The case reported from Mosler's clinic by Oette[44] may be mentioned here, though I might have included it among the more important cases. A girl aged twenty-three had fever with icterus. The leukæmic blood improved after six weeks, and six months later was "almost normal." The case is of great historical interest, and Oette's thesis of much value, but the case cannot now be compared with others. Chantemesse, in the discussion of Bezançon and Weil's case,[18] mentioned a patient of his who acquired erysipelas in the course of leukæmia.

Of the cases referred to above, there was a marked decrease of leukocytes to or near normal in 11, viz., those of Eisenlohr, Kraus, Wende, Froelich, Fraenkel (2 cases), Oette, Koermoczi, Dock, E. Mueller, Cabot. There was a relatively slight fall in 9, viz., those of Pal, Richter, H. F. Mueller, Weil, Thorsch, G. Heuck, Kovacs, Hart, Grawitz. No change or a rise in 3, viz., Mueller, Petit and Weil, Da Costa.

The cases differ so much in detail that it is difficult to make comparisons. Taking first streptococcus infections, we find that in Richter's case of facial erysipelas following puncture of the tympanic membrane, the leukocytes had fallen on the second day of the complication to 56,000 from the 320,000 of two weeks earlier. The spleen was smaller, and in three days more was 4 cm. less in length, 3 cm. in width. The leukocytes sank to 29,000 on the fourth day, but rose rapidly to 148,000 on the sixth day, along with the development of an abscess of the eyelid and bronchitis, and fell to 52,000 in six more days, while the general and local conditions improved.

In Weil's case of angina with streptococci in the blood, the lenkocytes fell during blood infection from 290,400 to 75,682 in four days; seven days later, 66,230. The author thought the angina had increased the leukocytes (the blood had not been examined before), which he estimated at 60,000 to 80,000. I can see no ground for this assumption.

In Kraus' case there was in the beginning a leukocyte count of from 360,000 to 420,000. The complication, a streptococcus and diplococcus infection of the bronchi with miliary tuberculosis, ran a somewhat obscure course, the blood symptoms being the only marked ones. After slight physical signs of bronchitis, blood-streaked sputum appeared, with fever and increased size of the spleen. The leukocytes were then 393,400, but fell to 251,600 in about seven weeks, during which there was erysipelas. Two weeks later the count was 240,000. In three weeks they numbered 390,000, in four weeks 504,000. The bloody sputum then contained the cocci mentioned. The sputum then ceased; there were no signs of pneumonia. In three days the leukocytes fell to 120,000, in eight days more to 4600, without myelocytes, mononuclear eosinophiles, mast-cells, and nucleated reds, but with many degenerated leukocytes. The spleen became smaller in the next few days. The leukocytes rose to 9000; death followed four days after the last count. Autopsy revealed pneumococci in the purulent exudate in the peritoneum and in the spleen and liver, bilateral pneumonia, purulent pleural exudates, pylephlebitis, and tuberculosis of bronchial glands, lung, larynx, peritoneum, and liver. The anatomical diagnosis of leukæmia could not be made. What part the various infections played is difficult to say, but the streptococci do not seem to have been so much concerned as the diplococci. The tuberculosis was probably too slight to be effective.

In one of Pal's cases of medullary leukæmia with bronchitis and erysipelas the leukocytes rose from 75,000 to 105,000 in two days. Tracheotomy was necessary, and death occurred a week later.

In Wende's case, lymphatic leukæmia with streptococcus infection, there was a marked fall, 45,000 to 600.

In Thorsch's case of pneumonia in lymphatic leukæmia (also cited by von Limbeck[51] and sometimes referred to as Zeissl's case) there was a rapid fall in the beginning from 119,000 to 43,500 by the fifth day. Next day there was an extension of the disease, and in three days more the leukocytes rose to 172,000 on the morning of the day of death, 133,000 in the afternoon.

Froelich's case was probably one of lymphatic leukæmia, though the author called it pseudoleukæmia. Under complicating pleuro-pneumonia the leukocytes fell from 66,667 (having been 309,000) to 8823 in the last week.

In Oette's case of chronic pneumonia the data are insufficient for analysis. He mentions two cases from the older literature showing that bronchopneumonia does not always alter the blood picture in leukæmia, as it had in his own case.

In chronic lymphocythæmia 2 cases have been reported complicated by pneumonia. In that of Grawitz the leukocytes, "already rather low," sank lower in the beginning and rose to a considerable height in defervescence. There was no change in the formula.

In Hart's case there was a fall of from 1,168,000 to 450,000 on the fourth day of pneumonia. Death occurred two days later.

The 2 cases of influenza cannot be compared with accuracy, because in 1, my own, the diagnosis was based on the anamnesis only. In Kovacs' case the leukocytes, only 67,000 at the highest count, though they had been higher, apparently, fell to 17,000 eleven days later. Six days later there were 33,000. The patient also had bronchitis, pneumonia, and otitis. In one of H. F. Mueller's cases the patient gave a history of influenza, not observed by the author, with diminution in the size of the enlarged glands, which regained the original size after the fever subsided.

The various cases reported as examples of sepsis complicating leukæmia cannot be compared with advantage, but some of them have points of interest that deserve mention. One of the first was the case of H. F. Mueller.[38] A man with lymphatic leukæmia, with 180,000 leukocytes, had a subperiosteal abscess in the right leg. A count made then, three weeks after the former one, showed 400,000 leukocytes. The glands were about a third their former size; the spleen was also smaller. Death ensued four days after the last count. In Cabot's case of sepsis in lymphatic leukæmia there was a sudden fall from 40,000 to 5661 in one week, and a progressive fall to 471 in nine days more. In Koermoeczi's case of myelogenous leukæmia with sepsis, originating in the nose and leading to hemorrhagic pericarditis without bacteriæmia, the leukocytes fell from 100,000 to 2000. In H. F. Mueller's case of myelogenous leukæmia there was sepsis following abscess from therapeutic injections. The leukocytes had already fallen from 406,200 to 246,900, influenza having been passed through. They then fell to 225,000 with the onset of sepsis, and in the following seven weeks reached 75,500. Pleurisy and pneumonia then developed, and ante-mortem, eighteen days after the last count given, there were 57,300 leukocytes. The spleen was smaller in the later stages; the leukæmic character of the blood was lost.

In both of Fraenkel's cases of acute lymphæmia, one of staphylococcus infection, the other colon infection, there was a marked fall from 123,000 to 600 in twelve days, and 220,000 to 1200 in sevendays.

In E. Mueller's case of acute lymphæmia with streptococci, staphylococci, and colon bacilli in the exudate in the pharynx, the leukocytes fell from 109,600 to 6800 in five days, 39,200 in the last twenty-four hours.

In Eisenlohr's case of typhoid-like infection, the leukocytes, enormously increased before, fell to almost normal. An attack of follicular angina was followed by an increase, which did not subside in the remaining four weeks of life.

In Pal's case of afebrile typhoid there was a fall from 991,000 to 650,000 in sixteen days, most of it in eight days. Death occurred a week later. Pal could not see that the typhoid infection (not suspected during life) had any influence on the blood or other clinical phenomena. Besides the typhoid there was jaundice, and a traumatic, suppurating hæmatoma.

In G. Heuck's case of empyema there was a variation of from 400,500 to 80,100, rising after thoracotomy to 169,800.

I have already mentioned H. F. Mueller's case, in which the leukocytes increased during infection. Two other similar cases have been recorded. In the case of Petit and Weil there was chronic lymphocythæmia. Bronchitis occurred, fatal on the sixth day, after diminution of the enlarged glands. The leukocytes increased in the period from two days before bronchitis to the last day from 202,238 to 398,866. Da Costa[37] mentions a case of splenomedullary leukæmia, in which, within ten days after the onset of peritonitis, the leukocytes rose from 245,000 to 400,000.

The cases just cited are of importance chiefly in a suggestion they offer. In all three the rise of leukocytes was discovered early in the complication; the patients died soon after. It is possible, of course, that a fall might have occurred after the rise had the cases ended less abruptly. The earliest period after complication has rarely been carefully observed and should be thoroughly studied in future.

From the foregoing it appears that in the great majority of cases intercurrent infections cause a decrease of the leukocytes in leukæmias of various kinds. The fall may be so slight as to leave the gross picture of leukæmia unchanged, but in about half the cases the white corpuscles fall to normal or below. It is interesting to note the extreme leukopenia that occurred in some cases: 600 in one of Fraenkel's, 1200 in another, 600 in Wende's, 471 in Cabot's, 2000 in Koermoeczi's.

Besides the leukocyte decrease, the organs, enlarged as the result of the leukæmia, became smaller. In some cases the organs became smaller later than the fall of leukocytes (Quincke[14]), sometimes earlier, in others simultaneously; sometimes the organs became smaller without diminution of leukocytes (H. F. Mueller, Petit and Weil). The diminution was sometimes very rapid. Quincke estimated the change in the volume of the spleen in one case at 100 grams a day, a loss that I think must have been exceeded in my own case. It is often difficult to distinguish between this change in the organs and that observed in some cases of leukæmia a short time before death. Sabrazès mentions a case in which cutaneous neoplasms became smaller during a terminal infection, but from the original report* I cannot see anything peculiar, especially as the patient was taking arsenic and quinine at the same time.

* Liffran, J. Contribution a l'étude de la leucocythémie aigue, Thèse, Bordeaux, 1898, p. 66.

Changes in the Red Blood Corpuscles.

Changes in the red cells have not been studied as carefully, perhaps, as they deserve in complicated leukæmias. Out of 18 cases in which the reports are full there was a rise in the number of red cells, simultaneous with the fall of leukocytes, in 8. The difference was often slight, but in 6 it was 500,000 or more (once 1,300,000) per cmm. (Lichtheim). In the other cases the rise was insignificant, or there was a fall. The latter was 500,000 or more in 4 cases; in 1 1,200,000 (Juenger). The great variations in the red count in leukæmia without complications should be borne in mind. A difference of a million or more may be observed in a short time independent of visible causes. The frequency of the rise in the red cells, while the leukocytes and other symptoms seem to indicate the opposite process, suggests a change in the blood fluid as the cause. The fact that 4 cases with marked rise occurred in tuberculosis (Lichtheim, Schmidt, Sturmdorf, de Roth) is interesting, but the cases do not offer a satisfactory explanation. Quincke noticed the unusual bloodlessness for leukæmia, post-mortem, in 1 of his cases. In my second case of tuberculosis the vessels were unusually full of blood.

The histological changes in the red corpuscles are interesting, but variable. Nucleated red cells are not always absent, as some have thought. In Richter's case they appeared during the complication. De Roth noticed many, including some in mitosis. In Juenger's case they were pretty numerous, but disappeared two days before death. In my case these cells were less numerous than before the complication, and increased as the leukocyte count regained a high point, but there were many, even at the lowest period, and often in mitosis. The condition of the red corpuscles should be carefully observed in future.

Qualitative Changes in the Blood, Especially in the Leukocytes.

The earlier observers were unable to notice the finer details in the cells, on account of the lack of methods. Mueller mentioned, in reporting his first case, that mitotic cells (myelocytes) disappeared almost entirely, and the leukocytes changed, so that the leukæmia seemed better, judging from the blood. Mueller's second case, with increase of the leukocytes, has often been misquoted. He himself admitted that no accurate examination of the blood cells had been made. He thought there might have been an increase of polynuclears, as occurs in sepsis, but he also thought the new cells might have been derived from the shrinkage of the enlarged glands, in which case they would hardly have been polynuclear.

Kovacs noticed in his case of influenza with slight decrease of leukocytes that the myelocytes disappeared almost completely, the eosinophiles also, the mitotic cells and nucleated reds completely.

There was an increase of polynuclear cells, so that the blood picture was that of leukocytosis. With the rise of leukocytes the marrow elements reappeared.

Fraenkel noticed no increase of polynuclear cells in his first case, in which, however, the examination was not thorough. In his second case all varieties were reduced.

Richter observed disappearance of mononuclear cells during the complication, with increase of polynuclears up to 90 per cent., the latter in the secondary rise with abscess. Before the complication the two classes had been about equal.

Thorsch, whose case appears to have been chronic lymphocythæmia, with mononuclear cells about 97 per cent., and no eosinophiles or nucleated reds, says that the changes were: mononuclears, 138,600; polynuclears, 1400 at one extreme and 40,585 to 4915 at the other, showing an absolute increase of polynuclears. But this was by no means such an increase as would cause distinct leukocytosis in a non-leukæmic subject, and before the complication, with 113,000 leukocytes at one time, there were 4520 polynuclears. Thorsch suggested that relative increase of polynuclear cells is observed by all in complicated leukæmia, and he made H. F. Mueller's case one of the number, but, as I have shown above, without sufficient basis. Hirschlaff* has a reported case showing that the polynuclears can increase markedly in leukæmia without infection.

In Lichtheim's case of tuberculosis with a fall of 250,000 to 8900, there was a relative increase of polynuclears, viz., from 50 per cent. to 90 per cent., which would amount to a slight increase above normal, but far below the polynuclear count at the height of the leukæmia.

In Baldwin and Wilder's case, without marked alteration of the blood count, there was no notable change in the leukocyte formula.

In Koermoeczi's case of sepsis, with a fall of from 100,000 to 7300, the eosinophiles, myelocytes, and mast-cells disappeared. The polynuclear neutrophiles numbered 75 per cent. (possibly 70 per cent.; there is an error in the report). Just before death counts of 3000 and 2000 were made, with slight increase of the lymphocytes, but no other change.

Adler[32a] examined the blood from Kraus' case, with special reference to the leukocyte formula. Kraus had reported disappearance of the myelæmic condition and the appearance of degenerated leukocytes. Adler shows in tabular form the fall and ultimate almost complete disappearance of the mononuclear neutrophiles (25.50 per cent., 100,514 cells to 0.40 per cent. and 18 cells), the complete disappearance of the basophiles and mononuclear and polynuclear eosinophiles. In the rise before the final fall there was an increase of lymphocytes and decrease of eosinophiles. The eosinophiles disappeared completely with the beginning of severe septic phe-

* Deutsche med. Wochenschrift, 1898, Vereins-Beilage, p. 162.

nomena, and the lymphocytes (small) increased to 40.80 per cent.; large lymphocytes, 1.80 per cent.; mononuclear neutrophiles, 0.40 per cent.; polynuclear, 58.80 per cent., the latter being only slightly increased relatively.

Bezançon and Weil noticed in their case of tuberculosis that the leukocytosis was polynuclear during the infection, instead of mononuclear; basophiles, mononuclears, and eosinophiles were few. There were no nucleated red cells, whereas before there were many, some of them in mitosis. Later, as the infection advanced, the leukocytes rose again (from 19,871 to 45,500), and myelogenous cells, with nucleated reds, increased. In the case of Petit and Weil there was no notable change in the formula. In the case of Weil the polynuclear cells were relatively as well as absolutely diminished; the eosinophiles also.

In Elsner and Groat's case there was an increase of polynuclears and lymphocytes, relatively, and a diminution of myelocytes, as the tuberculosis advanced. But not only in the number of leukocytes, at the lowest 121,000 cells, but also in the formula, the leukæmic character was preserved: polynuclears, 68; myelocytes, 17.5; lymphocytes, 6.5; eosinophiles, 5.2; many normoblasts and megaloblasts.

Sturmdorf observed in his case, in which the number of leukocytes was not much altered during the observations, that each rise in temperature was accompanied by an increase of polynuclears and decrease of myelocytes, "suggesting an intercurrent leukocytosis."

In Wende's case, with a drop of from 45,000 to 600 leukocytes, there was an increase of polynuclears of from 3.4 per cent. to 10 per cent., and a decrease of lymphocytes from 95 per cent. to 88 per cent. in nine days. There are some discrepancies in the author's figures, but they do not materially affect the statements.

In the case of Hirschfeld and Tobias, with a fall only to 110,937 (from 424,000), the polynuclear cells were not relatively increased; the myelocytes were lower then than when the count was above 400,000, but higher (11.5 per cent.) than when it was 300,000 (7.6 per cent.), and there were other variations, but as the author shows, by the counts of another leukæmic patient, the variations were no greater in the case of infection than are sometimes observed without it.

In Murrell's case there was a marked fall in the number of myelocytes, though the differential counts are unusual and cannot be readily compared with others. For example, the eosinophiles are given as 20 per cent. with counts of 20,000 and 29,000; none with 16,200; besides which it is said the myelocytes, 20 per cent., 44 per cent., and 7 per cent. on different days, were chiefly eosinophile.

Parker states that in the low count, 130,000, the polynuclears were relatively fewer than at the height of the leukocytosis, 70.8 per cent. and 57 per cent.; the myelocytes high, 25 as compared with 14; the other forms not notably altered.

Hart found no noteworthy changes in the blood in his case of lymphocythæmia.

Grawitz noticed no change in the formula, either in the fall in the beginning or the rise after the pneumonia or after a turpentine abscess with temporary low count.

In my own case the polynuclears were relatively and absolutely about the same as in normal blood. The lymphocytes were relatively and absolutely about normal, relatively higher than in the high stage, but absolutely slightly lower. The polynuclear eosinophiles were relatively and absolutely low, the mononuclear eosinophiles relatively lower than before, but still considerable, and even higher relatively than at later periods with excessive leukocytosis. The (Ehrlich's) myelocytes were relatively and absolutely low, but even at the lowest count, 9.6 per cent., higher than is usually found in any accidental myelocythæmia. Mast-cells were relatively as in other stages. Degenerated leukocytes were relatively about as high as in the first observation, but higher than they became later as the count rose. Nucleated red cells were relatively much higher than before, reaching 1 to 2.4 at one time, or absolutely 2090 per c.mm. One-fourth were megaloblasts, and a few of these were in mitosis. Nucleated reds were absolutely more numerous at the first count, 1 to 40, or 9074 per c.mm., with a few in mitosis. A few myelocytes also were in mitosis. The reds showed poikilocytosis, vacuoles, and variations in size, as well as polychromatophilia, but without notable changes from the earlier count. No Charcot crystals formed in blood kept for several weeks, and not until the leukocytes had risen to 35,000.

During the rise of leukocytes that began between two and four weeks after the fall was discovered the formula was altered by the relative decrease of lymphocytes, the relative increase of myelocytes, and a slight relative increase of eosinophiles of both kinds. The nucleated reds increased slowly. The large number of these cells during the low leukocyte stage is exceptional. It is possible that they were fewer or absent in the preceding two weeks immediately after the infection, and that they began to reappear in the stage of reaction, but the counts do not support this view.

It appears, then, that the changes in the leukocyte formula are not uniform, though there is a disposition for the leukæmic character to disappear more or less completely under the influence of infections, and for the polynuclears to increase absolutely as well as relatively.

When Does the Change Occur?

When the change occurs is a question that cannot be answered very fully, on account of the small number of cases in which the process could be observed from the beginning.

In Eisenlohr's case the glands and spleen diminished daily from the beginning of the infection and the blood changed simultaneously. As the glands and spleen enlarged again, the blood resumed its former leukæmic character. The decrease lasted fourteen days. One month after the decrease the blood showed proportions of 1 to 4.

In Kovacs' case the blood resembled that of leukocytosis nine days after the beginning of the infection. In twelve days the spleen was smaller and softer. On the tenth day there were few myelocytes; no nucleated reds. Three days later there was an increase, with many myelocytes, and in three more there were 33,000 leukocytes.

In Fraenkel's first case the whole process took place in twelve days. In his second one the leukocytes had fallen to 47,000 by the seventh day, 3800 by the eighth day, 1200 by the tenth day.

In Richter's case the leukocytes fell from 56,000 to 29,000 in two days, but two days later they were 148,000, and six more 52,000.

In Thorsch's case the lowest point was reached in four days. Death occurred three days later.

In Lichtheim's case there was a slow and steady decrease for two months, when death occurred.

In Koermoeczi's case, eight days after a count of 100,000, the leukocytes had fallen to 7300. The patient lived five days longer, with almost the same blood picture.

In Kraus' case the leukocytes fell quickly after infection, viz., from 120,000 to 4600 in one week. In five days more the leukocytes had increased to 9000, and in four more the patient died.

In Weil's case the fall from 270,000 to 75,682 took place in six days; in seven more the number was 66,230.

Elsner and Groat noted a gradual fall of 200,000 leukocytes in three months.

In Wende's case, sepsis in acute lymphocythæmia, the leukocytes fell in nine days from 45,000 to 1600. In Cabot's case the fall to subnormal took only sixteen days; in E. Mueller's case five days.

In Murrell's case there was a fall in three days of from 150,000 to 20,000. Then an increase six months later, and another fall from 167,000 to 16,200 within five weeks.

In my own case of influenza the fall of from 367,070 to 7500 probably occurred within two weeks, but there was no actual observation in that time.

In general, the fall occurs soon after the infection, more promptly in acute than in chronic infections. The cases of chronic infections, however, are too few and too diverse in character to enable us to draw sweeping conclusions. There are also too few cases observed from the beginning to ascertain the first effects of the infection (or intoxication). Perhaps these differ in various cases.

As regards changes in the formula, Hirschfeld and Tobias give a table showing that variations can be observed in the leukocyte formula quite apart from complications, especially notable in the polynuclear and myelocyte count. This will be confirmed by all who have followed up cases of leukæmia for some time, while changes in the gross number of cells, both red and white, are equally common, and often quite as much or even more marked than in some of the cases examined above.

A very interesting fact brought out in some of the cases, and one that I observed with particular care in my own, is the rapid rise of the leukocytes after a fall to normal, and with a great decrease in the size of the previously enlarged organs. Actual observation must, of course, be the final test of such a matter, but it is easy to understand how a chronic leukæmia may have a sudden increase of circulating leukocytes, including cells not found normally in peripheral blood, or how a so-called pseudoleukæmia may become leukæmic within a short time. These observations do not throw any light on the process by which the new cells get into the peripheral vessels, but they prove that a long time is by no means necessary for a great excess of leukocytes to appear in the peripheral capillaries.

The Effects of Various Processes Other than Infection on Leukæmia.

Finding such striking effects on the leukocytes from the influence of infectious disease, one naturally asks whether other diseases or intoxications may not have similar consequences.

Oette[44] studied the effect of fevers on the course of leukæmia, at the instigation of Mosler, as long ago as 1879, but he was limited by the greater obscurity then surrounding both fever and leukæmia, and did not materially advance the subject.

Freudenstein[31] re-examined it in 1895. He gathered many interesting facts regarding the fever of leukæmia from the early literature, besides the histories of ten of the earliest cases of infection studied here. He concluded that fever is a frequent (63 per cent.) but not constant symptom of leukæmia, and ascribed this to substances derived from broken-down leukocytes, but did not study the possible results of such processes on the leukæmia itself, doubtless because of the difficulties surrounding such an investigation.

Marischler[52] reported a case of lymphatic leukæmia complicated by a Grawitz tumor of the right kidney. There was repeated hæmaturia, considered at first as a result of the leukæmia, but later more properly ascribed to the renal tumor. The leukocytes fell from 96,000 October 16th, 84,000 November 25th, to 48,000 on February 27th, and then rose to 72,000 on the last day. The polynuclears rose from 15.60 per cent. (or 21.70 per cent. at the beginning of the hæmaturia) to 57.60 per cent. The mononuclears fell from 82.30 per cent. (or 76.20 per cent.) to 40 per cent. The difference was still more marked in the blood of the last day. The changes were, therefore, qualitative rather than quantitative. Marischler explained the changes as due less to the hemorrhage than to the carcinoma toxin, a view I do not think free from error. Marischler gives theoretic reasons, based on experiments, for his view, but the passage of a necrotic bit of tissue, 1.5 cm. by 0.25 cm., shows that the explanation by changes following loss of blood is very near. The author gives the literature of new-growths complicating leukæmia, the only genuine cases he could find being those of Whipham and Lannois and Regaud. In these no effect of the cancer upon the leukæmia was noted.

The literature of leukæmia contains references to cases in which reduction of leukocytes had taken place under the most diverse drugs, such as iron, arsenic and its salts, phosphorus, quinine, oxygen, etc.; but it is suggestive that the drugs that some have found most valuable have failed entirely in the hands of others, without perceptible reasons in the cases themselves. Most of the reports give such scanty details of the blood in the stage of recovery that they cannot be utilized at present. The literature is largely available in the study of Vehsemeyer.[53]

The first to report a careful study of the process were Toulmin and Thayer,[54] who noticed a fall of from 714,000 to 7500 leukocytes in twenty-three days in a patient taking arsenic. Two weeks later there were 9500 leukocytes. The leukocyte formula changed from:

Lymphocytes	0.96	to	6.9
Polynuclear	70.0	to	83.2
Transition	3.0	to	2.5
Eosinophiles	2.3	to	3.0
Myelocytes	23.5	to	4.0

showing a relative increase of lymphocytes and polynuclears. The myelocytes, though much reduced, were still notably high, 4 per cent.

Bramwell[55] mentions a case in which the leukocytes fell from 210,000 to 1600 in thirty-eight days under treatment with arsenic, CO_2, and oxygen, and remained below normal for a month. There was fever and an eruption from unknown cause, so that the case, perhaps, should be included among the infections. The formula was altered as follows:

	Sept. 28.	Oct. 9.	Oct. 15.	Oct. 21.	Nov. 4.
Polynuclear	69.0	70	91	75	62
Myelocytes	26.5	25	3	5	7
Lymphocytes	3.5	5	5	20	31
Eosinophiles	1.0	1+	1+	0	0

Cabot[56] and d'Allocco[57] have reported cases in which the leukocytes fell to normal or below, but, at least in the former case, myelocytes were always present, and in a degree that would in itself excite the suspicion of leukæmia, or, in the absence of acute symptoms, suggest some serious disease of the bone-marrow requiring careful observation.

McCrae,[58] however, published a case in which there was not only no leukocytosis, but no sign of medullary disease. A man, aged twenty-eight years, had medullary leukæmia with a blood count in the spring of 1898 of 2,680,000 red cells, 584,000 leukocytes. He was put on arsenic, and in August there were only 184,000 leukocytes, and the spleen was barely palpable. In September there were 9250 leukocytes. Arsenic was continued, but in November the leukocytes numbered 178,000. In December there were 98,000; in April, after taking 10-drop doses of Fowler's solution, 5000 per c.mm. The myelocytes numbered 20 per cent. to 23 per cent. in the high stage, but were absent in the low one. The polynuclear lenkocytes were 86 per cent. with 9250 leukocytes, normal with 5000. Mast-cells were present only once, in the relapse. Nucleated reds were absent after the first fall.

Taylor[59] has reported 3 cases in which the excessive leukocytes disappeared under the influence of arsenic. The improvement lasted for months, and then relapsed in all cases. A second stage of improvement followed in all; in 2 a third. The changes were qualitative at first, and varied both in quality and quantity at different times. In 1 case all qualitative changes disappeared, and a slight lymphocytosis was the only evidence of blood disease. In the other cases myelocytes persisted to the extent of 1 per cent. to 3 per cent., part eosinophilic. Taylor's discussion of this subject can be read with advantage by all who carry out experiments in the treatment of leukæmia. As in the case of infections, the low leukocyte count does not ensure recovery from the disease. This is shown by many reported cases, including the remarkable one of Saundby,[12] in which the white cells dropped from 540,000 to 8000 in eleven days, but death occurred in coma some weeks later.

It must be remembered that many of the patients whose cases are cited in the early part of this study were taking arsenic, sometimes in large doses, yet I think no one will ascribe the changes wholly or even in part to the drug in all cases. I may add that personally I have never seen a fall below 50,000 leukocytes in leukæmia from arsenic, but in only a small proportion of my cases was it possible to push the drug as it should be.

Under other drugs besides arsenic changes have been observed in the blood count in leukæmia. Von Jaksch[60] treated a patient with thyroiodin and cupric arsenate and noted a fall of from 295,000 to 560,000 to 28,000 in thirteen days, the blood at the latter count giving the picture of leukocytosis with few nucleated reds. The liver became smaller, even before the leukocytes fell. For five weeks the leukocytes were not above 100,000, but in six days reached the former high figure and remained there. Thyroiodin was also given during the rise. The formula two days before the lowest count was: polynuclears, 74.04 per cent.; mononuclear neutrophiles, 10.71 per cent.; polynuclear eosinophiles, 0.70 per cent.; mononuclear eosinophiles, 0.35 per cent.; small lymphocytes, 14.55 per cent.; large lymphocytes and transitional, 3.70 per cent. Basophiles were few at all times, and absent in the earlier examinations.

Pollitzer[61] reported a case of acute leukæmia, in which the leukocytes fell from 91,875 to 8500 in the course of seven days, while the patient was taking quinine in gram doses; fever continued; the spleen grew smaller. The patient died twenty-three days later. Post-mortem the picture was that of acute anæmia gravis with lymphoid hypertrophy of the spleen, intestinal tract, bone-marrow and lymph glands. The author attributes the effect to the quinine, but the fever and the fatal termination suggest that it was due to something else, either an intoxication from the products of cellular break-down or an infection.

In another case of Pollitzer quinine was used in 1.5-gram doses with a rise and subsequent fall, leaving the leukocytes higher than before. The author cites a case of Kuehnau and Weiss,[62] in which a patient with Hodgkin's disease was given pilocarpine and developed acute leukæmia. Sabrazès says that in a case of leukæmia with malaria quinine injections had a happy effect, not only on the malaria, but also on the course of the leukæmia.

Richter and Spiro[63] treated a patient with splenolymphatic leukæmia and apical tuberculosis with cinnamic acid. Intravenous injections of very small doses of this caused the leukocytes to increase within three hours from 170,000 to 560,000. There was also a slight increase of red cells. Polynuclear cells increased from 45 per cent. to 86 per cent.; mononuclears fell from 55 per cent. to 14 per cent.; eosinophiles, scanty before, increased, and nucleated red cells appeared, but the increase of leukocytes soon disappeared. In twenty-four hours the original number was reached; four days after the first injection the number was 46,000, and it then gradually rose to the former point. The process was repeated in two more injections. The spleen and lymph glands grew smaller; the general symptoms improved. The author points out that the experiment shows how much more intensely the diseased hæmatopoietic organs react to irritants than do normal ones, and he compared the results of his experiments with those in some of the cases studied in this paper.

A number of observations have been published on the action of organic extracts and bacterial products upon the leukæmic subject.

H. Heuck[64] at an early period gave tuberculin injections in a patient with leukæmia, who had slight signs in one apex, but no bacilli in the sputum, and no reaction to 5 milligrams of tuberculin. Doses of from 10 to 120 mg., in nineteen injections, caused reactions like those in phthisis. From the twelfth injection (60 mg.; the leukocytes were not counted before) there was a fall in the number of leukocytes each time, quickly returning, though not quite to the previous number; so that at the end of the observation the proportion was 1 to 48 instead of 1 to 57. There was general improvement, with diminution in the size of the glands.

Pal[29] also used tuberculin in a leukæmic patient, and noted a slight decrease of leukocytes after six hours, followed next day by a rise. In three days the number was 154,000 in place of 134,000, and the glands were larger, but the leukocytes fell to 103,000. A week later with 135,000 leukocytes the polynuclear cells were increased, the temperature and subjective symptoms worse.

Beitzke[65] [15] used tuberculin in 6 leukæmic patients in Quincke's clinic. The results were very uncertain, the injections not being continued long enough to permit conclusions to be drawn and other treatment being carried out at the same time. Two patients that gave most distinct evidences of improvement were taking arsenic.

Pollitzer[61a] gave tuberculin in a case of medullary leukæmia in doses of 2 to 200 mg., without reduction of leukocytes, but with increase in the size of the spleen and more marked cachexia. In a case of lymphatic leukæmia tuberculin was given for two weeks in doses of 2 to 64 mg., with a gradual but slight rise of leukocytes, without change in the formula.

Nuclein (Horbaczewski's) was also used by Pal in the case mentioned above, with a fall of leukocytes, but with enlargement of the glands. Pal purposely avoided marked reactions in his experiments, in order to prevent severe effects on nutrition. Pollitzer also used nuclein in both cases cited above. In the first 2-gram doses given for five days had no effect. In the other case there was a slow and immaterial fall, followed by a rise.

Jacob[66] used splenic extract in a patient with leukæmia, giving it subcutaneously at intervals of two to four days. The injections were followed by sweating, anxiety, and dyspnœa, symptoms that Jacob had observed in animals treated with organic extracts, and which he attributed to a leukocyte congestion of the lung capillaries. There was a slight rise in the number of leukocytes, after the early injections, followed by a fall to about half the number present before the experiment was begun. As there was an increased excretion of nitrogen in the urine, Jacob also concluded the injections increased the breaking down of leukocytes.

Here may be mentioned Franke's[67] attempt to use an extract of leukæmic glands. A packet of glands from a case of lymphatic leukæmia was rubbed up with physiological salt solution and kept sterile. Injected into rabbits in doses of 5 c.c. to 10 c.c. there were evidences of breaking down of leukocytes. On account of the patient's condition the treatment could not be carried out as intended.

From these few experiments we learn little more than the need of others, and also something of the practical difficulties of such experiments. The blood must be examined at short intervals after the treatment is given, differential counts must be made, and an almost limitless range of work may be found in studies of the cytolytic conditions at various stages. The careful observation of the body and the subjective symptoms and studies of the metabolism, as shown by the urine, are also desired.

There are still other cases on record that illustrate possibilities in leukæmia.

Strattmann[68] reported a remarkable case, in which a patient with enlarged spleen and leukocytes and red corpuscles in equal proportions underwent an exploratory operation on the supposition that the enlargement of the spleen was due to malignant disease. After considerable manipulation of the spleen for diagnostic purposes, and following massage of the organ in order to overcome possible bad effects of the manipulation, the removal was abandoned, and the patient made a good recovery, so that not only was the spleen smaller, but the blood count was 5,300,000 red corpuscles; leukocytes, 1500.

This may be contrasted with Parker's case, referred to in the early part of this paper. In this a patient with old tuberculosis and enlarged spleen, but negative blood count ("the large lymphocytes seemed more numerous"), was explored, with a view to removal of the spleen. Soon after this the blood was markedly leukæmic.

Here we may allude to Senn's[69] interesting case of leukæmia "cured by Roentgen rays." The symptoms of intoxication, such as high temperature, make one wonder whether there was an intoxication from the absorption of broken-down products of spleen and blood, or, perhaps, an accidental infection, and reports of other cases treated by the same method will be awaited with interest. It is to be hoped also that in such reports the blood will be fully described.

A full and satisfactory explanation of the changes observed in leukæmia under the influence of other diseases does not seem possible at present. We are still too much in the dark regarding the cause of leukæmia, the nature of thechanges in the tissues and the mechanism of the blood changes, and we are only beginning to learn something of the effects of infection and intoxication on the blood-forming organs and the circulating blood. The work done by Muir,[70 71] Dominici,[72] Werigo and Jegunow,[73] Rubinstein,[74] Lengemann,[75] Roger and Josué,[76] Weil,[77] Flexner,[78] Bunting,[79] and others opens up a most promising field, but at present does not go far in explaining the difficulties in this particular subject.

An early and natural explanation was that diseases associated with leukopenia, or without leukocytosis in ordinary cases caused in leukæmia a decrease of leukocytes. This might apply to miliary tuberculosis, or typhoid fever, such as Eisenlohr's case was supposed to be. But further reports not only opposed this view, but even led to the opposite one, viz., that diseases ordinarily causing lenkocytosis have an antagonistic effect in leukæmia.

Ortner[80] offered a plausible explanation, viz., consumption of the body, due to infection, but Beitzke pointed out some important objections. It does not account for the altered leukocyte formula often observed; the change sometimes comes on early, before the exhaustion of the body is evident; at other times leukæmia shows advanced wasting and cachexia without notable change in the leukocytes. H. F. Mueller's theory is attractive chiefly because of its obscurity. He suggested an "alterative" action, but in the present state of our knowledge this does not explain anything. The leukocytolytic theory of Fraenkel is also attractive. It seems borne out by the author's observations on degenerated leukocytes in his own cases, and the increased excretion of uric acid. It seems analogous to the rapid disappearance of certain tumors, some of which (sarcomata) closely resemble leukæmic growths, under the actions of poisons like arsenic, or those of certain infections, as erysipelas. Recently the chemotactic theory has become more prominent, and has received the support of Ehrlich, whose influence in the study of leukæmia is deservedly so great. Quincke's objection, that no evidences of transfer of leukocytes are present, might be explained by a rapid breaking down of the cells.

It seems to me the process in most cases is complex. Breakdown and consumption must occur in cases with severe cytolytic poisons, and in some must preponderate. In others chemotactic processes will be most important, and innumerable variations in the clinical course and the blood picture will probably depend partly on the kind, extent, and intensity of the intoxication, partly on the histological peculiarities of the new-growths, and the capacity of their cells to enter or be poured into the circulation. Thus, in acute lymphatic leukæmia, the changes will not be the same as in the chronic myeloid alteration of all the blood-forming organs.

Finally, the question as to therapeutic bearings must be met. It is easy to understand how many have looked upon the changes observed in cases cited above as evidences of healing. The most striking sign of leukæmia, the excess of leukocytes, disappears, and sometimes the spleen and lymph glands return to their normal size. Yet that the change is not wholly favorable appears from the fact that no case has really recovered. Most patients died while still under the influence of the process that was thought to have healed them, and, although some seem to have had their lives prolonged, none have lived longer than many leukæmics without such complications.

Weil has suggested that the action of the complicating infections is too "brutal," and this may be so, although the cases hitherto observed show considerable variation in severity. But, considering the hopelessness of the ordinary treatment of leukæmia, it seems that carefully planned experiments, either with bacterial products or organ extracts, might show a more safe and permanent result. I need not go into the details of such experiments, but may point out the necessity of thoroughness of the observations as an essential. Previous experience with the substances to be used, either on men or animals, is desirable, while a familiarity with the methods of blood examinations is indispensable.

BIBLIOGRAPHY

1. Virchow. Archiv f. path. Anat., Bd. ii. p. 587.
2. Bennett, John Hughes. Leucocythæmia, Edinburgh, 1852.
3. Bamberger, H. Verhandlungen der phys.-med. Gesellschaft in Würzburg, 1857, Bd. vii. p. 110.
4. Mosler, Friedrich. Die Pathologie und Therapie der Leukaemie, Berlin, 1872.
5. Hounsell, H. Strangways. Medical Times and Gazette, December 12, 1863.
6. Ollivier et Ranvier. Archives de physiol. norm. et pathol., 1869, pp. 407, 518.
7. Robin. Gaz. méd. de Paris, 1883, p. 333.
8. de Roth, Mlle. G. Contribution a l'étude de la leucémie et de ses complications, Thesis, Geneva, 1895.
9. Brueckmann, P. Ein Fall von Lymph-drüsen und Bauchfell-Tuberkulose kombiniert mit myel-lieno-lymphatischer Leukaemie, Inaug. Diss., Tübingen, 1896; also, Arbeiten a. d. path. anat. Inst. zu Tübingen, Bd. ii. p. 468.
10. Volpe, Angelo. Archivio internaz. de med. e chir., An. 12, 1896, 31 Mag., Fasc. 4, p. 161.
11. Musser and Sailer. Transactions of the Association of American Physicians, 1896.
12. Saundby, Robert. British Medical Journal, 1901, vol. i. p. 1.
13. Sabrazès, J. Hématologie clinique. Extrait de Comptes-rendus du Cinquième Congrès français de médecine, Lille, 1899; Paris, 1900.
14. Quincke, H. Tageblatt der 62 Versammlung Deutscher Naturforscher und Aerzte, 1889.
15. Quincke, H. Deutsches Archiv f. klin. Med., Bd. lxxiv. p. 445.
16. Lichtheim. Deutsche med. Wochenschrift, September 30, 1897, Vereins-Beilage, p. 193.
17. Schmidt, Hans. Beitrag zur Lehre von der Leukämie, Inaug. Diss., Göttingen, 1900.
18. Bezançon et Weil. Gaz. hebdom., 1900, p. 631.
19. Hirschfeld und Tobias. Deutsche med. Wochenschrift, 1902, p. 92.
20. Elsner and Groat. THE AMERICAN JOURNAL OF THE MEDICAL SCIENCES, March, 1901, p. 271.
21. Sturmdorf, Arnold. Ibid., August, 1901, p. 166.
22. Parker, G. British Medical Journal, May 10, 1902.
23. Murrell, W. The Lancet, London, July 19, 1902.
24. Stintzing. Tageblatt der 62 Versammlung Deutscher Naturforscher und Aerzte, 1889.
25. Juenger. Archiv f. path. Anat., 1900, Bd. clxii. p. 283.
26. Francksen, Bernh. Ueber die Complication der Leukaemie mit Tuberkulose, Inaug. Diss., Göttingen, 1892.
27. Baldwin and Wilder. THE AMERICAN JOURNAL OF THE MEDICAL SCIENCES, June, 1899, p. 656.
28. Eisenlohr, C. Archiv f. path. Anat., 1878, Bd. lxxiii. p. 56.
29. Pal, J. Jahrbuch der Wiener k. k. Kranken-Anstalten, V. Jahrg., 1896, II. Th. p. 5.
30. Richter, Paul Friedr. Charité Annalen, 1896, Bd. xxi. p. 299.
31. Freudenstein, Gustav. Ueber Fieber und fieberhafte Komplikationen bei pernic. Anaemie und Leukaemie, Inaug. Diss., Berlin, 1895.
32. Kraus, Emil. Prager med. Wochenschrift, 1899, Nos. 41 and 42; also, Beitr. zur inn. Med. Wien., 1900, p. 152.
32a. Adler, Emil. Zeitschrift f. Heilkunde (inn. med.), 1901, Bd. xxii. p. 221.
33. Mueller, H. F. Deutsches Archiv f. klin. Med., 1891, Bd. xlviii. p. 47.
34. Koermoeczi, Emil. Deutsche med. Wochenschrift, 1899, No. 47, p. 773.
35. Heuck, G. Archiv f. path. Anat., 1879, Bd. lxxviii. p. 475.
36. Kovacs, Friedrich. Wiener klin. Wochenschrift, 1893, No. 39, p. 701.
. Da Costa, John C. Clinical Hematology, Philadelphia, 1901, p. 263.
. Mueller, H. F. Deutsches Archiv f. klin. Med., Bd. l. p. 47.
37. Weil, E. Gazette hebdomadaire, Paris, 1900, No. 70.
40. Wende, Grover. THE AMERICAN JOURNAL OF THE MEDICAL SCIENCES, December, 1901, p. 836.
41. Cabot, R. C. Clinical Examination of the Blood, fourth edition, p. 177.
42. Fraenkel, A. Deutsche med. Wochenschrift, 1895, p. 677.
43. Mueller, E. Jahrbuch f. Kinderheilkunde, 1896, Bd. xliii. p. 130.
44. Oette, Max. Ueber den Einfluss gewisser Fieber auf den leukaemischen Process. Inaug. Diss., Greifswald, 1879.
45. Froelich. Wiener med. Wochenschr., 1893, p. 286.
46. Thorsch, E. Wiener klinische Wochenschrift, 1896, No. 20.
47. Grawitz, Ernst. Klinische Pathologie des Blutes, Berlin, 1902, p. 389.
48. Hart, T. S. New York and Philadelphia Medical Journal, August 1, 1903, p. 224.
49. Petit et Weil. Soc. med. des hôp., 1900, p. 398.

50. Rieder, Hermann. Beiträge zur Kenntniss der Leukocytose, etc., Leipzig, 1892.

51. von Limbeck, R. Grundriss einer klinischen Pathologie des Blutes, Jena, 1896.

52. Marischler, J. Wiener klin. Wochenschrift, 1896, No. 30, p. 686.

53. Vehsemeyer, H. Die Behandlung der Leukaemie, Berlin, 1894.

54. Toulmin and Thayer. Johns Hopkins Hospital Bulletin, 1891, vol. ii. p. 84.

55. Bramwell, B. Anæmia and Some of the Diseases of the Blood-forming Organs, etc. Edinburgh, 1899, p. 171.

56. Cabot, R. C. Boston Medical and Surgical Journal, 1894, vol. i. p. 277; and ibid., vol. ii. p. 507.

57. d'Allocco, O. Abstr. in Schmidt's Jahrbücher, 1899, Bd. cclxi. p. 206.

58. McCrae, T. British Medical Journal, 1900, vol. i. p. 760.

59. Taylor, A. E. Studies in Leukæmia. Contributions from the William Pepper Laboratory of Clinical Medicine, Philadelphia, 1900, p. 148.

60. von Jaksch, R. Prag. med. Wochenschrift, 1896, No. 21, p. 510.

61. Pollitzer, J. Wien. klin. Rundschau, 1899, p. 197.

61a. Pollitzer, J. Ibid., p. 385.

62. Kuehnau und Weiss. Zeitschrift f. klin. Med., Bd xxxii. p. 482.

63. Richter und Spiro. Arch. f. exp. Path. und Pharmakol., 1894, Bd. xxxiv. p. 289.

64. Heuck, H. Deutsche med. Wochenschrift, May 28, 1891, p. 746.

65. Beitzke, Hermann. Ueber Beeinflussung der Leukaemie durch complicierende Krankheiten, Inaug. Diss., Kiel, 1899.

66. Jacob, Paul. Deutsche med. Wochenschrift, 1894, No. 32.

67. Franke, M. Centralblatt f. inn. Med., February 8, 1902.

68. Strattmann. Deutsche med. Wochenschrift, 1899, Vereins-Beilage, p. 34.

69. Senn, N. Medical Record, New York, August 22, 1903.

70. Muir, R. Journal of Pathology and Bacteriology, 1901.

71. Muir, R. British Medical Journal, September 3, 1898.

72. Dominici, M. Comptes-rendus de la Soc. de biol., 1899, p. 721; 1900, p. 74.

73. Werigo, Br., und Jegunow. Archiv f. die gesammte Physiologie, 1901, Bd. lxxxiv. S. 451.

74. Rubinstein, H. Zeitschrift f. klin. Med., 1901, Bd. xlii. p. 161.

75. Lengemann, P. Beiträge zur path. Anat., 1901, Bd. xxix. p. 1.

76. Roger, H., and Josué, O. Suite des monographies cliniques, Paris, 1899, No. 21.

77. Weil. Gaz. hebd., May 2, 1900.

78. Flexner, S. University of Pennsylvania Medical Bulletin, vol. xv. p. 287.

79. Bunting, C. H. Ibid., vol. xvi. p. 200.

80. Ortner, N. Wien. klin. Wochenschr., 1890, p. 832.

CARCINOMA OF ABDOMINAL CAVITY; PUNCTURE OF INTESTINE DURING PARACENTESIS ABDOMINIS; PRESENCE OF CARCINOMATOUS FRAGMENTS IN ASCITIC EXUDATE.

REMARKS ON CYTODIAGNOSIS.

By Norman B. Gwyn, M.D.,

INSTRUCTOR IN MEDICINE, UNIVERSITY OF PENNSYLVANIA.

The following case is of interest as showing the difficulty of diagnosis of abdominal disease, the danger of even the most carefully performed paracentesis, and the value of microscopic examinations of exudate, etc.

Mrs. B., aged sixty-eight years, complaining of abdominal distention, dyspnœa, indigestion. Family history unimportant; acute Bright's disease twelve years ago, with apparent complete recovery as far as symptoms showed. Six months previously the patient noticed abdominal enlargement, which, being naturally corpulent, she attributed to fat, discovering soon, however, that fluid was present. Fluid increased, persistent discomfort after feeding developed, and, later, diarrhœa. The urine was markedly diminished, albumin and casts were present, and the patient became steadily weaker.

Examination revealed only ascites, hidden somewhat by a thick apron of fat; liver dulness present, as far as could be judged, in normal extent; œdema of legs, loud systolic apical heart murmur, slight dulness and few moist crepitations at base of lungs.

Patient had been tapped one month previously, eleven quarts of dark fluid being removed, a considerable amount of fluid blood coming away at finish of operation.

At the second tapping (the first while in our hands) twelve quarts of a bloody fluid were removed; no free blood flowed; liver dulness did not appear quite as extensive as normal; patient seemed much relieved after operation, and gastric symptoms abated.

Ten days later a third tapping brought away six quarts of fluid resembling that of the previous tappings, some gelatinous and granular material coming away just before removing the cannula.

The operation in each case was performed by a surgeon, local cocaine anæsthesia and incision through the skin between the navel and pubes preceding the introduction of the trocar; little if any pain was experienced by the patient; a large apron of fat reaching to the pubes interfered greatly with the drainage of the abdominal cavity.

In six hours after this (third) operation there was a complete collapse; temperature previously, 99° to 100° F., dropping to 97° F.

Tympanites developed quickly; abdominal pain and vomiting, rapid, weak pulse, and rising temperature made us suspect a bowel perforation and subsequent peritonitis. Death took place in three days. At no time after the first appearance of fatal symptoms did the patient's condition seem to justify any further exploration of the abdomen, and, as the examination of the fluid and material removed made the presence of cancer probable, such steps were deemed inadvisable in any case.

The clinical picture in this case was from the first obscure; the huge accumulation of fat present in the abdominal walls precluded any satisfactory examination; at times, even before twelve quarts of fluid were removed, fluctuation was indistinct; there was no anæmia, the withdrawal of so much fluid into the peritoneal cavity causing, in fact, a distinctly concentrated condition of the blood, as is sometimes seen; cirrhosis of the liver or carcinoma of some abdominal or pelvic organ were considered the most probable causes of the recurring ascites and associated symptoms.

The bloody appearance of the first fluid removed was suspicious of malignant or tubercular disease; neither suspicious cellular elements nor bacilli were to be detected. The second fluid removed was, on the contrary, suggestive from the outset. The colloid-looking lumps in the precipitate passing ready formed through the cannula must necessarily have been fragments of some tumor formation or material direct from the intestine; as a matter of fact, both substances were present. Further examination showed specific gravity, 1020; albumin, about 0.3 per cent.; sugar, 0. Microscopically fibrin, intestinal material, starch, vegetable fibres, meat fibres, and some bunches of leptothrix (proving that the bowel had been punctured) were readily seen.

The puncturing of the intestine in paracentesis abdominis, although always considered a real danger, must be considered as infrequent; in this case more than usual care had been taken; it is possible, of course, that portions of the intestines had become adherent in some part and presented resistance to the trocar.

The cellular elements in the exudate attracted our attention from the outset; quite numerous red blood cells were, of course, to be seen; distinct pus cells were few; on the other hand, epithelioid cells or cells resembling the larger lymphocytes were numerous, either single or grouped as in the drawing (4), showing fibrillar intercellular structure, and columnar cells in groups (3), evidently parts of distinct glandular structures, were in evidence. The arrangement and variety of these first-mentioned cells cannot be said to be diagnostic of carcinomatous conditions; similar-looking cells are present in tubercular exudates; their presence in masses, as in the figure, was suggestive and suspicious, more from its gross appearance than from the character of the individual cells; the distinctly glandular-looking cells, arranged in columns (3), could only be intestinal or from adenocarcinomatous new-growth.

The colloid masses referred to, on being teased out, gave the picture as shown in the figure and just described; it seemed certain thereafter that the cells of the exudate were the colloid elements. Hardened and prepared the colloid masses gave the picture shown in the drawing (1), which can be briefly described as "adenocarcinoma showing advanced colloid degeneration," probably from the suggestive follicular structures connected with the intestine.

The diagnosis of malignant disease in various parts of the body, by means of the character of the cells found in the exudate, has been for some time a rather fruitful field of speculation. We are at present, however, much nearer an accurate working knowledge on the subject, thanks to the careful work of Dock and others; but the readiness with which the earlier writers in the earlier microscopic days accepted various atypical cellular modifications as evidence of malignant disease is striking.

Quincke considered cells of large size in any number, either separate or grouped, as most suggestive; the presence of the glycogen reaction was considered to make the diagnosis almost certain.

Eichhorst makes the statement that "especially in cancer of the

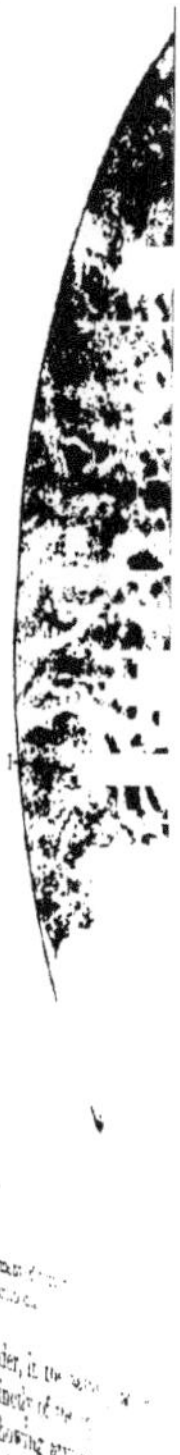

pleura we find in the exudate not rarely abundant fatty granular cells and cells with multiple nuclei," which are characteristic of cancer. Geigel and Voit were practically in accord with this view in 1895.

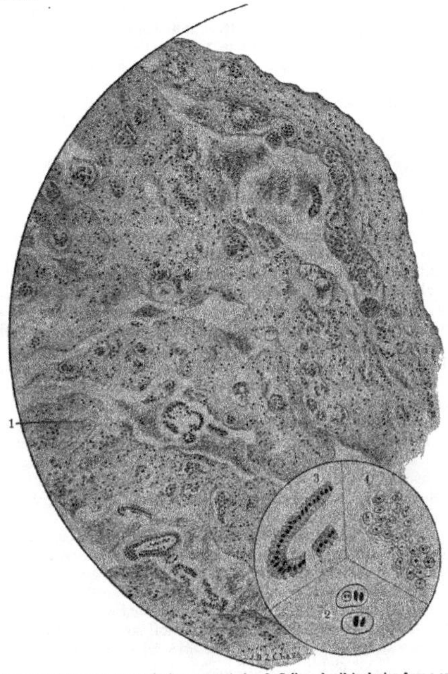

1. Fragment of tumor removed during paracentesis. 2. Cells and cell inclusion from a case of carcinoma recti. 3 and 4. Types of cells and arrangement found in fresh exudate.

Rieder, in the same year, in a detailed and well-illustrated article, is distinctly of the opinion that polymorphonuclear endothelial cells, cells showing atypical mitoses, vacuoles, and having a tendency to appear in clumps, are certainly malignant. Neelsen agrees with this view.

The description and illustrations of the cellular findings in malignant and other exudate, as given by Dock several years later, show clearly that these views must be taken cautiously, since all the cellular changes described by the observers as characteristic of malignant exudates were found by him in conditions distinctly not malignant, although, as he admits, in much smaller numbers.

Dock agrees with Rieder as to the possibility of distinguishing cancerous from tuberculous exudates from a consideration of the cellular constituents thereof. In the latter, as a general rule, according to both observers, the great variety of cells, the mitotic and amitotic figures are rare; a small cell, with the general characteristic of a lymphocyte, being more usually seen.

Warthin a few months later reports the ready diagnosis of a primary sarcoma of the pleura from the large number of spindle cells found in the exudate; these spindle cells differed rather materially from the ordinary fibroblast found in pleural exudate in not showing branching processes and in their regularly more oval-shaped nucleus; numerous symmetrical mitoses were also present. A comparison of these cells with those present in serous and fibrinous pleural and pericardial exudates and with normal pleural cells does show, in the gross, some difference, but certain characteristics are possessed by all. The great number of the spindle cells is probably the most suspicious character of the exudate in his case.

Hemmeter insists upon the regularity with which cells showing mitotic figures, symmetrical and asymmetrical, may be found in the washings from cases of carcinoma of the stomach.

A more complete microscopic picture and a certain diagnostic feature is presented in cases in which (as in ours) tumor fragments are removed during the simple operation of paracentesis or lavage. The reported instances of this happening are not numerous.

Steiner, Rieder, and Lenhartz give instances of recovery of tumor particles from ascitic fluid.

Prentess, Girvin and Steele found particles of malignant growths in pleural exudate; the fixed and stained specimens usually have shown very distinctly the nature of the new-growth; examination of the fresh particles is not always so certain, the cellular structure not being so clear. Ordinary small endothelial cells or lymphoid cells entangled in the fibrin coagulum of simple or tubercular exudates can present suspicious features when examined in the fresh state. Our own experience in cytodiagnosis has been of more or less interesting nature. In our cases of simple or supposed tubercular pleurisies it has been easy to demonstrate the preponderance of the lymphocyte-like cells described now as the most common cell in these conditions. The large endothelial cells, at times mononuclear, at times polynuclear, were regularly seen in small numbers.

In several fluids from spinal punctures, in which no pneumococci or other micro-organism could be demonstrated by stain or culture, but which were also negative for tubercle bacilli by inoculation, the same lymphocyte-like cell was the prevailing element.

No exudates due to the more common organisms, streptococcus, pneumococcus, or typhoid bacillus, have come under our observation since this paper was begun. It is now generally found that in such exudates the pus cell, the ordinary polymorphonuclear cell, is in excess.

In a gelatinous, chocolate-colored sputum from a patient with persistent cough and wasting, we were struck by the almost purely cellular condition of the material. Closer examination showed a total absence of the ordinary polymorphonuclear leukocyte, and the presence of such dense numbers of mononucleated round or oval lymphoid-like cells as to give the idea that one might be observing an extremely cellular tissue, such as sarcoma, rather than an exudate or secretion. These cells stained readily when fresh, were non-granular, the size of a medium-sized or large lymphocyte; no mitoses or multinucleated elements were made out; nucleated stains showed a reticulated, well-formed nucleus. The findings of the subsequent autopsy were given to be a "tumor of the lung." A further application of the cytodiagnosis was shown in the case of a patient suffering from an intermittent diarrhœa, associated with bloody, mucus-like discharge. Numerous mononucleated and multinucleated cells of epithelioid character were demonstrable, and were in themselves suggestive of a condition other than a simple inflammatory one, but the most suspicious elements were cells such as pictured in the drawing (2), with their cell inclusions. The association of these bodies with carcinoma and their supposed parasitic nature is now a matter of every-day discussion, and needs no comment.

I do not know of their being described previous to this in exudates, etc. Proctoscopic examination and subsequent history revealed malignant ulceration of the upper rectum.

We were singularly unfortunate in our cases in not being able to demonstrate mitotic figures, and hence the question of the diagnostic value of these figures in the cells of exudates cannot come into consideration. Steiner failed to find mitoses in his case. The condition of the new-growth, whether rapidly growing or not; various physical states, such as serous membrane irritation, probably account for the presence of these figures. I must agree with recent observers "that the presence in exudates of *many* cells showing mitosis will, in most cases, allow us to make a diagnosis of malignant disease;" such cells are certainly rarely present in other conditions, and then but in scant numbers. Small cells grouped in masses, as shown in the drawing (4), are suspicious, and were enough in our case to convince us of the malignant nature of the trouble. One does not often find such groups in simple conditions, nor could one readily explain their presence in such; masses of desquamated endothelial cells do not show the intercellular fibrous strands as in the figure; moreover, the large size of the endothelial cells would show their nature. Large, multinucleated, endothelial-like cells are more common in malignant disease, but are seen frequently in other conditions.

Cells of such glandular type and arrangement as found in our case, and pictured in the drawing (3), could not be passed over. In this instance not only the nature of the new-growth, but its situation or the situation of metastatic accidents is demonstrated.

One of our recent cases is of interest, and, at the same time, shows the limitations of cytodiagnosis. In this instance, a few days after an operation removing the right breast for what has been shown to be a cancerous degeneration of an adenofibromatous tumor, a pleural effusion, with fever, developed. Repeated aspirations (3) were necessary to relieve the patient. Subsequent metastasis, developing rapidly along the incision, led us to consider the condition as probably due to extension of the disease to the pleura. The fluid of the various tappings showed at no time, however, any cells suggestive of cancerous vegetation. On the other hand, the preponderance of 98 per cent. to 99 per cent. of small mononuclear lenkocytes was always evident. There has been no reaccumulation of fluid since the last aspiration eight weeks ago, the fever falling to normal after the first and remaining there. The cellular condition in this instance is suggestive of a tubercular more than a malignant or mechanical pleurisy.

One must certainly admit that considerable information and help may be derived from careful examination of exudates, etc., as to their cellular constituents. The presence of cells in any number should lead to more careful consideration of their type, arrangement, and nuclear condition.

In a majority of instances one may suspect malignant disease if large numbers of nuclear figures, typical or atypical, are present; their absence, on the other hand, by no means, excludes the possibility of malignancy. Occasional nuclear figures are to be found in other conditions.

Endothelial cells with many nuclei are probably but not certainly more numerous in cancerous exudates. Cells of exudate tending to appear in bunches or groups with intercellular fibrillæ (as shown in 4) are, to a degree, suspicious; apart from fragments of squamous epithelium and desquamated flakes of large endothelial cells, there are few conditions which would cause cells not of these varieties to appear in compact masses. Small groups of lymphocytes or pus cells, of course, are often seen.

Unusual cells of glandular or other type, or such as are depicted containing cell inclusions, must be given a significance of their own. The question of cytodiagnosis of tubercular and other exudates has been of late freely discussed, and it seems probable that tubercular exudates are more or less regularly associated with lymphocyte-like cells, particularly after the first few days.

Mechanical exudates show more often numbers of large endothelial cells, often in large plaques, the "placards" which Widal and Ravant consider pathognomonic of mechanical exudates or transudates.

Infectious pleurisies, etc., are found to have the polymorphonuclear leukocyte as the characteristic cell of their exudate.

BIBLIOGRAPHY.

Dock. THE AMERICAN JOURNAL OF THE MEDICAL SCIENCES, 1897, vol. cxiii.
Rieder. Deutsch. Arch. f. klin. Med., 1895, vol. liv.
Warthin. Medical News, New York, 1897, vol. lxxi.
Bahrenberg. Cleveland Medical Gazette, 1895-96, vol. xi.
Bogehold. Berl. klin. Woch., 1878, vol. xv.
Quincke. Deutsch. Arch. f. klin. Med., 1875, vol. xvi.
Lenhartz. Mikroskopie und Chemie am Krankenbett, Berlin, 1895.
Prentess. Transactions of the Association of American Physicians, 1893, vol. viii.
Girvin and Steele. Proceedings of the Pathological Society of Philadelphia, 1901, n. s., vol. iv
Bunting. Johns Hopkins Hospital Bulletin, July, 1903.
Musgrave. Boston Medical and Surgical Journal, March 5, 1903.
Steiner. Johns Hopkins Hospital Bulletin, October, 1901.
Widal and Ravant. Soc. de Biol., 1901, p. 648.

THE CLINICAL BEHAVIOR OF THE LYMPH GLANDS IN TYPHOID FEVER.

BY DAVID L. EDSALL, M.D.,
OF PHILADELPHIA.

So far as I can determine by examining the most important recent works on typhoid fever and by searching through any papers with suggestive titles, the statement that widespread enlargement of the lymph glands, recognizable clinically, occurs in typhoid fever has not been made. It is known that the lymphatic enlargement found at necropsy is not limited to the tissues in the intestine and to the glands in the direct path of the lymph stream from the intestine. Post-mortem findings of enlargement of the inguinal and the periœsophageal glands are sometimes noted; and lymphatic tissues that are even as distant from the intestines as are the tonsils occasionally show enlargement, and in some instances are probably directly involved in the typhoidal process. Indeed, typhoid fever plays its part so largely in lymphatic tissues that it is to be expected that it should, at times, produce widespread glandular enlargement, readily recognizable at post-mortem, particularly since the disease is well known to be a general bacterial infection and not a local process.

Clinically, however, in cases in which it is necessary to distinguish between typhoid fever and other diseases in which glandular enlargement is common, the discovery of many readily palpable glands is usually accepted as being a point in favor of the last-mentioned class of diseases and against typhoid fever.

In May, 1903, in the course of my services at the Episcopal Hospital and at St. Christopher's Hospital for Children, I encountered within two weeks 3 cases of rather peculiar nature,in which glandular enlargement was a point of some importance in the diagnosis. The first case was in a boy aged six years. In the course of typhoid fever, and while rötheln was prevalent, this child developed a rötheln-like rash and was found to have easily palpable glands in the occipital and the anterior and posterior cervical regions, as well as in the axilla and the groin; and subsequent observation showed that these glands exhibited a slight further increase in size and a distinct increase in number. The absence of any other new symptoms, the fact that the fever was dropping at the time and continued to decrease, the lack of any influence upon the patient's general condition, and the rapid disappearance of the eruption, without any trace of desquamation, led me to decide that this was merely an accidental rash.

In the second case, that of a boy, aged eighteen years, the presence of swollen and slightly ulcerated gums, with some excess of leukocytes, and with an absence of any distinctive evidence of typhoid fever, suggested the possibility of an early acute leukæmia. This patient showed a small number of readily palpable anterior and posterior cervical, axillary, and inguinal glands; and within a few days the palpable glands were found to be increasing in number, though not distinctly increasing in size. He soon developed spots and a Widal reaction, however; the leukocytosis disappeared, and he rapidly settled into a course of typical typhoid fever, no complication, except the mild grade of stomatitis, being discovered.

The nature of the third case still remains somewhat obscure, although I believe it was typhoid fever. In considering the possibility of syphilitic fever in this case, I found easily palpable anterior and posterior cervical, axillary, epitrochlear, and inguinal glands. The man denied the possibility of syphilis, however, and showed no primary lesion, and he had no subsequent manifestations of that disease. While he had no absolutely characteristic evidences of typhoid fever, that diagnosis remains the most probable.

These observations led me to make notes at various periods of the disease in a series of cases of typhoid fever. As a result, I think I may state without hesitation that in a considerable number of cases widespread glandular enlargement that is, to be sure, slight, but sufficiently marked to be discoverable clinically, occurs in this disease; and in some instances the glandular enlargement is as marked as that which usually occurs in certain other infectious diseases, and is usually looked upon as somewhat distinctive of those diseases.

The regions that I especially observed were the groin, the axilla, and the anterior and posterior portions of the neck. In some cases the condition of the epitrochlear and the brachial glands was also noted. In most cases the enlargement observed was very slight; it was sometimes so slight that I doubted whether it could be considered to be actual enlargement. The most common condition was the appearance of many glands about the size of buckshot or a little larger; these were, as a rule, especially easy to palpate in the axilla and the groin. Little attention was paid to such a condition of itself, as I appreciated the fact that glands of this size might readily have been present from the beginning and have become apparent only because of emaciation. Very frequently, however, I noted, during the course of the disease, the development in the axilla and the groin of glands that I have described in the notes as varying in size from that of small peas to that of hazelnuts, while in the neck they were often noted as being of the dimensions of small peas. In some of these instances such glands were present in small numbers on admission, but I noted a distinct increase in their number during the course of the disease. As a rule, the occurrence of glandular enlargement could be determined only by painstaking and deliberate examination; occasionally, however, it was sufficiently marked, especially in the axilla and in the neck, to be apparent upon rather hasty palpation. In the groin the conditions were not quite so patent, because most of these patients, as is so very common, showed here some old enlarged glands in the beginning; hence a little more care was necessary in this region, in order to determine whether these glands were enlarging and whether new ones were appearing.

I am, for several reasons, disposed to be very guarded in using my figures as to the frequency with which enlargement can be noted. In the first place, the number of cases that I have observed is too small to be distinctive. In the second place, the circumstances attending the observation of such cases are likely to lead one astray; that is, typhoid fever patients usually emaciate rapidly during the course of the disease, and then rapidly put on flesh after convalescence has begun. In consequence of this, glands already palpable would become more distinctly so; and others, not at first palpable, would appear as the result of the emaciation; while, when fat is being reacquired, the conditions are reversed. This tends to give one the impression that the glands are showing slight enlargement during the course of the disease, and that this enlargement is disappearing during convalescence. Furthermore, anyone that makes a practice of searching for small lymph glands will agree with me that in the most varied conditions a few may often be found high up in the axilla, while they are somewhat less easily and less frequently discovered in the anterior and posterior cervical regions, though common here. Naturally, also, the more frequently the search is repeated, the more often will glands be discovered and the greater will be the number found; hence, repeated search at various periods of the disease might give one the impression that the glands are increasing somewhat in number, when this is not the case. I have been careful to exclude, as far as possible, these sources of error, and have weeded out from the positive group the cases in which I thought that the notes of increase in the size or the number of the glands might have been due to mistakes in observation; but even after having done this, I am inclined to think that my figures show a greater frequency of the condition than is quite correct.

The total number of cases that I observed was about 60. Some of them, however, were seen only late in the course of the disease; and another group exhibited complications like furunculosis. The conditions in the former were not distinctive, and in the latter any glandular enlargement might readily have been due to the secondary infection. I have, therefore, excluded all these cases. This brings the total number down to 43. Of these, 7 at the time my service ended were still in such an early stage of the disease that the behavior of the glands during the course of the disease could not be determined properly, so that the cases in which satisfactory notes have been obtained number only 36.

In these 36 cases I observed the occurrence of glandular enlargement during the course of the disease in 25 instances; in 4 the conditions were doubtful, and in 7 there were no determinable changes in the glands.

At the time of admission, 12 of these 25 had enlargement of the peripheral glands other than the inguinal; they likewise had inguinal enlargement, but, of itself, this is, of course, of little interest. Twelve showed no enlargement of other glands than the inguinal, and in 5 of these cases no inguinal enlargement could be observed. Three of the last-mentioned 5 cases occurred in young boys. In the 1 case remaining of the 25 I have no notes made upon admission.

Notes during the course of the fever show that in 22 of the 25 cases there developed distinct enlargement of the axillary and the cervical glands; in 1 other case glandular enlargement, noted upon admission, distinctly decreased before the fever ended, while in the 2 remaining cases the condition of the glands was doubtful during the course of the fever. Although these 2 cases last mentioned were doubtful at this period, they are included among the positive cases because, in early convalescence, it was determined that there had been a decided increase in the size and number of the glands.

Upon discharge, 16 showed a distinct decrease in the glandular enlargement; in 6 it persisted about as it had been when last noted; in 2 there was, as mentioned, a distinct increase in the size of the glands, and in 1 the axillary glands were noted to be decreased and the cervical increased.

Of the 7 cases mentioned in which the notes covered too brief a period to allow of their inclusion in the above figures, 1 showed distinct decrease in the glandular enlargement within a week after admission (he had been ill twenty days when admitted), in 2 there seemed to be a distinct increase in the size of the cervical glands, and in 4 the notes were absolutely indistinctive.

While I have stated that I am not convinced that enlargement occurred in all the cases in which my notes indicate that it did, I have no question concerning most of the cases that I have included as positive, and there were certain cases in which the changes in the glands were so readily determinable that there could be no possible source of error in the observations. There were, for instance, three boys, aged between twelve and fourteen years, that upon admission showed, after the most careful search, no enlargement of any glands, except for a very few, about the size of buckshot, in the inguinal region. During the course of the disease these patients all developed many palpable glands, a few of the largest becoming the size of small hazelnuts, many reaching the dimensions of moderate-sized peas, and numbers of buckshot-sized ones becoming palpable. In two of these boys the glandular enlargement decreased decidedly during defervescence, even before the patient was being fed more freely, and hence before any flesh was being put on; and in both these patients the enlargement had practically disappeared before their discharge from the hospital. In the third case the enlargement, although it decreased somewhat, persisted until the time of discharge.

There were also several cases of relapse in which changes in the glands could easily be followed. In one of these it was noted that upon admission the inguinals only were enlarged. Within a week the cervical, axillary, and epitrochlear glands had become easily palpahle. Two weeks afterward, when the patient's fever had disappeared, the glands were found to have decreased markedly in size and number. Ten days later, after he had been for a week in a relapse, the enlarged glands were found to be much more numerous than they had been in the primary attack; and the number of these glands continued to increase up to the time of his discharge, which was somewhat premature. (Two weeks later, just after I left the service, this man was admitted in a second relapse.)

In another case there were no notes upon admission; but during the course of the disease the inguinal, axillary, and cervical glands were felt in moderate numbers and were the size of peas. At the end of an afebrile period of a week the axillary and the cervical glands had decreased greatly in size; the inguinals remained unchanged. Toward the end of a relapse of two weeks' duration the axillary and the cervical glands were found to be again as large as peas or larger, and to be much more numerous than they had been before. These glands had decreased to the size of buckshot before the patient's diet was increased, and remained in this condition at the time of his discharge.

In a third relapse-case only slight glandular enlargement, if any, could be determined to have occurred during the primary attack, while during the relapse there was distinct and general enlargement. Notes were not made with sufficient frequency during the course of these cases to determine definitely when the enlargement occurred. In some instances it seems to have appeared early in the disease, for a number of patients were admitted at the end of the first week with a large number of palpable glands, and this enlargement disappeared late in the course of the disease or during convalescence, indicating that it had been due to the attack of typhoid fever. In most instances, however, the enlargement appeared to develop—most strikingly, at least—in the latter part of the disease; and in a number of cases increased enlargement or the first definite enlargement was noted during early convalescence. As already indicated, it had, in the majority of cases, disappeared to a greater or less extent before the discharge of the patient, but in about one-quarter of them it persisted unchanged up to the time of discharge.

I at first thought that by carefully observing the glands it might be possible to learn some facts that would be of value in diagnosis. It seemed possible, for instance, that this might afford some help in distinguishing between typhoid fever and obscure cases of tropical malaria. There were a number of such cases in the wards during this period, and in 2 of these repeated searches for the plasmodium, even when instituted by a person so skilled as is Dr. Ghriskey, failed to show the parasites; although they were ultimately discovered. The glands in these patients were observed persistently, but showed no enlargement.

It likewise seemed possible that in acute tuberculosis glandular enlargement would occur less commonly and less rapidly and would not be widespread. Two cases of acute pneumonic tuberculosis were observed during this period in the ward; they showed no general glandular enlargement. Perhaps in disseminated tuberculosis and some other conditions the enlargement of the glands might be of interest in the diagnosis. On the whole, however, I believe that it is of little consequence in this way, for the enlargement in typhoid fever tends to occur late, and frequently so late as to be, for this reason if for no other, of no diagnostic importance; and it is also often so slight that it can scarcely be of much help. Furthermore, I do not believe that slight enlargement of the lymph glands, such as I have described as occurring in typhoid fever, can be of great importance in distinguishing this condition from other infectious diseases, for I am convinced that glandular enlargement occurs much more frequently in many infectious diseases than the common descriptions of these diseases would lead one to believe. This has recently been clearly shown by Schamberg to be true of scarlet fever and also of measles; and there is certainly a growing recognition of the fact that glandular enlargement is common in many of the other bacterial infections.

The possible bearing of the glandular enlargement upon prognosis has interested me somewhat, because, as I have already stated, the enlargement was in most cases observed rather late in the disease, a fact suggesting that it might have something to do with the production of immunity, instead of being merely an expression of general infection of the lymphatic apparatus with typhoid. The 43 cases that I have referred to all recovered, so that I can make no direct statement as to its possible bearing upon prognosis. During the time that these observations were being made there were three deaths from typhoid fever in the wards; but all these patients died of severe complications that had no direct connection with the severity of the typhoid toxæmia, and all these cases have been excluded from the list—two because they had furunculosis, and the other because I had no notes until toward the end of the patient's life. It is possible that more careful and more extended observation will show that the degree of the glandular enlargement may be made to influence the prognosis. This is, at any rate, suggested by the fact that the enlargement occurs most markedly as convalescence is approaching, as well as by the fact that the most marked enlargement of the glands was observed in several of the mildest cases. Furthermore, the behavior of the glands in several cases of relapse suggests this possibility. As stated, a limited glandular enlargement was observed in a number of cases during the primary attack; while during the relapses, which were followed by definite recovery, a much more marked enlargement occurred. The last-mentioned fact, however, indicates that glandular enlargement, unless quite marked and general, cannot have any important bearing upon prognosis, for readily discoverable enlargement may be followed by relapse.

I thought that the development of decided glandular enlargement, together with the usual signs of approaching convalescence, might afford some indication that the disease is actually about to terminate, and might be helpful in recognizing early the not uncommon cases in which the afebrile state is but slowly established or the disease is much prolonged. It cannot, however, prove of great importance in this way, as is indicated by the conditions just mentioned in connection with relapse; a recognizable and fairly considerable glandular enlargement may certainly occur, and yet be followed by a distinct relapse.

These observations concerning prognosis were suggested by the extensive discussion in recent years concerning the tissues active in the production of immunity. The behavior of the glands in the cases that I report has a certain degree of interest in this connection, although, of course, a limited one. The fact that the glandular enlargement occurred so generally in cases that ended in recovery and that it developed late in the disease, as convalescence was being established, seems to suggest that the lymphatic tissues were active in these cases in establishing immunity, and thus to add some support to the view that the lymphatic tissues play an especially active part in this function.

The chief interest in these observations, however, lies in their relation to diagnosis. Glandular enlargement, unless very marked, cannot be considered a strong point against typhoid fever, for enlargement of the degree that is, for example, usually seen in syphilis is not very uncommon in typhoid fever, and a somewhat lesser degree is very common.

RENAL DISEASE OF PREGNANCY AND RETINITIS ALBUMINURICA.

WITH REPORT OF A CASE.

By Leo Jacobi, M.D.,
of New York.

Many systemic manifestations of pregnancy are situated on the border line between the physiological and the pathological. Vomiting, œdema, hypertrophy of the heart, nervous disturbances, etc., are all illustrations of a fluctuating equilibrium. Still more important are the renal changes accompanying the condition, and these have, in the course of time, given rise to abundant discussion and discord; naturally enough, for no fixed line of demarcation can be traced between the normal and the pathological. Neither should this nonplus us, if we only recollect the gradual character of all fundamental transition, as between life and death, animal and vegetable, and many another.

It is granted by all that certain changes are found in the kidneys of the pregnant woman; but divergence of opinion begins the moment we ask, Are these changes organic and abiding, or merely functional and transitory? The practical bearing of the answer needs no emphasis, and yet a definite answer is not forthcoming.

Equally deplorable is the obscurity prevailing in respect to that most important result of renal disturbance—albuminuric retinitis—occurring in pregnancy.

The writer does not presume to deal exhaustively with these formidable problems. He wishes merely to report an interesting case and to indulge in a few warrantable inferences.

Mrs. Dora M., aged thirty-three years, a large, strong, and well-built woman; has been married thirteen years. The first conception took place soon after marriage. In the third month of this first pregnancy she sought the aid of a midwife, who performed criminal abortion. Since that time the patient suffered from a chronic inflammatory gynecological affection, for which she underwent repeated courses of treatment at home and abroad. Conception did not occur again for eight years, in spite of varied therapeutic measures directed to that end.

Four years ago she again went abroad, and her husband seized the opportunity for acquiring syphilis. He presented himself with a chancre and was properly treated from the start. He has remained well, at least to all appearances.

The wife returned soon after his infection, and, in spite of all admonitions, sexual relations were resumed. What seems to be noteworthy, the woman, who had been sterile for eight years, now conceived promptly. Though she never showed any manifestations of infection, the baby was born prematurely (eight months) in a macerated condition.

She now underwent varied but irregular antiluetic treatment with mercury, potassium iodide, and iodipin internally. Conception took place promptly, and one year after the first confinement she was delivered at full term of a macerated fœtus. In view of this renewed evidence of latent disease, she submitted to a course of specific treatment by subcutaneous mercurial injections.

After an interval of some two years she conceived again, the last menstruation having begun October 20, 1902. She enjoyed apparent good health up to April, 1903, when she first complained of severe headaches. She was instructed to send her urine for examination, but, the headaches having left her in the mean time, she neglected to do so.

Four weeks later she presented herself with a train of disturbances: nose-bleed, headache, vomiting, cough, dyspnœa, palpitation, diplopia, blurred vision, and impaired hearing. She passed but little urine and noticed that it foamed on passing (a sign of albuminous liquids noted, I think, by Hippocrates). Examination revealed the presence of considerable albumin. *The excretion of urea was diminished.* With the exception of slightly swollen eyelids, no œdema could at any time be discovered.

An ophthalmoscopic examination was made on June 1st by Dr. Schapringer, of this city, and his report stated the presence of "retinitis albuminurica."

The patient was now kept in bed on a milk diet and treated with hot baths and antiluetic as well as eliminative medication. No improvement followed, the condition becoming gradually but steadily worse. Muscular twitchings in the legs appeared from time to time, and, in addition to the uræmic manifestations (headaches, vomiting, insomnia), *a right-sided facial paralysis supervened.* Under these threatening toxæmic circumstances delay was fraught with danger, and the induction of premature labor was decided upon *ex consilio.* The patient was transferred to a private hospital and interference inaugurated on the morning of June 10th by packing the cervix with iodoform gauze. Slight pains appeared during the day and some bleeding took place—a welcome occurrence, in view of the high vascular tension. Twenty-four hours after the packing the cervix was sufficiently softened to permit rapid dilatation with the fingers under chloroform anæsthesia. The hand was now introduced, version performed, and the baby extracted without difficulty.

The puerperium ran an uneventful course, and on June 25th the patient returned home.

The child, a boy, weighing three pounds and five ounces, showed no signs of syphilis. He was tentatively placed in an incubator, but did not bear the latter well and had to be removed. Surrounded by hot-water bags, he lived two weeks.

Promptly following delivery a striking improvement became evident in the mother's condition. The vomiting, headaches, and a host of uræmic complaints ceased at once. She remained sleepless for two nights, but afterward slept soundly. Her appetite returned. Vision, which had been so dimmed that she could not recognize a person at her bedside, began to clear up noticeably, and by the end of the first week she was able to read large print. She passed an abundance of urine which, three days after delivery, contained only a trace of albumin.

The improvement of vision was henceforth progressive. An ophthalmoscopic examination made on July 20th showed only traces of the former white deposits on the retina. Some astigmatism was also found. With correcting glasses vision soon became perfect.

The facial palsy participated in the general recovery. After two weeks the effaced folds reappeared, largely restoring to the face its lost expression. The eye could be completely closed in three weeks. Drinking was soon no longer difficult owing to escape of fluids from the corner of the mouth. By the sixth week nearly all traces of the palsy were gone.

Examined three weeks after delivery the urine still showed some albumin, and does so to this day. We shall come back to this fact presently.

As will be granted, the case presents several noteworthy features. First, did the woman have syphilis? At no time were there any clear manifestations of the disease. This in itself is, however, no exceptional occurrence. Says Hutchinson: "Cases are innumerable in which a young wife remains in perfect health, never manifesting the slightest indication of disease, and yet bears an infant destined to show it." Such mothers, according to Colles' law, can suckle their syphilitic infants with impunity, while a healthy wet-nurse is in danger of infection. Some alleged exceptions to this law have been recorded and advanced in support of direct parental transmission with non-involvement of the mother. In the light of recent research,[1] however, Colles-Baumès' law appears to be *unexceptionally* valid, and the mother of a congenitally syphilitic infant is *without exception* and permanently immune against syphilis, not only of her own child, but against infection from any source whatever. Now, such a lasting immunity can be acquired, as in other infectious diseases, only by passing through an actual attack, since inheritance is able to confer no more than a transitory immunity,

[1] Rudolph Matzenauer. Wiener klinische Wochenschrift, February 12, 1903.

as plainly shown, for syphilis by authentic instances of *sub partu* infection (children infected with primary sores in passing through the genital tract of the mother). It would seem to follow, therefore, that every immune and apparently healthy mother has or has had latent syphilis. Such mothers not infrequently suffer at a later date from the tertiary manifestations, thus demonstrating *a posteriori* the correctness of the deduction. The important bearing of these considerations on prognosis and treatment is obvious. We may thus safely assume that our patient has passed through actual syphilis.

This inference is not without bearing on the nature of the facial paralysis in our case. Could the palsy have been luetic in origin? It involved both upper and lower peripheral branches. There was greater involvement of the lower, however. The affected eye could not be closed voluntarily without closing the other eye, while simultaneously with the latter its closure could be partially effected. The unaffected eye could be closed singly. This "sign of the orbicularis" has been looked upon by Board as pathognomonic of central paralysis, though Jacoby has found it present in peripheral palsies, and therefore inconclusive. W. M. Bechterew quite recently[1] has also observed the sign in peripheral facial palsies, but at a later stage, as a remnant of the affection. This illustrious author has demonstrated by experiments the value of the "orbicular sign" as pointing to a cortical or subcortical lesion. Winking in our patient was unaffected, both eyes participating in the act. Taste remained unimpaired.

In discussing the probable nature of the palsy, we must consider that slight hemorrhages into the retina and nose-bleed had occurred. Moreover, the time of appearance would rather lead to a non-specific explanation. The assumption seems to be most likely that a small central hemorrhage was responsible for the paralysis. Or, perhaps, the causative lesion was a localized œdema of the brain, as happens occasionally in uræmia. Finally, the palsy may have been purely toxic in character.

We now come to the most important aspect of our case, namely, the nature of the renal affection. Was it organic or was it functional? Did we deal with a genuine nephritis or with the so-called kidney of pregnancy?[2]

The existence of a nephritis antedating the last pregnancy is rendered unlikely by the anamnestic facts: not only were none of the corresponding complaints present, but the urine had been repeatedly examined by the attending physician and nothing disquieting had been found. It is thus safe to assume that the renal disturbance originated in the last pregnancy.

The kidney of pregnancy, according to Leyden, consists in anæmia of the organ with fatty infiltration of the renal epithelium, but without inflammatory changes. Attempts have been made to

[1] Obozrenie Psychiatrii, August, 1903. [2] Schwangerschaftsniere Leyden.

account for this anæmia by the vascular constriction consequent on reflex irritation from the pelvic organs, by direct pressure of the uterus, by mechanical retention of urine, etc. There is a growing tendency, however, to attribute the renal changes during pregnancy (together with certain changes in the liver) to the action of toxic metabolic products, the accumulated waste matter of maternal and fetal metabolism. That toxic substances are often the cause of renal lesions is sufficiently well established, and, reasoning by analogy, it is easily conceivable how in pregnancy the metabolic poisons may inflict an injury on the renal tissues. At first the impairment may be slight, but prolonged action or great intensity of the poison is likely to result in more serious damage, which may finally culminate in a true nephritis. It is quite plausible, furthermore, that the auxiliary factors mentioned above contribute their share to the result, for there is no doubt that the toxæmia of pregnancy is a complex condition. The possible cumulative effect of repeated pregnancies may be a matter of etiological speculation, as may also in our case the antecedent syphilis and the mercurial injections.

With the removal of the causes the renal insufficiency of pregnancy would naturally tend to subside or disappear, as we actually observe in many such instances after delivery. When, however, the renal lesion has become more pronounced, it is perfectly comprehensible that it should persist after the primary cause has been removed. As a matter of fact, it has long been noted that genuine nephritis not infrequently becomes superimposed on the kidney of pregnancy. Even Leyden, who considers the renal disturbance as merely functional, holds this opinion. But here, as so often, no fixed line exists between functional and organic, the interval being filled up by intermediate transitional forms.

In our case the presence of such symptoms as retinitis and paralysis would point to a graver renal lesion and render the persistence of the latter after delivery highly probable *a priori*.

This conclusion has, in fact, been borne out by subsequent observation of the patient. At the time of writing, six months after delivery, the albuminuria still persists, and the urine contains morphotic constituents indicative of renal involvement. Occasionally œdema of the eyelids is noted in the morning, and the woman complains at times of headaches, gastric distress, etc.

In view of this and the empirical observation that successive pregnancies cause more extensive retinal degeneration, future conception in our patient will have to be prevented *a tout prix*.

ON THE OCCURRENCE OF CYSTIC CHANGES IN THE MALPIGHIAN BODIES ASSOCIATED WITH ATROPHY OF THE GLOMERULUS IN CHRONIC INTERSTITIAL NEPHRITIS.

By Edwin Beer, M.D.,
of New York.

(From Prof. Chiari's Pathologico-anatomical Institute in Prague.)

During the past few years the Malpighian bodies of the kidney have been studied in greatest detail, not only in normal but also in diseased organs. Of the pathological changes, those associated with fibroid atrophy in chronic nephritis have, perhaps, been most thoroughly investigated. There is no doubt that this latter form of degeneration and atrophy of the glomerulus is well recognized, even though there are diverging views as to all the changes that precede the formation of the hyalofibroid spherical mass.

In the literature very little mention is found of another very frequent form of atrophy within the Malpighian body in the same disease, chronic interstitial nephritis, and it is to the histological pictures of this, as well as its relative frequency, that I hope to call attention in this paper.

In the literary synopsis which follows, it will be seen that the investigators of the early part of the second half of the last century, when thin sections and other refinements of technique were unknown, mentioned a cystic condition of the Malpighian bodies, whereas the recent writers ignore the condition. Rokitansky and Klebs, especially the latter, call attention to this in chronic interstitial nephritis, describing one phase of the change.

In the *Anatomie pathologique* (1879) of Laboulbène and in the *Histologie pathologique* of Cornil and Ranvier, published in 1884, the cysts that are found in chronic interstitial nephritis are discussed at some length. The frequent occurrence of these and their origin from uriniferous tubules they affirm, but they also mention as a rarity (Cornil and Ranvier) cystic developments from the Malpighian bodies in which the capillaries have almost entirely disappeared, just a few remaining attached somewhere along the wall of the cyst.

In the 1893 edition of Orth's *Special Pathology*, a cystic atrophy of the tubuli and Malpighian bodies in contracted kidneys and chronic interstitial nephritis is mentioned, but in the 1900 edition of his *Patholog. Anat. Diagnostik* he talks of these cysts as derived from tubules alone. Whether this is a change of view I do not know, but the fact that Baum, from Orth's laboratory, in 1900 published a paper in which he describes such a change in the Malpighian body as I am about to depict, and calls it a development anomaly or embryonic Malpighian body, suggests that in 1893

Orth's remarks were not intended to cover this peculiar pathological change, otherwise his pupil would have interpreted the picture in accordance with the earlier expressed views of Orth, or, at least, made some reference to the same.

In a picture in Dürck's *Atlas of General Pathological Histology*, p. 74, a cystic development from the Malpighian body is beautifully drawn. The lining membrane of the cyst is the typical wall of the Malpighian body—that is, Bowman's capsule—flat epithelium on a membrana propria; and at the right lower corner of the cyst are a few cells projecting into the lumen thereof, grouped irregularly about a bloodvessel. This cyst is filled with colloid, and is just the kind of cyst that is so commonly found in my researches. Dürck calls this a tubulus cyst. Otherwise little or no mention is found in reference to this change, except, perhaps, in Philippson's article (also in that of Beckmann), in which the former says he found hydrops of the Malpighian bodies similar to that seen in so-called congenital cystic kidney in kidneys of older people, but specifically states that there seems to be no relation between this and chronic interstitial nephritis (p. 556).

On the other hand, in Israel's (1889), Weichselbaum's (1892), Hamilton's (1894), Orth's (*Diagnostik*, 1900), Ribbert's (1901), Schmaus' (1901), Kaufmann's (1901), Ziegler's (1901), Langerhan's (1902), and Dürck's (1903) text-books the fibroid changes in the Malpighian bodies are discussed in more or less detail, but no mention of another—*i. e.*, cystic atrophy—is made. Weichselbaum, to be absolutely accurate, suggests such a possibility, while Ziegler and Ribbert mention the calcification in Malpighian body cysts that were described by Baum.

To avoid any mistake, I must mention here that the not uncommon macroscopic cysts lined with cuboidal epithelium, containing variously colored fluids and fluids of various consistency in chronic interstitial nephritis, are quite different from those to which I am about to call attention. These tubule cysts are very commonly visible to the naked eye, whereas the form that is derived from the Malpighian bodies is only occasionally so recognizable. If these latter are large enough to be seen by the naked eye, the microscopic examination alone can distinguish them from tubule cysts. Moreover, what I am describing has nothing to do with the small cysts that have been found in glomeruli that are undergoing the fibro-hyaline atrophy. These "cysts" are minute spaces made by the irregular growth of tissue within Bowman's capsule and scarcely deserve the name cyst. They involve a small part of the whole Malpighian body and are only an indication of irregularity in growth of the newly forming intracapsular tissue (Engel, Tschistowitch).

Here it must also be mentioned that the cysts that I am calling attention to have been interpreted as tubule cysts by some authors

—*e. g.*, Dürck—as seen in the illustration referred to previously. Orth and Baum have expressed somewhat similar views, while Cornil and Ranvier talk of most of these same cysts as tubule cysts in which the epithelium has been flattened out. In single sections, where remnants of the glomerulus are usually not seen projecting into these cysts, this view of their origin might seem justifiable. It is probably due to this misinterpretation that we find so little mention of a second form of atrophy of the glomerular structures in medical literature.

From the foregoing it will be seen that more or less complete descriptions of four different kinds of cysts derived from the kidney parenchyma in chronic interstitial nephritis are found in the literature. Two are referred to the Malpighian bodies and two to the tubules. Of the former, one is scarcely a cyst, while the other, of which very little mention is found in the literature, deserves that appellation, but has never been studied and clearly described.

Of the *so-called tubule cysts*, the two varieties differ most markedly, according to Cornil and Ranvier, Orth, and Baum, not to mention others, in the nature of their epithelium; in one these cells are more or less high and cuboidal, whereas in the other they are completely flattened out against a membrana propria.

The studies that underlie this article are based on twelve kidneys of chronic interstitial nephritis which were examined in serial section and thirty kidneys in single section (*i. e.*, non-serially), to determine both the origin and the development of the cyst in question and also the frequency of their occurrence. The serial sections demonstrated the origin of a *large number of cysts, those with "flattened epithelium," from the Malpighian bodies, by showing atrophic glomerular structures adhering to the wall of the cysts, and the study of the single sections from the thirty kidneys with chronic interstitial nephritis showed that cystic atrophy is a very common occurrence.*

In the usual non-serial sections of kidneys in which chronic interstitial nephritis is found, one sees cystic spaces filled with a more or less homogeneous substance. The walls surrounding this substance are made up of two elements, a basement membrane and a layer of epithelial cells attached to it. In some of these the epithelium is flat, so that only here and there a nucleus, with a small amount of flattened protoplasm surrounding it, is visible; while in others, again, the epithelium is arranged as in the uriniferous tubules, the nuclei being near one another and the cells to which they belong being more or less cuboidal in shape. These two kinds of cysts impress one as very different structures. The wall of the former is identical in structure with that of the Malpighian bodies—Bowman's capsule—while the wall of the latter reminds one of the uriniferous tubules. In addition to these cysts, one occasionally sees an altogether different picture. One finds a cystic formation and projecting into the contents of the cyst (Figs. 1 and 2) are tufts of capillaries, distinctly part of the glomerular tufts, but smaller in size than the normal capillary mass. The walls of these cysts are identical in structure with the walls of a normal Malpighian body, and, moreover, absolutely identical with the walls of the first of the above-described cysts—*i. e.*, flattened epithelium—whose nuclei are far apart (in usual sections), lying on a basement membrane.[1]

The size and general contour of these two "varieties" of cysts with walls of identical structure vary very much. In general, they are a little larger than the normal Malpighian bodies and more or less spherical. At times they are five to six times (in one plane) the size of the Malpighian bodies; at others even larger. They may be very irregular in shape, sending prolongations in between the tubules.

Of these two "varieties" the second is undoubtedly that to which Laboulbène, Cornil and Ranvier, and Baum refer, while the first is usually interpreted as a tubule cyst, despite the resemblance its walls bear to the normal Bowman's capsule and to the capsule of the cysts with small capillary glomerular tufts.

If these cysts that have been interpreted as tubule cysts with flattened epithelium are cut in serial section, in the majority of cases, one finds that at some spot attached to the wall and projecting into the lumen are some remnants of a glomerulus, very often one or more capillary vessels. In other words, those cysts with walls that resemble in their structure the walls of Malpighian bodies contain an atrophic glomerulus, so that in one or more sections one gets a picture such as the above authors have mentioned, while in all the other sections one gets the "variety" which has been interpreted as a tubule cyst with much flattened epithelium.

Having thus made clear the point that these cysts, so-called tubule cysts, are derived from the Malpighian bodies, I shall briefly point out the stages in this form of atrophy of the glomerulus, noting how both the capillaries and the visceral layer of Bowman's capsule behave in this process.

From a study of a great many sections in series, one can describe the various stages in this atrophy by a connected statement better than by describing in detail selected pictures. This I shall attempt in the following pages, repeating as little of what has been mentioned as accuracy will permit.

These cysts derived from the Malpighian bodies are, perhaps, most frequently found in the superficial cortical part of the kidney, and they vary, as just said, very much, both in their size and shape. They may be only slightly larger than a normal Malpighian body, but at times they are much larger and even visible to the naked eye. Their shape is most usually almost spherical, but it is not uncommon to find them very irregular in outline.

[1] As seen later other cysts of Malpighian origin show different remnants of the atrophying glomerular tufts, which are, however, rarely noted in non-serial sections.

The walls of the cysts are made up of flat epithelium lying on a basement membrane, absolutely identical with the structure of the normal Bowman's capsule. In serial section one finds any stage of atrophy between a fairly normal-looking capillary mass, smaller than the normal vascular tufts projecting into the cavity, to a single capillary vessel just projecting into the cavity of the cyst. At times not even this is seen, as detailed below. In the usual non-serial diagnostic section one more often finds no sign of the glomerulus, but occasionally, as in one of my specimens, one can see several cysts close together in one field (Fig. 1), in several of which one or two capillaries are visible. One can understand the whole process by finding these various stages in this atrophy of the capillaries from the cysts with fairly normal-looking capillary tufts of nearly normal size to those with only one or two vessels.

FIG. 1.

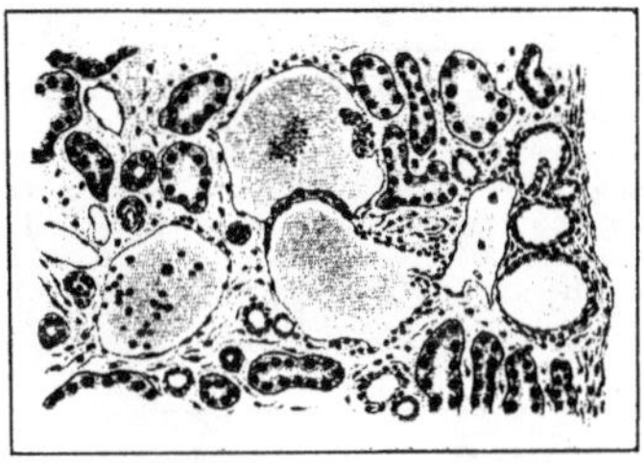

Shows directly under the kidney capsule three dilated tubules, and lying above these four Malpighian body cysts. Two of these show remnants of the glomerulus, the other two in this section show none. In two of the cysts, cells lie in the "colloid," in one fine granules of lime, and the fourth contains only the "colloid." (Drawn with 2 A. Zeiss.)

Rarer than these forms, of which the cyst with only a few vessels is the one most commonly seen in my serial sections, are those cysts that show no signs of glomerular vessels at all. Probably the relative frequency of one or the other stage of the atrophy in the glomerulus is dependent on the severity of the interstitial nephritis.

Not infrequently the visceral layer of Bowman's capsule, which now is fairly generally looked upon as a syncytium (Kölliker-Ebner), behaves in a very interesting way, which shows that the cells still retain individual characteristics, even if the theory of their syncytial life under normal conditions is true. In some of these Malpighian cysts in which the glomerular tufts are quite small, consisting of just a few capillaries, this visceral epithelial layer is very prominent, and each cell is distinctly visible (Fig. 4), their outline being definite and clearly distinguishable. In other cysts, though the nuclei stand out close together, as in the fetal kidney, the cell limits are indistinct (Fig. 3). Moreover, many of these cysts, where little or nothing of

FIG. 2.

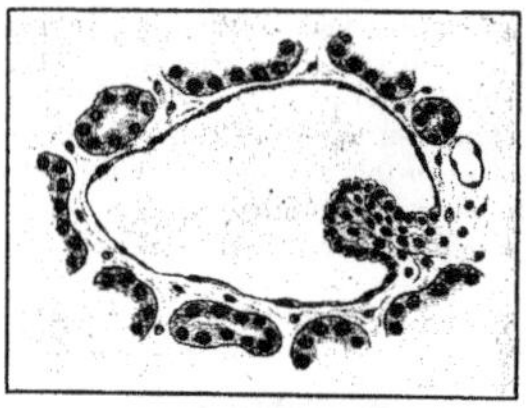

Shows similar cyst, but in this the cells of the syncytium have become individualized, each one being distinctly separable from its neighbors.

the capillaries remain, show small papillary excrescences covered with epithelium (Fig. 3), which, from their anatomy and the analogy they bear to other cysts, must be interpreted as a remnant of the syncytium supported on a tender branching framework of what

FIG. 3.

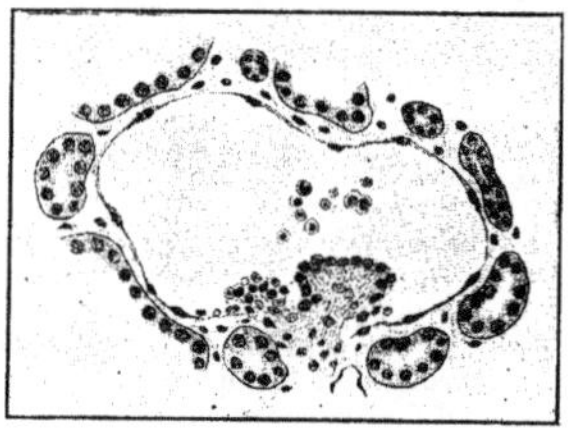

Shows similar cyst, in which the visceral layer of Bowman's capsule has become very prominent.

seems to be connective tissue. At times this more or less branched structure is attached to the cyst wall at both ends, dividing the cyst in some sections into two smaller cavities, which, however, communicate in the following sections of the series (Fig. 6).

The origin of this dividing, incomplete septum or bridge is seen in the following process: occasionally the glomerular tufts (Fig. 5) become attached to the parietal portion of Bowman's capsule, more

FIG. 4.

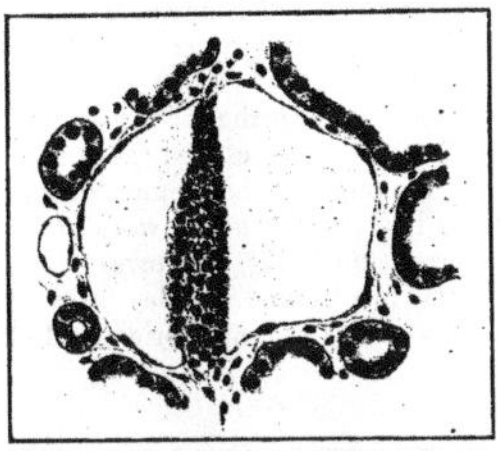

Shows similar cyst, but here the capillaries have disappeared, and the proliferated visceral layer of Bowman's capsule has covered the bridge with epithelium.

FIG. 5.

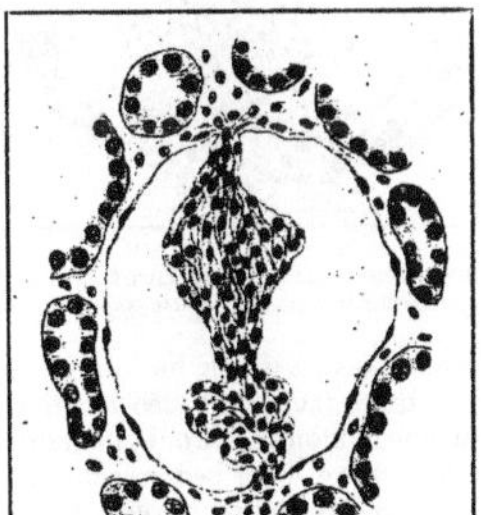

Shows another cyst in which the capillaries have become adherent opposite to the hilus. Pressure lines are distinctly visible running parallel from the hilus to the capsular adhesion.

or less opposite to the entrance of the artery of the glomerulus. The capillaries gradually undergo atrophy, so that in some pictures one can see a few capillaries running through the central part of the cyst, dividing it into seemingly two smaller cavities. With the proliferation of the visceral layer of the capsule, when the capillary atrophy becomes extreme, a mass of epithelial cells, on a connective-tissue framework, is found running through the cyst, dividing it into two more or less equal parts (Fig. 6). Whether these papillary bodies and the rejuvenescence and proliferation of the epithelium of the visceral layer of Bowman's capsule, that were just described, have anything to do with the production of kidney tumors, I am not in a position to state definitely. That such a possibility exists cannot be denied, and further investigation must determine the relation between these processes and those that lead to tumor—*e. g.*, adenomata formation. In this connection, it is of interest to note that Grawitz, in his criticism of the work of Weichselbaum and Greenish, who referred the latter structures—*i. e.*, adenomata—to the epithelium of the uriniferous tubules, said that he had seen pictures which suggested a Malpighian origin. Ricker saw a similar

FIG. 6.

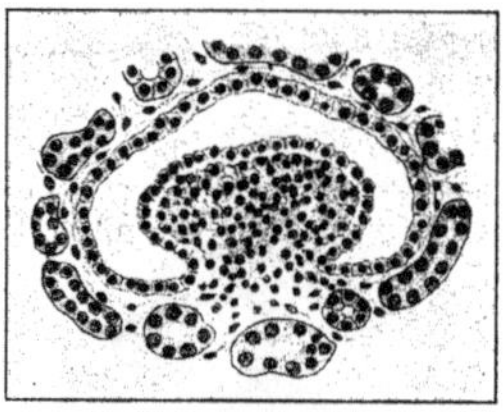

Shows a dilated tubule into which the growing connective tissue has pushed part of its wall, thus mimicking a Malpighian body cyst.

picture in an adrenal "rest," which he interpreted as a papillary growth. In view of these facts, and also in view of the fact that adenomata are not uncommon in chronic interstitial nephritis, this peculiar change that I have described in some of the Malpighian bodies that are undergoing the cystic atrophy must be kept in mind, and, perhaps, it will aid us in interpreting some of the new-growths of the kidney.

In all the cysts already described there is found some remnant of the glomerulus, but, in addition, one finds cysts of identical structure without any sign of the glomerulus projecting into their cavities. In these cysts the contents and the walls are of absolutely the same nature as those cysts which still show capillaries or the visceral layer of Bowman's capsule; and in single section the cysts that contain atrophic elements of the glomerulus and those that do not cannot be distinguished one from the other, unless the section happily strikes the plane of the atrophying glomerular structures in the former variety of cysts. Even then only serial section will make sure that no glomerular elements persist in the second variety of the above cysts. This absolute identity in structure between the cysts that contain glomerular elements and those that do not leave no doubt as to their common origin from the Malpighian body. The absence of all glomerular elements may be the final stage in the atrophy of the glomerulus.

That this process of cystic atrophy does not seem to be due to inflammation within the Malpighian bodies must be emphasized. No signs of inflammation either in the capillary tufts nor in the parietal layer of Bowman's capsule were ever seen, except, perhaps, in that form of atrophy in which the capillaries had become adherent opposite to the hilus. No marked signs of inflammation between capillaries and Bowman's capsule were seen even here, but the adhesion probably owed its origin to some such process. All the other pictures—the usual ones—point rather to a mechanical factor without the Malpighian body as the direct cause of this condition of cystic atrophy.

The contents of these cysts vary very much. The ground substance, if I may use that term, which fills them usually takes varying deep tints with eosin, stains yellow with Van Gieson, very faintly with hæmatoxylin, and similarly with alum cochineal, but still fainter after treatment with acids; in general, it has the characteristics of what is called "colloid." In this "colloid," which shrinks in hardening, leaving a more or less irregular space between it and the cyst walls, there are quite often various cells—leukocytes and epithelial—also not infrequently lime-salts, as I have described in another recent article in the *Journal of Pathology and Bacteriology*. It must be mentioned that in some of these cysts the fluid does not stain, but such cysts are quite rare and unusual in my experience. No indication of a direct change of the capillary tufts into this "colloid" were ever noticed, so that this, in all probability, is a product of secretion rather than a degeneration of previously normal protoplasm.

In looking for a tubulus contortus in connection with these cysts, it was the rule not to find any. Practically all of the cysts were blind, and this probably helps to explain their origin. Somewhat similar cystic Malpighian bodies are seen in congenital cystic kidneys without the "colloid" contents, and from the similarity in the picture and the fact that the tubuli contorti seem to be usually shut off, I think we can assume that the Malpighian body cysts in chronic interstitial nephritis owe their origin to a similar mechanical process, to obstruction in the efferent uriniferous tubule. Whether the very few cysts into which a tubulus contortus could be traced owed their origin to an obliteration or stenosis of this tubule some short distance from the Malpighian body, instead of directly at its origin from this body, I cannot state definitely. Perhaps, even in these there was a stricture at the insertion of the tubule into Bowman's capsule. It is of importance to note that where I found a tubulus contortus opening into a cystic Malpighian body, which in all my specimens I saw only a few times, the Malpighian body cyst was about the size of a normal Malpighian body.

What the nature of the process that leads to obstruction in the tubule is we can only guess at for the present, as it is almost impossible to imagine a method of investigating a stenosis of these channels. One would naturally think of the new connective tissue and its subsequent contraction, which is so characteristic of this form of nephritis, as the cause. It is of importance to state that I did not

FIG. 7.

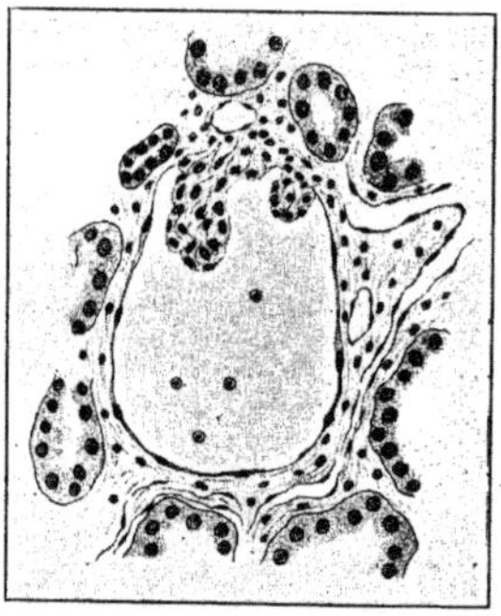

Shows Malpighian cyst with atrophic glomerulus flattened more or less against the cyst wall. Capillaries are still present. Contents of this cyst, cells and "colloid." (Figs. 2 to 7 drawn with 2 D. Zeiss.)

find any irregularity in the presence of new connective tissue about or near the cysts, but it seems likely that contracting bands at some distance might lead to occlusion of the tubuli contorti without being necessarily in absolute proximity to those tubules. Another method of closure might be within the tubule itself, as mentioned above, due to stricture formation. Perhaps future investigation will make these points clear.

Before leaving this general description I must state that although the signs of increased pressure within the Malpighian bodies were present in many instances they were scarcely the rule. In some cysts the remnants of the capillaries were spread out along one side of the wall, as if pressed and flattened there (Fig. 2). In the cases where adhesions had formed between capillaries and parietal layer of Bowman's capsule opposite to the hilus, the signs of pressure were even more distinct (Fig. 5); and the capillaries ran almost parallel to each other, being pressed together from the sides. The increase in size of the Malpighian bodies undergoing this cystic change and the frequent cystic prolongations between the tubules are also indications of a heightened pressure, as no signs of active proliferation of the capsule were visible in any case. That the increase of internal pressure must be very gradual in these closed-off Malpighian bodies is evidenced by the fact that most of the glomeruli undergoing this atrophy show no signs of active pressure in their general conformation.

From all the above it will be seen that in chronic interstitial nephritis the Malpighian body undergoes a change which is quite the opposite of the usually described "fibrohyalinization." This latter change most often depends on a vascular disturbance and leads to shrinkage of the whole structure, while the former, the cystic atrophy or degeneration, probably depends on a disturbance in the efferent uriniferous tubules, and leads to the formation of a cyst somewhat or much larger than the original Malpighian body. Both have in common the more or less complete destruction of the glomerulus.

As to the frequency of occurrence of cystic atrophy of the Malpighian bodies, the following table, based on sections from thirty different cases of chronic interstitial nephritis, will show. In each case one section was gone over and both fibroid and cystic Malpighian bodies were counted and arranged in parallel columns:

THIRTY CASES OF CHRONIC INTERSTITIAL NEPHRITIS WITH ENUMERATION OF GLOMERULAR CHANGES.

Cases.	Cystic atrophy.	Fibrohyaline atrophy.	Cases.	Cystic atrophy.	Fibrohyaline atrophy.
1	8	3	19	1	3
2	3	2	20	2	0
3	10	7	21	0	2
4	4	3	22	0	5
5	0	2	23	1	0
6	3	4	24	0	2
7 { in infarcted area	0	81	25	2	3
7 { in non-infarcted	4	1	26	6	0
8	2	1	27	3	3
9	4	1	28	1	3
10	0	2	29	2	2
11	2	1	30	3	4
12	1	1			
13	8	8	Totals	79	169
14	0	9			
15	4	0	Exclusive of infarcted		
16	2	2	area	0	81
17	1	13			
18	2	1		79	88

It will be seen that these two changes are almost equally frequently seen if we exclude the areas where infarcts appeared in the sections, for here the vascular change was the direct cause in the overproduction of the fibroid atrophy. But even if all these areas are included in our estimate, the proportion of cystic to fibroid changes is surely a large one and well deserving of more attention than it has received.

Looking a little more closely at these figures, it is evident that in these thirty single sections 248 atrophic Malpighian bodies were found. Of this total 79 were cystic and 169 were changed into the well-known fibrohyaline masses. Expressed in percentages, 31 per cent. were cystically changed, whereas the rest had undergone fibrous atrophy. If those sections in which no infarcts were noted were considered alone the percentage of cystic to fibrous would be considerably changed. From this point of view, 47 per cent. would be cystic and 53 per cent. fibrous atrophy.

It is also evident that in some sections no representatives of one of the two pathological changes may be found, and in other sections one form is more frequently seen than the other. A similar table could be made from the kidneys that were cut in serial section, and this emphasizes the fact that the above enumeration from single sections is absolutely reliable.

In closing I wish to emphasize the two most important facts that have been brought out in the preceding pages:

1. In addition to the well-known fibroid atrophy of the Malpighian body in chronic interstitial nephritis there is also a cystic atrophy.

2. Cystic atrophy is very common and in my cases almost as frequently seen as the fibroid change.

In closing, I wish to thank Professor Chiari for the material on which this work is based and for his many kindnesses while studying in his laboratory.

LITERATURE.

Beckmann. Ueber Nierencysten, Virch. Arch., 1856, p. 9.
Laboulbène. Anat. pathologique, 1879.
Cornil and Ranvier. Manuel d'Hist. pathologique, 1884.
Philippson. Anat. Untersuch. über Nierencysten, Virch. Arch. 1888, vol. iii.
Orth. Spec. Path. Anatomie, 1893.
Orth. Diagnostik d. Path. Anat., 1900.
Baum. Ueber punktförmige Kalkkörperchen, etc., Virch. Arch., 1900, p. 162.
Engel. Glomerulitis Adhesiva, Virch. Arch., 1901, p. 163.
Tschistowitch. Die Verödung u. Hyal. Entartung, etc., Virch. Arch., 1903, p. 171.
Dürck. Allg. Path. Histologie, 1903.

A PARTIAL STUDY OF ULCERATIVE ENDOCARDITIS.

By Beverley Robinson, M.D.,
of New York.

The subject of ulcerative endocarditis formed the thesis of Dr. Osler's Goulstonian Lectures in 1885. He begins them as follows:

"It is of use, from time to time, to take stock, so to speak, of our knowledge of a particular disease, to see exactly where we stand in regard to it, to inquire to what conclusions the accumulated facts seem to point, and to ascertain in what direction we may look for fruitful investigations in the future."[1]

It is with this spirit I have undertaken a renewed study of ulcerative endocarditis.

In 1898 Sir Douglas Powell delivered before the Royal College of Physicians of London "Lectures on the Principles which Govern Treatment in Diseases and Disorders of the Heart."[2]

In this third lecture he carefully considered those which specially dominate the treatment of ulcerative endocarditis. There he also reviewed the therapeutic measures likely to be of some use in the disease. He likewise gave a tabulated statement of the results of treatment by antistreptococcic serum, and of his own experience with yeast and with nuclein, after the method of Dr. V. C. Vaughn, of Michigan. In the Lumleian Lectures during the current year, Dr. T. R. Glynn[3] has again reviewed this subject and regarded it "mainly in its clinical aspects." He was influenced to do so because of its great clinical interest, and the fact that no disease presents itself under a greater variety and perplexity of forms. A very elaborate historic retrospect of our growing knowledge pertaining to the disease is at first dwelt upon. In it he cites Matthew Bailey, Morgagni, Senac, Corvisart, and Bouillaud. To the latter he ascribes the honor of associating ulceration of the cardiac valves with symptoms of typhoid fever. He shows how the "third period" was marked by a perfected bacteriological technique, and by the fuller comprehension of the biological characteristics of bacteria. Thus ulcerative endocarditis, which was formerly considered as a local affection, is now regarded as one of the complications of a general infection.

This malady, like the simple form of endocarditis, affects the lining membrane of the heart and especially the nerves. It is characterized by vegetations and is accompanied with loss of tissue. The ulceration may cause perforation of heart valves, or even of the septum or heart walls, under very exceptional conditions. With the ulceration we may find a limited area of suppuration. It is very rarely a primary affection, but ordinarily occurs as a complication of some infective disorder, or septic disease. No doubt this view explains how it is that the lesions of simple endocarditis often precede and are found in conjunction with those of the more advanced or far graver form of the disease. Between the latter and the benign malady there is, indeed, no essential anatomical difference, and they merely represent gradations, as it were, of more or less intensity.

Although cases which have developed primarily are occasionally observed, they are so infrequent as to have had legitimate doubt thrown on them. Osler reports one case in which at the autopsy no lesions were found other than those of ulcerative endocarditis.[4] In cases of obscure origin it is probable that the micro-organisms frequently enter the economy by the respiratory passages, and reach the heart in this way rather than through the digestive organs. Especially in cases of chronic heart trouble by reason of secondary congestion of the air-passages, the conditions become favòrable to bacterial invasiòn. An infective endocarditis originating in this way would occasionally appear to be of primary origin. (Glynn.)

On the other hand, ulcerative endocarditis occurs quite frequently as a complication of pneumonia. "In 16 cases of 100 autopsies in which this lesion was present, 11 were of this form."[5] According to Wells, the proportion in all cases of pneumonia is 3 per cent., while the percentage in fatal cases of the latter disease is 4 per cent. G. Studa's estimate of the relative frequency of ulcerative endocarditis in pneumonia is a much higher one (9 cases in 85 autopsies).[6] When it is found in this disease it appears to be exceptionally virulent, as numerous autopsies demonstrate. It is also seen in acute rheumatism. Anders[7] writes that the proportion is about 10 per cent. of the cases in which acute endocarditis appears. It may also occur as a complication of some eruptive fevers and in septicæmia. Vaccination has been followed by cellulitis and infective endocarditis. (Coleman.)

Cases are likewise due to dental caries and oral sepsis. When we consider the great number of cases of acute and subacute rheumatism we are called to treat, the number of those complicated with ulcerative endocarditis seems very small.

Ulcerative endocarditis often follows septicæmia of various origin, and is not uncommon in gonorrhœa. The intimate relations between some cases of gonorrhœa and ulcerative endocarditis have been established for more than twenty years, but it is only lately that these instances have been studied in a systematic manner.[8] A fatal case of this kind has been reported.[9] In some of these cases it has been impossible from the most careful local researches to discover the site of entrance of the infective disease. We should then turn to cultures made from the blood, and occasionally bacteria with the typical characteristics of gonococci will be shown.[10]

The cultivation should be made during life, and it may be confirmed at the autopsy from blood taken from the heart, or from the cardiac vegetations. For the cultivation it is not essential to take a great deal of blood, to dilute it much, or to make use of special media. It is now known, also, that the bactericidal action of the blood is less pronounced on gonococci than it is on pneumococci or the typhoid bacillus. The septic process that proceeds from the puerperal state is also a well-known source of grave ulcerative endocarditis. Although certain authors have described it as a complication of malaria, it is questionable whether such cases often occur. Among diseases which are occasionally complicated with malignant endocarditis I would cite measles, scarlatina, smallpox, erysipelas, and typhoid fever. In my experience such instances, with the exception of the latter disease, have not been seen, and even of this finding I have no available record.[11]

Cerebral complications are associated with it at times, particularly, as meningitis,[12] and this is especially true when the malignant endocarditis is found with pneumonia. I have observed one caseof obscure mental disorder in which the malignant endocarditis was shown to be "mural" at the autopsy, and no gross changes had taken place in the brain. Miliary abscesses have been found, however, in a number of instances. Once Jackson found an embolus of the artery of the Sylvian fossa, and Lartigau[13] reports a case of gonorrhœal origin, in which prior to death there was a sudden aphasic attack. The bacillus of influenza has also been detected in the valvular vegetations of ulcerative endocarditis. The cases observed were instances of the development of the disease upon a chronic cardiac affection.[14]

This fact is important as pointing to a demonstration of what has long been considered probable, namely, the vulnerability of the heart to the influenza poison. Ulcerative endocarditis occurred in 4 of de Batz's 20 cases, and a most interesting example has been recorded by Tickell. It has been observed during the influenzal attack, but most frequently in the convalescing period.[15]

A new organism of endocarditis, called micrococcus zymogenes, has lately been pointed out in a patient who died. The infarcts which accompanied this case are not stated to be other than bland; therefore it may be that the endocarditis itself belonged to the simple type. On the other hand, Maccullum and Hastings report a case caused by this organism, in which multiple septic infarctions in various viscera were found. Further, typical acute vegetative endocarditis was experimentally produced by intravenous inoculation in a rabbit and a dog, and the cocci were demonstrated in pure culture in the vegetations and in other parts of these animals after death. The micrococcus zymogenes is stated to be extremely minute, often elliptic in outline, usually found in pairs, is not motile, and stains with the ordinary stains.[16]

Although it is stated by some writers that the two forms of the disease, simple and ulcerative, never become one and the same, this affirmation is probably too positive. Litten believes that prompt response to the salicylates is characteristic of the benign form.[17] They may be used, therefore, with some measure of reliance to determine an otherwise doubtful diagnosis. Litten also criticises Lenhartz's views as to the fact that the finding of micro-organisms in the blood characterizes the endocarditis as septic. Very justly he remarks that if later the microbe of acute rheumatism be accurately determined, such distinction will be no basis to rest upon. In the septic-malignant form of Litten, suppuration occurs in thrombi and joints, which does not occur in the non-septic malignant form. He objects strongly to the term "ulcerative" endocarditis, but does not believe the time has come to make separations on the ground of the presence or differences of micro-organisms. Poynton and Paine consider that ulcerative and other forms are only different degrees of the same disease, and that benign forms may become malignant under the "influence of virulent breeds" of the common micro-organism of rheumatism. Ewart insists that, even though the practical identity of the organisms may not be proven, a very important clinical lesson is furnished. This essentially means that our efforts of prophylaxis in rheumatism should be strengthened, because in prophylaxis of this disease we also combat the development of most serious cardiac affections.[18] An equally important matter has already been insisted upon by Sir Douglas Powell in his Lumleian Lectures where he directs "attention to the necessity of observing certain prophylactic precautions during convalescence in rheumatic endocarditis" (*loc. cit.*, p. 1153). The lesions found may be in the heart, or other organs of the economy.

In Jackson's cases enlargement of the spleen was present in all but one instance. Leukocytosis was also regularly found, the leukocytes usually numbering from 16,000 to 20,000. This is an important point in the differential diagnosis from malaria, tuberculosis, and typhoid fever. The bacteria in the blood are important and have different forms. In 23 cases studied bacteriologically by Jackson "in 2 no cultures were obtained; in 2 there were micro-organisms which were not identified; in 8 streptococcus pyogenes was found; in 5, the pneumococcus; in 3, staphylococcus aureus; in 1, the colon bacillus; in 1, the streptococcus and staphylococcus; and in 1, the streptococcus with other organisms."

In the 38 cases discussed by Lenhartz, the author carried out bacteriological investigations in 28 cases. In 16 cases bacteria were found during life. They were principally staphylococci. According to Lenhartz it is usually comparatively easy to find the organism in the blood.[19] From the point of view of prognosis it is very desirable to differentiate between the various forms of ulcerative endocarditis. This may be accomplished by careful blood cultures during life. It is especially desirable at present, by reason of the more hopeful outlook of these cases. This seems to be proven partly by the results from treatment, partly by the data afforded by careful autopsies. Ewart, indeed, has stated, even in cases that resulted fatally, that evidences of repair in the local cardiac lesions could be shown. It may be remarked that there is little tendency in this process toward *cicatrization*, so that recovery may take place with little or no deformity of valves or orifices. (Wells.) The cardiac changes will depend upon the nature of the organisms which occasion them, and also upon the extent and duration of the disease. We do not find the same conditions in instances in which the process is wholly acute, and those where the acute disease is attached to former sclerotic changes of the valves. Usually we find vegetations on the valves. These are often found with an ulcerative process and small abscesses. According to Wells the distinguishing features of them are their massive character and broad base. Moreover, they do not extend often beyond the valves. The left heart is more frequently the site of the disease than the right. In regard to this point errors may be found in literature. Still the right heart is attacked oftener than in the benign form.

Mural ulcerative endocarditis is extremely rare. I have seen only one case, to which I have referred. The history of another one, hitherto unpublished, has been kindly given to me by my colleague, Dr. Van Horne Norrie. In rare instances the process may extend to the aorta and pulmonary artery. A secondary infective arteritis in various peripheral situations and in the different viscera, as a result of septic embolism from the heart, may also occur.[20] The vegetations are frequently small, especially when they alone are present. They are of gray or yellow color, and are situated on the margin or at the base of the valves. Under the microscope they are shown to be composed of numerous microbes, embryonic cells, and leukocytes. They also contain fibrin.[21] In many instances, however, the vegetations are larger and may become pedunculated. They have a markedly gray aspect also, or are covered with blood clot, and often show superficial or deep ulceration of tissue. In the latter case an aneurysmal pouch may be found. This pouch formation doubtless is due to blood pressure upon softened and degenerated valvular tissues. Sometimes the ulceration goes deep enough to make a perforation of the valve. Again, it extends to the chordæ tendineæ, beginning in the inflammatory stage, and separates later the valve segment completely. When this takes place we may have a flapping with each ventricular contraction of the detached valve against the auricle. Thus, secondary infection of the auricular walls is produced, and it is not uncommon to find warty growths here situated. In rare instances when the ulceration has enlarged and become still deeper, the septum or ventricular walls may be perforated. If the malignant endocarditis be caused by pyogenetic organisms it is not uncommon to find small abscesses in the valves, or, indeed, in other parts of the heart. These abscesses may rupture, sometimes with perforation of the heart walls, and then pus is found in the pericardial sac. It is also possible for small quantities of pus to be reabsorbed, and the evidence of this is found in old scar tissue, or calcareous deposits. In some cases, especially when malignant endocarditis is found in a patient suffering from chronic heart disease, the vegetations may be capped with calcareous incrustations. In very rare instances the deposit of lime salts may occur in acute cases.

The ulcerative condition of malignant endocarditis may possibly be confounded with that which follows the necrosis of former atheromatous deposits, or those incident to chronic rheumatic endocarditis of benign nature. A differential diagnosis may here be made, probably with the use of the microscope; but at times doubt may still remain. Osler, in an analysis of 209 cases, showed the proportion in which the different valves, the walls, and sides of the heart are involved. His report reads "aortic and mitral valves together, 41; aortic valves alone, 53; mitral valves alone, 77; tricuspid in 19; pulmonary valves in 15, and the heart wall in 33 instances. In 9 instances the right heart alone was involved; in most cases, the auriculoventricular valves."[22] In Strada's 85 autopsies the seat of the affection was in the left side of the heart alone in 6 cases, and in the right alone in 3 cases. In Jackson's 43 examinations post-mortem we find that "the aortic valves were affected in 9 instances; the mitral, in 15; both, in 10. The right side of the heart was involved 6 times, and the endocardium of the ventricle 3 times. In 5 of the aortic cases there was old endocarditis; it was present in 7 of the mitral cases. The malignant disease had become implanted upon the old disease."

The mechanical factor, however, is not considered essential by Lenhartz, and he has shown that fresh endocarditis does not always arise at the site of the old endocarditis if the latter is present. In Glynn's cases "the infective endocardial lesions were distributed as follows: the aortic and mitral valves were involved in 21 cases, the aortic in 10, the mitral in 15, and the endocardium of the ventricle alone in 1. The right side of the heart was involved in 6 instances" (*loc. cit.*, p. 1073.) Mural endocarditis is apt to affect either the upper portion of the septum of the left ventricle or the posterior wall of the left auricle.

According to the analysis of Kantback and Tickell, in 84 cases there were 51 males and 33 females; and in all but 16 cases old cardiac lesions were found. (Allbutt, p. 877.[23]) In Glynn's cases he found 65 per cent. of patients were males and 34 per cent. were females—"figures approximating those of Dr. Osler." The disease occurred, however, more frequently in young women than in young men. It was also remarked that the disease was likely to occur under conditions attended with general debility. In only

7 per cent. of the cases had an inflammation of the lungs preceded the endocarditis; in 11 per cent. of his cases the endocarditis originated in a recognized infective focus. The vegetations may become detached in larger or smaller masses and, carried by the circulation, form embolic plugs in different organs. Notably we find the kidneys and spleen affected; less frequently the brain and intestines are involved. The place where the embolic mass is arrested depends largely upon its size. While small emboli are more apt to be seen, it is not unknown to have a large artery completely obstructed. If the lungs contain infarcts, the embolic plugs originated in malignant endocarditis affecting the right heart. The embolic plugs are more or less numerous. In some cases where the malignant endocarditis is very pronounced and the ulcerative condition extensive, the autopsy does not show any embolic processes in the organs. They are also more or less irritating.

Consequent upon the degree of their infective nature follows the rapidity with which abscesses are formed. At the site of these abscesses it is not uncommon to find the arterial vessel already softened and ulcerated. Very many small abscesses are found at times in different organs of the body. Sometimes hemorrhage may be combined with the abscesses. Why in some cases the one is more frequent than the other is not positively known. (Strümpell, *Practice of Medicine*, 1901, p. 306.) Embolism was found to be "nearly three times as frequent in the infective as in the simple cases." (Glynn, p. 1076.) It is noted, contrary to the usually accepted opinion, that the so-called infarcts are not due to embolism, but are the result of "apoplexies" following the rupture of small bloodvessels, and made "specially liable to occur in severe passive congestion of the lungs."

The micro-organisms found in malignant endocarditis are pneumococci, streptococci, staphylococcus pyogenes aureus and albus, the gonococcus, and other organisms. The former are most frequently concerned, either alone or associated with others. The pneumococcus infection is more frequent in aortic endocarditis, the streptococcus infection in mitral endocarditis.[24] While in septic diseases malignant endocarditis is prone to occur, there are cases in which the valves are but slightly involved. In no case does the endocarditis form more than a part of the general septic condition. If, however, the heart is notably affected, it hastens very much the spread of the poison, and thus this organ becomes very important in the estimate of the gravity of the case. Of course, there is in these cases the local disease of which the malignant endocarditis is the result. This may be of the nature of an acute necrosis, a wound abscess, or puerperal disease, when there may be primary septic foci in the uterus, or its adnexa.

The etiology of the disease is varied. This is known. Many cases follow an infectious disease, especially pneumonia. This fact has been pointed out by Osler. Still there are cases which appear to be primary (Jackson), as no assignable or sufficient cause of their development can be discovered. All forms of endocarditis, whether ulcerative or benign, seem, according to later investigations, to be of parasitic origin.* This view had been entertained also by Bartel. According to this author, in cases of rheumatic origin the organisms soon die, and often are not discoverable, particularly in cases which have run a somewhat chronic course. There are, however, some cases which "are apparently not due to the direct action of micro-organisms." These are caused by thrombotic deposits, and are possibly the results of the action of bacterial toxins.†

In a peculiar case of endocarditis reported by Hopkins and Weir, in which death resulted from cerebral hemorrhage, we have one that "seems to belong to the group on the border-land between a septic and ulcerative endocarditis; all the emboli were simple, not septic."‡

Thayer and Lazear[25] have gone thoroughly into the subject of gonorrhœa as a cause of septicæmia and ulcerative endocarditis. In their paper they show that the discovery of the gonococci in the circulating blood and upon the cardiac vegetations was made by Blum in 1895. The endocardium may be directly attacked by the gonococcus, as the general infection may be the immediate cause of the local trouble.

Ulcerative endocarditis is a rare disease in childhood. When it does occur in childhood it does not differ essentially from the disease in the adult. One case is reported in an infant ten months old, by L. D'Astros,[26] which resulted fatally. This case followed diphtheria, and, as was shown at the autopsy, was the result of a staphylococcus infection. Cultures from the heart gave a pure growth of cocci. Holt[27] reports a case from Harris in a child four years of age. The lesion in this instance affected the right side of the heart and was secondary to a cardiac malformation. Another fatal case in a girl fifteen years old is described by Cantley. In this case the pulmonary valve was affected. On the other hand, Adams relates a case of recovery as one of only four hitherto reported under the age of fourteen years.§ The greater proportion of cases reported in early life have been over ten years of age. There are 25 or more of these (Holt), and although the right heart is occasionally affected, the disease, according to Lannois and Paris, seems usually to attack the aortic valves.[28] Loeb describes such a case where there were extensive lesions of this valve, and which followed gonorrhœa. The diplococci found had the morphological appearance of gonococci.

* Poynton and Paine. Medical and Surgical Society of London, April 8, 1902.
† Year Book, loc. cit.
‡ British Medical Journal, June 13, 1903, p. 1373.
§ Archives of Pediatrics, December, 1902.

While the authoritative cases of ulcerative endocarditis of rheumatic origin are infrequent, such cases are occasionally described. E. Berie[29] reports two such. The bacillus coli is rarely found and seldom exists as a cause. Still, cases are described both by Henchen and by Andrews.

The symptoms of malignant endocarditis vary very much in individual cases. Sometimes the signs pointing to endocarditis are very indistinct, or entirely absent. This is true particularly where the cardiac disease complicates another acute infectious and septic disease like pneumonia, empyema, or meningitis. Herzog, O'Donovan, and others report cases which appear to support this position. Not only is the difficulty of recognition very great by reason of the absence of distinctive signs, but also by the variety of clinical symptoms present. The latency of the disease is sometimes such that a diagnosis cannot be made in the beginning.* Gavala's case is an instance of this sort. In many cases during life there are no cardiac murmurs, and the diagnosis must be based wholly upon the symptoms.† Again, the symptoms may be most misleading and point to a very different disease, as in the two remarkable cases of N. Pitt,[30] in which symptoms at first appeared to be those of spinal disease. The complete absence of fever also in a given case is not an absolute reason for calling in question the diagnosis, as witness the fatal one reported by C. O'Donovan, without fever.[31] In very few cases of Glynn's patients were there rigors, and in some pyrexia was absent for days and weeks at a time. It may be remarked that the former part of this experience is certainly almost unique. The difficulties attending the diagnosis are sometimes insuperable, for trustworthy clinical indications may be wanting. (Glynn.)

In other instances where the malignant endocarditis is subacute or chronic, and complicates an endocarditis of rheumatic origin, it may show distinct signs and is quite easily recognized. In the former cases the autopsy alone reveals the nature of the disease.

Occasionally the differential diagnosis between rheumatic and acute infective endocarditis is practically almost impossible. There is a mild form of malignant, non-septic endocarditis which resembles in many particulars the grave form of septic endocarditis.‡ In this form, while the local symptoms are not dissimilar to those of simple endocarditis, the general condition is notably bad. In this form we have hemorrhages of the skin and mucous membranes, and emboli in various organs, and also joint implications. But though the joints are swollen and tender the inflammatory arthritis remains serous; it does not become purulent. In the graver cases of this type the patient will often succumb after a few weeks' illness to an aggravation of the general condition. On the other hand, the milder cases will often recover.[32] The severe malignant form of

* Jackson, loc. cit.

† British Medical Journal, May 19, 1900.

‡ Strümpell, p. 307.

endocarditis is almost invariably of septic origin. It is of distinct etiological origin as compared with the milder form referred to. It is characterized apart from cardiac symptoms by the formation of metastatic abscesses in different organs, with or without the accompaniment of hemorrhages. The malignant endocarditis and the metastatic abscesses are directly referable to micrococci; the parenchymatous swelling and changes of organs are the result of the transport of toxins. The microscopic investigation of the different organs often shows the march of the pathological process and how it originated in small foci where minute vessels are filled with micrococci, which later produce areas of cell necrosis, finally leading to suppuration. Because at times no origin at all is discoverable for this form of disease, it seems very obscure. Again, the disease is occasionally not seen by the physician until its later stages, and hence its diagnosis is rendered even more difficult. Very often a pronounced leukocytosis will help us recognize the disease, but the feature of greatest significance is the finding of micrococci in the blood during life. This has already been accomplished more than once. Further bacteriological investigations in this direction are most desirable. Some of these cases run a very chronic course, and one case is reported by Osler where the disease lasted over a year. The autopsy showed extensive vegetations and ulceration of the mitral valve (p. 704). The fever is not always remittent; it may be high and continuous. The rashes, under certain circumstances, may render the disease liable to be confounded with typhoid fever or cerebrospinal meningitis. The sweating is often most profuse. Jaundice is occasionally present and may render confusion with acute yellow atrophy of the liver possible. Cases, even the most acute, usually last a week or more, and yet the disease has been known to terminate fatally in forty-eight hours.

Ordinarily, malignant endocarditis is an intercurrent or secondary affection of some primary septic process. The symptoms of this primary state should not therefore be confounded with those belonging to one of its localizations. It is, however, frequently most difficult to differentiate them. Many of the febrile attacks, which occur in cases of chronic endocarditis and which are accompanied with grave symptoms, result in ultimate recovery. It is very difficult in these instances to be sure whether these cases belong to the benign or malignant variety of ulcerative endocarditis during the period of the acute attack. The fact of the recovery, of course, argues strongly in favor of the benign form, although the clinical symptoms closely simulate those of the graver disease.

As to whether an acute endocarditis will be simple or ulcerative may depend somewhat upon the number or nature of the bacteria transported by the blood. Yet as we find the same bacteria in both forms of disease, this position is not wholly tenable. It seems probable that the particular outcome locally, of the fixation of the bacteria, will depend more upon their virulence than any other one factor. It is also true that ulcerative endocarditis is liable to attack those persons suffering from exhausting diseases and the different cachexiæ. In some cases of ulcerative endocarditis the diagnosis is based mainly on the septic symptoms, and there is little or nothing in the local examination of the heart which will throw light on the case. On the other hand, a suddenly developed cardiac murmur, or a distinct and rapid modification of one already existing and showing previous valvular disease, will have great importance in diagnosis. It is necessary, therefore, in all suspicious cases, to make frequent and careful examinations of the heart, and to note all changes of rhythm which occur. The same is also true of the timbre of the murmur which may change at any time, and from being harsh and loud from the previous lesion may become soft and blowing by reason of the fresh disease which has developed. Combined with the heart symptoms are those of sepsis and embolism. The presence of fever and the numerous petechiæ or hemorrhages are always very significant; these symptoms being rarely combined in ordinary rheumatic endocarditis, sometimes the discovery of some evident cause of the septicæmia will bring light to an otherwise obscure case. Thus a foul vaginal discharge, which may be the result of an abortion in which the neck of the uterus has become abraded, will in this way prove satisfactory.

While chills, fever, and sweating point to septic fever, they do not fix the diagnosis of ulcerative endocarditis, and this must be done by examination of, and findings in the heart, or else by the changes due to emboli in the organs. Skin, urine, spleen must be frequently examined with this end in view. When other means fail to establish a diagnosis, an examination of the blood should be made. It is claimed that in most infections there is a decided leukocytosis, but in ulcerative endocarditis this statement is not always correct, according to Neussen, who says there is either an absence or possible decrease of leukocytosis.* On the other hand, Kelly dwells upon the importance in diagnosis of the presence of a moderate leukocytosis of the polynuclear variety. The latter also insists on the positive result of bacterioscopy of the blood. Likewise he attributes much value to the fact of the great instability of heart action, which may be noted in a very brief period. Some cases of ulcerative endocarditis may be readily mistaken for typhoid fever. In the latter, even though of severe type, hemorrhages in the skin are very rare. Moreover, we have earlier enlargement of the spleen, and pronounced abdominal symptoms, usually like tympanites, diarrhœa, distention, and rose spots. In all doubtful cases we should make the Widal test, and sooner or later we expect to get it in typhoid fever. The presence of this test would also help to

* Babcock. Diseases of the Heart, p. 181.

eliminate acute miliary tuberculosis, with which ulcerative endocarditis might be confounded. Unfortunately, the Widal test is not always absolutely reliable, even when present, to determine the differential diagnosis. One such instance is reported by Mathews and Moir,* where the Widal test was positive, thus confusing the diagnosis with one of typhoid fever. The autopsy showed that the disease was one of ulcerative endocarditis. Some instances, also, are reported, where the Widal test has proved negative. In other cases there has been a positive Widal reaction, and with different strains from one in twenty to one in two hundred. We thus perceive that this reaction is incapable at times of differentiating between these cases.†[33] The serum reaction in the differential diagnosis may be misleading in other instances, notably in septicæmia and acute tuberculosis. (Glynn.) Acute miliary tuberculosis may be differentiated frequently by the presence of tubercle bacilli in the sputum, and also by the preponderance of chest signs over those indicating a heart lesion.‡ I have had one case, unfortunately, of miliary tuberculosis of the lungs under my care, which resulted fatally, in which no tubercle bacilli were ever found, and in which the chest signs were changeable and uncertain for several weeks. In this case there was a soft, blowing murmur at the mitral orifice. There were, however, no hemorrhages of the skin, and no manifest symptoms pointing to emboli in the viscera. At one time there was slight hæmaturia, which made me somewhat suspicious of the renal condition. In a few days this cleared up, and I thought it was explained by renal hyperæmia, due to the febrile nature of the disease. The recurring chilly sensations, profuse sweats, and dyspnœa may occur in both diseases. The loss of flesh and strength may also be marked in both.

The temperature chart is probably more irregular and different in ulcerative endocarditis. Here again I have found it very difficult at times to pronounce in which direction I was carried by its careful consideration. As a rule ulcerative endocarditis may be readily distinguished from malaria by the discovery of the plasmodium in the blood, and also by the greater irregularity of the fever and chills which presents the septic type. In what Osler regards as a very remarkable sub-group of this type, the fever and chills may closely simulate regular attacks of quotidian or tertian ague. In those instances where there has been a previously well-marked malarial infection, the differential diagnosis would become additionally difficult. Again, and despite the affirmation of distinguished observers to the contrary, I have met with undoubted cases of malaria, as I believe, in which no malarial organisms have ever been found, and despite careful and repeated microscopic examinations of the blood by skilled observers.

* British Medical Journal, June 22, 1899.

† Lancet, March 22, 1902.

‡ Thompson. Practical Medicine, second ed., p. 319.

Occasionally chronic endocarditis, accompanied by a fever resembling that of typhoid or remittent fever, may lead to confusion in diagnosis. In these instances, however, embolic phenomena, septic or other, are not found. Moreover, these cases are often prolonged for several months, as in one of Bristow's, cited by Osler. In those cases accompanied with irregular fever, embolic phenomena and physical evidences of recent endocarditis with cardiac distress, and which run an acute course, it is sometimes most difficult to know whether ulcerative endocarditis is present or not. If the case goes rapidly to a fatal termination, as it often does, and we obtain an autopsy, of course the nature of the case can be positively decided. If, on the other hand, the fever, restlessness, cardiac distress, and local signs of heart lesions wholly disappear, and the patient recovers entirely, as in certain recorded instances of gonorrhœal endocarditis (Thayer and Lazear), we may still retain, perhaps, reasonable doubt as to our diagnosis.

The instances which are reported to recover are the less acute forms, and have usually been grafted more than once upon old sclerotic changes of the cardiac valves and orifices. In this category I should be inclined to put some of the gonorrhœal cases. These, however, as we know, are diagnosed at times more by cardiac changes than by septic symptoms.* The mechanical factor in the development of ulcerative endocarditis is not an essential one, inasmuch as the fresh endocarditis does not always arise at the site of the old endocarditis if the latter is present.† The distinction Lenhartz makes between chronic septic endocarditis and malignant rheumatic endocarditis, based on the presence in the former of micro-organisms commonly producing sepsis, is called in question by Litten on the ground of variability of bacteriological conditions, and he states that no distinction can be made on this basis. Stengel finds both classifications unsatisfactory.‡

In these instances much importance should be attached to the supposed etiological factor. If it be of the nature of articular rheumatism, chorea, or scarlatina, we would infer that we had to do with an endocarditis of benign type; if, on the other hand, we find in the antecedents some pus infection or focus of suppuration, puerperal processes, bone-disease, etc., we are prone to believe that ulcerative endocarditis has developed. Again, the febrile movement may be wholly absent, or else pursue a very mild and regular course. In the latter case it is probably due either to the acute endocarditis of simple type, or to the rheumatic cause. When either one gradually subsides the fever also disappears.

With the greatest possible care, however, on the part of the attending physician, the diagnosis of ulcerative endocarditis may be mistaken or overlooked, so frequently do the symptoms vary.§

* Allbutt, p. 882.
† Lenhartz. Gould's Year Book, 1903, p. 182.
‡ Loc. cit.
§ Thompson, p. 319.

Again, as I have pointed out already, there may be a complete absence of recognizable cardiac signs locally. In the acute classes resembling cerebrospinal fever, blood cultures do not help us very much to make an accurate differential diagnosis. If the spinal disease be of tuberculous nature, puncture of the spinal membranes and withdrawal of fluid may be of very great value in revealing the presence of tubercle bacilli. In the non-tuberculous variety, whether it has become suppurative or not, we may find the same organism that is discovered in ulcerative endocarditis, and of course our doubts are in that case not solved by this method of exploration.

The course of ulcerative endocarditis may be very brief. Indeed, it may be a very acute disease, last only a few days, and then terminate fatally. Such are the extreme and relatively rare instances. The more frequent ones are those where the disease has lasted several weeks. Its progress onward and downward may be continuous. On the other hand there may be periods of relative improvement followed by renewed exacerbations. The patients seem to improve for a time and subsequently relapse and return to the hospital in a worse condition. (Glynn.) When death actually occurs it is occasioned by the progress of the heart disease, which finally causes pronounced asthenia. Or again it is the prolonged general sepsis which apparently occasions the fatal outcome. There may be complicating pulmonary œdema or pneumonia, and in this way death occurs more rapidly. Sometimes it would appear that the term of life is closed essentially by reason of emboli in different organs—kidney, spleen, or brain.

An interesting case is reported by Babcock (p. 173 *et seq.*) following an attack of tonsillitis which after five months' duration terminated fatally. In this case, although clearly a septic one from the beginning, the pulse persisted at about the same rate (105), and there was a fairly continuous temperature with slight changes. There was present marked bulbous enlargement of the terminal phalanges of the fingers due to capillary dilatation. Unfortunately in Babcock's case there was no autopsy. Credé's ointment and antistreptococcic serum were employed, with the results perhaps of increasing strength for a while, and occasioning a slight reduction of temperature. The occurrence of emboli always renders the prognosis more serious. In addition to the mere mechanical results of these emboli in the different viscera we observe their septic consequences, which contribute to the speedy, fatal termination. Thus we find single or multiple septic abscesses in the spleen, liver, kidneys, and, indeed, throughout the body, and these are the evidences of general infection of the economy. Of course, death is the inevitable result, almost, of such a condition.

In general the treatment of ulcerative endocarditis is that of acute benign endocarditis with even greater precautions exercised about preserving the strength of the heart, noting that independently of the specially destructive tendencies of the disease to the cardiac valves and walls and the formation of abscesses locally in its structure the heart muscle is more likely to suffer from the effects of the toxæmia itself than in the relatively benign form of disease. The treatment may be regarded therefore as essentially symptomatic.

To combat general sepsis we should rely upon large and repeated doses of alcohol in the most palatable and useful form—*i. e.*, the best old brandy—alternating it with best champagne now and then for a day or two. The employment of alcohol in septic disease and in sufficient quantity is still heartily endorsed by many eminent clinicians and despite many and strong arguments made use of by its adversaries. Carbonate of ammonia is also possibly a useful adjunct to alcohol for a little while, in view of the thrombotic findings upon the cardiac valves which some autopsies reveal and by reason of the proofs we seem to have, clinically, of its action in lessening somewhat the tendency to such deposits or formations. The late Dr. Benjamin Ward Richardson insists forcibly upon this view as regards certain infectious diseases, notably diphtheria, and I have always believed with much reason. I am satisfied, however, that carbonate of ammonia is far more depressing even than alcohol if too long continued, and particularly in large, frequently repeated doses such as are so often insisted upon in clinical text-books of practice of medicine.

To abate or lessen the chills and the fever quinine is used by some with the idea that it will do so if given in doses of 5 to 10 grains three or more times daily. With our improved knowledge of the etiology and pathology of the disease such a view seems scarcely warranted. And when we think of the cardiac depression which may follow such doses, demonstrated many years ago by Binz, I find no adequate reasons for the use of the drug after this manner. The treatment of disease then, according to many, is practically that of septicæmia (Osler), and except the measures which we should rationally employ in all forms of endocarditis even the mildest.

Are there therefore no known measures which have any curative influence upon the march and termination of the disease itself? Dreschfeld speaks of having been useful by means of a combination of quinine and arsenic in 3 cases, 2 of which he reports.[34] In neither case, however, did recovery take place. Perhaps the prognosis of ulcerative endocarditis may become more hopeful with our improved forms of treatment; more so even than that of the cases of endocarditis which are regarded as relatively and less immediately dangerous.

With the progress of serotherapy and of intravenous medication this statement has become especially true during the past year. This progress is due to researches of pathologists who, like Poynton and Paine, have pointed out the parasitic nature of the disease.

Besides, several histories have been reported pointing to the favorable outcome of the disease through medication. Occasionally recovery may be expected. Clinical reports bear evidence of this, and besides it is more than justified by the results from autopsies.

The treatment of the disease has now definitely in view the killing of the germs. Two methods of medication have been tried —*i. e.*, the sera and the mineral germicides. They may be administered either internally by mouth or rectum, subcutaneously or intravenously. Later all three methods may be combined at the same time to hasten the cure.

As to the relative value of these remedies it is impossible to state at present. But each day seems to show how important has become the interactions between living and inorganic matter. In this line notably are the effects of radium on the tissues. The promulgation of the catalytic action of sera and albuminized metals is also related to our ignorance, but presuming this theory to be correct it would prove how useful the direct application of remedies may be to the cure of disease. An effort has been made to introduce antiseptic remedies in sufficient quantity into the system to exert at least a modifying influence upon the sepsis. (Babcock.) Among these the sulphocarbolate of soda in one-half drachm doses has been used by Sansom, and with such good effect that one patient was enabled to leave the hospital and remain away ten months before a fresh attack occurred. To the latter, however, she succumbed, and the autopsy justified the accuracy of the diagnosis by revealing cardiac valves permeated with micrococci.

Of course if antiseptic medication is to be of real service it must be employed in sufficient amount to affect the system thoroughly, and be continued for a considerable period. And here resides the danger with which we are all familiar, to-day more than ever, that in our efforts to destroy or neutralize micro-organisms and their toxins so pernicious to the economy, we may occasion great harm to the composition of the blood which would more than counterbalance any beneficial results from the use of antiseptic medication. This is especially true if we employ the hypodermic method. In illustration I would refer to the brilliant work of Barrows in the treatment of puerperal septicæmia, who at first seemed to have achieved a very remarkable triumph.

According to the latest laboratory experiments of J. M. Fortescue Brickdale,[35] injection of antiseptics produce no favorable results. This experience is corroborated by W. H. Park and W. A. Payne,[36] who state that in their judgment the use of plain salt and water intravenously will be found equally useful and less dangerous than diluted formalin injections.

On the other hand the use, clinically, of intravenous injections of antiseptics by Netter,[37] Maguire, Landerer, and Ewart, has been at times distinctly favorable. Further, Klotz narrates a case resulting successfully, in which colloidal silver was used hypodermically. After two injections there were rigors and no improvement; but after the third there was rapid decrease of fever and ultimate recovery.[38]

As Ewart remarks, forcibly, too rigid adherence should not be directed toward mere "germicidal potency" as a test for practical utility. It may be that intravascular antisepsis will prove delusory, but over and beyond is the great subject of intravenous medication which must remain as a very valuable aid to our methods of treatment. Inasmuch as the action of the antiseptic injections is not bactericidal, some other explanation must be given of their power for good. According to Netter this resides in a catalytic action much resembling the action of ferments, and depends upon a mysterious power of matter. In the discussion of Dr. Barrows' paper the majority seem to preserve an open mind as to the desirability of the treatment in any extensive way.[39]

O'Brien[40] has pointed out some of the dangers resulting from intravenous injections—*i. e.*, rigors, collapse, and respiratory embarrassment. In one case sudden death followed. As there was no autopsy a definite explanation could not be given. It is important to note that those who make use of these injections should be prepared to deal with sudden emergencies which may arise.

No doubt there is some comfort to be taken, as Babcock would have us believe, apparently, from the neutralization of the toxins found in the intestinal tract during the course of ulcerative endocarditis, and which doubtless, unless properly neutralized, tend to aggravate the original disease and prevent recovery. Among these so-called antiseptics used to modify favorably autointoxications from the intestinal tract, there are only a few in which I have at present even limited confidence. The best and least harmful which I have tried are small, repeated doses of beechwood creosote, the salts of bismuth, and wood charcoal. In a paper read before the New York Clinical Society about two years ago I directed attention in this connection to these drugs, and spoke favorably of their use as compared to others I had tried.

Up to the time of writing a certain number of cases have been treated by the antistreptococcic serum, and with more or less success. There is a certain degree of reason in the use of this serum, because it appears to be useful in other septic cases—notably puerperal septicæmia. It is also reasonable to employ it because streptococci are undoubtedly among the organisms which appear frequently infiltrated, as it were, in the cardiac valves at the autopsy of these cases. The serum itself, properly employed, does not cause injury to the patient, and again we find in the antitoxin treatment of diphtheria an analogy which makes us somewhat hopeful of this other new treatment. The outlook seems to be, therefore, that pathological sera will probably be more and more used. Antitoxins and immunizing sera have, indeed, more than one action, and, it has been demonstrated, may be useful in distinct diseases. The explanation of their effects may reside in a catalytic action not dissimilar to that of the albuminates of the metals. The intravenous route is the one now preferable for serotherapy, especially in the severer cases, and when subcutaneous injections have proved ineffective. To the former injections, despite disadvantages and dangers, we should recur hopefully.

Sir Douglas Powell reports three successful cases from the use of antistreptococcic serum, and emphasizes the fact that if it were employed earlier in the disease, and before a general dissemination of it in different organs had taken place, our results would be better. He also considers that in its use we must not expect benefit where organisms of another order, like pneumococci or gonococci, are present, but be hopeful and limit its use to those cases in which streptococci or staphylococci have been causative. If there be anywhere a purulent focus which surgery can reach it must be promptly dealt with and suppressed if possible. Otherwise we should expect continual accessions from this source of the toxic organisms whose influence we wish to combat. Hence, the employment of the antistreptococcic serum must remain useless. On the other hand, if the supply of toxic-bearing bacteria is stopped, and even though many of those already in the blood may be other than streptococci, this serum may prove very beneficial.

To obtain our best, most hopeful results treatment should be begun at an early date, or so soon as the diagnosis approaches a high degree of probability. There are, moreover, evident grades in the malignancy of different cases of ulcerative endocarditis, and it is impossible at first to pronounce as to the precise future course of a given case of the disease. The reported cases of improvement and recovery under more than one sort of treatment makes this fact very clear. Again, we should be encouraged from this standpoint to begin early treatment with the serum. It is always judicious and advisable also, to take blood in a doubtful case for the purpose of culture inoculation and other experiment, even though no profitable determination can always be made so as to fix, if possible, the cause of the disease. (Gibson, quoted by Babcock.) Great care must be taken that the blood obtained for bacteriological examination should not be contaminated. The staphylococcus albus, if found, is due to contamination, and is not the specific cause of the disease. The micro-organism which is most frequently found by cultivating the blood is the micrococcus pyogenes. It has been obtained in many cases of ulcerative endocarditis. If a patient with some valvular disease has irregular temperature, is anæmic, and streptococci are obtained from cultivation of the blood, a diagnosis of ulcerative endocarditis should be made, and the indication is to inject antistreptococcic serum. Blood examination should not be considered infallible as an aid to diagnosis and prognosis. As Bryant[41] writes in corroboration of Ewing's statement: "The examination having been performed, its results are to be interpreted only in the light of the fullest possible clinical information."

It would appear that ulcerative endocarditis of pneumococcic origin offers little hope for any beneficial result from this treatment. Let us hope that the day is not far distant when a suitable serum will be available for every kind of septic poisoning, no matter what the precise efficient bacterial cause may be. The modern researches of the Klemperer brothers and others give us renewed trust that our wishes may soon be realized. (Babcock.) From 3 cases reported by Babcock he is evidently disposed to make use of the antistreptococcic serum in any future cases he may see, even though the diagnosis may be somewhat doubtful, and provided other treatment has been used in vain. He remarks with justifiable emphasis: "Such cases are so desperate and the prospect of recovery so slight that I believe one is justified in resorting to whatever affords even a chance of benefit; and if an old preparation is employed there is not much danger of producing erythema or articular inflammation, and the remedy cannot prove more harmful than the disease itself, unchecked."* Successful results in the use of antistreptococcic serum in the treatment of ulcerative endocarditis have been reported by Sainsbury and by Pearce,[42] another also by Clarke.[43] The following case reported by Bryant[44] appears to me very convincing: "A boy, aged fifteen years, was admitted to the hospital suffering from mitral disease. He had had several attacks of rheumatism. His temperature was varied and running an irregular course, ranging between 98° and 101.5° F. When he first came under my care he had been in the hospital for nearly two months, and during the whole of the time his temperature had been raised and he had not had any manifestations of rheumatism or of tonsillitis. A bacteriological examination of the blood showed the presence of streptococci in pure culture. A few days afterward the temperature dropped to normal and remained normal. A subsequent bacteriological examination of the blood was negative. I considered this boy was suffering from infective endocarditis, that the acute process had subsided, and the streptococci died out."

In some cases of ulcerative endocarditis treated with antistreptococcic serum, while temporary benefit may result from its use, the result ultimately has been fatal. An instance of this kind is described by H. M. Cooper.† In this, as in other cases, it was thought if the serum treatment had been instituted earlier a successful result might have been obtained. Per contra, as regards the matter of the innocuousness of these injections, the following cases are interesting and important. B. M. H. Rogers[45] used five injec-

* Loc. cit., p. 797. † British Medical Journal, May 10, 1902.

tions of 10 c.c. each of antistreptococcic serum in a case of ulcerative endocarditis, in which pure cultures of streptococcus had been obtained from the blood. The injections caused violent pain, were without effect, and death occurred. Post-mortem cultures yielded streptococci. J. H. Abram[46] reports another case treated in a similar manner after streptococci had also been found in the blood. The case was fatal; but it was found after death that the streptococci had disappeared. The serum is believed to have caused this disappearance.

Cyril Ogle[47] indicates the value of antistreptococcic serum in cases in which the symptoms during life, or the post-mortem findings, showed ulcerative endocarditis. Of course, the cases are not favorable ones in view of the constant passage of the blood current over the surface of the affected organ—*i. e.*, the heart. Still, recovery is not incompatible with this grave infection when thus treated. In Dr. Ogle's table the successes amount to 31.5 per cent.; in Sir Douglas Powell's tables, to 25 per cent.[48] On the other hand, Nathan Raw used antistreptococcic serum in 5 cases without any beneficial results. And Glynn reports no information of an encouraging nature from Liverpool hospitals, and without success in 3 of his own cases. I find 1 successful case reported by Moritz,[49] in which antistaphylococcic serum was employed. Six injections of 5 c.c. were sufficient to dissipate the acute symptoms. When they were begun the patient had been ill during two months. In two weeks of treatment the temperature was normal. Six weeks later a heart murmur was present and the pulse was rapid. Still the man remained in good condition.[50] Other methods of treatment have also been followed by reported cures. One by Coleman which followed vaccination. Another from Hepburn in which the treatment was entirely symptomatic. In one instance the aortic murmur disappeared during convalescence. The treatment was by the Brand method and unguentum Credé.[51] Roussell[52] reports three recoveries. Another recovery of gonorrhœal endocarditis is from a paper of Lenhartz.*

The employment of yeast in the treatment of ulcerative endocarditis is referred to by Sir Douglas Powell, and 1 successful case out of 5 is reported by him. In the other case there was no appreciably good result. In one other instance where nuclein was employed there was a decided lowering of temperature. The remedy was employed subcutaneously. If yeast has any remedial value it is probably due to the nuclein or nucleinic acid it contains, as instanced by Vaughn. The latter may be used by mouth, rectum, or hypodermically, according to the strength and kind of preparation made use of. It would seem as though the curative action of the nuclein was essentially due to its power of increasing polynuclear white cells. These, as we know, are frequently more

* Loc. cit.

numerous in ulcerative endocarditis, and the germicidal properties of nuclein are explained by their additionally increased number. Many favorable reports, according to Babcock, have been made about the value of yeast-nuclein in the treatment of divers pus infections. And in view of these statements he was encouraged to give it a trial in a case of acute endocarditis complicating a follicular tonsillitis, possibly of rheumatic origin. During the period the remedy was taken the fever slowly abated. Despite this fact, however, the case terminated fatally. Latterly, Duckworth reports, in the Section of Medicine of the Fourteenth International Medical Congress (Madrid, April 25, 1903), a case of probable ulcerative endocarditis in which a treatment with fresh yeast and antistreptococcic serum hypodermically was employed without appreciable benefit. Subsequently, however, a cure was apparently effected by repeated injections per rectum of a mixed antistreptococcic serum, 10 c.c. being the dose employed.* "This case may be taken," writes Duckworth, "to illustrate the effects of a specially virulent quality or variety of the specific infecting microbe which commonly induces ordinary rheumatic symptoms, and may add support to the view of Poynton and Paine that infective endocarditis may sometimes be a primary affection due to a virulent form of the peccant matter of rheumatism."†

If all endocarditis should be properly regarded as infective, it is indicated to find our remedial agent among the class of antiseptic remedies. The most available and least objectionable is the one to make trial of. Amidst the rapidly increasing number of this class of remedies one will be ultimately found that is decidedly curative in many instances. Of course, in making use of the antiseptic remedy so as to influence the entire mass of blood and prevent the infection from being carried to and localized upon the endocardium, we should avoid strictly employing remedies which threaten the general health. At present, moreover, we make use of such remedies mainly in the treatment of the supposed virulent cases, and usually at a later stage of the disease when the outcome is almost surely fatal. In the far larger class of benign cases of endocarditis, and hence the more important ones, their progress is often not stayed by this or any other careful treatment soon enough. The result is they continue their onward insidious and disastrous march. If these cases were treated in the beginning by judiciously selected antiseptic remedies, it is to be hoped that eventually we should have fewer cases of both sorts, and mainly, I believe with Ewart,[53] of the ulcerative forms. Further, we should not be obliged to admit, as it seems to me, with the writer of the latest and most valuable treatise on diseases of the heart, "that the most the physician

* Lancet, May 2, 1903, pp. 1268, 1269; and Boston Medical and Surgical Journal, August 29, 1903, p. 238.

† British Medical Journal, May 23, 1903, p. 1195.

can do in the treatment of acute endocarditis is to aid nature by helping to maintain the vital powers that lie in nature's way."[54] Let us remember that recovery in an apparently desperate case is possible, and the future may bring improved methods both of serum and antiseptic treatment.

It may be well to add that the latest experiments upon animals seems to prove that the Aronson antistreptococcic serum is superior to the others, notably those of Marmorek and of Tavel. It is apparent, also, that to obtain the best curative effects the serum should be given intravenously. Also, treatment according to this method should be continued well into the period of convalescence, inasmuch as death occurs sometimes when all danger seems to have passed.

Finally, I would again insist upon the primary importance in all cases of beginning the use of the serum at an earlier date than hitherto has usually been done. Sometimes, not to say frequently, it has been employed when all curative methods must prove futile, as the economy is unable to respond favorably to that as to all other medication. Moreover, whenever the infection has lasted more than a very brief period much larger doses of serum are rendered necessary to produce similar curative effects. I shall not attempt to explain how the serum acts. Nor, indeed, is it positively known. Certainly it has no appreciable effect upon the growth of cocci in the culture tube, and it appears in final analysis merely, so far as our knowledge now extends, to diminish *virulence*, "for cocci which have been left for some time under the influence of the serum will no longer bring about hæmolysis."[55] The latest paper on the use of "antistreptococcic serum in the treatment of inflammatory rheumatism and other diseases" is to my mind very encouraging. It shows conclusively it is most efficient when given *early* in infectious disease; also, that it is useful in *diplococcic* infection. In Dr. G. H. Sherman's[56] cases "none of the patients developed heart complications, and complete recovery took place in a comparatively short time." This statement contradicts that of Osler—*i. e.*, "We know no measures by which in rheumatism the onset of endocarditis can be prevented."*

BIBLIOGRAPHY.

1. Medical News, March 21, 1885.
2. London Lancet, March 25, and April 2 and 9, 1898.
3. Loc. cit., April, 1903, p. 1153.
4. Practice of Medicine, 4th ed., p. 699.
5. Loc. cit., p. 700.
6. Progressive Medicine, September 1903, p. 79.
7. Practice of Medicine, 6th ed., p. 595.
8. C. S. Bull. Medical Record. December 20, 1902.
9. Johns Hopkins Hospital Bulletin, October, 1902.
10. Progressive Medicine; also Deut. med. Woch., May 22 and 29, 1902.

* Vide fifth edition, 1903, p. 705.

11. To show the extreme rarity, even with typhoid fever, I would cite Dr. Osler's medical clinic at the Johns Hopkins Hospital, where there never has been a case (written communication from Dr. W. S. Thayer, December 10, 1903). Very probable cases, in view of the symptoms during life, are occasionally met with. Even in fatal cases with characteristic symptoms, where no autopsy is obtained, doubt as to diagnosis may be urged, although in one of Dr. Thayer's cases such doubt would hardly be justified.

12. Wells says this complication is very frequent.

13. THE AMERICAN JOURNAL OF THE MEDICAL SCIENCES, January, 1901, p. 53.

14. Austen. Johns Hopkins Bulletin, 1899, p. 104.

15. American Medicine, October 17, 1903, p. 627.

16. Journal of Experimental Medicine, 1899, p. 521.

17. Journal of the American Medical Association, August 19, 1900.

18. Progressive Medicine, September, 1903.

19. Gould. American Year Book of Medicine and Surgery, 1903, p. 752.

20. Progressive Medicine, September, 1902, p. 128.

21. Allbutt's System of Medicine, vol. vi. p. 876.

22. Practice of Medicine, 4th ed., p. 701.

23. The vegetations themselves, although unrecognized during life, may have been present for a long while, as shown by autopsy.

24. Dessy. Boston Medical and Surgical Journal, September 1, 1898.

25. Journal of Experimental Medicine, January, 1899.

26. Rev. mens. des mal. de l'enfance. December, 1898.

27. Diseases of Infancy and Childhood. 2d ed. p. 622.

28. The exceptions to this rule would appear to be cases of gonorrhœal origin where the right heart is frequently involved (Thayer and Lazear).

29. Semaine méd., January 21, 1900.

30. Practitioner, November, 1898.

31. Medical News, July 23, 1898.

32. The duration in the fatal cases is only a few days or weeks, but in those that recover it is usually much more prolonged.

33. According to MacFarland there was in 4000 cases only 4 per cent. of error (Babcock, p. 182). If after sixth day of illness test is negative, typhoid fever may be properly excluded (Allbutt, foot-note).

34. Allbutt's System of Medicine, vol. vi. p. 884.

35. Lancet, January 10, 1903.

36. Medical News, April 4, 1903.

37. Bull. et mém. de la Soc. des hôp. de Paris, December 18, 1902, et seq.

38. Progressive Medicine, September, 1903, p. 81.

39. New York Medical Journal, January 31, 1903.

40. Lancet, October 11, 1902.

41. Ibid., February 7, 1903, p. 364.

42. Allbutt's System of Medicine. Loc. cit., p. 885.

43. Lancet, July 21, 1900.

44. Ibid., February 7, 1903, p. 364.

45. Ibid., June 10, 1899.

46. Ibid., February 25, 1899.

47. Ibid., March 14, 1903.

48. Ibid., April 25, 1903, p. 1153.

49. Serum therapie bei Endocarditis Maligna, St. Petersburger medicinische Wochenschrift, 1898.

50. In Moritz's case the diagnosis of the organism present had not been confirmed previously by a blood examination, although the evidence of implication of the valves seems to have been certain (Lancet, March 14, 1903, p. 723).

51. Philadelphia Medical Journal, January 12, 1901.

52. Ibid., February 23, 1901.

53. Progressive Medicine, September, 1902, p. 112.

54. Babcock, p. 198.

55. Medical News, September 5, 1903, p. 462.

56. American Medicine, October 17, 1903, p. 633.

NOTE.—Owing to the length of this paper, I am obliged to omit the histories of my cases.

In Bulletin of the Ayer Clinical Laboratory of the Pennsylvania Hospital, October, 1903, a unique case is reported of ulcerative endocarditis caused by Weichselbaum's meningococcus.

REMARKS ON GASTROSUCCORRHŒA AND TETANIC ATTACKS OCCURRING WITH CHRONIC ULCER OF THE STOMACH.[1]

By J. Kaufmann, M.D.,
of New York.

Ever since analyses of gastric contents have been made in order to study the function of the stomach and its disturbances mistakes have been made chiefly in two directions: certain functional disturbances which are really only symptoms have been stamped as diseases, and in explaining certain conditions too much stress has been laid upon secretory disturbances, the importance of motor disorders being underestimated. This applies also to the picture described as gastrosuccorrhœa. Although much has been written about this symptom-complex, there is still a great deal of confusion in regard to its correct interpretation, and it is therefore justifiable to consider once more whether this picture ought to be taken as an independent disease.

Reichmann was the first to apply the name "gastrosuccorrhœa" to a set of symptoms which are chiefly characterized by the presence in the fasting stomach of a fluid possessing all the chemical and physiological properties of gastric juice. The patients, who are generally emaciated, complain of pyrosis, eructation, and vomiting of highly acid matter, and suffer a great deal from gastric pains coming on after meals and during the night. Examinations of the stomach contents after test meals show hyperacidity and impaired digestion of starches. In the urine there is often a diminution, and sometimes even a total absence, of chlorides. In Reichmann's opinion the characteristic feature of this condition is the continual flow of gastric juice, not only after meals and during the process of digestion, but also during the intervals when the stomach of a normal individual should be empty.

Reichmann's publication aroused an extensive and lively discussion of the questions: Is gastrosuccorrhæa, as its name indicates, really a primary secretory disturbance, or is the accumulation of secretion in the fasting stomach the result of a motor insufficiency? Is gastrosuccorrhœa a disease *per se*, or is it merely a peculiar combination of symptoms which accompany other already well-known pathological conditions? A consensus of opinion on these questions has not as yet been reached.

There are two varieties of gastrosuccorrhœa—the periodic and the chronic. In the *periodic form* we have to deal with attacks of vomiting of gastric juice, coming on spasmodically and lasting from

[1] Read before the German Medical Society of the City of New York, April 8, 1902.

a few hours to several days. The condition has been attributed to a morbid overactivity of the secretory nerves of the stomach, which is regarded as a neurosis by itself, as a symptom accompanying hysteria or neurasthenia, or as a symptom occurring in the form of gastric crises in tabes and other spinal diseases. The remaining symptoms occurring with such attacks, pyrosis, headache, gastric pains, and vomiting, are classed as secondary manifestations. The same attacks have, however, been described by a number of other writers under different titles, the name depending upon the symptom regarded as being the most important. Thus, Leyden refers to them as "periodic vomiting;" Struebing classes them with disorders which he designates as "angioneurotic œdema;" Rossbach, who considers the increased secretion of hydrochloric acid as the chief factor in the condition, calls them "gastroxynsis." They are also found in descriptions of nervous diseases. Möbius, for example, associates them with migraine. I shall not further discuss this group of cases of periodic gastrosuccorrhœa, the pathogenesis of which is still very vague. The secretion of large quantities of gastric juice accumulating in the stomach independently of the ingestion of food may play an important role. However, all that has thus far been taught about the relation of the various symptoms to one another, and especially in regard to the point whether this increased secretion of gastric juice is the primary or only a secondary factor in the attacks, is still altogether hypothetical.

In *chronic gastrosuccorrhœa* the conditions are entirely different, since it is not of a nervous character, but is dependent upon anatomical changes of the stomach or duodenum. In these cases it can be demonstrated that the presence of fluid in the fasting stomach invariably means a motor disturbance, and that the view that chronic gastrosuccorrhœa is a disease *per se* is not well supported.

As has already been mentioned, Reichmann's theory was that the characteristic feature of the disease was the presence of gastric juice in the stomach at a time when the organ should be empty. According to his view, this accumulation of gastric juice occurs because the mucosa of the stomach secretes continuously without any apparent irritation, but solely in consequence of the morbid activity of the secretory nerves of the stomach.

Reichmann, however, did not overlook the fact that the presence of gastric juice in the fasting stomach could not be explained simply as a hypersecretion. In some of the cases described by him as much as a litre of fluid rich in hydrochloric acid could be expressed in the morning. In these cases there was undoubtedly an increased secretion, but this is by no means the rule. In a number of other cases the quantity found was decidedly less. The amount of hydrochloric acid contained in the fluid also varies. In cases where only relatively small quantities are found, or where the amount of hydrochloric acid is low, we cannot very well speak of increased secretion, especially as we do not know the quantity secreted by the normal stomach during a given time. The essential point, therefore, is not that there is an increased secretion, but is rather in the fact that this secretion is found in the stomach at a time when the organ ought to be empty.

The opinion was formerly held that the fasting stomach of a healthy individual was entirely empty. This view has since been somewhat modified, Rosin and Schreiber having reported that in systematically examining a large number of healthy individuals they often found gastric juice in the fasting stomach in varying quantities, sometimes reaching 40 c.c. Martius, Hemmeter, and others have confirmed these statements. The gastric secretion in these cases is explained as being the result of the stimulation caused by swallowed saliva and pharyngeal mucus.

However that may be, quantities of 50 c.cm. and over are surely pathological. Where such quantities are found it is possible that gastric secretion has been increased and kept up beyond the time required for digestion. But the fact that it is found in the fasting stomach can only be explained by the existence of some hindrance to its passage into the intestine. For, if motor function of the organ is normal, there is no reason why such increased secretion should not pass into the intestine just as well as other stomach contents.

The misinterpretation of these conditions was partly due to the singular confusion which followed the discussion of the meaning of gastric dilatation. I shall not enter into the discussion of this subject further than is necessary for understanding its relation to gastrosuccorrhœa. There is no reason for discarding the old, well-defined clinical picture of gastric dilatation. Its characteristic feature is that it is a combination of two conditions which must be distinguished: the enlargement of the organ and the stagnation of stomach contents. Enlargement of the stomach is an anatomical condition. Stagnation of stomach contents represents a functional disturbance—a motor insufficiency. A stomach with normal motor activity, no matter what its size, empties its contents during the night. Where this is not accomplished motor insufficiency is present.

The stagnating material may consist principally of solid food remains mixed with a larger or smaller quantity of fluid, or it may be chiefly fluid containing few or no solid particles. When solid particles are found, all authorities agree on the presence of stagnation. But when only fluid can be expressed from the fasting stomach, as is often the case in gastrosuccorrhœa, some authors maintain that the condition cannot be considered a stagnation, because no solid particles are contained in the fluid. To support this view, it was argued that in some of these cases certain symptoms generally associated with gastric dilatation were absent. It was claimed, for instance, that in cases where no lowering of the greater curvature could be demonstrated there could be no dilatation of the organ, and therefore no motor insufficiency.

In diagnosing dilatation of the stomach we must separately consider three things: (1) the size of the stomach; (2) its position, and (3) its mechanical ability.

Size and position of the stomach do not necessarily indicate its mechanical ability. A stomach may be very large and its greater curvature may be low, yet it may be motorily sufficient. In such a case we cannot speak of dilatation, but simply of a deeply situated, enlarged stomach—megalogastria. On the other hand, a stomach may be high and its motility be insufficient. This very condition is not infrequently found with gastrosuccorrhœa. We shall see later on that in these cases we have to deal with gastric ulcer. When the ulcer is situated at the lesser curvature and there are adhesions to the surrounding tissues, the stomach remains high, and in case of dilatation extends upward. In these cases I have frequently seen the fundus of a stomach almost reach the axilla in the dorsal position. When the lesser curvature is thus fixed the greater curvature may remain above the umbilical line, even in cases of pronounced dilatation with decided stagnation of the stomach contents. Hence, a high position of the greater curvature cannot be regarded as proving that in a given case no gastric dilatation is present, and, therefore, no motor disturbance.

Just as invalid is the argument that in certain cases of gastrosuccorrhœa no motor insufficiency was present because certain forms of fermentation were absent, particularly the gas fermentation. It is true that whenever there is stagnation in the stomach fermentation sets in. There are, however, various fermentations in the stomach, brought about by different organisms and leading to different fermentation products. The absence of any one form does not indicate that all fermentation is absent. By careful analysis some form of fermentation can always be demonstrated.

As for the statement that a motor insufficiency cannot be present when the stomach contents expressed in the morning do not contain food particles, it must be said that actual findings do not justify this conclusion. Reports of autopsies in such cases, where only fluid could be obtained without food particles, showed pyloric obstruction with ulceration. Also, it must be remembered how difficult it is to empty the stomach entirely when dilatation is present.

We may add that in the majority of cases this fluid actually contains food particles. If we examine the histories of typical cases, as reported by Reichmann and others, we find it especially stated that the fluid expressed from the fasting stomach contained varying amounts of food particles, principally starches, and also sarcinæ, which, beyond doubt, indicate motor insufficiency.

From the foregoing statements, therefore, we see that all arguments brought forward to explain the presence of larger quantities of gastric juice in the fasting stomach merely as a result of secretory disturbance without motor insufficiency are invalid. We must insist that the accumulation of acid fluid in the fasting stomach is always the result of motor insufficiency. This motor insufficiency may be due to atony of the stomach or to organic or spastic stenosis at its outlet.

Let us now consider the question: Is chronic gastrosuccorrhœa a disease *per se?* The fact that the presence of gastric juice in the fasting stomach always means a retention of secretion due to motor insufficiency does away with one argument often put forth in support of the theory that gastrosuccorrhœa is a primary and independent secretory disorder—the argument that the secretion of gastric juice takes place without the influence of direct irritation (stimulation by food), but purely as the result of the pathologically increased activity of the secretory nerves. For even small quantities of food particles are sufficient stimuli for the secretion of gastric juice, particularly when they lie directly on an ulcer, and when nothing but fluid is retained this stagnating fluid acts as an irritant. The more sensitive the mucous membrane the greater the quantity which it will secrete. The constant irritation of this stagnating fermenting fluid must in time increase the irritability of the mucous membrane and lead to anatomical changes.

Examinations of the mucous membranes in these cases, made at first by Korzynski and Jaworski, and later by Hayem, Hemmeter, Strauss and others, show a definite form of gastritis characterized by a destruction of the chief cells, the parietal cells remaining intact. There was often found a proliferation even up to the formation of polypi.

In opposition to the view which considers the gastritis a result of the permanent irritation by the stagnating masses, due to the motor insufficiency, some authors claim that the gastritis is the primary element of the whole process, and assert that the inflammation of the mucosa alone suffices to cause an abnormal irritability and an increased and continuous secretion of gastric juice. Even the development of gastric ulcer is attributed to this gastritis.

Granting that the gastritis plays an important part here, it seems to me that there is no reason for dwelling on the question whether the motor insufficiency or the inflammation of the mucous membrane is the primary disturbance. Both are factors in producing gastrosuccorrhœa; in some of the cases the motor insufficiency being the primary trouble, in others the gastritis.

However gastrosuccorrhœa is brought on, since we have seen that gastric juice in the fasting stomach always means a motor insufficiency, there can be no doubt that the stagnating secretion keeps up and increases the inflammation of the mucous membrane.

It is clear from the above explanation that where motor insufficiency and increased secretion go together a retention of gastric juice can take place. Such simultaneous occurrence of motor and secretory disturbance is often found during the course of various diseases of the stomach. Thus the presence of the gastric juice in the fasting stomach is a condition frequently observed in gastritis acida with atony, atony with secondary gastritis and hypersecretion, pyloric and duodenal stenosis resulting from adhesions or compressions, etc. It is obvious that in all these diseases gastrosuccorrhœa can only be considered as a symptom.

Some authors apply the term gastrosuccorrhœa to all cases where gastric juice is found in the fasting stomach. Others maintain that we ought to distinguish between the cases where the presence of gastric juice in the fasting stomach is only a symptom, and another well-defined group of cases for which they would reserve the term gastrosuccorrhœa. They claim that the presence of gastric juice in the fasting stomach does not justify a diagnosis of gastrosuccorrhœa unless the completely developed symptom-complex of Reichmann is also present. They regard this symptom-complex (Reichmann's disease) as a sharply defined, typical picture, showing, besides the characteristic presence of hydrochloric acid in the residual fluid, a number of other symptoms—pyrosis, vomiting, loss of flesh, and, most important of all, of severe pains occurring after meals and during the night.

If we now scrutinize this limited group of cases, in which the symptom-complex of Reichmann is fully developed, it must be said that even for this group no proof has yet been given that gastrosuccorrhœa occurs as a disease *per se*. In fact, whenever an operation or an autopsy has afforded an opportunity to gain an anatomical basis it has revealed ulcer or its sequelæ. Thus we see that even in these cases, which apparently are so well defined, gastrosuccorrhœa is only an accompanying symptom of a well-known disease—*i. e.*, gastric ulcer.

As long as we have no proof that gastrosuccorrhœa may occur as an independent disease we shall do well to regard it merely as a symptom. In this smaller group of cases in which the combination of symptoms given by Reichmann is completely developed and where severe gastric pain plays an important role, we shall not err if we regard it in every case as a symptom of gastric ulcer. If we look upon gastrosuccorrhœa in this light as a symptom, it becomes a valuable aid in diagnosing certain cases of gastric ulcer. Whenever we find a patient suffering from gastric pains coming on regularly after meals and especially at night, with or without vomiting, the presence of acid fluid even in small quantities in the fasting stomach indicates ulcer of the stomach. Hemorrhage and perforation, the most characteristic symptoms of ulcer, are observed only in a certain percentage of the cases. In the remaining cases gastric ulcer may present many different clinical forms, among which

Reichmann's symptom-complex stands out as a very characteristic and typical picture.

As a rule, in cases which develop gastrosuccorrhœa the ulcer is situated near the pylorus and causes a mechanical obstruction, generally by spasm of the pylorus. This spasm, which brings on severe pain, usually occurs after the greater part of the stomach contents have passed into the intestines. That frequent spasms do really occur here is proved by the finding of a strongly hypertrophie pyloric ring.

In the treatment of gastrosuccorrhœa it is of great practical importance to have clearly in mind the fact that the motor disturbance plays a more important role than the secretory, and, further, that the well-developed symptom-complex of Reichmann is not a disease *per se*, but a symptom of gastric ulcer. We accordingly treat the condition by freeing the stomach from its stagnating contents, also using methods usually resorted to in gastric ulcer. Cures by such treatment have often been reported, and my own experience is corroborative.

In cases which do not yield to methodical internal treatment for ulcer one should not hesitate to do away by operative interference with the hindrance at the pylorus, which is really the principal cause for the whole trouble. We are more apt to come to this decision when we are certain that we have to deal with ulcer and pyloric obstruction than when we regard gastrosuccorrhœa as a disease *per se*, caused simply by an increased irritation of the mucous membrane. In the literature there are descriptions and post-mortem reports of fatal cases of gastrosuccorrhœa which give one the impression that had the cases been diagnosed as ulcer with pyloric stenosis, and promptly operated upon, the patient could have been saved. In all the cases with Reichmann's symptom-complex which have come under my own observation and which were operated upon, the diagnosis of ulcer was confirmed.

I wish to describe one case in detail because it presents another interesting condition with which gastrosuccorrhœa stands in intimate relation, namely, tetanic attacks.

History. In May, 1898, the patient, aged forty-four years, stated that for the past two years he had suffered with heartburn and gastric pain of a dull and at times even intense character, occurring several hours after eating, but particularly at night. In the morning, before eating, he was troubled with a gnawing sensation in the stomach and gaseous distention; no vomiting; bowels regular. The trouble had been regarded as nervous dyspepsia and treated as such.

The patient was tall, thin, had a long thorax with healthy thoracic viscera, a flat abdomen and normal outlines for liver and stomach, the pyloric end being painful to pressure. Urine now and later throughout the whole course of the disease free from albumin and sugar and contained a moderate amount of indican.

Examination after test meal (tea and toast) showed moderate hyperacidity with impaired amylolysis. Alkalies and a suitable diet relieved the subjective symptoms for a few months, during which time patient gained six pounds. In the fall the symptoms returned with increased intensity, particularly the pains during the night.

Stomach analysis of November 19th showed strong hyperacidity. As ulcer had been suspected from the beginning, a treatment for ulcer was suggested, but again refused, as formerly. The patient did not place himself under treatment until the end of January, 1899, when the pain became so intense that it robbed him of sleep.

The first lavage (February 16th) showed a black fluid without food particles in the fasting stomach, so that there could be no more doubt as to the presence of an ulcer. From then on rest in bed. For four days nourishment exclusively by rectum—then in the morning Carlsbader Mühlbrunnen and, besides the enemata, milk per os, at first in small quantities, gradually increasing.

Since three weeks of this treatment gave but little relief from pain, and alkalies, bismuth, belladonna, codeine only relieved the patient temporarily, lavage was taken up and after the washing bismuth was introduced. The fasting stomach nearly always contained from 50 cm. to 100 cm., and occasionally more, of a strongly acid fluid, mostly stained with blood and often mixed with some remnants of food of the previous days.

The bismuth treatment alleviated the pain but little. Irrigations with silver nitrate (1:1000), which were begun two weeks later, also produced little effect. Changes in the milk diet (cooking with fine flour, peptonizing, sour milk) and a trial of thick gruels and soups gave no better results. On the contrary, during the second half of March the pain increased in intensity and duration. Since the rigidly applied internal treatment failed absolutely, operation was advised on March 24th, but had to be postponed several days for ulterior reasons.

During this time there was a decided change for the worse. Until then the quantity of fluid found in the fasting stomach had been relatively small, even when larger quantities had been ingested. During the middle of March, with the increase of pain, the amount of stagnating fluid became greater. From the 24th to the 29th signs of complete pyloric obstruction set in, with almost continual excruciating pains. Although smaller quantities of food were taken the amount drawn from the stomach increased; rapid diminution of urinary secretion, which so far had been plentiful; skin dry; emaciation more marked. Now, for the first time, a hard, painful resistance could be felt in the pyloric region.

March 25th. But little nourishment was taken; during the night, after most violent pains, for the first time there was vomiting of blood-stained fluid. In spite of the large quantity of the vomitus, and although nothing had been taken afterward, 750 cm. of fluid were withdrawn from the stomach in the morning of March 26th. During this day the patient took only 180 c.c. each of milk and Vichy. Yet in the evening, when the continual severe pain made it necessary to again introduce the stomach-tube, as much as 1100 c.c. of blood-stained fluid was obtained—that is, three times the quantity taken during the whole day. Upon standing a thin, reddish-film formed on the surface of this fluid, the remainder consisting of clear, light green liquid, with a very high percentage of hydrochloric acid.

During this last introduction of the stomach-tube violent vomiting set in, and with it appeared tonic spasms of arms and legs, both being stiffly extended, the fingers in obstetrician's position. The spasm lasted several minutes. Feeling of numbness in the extremities. Trousseau's phenomenon negative.

27th. A total of 600 c.c. of milk was ingested. In the evening a litre of sanguineous fluid of intensely acid reaction was removed. During the withdrawal of this fluid through the tube (this time without vomiting) both upper extremities became tonically extended, the fingers of the left hand were extended, those of the right in the position of a penman. The spasm relaxed slowly several minutes after the washing was finished. Lower extremities not affected this time. Trousseau's phenomenon negative.

28th. Condition improved. Pain diminished. Larger quantities of milk taken, and it passed into the intestine. Urinary secretion again reached 1000 c.c.

29th. Patient was taken to Dr. Lange's clinic. Lavage of the stomach at 11 A.M. One hour later sudden violent pain in the gastric region and symptoms of collapse. Pulse small; face pale; syncope; abdomen drawn in; liver dulness normal. All the abdominal muscles rigid as boards, several fibres standing out as sharp ridges above the level of the skin. Less pronounced cramps in the muscles of the trunk and extremities. The extremely painful tetanic contraction of all the abdominal muscles remained unchanged for hours, despite the injection of morphine and a mild anæsthesia from ether and chloroform.

Four hours after the perforation laparotomy was performed. The anterior wall of the stomach showed a flat, almost circular swelling, about 5 cm. in diameter, its firm edges extending downward to the greater curvature, and its right limit being still several centimetres removed from the pylorus. The serous covering of the swelling lay free in the peritoneal cavity, only its median edge being adherent to the omentum. Exactly in the centre of the swelling was a sharp-edged opening of the size of a pin-head; there was some turbid fluid in the neighborhood of the perforation.

A segment as broad as a hand was resected, which included the antrum pylori and the pylorus; suture of the stomach end; duodenal end joined to the posterior wall of the stomach by a Murphy button. The resected piece, cut open along the lesser curvature, showed on its inner surface an ulcer as large as a fifty-cent piece, with an uneven terraced surface, a very thin floor, and firm, undermined, wavy edges. Cut surface through this edge showed firm, white lines. Microscopically, adenocarcinoma. The pylorus thickened but patent. Microscopic examination of the pylorus showed greatly hypertrophied muscles, but no signs of carcinoma.

The healing of the wound progressed smoothly. Nourishment at first per rectum. Upon giving food by mouth recurrence of pyrosis and pain in the stomach; perhaps this can be partly accounted for by the retention of the Murphy button. These complaints, which were somewhat relieved by alkalies and washing of the stomach, manifested themselves after each meal, no matter what kind of food had been taken; and they continued to disturb the patient in the most annoying manner during the following months almost up to the time of his death.

An examination after test breakfast on May 25th again revealed considerably increased gastric secretion. Repeated examinations made after this date showed the continuance of hyperacidity for a remarkably long period, in spite of the development of metastatic tumors.

During the first few months following the operation the patient recuperated and gained in weight. In September the pyrosis and pain became worse again; all attempts to influence the secretion medicinally by means of alkalies, bismuth, atropine, etc., were fruitless.

At the end of September signs of decided stagnation set in, with intense pain and vomiting, so that stomach washings were again resorted to and continued until death, on November 19th, at first once a day, then with increasing stenosis, both in the morning and at night. Upon resuming the lavage the tendency to tetanic spasms recurred, and they were more or less pronounced until within a few weeks before death. They generally manifested themselves in extension of the fingers and hands, more rarely of the arms and legs, and lasted at times only half a minute, but occasionally several minutes.

As early as the end of May—two months after the operation—a distinct resistance could be felt at the umbilicus, and four weeks later hard masses were palpable in the abdomen to the right of and below the scar. They grew to be larger than a fist, pushing the abdominal wall forward. On September 23d, when these tumors had already gained very considerable size, the stomach contents still showed a very high percentage of hydrochloric acid. From the middle of October, however, the quantity of this acid decreased rapidly, and lactic acid appeared. From the end of October the large, fermenting residual masses smelt foul, almost fecal.

EPITOME. We have to deal here with a case of gastric ulcer which became carcinomatous in a comparatively short time. To be sure, the duration of the ulcer cannot be accurately determined. The symptoms of which the patient complained for several years had been regarded by competent physicians as manifestations of nervous dyspepsia. Cases of gastric ulcer which are diagnosed as nervous dyspepsia are by no means rare, and here we have another instance of it. But here, as in many other cases, it was the persistency of the pain that aroused the suspicion of the ulcer, which suspicion proved perfectly justifiable when lavage of the stomach showed sanguineous contents. Yet this ulcer had certainly existed some time before this proof was obtained, and had already involved the deeper layers of the stomach, for the operation, performed only six weeks later, showed an ulcer involving the whole thickness of the gastric wall, with firm, undermined edges, which had already undergone carcinomatous degeneration.

On looking back over the history of the case, therefore, we will not err if we presume that all the symptoms which the patient showed during the last three years of his life, including those taken for nervous dyspepsia, were caused by this ulcer, since during all that time the pains varied only in intensity, their character remaining the same throughout.

At the operation we found that the ulcer was situated several centimetres from the pylorus; the pylorus itself was patent and free from carcinoma, but showed greatly hypertrophied muscles.

This hypertrophy can be explained as a result of the frequent spasms which evidenced themselves clinically by the severe pains. The spasms occurred particularly during the night. For how long a period they had caused stagnation of the gastric juice, with or without food remains, cannot be determined, since for a long time the patient refused lavage. When we commenced to evacuate the stomach regularly in the morning the patient had already been in bed for weeks, living exclusively on a milk diet. In spite of these favorable circumstances, there were nearly always found in the fasting stomach quantities varying from 50 c.c. to 100 c.c. of very acid fluid, often containing food particles. Later the residual fluid became greater when the increase of pains in duration and intensity indicated longer spasms, and shortly before the perforation took place there set in under almost unceasing pains long-continued spasms, which caused extended periods of pyloric obstruction. It was this protracted period of pylorospasm which brought about the retention of the large quantities of excessively secreted gastric juice.

When cases like the one just described are considered without prejudice there can be no doubt that the main cause for the accumulation of such large quantities of gastric juice is given in the spastic stenosis which prevents the passage of the secretion into the bowels.

The more severe and the longer the duration of the spasm the larger the amount of fluid.

Tetanic Attacks. When the spastic stenosis in our case became more pronounced and large quantities of stagnating gastric juice were vomited or removed through the tube, tetanic attacks set in. These recurred in a milder form several months after the operation, when the increasing stenosis at the outlet of the stomach again required lavage. We find the same conditions in nearly all the cases of gastric ulcer with pyloric stenosis in which tetany develops: there is always the evacuation of large quantities of gastric juice, either by vomiting or through the tube. This points to the possibility that the withdrawal of such large quantities of chlorine which are not replaced causes certain changes in the system predisposing to the occurrence of tetanic attacks. We shall discuss this point later on.

In our case, as in many others, it was the lavage which furnished the direct irritation which reflexly brought on the spasm. Remarkable, however, is the severe and long-continued tetanic contraction of the abdominal muscles in connection with the perforation. Contraction of the abdominal muscles is, indeed, a well-known symptom of perforation into the abdominal cavity. In this case, however, where a strong tendency to spasm, perhaps due to the deficiency in chlorine, already existed, the perforation was the exciting cause for an extremely severe tetanic contraction of the entire abdominal wall.

It was Kussmaul who, in his famous article on the treatment of gastric dilatation by means of the stomach-pump, first described the occurrence of muscular spasm with pyloric stenosis. In some of these cases we have to deal with true tetany, which, as is well known, is characterized by increased mechanical and electrical irritability of the nerves and muscles. Other cases only resemble tetany, or else are epileptiform convulsions with loss of consciousness. The cases described by Kussmaul were pyloric stenoses, in which the frequent vomiting of large quantities of fluid led to a high degree of emaciation and decrease in the quantity of urine. He attributed the convulsions to the diminution of water in the organism, which was brought about by the vomiting of such large quantities of fluid and which led, as he reasoned, to the drying out of the nerves and muscles. This theory was not considered entirely satisfactory. It was claimed that there are other diseases of the gastro-intestinal tract in which an abundance of water is lost without the advent of tetany, and that in cases of tetany the introduction of water into the rectum did not prevent the attacks. Other explanations were, therefore, looked for.

Germain Sée believed that the convulsions were caused reflexly by the irritated nerves of the gastric mucosa. This so-called "reflex theory" explains only how the convulsions are brought on, without mentioning the predisposing element. We must remember, however, that the exciting cause, which may be of various characters, is only a secondary element; in order to bring on a tetanic attack a change in the irritability of the nervous system is required and is really the underlying cause of the whole trouble.

This predisposing element finds more consideration in a third hypothesis, which, thoroughly in accord with modern teaching, attributes the origin of the attacks to autointoxication. This theory is mainly advanced by French authorities, who assume that decomposition-products are formed in the stagnating stomach contents, which, when absorbed, act deleteriously upon the nervous system, and in this way lead to attacks.

However, in spite of diligent research, no one has yet been able to demonstrate such poisons, and Friedrich Müller, a supporter of the reflex theory, points out very correctly that tetany appears, not in cases where the fermenting stomach contents are finally absorbed, but only in those in which the stagnating masses are removed from the system either by vomiting or lavage.

Since the removal of great quantities of fluid from the body is actually the only objective finding which is regularly observed in these cases, it remains, after all, the most important point, and if properly interpreted, gives us a better insight into the origin of tetanic attacks than the purely hypothetical autointoxication theory.

Thus, going back to Kussmaul's first explanation, we must say, as this keen observer rightly maintained, that the great loss of fluid by vomiting or lavage brings about the changes in the system which cause the tetanic attacks. We would add, however, that these discharges deprive the system not only of large quantities of fluid, but also of large amounts of chlorides. For in these cases of gastric dilatation complicated with tetany we often find enormously increased gastric secretion. Since, as we have seen in the beginning, the pyloric stenosis prevents the excessively secreted gastric juice from passing into the intestine, it is removed by vomiting or lavage, and thus great quantities of hydrochloric acid become lost from the system instead of being again resorbed.

Bouveret and Devic claim that gastric tetany is observed exclusively in such cases of pyloric stenosis as are accompanied by excessive hypersecretion. This is not absolutely true. Though the instances are very rare, Fleiner, for example, reports cases in which no increase of gastric secretion was found. We will not investigate now the cause of tetany in these particular cases. Suffice it to say that in gastric tetany, as is the case with other spasms, different factors may contribute to the development of the attacks. In the majority of cases, however, it is a fact that large quantities of chlorine are lost from the body by the removal of the excessively secreted gastric juice. This is proved by the fact that in these cases the secretion of chlorine through the urine steadily diminishes, and finally ceases altogether.

To be sure, the disappearance of chlorides from the urine here is not an absolute indicator of the quantities really lost from the body. The organism holds on to its chlorine obstinately. When we limit the supply of chlorine by cutting it out of the food the quantity excreted in the urine becomes less, and finally disappears altogether. At the same time the secretion of hydrochloric acid with the gastric juice will stop, as was shown by A. Cahn in his experiments on dogs. The organism saves its chlorine by checking its secretion. In spite of the diminished secretion, there may still be a great deal left in the system. In gastrosuccorrhœa, however, the conditions are altogether different. Through the constant irritation to the mucosa here, causing the excessive secretion of gastric juice, large quantities of chlorine are constantly withdrawn from the blood, and since they are removed from the body by vomiting or lavage, reabsorption is prevented, so that the body suffers an actual loss of chlorine. At the same time these patients do not take the proper amount of food, and, therefore, not the proper amount of chlorine to make up for the loss. In other words, there is increased excretion of chlorine, and the amount ingested is decreased—a unique pathological condition which must lead to an impoverishment of chlorides in the system. We may well assume that this diminution of chlorine plays some part in the development of tetany.

In looking through the literature I find that Korszynski and Jaworski as early as 1891 already regarded the decrease of chlorine in the tissues as the probable cause of gastric tetany. It is remarkable that this view can nowhere be found quoted in the text-books, in the special articles on gastric tetany by Fleiner, Albu, and others, or in Frankl-Hochwart's monograph "On Tetany," in Nothnagel's series. Yet their theory is of great assistance for the treatment of that peculiar and dangerous condition.

Korszynski and Jaworski, following their theory, recommended the injection of large quantities of normal salt solution, subcutaneously or by rectum, in order to overcome the chlorine starvation in cases of gastric tetany.

Tetanic attacks are of serious import, and often lead quickly to a fatal issue. In the latest summary by Albu of these cases, forty in all, there were thirty-one deaths—*i. e.*, 77½ per cent. mortality. Their presence influences unfavorably the prognosis of an operation, and no operation should be undertaken in these cases before infusing large quantities of salt solution. This was done in our case before and after the operation, and it probably helped to bring about the favorable result, despite the presence of a perforation. To be sure, there were two other factors which favored the case: first, that the operation was performed only a few hours after the perforation; and, again, that the stomach had been washed shortly before the perforation occurred, thus preventing gastric contents from getting into the peritoneal cavity.

Albu claims that therapy offers no remedy which can either check or prevent a recurrence of the tetanic attacks. But, perhaps, as has been said before, it may be possible to end the attack by means of salt infusions. A recurrence can only be prevented by removing the cause. Their cause is, as we have seen above, motor insufficiency and the spastic or organic pyloric stenosis which hinders the passage of the more abundantly secreted hydrochloric acid into the intestines, thus preventing its reabsorption and depriving the system of large amounts of chlorine. In order to remove the cause the treatment should therefore be directed, first of all, against the motor disturbance. Whenever it is impossible to correct the motor insufficiency by internal means, it should be overcome by operation, either by pyloroplasty, gastroenterostomy, or resection, as the individual case may require. That is the rational treatment for gastrosuccorrhœa, as well as for tetany.

CHRONIC GASTRITIS DUE TO ALCOHOL.

By Nellis B. Foster, M.D.,
NEW YORK HOSPITAL.

In the large cities we are accustomed to see numerous cases of gastric disorders which can be traced directly to excessive and habitual use of alcoholic beverages. These maladies are very common in the low orders of society which make up the mass of hospital patients, and it was from this prominence of these affections that we became interested in them. It is, of course, well recognized that alcohol can produce a chronic gastritis, but the clinical differences of gastritis due to alcohol from gastritis of other causes is not at present so clear. At present we are concerned only with the secretory disturbances of the gastritis of alcohol. The methods of work were those ordinarily used in the routine examination of gastric contents, Ewald's test-breakfast of bread and unsweetened tea being given in the morning and expressed thirty minutes or an hour later. Free HCl was estimated by titration with $\frac{n}{10}$ NaOH, using dimethylamidoazobenzol and Günzborge reagent as an indicator, and phenolphthalein as an indicator in estimating the total acidity. Lactic acid was always tested for, as were the gastric enzymes.

The cases seen divide themselves into two classes: those presenting symptoms of gastritis and those without such symptoms. Of the first class but little need be said. The symptoms are familiar: nausea, with retching, on rising in the morning, and the vomiting, perhaps, of some mucus. These symptoms pass away after a couple of "drinks" to settle his stomach; then he is able to eat his breakfast, and is free from discomfort until the next morning. The gastric motility in these cases is considerably accelerated. The test-meal must usually be removed after forty-five minutes, at longest, in order to recover sufficient material for analysis. There is much mucus present, both free and mixed with food. Free HCl is usually absent. Total acids are low. Pepsin and rennin normal. The following case may be given as typical:

CASE XXI.—Man, aged thirty-four years; clerk. Family history and past history unimportant. Habits: drinks considerable whiskey; always a glass before breakfast. For last month or two the patient thinks he has averaged about one quart of whiskey per diem.

Present Illness. Has felt run down for some time, but with no special symptoms, however, except morning vomiting for several weeks. Ankles swell slightly, and is puffy under the eyes in the morning. No pulmonary, cardiac, or urinary symptoms.

Physical Examination. Normal, except for slight swelling of ankles. Urine: specific gravity 1024; no albumin or sugar; no casts.

Gastric Analysis. Ewald test-breakfast. Free HCl, 0; total acidity, 22; no lactic acid; enzymes present. Second analysis two days later shows same results.

The second class of these cases, those presenting no gastric symptoms, is of greater significance. The cases observed by the writer entered the hospital because of some malady other than gastric affections, and were recognized as possible cases of alcoholic gastritis on account of their habits or on account of the general alcoholic appearance. It was only after studying a number of the cases of chronic gastritis with pronounced symptoms that our curiosity was aroused concerning the gastric condition of those individuals who habitually use large amounts of alcoholic beverages, yet present no symptoms pointing to gastric disturbances. Hoping to obtain some light on this point, it has been our custom to make the routine gastric analysis on all of those cases that came into the hospital for any cause and whose appearance or history pointed to overindulgence in alcohol. The number of cases seen is now sufficiently large to permit of fairly accurate deductions. In contrast to the first class of cases there is no hyperkinesis, nor is there usually a great excess of mucus. The acid secretion being wherein morbidity is displayed, free HCl is always low, often absent, and in no case over 15. The average for our series is 5. The total acids are lowered, but not below the low normal limit. In other respects the gastric functions appear normal. The interest in these cases is mostly scientific, but there is, however, a practical application, namely, that one must be guarded in placing stress on the absence of free HCl in the diagnosis of stomach diseases unless free indulgence in alcohol can be excluded. The diagnosis of carcinoma of the stomach in the early stages is based upon a number of small data, the most significant of which is, perhaps, the continued absence of free HCl. The point to which the writer wishes to call attention is that in these cases of possible carcinoma without definite signs or symptoms a history of alcoholic habits casts great doubt on that diagnosis. A case of the kind may be cited:

G. W., male, aged forty-eight years, entered the hospital complaining of weakness, loss in weight, and indefinite and occasional distress in the epigastrium. History and physical examination pointed to no organic disease. Blood count, normal. Gastric analysis showed absence of free HCl (three analyses). No diagnosis could be made, and an exploratory operation was done, which disclosed a small tumor in the tail of the pancreas (possibly carcinoma); the stomach appeared normal. There appearing no cause for the absence of free HCl in the gastric analyses, the man was later questioned concerning his habits. He had always drunk two glasses of whiskey before breakfast, he stated, and occasionally a glass during the day.

Riegel, Ewald, and other observers have pointed out the relation of alcohol to chronic gastritis; we are able to find no references, however, to indicate that there is recognized a change in gastric secretion due to alcohol previous to the excitation of subjective symptoms. Such a change as we have described is not accurately a gastritis chronica because, while there is slight increase in the mucous secretion, it is not marked nor constant enough to bring the syndrome under that head. It is, however, the precursor of that condition; and its interest in differential diagnosis, we hope, will lead some one to confirm our results.

A DIFFERENTIAL STAINING OF THE BLOOD WITH SIMPLE SOLUTIONS.

By William Page Harlow, M.D.,
of Boulder, Colorado.

For the past year and a half the writer has been practically in daily use of some one of the methyl-alcohol-eosin-methylene-blue blood stains (Jenner, May, Grünwald and Wright's), and has experienced trouble at different times in obtaining a methyl alcohol that would, with one of the above powders, give results as satisfactory as with previous batches. Neither are the ready-for-use fluids furnished by the chemists uniform and always satisfactory in result. He believes this experience to be a common one with hæmatologists and physicians who are doing any considerable amount of blood work. Therefore, it seems permissible to call attention to a method giving a color picture similar to and recommended over the above because of:

1. The simple and less expensive solutions employed.
2. The easy technique and rapidity of staining.
3. The more uniform results obtained with stains and alcohols furnished from different manufactories and at different times.[1]

The solutions used are:

No. I. Eosin, 1 gram, in absolute methyl alcohol, 100 c.c.

No. II. Methylene blue, 1 gram; in absolute methyl alcohol, 100 c.c.

The procedure is:

1. A fresh-spread cover-glass (or slide) taken in the usual manner.
2. Dried in air only.
3. Preparation, held in self-closing cover-glass forceps, covered with as much eosin as it will readily hold without draining, allowing same to remain one minute.
4. Eosin rapidly decanted (shake off the surplus). Do not wash the spread in water, and do not allow it to become dry by evaporation.
5. The eosin moist specimen quickly covered with the methylene-blue solution, allowing to stand about one and one-quarter minutes (different blues require a few seconds more or less than this).[2]
6. Wash gently in ordinary pure water (best to wash or dip spread in a glass of water, rather than in a strongly running stream from tap).
7. Dry between layers of filter-paper and mount in balsam.[3]

The microscopic differential color picture shown by this method with the blood spread is as follows:

The Red Cells.

The hæmoglobin-holding cells, when normal, are a deep red, clean and evenly stained.

[1] The greater part of the work done by the writer was with Grübler's Pure French Eosin, the "B" Patent Methylene Blue, med. pur., and an absolute methyl Alcohol made by C. F. Kahlbaum, Berlin. Though recent experiments with other foreign-made stains, and an Eosin and a Methylene Blue furnished by Bausch & Lomb, and absolute Methyl alcohols furnished by Merck & Co., Eberbach & Son, Ann Arbor; E. H. Sargent & Co., Chicago, and Hynson & Westcott, Baltimore, have given quite uniform and very satisfactory results.

[2] It should be noted when the red blood cells are stained bluish that it is because of an understaining with the methylene blue, and that the eosin which is more or less loosely combined with the oxyphilic substances has not had sufficient time to neutralize the action of the methylene blue which has been added in excess. This variation in the time for counter-staining with the methylene blue has been found to be between one and one-quarter and two minutes in all the combinations that I have tried.

[3] Spreads dried in air may be kept unfixed, back to back, between folds of filter-paper for several months, and still give quite satisfactory staining results. A recent staining and examination of one-year-old unfixed spreads of malaria, leukæmia, and pernicious anæmia showed that the hæmoglobin-containing cell stained practically as well as when fresh—*i. e.*, anæmia, and all grades of polychromasia, nuclei, and the punctate basophilic granules of Grawitz are shown, as well as the malarial plasmodium. But in the colorless corpuscles the granules are not well differentiated, the nuclei, and basophilic substances only, being well brought out.

In the chloroses they are somewhat paler and show light to clear central areas.

In pernicious and other severe secondary anæmias, all grades of polychromatophilia, from terra-cotta, yellowish-brown, and greenish-yellow to a cloudy blue or purple are shown.

Small basophilic granulations are sharply brought out, being blue to deep purple in color, and found in cells the cytoplasm of which may show any grade of polychromatophilia.

The nuclei are deep blue, and, in the larger forms especially, the chromatin threads are clearly brought out.

The plaques, both in and out of the cells, are stained a lavender to dirty purple (but for the better study of the plaques, the simple staining of the unfixed spread for fifteen to thirty seconds with the methylene-blue solution alone is recommended. This is also good for all basophilic substances).

In the malarial plasmodium the cytoplasm is stained a bright light blue; the chromatin a deeper blue to purple; the segment walls are nicely shown, and the pigment appears as black dots or ovals.[1]

The Leukocytes.

Of the colorless polymorphonuclear granulated corpuscles, the neutrophiles generally show three or more quite dark-blue nuclei. The cytoplasm, taking a reddish tinge, is thickly studded with small violet to reddish granules, the whole apparently closely limited, as though by a cell membrane.

The oxyphiles, in a thickly spread blood specimen, are smaller than the neutrophiles, but in a thinly spread film usually appear larger than the neutrophiles. The nuclei, when there are three or more, as is often the case, are of the size and shape and stain the same as the nuclei in the neutrophiles, but more frequently there are two nuclei, oval or biscuit shaped, lying well apart in the cell, which are larger and stain a paler blue than the neutrophiles. The cytoplasm has a red tinge, if any, and is more or less loosely studded with large, glistening, rose-red granules that do not seem to be closely restrained, some often overlying the nuclei, others being entirely without the normal limits of the cell (the so-called "explosive" action after the drawing of the blood).

The basophiles generally are a little smaller than the neutrophiles, but vary in size to as large as the oxyphiles. The nuclei are often hard to differentiate from the cytoplasm, both being stained a pale blue. In some cases the nuclei are stained a deeper blue than the cytoplasm, are irregular in shape, and often eccentrically placed. But the coarse, spherical granules, varying in size from that of a

[1] The addition of one-half per cent. of sodium carbonate or lithium bicarbonate to the methylene-blue solution will give a better stain for the malarial plasmodium, but other structures are stained a little more blue than with the simple solution.

neutrophile granule to as large as fat-droplets, some staining a deep blue to purple or almost black, are distinctive.

The mononuclear granulated corpuscles or myelocytes stain about the same as the polymorphonuclear cells, having the same kind of granules. The nucleus is generally at one side and is round or oval, often showing two or more clear dots; and sometimes a fine reticular chromatin may be noted.

The neutrophilic myelocyte is the largest of this class. Its nucleus is large, often taking up more than half the cell, and is generally eccentrically placed. The cytoplasm is closely filled with violet-stained relatively small granules.

The oxyphilic myelocyte is a little smaller than the neutrophile. Its nucleus is stained a paler blue and generally shows little or no structure. The cytoplasm is of a reddish tinge, and the granules filling the same, sometimes partly overlying the nucleus, are large and quite uniform in size, and stain a glistening rose-red.

There appear to be two forms of the mononuclear cell, containing basophilic granules, though both may be of bone-marrow origin, and one an earlier form of the other.

The basophilic myelocyte (undoubtedly properly so classified because it is a mononuclear cell with basophilic granules, and can be demonstrated in normal and pathological bone-marrow) is a little larger than a polymorphonuclear neutrophile. It has a deep-blue staining nucleus located a little to one side of the centre. The cytoplasm is stained a lighter blue and is fairly well filled with basophilic granules about the size of the neutrophilic granules; these are stained a deep but real blue.

The other form, the origin of which has been attributed to the tissues and spleen, and classified as a mast-cell, is round or more often oval in shape, varying greatly in size—*i. e.*, from being but little larger than a red blood cell to as large as a neutrophilic myelocyte. The nucleus and cytoplasm are stained a pale blue and sometimes cannot be differentiated; others of these cells, however, will show a well-defined and cloudy to deep-blue staining, oval or lobulated nucleus. The cytoplasm is stained a pale, clear blue, and studded with deep blue to royal purple granules which differ somewhat in size and shape, but most of which are large and coarse, and oval, triangular, or cuboid in form.

The Non-granular Mononuclear Corpuscles.

The small lymphocyte is about the size of a red blood cell and stains in at least three different ways, under apparently normal conditions, and in the same specimen.

With this staining method, in one form, we see a small, nearly round cell with a relatively large pale-blue staining nucleus which may show two or more pseudonucleoli and a small amount of chromatin. The nucleus is apparently nearly surrounded by a crescent of cytoplasm which exhibits a band of reddish staining cytoplasm next to the nucleus, then outward from this a pale-blue shading to a dark-blue periphery, or the dark blue contiguous to the red.

In a second form this surrounding cytoplasm seems curled or pressed up around the nucleus, and we see a pale-blue nucleus surrounded by a very narrow band of deep-staining cytoplasm.

In the third form the cytoplasm seems to almost or entirely surround and cover the nucleus, and we get the same-sized cell, dark-blue staining, with nucleus usually not apparent; but often nodal thickenings of the cytoplasm give the appearance of granules.

In some cases of lymphatic leukæmia, where there is a great proliferation of these small lymphocytes, we may see a majority of the cells with the nucleus staining a hazy blue and the cytoplasm tinged with blue, or nearly clear.

The large lymphocytes are the size of or larger than a polymorphonuclear neutrophile. They have a larger nucleus and an absolutely and relatively larger amount of cytoplasm; otherwise the description of the first form of small lymphocyte will suffice, and in general they may be classed together.

The large mononuclears and transition forms may be considered together. They have a structureless light-blue staining nucleus, round or more often oval or indented (as kidney shaped), and with a relatively large amount of cytoplasm, which often is not stained and is barely discernible. In this there may be vacuoles and nodal thickenings, but no granules.

In a series of specimens lately examined, a number of cells that, with other staining methods, would have been classified as "large mononuclear" or "transition forms," showed the double coloring of the cytoplasm, and it seems quite probable that they are merely other forms in the chain of the lymphocytes.

There remain to be noted a group of mononuclear cells, product of the bone-marrow, and being either by-products (dying) or young cells intermediary in stage between basic cells and the corpuscles of peripheral blood. These have been noted as marrow cells (mark-zellen), stem cells (stamm-zellen), an earlier form of the mark-zellen and stimulation or irritation forms (Reizungsformen). These can be well classified together under the head of marrow cells. These are round cells about the size of the polymorphonuclear neutrophile. They all react to basic dyes only. In the young forms a nucleus is not noted, but we see a round cell staining quite deeply blue, being darker at the periphery. In this cell is a rough protoplasm having a "ground-glass" appearance, often two or more nucleoli or areas appearing vacuolated; and perhaps some granuloid areas due to thickened cytoplasm. In later stages a nucleus staining a little deeper blue than the surrounding cytoplasm is seen, otherwise with the same appearance as in the first stage.

In still later stages the cytoplasm may begin to take on a violet or reddish hue, and granules begin to appear, when we must class the cell as a myelocyte. All grades between the diffuse-looking stamm-zellen and the fully granulated myelocyte may be noted.

ON THE MECHANISM OF THE CONTRACTION OF VOLUNTARY MUSCLE OF THE FROG.

By Edward B. Meigs,
of Philadelphia.

As a first step in the search for a mechanical explanation of muscular contractility, it is necessary to have a definite idea of the change of form which takes place in a muscle fibre when it contracts. For various reasons I have used frog's voluntary muscle in nearly all of my experiments. It is well known that when a fresh frog's muscle is placed in distilled water it goes into a state

Fig. 1.

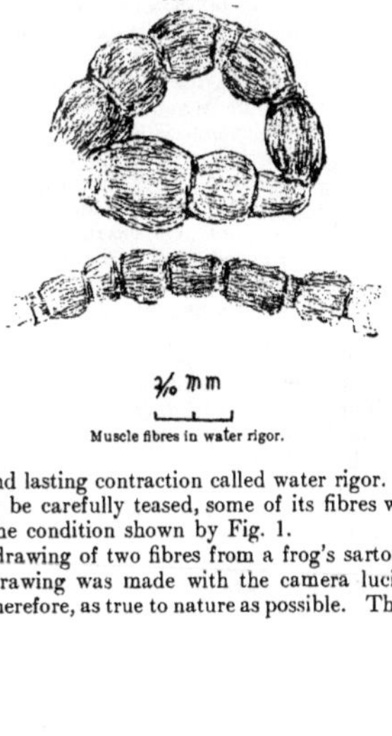

Muscle fibres in water rigor.

of complete and lasting contraction called water rigor. If a muscle in water rigor be carefully teased, some of its fibres will generally be found in the condition shown by Fig. 1.

Fig. 1 is a drawing of two fibres from a frog's sartorius in water rigor. The drawing was made with the camera lucida, and the outlines are, therefore, as true to nature as possible. The upper fibre has been bent almost into a circle by the teasing, while the lower one is nearly straight. The specimen from which Fig. 1 was drawn was prepared as follows: The sartorius was dissected from the thigh of a freshly killed frog and placed in distilled water for about ten minutes. It was then carefully teased in a little water on a glass slide, the excess of water was removed, and a drop of glycerin applied. The preparation was then covered with a cover-glass, which was cemented to the slide with asphalt. The teased fibres were examined under the microscope in water before the glycerin was applied, and they were then seen to present the same appearance as in the drawing, except that the distended portions of the lower one were as symmetrically globular as those of the upper one in the drawing. I do not know why the glycerin caused the irregularity of outline of the lower fibre without affecting the upper one.

I have treated a number of muscles in the manner described and I have almost always been able to obtain some fibres from each muscle in the beaded condition illustrated; but in no case have I found more than a small proportion of the fibres of a muscle in this state. The following, however, will show that the beaded is the true form of contracted muscle.

It is universally acknowledged that the contraction of muscle under electrical stimulation is the same as the normal contraction, and, therefore, if fibres can be shown to take the form of Fig. 1 when they contract under electrical stimulation, it must be admitted that the beaded form is the normal state of contracted muscle. It is not easy to observe beneath the microscope the change of form which frog's muscle fibres undergo during contraction due to electrical stimulation. If the muscle is large enough to be dissected out without damage, it is too large to allow its fibres to be seen clearly through the microscope. On the other hand, the least roughness in handling a small muscle destroys the irritability of all or of nearly all of its fibres. Besides this, the change from the uncontracted to the contracted form is so rapid that it throws the fibres under observation out of focus, and the contraction lasts at most only a few seconds, affording little time to get them in focus again.

I have found the sartorius to be the best muscle for this experiment. It is thin and flat and its fibres are parallel. If this muscle be carefully dissected from the thigh of a small frog and laid across the electrodes so that it can be observed through the microscope, the straight outlines of the fibres and the cross-striations can be distinctly seen. If now the tetanizing current be applied, the fibres will probably fly out of focus. But if they are quickly brought back into focus, it will be seen that their outlines are no longer straight, but that they have taken the beaded form.

After a muscle lying on a pair of electrodes with its ends unattached has been thrown into tetanus, it never again completely relaxes, but remains shorter and wider. This can be distinctly seen if the muscle be watched with the naked eye, and the fact is a great help in the observation of contraction. For, after the first application of the tetanizing current, the fibres, being already partially contracted, move to a much less extent with each subsequent application, and remain in focus, provided the objective used be of reasonably low power. If the tetanizing current be weak, and if it be applied for only short periods, the fibres may be seen with the microscope to contract and relax again and again, and the beading of the fibres can be seen to increase when the current is applied, and to diminish when it is removed. Of course, this beading of the fibres under electrical stimulation can only be seen at the cost of a good deal of care and trouble. I have again and again been disappointed by finding that the irritability of the fibres under observation has been completely lost; but I have repeatedly observed the increase and diminution of the beading on application and removal of the tetanizing current, and I have never seen a mere broadening of the fibres on application of the current and a narrowing on its removal.

It must be said, in passing, that the constrictions and bulgings of the contracted fibres cannot be regarded as "waves of contraction." As the bulgings do not entirely disappear on removal of the tetanizing current, it can easily be seen that they always occur at the same points. This seems to show that they are caused by definite structural peculiarities of the fibre. Moreover, the bulgings remain stationary during the flow of the current. It is impossible to conceive a stationary wave of any sort, and equally impossible to believe that "waves of contraction" could be present during tetanus, which is a state of complete contraction throughout the length of a muscle fibre.

It is, of course, difficult to observe the finer peculiarities of muscle fibres in tetanus. A whole muscle is an unsatisfactory object for microscopic examination, and the tetanus can last but a few seconds at most. As far as I have been able to discover, however, the appearance of fibres in tetanus is similar to that of the beaded fibres illustrated by Fig. 1. The important points of similarity are the disappearance of the cross-striæ and the great distance between the contiguous constrictions. The portion of a muscle fibre between two contiguous constrictions evidently contains many cross-striations, for the distance between two contiguous striæ is not more than a tenth of the diameter of the muscle fibre, whereas the distance between two constrictions is nearly equal to the diameter of the contracted fibre at its widest part.

It may be that observations similar to mine have been already recorded, but I have examined a good deal of the literature of the subject and have not been able to find any reference to the fact that frog's voluntary muscle fibres take the beaded form when they contract. Ranvier,[1] however, mentions the fact that the fibrils of insects' wing muscles often present the beaded appearance. But whether the facts have been recorded or not, they demand more consideration than they have hitherto received.

I shall now give what seems to me the most probable explanation of contraction. It is based partly on the observations recorded above, but the correctness of the observations is not affected by the probability or improbability of the explanation. I shall begin by showing that if the muscle fibre be assumed to have a certain mechanical

FIG. 2.

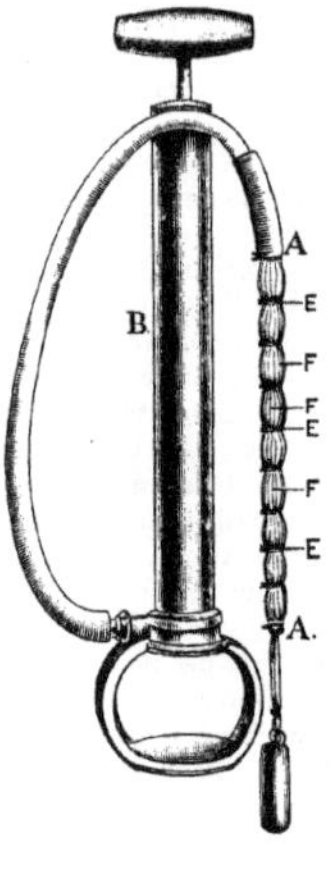

Fibre model.

FIG. 3.

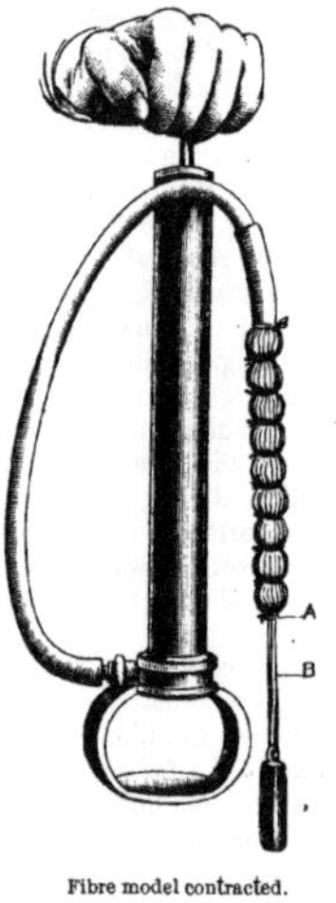

Fibre model contracted.

structure, the phenomena of water rigor may be explained on perfectly well-known mechanical and physical principles. I can best describe the structure by exhibiting drawings of a model.

Fig. 2 represents a model supposed to have the structure of a muscle fibre. *A A* is a tube of thin rubber, encircled at intervals by wire rings, *E E E*. Along the tube run inelastic cotton threads, *F F F*, each of which is attached to all of the wire rings. *B* is an

[1] Leçons d'anatomie générale sur le système musculaire.

air-pump, by which air can be forced into the tube *A A*. When this is done the model takes the form shown by Fig. 3. Each of the divisions of the tube between the wire rings tends to become spherical, the cotton threads are thrown into curves, and, as they are nearly inelastic, the whole structure necessarily shortens. The illustrations are reproduced from photographs of the model taken at equal distances from it, so that the relative dimensions are preserved; the distance between the lines *A* and *B* (Fig. 3) represents the amount of the shortening.

It will be necessary now to return a step and consider what are the most obvious changes that take place when a fresh frog's muscle is placed in distilled water. These changes may be summed up as follows: The muscle absorbs water, it contracts, and its fibres change from the cylindrical to the beaded form. It may be proved that the muscle absorbs water by weighing it before placing it in the water and afterward. It will be found to be heavier afterward. The contraction of the muscle is remarkable in several ways. It is very slow, for about fifteen minutes elapse before it is complete; it is almost exactly equal to the greatest contraction that can be obtained with the tetanizing current; and once complete it lasts indefinitely.

The absorption of water by the muscle may be explained by the laws of osmosis. The shortening of the fibres and their change of form are immediately explained if they are supposed to have a structure mechanically equivalent to that of the model. For if they had this structure, the water passing into them by the osmotic process would compel them to change from the uncontracted cylindrical form to the contracted beaded form, exactly as air forced into the model compels it to change from the form shown by Fig. 2 to the form shown by Fig. 3. When the osmotic process is complete there is no tendency for it to reverse itself, and the muscle therefore remains contracted for an indefinite time.

There is one mechanical fact which greatly strengthens the argument. It is a necessary part of the construction of the model that the distance between the wire rings should bear the same relation to the diameter of the tube as shown by Fig. 2. Suppose that all of the wire rings except those at the top and at the bottom of the tube were removed, and that the threads and the rest of the machine were left as before, a much greater amount of air would then have to be forced into the tube before the curvature of the threads and consequent shortening of the model was as great as in Fig. 2; for the whole tube would tend to take the form of a sphere, and before it could assume this shape the rubber at the middle would have to stretch enormously, and the diameter at that point would be very great. On the other hand, practically no shortening can be produced in a machine with its rings much nearer together than those of the model (Figs. 2 and 3). It is a striking coincidence that the constrictions of the fibres in Fig. 1, the constrictions of frog's fibres in electrical tetanus, and those of the fibrils of insects' wing muscles are all at just such distances that the greatest amount of shortening can be obtained with the least expansion in volume and with the least stretching of the fibre sheath.

The four preceding paragraphs may be summed up as follows: All of the phenomena of water rigor may be explained on perfectly well-known mechanical and physical principles, if it be assumed that the muscle fibre has the same structure as the model shown by Figs. 2 and 3. It is known that water passes into the fibres by osmosis while the muscle is going into water rigor, and if the fibres have the structure in question, this passage of water into them is sufficient to cause both the change of form and the shortening. As the phenomena of water rigor can be explained by so simple an assumption, I have thought it justifiable to make the assumption.

The fact that so few of the fibres of a muscle in water rigor can be found in the beaded condition is, of course, a strong counter-argument, but it must be remembered that distilled water is a reagent extremely destructive to muscular tissue. If the antenna of a living fresh-water snail be cut off near its base it will immediately contract. If it be then examined under the microscope in a little water, constrictions and bulgings are seen, not unlike those of the contracted muscle fibres. After a quarter of an hour the constrictions become much shallower and fainter, although the total length of the organ remains unchanged; and after half an hour or an hour they completely disappear. It seems quite possible that the constrictions of the muscle fibres are acted upon by the water in the same way as those of the snail's antenna. When it is added that fibres in electrical tetanus invariably present the beaded appearance, the fact that many fibres from muscles in water rigor do not present that appearance becomes insignificant.

If my explanation of water rigor is correct, it suggests very important conclusions. The structure which I have attributed to the muscle fibre is a highly specialized one, and it is apparently designed for the purpose of producing contraction. Besides this, it evidently acts when a muscle is thrown into tetanus by the electrical current, for fibres in tetanus exhibit the beaded form. The conclusion is inevitable that the structure in question is part of the mechanism of contraction.

To produce contraction in a structure like the model, it is necessary to increase the volume of the contents. There are only two ways in which this increase could be accomplished in muscle fibres. Either the contents of the fibres might expand or fluid might pass into the fibres from without. If contraction were caused by an expansion of the contents of the muscle fibres, it would necessarily be accompanied by an increase in the volume of the muscle. But it is known that the volume of a muscle does not increase during contraction, and it cannot, therefore, be supposed that contraction is due to the expansion of the contents of the muscle fibres. If, therefore, the muscle fibre contracts in the same manner as the model, it is necessary to suppose that its contraction is caused by the passage of fluid into it from without.

It is thus seen that a consideration of the phenomena of water rigor and of the change of form which frog's muscle fibres undergo during contraction leads to the conclusions that the fibres have a certain mechanical structure which causes them to contract when the volume of their contents is increased, and that the ordinary contraction of muscle is caused by the passage of fluid from the spaces between the fibres into the fibres. (For convenience, I shall hereafter call the spaces between the fibres the interfibrous spaces.) It may be asked whether this conclusion in any way helps to explain muscular contraction. I believe that it does, for the passage of fluid from one part of an organ to another is a process which is quite likely to be explained on the principles of inorganic chemistry. There are several analogous processes, such as diffusion and osmosis. And besides this, the passage of fluid from one part of an organism to another is probably the most widely distributed and elementary process in the organic world. Plants universally receive their nourishment and grow by this process; it may be observed in the amœba during the extrusion of a pseudopod; and in the higher animals it takes place in the digestive tract, in the vascular system, in the kidneys, and in all of the glands. Not only this, but there is good reason to believe that this process is the cause of the movements of the insectivorous plants[1] and of Mimosa pudica.[2]

The points of similarity between muscles and glands have received some notice from physiologists. Rosenthal mentions these similarities in the work quoted above (see pp. 212 and 213). They are: first, the fact that both muscles and glands are thrown into action by stimulation of their nerves, and, second, certain likenesses in the electrical reactions. The following experiment seems to show a striking histological similarity. If one of the voluntary muscles be dissected from a freshly killed frog and immediately frozen and cut into thin transverse sections the sections present the appearance of Fig. 4, which was drawn from such a section with the camera lucida.

The striking part of the appearance of Fig. 4 is the segmented ring of darker tissue which surrounds each of the fibres, and which resembles a layer of secreting cells. The fact that transverse sections of muscle prepared by the freezing process resemble sections of glandular tissue supports my hypothesis in the following manner: I have been endeavoring to show that the contraction of muscle is due to the passage of fluid from the interfibrous spaces into the

[1] Charles Darwin. On Insectivorous Plants, London, 1875, second thousand, p. 255.

[2] I. Rosenthal. General Physiology of Muscles and Nerves, London, 1881, pp. 2 and 3.

fibres. The activity of a gland is secretion, which consists in the passage of fluid from the interacinous spaces into the acini, whence it is discharged through the ducts. In other words, according to my hypothesis, there is a fundamental likeness between the function of a muscle fibre and the function of a gland acinus. And if, in addition to this, there is a strong histological likeness between the two tissues, the fact constitutes a considerable addition to the argument.

The appearance of Fig. 4 can always be obtained by the following method: A frog is killed, the sartorious is dissected out, frozen, and cut into sections without being put in any reagent, and all this is done as quickly as possible. The sections may be floated out in a 0.6 per cent. sodium chloride solution or in distilled water and examined with the microscope. They will then be seen to

FIG. 4.

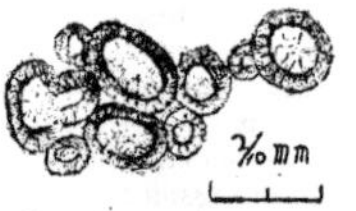

Cross-section of muscle prepared by the freezing process.

have the appearance of Fig. 4. Such sections may be preserved in glycerin. Alcohol produces a great decrease of the sharpness of the appearance. In very warm weather it is necessary to cool the frog with ice before killing it, and to dissect out the muscle and freeze it even more quickly than in cooler weather.

Whether the appearance presented by Fig. 4 or that of sections of muscles which have been preserved in alcohol or some other fixative, and have then been mounted by the paraffin or celloidin method, is more truly representative of the condition of frog's muscle during the life of the animal must be left to the judgment of scientific men. The answer to the question will depend on the answers given to two subordinate questions. First, Is the freezing process or is the alcohol and paraffin process likely to be more destructive? Second, Is the appearance of Fig. 4 or that of sections prepared by the alcohol and paraffin process more suggestive of mutilated tissue? In discussing the first question it must be said that frog's muscle may be frozen and melted again and immersed for a considerable period in 0.6 per cent. salt solution without losing its irritability.[1] The process by which the appearance of Fig. 4 is obtained can be completed within ten minutes of the death of the animal from which the tissue is taken, and no reagent capable

[1] American Text-book of Physiology, Philadelphia and London, 1901, 2d ed., vol. ii. pp. 58 and 162.

of destroying the irritability of the tissue is used. On the other hand, the alcohol and paraffin process requires many days for its completion, and any one of the reagents used is capable of destroying the life of the tissue.

It is difficult to discuss the question whether the appearance of Fig. 4 or that of alcohol and paraffin sections is more suggestive of mutilated tissue. Every histologist feels capable of judging from appearance alone which of two specimens of the same tissue is the more perfect, and yet it would be difficult for him to say on what he based his judgment. The distinctness of the outlines and the amount of differentiation in each of the specimens are, perhaps, the most important points to be considered. The sections illustrated by Fig. 4 certainly show more differentiation than the alcohol and paraffin sections. In Fig. 4 the fibres appear to be made up of two distinct parts, the central disk and the peripheral ring, and the latter is evidently divided into segments. In the alcohol sections each fibre appears as a nearly homogeneous disk. It is easy to imagine that the mutilation of a tissue whose true appearance was that of Fig. 4 might produce the appearance of the alcohol sections; but difficult to suppose that the mutilation of a tissue whose true appearance was that of the alcohol sections might produce the appearance of Fig. 4.

There is one difficulty which must be briefly considered before the conclusion of this discussion, namely, that the action of muscle is extremely rapid, whereas the process of the absorption of fluid is commonly regarded as a slow one. But the unusual conditions under which absorption takes place in muscle must be kept in view. The largest muscle fibres are in reality the merest threads, each of them is entirely surrounded by fluid, and there is, therefore, in every muscle a very large surface exposed by the fibres in comparison to the small amount of fluid to be absorbed by them. The finest cotton thread is exceedingly thick in comparison with even the largest frog's muscle fibre, and yet a cotton thread cannot be dipped in water for a fraction of a second without becoming saturated. The saturated thread has absorbed at least half its volume of water, and this is much more proportionally than would be required to cause complete contraction in a muscle fibre with the structure of the model. But a stronger argument can be adduced against the assumption that the contraction of muscle cannot be due to the movement of fluids because the fluids cannot be conceived to move sufficiently rapidly. If nothing further be conceded regarding the constitution of muscle than that it is composed of solids and fluids, it must be admitted that the fluids move whenever the muscle contracts; and the fluids could surely be moved by chemical processes as rapidly as by the movement of the solid parts of the muscle.

If I knew nothing further about muscle than that it was composed of solids and fluids and had the power of movement, it would seem to me much more likely that the movement of the fluids caused the movement of the solids than that the movement of the solids caused the movement of the fluids. The former is the case in every machine made by man for the purpose of converting chemical into mechanical energy.

I realize that my conclusions are opposed to the latest results of scientific research, in so far as these seem to show that muscle fibres are composed of fibrillæ. If frog's muscle fibres are composed of fibrillæ, which are independently capable of contraction, the whole of the foregoing argument falls to the ground. I hardly dare to urge my own observations against those of such an authority as Rollett, and yet everything that I have seen seems to me opposed to the view that the muscle fibres are composed of fibrillæ. The appearance of the cross-section of frog's muscle, of which a drawing has been submitted, goes to show that fibrillæ do not exist in frog's muscle; and the beaded appearance of contracted fibres, whatever construction may be put upon it, seems to favor the idea that the fibre is the contractile unit. It may be urged that most of the work which tends to prove the existence of fibrillæ has been done with other muscle than the voluntary muscle of the frog, and the evidence favoring the existence of fibrillæ in frog's muscle is very unsatisfactory. It depends on the appearance of the muscle and on certain results to be obtained from specimens hardened in alcohol. Leaving aside the argument that appearance alone can never be a very satisfactory indication of mechanical structure, it must be conceded that the exact appearance of the interior of a fresh frog's muscle fibre is not very accurately known. Great amplification must be used to see the details of the structure which are supposed to represent fibrillæ, and with a high power little more than the upper surface of a thick frog's fibre can be sharply seen. As for the fact that frog's fibres may, after a long immersion in alcohol, be teased into much smaller fibrillæ, there is no evidence to show from which part of the fibre these fibrillæ come. They may be merely portions of the fibre sheath. And there is a good deal of direct evidence to show that the interior of fresh frog's muscle fibres is in a fluid or semi-fluid state.

Sir Michael Foster[1] mentions the classic instance of the nematode worm seen making its way through the centre of a fibre. And Rosenthal[2] says: "It can be shown that a muscle fibre when recently taken from the living animal must, in reality, be of a fluid, or, at least, of a semifluid nature. So that it is impossible to affirm that either the discoid or the fibrilloid structure actually exists in the muscle fibre itself; it must rather be assumed that both forms of structure are really the result of the application of reagents, which

[1] M. Foster. Text-book of Physiology, London and New York, 1891, 5th ed., part i., p. 95.
[2] General Physiology of Muscles and Nerves, London, 1881, p. 14.

solidify the originally fluid mass and split it up in a longitudinal or transverse direction."

It will probably be a long time before an adequate comprehension of the mechanism of muscular contraction is attained, and it is not to be expected that the subject could be completely elucidated within the limits of a single paper. I have simply pointed out the explanation which, after a consideration of the various facts, would seem to be the most likely one.

OBSTRUCTION OF THE CENTRAL RETINAL ARTERY.[1]

REPORT OF A CASE.

By William T. Shoemaker, M.D.,

of Philadelphia.

The question of embolism versus thrombosis of the central retinal artery has for a great many years been discussed and argued until it might be said to be almost threadbare; and, curiously enough, many of the best observers have titled their cases embolism, while declaring their belief in probable thrombosis. That this question is still an unsettled one in medicine is sufficient apology for further contributions.

The following case I believe to be one of lateral thrombosis of the central artery of the retina. The evidence to be adduced, though not conclusive, strongly favors such a diagnosis.

F. W., aged seventeen years, twister in a mill, came to the Eye Clinic of the German Hospital November 18, 1903, with history as follows: One week ago, while returning home from a matinee, she suffered a sudden attack of partial blindness in the left eye. This was described as everything becoming black before O. S., except in the lower field, where vision remained. Subjectively she noticed that the top of the head of a person looked at was not seen. The condition did not improve, but, on the contrary, she thinks became worse in the succeeding few days. The attack was neither preceded, accompanied, nor followed by vertigo, headache, or any physical discomfort whatever. An interesting event in the history of the attack which must be considered, though it is, perhaps, a little sensational, is the following: The play which she witnessed was an extravagant melodrama, in which the heroine, during the third act, became suddenly blind, and continued so until the end of the play, with dramatic effect. The patient was much impressed, and, as she expressed it, could not get the afflicted heroine out of her mind. While thinking of this accident, she had proceeded but three squares from the theatre when her own trouble commenced.

[1] Read before the Ophthalmological Section, College of Physicians, December 15, 1903.

Her family history is good. Her father and mother are living and well. She is the third of eight children, the oldest twenty-one years, the youngest three years; all living and healthy, except the seventh, who died in infancy. Her personal history is good. She had scarlet fever, measles, and whooping-cough in childhood; she has never had rheumatism, has no intestinal nor digestive disturbance; shows no evidence of syphilis, congenital or acquired. She menstruated at thirteen and has done so normally since. Two years ago she had typhoid fever, and was probably quite ill. At the present time she is well developed, of good color, and apparently well balanced. She seems to be in no way neurotic. She experiences some shortness of breath after sudden exertion, such as running up stairs.

Dr. Henry F. Page examined her heart November 27th; in his report he states: "Patient well nourished, color good, mucous membranes normal in appearance. Radial pulse soft, receding, and slow. Pulse rate 63. Inspection of chest shows slight bulging of left side, due probably to a slight degree of lateral curvature. Apex-beat not visible, but determined normal by palpation and auscultation. Slight pulsation of vessels of the neck. Fine thrill felt over carotids. Soft, blowing, systolic murmur heard at aortic and pulmonary orifices transmitted to the carotids." As a result of his examination, he believes the murmur present to be functional in character.

A complete analysis of the urine was made in the chemical laboratory of the Medical Department, University of Pennsylvania, by Dr. John M. Swan. It is not necessary to read the figures; suffice it to say that the patient has nephritis, and is eliminating much less nitrogen, sulphates, and phosphates than normal. The albumin is less than 0.025 per cent. by Esbach's method; the casts are hyaline and very few in number. There is no sugar.

Upon admission, both eyes, conjunctiva slightly injected, pupils equal, irides freely active to light. Movements of eyeballs free in all directions. Central vision: O. S. (affected eye), 5/7.5. V. O. D., 5/5.

Ophthalmoscopic Examination. O. S., media clear disk margins everywhere blurred, but more so below. There is a diffused area of ischæmic infarction, mostly below, but especially marked in a localized patch about the size of the disk, situated 1 d. d. down and out. Into this patch runs an obliterated vessel from which has been a small extravasation. The lower temporal artery from its exit to a turn 1 d. d. from the disk is reduced to a thread; from there on it is of good size. A small branch from this artery running through the infarcted area is filiform, but peripherally recovers a normal diameter. Directly off the disk below are three small, indistinct, flame-shaped hemorrhages. Most of the arteries and veins are reduced in size; they all taper as they enter the disk, and many of them show a most irregular contour varying with diameters. The light streak on the smaller vessels is absent, and on the larger is diminished in brilliancy, but continued far to the periphery. The light streak on a few of the upper ones is beaded. The vessels are nowhere tortuous, and peripherally they seem normal. The macular region shows a number of reflexes, streaked and radiating. The appearance here is granular, but there is no cherry-red spot. The porus opticus is enveloped in an impenetrable mist. Pressure on the eyeball causes a complete blanching of the disk, with not a vessel on the disk to be seen.

There is a little variation from the usual arrangement of the vessels. The majority of them, for instance, seem to come from the superior branch of the first bifurcation, there being at least seven from this source against three or four from the inferior branch. Among those

FIG. 1.

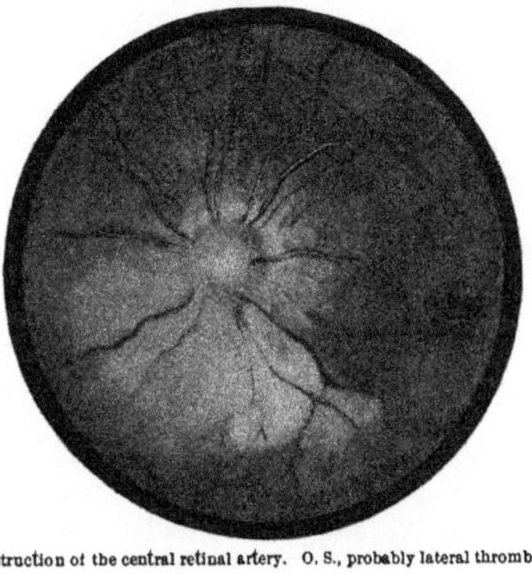

Obstruction of the central retinal artery. O. S., probably lateral thrombus.

first mentioned is a large artery running directly outward and curving above the macula, in close proximity thereto. This vessel, although it points to the lower retinal artery, probably belongs to the upper system because it passes above the macula and supplies the upper outer fundus.

O. D. is normal ophthalmoscopically, but shows the same arrangement of the vessels. The upper fundus is much more vascular than the lower, and there is also a large macular artery, but in this eye it is a branch of the inferior system. There is in both eyes a tendency to lateral distribution of the vessels.

Dr. Buchanan, who has followed this case with me from the start, and who has been of great assistance in its preparation, has made the water-color sketch, which shows well the condition about ten days after the attack. The rough sketch of O.D. shows the arrangement of the vessels in that eye.

Subsequent changes noted at intervals of two or three days have all been in the direction of increasing haziness of the retina (secondary œdema), enlargement of the veins and some increase in the diameter of the arteries. The small hemorrhages have disappeared. The infarcted area has become less pronounced by contrast. Vision gradually reduced until seven days after the first note it was 5/15. Since then it has improved, and at the present time it is 5/10.

Fig. 2.

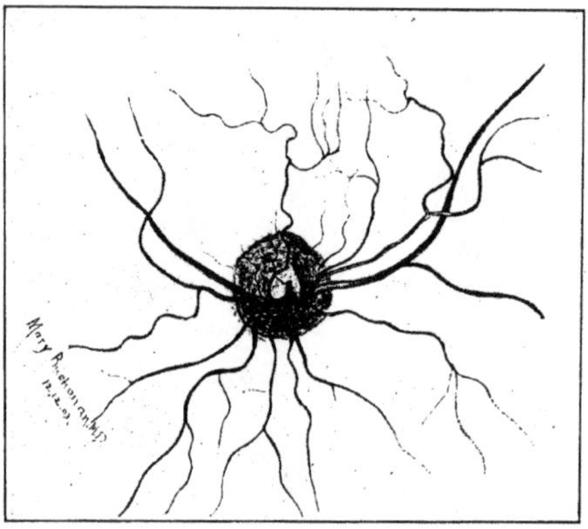

Vascular arrangement of fundus. O. D.

November 25th. Two weeks after the attack a punctate deposit appeared on the posterior surface of the cornea, rather general in distribution, with a tendency to conical formation. This deposit has almost entirely disappeared. Fine vitreous opacities are now present. There has been no alteration in tension. The fields correspond to the fundus condition.

The clinical signs of thrombosis as given by Priestley Smith, in 1884 (*Ophthalmic Review*), and which might be said to have become classic, are:

(*a*) Previous attacks of transient blindness in the affected eye.

(*b*) Simultaneous attacks of transient blindness in the fellow-eye.

(*c*) Previous or subsequent attacks of transient blindness in the fellow-eye, especially if conditions of the attack were the same in the permanent as in the transient attacks.

(*d*) Signs of disturbance of the cerebral circulation at the onset of the blindness—dizziness, faintness, headache.

In the history of the present case there are no points of correspondence with the above, but investigation along other lines would seem to make questionable the necessity for any one of these signs in establishing a case of thrombosis. It is true that with these clinical signs the case is probably thrombosis, but, with any or all absent, thrombosis is not to be excluded. In other words, when positive they are strong, and when negative they are weak. This case has been

FIG. 3.

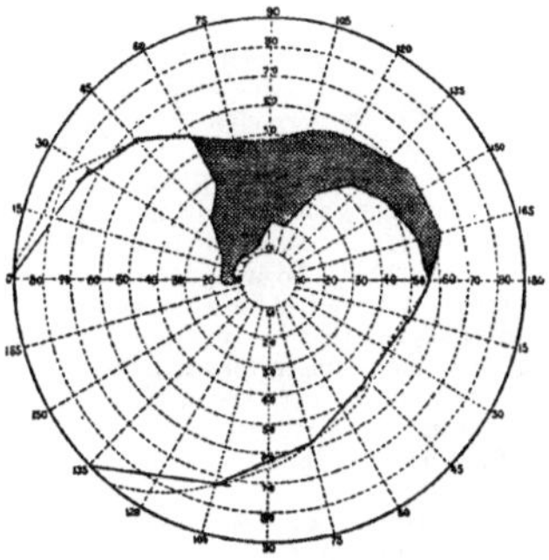

Field. O. S.

studied therefore more from the side of general medicine and general pathology than from the clinical.

There are three important causative factors in the coagulation of blood within the vessel wall during life, two or all of which are for the most part essential.[1] These factors are alteration in the blood current, changes in the vessel wall, and alteration in the blood.

Ludwig Gutschy, in a recent article in the *Beiträge* for pathological anatomy and general pathology, has arrived at conclusions as to thrombus formation which seem to be of service in considering cases such as the one here reported. The first change he declares is one of separation; the fibrin separates from the blood plasma, forming a jelly-like mass, which adheres to the vessel wall, and

[1] Stengel. Text-book of Pathology.

which he calls the *primary fibrin membrane.* Upon this membrane, which is sticky, leukocytes collect, the resulting mass being a white thrombus. T. Wharton Jones[1] has found that on pressing the neck over the artery or vein firmly with a blunt point, an agglomeration of colorless corpuscles, with a few red ones, held together apparently by coagulated fibrin, occurs, adheres to the wall of the vessel, and more or less completely obstructs it at that place.

Returning now to the three factors more or less essential for thrombosis; under the first, or alteration in the blood current, we have to consider anything which slows the blood current, such as weakness of the heart, narrowing of the bloodvessels, or pressure on the vessel wall. I think it can be demonstrated that the blood current in this case was very much reduced in velocity, especially in the central retinal artery. Normally the blood travels in the carotids from 300 mm. to 500 mm. per second, and in the very small arteries it travels but a few mm. per second.[2] The external diameter of the central retinal artery is about $\frac{1}{10}$ mm.; it is therefore a very small artery, and has a very small lumen. Dr. Page's examination shows the pulse to be soft, receding, and slow, with a rate of 63 per minute. His examination was made under the usual conditions which tend to excite the patient and accelerate the heart-beat. If now the velocity of the blood in the radial artery is reduced below the normal to the extent shown by a pulse of 63, what must be the reduction in the central artery of the retina if we take as a standard Foster's figures just given? Furthermore, the axial stream in which the red cells travel is much quicker than the peripheral stream of plasma next the vessel wall. Here is certainly a condition favoring the separation of fibrin from the plasma, and the formation of Gutschy's primary fibrin membrane.

The next factor in thrombosis is alteration in the vessel wall. The patient has nephritis; it might, therefore, be said that she has endarteritis, arteriosclerosis, etc., but it is not likely, however, much as it would simplify things, if she had. Some change in the bloodvessel wall is very desirable for the purposes of this paper. This want is to be supplied by the bifurcation of the vessel. The point of bifurcation of the central artery of the retina—that point projecting in midstream, as it were—must necessarily stand more opposed to the onward flow of blood than the unobstructed wall. Such a mechanical arrangement causes a sudden halting of the stream with consequent embarrassment of some of the elements. Under these circumstances, and with an abnormally slowed current, the abovementioned changes of separation might well take place. This might also be favored by some individual peculiarity in the angle and form of bifurcation. This case shows peculiarities in the vessels of the

[1] Guy's Hospital Reports, series 2, vol. vii. pt. i.

[2] Foster's Physiology.

fundus, and it is not unreasonable to think that the vessels are also peculiar farther back. In support of this explanation is the experiment of Wharton Jones.

Changes in the blood itself have not been found. Two analyses were made by Dr. George P. Mueller, the second including an estimation of the fibrin. The first count gave: hæmoglobin, 100 per cent.; red cells, 4,650,000; white cells, 7650. Second count: hæmoglobin, 80 per cent.; red cells, 4,430,000; white cells, 5800. No increase in fibrin. Differential, normal.

This was somewhat of a disappointment as a functional heart murmur, which this undoubtedly was, is not usual with normal blood. My brother, Dr. Harvey Shoemaker, suggested that the blood quantity of the patient might be reduced as a whole. Cabot is authority for the existence of this condition. He has found it in typhoid fever, and attributes it to a concentration of the blood. There is no concentration of blood in this case, unless such coneentration is offset by anæmia, for there is no increase of corpuscular elements, the ratio remaining unchanged.

Clinically the case suggests the following points: From the changes observed in the fundus I would locate the obstruction laterally in the central artery near or at the bifurcation and passing into the lower branch. If the lower arterial system alone were involved, there should be no changes in the upper vessels other than those brought about by doing extra duty or carrying more blood. But they were changed in size, contour, and light streak. An embolus to produce this condition would have to be of that rare variety in which the plug straddles the bifurcation. That the macular region was not more affected is attributed to the peculiar arrangement of the vessels described above. The more normal condition of the vessels at the periphery, and the subsequent return of some of them to their normal calibre are changes described in many of the reported cases of obstruction, and in the absence of any opportunity for collateral circulation in this locality have been thought to be due to backward flow from loss of *vis a tergo*. The keratitis and vitreous opacities are inflammatory, natural results of this condition. The white area so characteristic in these cases, is pathologically infarction, and not œdema, as invariably called. Secondary œdema does occur, but I am told reaches only to the edge of the infarcted area. The process is one of starvation.

Treatment. For the general treatment of cases of retinal artery obstruction, it is *important* to determine, if possible, whether or not the obstruction is thrombosis. Against embolism we are helpless, and the other eye will suffer or not, as fate ordains. But if the conditions contributory to thrombosis, as above outlined, can be established, they should be treated until they disappear.

Local treatment to be of any service must be immediate, and that these cases are sometimes seen early is shown by one of embolism which Dr. de Schweinitz had under observation twenty minutes after the attack.

Now, as to the immediate treatment of arterial obstruction in the eye, whether from embolism or from thrombosis, I am convinced that pressure massage, which has been strongly advised by most writers, is irrational and should not be practised. Pressure on the eyeball stops what flow of blood still exists, and produces the most favorable conditions for further agglutination and accretion. It tends to fortify the obstruction. Surely the indication is to increase the force of the circulation without causing vasoconstriction or to increase the heart action and dilate the peripheral circulation. The drugs of one class will do this, viz., the *nitrites*, and best among these are nitroglycerin and nitrite of amyl. These drugs cause rapid heart action and a dilated peripheral circulation. Gifford has recommended nitrite of amyl. The use of any vasomotor constrictor, which will cause the artery to contract and thus hold tighter the thrombus or embolus, is clearly out of place.

But better than any drug, it seems to me, would be forced muscular exertion, such as running or climbing stairs. In this way the heart could be accelerated, and the peripheral circulation, if affected at all, dilated. Had my patient been enough frightened to run home, I believe she would have been benefited.

Another therapeutic procedure which might be indicated in some cases, and probably was in this case, is hypodermoclysis, or the injection of large quantities of fluid into the cellular tissue of the body for the purpose of rapid absorption into the circulation. Likewise the intravenous injection of saline solution should constitute a part of our resources.

The prognosis of these cases is well known, and I have nothing to add.

EMPYEMA OF FRONTAL SINUS, FOLLOWED BY EXTRADURAL ABSCESS AND ABSCESS OF FRONTAL LOBE; OPERATION AND DEATH FROM HYPOSTATIC CONGESTION OF THE LUNGS.

By Paul S. Mertins, M.D.,
MONTGOMERY, ALA.

Abscess of the brain resulting from empyema of the frontal sinus is a sufficiently rare condition to demand the report of cases. The case which I here present is that of Mr. W. D. L., a boilermaker, aged about forty years, who came to the office of Dr. M. L. Wood, September 8, 1903. For the past six months or more he has suffered from violent headaches, which have steadily increased in severity.

Within the last three days a swelling, the size of a goose-egg, has appeared in the region of the glabella. It was white, fluctuating, and very tender, and a harder rim, consisting probably of thickened periosteum, could be felt around its margin. On inquiry, a history of syphilis sixteen years ago was obtained. Two years ago he received a blow from a hammer on the top of his head, from which he was unconscious for several days.

The abscess was incised by Dr. Wood, and about one ounce of foul, dark-colored pus evacuated. The patient experienced complete and immediate relief of pain. He was instructed to go home, make hot applications to his head, and to return on the next day. On the third day the pain returned, and the patient noticed that when he held his head forward the flow of pus increased, and the pain became less. During the night of September 13th the pain grew more severe, the patient vomited several times, and had three convulsions. He was seen by Dr. Baker, who administered chloroform and morphine.

I saw Mr. L. on the following morning in company with Dr. Wood. He was in bed and seemed to be suffering greatly. His cerebration was slow, but relevant. No paralytic phenomena were observed. His pupils were small, equal in size, and reacted well. The eye movements were good in all directions. His breath was very foul, and the tongue, which was heavily coated, was protruded slowly in the centre line. His hand-grasp was strong, alike on both sides. His patellar reflexes were lively. No rigors have been noted. The ears were normal. The anterior end of the middle turbinate was greatly swollen. Temperature, 97.5° F.; pulse 78; respiration 20. His intimate friends stated that he has been considered stupid for a year or more, but his employer considered him an excellent workman.

On probing the wound necrosed bone was found, and in several places the probe seemed to enter the cranial cavity. A diagnosis of extradural abscess was made, and the patient was admitted to St. Margaret's Hospital for operation.

Operation September 14, 1903, at 3.30 P.M., under chloroform narcosis, Drs. Wood, Baker, and Pollard assisting. I performed the following operation: A three-inch incision was made in the integument of the forehead, through the seat of the abscess. The pericranium, which had been dissected from the bone by the abscess, was held back by retractors, and an area of necrosed bone, the size of a silver dollar, was exposed. It was of dark-brown color, and presented the appearance of a pepper-box top, from the numerous fistulæ through which pus oozed at each respiration. A half-inch trephine was applied to the centre of the necrosed area and a button removed. An extradural abscess, containing about one ounce of pus, was found. The trephine opening was enlarged with rongeur forceps to the size of a dollar. The dura was found adherent to the frontal bone all around, and formed the bed of the abscess. Removing the necrosed bone opened the left frontal sinus, and about one-half ounce of pus was found in it. The right frontal sinus on being opened was found to be healthy. The wound having been irrigated with a boracic-acid solution, the dura was examined. It appeared to be very thick, was of a dirty yellowish color, and pulsated only on the left side. No fistulæ could be found. A hollow needle was introduced on both sides, with negative result on the left side, but with the finding of four or five drops of pus on the right side as the needle was withdrawn. The needle was repeatedly reintroduced on the right side, but pus could not again be found. The wound was irrigated and an iodoform gauze dressing applied. The patient was sent to the ward at 4.45 P.M. in good condition. One-half grain of morphine was administered. During the night he became delirious, tore off the dressings, and was kept in bed by an attendant.

September 15th. The patient's general condition was good; his mind, though much clearer than before the operation, was not entirely clear. He was in a nervous condition, and picked at the dressing constantly. The wound was dressed. The right side of the brain did not pulsate. The patient complained of no pain. Iodide of potash, 10 grains thrice daily, to be increased to 30 grains, was ordered, in view of the history of syphilis. Bromide of potash, 20 grains every four hours, for nervousness.

The wound was dressed daily. His bowels were obstinately constipated, and cathartics were necessary to obtain a movement. His urine was frequently passed involuntarily. This condition of irritability and semistupor continued. On September 23d a transient paresis of the right internal rectus was noted, and examination of the eye-grounds showed an optic neuritis on the right side. On September 24th, as the patient seemed to be in a more than usually stupid condition, and was unable to answer questions, I decided to aspirate the right frontal lobe again.

Second Operation. Drs. Wood and Baker were present. No anæsthetic was used. On introducing the aspirating-needle into the right frontal lobe at a depth of three-quarters of an inch, it was felt to enter a cavity and pus flowed into the aspirator. A small pair of scissors was entered by the side of the needle and the blades separated. About one and a half ounces of creamy pus and yellowish lump of broken-down brain tissue were evacuated. The cavity was gently curetted, and an iodoform gauze drain inserted. The patient's condition showed an immediate improvement. His mind became much clearer, and for the first time he spoke without a question being asked. His pulse rose from 78 to 100 beats per minute.

The accompanying chart gives the patient's pulse, respiration, and temperature while in the hospital.

The patient's condition continued to improve slowly. The abscess cavity grew smaller and the discharge less. Granulations began to cover over the exposed dura. His appetite continued good and his mind clear. The wound was dressed daily.

On the evening of September 30th I found a marked change in the patient's condition. His mind was less bright and his answers were much slower. His temperature was 102° F., pulse 98, and respiration 24. The wound was in good condition and draining freely. Examination of the chest showed a hypostatic congestion of the inferior lobe of the right lung; and the nurse informed me that during the afternoon the patient had coughed up several mouthfuls of blood. Strychnine $\frac{1}{30}$ grain and brandy $\frac{1}{2}$ ounce every four

FIG. 1.

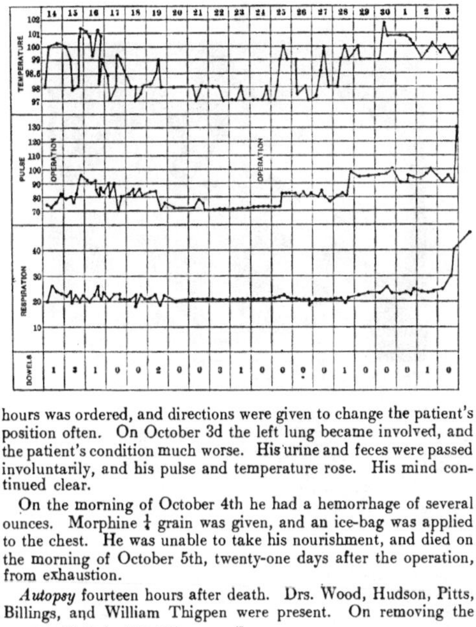

hours was ordered, and directions were given to change the patient's position often. On October 3d the left lung became involved, and the patient's condition much worse. His urine and feces were passed involuntarily, and his pulse and temperature rose. His mind continued clear.

On the morning of October 4th he had a hemorrhage of several ounces. Morphine $\frac{1}{4}$ grain was given, and an ice-bag was applied to the chest. He was unable to take his nourishment, and died on the morning of October 5th, twenty-one days after the operation, from exhaustion.

Autopsy fourteen hours after death. Drs. Wood, Hudson, Pitts, Billings, and William Thigpen were present. On removing the scalp a depressed fracture, the size of a hammer-head, and about one-half inch deep, was found on the left parietal bone, near the sagittal suture. An opening the size of a match-head was found at the bottom of this depression. The bone was healthy, and this was probably the result of the blow received two years ago, from which he was unconscious for several days. On removing the calvarium the dura was found to be adherent around the original trephine opening, both to the bone and to the brain. It was also adherent to the bone at the point of the depressed fracture. The membranes appeared normal, and no increased amount of cerebrospinal fluid was noticed. The brain appeared normal, except at the point of operation, where an opening, 1 cm. in diameter, was

FIG. 2.

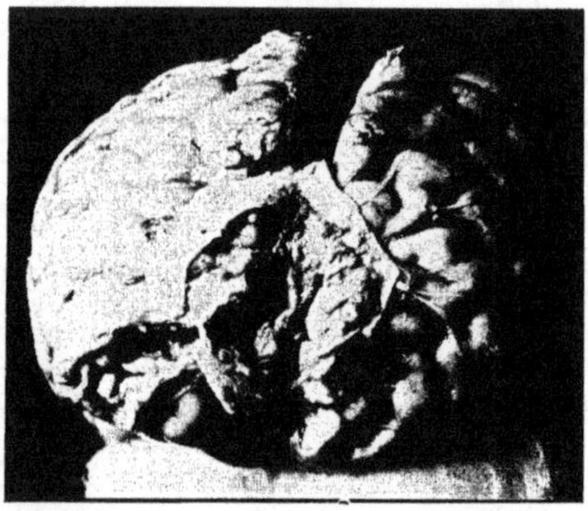

Photograph of brain, showing opening of abscess and adherent dura.

found leading into an abscess cavity. The longitudinal sinus was found normal. The brain was placed in a solution of formalin to harden. On opening the thorax the heart was found normal. Both inferior lobes of the lungs were found to be in a condition of hypostatic congestion, and on section of the right lung a cavity the size of a walnut, filled with clotted blood, was found. Old adhesions were found on the left side, between the pleura of the lung and diaphragm. The abdominal cavity was not opened.

The photographs of the hardened brain show the location and size of the abscess. In the photograph of the entire brain the dura has been left adherent to the brain about the abscess opening, showing that the abscess was well walled off. The opening into the abscess is seen as a dark spot on the right side. The small rupture in the brain was made in removing the skull-cap. In the sagittal section the depth of the abscess, one and one-half inches, is seen. In this section the abscess was found to be well walled off by a thick lining membrane. The brain tissue about the abscess was in a nearly normal condition.

The dark area below the abscess is an extravasation of blood.

FIG. 3.

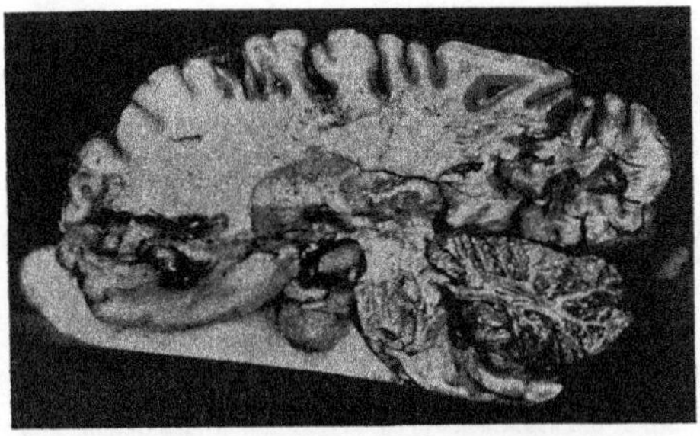

Anteroposterior section of brain, showing depth of abscess cavity, a part of lining membrane, and hemorrhagic focus below abscess.

REMARKS. From the condition of the brain at autopsy, I think we have every reason to believe that this patient would have recovered from his abscess. The pulmonary complications were, without doubt, the cause of death. The abscess was the direct result of the empyema of the frontal sinus. The posterior wall of the sinus was necrosed and a fistulous tract was found from the sinus to the extradural abscess. This case is similar to that of Roth[1] in many respects; an external abscess was found, an extradural abscess and abscess of the left frontal lobe. His patient died. Macewen[2] reports a case of abscess of the frontal lobe with recovery. This case was, however, of traumatic origin. Professor G. Killian[3] discusses three other cases of intracranial complications following empyema of the frontal sinus, namely, those of Carver,[4] L. Müller,[5] and E. Fraenkel.[6]

[1] Wiener klinische Wochenschrift, 1899, No. 14, p. 383.
[2] Pyogenic Diseases of the Brain and Spinal Cord.
[3] Archives of Otology, August and October, 1901.
[4] British Medical Journal, June 16, 1883.
[5] Wiener klinische Wochenschrift, 1895, p. 194.
[6] Virchow's Archiv, vol. cxliii. p. 80.

CHONDRODYSTROPHIA FŒTALIS.*

By P. W. Nathan, M.D.,
of New York.

The majority of chondrodystrophic individuals are either born prematurely or born dead at term. The affection is, therefore, a very serious fetal disease, with a high mortality. Those infants which are born alive are usually very weak, and for some time life is precarious; should they, however, survive this critical period, they seem to grow stronger, and later they are *no* weaker than normal infants of the same age.

The nature of the affection thus accounts for the fact that up to the present time practically all the reports of cases have simply contained post-mortem findings. The earlier observers contented themselves with a description of the external characteristics; and these they found so closely analogous to those found in rachitic infants that they found no hesitation in classing the two conditions together. Thus the disease became known as an antenatal prototype of rachitis, being sometimes called congenital rachitis, sometimes fetal rachitis.

The earliest published case dates back as far as 1791, when Sömmering[1] reported his post-mortem findings of a case of fetal abnormality, which he did not attempt to classify. From his description, which is fairly accurate, there can be no doubt as to the nature of the condition. The bones are said to present the characteristic rachitic abnormalities; the fœtus is obese; the extremities are much too short, and much bent and deformed. In 1836 Busch[2] gave a very accurate description of a case, which he called congenital rachitis. He notes all the salient features which characterize these cases, viz., very large head; short, deformed extremities, with hard skeleton, large epiphyses, so-called rachitic rosary, rachitic pelvis, and general obesity. Following him numerous writers gave more or less accurate descriptions of cases which, in the light of our present knowledge, may be considered cases of chondrodystrophia fœtalis.

The majority of these writers, however, drew their conclusions as to the nature of the abnormality from the more or less cursory examination of a single case; and it was not possible, until the publication of the more extensive and careful observations of H. Mueller[3] (1860), to formulate a distinct and coherent idea of this singular affection. H. Mueller's researches, which are remarkable for their accuracy and insight, may be said to have formed the basis for all future investigation. He showed decisively that chondrodystrophia is a disease of the primordial bone cartilage; that it has nothing in

* Read before the Orthopedic Section of the New York Academy of Medicine, Oct. 16, 1903.

common with rachitis, and that the inhibition of the growth of the long bones, which is the most prominent characteristic of the condition, is due to a disturbance in the row formation of the proliferating cartilage cells. The examples which he first examined occurred in calves, but he re-examined the cases previously published by Virchow as congenital rachitis and congenital cretinism, and found that in man the pathological phenomena are identical.

Some time afterward (1873) Urtel[4] carefully examined a still-born child macroscopically and microscopically, and his findings were identical with those of Mueller in the principal features; he hesitates, however, to place his case in the same category, because they differ in some particulars. Later investigation has proved his hesitation unwarranted.

The further development of our knowledge of chondrodystrophia fœtalis we owe to Eberth,[5] Schidlowsky,[6] Kirchberg,[7] Marchand,[8] but above all to Kaufmann,[9] who, having special opportunities for investigation (he had thirteen cases), was enabled to clear up many points in the pathology.

External Appearance. The appearance of a chondrodystrophic fœtus is characteristic. The head is very large and appears still larger in contrast with deficient length of the fœtus as a whole. Both upper and lower extremities are too short. The arms do not reach the waist-line, and the lower extremities are so short that decentralization of the body is produced. Thus, the midpoint between the crown of the head and the soles is not, as it should be in normal infants, at the navel, but above it; in many cases as high as the xiphoid cartilage. The extremities, moreover, are bent and deformed, and occasionally fractured. All the epiphyses appear more or less enlarged, and those of the ribs produce the so-called rachitic rosary. The skin and subdermal tissues are hypertrophied, causing an exaggeration of the natural skin-folds; the abdomen is prominent, and the fœtus as a whole appears very obese. There is frequently epicanthus; the lips, eyelids, and tongue are thickened, and the latter protrudes from the mouth.

The anomalies of the skeleton give the fœtus that peculiar appearance which has long been known to be characteristic of rachitis, and which has led so many observers into the error of associating these two conditions. But aside from the pathological differences, which will be spoken of later, the peculiarity of the head and face in chondrodystrophia fœtalis should lead one to suspect that, similar as are the other external phenomena, these at least are peculiar to another affection.

As has been pointed out, the head is abnormally large; indeed, it is so large that its circumference equals the length of the body, and in many cases exceeds it. The distinguishing characteristic, however, is the decided prognathus, with marked retraction of the nose, and, in some cases, flattening of the whole nasal region. The latter abnormalities very much resemble those of infantile myxœdema, and where, as is usually the case, they are associated with thick lips, protruding hypertrophied tongue, epicanthus, and prominent abdomen, the resemblance to the congenital cretin is so close that without a microscopic examination of the bones, or a clinical history, the two conditions cannot be differentiated.

Pathological Anatomy. Before proceeding to the discussion of the pathological changes at the base of the skull, a few words as to its anatomy and development are necessary.

Upon the development of the base of the skull depend the peculiarities in the shape of the head and the physiognomy. Most important in this respect is that portion of the base of the skull which Virchow designated the os tribasilaris, and Hyrtle the fundamental bone. This bone is composed of the basilar process of the occipital bone, the os basilaris posterius, and the two portions of the body of the fetal sphenoid, the os basil. ant. and os basil. med. These three parts of the compound bony os tribasilare are, in fetal life, separated by synchondroses, the synchondrosis intersphenoidalis and the synchondrosis spheno-occipitalis, which at birth are only partially ossified. Normally the synchondrosis intersphenoidalis is ossified at birth or soon thereafter; the synchondrosis spheno-occipitalis, however, remains patent until at least the thirteenth year, and complete synostosis occurs between the eighteenth and twentieth years. The growth of the base of the skull depends upon the persistence of these synchondroses; synostosis or even a disturbance in their development therefore produces a shortening of the base of the skull. As deficiency in the length of the base of the skull always causes prognathus, the relation of the above-mentioned synchondrosis to the prognathus is evident. In the case of so-called congenital cretinism, which Virchow[10] used to demonstrate this fact, there was complete synostosis of the synchondroses os tribasilare, but he did not claim that synostosis was necessarily present in every case of prognathus. On the contrary, he laid particular stress upon the fact that not alone synostosis, but any deficiency in the length of the base of the skull would cause this anomaly. The writers following him, however, assumed that synostosis was the cause of prognathus in all cases; and this opinion was generally held, though the observations of Klebs,[11] His,[12] Marchand and Paltauf[13] were opposed to such an assumption. In his examination of thirteen cases of chondrodystrophia Kaufmann was enabled to settle this question definitely; he found that not alone premature synostosis of the os tribasilare, but *any* inhibition of the growth of the os tribasilare or inhibition of the growth of any of the bones at the base of the skull causes prognathus. He found that synostosis of the os tribasilare was present in many cases of chondrodystrophia fœtalis, probably in the majority of them, but in a certain number the synchondroses are patent. Moreover, Kaufmann showed, by careful measurements of all the bones at the base of the skull, that though the os tribasilare is a very important factor in its growth and development, it is not the only factor; for in some of his cases there was retraction of the root of the nose, though the os tribasilare was of the normal length. Even in those cases in which the os tribasilare is shortened or synostosed, it must not be assumed that this is the only part which is instrumental in causing the prognathus; not infrequently the bones anterior, the ethmoid, and nasal are also involved, either taking part in the shortening or, as occasionally happens, being entirely responsible for it (Kaufmann's Case XI.).

Another peculiarity of the base of the chondrodystrophic skull, first pointed out by Virchow, is a reduction in the angle formed at the junction of the basilar process of the occipital bone and the body of the sphenoid. Virchow called this condition kyphosis of the saddle angle.*

We must, therefore, conclude that the conditions which are active in causing the peculiar physiognomy in chondrodystrophia fœtalis vary within rather wide limits. They may be enumerated as follows: 1. Most frequent is premature synostosis, and consequently inhibition of the growth of the os tribasilare, with or without shortening of the bones anterior. 2. Shortening of the os tribasilare, patent synchondroses, varying degree of shortening of the bones anterior. 3. Decided shortening of the ethmoid and nasal bones, with slight or no shortening of the os tribasilare, and patent synchondroses. With these is associated a change in the saddle angle (kyphosis) of varying extent.

The bones of the skeleton present a variety of changes. They are always shortened and apparently thickened. In only a small percentage of cases, however, are the bones really thickened; as a rule, the apparent increase in thickness is due to the shortening, which changes the ratio between the length and thickness. The same is true of the epiphyses, which always appear larger than normal, though they are really enlarged in only a certain percentage of cases. In some cases, however, the epiphyses are enormously enlarged.

Sections of the long bones show that the pathological change occurs primarily in the growing cartilage. This portion of the bone, though it shows a variety of changes, is invariably affected in every case. The vascularity is always increased, but its size and consistency vary in different instances. According to the latter, Kaufmann distinguishes three distinct types: First, the epiphysis is not enlarged and the consistency is normal; second, it is absolutely enlarged, and the consistency may or may not be changed; third, the cartilage is softened.

The microscopic examination of the bones shows changes in the growing cartilage which correspond to the gross changes just enu-

* Normally the saddle angle increases from the third fetal month until birth, when it is 155°; thence it diminishes to puberty.

merated. There is, however, one change which is constant and characteristic. This is the more or less complete inhibition of the normal row formation of the proliferating cartilage cells in the preparatory stage of ossification. The limitation of row formation is not, however, the same in all cases; though it is never absolute, in some cases it is almost so, and there is only a suggestion of row building in isolated areas of the ossifying zone. On the other hand, there are others which may, with propriety, be called mild cases, in which the row formation occurs, though the rows are stunted and rudimentary, inconstant, and irregular. Between these two extremes all gradations occur.

In the class of cases referred to as type one, which shows no increase, but rather a diminution in the size of the epiphyseal cartilages, besides the limitation in the row formation, there is also an inhibition of the proliferation of the cartilage cells. For this reason Kaufmann designates this type of cases chondrodystrophia fœtalis hypoplastica. In contrast to these is type two; here, though the row formation is rudimentary, the cartilage cells, instead of showing defective proliferation, are, on the contrary, enormously increased in numbers, and very closely packed together, causing the characteristic enlargement of the epiphyseal cartilage. This type Kaufmann designates chondrodystrophia fœtalis hyperplastica. The intercellular substance of the cartilage other than increased vascularity shows no change in the two types of the disease just described; in the third type, however, this is also abnormal. Here the cartilage has softened, in the severer cases quite extensively so, and the epiphyses appear as more or less completely gelatinous and very vascular masses, with variable dimensions. The intercellular substance is distended and forms an irregular network, in which cells of varying size are irregularly distributed. These cases Kaufmann designates chondrodystrophia fœtalis malica.

Thus, according to Kaufmann, we have three distinct types of chondrodystrophia fœtalis, viz., chondrodystrophia fœtalis hypoplastica, chondrodystrophia fœtalis hyperplastica, and chondrodystrophia fœtalis malica. Between these three types the rudimentary row formation is the connecting link, for it occurs in all of them, and is, therefore, the most characteristic and uniform change. Moreover, it must not be supposed that the three types occur perfectly distinct as individual cases; all three types may be found in the same individual in the various epiphyses, though one type usually predominates in a given case.

These pathohistological changes occur in all the bones subject to enchondral ossification, and they readily account for the dwarfism of not alone the long bones of the skeleton, but also for the shortening of the base of the skull and the resultant cretin physiognomy. The variation in the intensity of the process and its modifications, evidently, cause the variation in the conditions found in the latter region. Thus, the prognathus may be due to the hypoplastic, the hyperplastic, or the malic process; any one of which may affect the cartilaginous skull in its entirety or one or more of the primordial cartilages more than others. With the cessation of the row formation, further bone development becomes impossible, and, as a result, ossification takes place, which may or may not be complete, according to the severity of the pathological process. Hence we find all gradations, from complete synostosis of the primordial skull vertebræ (os tribasilare) to only slight shortening, with patent synchondroses. In the malic form of the disease the affected primordial cartilages are soft, the ossification centres are rudimentary or even absent, and in the severer cases growth ceases entirely.

Synostosis of the synchondroses os tribasilare is, therefore, not, as the earlier writers assumed, necessarily present in all cases of chondrodystrophia fœtalis. Nor is the os tribasilare shortened in every case; so that the absence of either or both of these conditions does not decide the doubt, if any exists, that we have chondrodystrophia fœtalis before us in a given instance. All the bones at the base of the skull, which develop from cartilage, must be measured, and should the diagnosis still remain doubtful, it can always be cleared up by the microscope.

Besides the disturbance in the proliferation cartilage cells, there are still other peculiarities of the chondrodystrophic skeleton revealed by the microscope. It is found that the deposition of the calcium salts, no matter how great the abnormalities in the cartilage, goes on in a perfectly normal manner; the line of calcification is always found to be fairly regular, and the formation of ostoid tissue and its ossification is typical. Still more remarkable, considering the gravity of the pathological process in the cartilage, is the fact that periosteal bone formation goes on in a perfectly normal manner. Not alone this, but all the bones or parts of them which are formed and ossified very early in fetal life, or directly from connective tissue, pursue their normal course of development and show no abnormality. Thus the clavicle was found to be normal in length and other respects in all the cases reported; so also the bones of the cranial vault and all other bones similarly developed. In the long bones the normal development and ossification of the periosteal bone stands out in sharp contrast to the short and defective enchondrium, and the change in the ratio of the row gives rise to the appearance of thickening, to which attention has been called.

A very remarkable and interesting phenomenon which occurs in a great many and at some point in the skeleton in all cases of chondrodystrophia is what the Germans call the periosteal lamella. This very peculiar formation, which was first described by Urtel as it occurred in a human fœtus, later by Eberth in the calf, and subsequently by nearly all authors on this subject, consists of a layer of connective tissue emanating from the periosteum, from which it pushes its way between the epiphysis and diaphysis toward the axis of the bone. Thus the epiphysis and diaphysis are separated more or less completely from each other. The periosteal lamella, which for reasons which will appear later I shall call the periosteal inclusion, varies in extent in the different cases and in the various parts of the skeleton in the same case. In the majority of instances it begins in the periphery as a distinct band, but gradually diminishes in breadth toward the axis of the bone, where it disappears. It is often apparent macroscopically, forming a distinct wall at the epiphyseal line, but it varies to a considerable extent, and not infrequently is only visible with the aid of the microscope. The breadth and the depth from the periphery usually correspond, so that when it is narrow it only invades the bones for a short distance, leaving a considerable portion of the axis free.

Microscopically, it can be seen that the cartilage cells adjacent to the periosteum inclusion run parallel with it, and assume a spindle form. The intercellular substance of the cartilage is fibrillated, and thus the transition between the inclusion and the cartilage is very gradual, at times almost imperceptible. On the diaphyseal side the conditions are liable to some variation. In some instances the inclusion undergoes ossification, with the formation of true bone, in a manner exactly similar to that which occurs under the normal periosteum (Urtel,[4] Hoess,[14] Eberth,[5] Bode,[15] Sturp,[16] and others). In others, as in Kaufmann's Case II., the inclusion is surrounded by cartilage on both sides.

The relatively greater production of periosteum, as compared with the enchondral growth, is considered by all authors as the underlying cause of the periosteal inclusion. The manner of its production, however, is subject to some difference of opinion. Some authors (Urtel, Hoess) consider it due to an invasion of the cartilage by a periosteal process, due to an active local proliferation of the periosteum; and Kaufmann considers his Case II., in which the inclusion is surrounded by cartilage on both sides, as demonstrative of such a manner of production. It is difficult, however, to understand why the periosteum should proliferate excessively in a given locality without assignable cause. Eberth's explanation seems more plausible; he believes that the inclusion is due to the overgrowth of the epiphysis beyond the peripheral diaphyseal line, causing an involution of the periosteum, which subsequently proliferates. Kirchberg and Marchand also attribute the cause to an involution of the periosteum, but they consider this involution due to a continued growth of the periosteum, without a corresponding increase in the length of the bone.

Personally, I believe that all these conditions, and not a single one alone, are, to some extent, responsible for the formation. I imagine the process of development to be somewhat as follows: The epiphysis enlarges until it grows beyond the peripheral diaphyseal line, thus causing an involution of the periosteum at the point where the epiphysis and diaphysis join. Subsequently the diaphysis grows in thickness, but not in length, so that the fold of periosteum, instead of being eradicated (as it would be if the growth in length and thickness were in the normal ratio), becomes more pronounced, and is included between the adjacent surface of the epiphysis and diaphysis. The inclusion continues to act as periosteum; it therefore proliferates, forms ostoid tissue and true bone.

The periosteal inclusion, by its encroachment upon the epiphyseal line, necessarily precludes growth in length; and Kaufmann believes that this cessation of growth is analogous to that experimentally induced by injury or removal of the intermediate epiphyseal cartilage. But it must not be hastily decided that the cessation of growth is always absolute; in some cases the inclusion is very rudimentary, leaving a considerable portion of the axis of the bone free, and here the row formation, though defective, may still go on. It is only in those cases in which the periosteal inclusion is very extensive and undergoes ossification, thus causing synostosis of the epiphyseal synchondroses, that growth is definitely concluded. (Examples of such a condition occur in the os tribasilare and also, but less frequently, in the long bones.) Naturally, the earlier in fetal life the disease begins the more rudimentary is the row formation, the more complete the periosteal inclusion, and the more limited the growth of the long bones.

Thus, from an anatomical point of view, chondrodystrophia fœtalis is a well-defined morbid condition, and if we bear in mind its salient features, there can be no difficulty in differentiating it from other affections. The characteristic signs are defective growth of the enchondral skeleton, including the base of the skull and the pelvis, which, upon microscopic examination, is found to be due to the rudimentary row formation of the proliferating cartilage cells and the periosteal inclusion. In contrast to this is the normal ossification and the normal development of the periosteal and membranous bone. With postnatal rachitis it has absolutely nothing in common, except the apparent enlargement of the epiphyses, the prominent abdomen, and the occasional bowing of the legs; the latter is due to entirely different causes, which cannot be discussed here. Osteogenesis imperfecta, with which it has been confounded, differs from it in all the essential details. Here the salient pathological condition is a deficiency of ostoid tissue and defective ossification; the bones are of normal length, and the skull and all the other morbid changes of chondrodystrophia fœtalis are absent. Osteoporosis and osteosclerosis may both occur as complications of chondrodystrophia, but when present they are always secondary to the changes already described, and not pathognomonic.

Before closing our review of the pathology of this very interesting condition, though time presses, I cannot omit a few words as to the

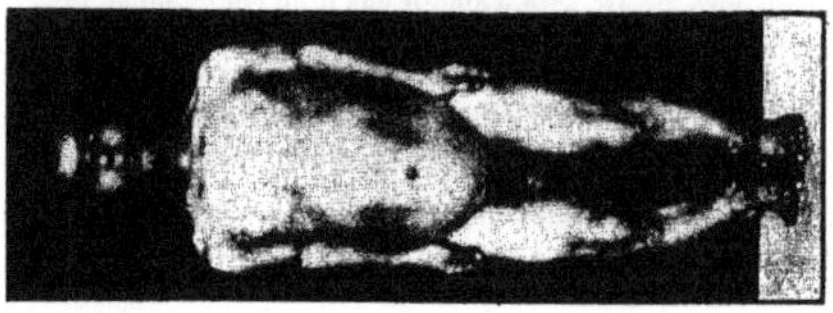

FIG. 1.

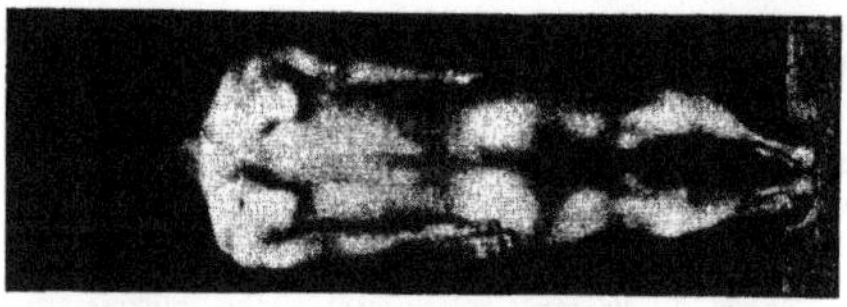

FIG. 2.

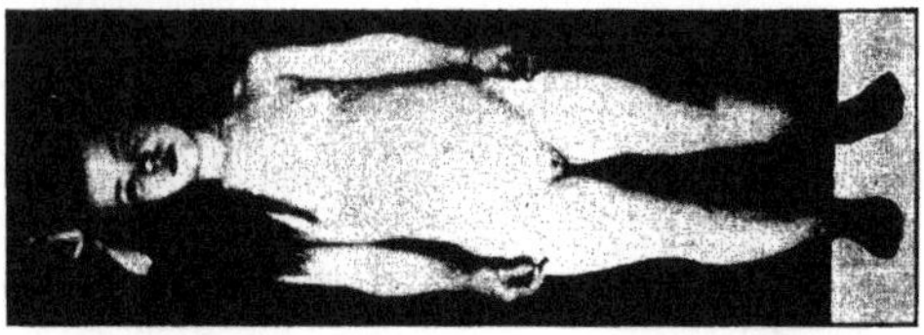

FIG. 3.

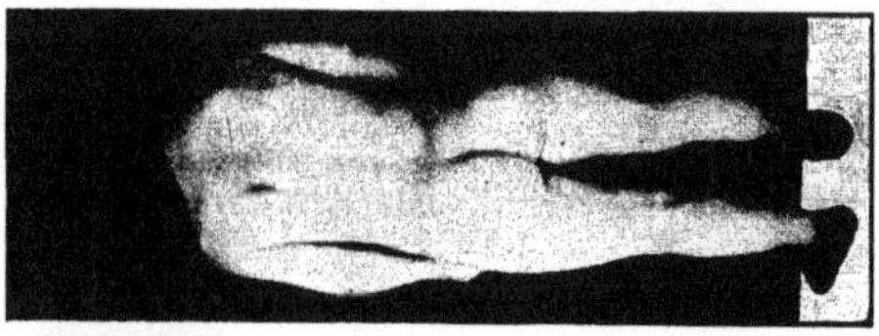

FIG. 4.

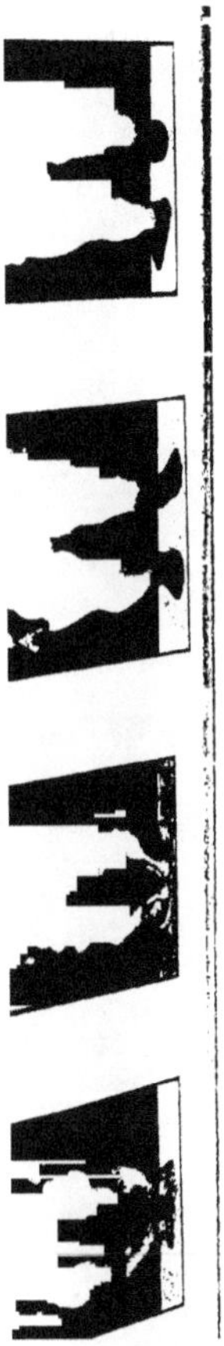

pathogenesis. Mueller, Eberth, and a large number of authors consider the nature of this anomaly analogous to that of congenital cretinism. However, though the skin and skull lesions lend some support to this view, clinical experience and the pathological anatomy teach us that the two diseases have nothing else in common. I think the changes in the skeleton and in the subdermal tissues point very distinctly to a constitutional anomaly, which, though not exactly analogous to that of congenital cretinism, nevertheless acts upon fetal organism in a similar manner; that is, by disturbing the metabolism in some unknown way.

Clinical Aspect of Chondrodystrophia Fœtalis. As has been said, the majority of infants with chondrodystrophia is born dead. But the disease is not nearly so uncommon as some authors would have us believe; and to judge by the number of living examples to be found in the literature, and my own experience, it is not necessarily fatal. Quite a number of isolated cases have been reported, and recently Kassowitz[17] has described seven cases which came under his own observation. I have had the opportunity to examine eight cases, a number of which I still have under observation. One I have re-examined after an interval of several years (Case IV.); he was shown by Dr. C. Hermann, in the Pediatric Section of the Academy some time since. I show you his photograph, with that of Case V. Moreover, I have seen a number of adult cases walking about, and though I had no opportunity to examine them more closely, their appearance was so characteristic that I do not hesitate to classify them. All my cases were seen within the last three years, and it is for this reason that I consider chondrodystrophia not nearly so uncommon as has been supposed; and I believe this statement will be borne out by general experience when the knowledge of this disease becomes more universal.

The general appearance of a chondrodystrophic infant differs very slightly from that of a fœtus with the same disease. They are dwarfs, with a large head, and very short, often bowed, extremities. In infants the abdomen is very prominent, as are the epiphyses, and there is obesity, but in the older cases these symptoms, though present, are not nearly so distinct. The head is large; in the younger individuals its circumference equals the length of the body in measurement, and there is a decided prognathus, which is accented by very marked retraction of the root of the nose, or flattening of the whole nasal region. The hair on the head is abundant, fine and soft, in my cases never coarse or brittle.

The lower extremities are always too short, being entirely out of proportion to the length of the trunk. This causes a decentralization of the body and tends to give these individuals a very characteristic, at times ludicrous, appearance, and very readily distinguishes them from other dwarfs; for in cretinism, or in the so-called idiopathic dwarfism, the extremities and the trunk are both shortened and are not out of proportion. The disproportion between the trunk and extremities in chondrodystrophia is readily demonstrated by measuring the height of the individual, first standing, then sitting. Measured in this way, my cases showed this peculiarity very distinctly:

	Height standing.	Height sitting.
Case I.	21½ inches.	15½ inches.
" II.	28½ "	18½ "
" III.	23 "	14¾ "
" IV.	45 "	29⅛ "
" V.	47⅛ "	30 "

The decentralization is also very well demonstrated by comparing the distance between the crown of the head and the umbilicus to that between the umbilicus and the sole of the foot. In the normal newborn infant these are the same, but as the child grows the distance between the umbilicus and the soles increases much more rapidly than the other, and exceeds it more and more as the individual grows older. In chondrodystrophia the midpoint of the body is not at the umbilicus at birth, but above it, sometimes as high up as the xiphoid cartilage, and this disproportion or decentralization of the body continues throughout life.

The upper extremities are also too short; they do not, as in the normal individual, reach to the hips. The fingers and toes are short, and, in fact, the conditions found in the living subject are exactly what the pathological anatomy would lead us to expect.

During early life these individuals are obese, and the natural skin folds are exaggerated, but as they grow older the obesity gradually disappears. In all the cases I have examined, and as far as I can tell from the reports of other cases, the skin is never harsh and scaly, and the development of the hair on the head and other parts of the body is perfectly normal.

The mental faculties are always intact; these children are not sluggish and somnolent, but bright, taking an intense interest in their surroundings and learning to talk as readily as other children. If the older individuals are backward in their studies, it is more because they are apt to be kept from school because of their small size and peculiar appearance than from lack of intelligence. They begin to walk late, as a rule, and those cases with complicating osteoporosis do not do so for a long time; but when they have learned to walk their gait is in no way peculiar or unsteady.

Like all infants with congenital abnormalities, they usually present some other congenital defects. The most frequent of these is inguinal hernia and a highly arched palate. In some of the postmortem findings dislocation of the hips is noted, but I have not been able to trace a direct causative relation between chondrodystrophia and the ordinary cases of congenital dislocation of the hip which we see in practice. Kassowitz attempts to bring them in connection, but I can hardly agree with him when he considers the fact that patients with congenital dislocation of the hip are liable to other congenital malformations, such as epicanthus, highly arched palate, etc., as an indication of a connection between the two abnormalities. As I have pointed out, all individuals with one congenital malformation are very apt to have others. Moreover, I have carefully examined some twenty cases of congenital dislocation of the hip without being able to find any trace of chondrodystrophia. I must not, however, be understood to deny the possibility of the occurrence of dislocation of the hip in chondrodystrophia; I simply deny its causative relation to congenital dislocation of the hip in general.

Kassowitz also groups chondrodystrophia with mongolism and myxœdema. In practice there is hardly any danger of confounding these affections. The mongols are idiots, without any disproportion of the skeleton, and with a characteristic mongolian physiognomy, which is absolutely distinct from that of chondrodystrophia. Myxœdema is very readily distinguished from it; there is always mental defect; there are the skin and hair changes, and the disproportion between the extremities and the trunk is not present. That all three diseases have the abnormalities which are apt to appear in all congenitally abnormal individuals is certainly no reason for grouping them together, though Kassowitz very naïvely considers this a scientific classification. That this disease, like cretinism and some others, antenatal and postnatal, may be caused by a disturbance of the metabolism can, in the light of our present knowledge of the normal metabolism, be neither positively affirmed nor denied. In chondrodystrophia the thyroid gland and the organs other than the skeleton show no change perceptible to us, and we must confess that the pathogenesis of this, as well as of nearly all other diseases, is still unexplained.

Of the etiology we know nothing. In one case a chondrodystrophic mother is said to have given birth to an infant similarly affected, but in all others we have nothing upon which to base a surmise as to the cause of this disease. To judge by the cases reported, the female is somewhat predisposed, though my own cases are equally divided between the two sexes.

MEASUREMENTS.

(Cases VI., VII., and VIII. were not accurately measured.)

	Case I.	Case II.	Case III.	Case IV.	Case V.
Age	16 mos.	4½ yrs.	9 mos.	14 yrs.	14 yrs.
Sex	Male.	Female.	Male.	Male.	Female.
Height standing	24¼ in.	28½ in.	23 in.	45 in.	47⅛ in.
" sitting	15½ "	18½ "	14¾ "	29⅛ "	30 "
Circumference of head	17½ "	20½ "	17⅝ "	19⅞ "	
Length from crown to umbilicus	....	14 "	12½ "	....	21 "
" " umbilicus to sole	....	14½ "	10½ "	....	26 "
Ant. sup. spine to ankle	7¼ in.	13¼ "	9½ "	18½ in.	20¾ "
Femora	....	6 "	9¼ "	10¾ "	
Tibiæ	R. 3½ in.	R. 6¼ "	R. 14⅛ "		
"	L. 3¼ "				
Arms	3½ "		.....	6½ "	
Forearms	3½ "			6½ "	

Literature.

1. Sömmering. Abbildungen u. Beschreibungen einiger Misgeburten, etc., Table XI., Mains, 1791.

2. Busch. Zeitschrift f. Geburts. und Gynäkologie, 1899.

H. Mueller. Würzberger med. Zeit., Bd. i. 1860.

3. Urtel. Ueber Rachitis Congen., Diss. Halle, 1873.

5. Eberth. Festschrift, Leipzig, 1878.

6. Schidlowsky. Ueber sogenannte foetale Rachitis, Diss. Berlin, 1885.

7. Kirchberg. Ibid., Diss. Marburg, 1888.

8. Marchand u. Kirchberg. Ziegler's Beiträge, Bd. v.

9. Kaufmann. Untersuchungen ueber die sogenannte foetale Rachitis (Chondrodystrophie Foetalis), Berlin, 1892.

10. Virchow. Gesammte Abhandlungen, 1852.

11. Klebs. Archiv f. experim. Path., Bd. ii.

12. His. Cited by Kaufmann.

13. Paltauf. Ueber d. Zwergwuchs in anatomischer und gerichtaerztlicher Beziehung, Wien, 1891.

14. Hoess. Ueber foetale Rachitis, Diss. Marburg, 1876.

15. Bode. Virchow's Archiv, Bd. xciii.

16. Sturp. Untersuch. u. foetale Rachitis, Diss. Königsberg, 1887.

17. Kassowitz. Myxodoeme mongolismus u. Micromelie, Wien, 1902.

A full list of the literature is given by Kaufmann, also by Schmidt, Lubarsch's Ergebnisse der Algemeine Pathologie u. pathologische Anatomie, Jahrg. iv. 1897.

LEUCONYCHIA STRIATA ARSENICALIS TRANSVERSUS.

WITH REPORT OF THREE CASES.

By Charles J. Aldrich, M.D.,

LECTURER ON CLINICAL NEUROLOGY AND ANATOMY OF THE NERVOUS SYSTEM, COLLEGE OF PHYSICIANS AND SURGEONS, CLEVELAND; NEUROLOGIST TO THE CLEVELAND GENERAL HOSPITAL AND DISPENSARY; NEUROLOGIST TO THE CITY HOSPITAL.

Five years ago at the Cleveland City Hospital, while examining a woman suffering from a very severe arsenical neuritis, I was struck by the observance of a peculiar white transverse line occupying the middle of the outer third of the finger-nails of each hand.

Taking into consideration the fact that the nails grow more rapidly following arsenical poisoning, I was able to estimate that these white lines corresponded to the time when, with suicidal intent, she had taken a teaspoonful of "Rough on Rats," which is well known to contain a large quantity of arsenic. The white streaks were about one-sixteenth of an inch in width, quite regular, with fairly sharp margins, and occupying an identical position on each nail. They were slightly larger on some nails than upon others and a little wider in the centre than near the margins; extended from side to side, forming a crescentic band, with the convexity directed to the free margins of the nail, and presenting a curve identical with that of the lunula. The markings were less plainly seen upon the toe-nails. Her body was covered with branny exfoliating dermal scales; much of the hair had fallen, and the palms and soles showed some kera-

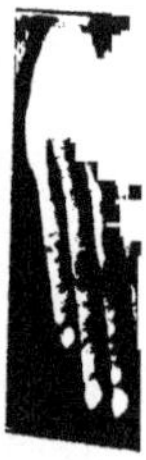

tosis. At that time I looked through the literature very carefully, but was unable to discover any reference whatever to such lines occurring in arsenical poisoning, and while I felt positive that in my case they were caused by the mineral, yet decided to wait for further confirmation of that opinion.

About twelve months following the observation of this case I was consulted by a man with an undoubted neuritis, who had been referred to me by Dr. F. W. McLean, of Elyria, and who gave the following history:

He had suffered a very violent attack of "stomach difficulty" about three months preceding his visit to me. He says the vomiting was so violent that the vomitus contained blood. He did not suffer any marked cramps in the legs or arms. Shortly after he began to grow weak in his legs, and at last was barely able to get about with two canes.

FIG. 1.

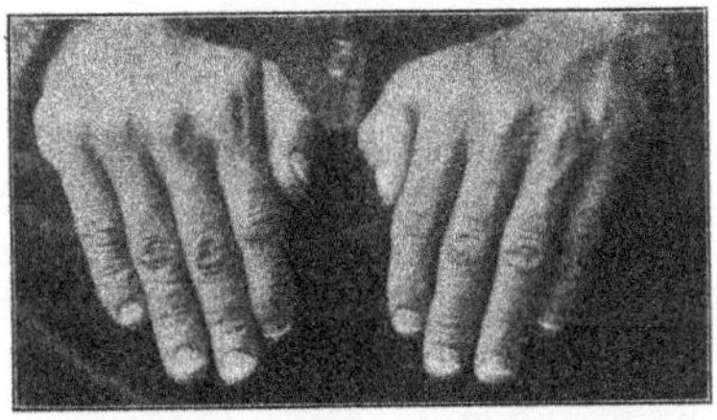

On examination I found he was ataxic, had a partial double foot-drop, absent knee-jerks, some loss of sensation, no pigmented spots or keratosis, no loss of sphincter control. In short, he had all the symptoms of a multiple neuritis. Inspection of his nails showed the characteristic transverse streaks as described, and as illustrated in this rather poor photograph (Fig. 1). It does not show the striation plainly. After talking with the patient some little time, during which he asked my opinion, I told him I thought he would probably recover from the neuritis, and that the neuritis was undoubtedly due to poisoning. At first he demurred, but after a little conversation told me that he believed he had been poisoned, but offered no explanation except that he was positive that it was arsenical poisoning. After urging upon him the necessity and the perfect safety of giving me his confidence, he confessed to having taken a large dose of white arsenic, but stated that it immediately produced vomiting, and ultimate recovery took place, save his nerve inflammation.

In May, 1899, Dr. George Gill, of North Ridgeville, Ohio, referred to me a patient giving the following history:

F. S., male, white, aged twenty-nine years; has a wife and two healthy children. The wife is healthy; one induced miscarriage seven years ago. Patient gives a history of good health in early childhood; in early manhood gonorrhœa, but no history of lues. I cannot learn that he has had any other sickness. He uses tobacco and drinks to excess. He states that one night about three months ago, on returning home from a debauch, he concealed a bottle of whiskey beside a hedge-row near his house. Becoming thirsty about 1 o'clock the next day he sought the bottle and took a large drink. In a short time he began to suffer extremely from pain in the stomach, vomited almost continuously, had cramps in the legs and arms, and became unconscious. His vomiting continued until 10 o'clock the following day. He remained in bed three days, and then got up, feeling very weak and still suffering from occasional attacks of vomiting and colicky pains in the abdomen. Six weeks later he began to feel tired, sore, and lame; the legs grew weak, the arms and hands felt heavy, weak, and numb. There was no loss of bladder power, but considerable diminution of sexual power. He unhesitatingly expressed to me the opinion that his uncle, with whom he had had trouble, had put poison in the whiskey.

Examination. Patient is a fair-sized man, walks with canes, gait ataxic; partial double foot-drop; station is not good, in fact, without his canes he is unable to stand with the eyes open. Both knee-jerks are absent, wrist-jerks and elbow-jerks are also absent. He is slightly anæsthetic throughout the lower limbs, which anæsthesia grows more marked as the extremities are approached. He is proportionately more analgesic than anæsthetic. The fingers are slightly anæsthetic; he is unable to button his clothing well or to handle small objects. There is no tremor. The hand-grasps are equal and weak, registering thirty-six. There are no scars or spots on the body, and in fact nothing else abnormal is noted, except a white, slightly crescentic transverse streak on each finger-nail; the convexity of the crescent is directed toward the free margins. These streaks were so strikingly like those of the related cases that I immediately informed him that his stomach attack was due to arsenical poisoning. It was at this time he told me about the whiskey, adding that he thought his uncle had poisoned him. Shortly after this, in answer to some inquiries regarding the case, I received a communication from Dr. Gill, who informed me that the man had made a confession, which was corroborated by his wife, that he had taken a quantity of "Rough on Rats," with suicidal intent.

The accompanying black and white drawing (Fig. 2) affords an exact representation of the condition of his nails, and, indeed, the appearance common to each of the three cases observed. There were no transverse ridges on the nails, nor furrows; the lines were, in longitudinal relation at about the point which we would expect them to occupy from the outward growth of the nail since the poison-

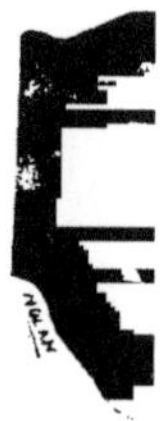

ing. His toe-nails also showed faint markings, but no keratosis was present on the palms or soles.

I was about to publish these cases when I noticed the report of a case of arsenical neuritis by Dr. Florence Sabin, in the May number of the *Johns Hopkins Hospital Bulletin*, 1901, in which a white line running transversely across each finger-nail was referred to. In answer to a letter to Dr. Sabin, I received the following reply:

"Your note in regard to the white lines in the nails in cases of arsenical poisoning has interested me greatly. I do not know of any references in the literature, and Dr. Osler says that he does not. Dr. Osler expressed himself as anxious to see the photographs of your cases."

Fig. 2.

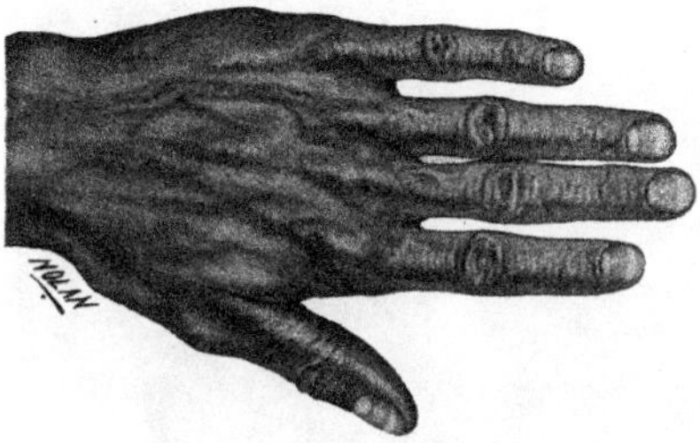

Since the observation of a large number of cases of arsenical neuritis reported as occurring in beer-drinkers throughout England, and especially about Manchester, I have had considerable correspondence in reference to the condition of the nails with the English physicians observing those cases.

In April, 1901, Dr. Nathan Raw, of Manchester, wrote me that he had observed changes in the nails, particularly the toe-nails. He states that they were often markedly transversely ridged, but does not refer to any white lines. He very kindly sent to me the photograph (Fig. 3).

Dr. Leslie Roberts, of Liverpool, writes me that he has not met with such changes herein described, and says, "Temporary arrest of nutrition and formation of air-cavities may produce various markings on the nails."

Dr. Ernest S. Reynolds, of Manchester, who was first to discover and point out the nature of arsenical poisoning due to beer-drinking in England, has very kindly written me under date of May 2, 1903, as follows:

"The white transverse streaks on the nails of cases of arsenical poisoning had already been noted and described by me. (See *Lancet,* January 19, 1901.) Also, you will there find an account of several parallel transverse streaks which I stated would almost suggest a series of drinking debauches.

"I am much obliged for your letter and much interested in it, as it corroborates my own observations. At the time a well-known skin specialist told me he did not think that the transverse streak had anything to do with the arsenical poisoning, but I observed it too frequently for it to have been a mere coincidence."

Fig. 3.

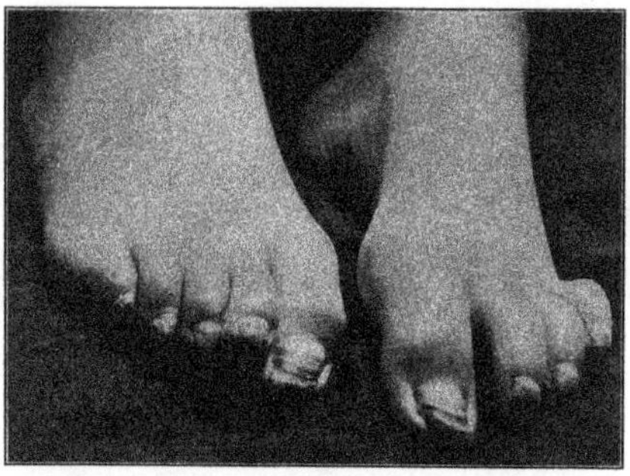

Referring to Dr. Reynolds' article, which appeared in the *Lancet,* January 19, 1901, page 68, in the clinical description, and under the subhead "Nails," I find the following:

"In many cases the nails are affected. After the patients have stopped taking the beer for some weeks the best appearances are seen, for then there is a transverse white ridge across the nails; proximal to this the nail is normal, but distal to it the nail is whiter, cracked, thin, and toward the tip almost papery, and much flattened. In some cases there has been a series of parallel transverse ridges on the nails almost suggesting a series of week-end 'drinking bouts.' The deformed nails, of course, break easily."

It is to be observed that Dr. Reynolds speaks only of "a transverse white ridge." In my cases and also in Dr. Sabin's there was no well-defined groove or ridge. This difference is possibly due to the fact that his cases were subjected to more prolonged and chronic poisoning by the arsenic. I am nevertheless certain that they are both evidences of arsenical poisoning.

It is possible that careful observation will show that these peculiar markings on the nails quite constantly follow severe acute arsenical poisoning, and I believe they depend upon the serious alteration in the nutrition incident to the profound shock of the poisoning, aided, perhaps, by the specific effect of the arsenic, since I have observed three cases of arsenical neuritis from slow poisoning in which there were no streaks, although the nails were ridged, particularly the toe-nails; nor did I observe in the cases of chronic poisoning that the nails were flecked with little white spots, which are vulgarly called "flowers" or "lies;" they were transversely ridged, pale, brittle, and papery. I do not believe that it is the profound nutritional disturbance alone which produces these transverse lines, since in neither of three cases of severe corrosive poisoning observed after seeing the first case of arsenical poisoning here recounted did white lines develop on the nails; nor has a diligent search through the literature revealed any observations of such changes in the nails following other severe poisoning. It is possible that the arsenic has some specific effect upon a plane of newly developed nail cells within the matrix, and as a result the normal keratinization fails to become physiologically complete.

If my contention is just we have in these nail-markings important corroborative evidence of poisoning by arsenic. The occurrence of these bands following arsenical poisoning is sufficiently established to warrant the use of the term leuconychia striata arsenicalis transversus.

When I began a search of the literature for observations upon the nails it was with some surprise that I found that these transverse white lines had been observed, carefully described, and figured by several authors, but none, excepting Reynolds, ascribed them to arsenic. One recorded case seems to show that they may appear as a congenital anomaly; other observations that they may present, as it were, an unguinal record of a severe illness.

While leuconychia punctata is frequently observed, one may obtain some idea of the rarity of leuconychia striata by the statement of Jules Heller,[1] in his recent work on *Diseases of the Nails*, that it is so rare that but two cases have been thus far reported. In justice to the literature, it is only right to state that Heller is afflicted with the usual literary myopia of German writers, as the following references will evidence:

Reil,[2] in 1792, and Bean,[3] in 1846, published observations upon peculiar changes in the nails due to fevers; also Murchison, in his exhaustive treatise on fevers, alludes to these markings and changes in growths.

Dr. Langdon Down[4] observed two sets of white lines extending transversely over the nails on the fingers and toes of a man who had experienced two attacks of poor health, in each case the lines corresponded with the occurrence of the attack.

Prof. Alfred Vogel,[5] in 1870, and again in 1873, in thorough German fashion, discussed the question of nail changes following fevers, and figured several cases of the white transverse lines in the nails which appeared after typhus fever.

I found a description by Longstreth[6] of transverse white bands extending over the surface of the nails, which appeared after each exacerbation of a case of relapsing fever, recording, as it were, each relapse.

Da Costa[7] also has described such bands appearing after a relapse of typhoid fever, and gives a beautifully colored illustration of a hand the nails of which are traversed with several white bands, each corresponding to a relapse of the typhoid from which the patient had suffered.

Dr. Morrison,[8] of Baltimore, has described a case of transverse white bands on the nails, under the title of "Leucopathia Ungninum," occurring in an otherwise healthy young woman. There appeared a number of these white lines extending from one lateral nail margin to the other, and were about one-sixteenth of an inch apart. No cause for their origin could be ascertained.

Dr. E. J. Stout[9] has reported a case where it appears that a negro had presented such white bands on his nails from birth.

Heidingsfeld,[10] of Cincinnati, has contributed considerable to this subject in a very able article, "Leucopathia Unguinum." He has observed seven well-marked cases of leuconychia striata and nearly double the number of slighter degree. While he does not clearly state that all were due to injudicious use of the cuticle-knife, a "new and somewhat American instrument," I assume, in absence of any mention of other cause operative in his personally observed cases, that each had its origin in tinkering vanity.

He is inclined to disagree with Heller and about all other writers upon the extreme rarity of leuconychia striata. His personal experience hardly warrants his contention, but rather convinces the reader that a very modern use of the cuticle-knife, a comparatively new and certainly vicious instrument, or an unskilful use of it in Cincinnati, is the explanation of his frequent observations. He has made some very interesting and valuable discoveries as to the pathological histology of these striations which seem to overturn the accepted theory of air infiltration. I give his conclusions in his brief recapitulation:

"Leuconychia is the result of some pathological change of structure of a plane of nail-cells, approximating a failure of the affected cells to undergo normal physiological keratinization.

"The cause may be trauma, malnutrition, febrile diseases, neuroses, or any agency which disturbs the growth, development, or keratinization of the matrix cells in their change to nail-structure.

"An infiltration of air is absent, and there is no rational physiological basis for such a theory."

I have given these references to the literature at length for two reasons: First, to show that a thorough search reveals but little upon the subject; a few cases occurring in connection with fevers, some from traumatism; a very few of unexplained origin, and none ascribed to arsenic but by Reynolds. Secondly, as an aid to the diagnosis. Since, if in the presence of such nail changes as here described and illustrated we can exclude congenital anomalies, traumatism, severe illness, especially the acute specific fevers, particularly typhoid, relapsing and typhus, we will be warranted in suspecting arsenical poisoning. And if other corroborating evidences, such as violent unaccountable vomiting, abdominal pain, cramps in the legs and arms, and neuritis can be obtained, I believe we can positively assert that poisoning by arsenic has taken place. And allowing for the rapid growth of the nail following arsenical poisoning, and giving seven months for complete nail-growth, from the position of the white band, we can quite accurately estimate the time of the poisoning.

References.

1. Heller, Julius. Krankheiten der Nagel, Berlin, 1900.
2. Reil. Memorabilia Clinicorum, Fascicul , 3 Halae, 1792, p. 206.
3. Beau. Archives générales d. médecine, Août, 1846, 4e ser., tome xi. p. 447.
4. Langdon Down. Transactions of the Pathological Society, 1870, vol. xxi. p. 409.
5. Vogel. Die Nägel bei Fieberhaften Krankheiten, Deut. Archiv f. klin. Med., 1873.
6. Longstreth. Transactions of the College of Physicians of Philadelphia, 1877, 3d series, vol. iii. p. 113.
7. Da Costa. Relapses in Typhoid Fever, Transactions of College of Physicians of Philadelphia, 1877, 3d series, vol. iii. p. 101.
8. Morrison. Medical News, 1887, vol. li. p. 430.
9. Stout. Quoted by Van Harlingen and Stout. System of Genito-urinary Diseases, Syphilology, and Dermatology. Edited by Prince A. Morrow, New York, 1894, vol. iii. p. 904.
10. Heidingsfeld. Leucopathia Unguinum, Journal of Cutaneous and Genito-urinary Diseases, November, 1900.

Other Literature.

De Frankenau, G. F. Frankus. Onychologia curiosa sive de unguibus, Jenae, 1646.

Unna. · Histopathologie der Hautkrankheiten, 1895.

Joseph, M. Leuconychia totalis, Dermatolog. Zeitschr., 1898.

Bielschowsky. Jahresber. f. Vaterl. Kultur, 1890.

Collineau and Thibierge. Annales de Dermat., 1897.

Leyden, E. Ueber Multiple Neuritis, Charité-Annalen, B. V.

Unna. Uber das Wesen der Verhornung, Monatshefte f. Dermat., xxiv.

Joseph, Max. Haut Krankheiten, Leipzig, 1892.

Columbini. Un caso die Leuconychia, Rif. Med. Napoli, 1894, x.

Jackson. Diseases of the Skin.

Hardaway. Manual of Skin Diseases.

Echeverria, E. Ein histologisches Beiträg zur Kentniss des gesunden und Kranken Nagels. Monatshefte f. Prak. Derm., Bd. xx.

Duhring. Cutaneous Medicine, Part I., p. 50.

Duhring. A Case of Tricophytina Unguinum, Med. and Surg. Reporter, 1878.

Kobner. Onychomycosis tonsurans, Virchow's Archiv, 1861.

A CASE OF PRENATAL APPENDICITIS.

By W. Fred. Jackson, M.D., C.M.,

STAFF SURGEON TO THE BROCKVILLE GENERAL HOSPITAL, AND TO THE ST. VINCENT DE PAUL HOSPITAL, BROCKVILLE, ONTARIO.

This case, being of a very unusual nature, is presented as a contribution to our knowledge of this interesting and prevalent disease.

A female child, fully developed and well nourished, died at 5.30 P.M. from symptoms of metallic poisoning. At the hour of death the child had barely completed forty hours of natal life. At 12.30 P.M. the attending physician saw the infant, and it was perfectly well. Another physician was called hurriedly at 5.15 P.M. the same day, and found the infant collapsed and with a greenish-blue froth issuing from its mouth. This froth and accompanying fluid stained the garments a deep chemical blue. The supposition is that the child died of poisoning by the administration of a blue tablet of bichloride of mercury with citric acid.

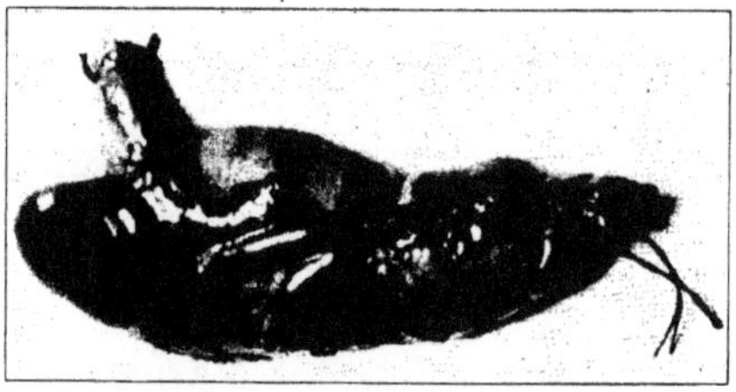

A post-mortem examination, which I as Coroner ordered, brought to light the condition of the appendix, as shown in the accompanying illustration, which is taken from a photograph of the specimen.

The appendix is much elongated and congested, lying upon the cæcum, and bound down upon it by numerous and firm adhesions. The surfaces of the appendix, where it is reduplicated upon itself, are firmly bound together. The small intestine and the colon below the ileocæcal opening present no evidence of inflammatory action.

The mother's labor was regular and without incident. The delivery was accomplished with the forceps without injury to the child. The infant was lusty and strong, and apparently perfectly well up to a very short time of its death. How the blue tablet was administered to the child, or by whom, has not been demonstrated.

It seems that the inflammatory condition, as evidenced by the thickened and congested appendix and firm adhesions, must have occurred previous to the child's birth. The more so, as the inflammation was evidently in the stage of resolution.

LUXATIO ERECTA.

By George Tully Vaughan, M.D.,
of Washington, D. C.

Luxatio erecta, a variety of subglenoid dislocation, is so rare that the following case is of interest:

J. M., white, male, aged sixty-six years, barkeeper, was admitted to Georgetown University Hospital October 4, 1903, having just been injured by being struck by a street car. On examination the patient's left elbow was seen pointing upward at an angle of forty-five degrees, the forearm was flexed, with the hand hanging down, dorsal surface toward the patient's face.

The patient could not lower the elbow, even to a horizontal position, although the elbow could be moved inward toward the head to a vertical position without pain. The forearm was placed by me on the top of the patient's head, and the typical attitude of a case of luxation erecta was presented. The head of the humerus was easily felt low down in the axilla. Reduction was effected without trouble after about one minute's extension—seizing the arm with the right hand just above the flexed elbow and making extension upward and slightly outward, while the fingers of the left hand were used to press the head of the bone upward.

No anæsthetic was used and the manipulations were attended with little or no pain.

The patient was last examined November 4, one month after the injury. He could abduct the arm well from the side and carry it across the chest, so as to place the fingers on the opposite shoulder. Flexion of the fingers was possible, but the grasp was quite feeble; extension of the fingers or of the wrist was impossible; there was well-marked "wrist-drop."

He said the fingers felt slightly numb, though rough tests with a pin indicated no difference in the two hands. Flexion and extension of the forearm and abduction and adduction of the arm were well performed.

This variety of subglenoid dislocation of the shoulder was first reported in 1859 by Middeldorpf and Scharm, and up to 1899 Stimson had collected only 9 cases, which, with Middeldorpf's, made 11 cases in all. Of 539 shoulder dislocations observed at St. Thomas' Hospital no case of luxatio erecta was recorded (Makins).

Krönlein reports 3 cases of luxatio erecta in 207 dislocations.

In 400 dislocations Bardenheuer met with no case of luxatio erecta, but saw 2 cases in which the arm was abducted slightly beyond a right angle with the body—luxatio horizontalis—a variety of *subclavicular* dislocation.

REVIEWS.

A Manual of Operative Surgery. By Sir Frederick Treves, Bart., K.C.V.O., C.B., LL.D., F.R.C.S. Second edition. Revised by the Author and Jonathan Hutchinson, Jr., F.R.C.S. 2 vols. Philadelphia and New York: Lea Brothers & Co.

In reviewing a new edition of a work so widely known and so deservedly esteemed as this, it is of chief interest to note the additions and omissions, the changes of opinion, or the confirmation of earlier views wrought by ten years' experience.

In Chapter I. the most noteworthy change is the substitution in place of the remarks on "Cleanliness" of an article on the "Preparation of the Skin." There is perhaps no point in antiseptic technique as to which so much difference of opinion prevails as this, and the method described by the author, who prefers as the chief germicide a 1:500 alcoholic solution of mercuric potassium iodide, is not, so far as we know, employed in this country, and is worthy of trial.

In Chapter II. the chief addition is as to matters of *dress*. In this connection the author will probably be regarded by many American surgeons as unduly conservative, and only time and experience will show whether or not he is right. In the mean while his remarks will bring comfort to those operators who doubt the necessity of some of the elaborate precautions now fashionable.

Chapter III., on "The Operating Room," has been expanded and fully illustrated, and now includes a section on "Operations in a Private House," as to which the statement is made that "provided that the greatest care is exercised, there is no reason why as complete asepsis should not be secured in the patient's room as in the most elaborately fitted hospital theatre."

This may be true, but as it is added that "it is in the first place essential that the house be in a perfectly sanitary condition, and as it appears to be an article of the householder's faith that the hygienic state of his or her premises is exceptionally perfect, it is well that the building should be examined by a skilled person without the residential bias;" and that it is desirable that "the room should be quiet, light, and well ventilated," that its windows look toward the south; that it should not be near a water-closet; should have an open fireplace, and should have as little gas burned in it as possible, it is apparent that the author practically shares the widespread prejudice of surgeons in this country against operations in private houses.

In Chapter IV., the directions for the sterilization of sponges by formaldehyde—misprinted "formal aldehyde"—would seem unnecessary in view of the almost universal preference—which the author shares—for gauze pads.

The omission of the page devoted to an explanation of the abandonment of the steam spray marks one of the milestones in the advance of antiseptic technique. It seems now as if long before 1891—the date of the first edition—the "fort mit dem spray" of the German surgeons had been accepted everywhere.

In Chapter V. a little concession to "blunt dissection" is noticeable, and the teaching seems more in accord with the practice of to-day than the earlier and practically absolute prohibition of such dissection.

On page 71 we note one of the few misprints that we have noticed, viz., "gauge drain" for "gauze drain."

In Chapter VI. the most important addition is found in a paragraph which indicates a change in the methods of wound treatment, and expresses unqualified preference for the practice of keeping the wound absolutely dry from beginning to end. "Micro-organisms cannot grow without moisture, and moist dressings and washing of the wound provide this medium." The details of treatment of an abdominal incision are given, and the author adds: "In my experience no method of dealing with wounds has given such uniformly successful results as this."

In Part II., dealing with the Ligature of Arteries, the previous unqualified opinion that "the best ligature material on the whole is chromicized catgut" has become: "There is considerable choice in the form of ligature used. . . . Kangaroo tendon, catgut, and soft silk of medium thickness may all be recommended."

The author's opinion in favor of the intraperitoneal ligation of the common iliac has been strengthened by further experience. He adds a quotation from Mr. Makins' article on that subject calling attention to the greater anatomical difficulties that surround the ligation of the left common iliac as compared with the operation on the right side.

In Part III., as an addendum to the article on Meckel's ganglion, Mr. Hutchinson—the co-editor of this edition—says: "It is possible that an intracranial resection of the superior maxillary trunk—performed in a similar way to removal of the Gasserian ganglion—may prove to give more lasting results than the operations described."

The article on the Excision of the Gasserian ganglion has been much expanded and the positive statement that "excision of the ganglion by the temporal route is by far the best method, as it offers a good prospect of permanent cure, and leaves hardly any deformity of the face," is fully justified by the experience of the last few years. The omission of Cushing's method is accounted for (apparently by the co-editor) with the statement that "it is largely a return to the old pterygoid route, involves division of the zygoma, and appears to have nothing to recommend it." Cushing's method is, however, not largely a return to the pterygoid route, and, in the opinion of many surgeons who have employed it, has very much to recommend it. The division of the zygoma is perhaps the least essential part of the method.

In the admirable section on Amputations the only addition to the statistics that we have noticed is a paragraph giving the result of ninety-four major amputations at the London Hospital from 1890 to 1900, with eleven deaths (Mr. Hutchinson). A wider survey of operative results in these cases during this important decade would, we believe, have been of interest and value, although this is not meant in criticism of the mortality (12 per cent.) in this series, which is very creditable.

In the chapter on Interscapulothoracic Amputations no mention is made of the desirability, in some cases of malignant disease, of removing the entire clavicle instead of only the outer two-thirds (Le Conte).

In amputation of the leg the old term as to the "place of election" —a point "about a hand's breadth below the knee-joint"—is employed, although, in this country at least, the point of election has, with the improvement of prosthetic apparatus, descended at least to the junction of the lower and middle thirds of the tibia. No mention is made of an operation now in favor with many American surgeons, in which the tibia is sawn twice, so as to secure a periosteal flap without disturbing the relations of vessels, nerves, and muscles, and so as to prevent the adhesion of the latter to the bone and minimize bone atrophy. It is warmly recommended (Matas, White) and has stood the test of experience.

In the section on Ununited Fracture it is correctly said that "as a practical measure the wire is a delusion and a snare, so far, certainly, as the long bones are concerned;" but when it is added that "the various forms of apparatus in which plates of metal are secured (outside the skin) to the fractured bone by long screws" are "equally fallacious and more dangerous," it would seem impossible to American surgeons that the author—or the co-editor—could be practically familiar with the ingenious Parkhill bone-clamp, here universally regarded as the best of all mechanical devices for securing fixation of the fragments of the long bones after resection of their ends in cases of non-union. The published results obtained in this country amply demonstrate both its safety and its utility.

Volume II. shows fewer alterations or additions. The excellent section on Plastic Surgery remains largely unchanged.

We found no mention of intubation of the larynx in croup or diphtheria. The value of this procedure has been sufficiently demonstrated to justify its inclusion in a work of this comprehensive character, while it can scarcely be dismissed, as might catheterism, as belonging rather to the field of minor surgery.

In describing the operations for hypospadias it would seem as though less space might be given to the elaborate description and illustration of Duplay's and Anger's operations, and more to the very excellent method of Wood, which is criticised, it would seem, on theoretical grounds, and not as a result of practical experience. In the writer's hands the preputial integument has yielded most satisfactory results when used to form the principal flap in this operation, and no trouble has been experienced with "œdema of the lax subcutaneous layer."

A word of caution has been inserted in regard to the term "complete excision" in describing thyroidectomy, attention being called to the absolute necessity of leaving behind some portion of the thyroid gland in all such operations.

In dealing with the surgical accident of the entrance of air into divided veins, the immediate treatment by filling the wound with fluid and expressing air from the chest by direct pressure is described, and the suggestion that air should be sucked out of the right auricle by a catheter passed into the heart is very properly spoken of as "preposterous." When, however, the author adds, "the advice given in nearly every text-book that artificial respiration should be resorted to is almost as silly; there is not too little air in the thorax, but too much," he does not seem to realize that the forcible compression of the thorax to expel the air is only a form of artificial respiration; that the pulmonary circulation must be re-established because otherwise the left heart remains collapsed from want of blood; and that artificial respiration offers the best means of meeting this tremendously urgent indication.

In the chapter on Abdominal Section a useful summary of the arterial supply of the abdominal wall has been added. The statement that the ileocæcal valve corresponds to the spinoumbilical line and that the root of the appendix will be placed more than one inch lower down, and perhaps internally to it, is of interest, but cannot be regarded as demonstrated by the researches of Dr. Keith, to which the writer alludes, and which at present lack confirmation, as does the further statement that the ileocæcal valve in a normal person is usually tender to pressure. The practical importance of the matter is obvious; there are reasons for believing that it is a fact and that it serves to explain some of the too frequent cases in which tenderness elicited by pressure in this region has constituted the chief indication for operation which has revealed a normal appendix.

In addition to the chapter on the Operative Treatment of Enlarged Prostate, the author—or the co-editor—says that castration and vasectomy in this condition "have been practically abandoned." Mr. Reginald Harrison has reported 100 cases of vasectomy, in every one of which some degree of improvement resulted; and Rovsing, of Copenhagen, has recently (1902) reported 40 cases, of which 27 were cured, 9 relieved, and 4 unimproved. There were no deaths, and he adds, "I should, under no circumstances, feel myself justified in undertaking the total extirpation of the prostate in a patient in whom I had not done a vasectomy, which, in many cases, gives such extraordinary relief." The operations in question have certainly not yet reached their ultimate position in the estimation of the profession. It may be that they will be entirely discarded, but it would seem as though after the expiration of the inevitable period of indiscriminate employment of a novelty (of which Treves has himself complained in relation to the appendix) there would still be a restricted field of usefulness for them remaining; and that the statement that the operations are now practically abandoned is not fully borne out by the facts while men of the professional position of Harrison and Rovsing are still using them.

In the preliminary remarks upon operations on the kidney no mention is made of the two layers of the fat surrounding the kidney (Gerota), recognition of which is of practical value in approaching that organ during an operation.

In describing abnormalities of the kidney, Mr. Morris' more recent figures have not been given; they would, for example, increase the cases of absence or extreme atrophy of one kidney from 1 in 4000 to 1 in 2400 cases. The remaining statistics on this subject are similarly incorrect.

These are all, however, minor matters. The book, as a whole, has not yet been supplanted or replaced by any other single work on the subject in respect to the excellent average judgment that has been displayed in the difficult task of selecting from among thousands of varying procedures those most worthy of description, and in respect also to the simple, clear, straightforward manner in which the information thus gathered has been conveyed to the reader.

J. W. W.

THE PRINCIPLES AND PRACTICE OF SURGERY: DESIGNED FOR STUDENTS AND PRACTITIONERS. Lippincott's New Medical Series. By GEORGE TULLY VAUGHAN, M.D., Assistant Surgeon-General, Public Health and Marine Hospital Service of the United States; Professor of the Principles and Practice of Surgery, Georgetown University. Philadelphia and London: J. B. Lippincott Co., 1903.

THE time has passed when it is possible for an author to present comprehensively in a small single volume the general surgery of to-day, and yet there is a constant demand for such books on the part of the medical student and the man engaged in the general practice of medicine. It was with the idea of supplying this demand that the present work was prepared. It offers to the reader a condensed, and in most respects a thoroughly satisfactory, presentation of general surgery. The book is quite readable and comprehensive as far as possible in its limited space. It possesses, as such books always do, its points of weakness as well as its points of strength.

In our opinion the chapter on Anæsthetics is distinctly weak, since we feel that this is a subject so little taught in our medical schools that when the student turns to his text-book he should be able to find there all the necessary information regarding anæsthetics, and particularly as regards the method of their administration. The author speaks of bromide of ethyl as a general anæsthetic, although this agent is but little used at present, but he makes no mention whatever of chloride of ethyl, which is being so extensively employed for short operations and as a preliminary anæsthetic to ether. We think also that in the chapter on Fractures too little stress is laid upon the necessity of massage and movement, and particularly is this omission noticeable in the discussion of fractures of the lower end of the radius. We heartily approve of the author's teaching as regards the treatment of strangulated hernia, though we believe that, whenever possible in operating for this condition, a radical cure should be sought rather than the simple reduction of the hernia by the older methods of performing herniotomy. The chapters dealing with Genito-urinary Diseases are more complete than is usually found in single-volume text-books on general surgery.

A general criticism which we feel we must make of this work is the fact that the author has devoted too much space to the older methods of treatment and too little to recent and generally accepted methods, although it is possible that this is wiser in a work intended chiefly for students and general practitioners.

The illustrations are many of them old, although there are also many reproductions of interesting photographs. G.

A Portfolio of Dermochromes. By Professor Jacobi, of Freiberg im Breslau. English adaptation of the text by J. J. Pringle, M.B., F.R.C.P., Physician to the Department for Diseases of the Skin at the Middlesex Hospital, London. London: Rebman, Limited, 1903.

The portraits in this atlas, as in a recent French one, have been made entirely after models, the great majority after those in Neisser's collection at Breslau, the remainder after models in the collections of Lassar and Lesser, of Berlin; Hennig, of Vienna and Baretta, of Paris. A new color-printing process, called *citochromy*, has been employed in their production, for which is claimed absolute accuracy in the reproduction of colors. While the claim of *absolute* accuracy is hardly justified, the appearance of these portraits indicates that the process is much in advance of any of those hitherto employed; we have rarely, if ever, seen more accurately colored pictures of diseases of the skin. The two parts of the atlas thus far published contain 78 portraits on 42 plates, the diseases represented being for the most part selected from among the commoner affections of the skin. The more important and interesting rarer diseases, however, are not omitted, there being excellent portraits of Raynaud's disease, actinomycosis, and anthrax.

Among the plates which especially deserve notice on account of their excellence are those representing various forms of psoriasis, particularly psoriasis gyrata, lupus vulgaris, lupus erythematosus, pityriasis rosea, pityriasis rubra pilaris, and the exanthemata. Two portraits, one representing variola, the other varicella in the adult, are very instructively placed side by side on the same plate. The portrait of scarlatina is most accurate in coloring, but measles is not so successfully represented.

And just here seems the place to say that we have frequently wondered why portraits of the exanthemata do not find a place in *every* atlas of diseases of the skin, since in no class of affections do blunders in diagnosis occur more frequently and result more disastrously.

As the atlas is not designed by its author to take the place of a text-book, the text is considerably condensed. The symptoms of the various diseases portrayed are succinctly and clearly given together with a brief outline of the diagnosis and treatment.

While portraits and models, however well made, can never altogether replace the study of the living subject, portraits as accurate in drawing and coloring as these make very efficient substitutes, and must prove of the greatest service in the recognition of diseases of the skin to those whose clinical opportunities are limited.

M. B. H.

A Text-book of Pathology. By Alfred Stengel, M.D., Professor of Clinical Medicine in the University of Pennsylvania; Physician to the Philadelphia Hospital; Physician to the Pennsylvania Hospital. Fourth edition, thoroughly revised. Philadelphia, New York, and London: W. B. Saunders & Co., 1903.

That pathology and clinical medicine are intimately related is shown by the fact that one so widely known as a clinician should be so widely read as a pathologist. The usefulness and popularity of this book, especially to the practitioner, is evident when one considers that four editions have been called for within a period of five years. The book is so well known to pathologists in general that a detailed description is unnecessary. In the present edition numerous revisions and additions have been made, notably in the sections upon typhoid fever, tuberculosis, yellow fever, dysentery, and in the discussions upon diseases of the blood. A short account is given of the latest theories of immunity. In many places the results of the most recent researches in pathology are alluded to, but, as in the earlier editions, references are intentionally omitted. A very wide range of subjects is dealt with and throughout the book special attention has been paid to physiological pathology. In this respect and in many other ways the book is essentially a clinical pathology. An appendix has been added in which one finds a description of the generally accepted methods of pathological and bacteriological technique, and the book justifies in every detail the position which was accorded the former editions. W. T. L.

MANUAL OF THE DISEASES OF THE EYE. FOR STUDENTS AND GENERAL PRACTITIONERS. By CHARLES H. MAY, M.D., Chief of Clinic and Instructor in Ophthalmology, College of Physicians and Surgeons, Medical Department, Columbia University, New York, 1890–1903; Ophthalmic Surgeon to the French Hospital, New York; Consulting Ophthalmologist to the Red Cross Hospital, New York; Adjunct Ophthalmic Surgeon to Mt. Sinai Hospital, New York, etc. Third edition, revised, with 275 original illustrations, including 16 plates, with 36 colored figures. New York: William Wood & Co., 1903.

THIS work contains a clear and terse account of the present state of ophthalmology, so far as this is possible in a book of its size. The reader is never left in doubt as to the writer's meaning. It is easy reading, and we know upon the authority of a famous writer that "easy reading is—hard writing." The author has succeeded in saying enough and not too much, which, as he rightly states in the preface, is the "great difficulty in preparing a book of this sort." Sanity of view characterizes it throughout. One would have to make a somewhat minute search to discover opinions opposed to views now generally held by practical ophthalmologists. We are somewhat surprised at the very little stress laid upon the salts of silver in the treatment of purulent ophthalmia.

This is one of the few books which recognizes that a portion of the accommodation must be kept in reserve during near work, but under the directions for prescribing glasses for presbyopia we do not find that the author is consistent therewith. He subtracts the total accommodation from the amount required for near work and makes good the deficit by glass, allowing no part of the accommodation to be held in reserve.

A high place (but not too high) is given retinoscopy as an objective test of refraction. In competent hands this is unquestionably the most accurate objective method known, rivalling the best results obtainable by the subjective method under the most favorable conditions. In certain cases it is the only reliable method of determining the refraction. The ophthalmometer is accorded its proper subordinate position in the statement that "it is of service when used in connection with other tests." A mydriatic is recommended in all cases of children and young adults in estimating the refraction. Homatropine is declared to be "*sufficient for all practical purposes*," an opinion with which the reviewer entirely concurs from daily experience.

We note with satisfaction that heterophoria is relegated to a very subordinate place, as in our opinion it deserves. We think that more than enough is granted when neurasthenia, disturbances of digestion and nutrition are set down as possible results of muscular error, even in predisposed individuals; operation is only recommended as a last resort. Disappointment and aggravation of symptoms are truly stated to frequently follow this treatment. The author evidently has little belief in partial tenotomies and advancements. T. B. S.

MANUAL OF MEDICINE. By THOMAS KIRKPATRICK MONRO, M.A., M.D., Fellow of and Examiner to the Faculty of Physicians and Surgeons, Glasgow; Physician to Glasgow Royal Infirmary and Professor of Medicine in St. Mungo's College; formerly Examiner in the University of Glasgow and Pathologist to the Victoria Infirmary. Philadelphia and New York: W. B. Saunders & Co. London: Baillière, Tindall & Cox.

DR. MONRO's book should serve admirably the purpose for which it is primarily intended: that of a text-book for students. He has accomplished successfully the difficult task of condensing into a volume of moderate size the enormous mass of facts which makes up our present knowledge of internal medicine. The work throughout shows painstaking care in the classification and arrangement of these facts and in their concise and lucid presentation.

In arrangement it does not differ materially from the usual plan of the larger treatises. The space has been judiciously divided, and each section receives its due consideration. This same sense of proportion is seen also in the space allotted to the individual diseases and to their subdivisions of etiology, morbid anatomy, symptomatology, diagnosis, and treatment.

The value of the book to students is considerably increased by the prefacing of most of the sections with introductory chapters upon the topographical anatomy, general symptomatology, and methods of examination of the subject in hand.

The section on Diseases of the Nervous System merits especial commendation for its completeness and for the clearness with which the subject is treated.

Somewhat less full and satisfactory are the chapters upon Diseases of the Stomach. For some reason the subject of Hemorrhage from the Stomach is not considered, although a corresponding chapter appears under Diseases of the Intestines. The somewhat surprising statement is met that epithelioma is one of the four anatomical types of cancer of the stomach!

In addition to the sections usually found in text-books on medicine there is a short but adequate one on Diseases of the Skin.

L. A. C.

A Surgical Hand-book for the Use of Students, Practitioners, House Surgeons, and Dressers. By Francis A. Caird, M.B., F.R.C.S. Ed.; Assistant Surgeon, Royal Infirmary, Edinburgh; and Charles W. Cathcart, M.B., F.R.C.S. Eng. and Ed., Surgeon Royal Infirmary, Edinburgh. With very numerous illustrations. Twelfth edition. London: Charles Griffin & Co., Limited. Chicago: W. T. Keener & Co., 1903.

As the authors say in their preface, they have endeavored to make this little work of some three hundred pages as practical as possible and as thoroughly in keeping with modern surgical methods as the size of the volume will permit. The mere fact that it is in its twelfth edition is a warrant as to its popularity, at least on the other side of the water. In this edition a number of methods of treatment which are now seldom used have been dropped, and instead have been inserted accounts of the latest technique. It is really worthy of note the amount of useful information the authors have been able to put in such a small book, preserving at the same time the necessary clearness of description.

All minor surgical operations are fully covered and many major ones, while the chapters on dressings afterward and emergency work are most admirable. The illustrations are mostly woodcuts and are diagrammatic, but are clear and show well what is intended. They are very numerous. Special chapters on Surgical Electricity, Massage, Urine Examination, and Post-mortems seem a little out of place in a work of this character, but are well written and of interest. Written, as it is, as an aid to hospital internes and students, it is excellent and to be highly commended.

G. M.'C.

THE MEDICAL EPITOME SERIES. ANATOMY: A MANUAL FOR STUDENTS AND PRACTITIONERS. By HENRY E. HALE, A.M., M.D., Assistant Demonstrator of Anatomy, College of Physicians and Surgeons, Columbia University, in the city of New York. Series edited by V. C. PEDERSEN, A.M., M.D. Illustrated with 71 engravings. Philadelphia and New York: Lea Brothers & Co., 1903.

THE books of this series are designed by the editor to represent more than the mere quiz compends—to be, in fact, brief manuals of condensed useful information on their respective subjects.

They have, however, for quiz purposes, a list of questions at the end of each general division which serves rather as a guide to the quiz-master than to furnish him actual questions and answers, as is often done, and in which case the continuity of the text is interrupted. This work on Anatomy is clear, concise, and presents more than the mere essentials of human anatomy. It is well written and well printed, while the illustrations are most excellent—far better than those usually seen in short works of this character—and the explanatory notes are clear and well adapted to show the desired point. It is a very good and useful little book. G. M. C.

A TEXT-BOOK UPON THE PATHOGENIC BACTERIA. FOR STUDENTS OF MEDICINE AND PHYSICIANS. By JOSEPH MCFARLAND, M.D., Fourth edition, rewritten and enlarged. Philadelphia, New York, and London: W. B. Saunders & Co., 1903.

DURING the five years which have passed since the last revision of Dr. McFarland's book much new material has been collected, and the present edition shows the care with which this material has been added and welded into the text. The many references to literature give the book a certain value. The subjects of infection and immunity have been expanded at some length and in places detailed descriptions are given of recent work along these lines of investigation. The chapters upon the pathogenic bacteria are arranged under four main heads: (*a*) "Phlogistic Diseases," including "Acute Infective Inflammations" and "Chronic Inflammatory Diseases;" (*b*) "Toxæmias;" (c) "Bacteremias" and "Miscellaneous Diseases." Each chapter represents a consideration of the disease or pathological processes caused by that organism, as well as a description of the organism itself. When necessary, closely allied bacteria are also discussed. Since the book deals simply with bacteria, the parasites and protozoa are necessarily omitted. Revisions and additions have been made in various portions of the text, and the present edition will perhaps attract even more attention than the previous ones. W. T. L.

PROGRESS

OF

MEDICAL SCIENCE.

MEDICINE.

UNDER THE CHARGE OF

WILLIAM OSLER, M.D.,

PROFESSOR OF MEDICINE, JOHNS HOPKINS UNIVERSITY, BALTIMORE, MARYLAND,

AND

W. S. THAYER, M.D.,

ASSOCIATE PROFESSOR OF MEDICINE, JOHNS HOPKINS UNIVERSITY, BALTIMORE, MARYLAND.

Ochronosis: The Pigmentation of Cartilages, Sclerotics, and Skin in Alkaptonuria.—OSLER (*Lancet*, January 2, 1904, p. 10) reports two cases of ochronosis in patients also suffering from alkaptonuria. This rare condition was first described and named by Virchow in 1866. A man, aged sixty-seven years, died of aneurysm, and at autopsy it was found that there was a remarkable blackening of the cartilages of the whole body. The color was coal black, not ochre-colored or yellow. It was more than an ordinary melanosis. Previous to Osler's two cases there have been only seven instances reported in the literature. Two of these cases had melanuria, and in one of them it was definitely stated that the patient did not have alkaptonuria. The seventh case was reported by H. Albrecht in 1902, and to him is due the credit of first suggesting the association of the condition with alkaptonuria. The urine of his case was dark-colored and reduced copper-sulphate solution, but no homogentisic acid was definitely demonstrated in it. The necropsy in this case showed a general ochronosis. A point of special interest was the gray-blue color of the inner part of the ears, as if due to dilated veins.

Osler's two cases of ochronosis are of especial interest in that the condition was recognized clinically, owing to the pigmentation of the sclerotics and cartilages of the ears, and in one by a remarkable ebony-black discoloration of the skin of the nose and cheeks. Both of these cases had previously been reported as instances of alkaptonuria, the urine of both showing all the features characteristic of this anomaly. The two pa i s were brothers. The first is a man, aged fifty-seven years, and thenpigmentation now presents the following distribution: The exposed portion of the sclerotics of both eyes show areas of deep-black pigmentation. The cartilages of both ears, particularly the concha and antihelix, exhibit a remarkable blue-black discoloration. Of particular interest in this case is the fact that over the nose and cheeks there is a butterfly-shaped area of black pigmentation of the skin. The pigmentation closely simulates the appearance of powder marks. The involvement of the skin has not been previously recorded. The pigmentation had been observed for eight years and it had gradually deepened. The other brother, aged forty-nine years, presented similar pigmentation of the sclerotics and ears, although in a less marked degree. He recently died of some cardiac affection, but no autopsy was obtained. Both patients had had alkaptonuria for many years, and there was no question but that the pigmentation was that of ochronosis. Alkaptonuria heretofore had been recognized clinically only by the urinary changes. These observations leave little doubt that ochronosis is a part of the malady. At least one of the previously reported cases of ochronosis was proven not to be an alkaptonuric, and A. E. Garrod suggests that there may be two distinct classes of the condition.

Multiple Myeloma (Myelomatosis) with Bence-Jones Proteid in the Urine (Myelopathic Albumosuria of Bradshaw, Kahler's Disease).—F. Parkes Weber (*Journal of Pathology and Bacteriology*, December, 1903, p. 173) reports a case of albumosuria in association with multiple myelomata. The patient was a man, aged fifty years, with a definite luetic history. He complained of pain in his loins and of stiffness in the small joints of his hands. Later the upper part of his back began to bend, so that he always stooped. There were no localized outgrowths projecting from the bones, as has been observed in many of the cases reported. The urine contained the so-called Bence-Jones bodies. It coagulated at about 58° C., at a temperature much lower than ordinary albumin does; the precipitate almost completely dissolved on raising the urine to the boiling-point, and completely on adding acetic acid, and reappeared on cooling. An interesting feature was the fact that the proteid was occasionally precipitated spontaneously and caused the urine to be turbid when freshly voided. The autopsy showed that there were no localized bone tumors, but that there was a diffuse myelomatous involvement of the marrow of all the bones examined. There was a chronic ulcer of the duodenum, which has led to a severe hemorrhage, causing death.

The presence in the tumor cells of certain granules and globules of various sizes constituted a striking histological feature in the case. Prof. R. Muir, of Glasgow, who examined the growth, expressed his opinion as follows: "That the tumor is formed by a special and characteristic type of cell, which is probably derived either from the neutrophilic myelocyte or its predecessor; that the cell produces in its protoplasm, in a granular form, a substance which is closely allied to, though not quite identical with, the substance of the neutrophile granules; and that this substance is formed in excess and may form larger granules by confluence of the smaller, the larger globules sometimes becoming free."

The nature of the Bence-Jones bodies is considered at some length. The view advanced by Magnus-Levy, that it is a non-assimilated digestive proteid, is opposed, because in this case alteration of the diet had no effect on the excretion of the albumose, and as much was eliminated during the night as during the day. The view that this proteid is produced in the bone-marrow is supported, and the suggestion is thrown out that the curious granules found in the specific cells of the tumor may possibly be its source.

Weber has collected the cases of Bence-Jones' albumosuria from the literature, and finds that, including his own, there have been thirty-five undoubted instances recorded. In addition to these there were four doubtful cases.

Family Diabetes.—Martinet (*La presse médicale*, February 10, 1904, p. 94) reports that in June, 1900, a man, aged forty-eight years, consulted him for symptoms which proved to be those of diabetes mellitus. The disease had followed an attack of influenza contracted in the previous February. The patient's father had died of diabetes also.

Several months later the writer was consulted by the patient's wife, a woman aged forty years. She was found to have exophthalmic goitre. The examination of the urine showed a large amount of sugar present. Martinet considers this a typical case of *conjugal diabetes*, although some objection might be taken to this opinion, owing to the not infrequent occurrence of glycosuria in exophthalmic goitre. He states that he observed four cases of conjugal diabetes in his practice during the year 1903, and does not believe that the condition is extremely rare.

At the beginning of this year the mother of the first patient, aged sixty-six years, came under treatment for a phlegmon on the right hand, which developed very rapidly after being pricked with a needle. The examination of this patient's urine also showed abundance of sugar. She lived with her son.

In this family the patient, his mother, and his wife had diabetes and his father died of the disease. The writer lays down the following axiom: If one discovers diabetes in one or several members of a family, the urine of all the other members should be examined for sugar, especially if the various members live together.

The Reactions of the Blood in Diabetes Mellitus: A Contribution to Our Knowledge of the Thermolabile Complements.—Sweet (*Journal of Medical Research*, October, 1903, p. 255) carried out a series of experiments with the view of ascertaining, if possible, the cause of the abnormal susceptibility of diabetes to infectious processes. The experiments were made on the blood of dogs rendered diabetic by the extirpation of the pancreas. The washed red cells of guinea-pigs and rabbits were used for testing the hæmolytic activity of diabetic dogs' serum. His experiments seem to afford the first adequate explanation for the frequency of infections in diabetes mellitus.

The writer's more important results may be summarized as follows: The complete removal of the pancreas from dogs, which causes a true diabetes mellitus of a severe type, is followed by a marked decrease of the hæmolytic activity of the diabetic dog's serum for both rabbit's and guinea-pig's erythrocytes. The diabetes caused by the complete extirpation of the pancreas is further characterized by what is to be interpreted as a complete loss of the normal bactericidal property of the serum of the dog. This he demonstrated conclusively for *B. coli communis*, *B. typhi abdominalis*, and for *B. dysenteriæ*. The demonstration of the decrease of bactericidal power of the diabetic serum for *staphylococcus pyogenes aureus* was not so conclusive, for the reason that the normal serum of the dog has very little if any bactericidal effect upon this organism. The decrease of the hæmolytic activity of the serum of the diabetic dog is due to loss of hæmolytic complements. The loss of bactericidal power is, from analogy with the hæmolytic phenomenon, doubtless to be interpreted as due to a loss of bacteriolytic complements. The complete removal of the pancreas is as necessary to this loss of complements as it is to the production of a diabetes. The complete removal of the pancreas does not deprive the organism of its power to react to the inflammatory process by an increase of the complementary substances. The loss of the complementary substances in diabetes melli us points conclusively to the fact that no relation exists between the leukocytes of any type and the production of the complements.

SURGERY.

UNDER THE CHARGE OF

J. WILLIAM WHITE, M.D.,

JOHN RHEA BARTON PROFESSOR OF SURGERY IN THE UNIVERSITY OF PENNSYLVANIA; SURGEON TO THE UNIVERSITY HOSPITAL,

AND

F. D. PATTERSON, M.D.,

SURGEON TO THE X-RAY DEPARTMENT OF THE HOWARD HOSPITAL; CLINICAL ASSISTANT TO THE OUT-PATIENT SURGICAL DEPARTMENT OF THE JEFFERSON HOSPITAL.

On the Use of Rubber and Thread Gloves.—GOEPEL (*Centralblatt für Chirurgie*, 1903, No. 42) states that in view of the fact that rubber gloves tear very easily and that thread gloves are very permeable, it is a good procedure to wear the latter over the former, which not only prevents the slipping of instruments, etc., but also has the following advantages: 1. It is a greater safeguard against infection, either of the patient by the operator or *vice versa*. 2. The hands can be used more freely and easily. 3. The gloves can be rapidly changed should necessity require. 4. The use of the thread glove does quite away with the slipperyness of the rubber, and so ligatures may be tied more easily and securely. 5. The thread gloves can be easily removed in any case where their roughness might injure the tissue and then be replaced when the danger is passed. 6. The time of the operation is shortened. 7. By their use repeated washing of the hands becomes unnecessary, as the gloves can be scrubbed while on the operator's hand, and this prevents chapping or eczema in those cases where the hands are very sensitive.

Three Cases of Rupture of the Intestines without External Lesion.—SENEREANO (*Bull. et mém. de la Soc. de chir. de Bucharest*, 1903, Nos. 3 and 4) states that during the past year he has had three such cases present themselves for treatment, respectively, twelve hours, twenty-four hours, and thirty-eight hours after the receipt of the injury. The first patient had an old and reducible right-sided hernia, and gave a history of having received a sharp blow in the right iliac fossa. He entered the hospital on the next day, and in the afternoon was given a purgative. The next day he was in a very grave condition, presenting the symptoms of an intestinal lesion, but nothing characteristic. An exploratory incision was made as for hernia or appendicitis; the hernial sac was found empty and there was no strangulated intestine. The incision was then enlarged, the cæcum and appendix were found to be normal, but the entire abdominal cavity was filled with intestinal contents, and 25 cm. from the cæcum was a perforation which admitted the little finger. This was closed, thorough lavage of the abdominal cavity was then performed and the wound closed; the patient made a good recovery. The second case had an old and reducible hernia upon the left side. He was kicked in the abdomen by a horse and twenty-four hours later was admitted to the hospital. Upon operation on the third day, it was found that there was a perforation of the small intestine, and that the abdominal cavity was filled with intestinal contents. The perforation was closed, the abdominal cavity irrigated, and then the wound closed. The patient recovered. The third patient had no hernia, but had received a blow upon the abdomen, which was opened in the median line. Two perforations were found near the cæcum about 8 cm. apart. They were closed and the abdomen washed out. This patient also made a good recovery.

Actinomycosis of the Liver.—Auvray (*Revue de chir.*, 1903, No. 7), after an admirable and exhaustive review of the subject, states that medical treatment by the iodide of potassium has proven to be of no value in these cases. Although the number of cases is small, still, it may be well said that this treatment has been followed by good results when the disease is localized elsewhere, and in every case it would seem to be a valuable adjunct of the surgical treatment. The author reports the surgical treatment of six cases in which the liver was involved, but it is to be regretted that some of these reports are quite incomplete as regards the exact operative procedure in the individual case. These cases all presented some form of abscess, and there are three ways of reaching and evacuating such a purulent collection: 1. By way of the abdomen, the usual method. 2. The thoracic route. 3. The lumbar route. In four of the cases the abscess was opened through the abdomen, in some the operation merely consisted in a simple incision of the abdominal wall, while in others a formal laparotomy was necessary, with a resection of the ribs in an effort to discover the exact point of the infection. The only complication during these operations was in one case in which there was an abundant hemorrhage. The lumbar route was used in only one case; the incision was made parallel to the last rib, and then the abscess was punctured with a trocar and evacuated. The thoracic route was followed in one case without a previous resection of the ribs. These six cases were all eventually fatal, but not as the result of the operative interference; the results might have been better had the operations been performed earlier—in other words, before the formation of an abscess.

Suture of the Patella: A Practical Study Based upon Seventy Operations.—Lucas-Championniere (*Archives internationales de chirurgie*, 1903, No. 1) states that the first antiseptic operation of suturing of the patella was performed by Cameron, of Glasgow, in

1877. At this time Lister also reported his first case, and in 1883 he was able to note six more, and clearly showed that this new method of treatment was followed by a perfect recovery, whereas in the past the condition had been looked upon as being of necessity followed by lameness. In view of the fact that fracture of the patella is comparatively rare, the author's experience of seventy cases is quite remarkable. A study of these cases shows that the only rational method of treatment is a free incision of the joint; the evacuation of its morbid contents, such as blood; the accurate apposition of the fragments by suture, and then the repair of the torn synovial membrane, and this is the only way in which good union can be secured. The best suture material is silver wire, which is in itself antiseptic. Care should be taken to have absolute asepsis, and the joint should be thoroughly flushed out with a 5 per cent. solution of carbolic acid. The best time to operate is either two, three, or four days after the accident, and not within the first twenty-four hours. The wound should be drained for four days, and there should be passive motion at each dressing. The patient should be allowed to walk in from ten to fifteen days. In conclusion, the author reports in detail many of the more interesting and complicated cases of the series.

THERAPEUTICS.

UNDER THE CHARGE OF

REYNOLD WEBB WILCOX, M.D., LL.D.,

PROFESSOR OF MEDICINE AND THERAPEUTICS AT THE NEW YORK POST-GRADUATE MEDICAL SCHOOL AND HOSPITAL; VISITING PHYSICIAN TO ST. MARK'S HOSPITAL.

Light Therapy.—DR. KELLERMANN considers that the use of dark-blue incandescent light produces excellent results when locally applied in neuralgia and eczema, and his statistics seem to prove his assertion. He also states that the treatment may be applied in leg ulcers. The duration of each treatment is not more than fifteen minutes and the number of sittings should not be more than four per week. He believes that the beneficent effect is due chiefly to the action of dry heat, and that the chemical or specific action of the light rays plays a very subordinate part in producing the result. His article contains a report of numerous cases which have undergone the treatment.—*Zentralblatt für die gesamte Thérapie*, 1904, No. 1. p. 16.

Serum Therapy in Plague.—DR. VICTOR GODINHO, in his plague service at the hospital in San Paulo, Brazil, has employed a serum made after the manner of the plague serum prepared at the Pasteur Institute, and reports upon its use as follows: The minimum dose injected was 150 c.c. to 200 c.c. When injected during the evolution of the disease no abortion of the malady took place and the buboes appeared as usual, but their pain was lessened and sudorific crises and defervescence by lysis were produced. Intravenous injections of 20 c.c. to 40 c.c. of the serum would cause a rise in temperature of a degree, followed by abundant perspiration and a fall of two or three degrees. In some patients it seemed as if the crisis of the disease was brought about by the serum, since the temperature fell and did not rise again after its use. Certain transitory symptoms, such as chill, agitation, dyspnœa, cyanosis, vomiting, etc., were caused by the injections. When administered before the third day of the disease the serum almost always brought about a cure in adults, but did not influence the development or the suppuration of the buboes. The course of the disease being much more violent in children makes it imperative that the serum should be used as early as possible. The occurrence and course of pneumonia as a complication did not seem to be influenced by the serum. Those suffering from the septicæmic form of the disease bore the serum well, but its good effects were less marked than in those affected with the bubonic type. Lastly, the serum did not prevent the termination of the disease by cachexia. In conclusion, the author states that the use of the serum, like that of diphtheria antitoxin, results favorably in certain cases, but not in all.—*La presse médicale*, 1904, No. 8, p. 60.

Suprarenal Opotherapy.—Dr. A. Goy states that in connection with this subject the following conclusions have been reached: 1. That the administration of the suprarenal extract slows the pulse by stimulating the pneumogastric. 2. That it strengthens the cardiac systole by direct stimulation of the heart muscle and by stimulation of the cardiac ganglia. 3. That it causes an increase in blood pressure due to contraction of the capillaries through stimulation of their vasomotor nerves and muscle fibres and by action upon the vasomotor centr . 4. That it blanches and causes an anæmia of the tissues. The primary therapeutic application of the extract is in Addison's disease and in the treatment of certain symptoms of suprarenal insufficiency. In Addison's disease in a short time the extract causes a diminution in the pigmentation and a rapid increase in body weight. In experimental physiology the extract has been employed as an intravenous injection as an heroic remedy in animals in chloroform syncope. An important consideration is that the preparation used should be of definite strength. —*Revue francaise de médecine et de chirurgie*, 1904, No. 3, p. 64.

The Treatment of Hepatic Colic.—The indications to be met in this condition are these: to relieve the pain; to bring about a favorable issue of the crisis by facilitating the passage of the calculus; to prevent complications. The pain may be relieved by the hypodermic use of morphine in connection with atropine. This latter should be most carefully given when there is tendency to collapse. To patients who bear morphine badly chloroform to the obstetrical degree may be given, or if there is no vomiting the following formula: Chloral hydrate, 2; syrup of peppermint, 30; chloroform-water, 100. Dose, two dessertspoonfuls every quarter-hour until relieved. When the stomach is intolerant the chloral may be given per rectum, thus: Chloral hydrate, 2 to 3 parts dissolved in 10 parts boiling water mixed with the yolk of an egg, to which mixture 1 part of wine of opium and 200 parts of milk are added. Ether and turpentine, on the one hand, and olive oil and glycerin, on the other, are the remedies most usually employed to facilitate the passag of the stone. The latter agents are preferable. The great difficulty is to overcome the repugnance of the patient to the olive oil. Toward this end the oil may be stirred up with a little beer, or to it may be added a little menthol or a few drops of essence of bitter almonds or anise. The quantity of the oil should be from four to eight ounces. Glycerin is more acceptable to the patient, but less effective. Finally, the spasm of the bile-ducts may be relieved by the application of hot-water bags to the abdomen. Of the complications of hepatic colic, the most formidable is heart-failure. To combat this it is wise to substitute for the atropine, so frequently given with the morphine, a heart stimulant, such as sparteine. Chloral should not be given where collapse is threatened, and in this juncture hypodermic injections of camphor in olive oil are useful. To prevent accidents to the biliary passages, we should avoid the use of purgatives and suspend food until the pain has ceased for several hours. Rupture of the bile-passages necessitates immediate surgical interference.—*Revue francaise de médecine et de chirurgie*, 1904, No. 5, p. 115.

Iodized Oil in Simple Goitre.—DR. DUBAR reports two cases of simple goitre in young girls which he has treated by injections of oil containing 40 per cent. of iodine. He injected very slowly at intervals of about one week fifteen drops of the oil into the substance of the gland. Each injection was made into a different part of the gland, and while in no case was there any unpleasant reaction, two or three of the injections were followed by the appearance of a small, firm node showing no signs of inflammation. These eventually disappeared. In one patient, after a series of nine injections, the size of the goitre was diminished by three-fourths of an inch. In the other six injections resulted in a diminution of nearly one inch, and a series of four more injections caused a total shrinkage of nearly an inch and one-half.—*Le progrès médicale*, 1904, No. 4, p. 50.

Sodium Bicarbonate in Gastropathies and Other Diseases.—M. HENRI HUCHARD, in a paper upon dyspepsia, deals at length with this therapeutic agent. In anorexia he believes it to be indicated in small doses (3 to 5 grains), since, taken a half-hour before eating, it increases gastric secretion and excites the contractility of the stomach. In this connection he considers it far preferable to the bitters. In hyperchlorhydria, since here we have an excess of gastric secretion, the drug should be prescribed in large dosage at the end of the period of digestion, at about the time when the gastralgia is likely to appear—that is to say, about two or three hours after the meal. In this condition the author gives 4 or 5 drachms daily of the salt for several weeks at a time, and finds no resulting evil effects; on the contrary, oxidation and metabolism are favored, and an increase in body weight often takes place. The gastric crises of tabes, when these are accompanied by hypochlorhydria, respond well to sodium bicarbonate given in doses of 5 drachms per day. Also the drug produces excellent results in the migrainiform affection termed nervous gastrotoxia. Undoubtedly, when the drug is given improperly, various bad effects may follow; even anæmia may be produced, but these results are not to be considered the fault of the alkali, but of the prescriber. Sodium bicarbonate is the remedy *par excellence* in diabetes, in the prevention of coma, which condition is characterized by a true acidæmia. The dosage in this disease should be at least 2.5 drachms daily, and where coma actually exists as large a quantity as 3 ounces may be given. In dermatoses, especially those of arthritic origin, alkaline medication has a distinct sphere, and in such conditions the bicarbonate is indicated in doses of 3 or 4 drachms per day. In biliary lithiasis and hepatic colic there is, in the author's experience, no surer method of cure than regular alkaline medication employed in massive doses.—*Revue de thérapeutique*, 1903, No. 2, p. 37.

The Treatment of Thrush.—DR. MERLETTI has found that the treatment of this affection by successive applications of hydrogen dioxide and sodium borate solutions is to be recommended. These two agents produce an abundant froth, which acts rapidly upon the *oïdium albicans*. The author has employed this procedure in a great number of cases, and is convinced that, when repeated three times every twenty-four hours, it will bring about a cure even in marked cases of the confluent type of the disease. If the treatment is instituted at the beginning of the affection two or three applications are sufficient to stop the growth of the fungus.—*Journal de médecine de Paris*, 1904, No. 4, p. 31.

OBSTETRICS.

UNDER THE CHARGE OF

EDWARD P. DAVIS, A.M., M.D.,

PROFESSOR OF OBSTETRICS IN THE JEFFERSON MEDICAL COLLEGE; PROFESSOR OF OBSTETRICS AND DISEASES OF INFANCY IN THE PHILADELPHIA POLYCLINIC; CLINICAL PROFESSOR OF DISEASES OF CHILDREN IN THE WOMAN'S MEDICAL COLLEGE; VISITING OBSTETRICIAN TO THE PHILADELPHIA HOSPITAL, ETC.

The Induction of Labor for Contracted Pelves.—In the *Archiv für Gynäkologie*, Band lxx., Heft 3, 1903, HAHL gives the result of 84 cases in the Obstetric clinic of Helsingfors in which labor was induced for contracted pelvis. His statistics cover the practice of the Clinic for thirty-two years and the cases occurred among 23,000 patients. The relative frequency of the operation was one in 274 confinements, or 0.365 per cent. In Leopold's clinic the operation was done once in 131 patients, and in a subsequent series of cases once in 151 patients. Braun's statistics give one in 441 patients; Chrobak one in 627; Pinard one in 150, and Walter one in 165.

The smallest true conjugate in these cases were 7 cm. in three and 7.5 cm. in one case, a flattened and symmetrically contracted pelvis. The earliest period of gestation at which pregnancy was interrupted was thirty weeks in one case, and the latest thirty-eight weeks in seven cases. The average was from the thirty-fifth to the thirty-sixth week.

In seven cases the fœtus was in a transverse position. This was corrected by version or spontaneous evolution. The complications which occurred during the labors were transverse presentation in 5 cases, breech presentation in 2, prolapse of the cord in 3, lateral placenta prævia in 1, and threatened rupture of the uterus in 1; 29.76 per cent. of the cases terminated in spontaneous birth; 70.24 per cent. required operation. Version was done most frequently and then forceps. Craniotomy was performed but twice, or 3.38 per cent.

The results of this series of cases were as follows: The maternal mortality was 2.38 per cent. from all causes. From septic infection alone the mortality was 1.19 per cent. The maternal morbidity was 7.23 per cent. Of the 84 children, 75 per cent. were born living and 25 per cent. were stillborn; 59.52 per cent. were discharged living from the hospital, while 13 of the 63 children born living died in the hospital during the first two weeks. Of the children who left the hospital living, 84 per cent. survived for a year, which was one-half the entire number of children born alive.

Mechanical Dilatation of the Cervix during Pregnancy and Labor.—DE SEIGNEUX (*Archiv für Gynäkologie*, 1903, Band lxx., Heft 3) criticizes Bossi's dilator because it has no pelvic curve, cannot be taken apart for cleansing, and cannot readily be shifted to vary the line of application of its force during its use. To correct these faults, he has invented an instrument resembling Bossi's in its general principles, having a pelvic curve and which can be taken apart for cleansing and whose branches are so placed upon the joints that they exercise force in various directions. He reports seven cases in which his instrument was used by himself and others with satisfaction.

Prolapse of the Placenta from its Normal Situation.—In the *Archiv für Gynäkologie*, 1903, Band lxx., Heft 3, KAYSER reviews extensively the literature of this subject. He finds in the records of the Clinic at Dresden no case of prolapse of the placenta recorded in 22,000 births. In the Clinic at the Charité there was recorded no case in 42,800 births. On examining the records, a case of version with bleeding is described which must have been a prolapse of the placenta. A few cases collected from the literature are quoted in which this accident happened.

His own case was that of a multipara, aged thirty-three years, who had a considerably contracted flattened pelvis. Eight hours after the rupture of the membranes, the head presenting, fetal heart sounds became much less frequent. On examination, the placenta was found presenting at the internal os, although formerly it could not be discovered. There was slight hemorrhage. Prolapse of the placenta was diagnosticated and version was performed, which was accompanied by a slight discharge of blood. The fœtus was not extracted, but was allowed to remain in the uterus in the hope that labor pains would come on. Fifteen hours after the performance of version the patient was found in collapse and shock. The cervix was incised. The body of the child was delivered with difficulty and the head was delivered by craniotomy. The patient died during the operation. Upon autopsy the attachment of the placenta had been at the fundus of the uterus. A transverse rupture of the uterus was found on the anterior wall of the cervix, while upon the right side was discovered a dermoid cyst. It was Kayser's belief that the rupture of the uterus occurred while an assistant made strong pressure upon the after-coming head in an effort to press it downward into the pelvis.

From the cases reported and from his own, Kayser deduces the following conclusions: In the presence of prolapse of the placenta with hemorrhage, delivery is imperative. A high degree of pelvic contraction forbids the performance of version. Embryotomy is usually indicated.

If hemorrhage be absent and the child be living, an effort should be made to save its life. Delivery should then be conducted in the manner least dangerous for mother and child. If the child is dead and the pelvic measurements are normal, immediate interference is unnecessary.

A Contribution to the Etiology, Symptomatology, and Treatment of Ectopic Gestation.—Runge (*Archiv für Gynäkologie*, 1903, Band lxx., Heft 3) reports 233 cases of ectopic gestation from the Charité and Polyclinic in Berlin. There were 125 cases of recognized pregnancy and 108 cases of hæmatocele. Among the cases of pregnancy, 73 were tubal abortions, 47 ruptures of the tube, and 5 intact tubal pregnancy. Among the unusual cases were one treated by posterior colpotomy in which the tube was removed with the ovary; one case of interstitial pregnancy; one case of ectopic gestation in which a living child was delivered by abdominal section, the child surviving and the mother afterward dying from purulent peritonitis, and one case of tubal abortion with suppuration.

So far as the results were concerned, from the 73 cases of abortion, 36 recovered without operation and 36 recovered after operation. One case died after operation. In 47 cases of rupture of the tube, five were treated without operation and recovered. Forty-two were operated upon, of whom 31 recovered and 11 died. This gives a mortality of 1.4 per cent. in tubal abortion, and 23.4 per cent. in ruptures of the tube. Eight of the deaths resulted through anæmia from hemorrhage and 3 from septic infection. In one case the cause of death could not be distinctly made out. The entire mortality for cases of rupture, excluding those dying upon the operating table, was 6.4 per cent.

In 108 cases of hæmatocele, 37 were treated by operation; 25 of these were done by incision through the posterior wall of the vagina. Seventy-one cases were treated without operation, and of these one died. This patient perished from purulent septic peritonitis. One patient died after operation from infection of the hæmatocele.

Runge's conclusions in the study of his cases are as follows: He believes that the principal causes for tubal gestation are infection during the puerperal period and gonorrhœa. It is, however, true that women who have not been previously pregnant are not exempt from ectopic gestation. A period of sterility in most cases precedes the period of ectopic gestation. Tubal abortion and rupture occur most frequently from the first to the third month of pregnancy. In these cases operation is to be undertaken when conditions threatening life arise, when the tumor increases rapidly in size, when the general condition of the patient grows worse and resorption of the tumor does not occur, and when the patient has long-continued fever. Abdominal section without drainage is best for these cases and the placenta and fetal sac should be removed entire if possible. Only those blood clots which can be readily reached should be removed unless the blood is decomposed and infected. In view of the risks of abdominal pregnancy, it is not well to wait until the child is viable.

Hæmatocele should, if possible, be treated without operation. The method of election is by incision of the posterior vaginal wall, abdominal section being reserved for those cases in which the tumor is large and in which it cannot safely be reached through the vagina.

The Morbidity of the Puerperal State in Cases Complicated by the Birth of a Macerated Fœtus.—KOTHEN (*Archiv für Gynäkologie*, 1903, Band lxx., Heft 3) reviews the literature of the subject, in which he has collected 358 cases of labor complicated by death and maceration of the fœtus. In 34 of these cases some complication arose during the puerperal period. A morbidity of about 10 per cent. was observed. The second series of 274 cases was observed, 157 of which made normal recoveries, although the fœtus had been considerably decomposed. Spiegelberg ascribed morbidity in these cases not to the death of the fœtus, but to outside contamination in the conduct of labor. Klein injected into animals an extract of the tissues and organs of a fœtus which perished about fourteen days before its birth. Two animals died after such injection. The symptoms of death were those of toxæmia, as the injected material was proved by culture to be sterile of bacteria.

Kothen's cases were 70 in the Clinic at Giessen. Fever was considered present when the patient's temperature rose above 99.5° F. at any time. In 14 of these cases, or 20 per cent., the temperature rose. In 27.1 per cent. some abnormality followed the birth of a macerated fœtus. In comparison with the general morbidity of other puerperal patients, the death and maceration of the fœtus increases the complications of the puerperal period by 10 or 11 per cent. In none of these cases was the death of the mother traceable to a macerated and dead condition of the fœtus.

Kothen concludes from a study of this subject that an increased morbidity of from 10 to 11 per cent. over the ordinary morbidity of labor and the puerperal state is observed in cases where the fœtus is macerated. A foul condition of the lochia is apt to be present in these cases.

GYNECOLOGY.

UNDER THE CHARGE OF

HENRY C. COE, M.D.,

OF NEW YORK.

ASSISTED BY

WILLIAM E. STUDDIFORD, M.D.

New Method of Ventrosuspension.—BARDESCU (*Zentralblatt für Gynäkologie*, 1904, No. 3) describes the following method of suspension of the uterus: The uterus is drawn upward with a volsellum after the separation of adhesions. An incision is made through the fascia and rectus muscle on either side of the wound, and each round ligament is seized in turn with a bullet-forceps and the loop is drawn through the opening and secured with four catgut sutures. The fascial edges are then united, after which the loops are sutured together in the median line. The patient is kept on her back for ten or twelve days, the urine being drawn by catheter until the third day.

Care should be taken not to elevate the fundus uteri above the symphysis, or to approximate it too closely to the abdominal wall, in order to preserve the normal relations and mobility of the organ.

Causes of Sterility.—In a discussion of this subject before the Dutch Gynecological Society (*Zentralblatt für Gynäkologie*, 1904, No. 3) KOUWER stated that in 700 private cases sterility was noted in 101, 11 being due to impotence in the husband. The speaker had been successful in treating less than one-half of the cases in which this was the main symptom for which relief was sought (24).

Treub had noted 39 cases out of 188 in which the husband was at fault. In 80 cases occurring in married women where the semen was examined, he found azoöspermia in 25 and oligozoöspermia in 12. The speaker said that he always examined the husband's semen if possible.

Lysol Poisoning.—HAMMER (*Münchener med. Wochenschrift*, 1903, No. 21) reports several cases in which intrauterine injections of lysol solution were followed by unpleasant results. From experiments on animals, he concluded that the use of strong solutions was not advisable. In a puerperal case fatal thrombosis occurred from the entrance of lysol into a vein (the strength of the solution was not stated).

Torsion of the Uterus.—PETIT (*Semaine gynécol.*, June 30, 1903) reports a case of laparotomy for severe dysmenorrhœa and menorrhagia in which adhesions confined to the left side of the pelvis had caused a half-turn of the uterus around its long axis from right to left, so that the right adnexa were situated behind the left broad ligament below a cystoma of the left ovary.

A New Method of Preventing Ventral Hernia.—NIKONOW (*Jour. akus. i Shenbolesnej; Zentralblatt für Gynäkologie*, 1904, No. 3) reports a series of cases in which the following procedure was adopted: In opening the abdomen an incision was made about two inches to one side of the median line. After opening the anterior layer of the sheath of the rectus, the muscle is separated by blunt dissection and is drawn outward so that the posterior layer and peritoneum can be incised in the median line.

At the close of the operation the peritoneum and posterior fascial edges are closed separately, then the muscle is replaced and the anterior layers of the fascia and skin are sutured. The writer believes that this is a sure way of preventing subsequent hernia.

Results of Vaginal Hysterectomy for Cancer of the Uterus.—FLAISCHLEN (*Zentralblatt für Gynäkologie*, 1903, No. 52) reports a series of 48 cases in which the cancerous uterus was removed per vaginam. Four patients died from the operation; recurrence occurred in 24. Seventeen were living after an interval of eight years; 12 were free from recurrence after ten years; 9 were well after thirteen years. The writer contrasts these results with Pozzi's pessimistic statement that out of 204 cases he could report only 2 permanent cures, and believes that his favorable statistics are explained by the fact that in every instance an early diagnosis was made. This supports Winter's statement that the success of the surgical treatment of uterine cancer in the future will depend more on the early recognition of the disease than on the radical nature of the operation, and, in the writer's opinion, proves that radical abdominal hysterectomy will not supplant the vaginal method.

Comparison of Vaginal and Abdominal Hysterectomy for Cancer.—OLSHAUSEN (*Zeitschrift für Geb. u. Gyn.*, Band l., Heft 1) reports 206 vaginal hysterectomies for cancer with 15 deaths, and 4 abdominal with 1 death during the years 1901 and 1902. He prefers the vaginal route until statistics extending over five years shall prove that the results of the abdominal method are better. The fact that Wertheim hopes that from 15 per cent. to 18 per cent. of his cases will be permanently cured by the radical operation does not convince the writer, as his own cures have been 18 per cent.

Conservative Surgery of the Adnexa.—TREUB (*Annal. de gyn. et d'obstétrique*, 1903, No. 5) deprecates hasty resort to a radical operation in cases of adnexal disease, since these rarely result fatally. In 612 cases of salpingo-oöphoritis a more or less complete cure was obtained in 80 per cent. by non-surgical treatment—rest, ice-bags, hot douches and tampons. The mortality after radical operations is from 5 to 6 per cent., and patients are not always relieved of pain, aside from the fact of subsequent climacteric disturbances.

The writer performs posterior section when possible, and when the abdomen is opened always tries to preserve portions of tubes and ovaries, except in cases of tuberculosis, when he extirpates the uterus with the adnexa.

Premature Menopause.—SIREDEY (*Comptes-rend. de la Soc. d'obstétrique de gyn. et de paed.*, December, 1903) reports 5 cases in women whose ages ranged from twenty-two to thirty-five years. Three were in good health; in one menstruation ceased after typhoid fever, though no direct causal relation could be establ shed. One patient subsequently developed diabetes, from which she died. In all menstruation had previously been somewhat scanty, and three had been sterile. Climacteric disturbances were slight. The usual anatomical changes, especially atrophy of the cervix, were well marked. Treatment in true cases of premature menopause is useless.

The Adnexa in Cases of Uterine Fibroids.—DANIEL (*Revue de gyn. et de chir. abdom.*, 1903, No. 1) found pathological changes in 59 per cent. of the cases which he observed. Catarrhal salpingitis was present in one-fourth of the operations, pyosalpinx and pachysalpingitis in others. Hydrosalpinx and hæmatosalpinx, tuberculosis of the tubes, and ectopic gestation were all noted.

The ovaries were more frequently diseased than the tubes (40 per cent.), cystic degeneration, cystoma, and abscess being most common. The writer attributes the adnexal changes to three causes, viz.: 1. Infection. 2. The "fibromatous diathesis," marked by vascular changes which lead to hyperplasia of fibromuscular tissue. 3. The presence of the uterine fibroids, which causes obstruction in the tubes, with resulting hydrosalpinx or hæmatosalpinx.

Notwithstanding the relative frequency of tubal and ovarian disease accompanying fibroids, this is frequently unrecognized before operation. It should be suspected if the patient complains of pains in the ovarian regions, since these are caused by fibroids only when the latter are impacted. Sterility in women with fibroids is usually due, the writer believes, to disease of the adnexa.

Pyosalpinx Complicating Uterine Fibroids.—STRASSMANN (*Zentralblatt für Gynäkologie*, 1904, No. 4) reports 3 cases (2 of his own and 1 of Lomer) in which pyosalpinx accompanied calcified fibromyomata. He believes that there is a direct causal relation between the two conditions. While the tubes may be infected as the result of septic or gonorrhœal endometritis occurring in a fibroid uterus, pus is rarely found at operations. He infers that prolonged pressure of hard uterine tumors is apt to cause occlusion of the tubes, with the subsequent formation of pus (if bacteria are present) just as occurs in the case of renal calculi.

The Adnexa in Cases of Fibroid.—DANIEL (*Revue de Gynécologie*, Band vii., Heft 2–4) finds that in 207 cases only one-third of the cases of diseased adnexa in connection with fibroid uteri were due to infection. In over one-half there was a diffuse genital "fibromatosis," due to vasomotor or reflex influences. In some cases pressure may be the cause of adnexal disease, as in unilateral hydrosalpinx. The diagnosis is aided by the presence of ovarian disturbances, pressure in the bladder and rectum and symptoms of torsion; 3.68 per cent. of the fatal cases are due to adnexal complications.

Fibroids and Sterility.—AUSTERLITZ (*Prager med. Wochenschrift*, Nos. 23 and 24, 1903) among 339 cases of uterine fibroid found primary sterility in 20.23 per cent. and secondary in 21.25 per cent., as compared with 4.17 per cent. and 13.68 per cent. in women without such neoplasms. The writer was unable to demonstrate whether sterility was directly due to fibroids or not; 51.2 per cent. of women with interstitial tumors were primarily sterile; 22.2 per cent. of the mixed variety; 16.9 per cent. subserous, and 12.7 per cent. submucous.

Appendicitis and Dysmenorrhœa.—MÉRIGOT DE TREIGNY (*Revue prat. d'obstétrique et de gyn.*, 1903, No. 12), in reporting a case illustrating the difficulty of diagnosis between these conditions, quotes from Legendre to the effect that intestinal troubles are apt to be aggravated during menstruation, pain being localized, especially over the appendix. The muscular rigidity characteristic of appendiceal inflammation may be present. The pains sometime cease at once after the discharge of mucus from the bowel. The symptoms simulate those of recurrent rather than acute appendicitis, and the pain is apt to shift from McBurney's point, while the patient's general condition is not such as to suggest the presence of peritonitis.

In the case reported by the writer a girl, aged eighteen years, had severe abdominal pain during menstruation, with obstinate constipat'on. The pains were sometimes localized over the appendiceal region, although they were again equally severe over the left lower abdomen. They were generally relieved by laxatives. As they became intermenstrual and were evidently of intestinal origin, an incision was made over the appendix, which was found to be thickened and adherent. After its removal the pains disappeared; the patient married and had a normal confinement. The writer raises the question whether so-called intermenstrual pain may not often be of appendiceal origin.

OPHTHALMOLOGY.

UNDER THE CHARGE OF

EDWARD JACKSON, A.M., M.D.,
OF DENVER, COLORADO,

AND

T. B. SCHNEIDEMAN, A.M., M.D.,
PROFESSOR OF DISEASES OF THE EYE IN THE PHILADELPHIA POLYCLINIC.

Resection of the Cervical Sympathetic Ganglia in Glaucoma.—Wilder, Chicago (*Annals of Ophthalmology*, January, 1904), gives a summary of 68 operations, 7 by himself. Of these operations, 38 were for simple glaucoma, 16 for chronic inflammatory glaucoma, 4 for subacute glaucoma, 3 for acute glaucoma, 4 for absolute glaucoma, 2 for hemorrhagic glaucoma, 1 for buphthalmos; 5 operations were preventive, in none of which has glaucoma occurred. One death occurred. Of the 38 operations for simple glaucoma, 14 gave no improvement whatever, 5 were temporarily improved for periods from fifteen days to eight months, but had recurrent attacks that necessitated iridectomy or caused loss of the eye; 15 were improved as long as they were under observation for periods of from two months to two years. Of these, 3 were stationary, 1 died, 6 remained unimproved after iridectomy, but improved after sympathectomy.

Of the 16 operations for chronic inflammatory glaucoma, 4 were improved, 3 temporarily, 3 remained stationary, and 6 were unimproved. Of the 4 operations for subacute glaucoma, 3 were improved and one temporarily. Of the 3 operations for acute glaucoma, 1 improved, 1 improved temporarily, and 1 remained stationary. Of the 4 cases of absolute glaucoma, 1 was improved, 3 unimproved. Both of the cases of hemorrhagic glaucoma were improved. The case of buphthalmos was improved.

The results in this series of cases do not seem as favorable as those presented by some others; thus Rohner reports 79 improved of 114 operated on. However, there seems a field for this operation, for cases have been reported in which sclerotomy and iridectomy had failed and in which sympathectomy reduced tension and improved vision.

The simple chronic form seems the most suited next to the hemorrhagic. If the operation is to be performed at all Abadie's rule holds:

In acute and subacute glaucoma, iridectomy first; if that fails, sympathectomy; in simple glaucoma myotics twice a day; if in spite of them the vision fails, sympathectomy.

Toxic Amblyopia Caused by Wood (Methyl) Alcohol.—BULLER, Montreal (*Montreal Medical Journal*, January, 1904) reports 3 cases of this lately described affection. The amount taken was about a wineglassful; in the third case three such doses were taken. In cases 1 and 2 the vision was reduced to counting fingers from three to eight feet. In Case 3 the vision was about a quarter of normal and improving. In each of the cases there was, as usual, improvements with quick relapses. In all 3 cases there was evidence of optic atrophy; the third showed only slight pallor of the papillæ.

The pathogenesis of wood alcohol blindness is still a matter of dispute, some holding that the primary lesion is in the retrobulbar portion of the optic nerve and others that it is in the macular region of the retina. Buller considers the optic nerve to be primarily at fault.

Wood alcohol is used in many trades and manufactures, and as even working with materials largely containing it, such as varnish, can induce poisoning from the vapor alone, the public should be informed of the dangers to sight from this substance.

Delirium after Eye Operations.—FINLAY, Havana (*Archives of Ophthalmology*, January, 1904) reports a case of violent delirium following extraction of cataract in a woman sixty-six years of age. Operation of the second eye was followed by nervousness but none of the excitement of the first. Atropine not having been used, could be excluded as the cause, and so could darkness, the patient being in a ward where there was a superabundance of light and air. Alcoholism was not a factor. The twenty-four hours' urine was found to be remarkably scanty and the proportion of urea considerably diminished. Traces of sugar and albumin were also present.

Finlay considers this case as confirmatory of Fromaget's view that such delirium is the result of an autointoxication most often uræmic, in accordance with the views expounded by Regis and Lavaure in 1893 with regard to delirium following operations in general, the source of the intoxication being endogenous or exogenous.

Acute Dacryoadenitis.—INMAN, House Surgeon, Royal London Ophthalmic Hospital (*Reports*, October, 1903), reports 10 cases of this affection observed at the hospital in two years, a rather extraordinary number, considering the experience of others; thus Arlt in his "Lehrbuch," 1853, says he has never seen a case; Powers asserts in 1886 that the indices of the Royal London Ophthalmic Hospital Reports make mention of only one case of abscess of the lacrymal gland. Hirschberg states that among 22,500 recorded cases of diseases of the eye, he met with but one case of suppurative inflammation of the gland.

The cases of this disease described in literature divide themselves into two main groups: (1) Those in which the affection of the lacrymal gland is associated with mumps. The main features are: it is usually bilateral and suppuration does not occur. (2) Those in which there is no connection with mumps, the main features being that it is usually unilateral; suppuration may or may not occur. It is a disease of the young, although it may occur at all ages. Of the writer's 10 cases—6 males, 4 females—the average was sixteen years, youngest three years, oldest thirty-seven years. The left side was more frequently attacked than the right; thus in this series, 9 out of 10. No cause can be assigned for this marked difference. The connection of this disease with mumps has been noted, though in this series of cases only one was so associated. The lacrymal sac was invariably healthy.

The symptoms are: beginning with a series of sensations of stiffness in the outer part of the upper lid, there is some pain and redness, with slight injection of the conjunctiva. The pain increases with the progress of the disease accompanied by marked œdema of the ocular conjunctiva on the outer side out of all proportion to the conjunctival inflammation accompanying it. The lacrymal gland shows distinct enlargement and induration; the vessels lying upon it are swollen and tortuous; there is moderate malaise and slight fever reaching 100° F. as the highest. As the disease progresses the eye becomes completely closed and the upper lid cannot be raised voluntarily, while eversion of the lid is extremely painful. The disease may be confounded with orbital cellulitis. This probably accounts in part for the rarity of recorded cases.

The outcome is favorable. The treatment is simple, consisting of hot fomentations with free incision to evacuate pus when such can be detected.

OTOLOGY.

UNDER THE CHARGE OF

CLARENCE J. BLAKE, M.D.,

OF BOSTON, MASS.,

PROFESSOR OF OTOLOGY, HARVARD UNIVERSITY.

ASSISTED BY

W. A. LECOMPTE, M.D., E. D. WALES, M.D., AND D. H. WALKER, M.D.

The Limits of Variation in the Depth of the Mastoid Antrum.—Philip D. Kerrison (*Archives of Otology*, June, 1903) gives some interesting results obtained from making sections of a large number of temporal bones to find out the maximum depth of the antrum to which one can proceed with safety. Politzer gives 15 mm. as a maximum depth, while Schwartze and Broca give 25 mm. and 29 mm., respectively. The author examined thirty bones to discover if any relationship exists between the length of the posterior canal wall and the depth of the antrum. The distance in millimetres between the spine of Henle externally and the inner border of the meatus was measured, then sections through the antrum were made and the distance between the antrum and the mastoid process was taken. In the thirty bones examined the length of the superior canal wall varied from 12 mm. to 18 mm. and in the same bones the depth of the antrum varied from 6 mm. to 15 mm. The deepest antrum measured 15 mm., this extreme depth occurred in the bone in which the length of the posterior canal wall measured 18 mm. Emphasis is laid upon the fact that the depth of the antrum is invariably less than the length of the posterior canal wall and never exceeds 15 mm.

Broca directs that the antrum be opened in the centre of a square, the anterior border of which is 5 mm. behind the spine of Henle. This point is the thickest part of the mastoid process and naturally the antrum would lie at an unusual depth.

The author also calls attention to the location of the facial and the semicircular canals.

Facial Paralysis.—NORTON L. WILSON (*American Medicine*, vol. vii., No. 7). In addition to its comprehensive review of the subject, this paper contains material of interest to the otologist, both on account of questions of function of the nerve and its branches and of lesions in its course, either secondary to causative conditions in the middle ear or differentiated from them.

The so-called first branch of the facial nerve is the stapedius, supplying the muscle to the stapes; the so-called second branch is a twig to the pneumogastric which, apparently, comes off the facial trunk just above the chorda tympani. This, like the other filaments to the ganglion, is sensory, and undoubtedly goes to the geniculate ganglion, being a part of the *pars intermedia*. The chorda tympani, considered the last branch of the facial in the Fallopian canal, is nothing more nor less than a continuation of the *pars intermedia*, supplying the anterior two-thirds of the tongue with taste. There is, therefore, but one branch in the facial canal which actually comes directly from the nerve, namely, the stapedius, the other branches being all sensory and probably a part of the *pars intermedia*.

In a case of lesion external to the stylomastoid foramen, the paralysis of the facial muscles, including the orbicularis and frontalis, is not associated with disturbances of the senses of taste and hearing.

If the lesion occurs in the lower half of the facial canal, there is, in addition to the facial paralysis, loss of the sense of taste in the anterior two-thirds of the tongue on the affected side and a diminished secretion of saliva, the lesion involving the chorda tympani and twig from the glossopharyngeal nerve.

If the lesion is in the upper half of the canal so that the stapedius is involved and not the ganglion, there is, in addition to the symptoms above named, an abnormal acuteness of hearing, for tones of high pitch especially, because the paralysis of the stapedius permits the unhindered contraction of the tensor tympani, and a correspondingly increased tension of the sound transmitting apparatus of the middle ear.

Concomitant paralysis of the soft palate is usually attributed to involvement of the superficial petrosal, assuming that this nerve comes from the geniculate ganglion. In this opinion the writer does not concur, regarding these filaments as sensory and not motor, and that it is the fifth nerve which innervates the palate, and which is, therefore, the nerve involved when the palate is paralyzed. In support of this contention is the case of a man who fell a distance of eighteen feet, and was picked up unconscious, bleeding from both ears. The hemorrhage from the ears continued for two days, and he was apparently totally deaf, both to sounds aerially conveyed and to the tuning-fork, by bone-conduction. The left side of the face was paralyzed, and there was complaint of tinnitus and vertigo. There was a fracture of the base of the skull involving both eighth nerves and the seventh nerve of the left side. There was no sense of taste in the anterior two-thirds of the tongue on the left side, and on this side, also, the salivary secretion was apparently diminished. The uvula and soft palate were normal. Contractility of the muscles of the left side of the face was lost for the faradic current, but was apparently increased for the galvanic current.

Were the geniculate ganglion involved and the general contention correct, the soft palate would have been affected, but in this case it was normal.

Where the cause of a facial paralysis is of otitic origin, attention must be directed to the cause, and the importance of the electric reactions, both as symptoms and as prognostic indications, must be duly regarded. Electric changes soon develop in paralyzed muscles, and the reaction of degeneration, partial or complete, appears in four or five days after the paralysis occurs.

Electricity should not be applied, except to ascertain the excitability of the muscles, until the end of the third week. One month after the paralysis has occurred, electricity and massage should be used regularly and systematically. If the muscles respond to faradism, that current should be used; if they do not, galvanism should be used, but only with the galvanometer, in order that the strength of the current may be known and gradually increased if necessary.

Einige Versuche ueber die Uebertragung von Schallschwingungen auf das Mittelohr.—Nagel and Samoyloff (*Archiv für Physiologie*, 1898; *Archiv für Ohrenheilkunde*, November, 1903) state that the graphic demonstration of the movements of the drumhead, in response to sound waves or the use of the membrane as a manometric capsule for the same purpose, presuppose some approach to normal flexibility. This is attainable either through the use of fresh specimens or by the infiltration of the tissues of the membrane with substances which serve to conserve its mobility.

For the grosser forms of graphic demonstration, drumheads thus conserved will give good service for a considerable time, months or even years, and may be used also as manometric capsules for demonstration of their movements by actuation of an illuminating gas current feeding a sensitive flame, but never so satisfactorily as the membrane of a freshly killed animal or the normal membrane *in situ* in the living subject.

The latter method consists in making the external auditory canal a closed chamber by means of a stopper having two openings, one by which the illuminating gas enters the canal and the other by which it passes on to the lighted gas jet.

Actuation of the drumhead by singing, speaking, or by communication of sounds conveyed through the bones of the head, are transmitted to the gas current in the external canal and made manifest in the movements of the sensitive flames, care being taken to guard the latter from the extraneous influence of sounds aerially conveyed.

In their experiments Nagel and Samoyloff have used, as a gas chamber, not the external canal, but the tympanic cavity of freshly killed animals and of the living subject. In the former instance the illuminating gas was introduced by means of a fine trocar passed through the Eustachian tube, while exit to the burner, a platinum tip with a minute opening, was afforded by a drillhole through the thin floor of the tympan and the insertion therein of a small rubber tube. In the living subject a tube with a T-shaped outer end was passed into the Eustachian tube, one end of the "T" connecting with the gas supply, and the other, by means of elastic tubing, with the burner.

Under these conditions sounds conveyed to the drumhead through the external canal and the vocalization of the subject of the experiment, even when only a light whispering voice was used, gave much more detailed representation in the flame than that afforded by the König manometric capsule with a rubber membrane.

Experiments were also made in reference to the question of cranio-tympanic sound transmission, but, although in themselves interesting, they seemed to have failed to negative the idea of the cranial passage of sound waves direct to the internal ear.

A vibrating tuning-fork, the influence of which upon the flame when held opposite the external canal had been noted, was placed with its stem upon the skull and the character of the flame effect compared with that produced when the external ear was firmly closed, the reaction of the flame, in the latter instance, being much increased.

That the term *craniotympanic*, as referred to the participation of the sound-transmitting mechanism of the middle ear in conveyance to the labyrinth of tones transmitted to the cranial bones is justifiable was shown by another experiment, in which, the vibrating tuning-fork having been placed upon the skull at the point previously found to give the greatest flame reaction, quicksilver or melted paraffin was poured into the external canal, effectively damping the movement of the drum-head. Under these circumstances the craniotympanic reaction was entirely wanting, the sensitive flame showing no movement whatever. On removal of the quicksilver or paraffin the flame immediately responded to the tone of the vibrating tuning-fork.

HYGIENE AND PUBLIC HEALTH.

UNDER THE CHARGE OF

CHARLES HARRINGTON, M.D.,

ASSISTANT PROFESSOR OF HYGIENE, HARVARD MEDICAL SCHOOL.

Measurements of Relative Humidity in Offices and Dwelling-houses in Winter.—An interesting proof of the statement that the air of heated houses in winter surpasses in aridity any climate in the world is given by G. A. LOVELAND (*Engineering News*, December 10, 1903, p. 925), who relates that in consequence of the evident effect of dry air on the furniture in the United States Weather Bureau Office in Lincoln, Nebraska, which is heated by steam radiators, a consecutive record of the relative humidity was made during the following winter. The observations, made by means of the sling psychrometer, were taken usually twice a day, but sometimes four or five times, and occasionally but once. They showed that during the whole winter the air was exceedingly dry. During the coldest month, February, with a mean temperature of 19.2° F. above zero, the average relative humidity of the office air was but 15.3 per cent. The extreme range was from 7 per cent. to 25 per cent., but only once was the relative humidity higher than 20 per cent., and only once did it fall below 10 per cent. In December, with a mean temperature of 22.6° F., the average relative humidity indoors was 18.6 per cent., and in January, which was the warmest month, with a mean outdoor temperature of 26.8° F., the indoor humidity was 21 per cent. The office temperature during the three months averaged slightly below 70° F. The mean relative humidity outdoors was 77.4 per cent. in December, 73.4 per cent. in January, 77.9 per cent. in February, and 76.2 per cent. for the three months, against but 18.3 per cent. indoors. These results led to further experimentation in a double house, the two halves of which were heated by furnaces of the same size, pattern, and make. The water-pan of each furnace had a capacity of twenty quarts. In one house the amount of water evaporated was determined each day at noon and was found to be but two quarts; in the other the pan was left empty for purposes of comparison. It was found that the difference in relative humidity in the two was so very slight (about 1 per cent.) that the value of the water-pan was not established. After seventeen days' observation the amount evaporated daily was increased to five and nine-tenths quarts by placing pans of water in each of the registers of one house. This resulted in increasing the relative humidity of that house 2.4 per cent. over that of the other. Additional pans were then placed in the cold-air box, whereby the amount of water evaporated daily was increased to ten quarts, but even then the difference in humidity was but 2.2 per cent. Taking into account the probable rate of natural ventilation, it was reckoned that it would require from seventy to one hundred and fifty quarts of water, or possibly more, per day to maintain the relative humidity as high as it was outside, the difference between inside and outside temperatures being from 35° to 50° F., as is the case in winter in Nebraska. In the first period of the experiment the outside and inside relative humidities were, respectively, 68.2 per cent. and 36.2 per cent.; in the second they were 73.8 per cent. and 35.8 per cent.; and in the third, 66.8 per cent. and 29.1 per cent. The average outside and inside temperatures during the three periods were 39.4° F. and 72.1° F., 39.3° F. and 70° F., and 33.3° F. and 69.9° F.

(By means of the "humidifier," which presents to the hot air issuing from a register a surface of wicking kept saturated with water, the relative humidity of the air of a room can be maintained at over 50 per cent., according to Dr. H. J. Barnes, of Boston, who brought it to public notice. In a large office building in Boston the air is maintained at about 50 per cent. relative humidity by means of steam injected into the hot air in the stock-room, from which the air is distributed to the various rooms. The amount of water thus vaporized in a ten-hour workday is no less than 675 gallons.—C. H.)

Shellfish and Typhoid Fever.—It is the belief of Dr. J. T. C. Nash (*Journal of State Medicine*, December, 1903, p. 70) that sewage-contaminated shellfish have played a very large if not a leading part in the general incidence of typhoid fever in England. Prior to the advance in sanitary administration, the chief factors in the incidence of the disease were undoubtedly polluted water and infected milk, but to-day these sources have been so attacked that, as compared with fifty years ago, the relative amount of typhoid has diminished considerably. Yet during the past ten years no improvement, but, on the contrary, a tendency to increase, has been observed, in spite of all sanitary effort. No notable instance of epidemic water-borne typhoid has been observed since the Maidstone and Worthing outbreaks, and milk-borne typhoid has been more uncommon; but yet there appears to be an apparently irreducible minimum of typhoid, with an actual slight increase in prevalence. The reason for this is, in his opinion, that sufficient attention has not been given to the consideration of cleanliness of other foods than milk, for otherwise, the mouth being the portal of infection, localities provided with pure water would not have an undue amount of the disease. An infected water-supply causes a widespread epidemic; an infected milk-supply produces the disease among the customers of the particular dairies involved; but when an outbreak occurs where both the water and the milk are above suspicion, there must be some other common source. Polluted soil may be expected to act as a vehicle of infection only by the surface soil becoming pulverized and blown about by the wind, so that it is deposited on articles of food or directly in the open mouth; but surface soil, owing to the action of direct sunlight, dryness, and the ordinary soil bacteria, is not a favorable habitat for the typhoid organism, which, however, finds more favorable conditions in the deeper layers, where there are fewer saprophytes, more moisture, and less light. Yet it must be admitted that aerial infection from polluted surface soil is an occasional factor. On the other hand, contaminated foods are obvious and most probable sources of infection, especially in the case of those which are obtained in polluted water, such as shellfish, water-cress, etc. He believes that a very considerable proportion of cases of typhoid in England is due to sewage-contaminated shellfish, and in substantiation he asserts that out of 105 cases noticed in his district in 1902, he traced some connection with shellfish in at least 82. He cites the fact that at a well-known seaside resort (presumably Brighton) about 30 per cent. of the cases of typhoid that have occurred for some years past have been attributed to this cause, and that at another, where the disease was unduly prevalent in 1898 and 1899 and was attributed to polluted mussels, the stopping of the sale of the mussels the next year was followed by a marked diminution in the number of cases reported. Owing to the bringing about of diminished consumption of shellfish, on the one hand, and of better methods of laying and cooking and of greater care in obtaining supplies from purer layings, on the other, a very decided diminution in the incidence of the disease has occurred in his own district. By careful inquiry, he estimates that rather less than more than 5 per cent. of the population of that district are eaters of shellfish; and working out for typhoid fever the standard ratios during 1902 per thousand persons in each section of the population, he calculates that for the entire population the attack-rate was 3.28 per thousand; for the shellfish-eating section, reckoned as 5 per cent. of the population, it was 51.25; and for the remainder, only 0.75. Among the shellfish vendors and their employés, he calculates the attack-rate at no less than 160 per thousand. Furthermore, the seasonal incidence of typhoid fever in the country generally is at its lowest in May and June, which months are the close season for English and French oysters. During these months, also, cockles and mussels are not in their prime, and hence are less eaten than at other times. In addition to necessary legislation concerning supervision of all shellfish layings and cultivation beds, he recommends for the diminution of the apparently irreducible minimum of typhoid fever the avoidance of all contact with shellfish, except such as are beyond suspicion of sewage pollution, the avoidance of uncooked vegetables which have been subjected to manurial pollution, the early removal to hospital of all cases of the disease, careful and constant attention to effective disposal of sewage and all forms of refuse, and general cleanliness of all food supplies, especially shellfish and watercress.

According to an editorial in the *Journal of the American Medical Association* of January 23, 1904, a careful investigation by the Health Board of Orange, N. J., of a recent increased prevalence of typhoid fever, exonerated the water-supply of the city as the cause thereof, and led to the conclusion that the outbreak was due to the consumption of oysters procured from infected beds.

Concerning Yellow Fever.—DR. L. O. HOWARD (Supplement to *Public Health Reports*, November 13, 1903) observes that, although the actual localities in which the *stegomyia fasciata* has been found are comparatively small in number, both in the United States and in other parts of the world, we have sufficient facts on which to base a sound generalization, both as to probable actual occurrence and as to the regions in which the species will readily establish if once introduced. All the occurrence within the United States, except at Nashville, fall within the limits of what are known as the tropical and lower austral zones, which include practically all the southern United States which border on the Atlantic Ocean and the Gulf of Mexico, with the exception of those portions of Virginia, North Carolina, South Carolina, Georgia, and Alabama which constitute practically the foothills of the Appalachian chain, namely, Western Virginia and North Carolina, the extreme northwestern corner of South Carolina, the northern part of Georgia, and the extreme northeastern corner of Alabama. The lower austral zone includes also the western half of Tennessee, the western corner of Kentucky, the extreme southern tip of Illinois, the southeastern corner of Missouri, all of Arkansas except the northern portion, the southern portion of Indian Territory, Southern Arizona, some of Northern Arizona, and southern strips in Utah, Nevada, and California. In the greater part of this territory and where the climate is not too dry, the *stegomyia fasciata* probably exists; and in all the rest of this territory where the climate is not too dry, it will undoubtedly flourish if once introduced. We may expect to find it everywhere in the moist tropical zone, or, at all events, when introduced at any point within the low, moist tropics, it may be expected to establish itself. It is noted that the geographical distribution of the yellow fever mosquito corresponds rather well with that of the Texas cattle tick.

The French Yellow Fever Commission, composed of Marchoux, Salimbeni, and Simond, which has pursued the study of yellow fever at

Rio de Janeiro for more than a year, reports (*Annales de l'Institut Pasteur*, November, 1903) that all the conclusions of Reed and his associates have been confirmed in every particular. Otherwise, its work has been unproductive. DR. G. SANARELLI (*Il Policlinico*, November 21, 1903), however, still opposes the idea that stegomyia is a necessary factor in spreading yellow fever, and asserts anew the importance of the part played by *B. icteroides*.

In a communication to Surgeon-General WALTER WYMAN (*Public Health Reports*, January 15, 1904), under date of December 18, 1903, the members of Working Party No. 2, Dr. M. J. Rosenau, chairman, report that from their studies at Vera Cruz, Mexico, during the summer of 1903, they are unable to corroborate all the findings of Working Party No. 1, having found phases of the organism *myxococcidium stegomyiæ* in normal mosquitoes.

The fact that it has been proved beyond doubt that the female *stegomyia fasciata* serves as an intermediate host and conveys the poison of yellow fever to non-immunes has led the Louisiana State Board of Health to promulgate the following recommendations (*Public Health Reports*, February 5, 1904): 1. The patient shall be put under a bar and the room properly screened, and all mosquitoes destroyed. 2. The house shall at once be closed and fumigated with pyrethrum powder, 4 ounces to 1000 cubic feet. Intoxicated mosquitoes must be swept up and burned. In case house is not occupied, sulphur should be used, 7 pounds to room, etc. Fumigation must be repeated every fourth day for three or four times. Commence all over with every new case of fever. 3. Every house or outhouse shall be so fumigated for a distance of 100 yards in every direction from the infected house. Fumigation repeated every fourth day for three or four times. 4. Great care to be exercised to prevent new mosquitoes from entering the infected room. When they do so, they must be killed and burned. 5. All cisterns in infected area must be screened or coal-oiled. 6. All vessels containing water must be emptied; pools and ditches drained and coal-oiled. 7. All drains, sinks, and privies are to be liberally sprinkled with coal-oil every third day for a period of eighteen days. Repeat after every new case.

PATHOLOGY AND BACTERIOLOGY.

UNDER THE CHARGE OF

SIMON FLEXNER, M.D.,

DIRECTOR OF THE ROCKEFELLER INSTITUTE FOR MEDICAL RESEARCH, NEW YORK.

ASSISTED BY

WARFIELD T. LONGCOPE, M.D.,

RESIDENT PATHOLOGIST, PENNSYLVANIA HOSPITAL, PHILADELPHIA.

A Note on Experimental Arterial Atheroma.—Attempts have been made by several investigators to produce atheroma of the aorta in animals by intravenous injections of bacteria or bacterial toxins. In some cases the aorta was previously injured. Crocq has reported negative results, while Thérèse and Pernice were only able to produce very slight microscopic lesions in the wall of the aorta. Boinet and Romary have described small, raised areas in the aorta, which, on microscopic examination, had the characters of gelatiniform plaques. They believed these areas were the result of bacterial infection of the arterial wall. Josué has observed the formation of true calcareous plates after repeated injections of adrenalin. GILBERT and LION (*Arch. de méd. exp. et d'anat. path.*, 1904, T. xvi. p. 73) describe lesions in the aorta which they found in two rabbits after repeated intravenous inoculations of both living and killed cultures of a paracolon bacillus. In these experiments the artery did not receive any previous injury. One animal was allowed to live six months, the other ten months, after the primary inoculation. The middle coat of the aorta was the one affected, and the lesion consisted in a sclerocalcareous transformation. In another series of experiments the aorta was injured, and later cultures of typhoid bacilli were inoculated intravenously. After a few days the animals were killed. An acute aortitis was found at the site of trauma. The authors conclude that it is possible to produce atheroma of the aorta and acute aortitis in animals by intravenous inoculations of bacteria and bacterial toxins. This may take place with or without previous injury to the arterial wall.

Scarlet Fever, Protozoan-like Bodies Found in Four Cases.—MALLORY (*Journal of Medical Research*, 1903, vol. x. p. 483) has found in four cases of scarlet fever certain bodies which in their morphology strongly suggest that they may be various stages in the developmental cycle of a protozoan. They occur in and between the epithelial cells of the epidermis and free in the superficial lymph vessels and spaces of the corium. The great majority of the bodies vary from 2 to 7 microns in diameter, and stain delicately but sharply with methylene blue. They form a series of bodies, including the formation of definite rosettes with numerous segments, which are closely analogous to the series seen in the asexual development (schizogonia) of the malarial parasite, but, in addition, there are certain coarsely reticulated forms which may represent stages in sporogonia, or be due to degeneration of other forms. The bodies were not found in the blood, lymph nodes, or any of the internal organs. The possibility of these bodies being artefacts or degenerations can be effectually excluded. If they are protozoa they must have some causal relation to scarlet fever, for were they normal or occasional inhabitants of the skin, their presence could hardly have been overlooked in the extensive work which has been done on the skin. Though the author believes that these bodies are protozoa and have an etiological relationship to scarlet fever, he does not claim that such a relationship has been absolutely proven. He proposes the name of "cyclaster scarlatinalis" for the organism.

Tuberculosis of the Tonsils in Children.—The belief has steadily been gaining ground that the tonsils are one of the most important channels by which the tubercle bacillus enters the system during childhood. A comparatively large number of cases in which tubercle bacilli or tubercles could be demonstrated in the tonsils of adults have been recorded, but only a few observers, especially Friedmann and Latham, have confined their attention to the study of the tonsils in children. KINGSFORD (*Lancet*, 1904, vol. i. p. 89) has examined the tonsils of seventeen children under five years of age, which at autopsy showed tuberculous lesions in various parts of the body. Tuberculosis of the tonsils could be demonstrated microscopically in seven of these cases, but in only one was there any evidence that the tonsillar infection was primary. In the other cases the infection probably took place by means of the blood stream or expectorated sputum. The author concludes that though tuberculosis of the tonsils is fairly common, the process is rarely primary in the tonsils. If the tonsils are tuberculous the cervical glands are also affected, but it may happen that the infection enters the body through the tonsils and reaches the cervical glands without leaving a demonstrable lesion in the tonsils themselves.

The Pathological Anatomy of "Paratyphoid Fever:" Report of a Fatal Case with Bacteriological Findings.—WELLS and SCOTT (*Journal of Infectious Diseases*, 1904, vol. i. p. 72) have collected the pathological and bacteriological reports of four fatal cases of paratyphoid fever. They describe in detail the history, bacteriology, and pathological findings of a fifth case. The case was one simulating typhoid fever, but giving negative Widal reactions throughout the course. The spleen was palpable, rose spots were present over the abdomen, and twice blood was passed in the stools. There was absence of depression, little or no delirium, and a relatively high pulse rate. At autopsy the general pathological picture was that of an acute infection. In the ileum, a short distance above the ileocæcal valve, an extensive ragged ulceration was found; the ulcers bore no relation to the lymphatic apparatus and appeared entirely dissimilar to the ulceration of typhoid fever, inasmuch as they were quite superficial and showed lack of infiltration. They resembled much more the ulcers of dysentery. There was no swelling either of the mesenteric or retroperitoneal lymph nodes. In sections the ulcers in the ileum looked entirely different from typhoid ulcers, particularly in the absence of infiltration and hyperplasia of the lymphoid follicles. The mesenteric lymph glands also showed total absence of congestion or lymphoid swelling of the lymph follicles and sinuses. A few foci of necrosis were seen in the liver. They were noticeable for their lack of endothelial cells. The spleen showed congestion with the presence of large endothelial cells containing golden-brown pigment. Cultures from the spleen and kidney gave a pure growth of paratyphoid bacilli. With the serum of a rabbit immunized against Buxton's paratyphoid bacillus, they agglutinated in dilutions of 1:40,000. The serum did not react toward typhoid or colon bacilli. The authors conclude that paratyphoid infections are accompanied by changes quite different from those of typhoid fever. The intestinal lesions are variable, and there is little anatomically to differentiate this type of infections from other septicæmias.

Influence of Splenectomy on the Leukocytes of the Blood of the Dog.—NICOLAS and DUMOULIN (*Jour. de phys. et de path. gén.*, 1903, T. v. p. 1073) conclude, from a study of the blood in two splenectomized dogs, that after splenectomy there is an increase in the number of white blood cells, and that this increase persists for some time after the operation, but eventually, perhaps after months, returns to the normal. There is an immediate diminution in the number of leukocytes, followed by a transient elevation of these cells. This finally gives place to a marked and persistent decrease in the relative number of lymphocytes. The authors believe that this observation is important, inasmuch as it suggests that the spleen plays some part in the genesis of the lymphocytes. The polymorphonuelear leukocytes show a slight variation and are usually relatively increased. A marked eosinophilia occurred in one of the two dogs.

Changes in the Power of Absorption of the Animal Peritoneum Brought about by Intraperitoneal Injections of Adrenalin.—It is well known that the application of adrenalin to mucous surfaces causes anæmia, owing to the contraction of the capillaries. EXNER (*Zeitschrift für Heilkunde*, 1903, Bd. xxiv. p. 302), applying this principle to serous surfaces, experimented with adrenalin to study its effect when, injected intraperitoneally, upon the absorbing power of the peritoneum. Guinea-pigs and rabbits received intraperitoneal injections of adrenalin. Subsequently, when strychnine, potassium cyanide, physostigmine, and indigo were given into the peritoneum, the onset of toxic symptoms from these drugs or their absorption was much delayed over the control animals. With potassium iodide, the time required for its appearance in the urine was the same in normal animals and animals which had received adrenalin intraperitoneally. To determine whether the adrenalin injections affected the absorption through the bloodvessels or lymphatics, a fine emulsion of paraffin in gum arabic was used. The absorption of this substance was much retarded by previous intraperitoneal injections of adrenalin. By staining the diaphragm with silver nitrate, the structures described as stomata appeared less numerous in the adrenalin animals than in the normal animals. It was, therefore, thought that absorption through the lymphatics alone was retarded by adrenalin. Adrenalin injections had a very marked retarding effect upon the extension of bacteria from the peritoneum into the circulating blood.

From the results of these experiments, the author suggests that in operations for peritonitis a very material benefit might be derived by previously injecting adrenalin into the peritoneal cavity. By this procedure it is possible that the absorption of bacterial toxins from the peritoneum might be lessened during the manipulation of the intestines at operation.

Notice to Contributors.—All communications intended for insertion in the Original Department of this Journal are received only *with the distinct understanding that they are contributed exclusively to this Journal.*

Contributions from abroad written in a foreign language, if on examination they are found desirable for this Journal, will be translated at its expense.

A limited number of reprints in pamphlet form will, if desired, be furnished to authors, *provided the request for them be written on the manuscript.*

All communications should be addressed to—

DR. FRANCIS R. PACKARD, 1831 Chestnut Street, Philadelphia, U. S. A.

THE

AMERICAN JOURNAL

OF THE MEDICAL SCIENCES.

MAY, 1904.

ON THE SURGICAL IMPORTANCE OF THE VISCERAL CRISES IN THE ERYTHEMA GROUP OF SKIN DISEASES.

BY WILLIAM OSLER, M.D.,
PROFESSOR OF MEDICINE, JOHNS HOPKINS UNIVERSITY, BALTIMORE.

THE possibility of mistaking these visceral crises for appendicitis or intussusception or obstruction of the bowel, and handing the patient over to the surgeon for operation, is by no means remote. In Case II. of my series[1] one attack was unilateral, and of such severity that the physician who was called in, knowing nothing of the previous history of the case, diagnosed renal colic. In Case XX. the child was admitted to the surgical wards supposed to have appendicitis. Fortunately the skin rash was noticed, the pain subsided, and he was transferred to the medical wards. The association of the colic with the passage of blood *per rectum* may, of course, lead to the diagnosis of intussusception. In the January number of the *British Journal of Children's Diseases*, vol. i., No. 1, Dr. G. A. Sutherland reports the case of a boy, aged five years, who, eight days before admission, had been seized with severe abdominal pain and vomiting. After continuing intermittently for four days the attack passed off, but recurred two days later in a more persistent manner. The day before admission the motions were blood-stained. The boy looked very ill; the abdomen was distended, and he had recurring attacks of severe colic. The temperature was normal. The next day the abdomen was more distended and palpation was impossible. It was decided that the symptoms indicated obstruction from intussusception. The abdomen was

[1] THE AMERICAN JOURNAL OF THE MEDICAL SCIENCES, January, 1904.

opened and the sigmoid flexure was found much distended; "on going over the small intestine a part of the bowel about five inches long was found, which was dark in color, evidently from extravasated blood, and with thickened walls." There were no other hemorrhages visible. The boy reacted well from the operation, and for the next five days he had only occasional pains. He then for the first time had a skin eruption, with albumin in the urine, and the diagnosis was cleared up.

In a second case reported by Dr. Sutherland, a girl, aged seven years, was admitted to hospital with Henoch's purpura. She had a prolonged illness with the usual attacks of abdominal pain, vomiting of blood, melæna, albuminuria, and hæmaturia. She gradually recovered, and three months later was readmitted with a recurrence of all the symptoms. The pain was more severe, referred to the umbilicus, spasmodic and colicky in character. There were hemorrhages similar to the previous attack. She died in a general convulsive seizure. The temperature was 104° F. There was acute general peritonitis and intussusception of the cæcum and part of the ileum into the colon. The involved portions of the intestine were black and hemorrhagic and gangrenous. As Dr. Sutherland rightly surmises, the fatal attack was induced by hemorrhage into the wall of the colon, leading to paralysis of the affected part and to increased muscular contraction, with colic, in the adjoining part of the bowel. As a result of these strong muscular contractions the sound part of the intestine became invaginated into the paralyzed and hemorrhagic portion.

In the same journal there is reported by Mr. Harold Burrows a case in which laparotomy was performed. A boy, aged eleven years, was admitted to the Bolingbroke Hospital July 6th with a diagnosis of obstruction from intussusception. After feeling out-of-sorts for ten days, on the morning of the sixth he was seized with violent pain in the abdomen and vomiting, and shortly afterward passed blood, the vomitus being dark brown, with a fecal odor. There was general tenderness of the abdomen; no distention; no lump. The abdominal muscles were held rigid. The patient was examined under an anæsthetic, and it was decided to operate. A few inches from the ileocæcal valve the ileum showed small petechial hemorrhages and some irregular patches of congestion. The peritoneum over these parts was sticky and had lost its gloss. On the following day the patient was free from pain, but it was then noticed that there was a skin eruption. From the history the boy had had on June 26th, eleven days before admission, some arthritis and a skin rash.

The following case, at present in my wards, is a further illustration of the surgical importance of this group of cases.

Lena F., aged seventeen years, admitted for the first time December 1, 1903. The patient was seen by Dr. McCrae in consultation with her attending physician. She was in bed, rolling about with the pain, and at times assumed very curious positions, getting in the knee-elbow position and crouching and bending, very rarely staying very long in any one place. The pain was evidently of great severity, paroxysmal in character. Examination of the abdomen was negative. There was no tenderness anywhere on pressure; no resistance. The knee-joints were slightly swollen and quite tender. There was no skin eruption; no fever. She had had large doses of morphine hypodermically, which only relieved the pain for a short time. The association of the arthritis made Dr. McCrae suspicious of the form of abdominal colic associated with skin lesions and nephritis. She was removed to the hospital with some difficulty.

The history obtained was as follows:

She had been a healthy girl. The family history was excellent except that the mother was very neurotic. There was no rheumatism in the family. She had been very well as a child and had grown and thriven. Six months before admission she had her first attack of pain in the abdomen, which every week or two had recurred and had been very severe. The attack was usually associated with vomiting. It had no relation to food, never associated with jaundice; no chills. The bowels were obstinately constipated. The attacks recurred with great severity, and on August 3d an exploratory operation was made at the City Hospital—an incision in the upper part of the abdomen. The gall-bladder was found to be clear and there was no sign of gastric ulcer; no appendicitis. Three weeks after the operation the attacks recurred, and she has had a number of very severe paroxysms. On admission she was a healthy-looking, well-nourished girl. The abdomen was not distended; no special tension; palpation could be made readily in all regions and was negative. Examination of the thoracic organs was negative. The knee-joints were a little swollen and tender, not red. Examination of the gastric juice on two occasions showed nothing special. The stools were searched carefully without finding anything abnormal. For the first few days after admission she had attacks of pain lasting from one and a half to two minutes, colic-like in character, readily controlled with codeine. She vomited on December 1st. There was no special change in the leukocytes. The count on admission was normal; coagulation time three minutes. On December 5th she had slight bleeding from the nose. On the 6th there was a trace of albumin in the urine, which persisted, and toward the close of her stay in the hospital there were a few hyaline casts. There was no skin rash. The knee condition rapidly disappeared. She was discharged December 15th, very much improved.

She was readmitted January 28, 1904. She had been very much better, but she had had slight attacks. On January 25th the colic became very severe and she had much nausea. She had had recurring attacks of bleeding from the nose, and once, she said, bleeding from the gums. There had been no skin eruption. The knee-joints became swollen and painful shortly after admission. The leukocytes were 12,500. The urine on the 29th (catheterized specimen) was smoky, and contained albumin in small amount, a few red corpuscles, and numerous hyaline casts. She remained in the hospital for nine days; the pains lessened, and she improved in her general condition.

The practical lessons to be drawn from these three cases in which laparotomy was performed are: first, that in children with colic the greatest care should be taken to get a full history, which may bring out the fact of previous attacks, either of skin lesions, of arthritis, or of intestinal crises; and secondly, to make the most careful inspection of the skin for angioneurotic œdema, purpura, or erythema. It is also to be borne in mind that recurring colic may be for many years the sole feature of this remarkable disease, as in Cases XVII. and XXVII. of my series, in which the obscurity of the attacks of colic was not cleared up until the final appearance of skin lesions. In the case here reported the intestinal crises, in combination with arthritis and the renal features, leave no doubt as to the diagnosis. In her next attack there may be purpura or angioneurotic œdema, or an acute nephritis may occur alone. The colic is the most constant of the visceral manifestations, occurring in twenty-five of the twenty-nine cases in my series. So far as I know, it is never dangerous. In no case recorded has death resulted, I believe, from intestinal causes. The examination in the cases of Dr. Sutherland and Mr. Barrows confirms the view that the colic is due to infiltration of the intestinal wall with blood and serum.

CHANGES IN THE INTERCOSTAL MUSCLES AND THE DIAPHRAGM IN INFECTIVE PROCESSES INVOLVING THE LUNG AND PLEURA.[1]

By W. M. L. Coplin, M.D.,
PROFESSOR OF PATHOLOGY, JEFFERSON MEDICAL COLLEGE, PHILADELPHIA.

(From the Laboratories of the Jefferson Medical College Hospital.)

So far as the writer is aware, no important study has been undertaken of the relation, if any, existing between the intercostal muscles and inflammations of the lung and pleura, or of either alone. An examination of the most important text-books on medicine and pathology discloses no reference to characteristic anatomical changes in the intercostal muscles or nerves in any of the conditions under consideration.

[1] Read before the Pathological Society of Philadelphia, January 28, 1904.

Aufrecht,[1] in a most exhaustive article on pneumonia, notes the occurrence of severe intercostal pain and pain in the abdominal muscles, both of which are attributed to the cough, and this seems to be the view held by other observers. It is reasonable to assume that the cough induces muscular soreness, comparable to the soreness resulting from any other form of muscle fatigue, but, in some cases at least, muscle pain and tenderness may depend upon demonstrable lesions in the affected tissues.

Rosenbach,[2] in his elaborate article on pleurisy, speaks of atrophy of the thoracic muscles and antagonistic muscles, and briefly refers[3] to the fact that changes occur in the costal pleura and intercostal muscles during perforation.

Again,[4] without any special detail as to the character of the lesions, he refers to degeneration of the thoracic muscles in acute and chronic pleurisies. The same writer notes that certain of the sensations apparently arising in the intercostal spaces resemble muscle pain,[5] and that in large exudations where muscles and pleura are "much involved," the intercostal depressions are obliterated, so as to admit of deep pressure. He does not refer to these phenomena as indicating a period of relaxation in the muscle, although that seems to be the probable explanation.

In an editorial note Musser refers to a case in which pleurisy and intercostal neuralgia were concurrent. In the first week signs of pleurisy dominated; in the second, third, and fourth weeks intercostal neuralgia was most evident. An herpetic eruption developed along the course of the ninth intercostal nerve.

Rosenbach[6] refers to marked dyspnœa if there be much pain in the thoracic muscles, and speaks of rheumatic pains in these muscles as accompanying dry pleurisy. In common with other observers, he[7] notes the respiratory asynchronism evinced by delayed excursion on the affected side. The chest deformity associated with contracting thorax, he says, may be due to degenerated and contracted muscles[8] and the intercostal spaces may be obliterated, the ribs overlying each other like tiles on a roof.

The same writer[9] is of the opinion that in affections of the thoracic muscles, such as rheumatism and intercostal neuralgia, contraction of the intercostal muscles may give rise to conditions that simulate dulness; at just this point it might be well to note that œdema, perivascular infiltration, and lipomatous change of the intercostal muscles would, theoretically, favor the same result. With full recognition of his entire unfittedness, it is not the writer's purpose to discuss the influence of the alteration in the intercostal tissues on physical signs, but any of the mentioned changes in the intercostal

[1] Diseases of the Bronchi, Lungs, and Pleura, Nothnagel's Encyclopedia, 1903, p. 455.
[2] Ibid., p 826. [3] Ibid., p. 830. [4] Ibid., p. 832. [5] Ibid., p. 845.
[6] Ibid., p. 849. [7] Ibid., p. 852. [8] Ibid., p. 853. [9] Ibid., p. 856.

muscles would presumably influence the percussion note and probably modify the auscultatory sounds.

With regard to the pseudopleural friction sound, called by the French *bruit de cuir neuf*, Rosenbach[1] accepts the condition as a muscle phenomenon, and it is not improbable that other pseudopleural friction sounds are, at least in part, of muscle origin. As will be shown later, pleurisy may be complicated with a myositis, and it would be of great interest to know if any friction sound results from movement in muscles the seat of inflammation. This could be determined, probably with great accuracy, by auscultation of muscles so situated as to exclude the probability of friction sounds arising from any other cause. It is well known that œdema of collagenous membranes, such as tendon sheaths, may give rise to friction sounds, and it is not impossible that the septal fibres or septal membrane between the external and internal intercostals, and possibly the movement of fibre sheaths or bundles, one upon another, might give rise to such friction.

Przewalski[2] calls attention to the narrowing of the intercostal spaces and increased resistance to intercostal digital pressure in all of 19 cases of pleurisy, 14 of which were serous and 5 suppurative. The sign is most easily elicited in children. He regards this narrowing of the intercostal spaces and fixation of the intercostal muscles as characteristic of pleurisy and analogous to *les attitudes fixes des membres* in inflammations of the joints. He does not seem to have suggested that the phenomenon he observed could have depended upon architectural change in the muscles of the area to which he draws special attention.

Although Rosenbach[3] speaks of extension by contiguity from pleura to peritoneum, the anatomical changes in the diaphragm accompanying such extension received no specific notice. The only study of the muscles of respiration in pneumonia and pleurisy with which I am familiar is that by Rohrer.[4] This observer made a careful study of the diaphragm in pneumonia, pleurisy, and pericarditis, and shows that in pneumonia and pleurisy an interstitial myositis of the muscular portion of the diaphragm adjacent to the area involved, whether it be pleura, pericardium, or peritoneum, frequently results. His studies include only lesions of the muscle areas of the diaphragm; he makes no reference to any involvement of the tendon. His excellent paper is illustrated by a number of exceptionally good photomicrographs of the condition that he describes. This phrenitis or diaphragmitis, Rohrer believes, may result from (1) direct extension, (2) extension by the lymphatics, and (3), though rarely, hæmatogenous infection.

[1] Diseases of the Bronchi, Lungs, and Pleura, Nothnagel's Encyclopedia, 1903, p. 864.
[2] Centralbl. f. Chir, 1902, vol. xxix. p. 377.
[3] Ibid., p. 830.
[4] Maryland Medical Journal, September, 1902, No. 9, vol. lxv. p. 391.

PERSONAL OBSERVATIONS. The writer has studied the intercostal muscles in 7 cases; 2 of these were croupous pneumonias with plastic pleurisies, the pneumococcus being isolated from the lung and pleural effusion. Two were tuberculous lesions of the pleura; one of them a direct extension of tuberculosis to the pleura from a large area of recent tuberculous pneumonia in the presence of a dense fibrous adhesion, irregular in outline, 12 cm. in length anteroposteriorly, and possessing a maximum breadth of 6 cm., situated immediately over and involving the lower portion of the upper lobe of the right lung; the anterior margin of the sclerotic area corresponding to the costocartilaginous junction. The other case was a frank tuberculous serofibrinous pleurisy, acute in time, the tubercle bacillus being demonstrable in films from the exudate, and the condition associated with a number of chronic tuberculous lesions of the lung, some of which were fibroid, partly encapsulated, others evidently more recent. Two other cases were acute pneumococcal pleurisies, one in a child (seven years), the other in an adult, and associated with pericarditis. The seventh case was a chronic empyema, for which Professor Keen performed an extensive resection of the thoracic wall.

In both cases of croupous pneumonia the diaphragm was also examined. One case showed the acute leukocytic infiltration similar to that described by Rohrer, with, at points, evident beginning abscess formation. This is evinced by areas of necrosis extending the breadth of six to eight muscle fibres, the necrotic detritus being richly infiltrated with polymorphonuclear and hyaline leukocytes. At such points, by appropriate staining methods, organisms possessing the morphology and tinctorial characters of the pneumococcus can readily be demonstrated. The change not mentioned by Rohrer, but clearly made out in this case, is an evident involvement of the lymphatic tracts of the tendon of the diaphragm. Sections of this tissue show irregular columns of leukocytes arranged parallel with the fibres and sometimes so solidly grouped as to constitute almost an injection of what appears to be a lymph vessel. Within the muscle area and occasionally in the tendon the fibrin content of the exudate can be demonstrated satisfactorily by Weigert's fibrin stain.

Fragmentation of the muscle fibres and the appearance within them of phagocytic leukocytes would indicate that an attempt was being made to clear up the areas of necrosis by the ordinary process for the removal of necrotic tissue. In this particular instance I have found no evidence of further effort at repair. The acuteness of the process probably explains this finding. The change in the muscle, so far as can be determined from the examination of a single specimen, is restricted to the side involved. In the tendon, however, the lesion is a little more diffuse. The diaphragm in the other case of pneumonia and also the intercostal muscles in the same case show practically no structural alteration, at least nothing that could not be attributed to such variation in spacing of fibres and in size as might be found in any muscle. The changes found in the other 5 cases may be grouped together with the case of acute tuberculous pleurisy. They were not marked. In another case the lesion is much more advanced, and later will be described in detail. In the two acute pneumococcal infections engrafted on catarrhal pneumonia, the lesions are evident and clearly recent; the one chronic case must be considered separately.

The number of cases examined is, of course, too small to determine with accuracy, and, to the satisfaction of the critical observer, the exact order in which the lesions occur. Probably the following order will require revision upon more extended observation; it is at present submitted more for the purpose of indicating the character of the lesions found than with the idea of definitely establishing the chronological order in which the processes occur:

1. Muscle fibres showing marked granular change, inadequate tingibility, and unsatisfactory stain reaction, such as commonly observed in granular tissues, can be recognized in all cases. It is not clear that this granular degeneration or cloudy swelling can be attributed to inflammation in the adjacent serosa, as it closely resembles, indeed, is probably identical with, the cloudy swelling observed in muscles as a result of infectious processes where apparently the toxin is acting through the blood. It would, therefore, seem wise to regard this change as a part of an alteration affecting the general musculature, the intercostals, in common with other muscles, manifesting their share in the change induced by the systemic action of toxic bodies.

2. With this alteration probably begin the changes that are incident to the involvement of and extension from the adjacent serosa. Muscle fibres are dissociated, the separation in some instances being quite distinct. The presence of a granular acidophilic deposit around the muscles and interfascicular connective tissue indicates that we are dealing with an œdema; but few leukocytes can be seen in this stage. The muscle cells stain poorly; the connective tissue does not respond with its wonted activity to the usual connective-tissue dyes. The component cells are swollen and granular, and occasionally a faint network of fibrin can be demonstrated at selected points. There is not, however, in this stage, any conspicuous addition of a fibrin-containing substance. With this condition, bands, groups, and bundles of muscle fibres may be seen showing a change that, so far as I can observe, cannot be differentiated from the hyaline, vitreous, or diaphanous degeneration described by Zenker, known to occur in the muscles of the abdominal wall in typhoid, and now recognized to be a much more widely distributed lesion often found in other conditions. In these hyaline areas muscle fibres often appear to coalesce, so that the hyaline change seems to include the interfascicular tissue as well as the

muscle fibre. Whether this change be a secondary degeneration or necrosis, probably our present methods are inadequate to determine. That it is not identical with coagulation necrosis containing fibrin can easily be established by the absence of fibrin in some areas where the process now under consideration is conspicuous; we are familiar with processes clearly necrotic and closely resembling, if not identical with, the change now under consideration, that could not, with propriety, be grouped with the necroses. As this, however, is neither the time nor the place to enter into the academic discussion as to what constitutes necrosis and what degeneration, it does not seem necessary to consider further the change present, the appearance of which is fairly well reproduced in Fig. 1.

FIG. 1.

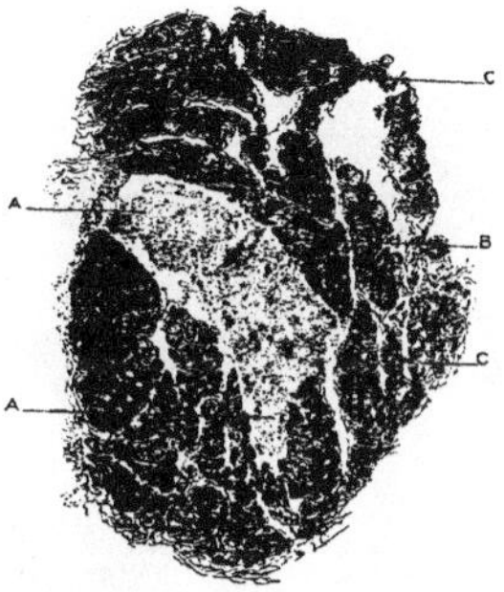

Intercostal muscle, transverse section, from a case of epipneumonic pleurisy, showing area of necrosis. Tissue fixed in Zenker's fluid; hæmatoxylin and eosin stain. A, A. Necrotic area in some portions of which the shadowy outlines of muscle fibres may still be distinguished, B. A few mononuclear leukocytes, mostly of the lymphoid type, aggregated on the margin of the necrotic area. C, C. Fragmenting vacuolated fibres, of which several can be seen in the field.

3. It seems reasonable to assume that the stage now to be described is preceded, at least in some instances, by the alterations mentioned above. The dissociation of the fibres, the granular material, the areas of hyaline change, can still be recognized, or at least appearances of their having been present may be more or less fully identified. In this stage there is a leukocytic infiltration of the muscle similar to that shown in the photographs illustrating Rohrer's article. The leukocytes present in the specimen studied are mostly of the mononuclear type, many of them corresponding to the large lymphocyte or hyaline cell; the polymorphonuclears have not been exceedingly numerous; eosinophiles have not been identified in the altered areas. The dissociation, fragmentation, granularity, and necrosis of the muscle fibres are in this stage very much more evident. It is a diffuse process; some of the fibres appear to suffer

to a marked degree, almost amounting to a necrosis, while others but slightly altered may be seen immediately adjacent, in a way resembling very closely the myocardial degenerations that have been described in various infectious diseases. (See Fig. 2.) Fibrin is abundantly present; bacteria may be conspicuous, while in the preceding forms they were at most but scanty and usually absent. There is in this stage no difficulty in the identification of organisms that in the pneumonias and epipneumonic pleurisies may, with reasonable certainty, be considered pneumococci. Sometimes the bacteria are grouped in the spaces between the muscle fibres in such a manner as to indicate dissemination along a lymph vessel, possibly only a larger lymph space.

FIG. 2.

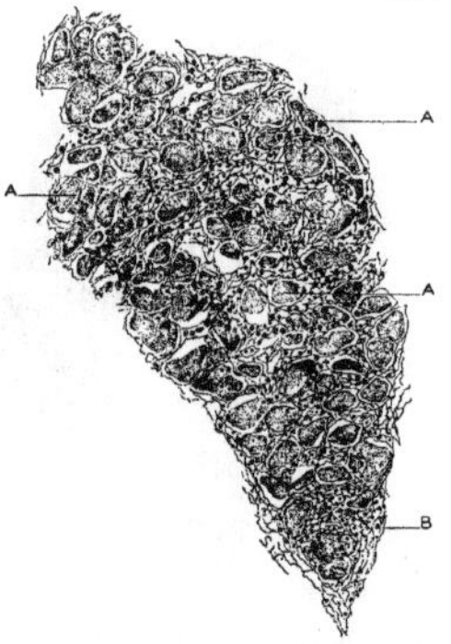

Intercostal muscle, transverse section, from a case of epipneumonic pleurisy, showing dissociation of fibres, interfascicular leukocytic infiltration, and slight fibrin formation. Tissue fixed in Zenker's fluid; hæmatoxylin and eosin stain. A, A, A. Granular and fragmented muscle fibres B. Accumulation of leukocytes and fibrin around and extending between the muscle fibres. In some areas the change is more marked than in others, and at points many polymorphonuclear leukocytes can be seen.

It has not been possible to secure specimens showing what might be looked upon as the next stage, and as to the ultimate outcome, should the patient recover, it is not possible at the present time to offer any unassailable opinion. Evidence of abscess formation is usually absent; the process seems more diffuse, but one could easily appreciate that the small necrotic areas infiltrated by polymorphonuclear leukocytes are really microscopic abscesses, such as can readily be demonstrated in the diaphragm. Our knowledge of the pathology of muscle inflammations leads us to infer that with the subsidence of active infection the necrotic muscle fibres would be removed by phagocytic cells (myoclasts); the interfascicular exudate would undergo absorption, and, with the formation of a certain amount of fibrous tissue, there would eventually result a moderate degree of muscle sclerosis. It therefore seems reasonable to assume that where the disease lasts a sufficient length of time—where, in other words, the infection is permitted to continue—the changes between the stages just described and the conditions found in the specimen examined and reported below would fall under the head of subacute or chronic sclerosing myositis, which, toward the end, would give rise to the picture presented in the following case.

For the privilege of reporting this case I am under particular obligation to Professor Keen, who kindly placed at my disposal his notes and description of the operation, from which I summarize as follows:[1]

F. A., male, aged twenty-two years. Admitted to the Jefferson Hospital on June 11, 1903. Patient of Dr. Boyer.

Left-sided pleurisy of six years' duration, terminating in empyema. Upon admission to the hospital the left side of the chest was fuller than the right. The intercostal spaces obliterated. Mediastinal organs displaced to the right. June 9, 1903, aspiration; three quarts of yellowish pus withdrawn. On June 16th Dr. Stewart excised two inches of the seventh rib on the left side at the anterior axillary line, opened the pleural cavity, evacuated a large quantity of greenish-yellow, turbid fluid, and inserted two drains. Bacteriological examination by Dr. Rosenberger at this time showed cultures of the micrococcus pyogenes aureus and albus. The urine contained albumin, hyaline and granular casts. Under drainage the patient improved and left the hospital on June 28th. Daily irrigation of the cavity was practised for some time before leaving the hospital. He was readmitted under Professor Keen's care on October 26th. The heart was still displaced somewhat to the right; the left side of the chest was still flat; diminished resonance over left lung, with respiratory sounds diminished in upper and absent in lower half of organ. Urine contained trace of albumin, but casts were not detected. Tubercle bacilli were not found in the discharge from the pleura. Pneumococci noted as absent. Staphylococcus pyogenes aureus still present, and an organism possessing the morphology and tinctorial characters of the diphtheria bacillus, but without pathogenic action for animals, was obtained in studies made by Dr. Rosenberger.

On November 4th Professor Keen again submitted the patient to operation, and the following record is from his notes:

"I made the usual large flap extending from the second rib, with a broad sweep under the arm down to the level of the seventh rib, and backward between the scapula and the spine. The entire thickness of the chest-wall, including a greatly thickened pleura, was then removed from the third to the seventh ribs, inclusive. The pericardium and pleura were exposed. I made no attempt at decor-

[1] The physical signs were characteristic and need not be detailed.

tication, but only curetted the parts thoroughly, because the patient's condition was bad, with his heart pushing over to the right side, the left lung of very little use, and the right hampered by the displacement of the heart and the left lung; the operation was finished as rapidly as possible; after replacing the flap, which left a large opening at the lower portion, and packing some iodoform gauze to check the slight oozing, the wound was closed.

"On December 2d there were evidences of a beginning œdema of the lungs; he rapidly failed and died on the 4th."

No autopsy was obtained.

The specimen removed came to the laboratory for study and was submitted for examination to Dr. Ellis, Demonstrator of Morbid Histology, whose report is as follows:

"The specimen consists of a number of pieces of ribs varying from 2 cm. to 9 cm. in length, to which are attached masses of tissue; portions of this tissue are grayish in color, dense, and apparently fibrous. The surface of some of the masses is yellowish or yellowish-gray and shows areas of necrosis. Small fragments of muscle are also attached.

"The soft parts were fixed in Bensley's fluid, dehydrated, cleared, and infiltrated with paraffin. Sections were cut and stained by the usual laboratory methods.

"Microscopic examination shows the majority of the sections to be made up of fibrous tissue, most of which is in the early stages, though certain parts are quite dense. The margin of the sections bordering the most recent fibrous tissue is composed of embryonic and granulation tissues in which are numerous polymorphonuclear leukocytes. Beneath this formative zone is fibrous tissue in various stages of formation. Some of the sections contain considerable striated muscle, which has undergone pronounced changes. Certain areas show a high degree of fatty infiltration, while in others this is associated with a marked increase of the fibrous tissue. The latter change is for the most part fairly recent in point of time. The muscle fibres show varying degrees of atrophy. Vacuolization and fragmentation of the fibres are also seen."

It will be observed that this specimen shows marked atrophy and advanced destruction of the muscle fibres, with intercalation of newly formed and forming fibrous tissue with, at points, advanced substitutive lipomatous infiltration. It seems reasonable to assume that the long-continued infection of the pleura has given rise to this alteration in the intercostal muscles. These structures in this specimen show no evidence of an existing infection. The process has assumed a very much more chronic type manifested by the development of formative tissue in the intramuscular septa and in the interfascicular spaces. Necrotic processes are no longer active in the muscles. Fig. 3 represents a small area from this specimen, and shows to advantage the essential changes in the muscular tissue.

PATHOGENESIS. It seems to the writer that the cause of these changes in the intercostal muscles is clear. Feiner has shown that after injecting fluids containing suspended granules into the pleura the extraneous matter may be demonstrated in the costal pleural lymphatics, and that but little resorption takes place through the pulmonary pleura. When we consider the fact that in inflammations of the lung and pleura the interlobular and intralobular lymphatic systems can be seen engorged with products of absorption from the lung principally, we can understand how the parietal or costal lymphatic system must necessarily care for the major part of the drainage from the pleural cavity. This being the case, toxic materials passing off by this route are brought in close proximity to the inter-

FIG. 3.

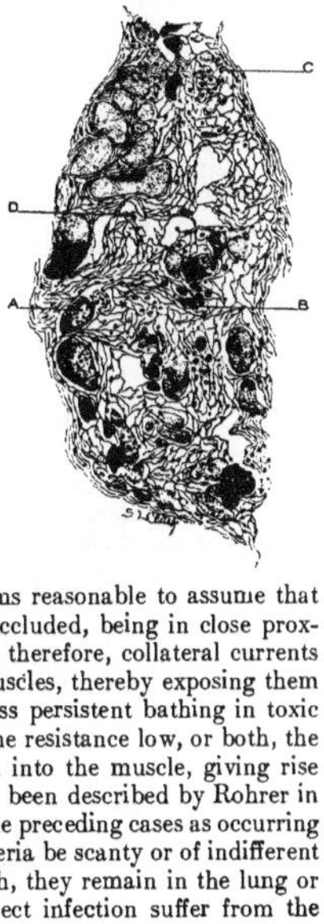

Intercostal muscle, transverse section, from a case of suppurative pleurisy of several months duration, showing advanced fibrosis and lipomatous change. Tissue fixed in Zenker's fluid; hæmatoxylin and eosin stain. A. One of several granular fibres, some of which are fragmented and undergoing absorption. B. A small group of greatly shrunken muscle fibres. C Relatively large mononuclear cell, not very abundant but commonly associated with fibroblastic elements. D. The leader from this letter passes between two imperfectly preserved fat bodies, a number of which are present in the newly forming or formed fibrous tissue. The fat content is scanty in the particular field from which this drawing is made.

costal muscles and diaphragm; it seems reasonable to assume that direct lymphatic paths may become occluded, being in close proximity to the centres of irritation, and, therefore, collateral currents must form through the intercostal muscles, thereby exposing them to the dangers induced by more or less persistent bathing in toxic lymph. If the infection be active or the resistance low, or both, the pathogenic organisms may be carried into the muscle, giving rise to suppurative processes, such as have been described by Rohrer in the diaphragm, and figured in one of the preceding cases as occurring in the intercostal muscles. If the bacteria be scanty or of indifferent activity or the patient's resistance high, they remain in the lung or pleura, and the muscles escaping direct infection suffer from the toxic action only.

Where the irritation extends over a considerable length of time and granulation tissue with its protective influence against infection clothes the costal pleura, or where newly formed collagenous tissue is intercalated between the muscle and the altered serosa, then products reaching the muscle would probably be less active or materially modified toxins without evident bacteria. Here, then, results the chronic sclerosing change comparable to that seen in the muscles adjacent to tuberculous areas elsewhere in the body, as, for example, around tuberculosis of the hip, vertebræ, etc. In the more acute stages of the process the degenerative and necrotic change seen in the muscles may be attributed to the action of the toxins, passing through the lymphatics of the muscles or diffusing into the muscle tissue. In the later acute cases bacteria themselves enter. In the cases of longer duration there might occur a chronic suppurative interstitial and parenchymatous myositis, but probably the patient would not survive an infection of this type, except purely as a local manifestation. The chronic alteration of importance is the sclerosing process by which the muscle is in part or almost wholly replaced by newly formed fibrous tissue in which fatty infiltration or lipomatous substitution almost constantly occurs.

The influence of the changes already described on the thoracic wall so fully suggest themselves that a detailed consideration need hardly be given. The clinician will at once think of the modifications in physical signs—muffling and alteration in auscultatory sounds depending upon increased density of the thoracic wall—brought about by any of the changes described, including serous infiltration, cellular accumulation, as well as fibrous and lipomatous change in the intercostal muscles; the influence of the change upon the function of these muscles will also be apparent. Even slight myositis is associated with rigidity, a more or less successful attempt at fixation, and this fully accords with the recognized clinical data.

A large amount of space might profitably be devoted to consideration of the influence of the change upon respiration, but as this is evident, I need but touch upon this point. Hamberger's observations on the functions of the intercostal muscles in respiration has received general acceptance, and has been corroborated by the studies of Newell Martin and Hartwell, Masoin, and R. du Bois-Reymond.[1] The fact that the internal muscles are actively operative in respiration only when the function is labored renders more important the alterations now under consideration, because with alterations in the diaphragm, the principal muscle of respiration, and with the influence of intoxication upon the respiratory centres, and satisfactory evidence of narrowing of the intercostal spaces, as suggested by Przewalski, it becomes at once clear that structural alterations

[1] The details of muscular action in respiration are fully considered by Starling in Schäfer's Text-book of Physiology, vol. ii. pp. 274–280; he also cites the authorities to whom I refer.

in these muscles must materially influence the alterations in chest volume upon which air intake so largely depends. The fact that the external intercostal muscles are but slightly involved and often escape does not modify this observation, because physiologists are fully familiar with the fact that opposing muscles are reciprocally influenced. Mention should be made of the influence of sclerosing myositis in the production of costal fixation in the chronic cases; whatever views may be entertained with regard to the inexpansibility of lungs long atelectatic, the condition of the ribs as regards motility cannot be ignored. The fixation of the affected side in acute cases may be, as is usually held, reflex, but it may also depend upon the spastic fixation of muscles (intercostal and diaphragmatic), the seat of pronounced architectural change.

Structural alterations in the intercostal muscles possibly clear up to some extent the observations that intercostal rheumatism, intercostal neuralgia, etc., are complicating or associated phenomena of pneumonia and pleurisy. In this connection there are several factors in this field that the writer appreciates are not worked out. Probably the most conspicuous is alteration of the nerves. Some of the sections show nerves that appear œdematous. In none of them has any cellular infiltration been observed. The tissues have not been prepared suitably for the demonstration of myelin degeneration, and this question must be taken up with some detail later. I might at this point, however, say that sections show, what histologists so far as I know do not mention, namely, that nerve filaments or even relatively large trunks can be seen coursing between the internal intercostal muscles and the adjacent pleura. They are so situated as to expose them to all the toxic substances permeating the adjacent muscle. In one block of tissue from an acute case two relatively large nerve bundles can be seen immediately below the serosa imbedded in a small cushion of fat; the epineurium touches the serosa, and a vessel lying in immediate proximity contains, on transverse section, seventeen erythrocytes, two polymorphonuclear leukocytes, and one hyaline cell—presumably a local leukocytosis. The nerve bundle is retracted from its sheath, on the inner aspect of which can be recognized transverse sections of two capillaries containing red cells, but no leukocytes; there is no leukocytic infiltration of the sheath or nerve. Another specimen contains a longitudial section of a nerve that at one point shows a suggestion of cellular infiltration and contains a widely dilated capillary. Such axis-cylinder stains as have been applicable to Zenker material demonstrate no noteworthy change in the myelin sheaths and axis-cylinders of the nerves, but, as usual in such material, myelin stains have proved unsatisfactory.

The foregoing offers no sufficient anatomical basis for the conclusion that the nerves suffer; nevertheless, I am satisfied that in such instances as the one narrated they cannot long escape. Their perilous situation exposes them to the noxious influences of infection, toxic bodies, and other coincidents of inflammation, to the action of which nerve elements are conspicuously susceptible. It would be interesting to know if the clinicians have observed any paralytic phenomena that indicate a toxic degeneration or neuritis involving the phrenic nerve or motor branches to the intercostal muscles. Alteration in the sensory fibres is strongly indicated by certain of the clinical factors; will the clinicians kindly advise us what, if any, symptoms or physical signs point to motor involvement? I feel reasonably certain that there is no sufficient reason why the motor nerves should escape.

An extremely important point to be determined is whether there are any lymphatic ways corresponding to intercostal spaces in which this change is most marked. While I have no information that would justify a positive conclusion upon this point, the fact that well-marked changes may be seen in one area of an intercostal muscle, and the block of tissue from an adjacent neighborhood fails to show the alteration, leads to the belief that the lymphatic course or tract should merit special consideration, and it appears that in a very general way only have the anatomists and histologists solved this problem. Possibly we have, in what might be called pathological injection of the lymphatic spaces and vessels, an important adjuvant in the study of the lymph courses. I have had no opportunity to study the changes in the lymph trunks draining the costal pleura; such a study, based upon experimentally produced inflammations of the lung and pleura, is needed.

An important question suggested by Dr. Riesman is what would the intercostal muscles of the sound side show? In one of the cases of pneumococcal pleurisy the muscles of the other side escaped, or at least showed no structural change. I am not inclined to believe that the opposite side is involved, unless thrombosis of the costal lymphatics of one side might lead to an anastomotic current passing to the other; such spanning of the mediastinum would seem improbable.

Another point upon which these studies are inadequate is the frequency with which the intercostal involvement occurs. Five of the seven cases studied are Philadelphia Hospital patients, and those familiar with the Blockley morgue know that we may draw incorrect conclusions as to the frequency of concurrent conditions, because we are dealing with a class in whom coincidence of pathological processes is a conspicuous feature.

Kuettner[1] has made an exhaustive study of the perforating lymphatics of the diaphragm. He shows that the drainage territories of the diaphragm are such that abundant opportunity is

[1] Thirty-third Congress of the German Surgical Society, June, 1903; Centralbl. f. Chir., 1903, No. 36; Beiträge z. klin. Chir., Tübingen, vol. xl., No. 1.

afforded for transdiaphragmatic infection, and has so worked out the lymph paths as to show that while each half of the organ possesses its own lymphatic field communicating with other parts by way of lymph nodes only, all parts of the diaphragm possess anastomotic communication with the pleura and peritoneum. The anterior and posterior lymph vessels communicate and drain in common into certain glands; some of these vessels vertically transverse the diaphragm twice in coursing over it. Taken with the studies of Rohrer and my own observations, it seems that Kuettner's work forms the necessary link in completing our already fairly full comprehension of the possibilities of transdiaphragmatic infections. That a juxtaposed abdominal viscus may infect the pleura or pericardium (*e. g.*, hepatic, splenic, and perirenal abscesses and gastric ulcer) has long been common property, but that lesions of a finer texture may be recognized, and that the four great serous cavities are really intercommunicating lymph spaces, is within recent times leading to deductions some of which may be important. Is it possible that the pneumococcal inflammations of the peritoneum (even when primary) may be transdiaphragmatic infections, the lung and pleura escaping in some cases? The frequency with which the ribs suffer typhoidal osteomyelitis is suggestive, and if, as Fraenkel holds, the typhoidal spondylitis is really a bacillary infection of the cancellous tissues of the bodies of the vertebræ, the demonstration of abdominal and thoracic lymph systems as so closely allied threatens, as the result of a minor disclosure, to lead one into a labyrinth of unjustified speculation.

It is not the purpose of this paper to consider transdiaphragmatic infections, the passage of fat-necrosing substances through the diaphragm, and cancerous extension from peritoneum to pleura, or the reverse; these subjects have recently been studied by von Brunn[1] and Jensen,[2] in pneumococcal peritonitis; by Henle,[3] in an article on "Pneumonia and Laparotomy;" by Truhart,[4] in considering intrathoracic fat-necrosis in disease of the pancreas, and by Tilger,[5] in pleurisy and peritonitis; Kuettner[6] discusses and gives most of the references. The demonstration of lesions in the tendon of the diaphragm is only a minor extension of Röhrer's observation.

In conclusion, I wish to express my appreciation of the kindness of Professor Keen, and Drs. Rosenberger, Ellis, and Funke, for p aid in the preparation of material upon which this paper is [illegible]

[1] Beiträge z. klin. Chir., Bd. xxxix., Heft 1, p. 94.

[2] Langenbeck's Archiv, Bd. lxx., Heft 1, p. 95.

[3] Ibid., Bd. lxiv., Heft 2.

[4] Pankreas Pathologie, 1902.

[5] Virchow's Arch., Bd. cxxxviii. p. 499.

[6] Loc. cit.

A CLINICAL REPORT OF THREE CASES OF INJURY TO THE LOWER SPINAL CORD AND CAUDA EQUINA:

WITH REMARKS UPON PERONEAL PALSY DUE TO A LESION IN THE EPICONUS, UPON INCREASE OF THE PATELLAR TENDON REFLEXES FROM A LESION BELOW THE LUMBAR SEGMENT, AND UPON A RARE FORM OF BROWN-SÉQUARD PARALYSIS RESULTING FROM A LESION OF THE LOWER END OF THE SPINAL CORD.[1]

BY THEODORE H. WEISENBURG, M.D.,

INSTRUCTOR IN NERVOUS DISEASES AND IN NEUROPATHOLOGY, UNIVERSITY OF PENNSYLVANIA; ASSISTANT NEUROLOGIST TO THE PHILADELPHIA HOSPITAL.

(From the service of Dr. Wm. G. Spiller, Philadelphia and Polyclinic Hospitals.)

THE following three cases are reported because of their unusual symptoms. The first case presents bilateral peroneal palsy with typical steppage gait due to a lesion in the epiconus—*i. e.*, that portion of the spinal cord between and including the fifth lumbar and first and second sacral segments. Peroneal palsy is almost always due to a peripheral lesion. The second case is one with increased patellar reflexes with a lesion in the cauda equina, below the reflex arc for the knee-jerk. This condition has not been heretofore dwelt upon. The third case is interesting because of a form of Brown-Séquard paralysis peculiar to cases of unilateral lesions in the lower end of the cord. In this type motion and sensation are affected in the same lower limb, while sensation in the external genitalia and perineum of the opposite side is also disturbed.

CASE I.—J. K., aged thirty-five years, laborer, while walking on a railroad track was struck by an engine going at a moderate rate of speed. He was struck in the middle of the back and was thrown about thirty-five feet. He was picked up in an unconscious condition, and when admitted to the University Hospital two hours afterward consciousness had returned. He had always been healthy up to this time (January 5, 1901). His family history and past history are negative. Examination on admission showed numerous lacerations of the head, ears, a broken nose, and subconjunctival ecchymosis. The back in the mid-dorsal and lumbosacral region was contused, but no fracture or dislocation of the vertebræ could be made out. The man complained of intense pain in the back and of a burning sensation in his feet, which was aggravated by pressure. There was complete motor paralysis of his lower extremities. Vesical control was lost. No rectal disturbances were present. Examination

[1] Read before the Philadelphia Neurological Society, October 27, 1903.

three days after the injury by Dr. Potts gave the following results: The patient can voluntarily contract the quadriceps and adductor muscles of either thigh. He is able to raise the thigh slightly from the bed. No atrophy is noticeable in the lower extremities. All muscles respond to the faradic current. All the reflexes in both lower extremities—*i. e.*, the patellar jerk, Achilles jerk, and ankle clonus—are absent. Plantar irritation produces no movement of the toes. He cannot pass his urine voluntarily, but knows when his bladder is full. To-day he defecated voluntarily. Sensation for touch, pain, and temperature is lost over the dorsum of both feet, and on the outer side of both legs to the knees. He complains of an intense burning and numb feeling in both feet, especially marked when pressure is applied. He does not know when his toes are moved. A beginning bed-sore is found over the sacrum.

A note made twenty-five days after the injury states that vesical control was normal. Examination by Dr. Potts a month after injury gave the following results: the patellar jerks are still absent. The Achilles jerk is present on each side and is marked more on the right. Plantar irritation produces a doubtful extension of toes on both sides. The muscles are flabby and somewhat atrophied. No change in electrical reactions is found. Sensation is about the same as at the previous examination. From this time on his condition gradually improved, the patellar jerk on the left side returned two months later. Six months after the injury he was able to be out of bed and could walk with the aid of crutches, at which time it was noticed that he had a typical "steppage" gait. He left the University Hospital (April 30, 1902) and could then walk without the aid of a cane, and was admitted later to the nervous wards of the Philadelphia Hospital, service of Dr. William G. Spiller.

Examination on September 30, 1903, by me showed a wasting of the buttocks and of both lower extremities, more marked on the right side, there being a difference of one inch above and one-half inch below the knees. He lies with both extremities strongly abducted. Motor power is diminished on the right side more than on the left. The flexors of the right thigh are weak, while power of adduction of both thighs is greatly diminished, and more so on the right side. He can flex and extend the toes slightly, but no movements are possible at the ankle-joints, and he has bilateral foot-drop. The patient walks with a swinging step, lifting his foot high from the ground, and has a distinct steppage gait.

The cremasteric reflex is prompt on either side. The left patellar tendon reflex is much exaggerated; on the right side, however, there is no movement of the leg on the thigh from tapping the patellar tendon, but a strong contraction of the quadriceps muscle can be easily felt. Ankle clonus is prompt and persistent on both sides. Babinski's sign is present on either side. There is a hypæsthesia for all forms of sensation over the dorsum of both feet, extending on the outer side of both legs to the knees. Bladder and bowel control are normal. All the muscles of the lower limbs respond to the faradic current.

The lesion in this case was most probably a hemorrhage into the spinal cord or a traumatic myelitis between the fourth lumbar and third sacral segments of the spinal cord. The absence of bladder, rectal, and sexual disturbances shows that the conus medullaris, arbitrarily put by Raymond between the beginning of the filum terminale and the third sacral segment, and including that segment, and that the fibres in the lateral columns controlling these reflexes are intact. The paralysis involves principally the peroneal group of muscles on either side, while the adductors and flexors of the thighs, especially on the right side, are paretic; in addition, there is a weakness of the glutei. The cells in the anterior horns of the spinal cord controlling these muscles have been placed by various authors between the fourth lumbar and third sacral segments, some writers placing the centres for the adductors and flexors as high as the third lumbar segment. The upper limit of the lesion is shown by the presence, in fact, the exaggeration of the patellar tendon reflexes and the preservation of the cremasteric reflex, these reflexes showing the integrity of the fourth lumbar segment and the lumbar segments above.

The case affords evidence that the cremaster reflex arc must have its spinal portion above the fourth lumbar segment, and that it is not in the sacral cord, as some writers have taught, and that the reflex arc for ankle clonus must be below the second sacral segment. The preservation of the bladder, rectal, and genital reflexes seems to indicate that the white matter of the lateral columns is not seriously affected, even in the lower lumbar and upper sacral cord, and that the lesion must be almost confined to the gray matter.

Minor,[1] of Moscow, pointed out in 1901 that just such a symptom-complex always occurs in lesions involving the gray matter of this area—*i. e.*, the fifth lumbar and first and second sacral segments. In such cases the paralysis always involves the distribution of the sacral plexus, and the peroneal group of muscles is most affected and the paralysis of these muscles lasts the longest. In some of his cases there was paresis of the flexors and adductors of the thigh. The negative symptoms were preservation of the patellar reflexes and absence of bladder and rectal disturbances. He called this region of the spinal cord the epiconus.¶ Similar observations have been recorded by others, Remak,[2] Wagner and Stolper, Kötter, Barth and Hartmann, and Erb, but none by English and American writers, so far as I know. The important feature of these cases is

[1] Deutsche Zeitschr. f. Nervenheilkunde, 1901, p. 334.
[2] Quoted by Daus., S. Monatsschrift f. Psych. u. Neurol., B. xiii., H. 5, S. 394, 1903.

the involvement of the gray matter of the fifth lumbar, and first and second sacral segments with integrity of the white matter.

CASE II.—J. C., aged thirty-one years, white, laborer, was admitted to the Philadelphia Hospital July 13, 1903. He was shot June 8, 1903, in the left buttock with a thirty-eight calibre Colt revolver about ten feet away, the ball entering and perforating the left fifth lumbar vertebra, as was shown afterward by the x-rays. The course of the bullet was downward and to the right; the ball, however, has not as yet been located. The patient could not walk during the first two weeks and had no control of the bladder or rectum. Examination by Dr. Spiller, July 18, 1903, one month after injury, showed that voluntary power in the lower limbs was nearly normal, except in the flexors of the right foot. Both patellar jerks were a little prompter than normal. The Achilles jerk was absent on either side, and Babinski's sign was absent, there being no movement of the toes in either direction. There was an area of greatly diminished sensation for touch and pain over the right buttock, extending about three or four inches from the median line, and in a narrow zone back of the right thigh and back of the right leg, and on the outer side and sole of the right foot, corresponding, according to Kocher's diagram, with the distribution of the second, third, and fourth sacral segments. The sensation in the left lower limb was normal. He had incontinence of the bladder and bowel.

Examination by me October 11, 1903, three months after the injury, showed the patient's condition to be much improved. The flexors of his right foot were still weak and he could not rotate outward his right thigh as well as he should. The right buttock was flat, there being atrophy of the glutei. Sensation was about the same as at the previous examination, with the addition of a hypæsthesia of the right side of the scrotum and penis.

Both cremasteric reflexes were present, and both patellar tendon reflexes were distinctly increased. No Achilles jerk nor Babinski's sign was obtained on either side. He could hold his urine, but the power of the bladder was still diminished. He was constipated, and after a purgative could not control the rectum. All the muscles responded to the faradic current, except the right glutei, there being also no response in these muscles to the galvanic current.

The lesion in this case must have implicated the cauda equina, as the bullet entered at the fifth lumbar vertebra, and its course was downward. The interesting point of this case, and the one I wish to call special attention to, is the increase of the patellar tendon reflexes when the lesion was below the reflex arc. I have been unable to find any reference to this condition in the literature at my command, except in Thorburn's[1] contribution to the *Surgery of the Spinal Cord.* This author mentions the following cases with increase

[1] Philadelphia, Blakiston & Son, 1889.

of the patellar reflexes, but pays no special attention to this subject. One case I have found also reported by Franz Volhard.[1]

First case, cited by Thorburn from Kirchoff: backward crushing of the first lumbar vertebra causing a degeneration of the fourth and fifth sacral segments, the only symptoms being paralysis of the bladder and rectum and increased patellar reflexes. Sexual and sensory changes are not mentioned.

Second case: a partial compression of the cauda equina about the level of the last lumbar vertebra, causing severe neuralgic pains in the sciatic and pudic distributions, a weakness of some of the muscles of the lower limbs, but no complete paralysis and no anæsthesia of the limbs. The bladder and rectal functions were paralyzed. The patellar reflexes were slightly exaggerated, but there was no ankle clonus.

The third case is cited by Thorburn from Oppenheim, and was one of fracture of the first lumbar vertebra, causing a myelitis of the conus medullaris. There was a slight weakness of the calf muscles, otherwise no loss of power or atrophy. Anæsthesia was limited to the peroneal region and buttocks. There was paralysis of bladder and rectum. Here also the knee-jerks were exaggerated, but there was no ankle clonus.

The fourth case, by Volhard, of a tumor of the cauda equina, as proved by necropsy, with motor and sensory symptoms, absent Achilles jerks, and weakness of the plantar reflexes, but both the patellar reflexes and the cremasteric reflexes were exaggerated.

In all four of these cases, therefore, the exaggeration of the patellar reflexes was probably caused by lesions *below* the reflex arc.

It is difficult to find a satisfactory explanation for such a phenomenon as this, but evidently the patellar reflex arc is in some way thrown into a state of excitation in these cases. No writer has made this a subject of careful study, and it seems therefore important to emphasize the fact that a reflex may be increased by a lesion in the spinal cord below the portion in which the reflex arc is represented. Considerable evidence is offered that in the nervous system there are both depressomotor and excitomotor fibres for the different reflexes, these having their origin in the brain; and it may be that other excitomotor fibres exert their influence on segments above those in which these fibres arise. We know that spinal roots on entering the cord give off descending branches that pass downward in the posterior columns; the function of these fibres is entirely unknown, but we must assume that in some way they affect the function of the lower segments. It is probable that in a similar manner the lower spinal segments exert some influence over higher spinal segments, and there is no doubt whatever that in the anterolateral columns degeneration of short fibres occurs upward. It is

[1] Deutsche med. Wochen., 1902, No. 33.

presumable that these fibres exert some control over higher segments than those in which they arise, and in this way possibly cause an exaggeration of tendon reflexes.

CASE III.—S. W. was admitted to the Polyclinic Hospital July 15, 1903. He fell down an elevator-shaft from the eighth floor, a distance of about 120 feet. He was not unconscious, but sustained a fracture and displacement of the second lumbar and twelfth thoracic vertebræ, as determined by the x-rays several days afterward.

Examination by Dr. Spiller on the following day gave the following results: The right lower limb was completely paralyzed. Voluntary power in the left lower limb was almost normal; some weakness, however, was present in the flexors of the left thigh. The patellar jerks, Achilles jerks, Babinski's reflex, and ankle clonus were not obtained on either side. The cremasteric reflex was lost on the right side, but prompt on the left side. The bladder and bowel control was lost. The whole right leg felt numb. Sensation did not appear to be lost entirely in any part, but touch and pain sensations seemed impaired in the right thigh, both front and back, over the right buttock and the right side of the scrotum. The sensation of the left lower limb was normal.

Examination by me August 10, 1903, one month afterward, showed no appreciable change, except that by reinforcement a slight movement of the leg on the thigh was obtained on tapping the left patellar tendon. The whole right leg seemed wasted. He could flex the toes slightly, and bladder and rectal control was better. From this time on the patient improved steadily, and was discharged from the hospital September 1, 1903, about two months after admission.

Examination at present, three months after injury, gives the following results: The patient is able to walk without the aid of crutches, although still weak. The left lower limb seems normal. The right lower limb is generally wasted as compared with the left lower limb. All movements of the toes, ankle, knee, and hip on the right side are possible, although not quite normal. The patellar tendon reflexes, Achilles jerk, and ankle clonus are absent on either side.

Plantar irritation produces no movement of the toes. The cremasteric reflex is absent on the right and prompt on the left side. There is no absolute loss of sensation in the right lower limb, but he does not feel touch and pain as well as he should, and he complains of numbness in the anterior part of the thigh and foot. The bladder, bowel, and sexual functions are still impaired. Sensation is normal over the left lower limb, but touch and pain sensations are diminished over the left half of the penis and scrotum.

The interesting feature of this case is the Brown-Séquard symptom-complex, as shown by the weakness of the right lower limb and the hypæsthesia for touch and pain in the same lower limb, while on the other side there is hypæsthesia for the same forms of sensation over the left side of the penis and scrotum. The lesion must have been a traumatic myelitis of the right side of the spinal cord or an intramedullary hemorrhage, sufficiently high to involve some of the motor and sensory fibres of the same side supplying the right lower limb, but not high enough to involve the sensory fibres supplying the left lower limb after their decussation to the opposite side. It has been shown that the sensory fibres of the pudendal plexus decussate lower in the spinal cord than do the sensory fibres supplying the lower extremities. This case seems to prove this view to be correct,

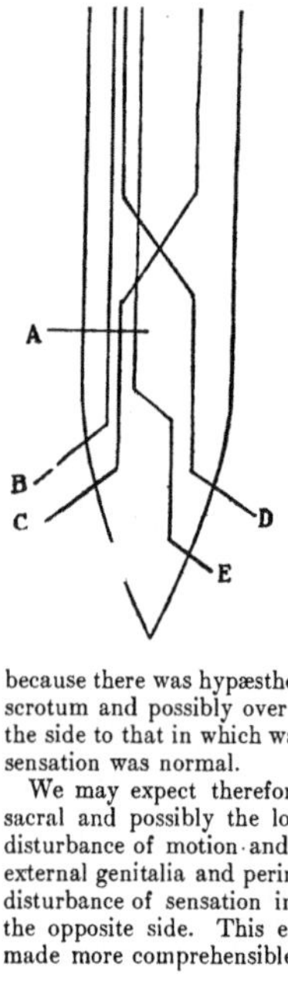

Diagram showing the motor and sensory fibres implicated within the spinal cord in Case III. A. Unilateral lesion implicating the lumbar and sacral regions below the line represented by A. B. The motor fibres of one side of the cord for the innervation of the lower limb. C The sensory fibres from the same lower limb, decussating above the lesion. E. The sensory fibres from the perineum and external genitalia of the opposite side, decussating below the lesion. D. The sensory fibres from the opposite lower limb, decussating above the lesion.

because there was hypæsthesia for touch and pain over the penis and scrotum and possibly over the perineum on the left side, opposite the side to that in which was the lesion, while in the left lower limb sensation was normal.

We may expect therefore in a case of unilateral lesion in the sacral and possibly the lower lumbar region of the spinal cord, disturbance of motion and sensation in the lower limb and in the external genitalia and perineum on the same side as the lesion, and disturbance of sensation in the external genitalia and perineum of the opposite side. This explanation for this symptom-complex is made more comprehensible by the accompanying figure. This is a form of Brown-Séquard paralysis, but very different from that occurring when the lesion is higher in the cord.

This interesting symptom-complex was first described by Wernicke[1] in 1891. Later, Mann[2] described more fully the same case, and added a similar one of his own. So far as I know these two are the only previous cases on record. A short abstract of these cases is given below:

Case I.—Patient, aged thirty-two years, had not had syphilis, and previously had been healthy. One evening he complained of intense pain in the back and a weakness in the left lower limb. This increased so that he could not use his leg at all. Pain disappeared shortly and paresis improved. Six months after this he presented a flaccid paralysis of the left lower limb; the only muscle acting was the iliopsoas. All the reflexes were lost. He never had bladder, rectal, or sexual disturbances and no pain in his left leg. Sensation for pain and temperature was diminished in the left lower extremity as compared with the right lower extremity. On the right side sensation for pain and temperature was diminished over the scrotum, penis, and perineum. No motor weakness was found in the right leg.

Case II.—Patient fell three metres, landing on his buttocks. This resulted in a paralysis of the left lower limb, loss of sexual, bladder, and rectal control. One year after the injury the gait was spastic and paretic, the left leg being dragged on the floor. There was weakness of both lower limbs, much more marked on the left side; the patellar reflexes and Achilles jerks were much increased, but more on the left side. Ankle clonus was not obtained. Both lower limbs were flaccid on passive movement. On the left side there was hypæsthesia for pain and temperature up to the inguinal region anteriorly and iliac crest posteriorly. Touch sensation was normal. The right half of the penis, rectum, and perineum were hypæsthetic to pain- and temperature-sense.

Another interesting feature of my third case is the almost complete restoration of motion in the right lower limb, following probably a traumatic myelitis. In another case which I had the opportunity of seeing through the kindness of Dr. Spiller, paralysis in all four extremities following a jump out of a third-story window existed. Thirteen months after the injury examination showed hardly a trace of paralysis. Such cases as these show the wonderful recuperative powers of the spinal cord when destruction is not complete at any one level.

[1] Sitzungsberichte der schlesischen Gesellschaft f. faterländische Cultur. Sitzung vom 6 Februar, 1891, ferner Gesammelte Aufsätze, p. 300.

[2] Deutsche Zeitsch. f. Nervenheilkunde, vol. x.

THE RELATION OF TYPHOID FEVER TO TUBERCULOSIS.

By James M. Anders, M.D., LL.D.,

PROFESSOR OF MEDICINE AND CLINICAL MEDICINE AT THE MEDICO-CHIRURGICAL COLLEGE; VISITING PHYSICIAN TO THE MEDICO-CHIRURGICAL HOSPITAL; CONSULTING PHYSICIAN TO THE JEWISH HOSPITAL, ETC., PHILADELPHIA.

It is well known that typhoid fever and acute tuberculosis may be rarely associated, and form, so to speak, a composite clinical picture. More commonly, typhoid fever develops in the course of chronic tuberculosis. When acute miliary tuberculosis and typhoid are concurrent, the former disease is, as a rule, secondary to the latter, although it must be recollected that an old tuberculous focus usually co-exists.

In other words, these are cases in which persons with either an active chronic tuberculosis or a latent encapsulated focus contract typhoid fever. It may be assumed that the reaction of the tissues is incomplete; that the resisting powers are defeated and the bacilli liberated under the influence of the typhoid infection. It is also clear that forms of acute tuberculosis are not likely to supervene when there is present a thick, dense limiting wall as in old cases that are practically cured.

This paper deals principally with typhoid fever complicated with acute miliary tuberculosis and acute pneumonic phthisis. It is important to bear in mind that the typhoid process is responsible, in the manner explained above, for the rapid dissemination of the tubercle bacilli or the conversion of chronic into acute tuberculosis.

It must be admitted that rapid infection of the lungs with tubercle bacilli from without may also occur in the course of typhoid fever and acute pneumonic phthisis result as a complication, the primary infection serving as a predisposing condition. Indeed, in at least 4 of the six cases of combined typhoid and acute tuberculosis reported below, the latter affection assumed the pneumonic type, and some of these at all events may have been due to this mode of infection. Moreover, it must be recollected that when typhoid fever arises in subjects of arrested pulmonary tuberculosis and is complicated with bronchopneumonia (as was true of Case II. of my series) the inflammatory changes occasioned by this complication may break down the protecting wall and allow of the distribution of the tubercle bacilli throughout the lungs as well as to other and more remote regions by means of blood and lymphatic metastasis.

It does not appear that a chronic tuberculous process predisposes markedly to typhoid fever, judging from the comparative infrequency of enteric fever in the course of that common disease. Thus out of a totality of 249 autopsies in cases of typhoid fever, only 19 (7.6 per cent.) showed the presence of old tuberculous lesions. Per contra, the former widespread opinion that typhoid fever predisposes to tuberculosis receives no support from my observations, as will be shown hereafter.

Eshner[1] has reported a case of triple infection—pulmonary tuberculosis with intercurrent typhoid fever complicated by pneumonia—and, bearing upon the subject of the occurrence of typhoid fever in the course of tuberculosis, he makes the following statistical quotations: "Among 2000 fatal cases of typhoid fever examined after death at Münich, Hölscher noted 108 (5.4 per cent.) of tuberculosis in various situations, and he quotes Gruber as having noted, among 710 fatal cases of typhoid fever, 22 (3.3 per cent.) complicated by old tuberculosis of the lungs. Bettke, among 1420 cases of typhoid fever at Basle, noted 23 (1.6 per cent.) in tuberculous subjects; while Dopfer noted tuberculosis in 46 (5 per cent.) among 927 cases of typhoid fever."

No allusion is made to the association of acute forms of tuberculosis with typhoid fever in these statistical representations. M. Forget[2] affirms that persons suffering from pulmonary tuberculosis are rarely attacked by typhoid fever, and regards the former as preservative against the latter.

The question of the diagnosis of these combined affections is of the utmost importance from the standpoint of prognosis, the outlook in pure typhoid being generally hopeful. I have also endeavored to determine the incidence of the hybrid affection—typhoid fever and acute tuberculosis—which, as will be shown hereafter, is fortunately extremely rare. The writer has recently met 2 cases in his hospital practice in which these two leading affections appeared to be concurrent. The post-mortem records of the Philadelphia and Episcopal Hospitals for the last ten years have been carefully examined with reference to the question of the relation of typhoid fever to tuberculosis, and the results have been tabulated as follows:[3]

	Total number of cases showing typhoid lesions.	Number of cases showing both typhoid and tuberculous lesions.	Number showing		Variety of acute tuberculosis.
			typhoid and chronic tuberculosis.	typhoid and acute tuberculosis.	
Philadelphia Hospital.	90	11	10	1	Acute miliary tuberculosis.
Johns Hopkins Hospital.	80	4	3	1	Acute pneumonic phthisis.
Episcopal Hospital.	79	8	6	2	Acute pneumonic phthisis and miliary of lungs and pleuræ.
Summary	249	23	19	4	

[1] Philadelphia Medical Journal, March 25, 1899.

[2] Quoted by Murchison, The Continued Fevers of Great Britain, third edition, London, 1884.

[3] The writer desires to make grateful acknowledgment to Dr. Wm. Egbert Robertson and Dr. Ralph H. Spangler for kind aid in collecting statistical data.

Cases illustrative of combined typhoid and acute pneumonic phthisis and acute miliary tuberculosis.

CASE I.—L. B., aged twenty-five years, colored, unmarried, and by occupation a domestic; no history of the use of alcohol, but has had syphilis and one miscarriage; menstruation was regular as a rule.

Family History. Father deceased of unknown cause; mother of pneumonia; patient statedth at she was sick all of last winter; she died in spring; patient had never had any brothers or sisters.

Personal History. Whooping-cough, measles, and mumps as a child; at eighteen years had an attack of rheumatism lasting two weeks and making good recovery. Colds and "coughs" have been common during second decade of life; also sore throat, and much headache.

Present Illness. August 23d went to Cape May and contracted a "cold," which became persistently worse, and she was obliged to betake herself to bed. On September 8th patient was admitted to the female wards of the Medico-Chirurgical Hospital with a cough, pain in her left axillary region, fever, etc.

Physical Examination. Young colored woman, medium size, with poor development and slightly emaciated. There are visible a considerable number of punched scars on the anterior surface of leg. Knee-jerks normal; sensation normal; eyes, liver, and heart also normal. Spleen somewhat enlarged; consolidation of lower lobe of left lung, with a small cavity in left upper lobe.

September 18, 1903, 5 P.M. On account of the splenic enlargement the blood was tested for the Widal reaction, and it responded positively. A sero reaction was also obtained on September 20th and again on September 30th; the diazo reaction was present; considerable enlargement of spleen. Cardiac impulse weak and diffuse pulsation felt over region of left auricle. Slight increase of dulness over same region, but no murmur detectable. Patient much distressed; feels certain that death is at hand. Has at no time been delirious, but symptoms of motor irritation were noted as tremor of upper lips and hands.

Blood Examination. Hæmoglobin, 75 per cent.; reds, 4,680,000; whites, 9400.

Urine Examination. Granular casts; albumin, a trace; specific gravity, 1012.

21*st.* *Sputum Examination.* Tubercle bacilli present; also elastic tissue.

There would appear at first sight to be no doubt as to the coexistence of typhoid fever and acute pneumonic phthisis in this case. The earlier examinations of the patient after admission into the hospital all seemed to indicate tuberculosis; the sole feature that directed attention to the typhoid infection was some considerable splenic enlargement—a more marked increase in size than I had ever seen in pure acute pneumonic phthisis. This fact suggested the making of a blood examination for the Widal reaction and led to the discovery of the associated disease—typhoid fever. Other symptoms of enteric fever, however, developed subsequently.

Case II.—J. S., aged twenty-eight years, a Polander, single, laborer, was admitted to the Medico-Chirurgical Hospital October 29, 1903. The family history proved negative, and the same is true of his previous personal history. Patient was well developed and well nourished on admission; he was rational, though considerably prostrated and temperature 102° F.; spleen enlarged and two rose-colored spots visible. In addition, there are noted bluish spots, the "taches bleuatres" of the French writers, ranging from one-third to one-half inch in diameter and scattered over the entire body; they do not disappear upon pressure. A noticeable enlargement of the postcervical or epitrochlear glands can be detected; the penis shows an old linear scar beneath the frenum. There is slight rigidity of neck, but no tenderness along spine, scalp or head; the conjunctivæ are injected, the pupils slightly dilated. The gums are inflamed at the teeth, and bleed upon the slightest touch, and the pharynx is the seat of a decided catarrhal irritation. Numerous moist rales are heard over both lungs, more especially at right base, where the breath sounds are also bronchovesicular, showing lobular infiltration. Heart normal, although pulmonic sound is slightly accentuated. The spleen is enlarged; the abdomen not tender, but somewhat tympanitic with gurgling to pressure in right iliac region.

November 4th. General symptoms increased in severity; eruption characteristic and abundant; had rigor previous night, and later slight intestinal hemorrhage. The physical signs indicate resolution in right lower lobe of the lung. A bandage applied to right elbow after taking a blood culture produced ecchymosis of right forearm. Has marked hiccough, and is delirious.

12th. The physical signs indicate an area of consolidation in left lung near the base, and also one on right side at angle of scapula (bronchopneumonia). The sputum is tenacious, and decidedly hemorrhagic, and has been so for twenty-four hours; it shows no tubercle bacilli but streptococci and staphylococci. The urine analysis revealed the findings of an acute hemorrhagic nephritis.

15th. Small mass is noted in lower right quadrant of abdomen, below (?) the seat of the appendix. It is soft and presents fluctuation, and is slightly painful to touch.

18th. Patient's general condition has improved, although a large hemorrhage occurred last evening, accompanied by the usual drop in temperature. The palpable mass in abdomen is still present without change; the surgeon refuses to operate on account of extensive bronchopneumonia. The sputum is viscid, and tinged with specks of red blood. Signs of resolution slowly progressing in right lung.

December 10*th*. Since former note, numerous examinations of the sputum were made, with the same result as noted above. The Widal reaction was noted a few days after admission, and on several occasions during the course of the illness; the diazo reaction was also present.

11*th*. The physical signs indicated the presence of a small cavity in the left interscapular space. It was thought that an abscess had developed, but the sputum examination on the following day showed the presence of numerous tubercle bacilli for the first time, but subsequently they were constantly present and the temperature became hectic in type. The conclusion was now inevitable that tuberculosis had probably been associated with typhoid fever, and only declared itself during early convalescence.

The next case herein reported occurred in the Philadelphia Hospital, and is taken from the post-mortem and clinical records of that institution; it is the only instance of combined diseases under consideration out of 90 autopsies on cases of typhoid fever and on all cases of acute tuberculosis covering a period of ten years.

CASE III.—G. K., aged twenty-one years, white, single, laborer, admitted April 18, 1899. The history sheet was lost, but a few ward notes were found; the temperature averaged from 102° to 103.2° F., pulse 72, later frequent; respirations about 26; the spleen was enlarged, the abdomen was tympanitic and diarrhœa was present; sero reaction present; tubercle bacilli absent at first, later found; no mention of rose spots. Condition grew progressively worse, and patient died May 21, 1899.

The autopsy showed intestinal perforation with adhesions to the omentum. Typhoid ulcers in large intestine cicatrizing; also ulcers about the valve with swollen solitary follicles. Peyer's patches in stage of infiltration and ulcers very numerous.

The left lung is almost entirely free from pigmentation; the anterior portion of lung normal, except a few tubercles scattered through the apex; posteriorly, there are patches of pneumonia, involving about one-half the depth of the entire posterior portion of lungs. Right lung: upper lobe, normal; middle lobe is tubercular throughout, being consolidated to a considerable extent with many tubercles; lower lobe shows hypostatic pneumonia almost throughout.

The post-mortem records of the Episcopal Hospital furnish two instances of combined typhoid fever and acute tuberculosis, as follows:[1]

CASE IV.—J. McI., aged eighteen years, single, was admitted to the medical wards of the Episcopal Hospital August 30, 1898, and died September 12, of the same year.

The clinical diagnosis was typhoid fever with perforation. The

[1] The writer regrets that no clinical notes of this case are available.

autopsy, however, showed acute miliary tuberculosis in addition to the typhoid lesions with perforation. Both lungs were studded throughout with miliary tubercles, but there was no consolidation. The spleen was enlarged, and the small intestines presented typhoid lesions in the usual seat associated with marked hyperæmia. Perforation had taken place in the ileum, around which there was an adhesive, localized peritonitis. Many of the lesions were about to show necrosis.

CASE V.—On admission, the diagnosis of typhoid fever accompanied the patient, but the clinical diagnosis during the stay in the hospital was pulmonary tuberculosis and tubercular bacilli were found in the sputum. The case proved fatal, and loculated, serofibrinous, and hemorrhagic pleurisy was noted at autopsy; also caseous deposits and miliary tubercles throughout lungs and pleura, while the intestines presented typical typhoid ulcers. In this instance of combined typhoid fever and acute tuberculosis both affections had been, although at different times, diagnosticated during life, but their association was not recognized.

CASE VI.—Osler has informed me that out of a total of 80 autopsies of cases of typhoid fever at the Johns Hopkins Hospital, one showed acute tuberculosis starting in as an acute pneumonic condition.

It is evident from the foregoing statistical facts including the reports of the 5 cases, that combined typhoid infection and acute tuberculosis, as stated above, is rare. Thus acute tuberculosis was associated in 1.6 per cent., and chronic tuberculosis in 7.6 per cent. of the cases of typhoid that came to autopsy. I have not included case histories (except Nos. 1 and 2), unsupported by post-mortem proof, for the reason that the chances of error in diagnosis are exceedingly great, as will appear hereafter.

It is said that when tuberculosis and typhoid fever are associated together in the same case, the former may dominate the scene and cause the Widal reaction either to disappear or to fail to appear. For this reason, certain cases of the combined disorders may be readily overlooked.

E. Kraus[1] found in 1 case that a complicating pneumonia caused the sero reaction to disappear just one day prior to the death of the patient. The post-mortem revealed the lesions of typhoid and lobar pneumonia in combination. It would appear from this fact that the serum of some other disease like pneumonia and acute tuberculosis may prevent the reaction of the typhoid bacilli. It is possible that the sero reaction of typhoid fever is sometimes also delayed on account of interfering complications, or again, it may be temporarily absent in the course of a given case for the same reason. A careful study of the cases reported in the literature will reveal

[1] Zeit. f. Heilk., Bd. xxi., H. 5.

much evidence to support this view. Thus cases complicated with appendicitis at times, as I know from personal observation, do not show the Widal reaction until the complication is removed by operation.

Conversely, F. Lobiesen[1] examined the blood of 151 patients who did not have typhoid fever, but were admitted into the hospital with that diagnosis or suspected enteric fever. Of these 4 gave a positive reaction at 1 to 25, and 3 died, showing respectively acute miliary tuberculosis, retroperitoneal abscess and calculous pyelitis with tuberculous meningitis. He, with Fiocca,[2] concludes that a positive diagnosis can be made when the reaction occurs with a dilution as great as 1:50. Now, in Case I. of my series the blood examinations were made by the Bacteriological Department of the Bureau of Health, where the higher dilutions (1:40 to 1:50) are employed. It was deeply regretted that no autopsy was allowed, and yet, as stated above, there can be little room for doubting the coincidence of typhoid fever and acute pneumonic phthisis in view of the three positive sero reactions at intervals of several days. There was absolutely no history of previous typhoid infection.

If the Widal reaction can be relied upon to differentiate typhoid fever from acute tuberculosis with absolute certainty, then these two diseases were associated in this instance. In 2 of the cases reported below, however, in which the sero reaction occurred, the necropsy failed to show any typhoid lesions.

A number of recent observers have found that icteric serum was possessed of a certain amount of agglutinizing power. The subject has just been carefully reviewed by E. Libman.[3] He quotes Koehler, who found in 8 cases of icteric diseases of the liver an agglutination reaction in 6. The highest dilution in which he obtained the reaction was 1:40; very rarely 1:50, and once it was only 1:10. Koehler experimented with the bile of rabbits which had slight agglutinizing power; also with that of dogs, and this manifested a decided agglutinizing potency (even up to 1:160).

Libman[4] made observations upon ten specimens of human bile, either normal or from cases of typhoid fever, chronic pancreatitis or cholelithiasis, and in no instance could he get a positive Widal reaction. Sailer[5] reports 3 cases of intense jaundice, all of which failed to give the sero reaction. The time has arrived when a *slight reaction* in a dilution of 1:50 is not to be regarded as a positive Widal reaction.

It is admittedly difficult to interpret the clinical phenomena of the combined diseases during life. All of the cases that came to autopsy showed that the clinical diagnosis was either incomplete

[1] Zeit. f. klin. Med., D. V. L. 111, Heft 1 und 11.
[2] Il Policlinico, November 1, 1900.
[3] Medical News, January 30, 1904.
[4] Loc. cit.
[5] Transactions of the Philadelphia Pathological Society, 1902, p. 258.

or erroneous. In Cases I. and II. (see *ante*) acute pneumonic phthisis was associated with typhoid fever, and in the former a lobar type of consolidation occurred, while in the latter it was a bronchopneumonic type.

The question of the effect of acute tuberculosis upon the course of typhoid fever is one of considerable interest. It was observed in Case I. that the typhoid fever was apparently uninfluenced by the tuberculous process. Indeed, it may be said that the symptoms of typhoid were distinctly in abeyance. In Case II. the clinical features of typhoid were intense and the course prolonged, and yet this disease was a thing of the past before the tuberculous process reached the stage of cavity formation, and tubercle bacilli found in the sputum.

The temperature-curve in the combined cases resembled closely that of typical typhoid—at all events until the typhoid process had spent its main force. On the other hand, the pulse partook during the fastigium more of the character of that seen in acute tuberculosis than of typhoid fever, being rapid and feeble.

The diagnosis of the combined affections may be assisted by remembering that the characteristic typhoid symptoms usually manifest themselves before the diagnostic evidences of acute tuberculosis. This is particularly true of the cases in which the pneumonic type of a tuberculous process is associated with typhoid. Here the diagnosis cannot be completed, as a rule, until tubercle bacilli are discovered in the sputum usually after the lapse of weeks. In my cases no tubercle bacilli were detected until the physical signs denoting apical cavity formation were noted. In this connection, attention should again be called to the fact that in the majority of the cases the associated tuberculosis assumes the form of acute pneumonic phthisis, according to the results of my collective investigations. Certain forms of acute tuberculosis were commonly mistaken for typhoid fever, such as acute miliary tuberculosis and the acute pulmonary varieties, as the reports of the following cases will illustrate:

In November, 1901, I had under my care a patient in the Medico-Chirurgical Hospital suffering from typhoid fever, and who gave a strong family history of pulmonary tuberculosis. The case began with pleuritis, accompanied with moderate effusion. The diagnosis of tuberculous pleurisy was provisionally made, but after the lapse of ten days true typhoid symptoms supervened, while the effusion was slowly and gradually absorbed. Recovery ensued.

An interesting and instructive case is recorded by Osler,[1] in which for nearly two weeks tuberculous pneumonia was suspected on account of apparently clear physical signs and the family history. Later, the true typhoid symptoms appeared and became well

[1] Studies in Typhoid Fever, series 3, p. 464.

marked, although the Widal reaction was not present until the end of the third week.

The following two case histories bearing on this point have been taken from the clinical and post-mortem records of the Philadelphia Hospital:

CASE I.—S. R., aged twenty-two years, Polander, occupation laborer, was admitted to the medical wards of the Philadelphia Hospital April 26, 1902; a chill one week before, followed by dyspnœa, cough, bloody expectoration, intestinal disturbance, and mental dulness. No family history obtainable. The physical examination showed coated tongue, dicrotic pulse, broncho-vesicular breathing, and impairment of resonance over lower lobes. The abdomen was distended and tympanitic; spleen enlarged; few suspicious rose spots observed; temperature ranging from 102° to 104° F.; pulse 66 to 100; no positive Widal reaction; diagnosis of pulmonary tuberculosis was made during life.

The autopsy revealed typical typhoid ulcers, acute splenic tumor, parenchymatous degeneration of the liver and kidneys, and congestion of the lungs. On section, the lung texture showed slight increase of consistency, but crepitation was everywhere present. Typhoid ulcers were found in the ileum, and several large ulcers in the cæcum.

CASE II.—C. S., aged thirty-six years, a patient in the medical wards of the Philadelphia Hospital, died February 6, 1902. The history of the case was as follows: Ill three weeks with chill, cough, slight expectoration, occasional vomiting, some abdominal pain, diarrhœa, with bloody stools twenty-four hours after admission; temperature 104° F. Patient passed into the typhoid state, but no rose spots and no splenic enlargement was detectable. On percussion the bases of the lungs showed dulness, and on auscultation crepitant rales were heard over both lungs. A trace of albumin was found in the urine; the sputum showed no tubercle bacilli; Widal reaction not mentioned. The diagnosis during life was acute tuberculosis.

The post-mortem revealed typhoid ulceration of the intestines, acute splenic tumor, hyperplasia of mesenteric and other lymph glands, œdema of lungs and apparent parenchymatous degeneration of the kidneys. The lungs, it may be mentioned, showed increased consistency, and on section a dark and blood-stained fluid exuded upon pressure; no evidence of consolidation, and bronchial lymph glands negative.

Typhoid fever may be mistaken for tuberculosis, as shown by the following illustrative cases:

CASE I.—J. P., aged twenty-five years, colored, laborer, admitted April 23, 1899; family history negative; had malaria one and pneumonia three years previously. Present illness began two weeks ago with typical prodromes of typhoid; a few days later was seized with pain in left side, and cough with slight expectoration. The above symptoms lasted until admission, after which he had two or three stools daily; also high temperature of irregular type; pulse small, frequent, and little tension; slight albuminuria; a few dry rales at end of inspiration. The Widal reaction was present and a few tubercle bacilli were found in sputum. The clinical diagnosis had been typhoid fever and tuberculosis.

The patient died twenty-eight days after admission, and the necropsy showed only tuberculous lesions, the intestines being normal (not injected even); tuberculosis of the mesenteric, retroperitoneal and periaortic lymph glands, and a small nodule in the liver. Miliary tuberculosis in lungs and spleen. Pathological diagnosis was chronic followed by miliary tuberculosis.

It will be noted that the sero reaction was found in this case without the presence of any discoverable typhoid lesions. It must be recollected, however, that cases of typhoid septicæmia occur in which there may be an utter absence of characteristic intestinal ulcers. It is with considerable unreadiness that I place on record this case and the following, both of which tend to disprove a dictum which has been generally accepted, while searching for data to show the interrelation of these affections.

Case II.—H. M., aged twenty-four years, occupation brakeman, was admitted to the male medical wards of the Philadelphia Hospital August 2, 1903. Family history negative; the patient had always been healthy except that he contracted syphilis two years previously. He was a confirmed alcoholic and an excessive smoker. On admission, was thought to be intoxicated, and taken to the "drunk ward," but the symptoms and appearance did not portray drunkenness; he was semiconscious, although in muttering delirium. It was learned that he had been indisposed for two weeks with anorexia, headache, increasing prostration. The spleen was slightly enlarged; the diazo reaction negative, Widal positive, and a few suspicious spots were noted on the back; the physical signs seemed to indicate lobar consolidation, and the respirations were as high as 40 per minute. A clinical diagnosis of typhoid fever complicated with pneumonia was made.

The patient died August 12, 1903. An autopsy revealed encysted pleural effusion and miliary tuberculosis; the intestines showed no macroscopic changes.

Case III.—C. H., aged twenty-five years, admitted to the Philadelphia Hospital March 20, 1900. Nothing could be gleaned regarding either the family or personal history. Said to have been ill two weeks, beginning with headache, malaise, diarrhœa, and high fever, but no cough. Physical examination shows tenderness, and gurgling in right iliac fossa, splenic region tender, but spleen not palpable. On sixth day after admission he became delirious, spat up a couple mouthfuls of blood; next day passed a quantity of dark blood with stool. The urine contained both albumin and tube casts; the temperature ranged from 101° to 102° F. for six days, then from 99° to 100° F. until death, which occurred March 28, 1900.

The clinical diagnosis was typhoid fever. Post-mortem examination revealed acute tuberculosis; left lung rather firm, but crepitant throughout; no tuberculous cavity or nodes. Right lung at apex showed marked tuberculous change; spleen normal in size; the intestines showed numerous tuberculous ulcers.

CASE IV.—C. L. G., female, aged thirty years, died April 9, 1899, at the Episcopal Hospital (no bedside notes obtainable). A clinical diagnosis of typhoid fever was made, but the pathological findings showed the following: Lungs riddled with miliary tubercles, although no source of infection was discoverable; neither caseation nor cavities were observed. Bronchial glands slightly enlarged, but not broken down; the spleen weighed 6½ ounces, was very soft and friable, with some miliary tubercles scattered through its surface. The intestines were perfectly normal; the peritoneal surface of the bladder and uterus was studded with a few tubercles.

CASE V.—Patient was admitted to the medical wards of the Episcopal Hospital believed to be suffering from typhoid fever. The disease ran an acute course and proved fatal. At autopsy, miliary tuberculosis following chronic pulmonary tuberculosis, with cavity formation in lungs and also intestinal tuberculosis, was found.

CASE VI.—On admission, this case was diagnosticated as typhoid fever, but had typhoid six years previously. The Widal reaction was present; leukocytes, 10,400. Blood cultures were made, but did not show typhoid bacilli, and lumbar puncture failed to elicit fluid. The necropsy showed acute meningitis, especially at the base, associated with pleural adhesions, cavities in both lungs, and tuberculous ulcers in the intestines.

The question here arises, Was the Widal reaction in this case due to the attack of typhoid fever which had occurred six years previously?

Osler[1] has reported 3 interesting cases of the sort in which at the outset typhoid fever was strongly suspected, although the positive signs of this disease were absent, and the certain features of pulmonary tuberculosis finally supervened. In 1 of the cases, as is usual, rapid progress was made during lactation and the fever was mistaken for typhoid.

While it is important to recognize these two leading affections when combined, remembering the extreme rarity of the association, it becomes a matter of greater clinical importance to distinguish between typhoid fever and the various forms of acute tuberculosis, since they are so commonly confused with one another. Acute miliary tuberculosis may simulate typhoid fever so closely as to

[1] Loc. cit.

offer the greatest clinical difficulty. The absence of the Widal reaction, of the characteristic eruption and of the comparatively slow pulse in miliary tuberculosis, are to be especially noted. On the other hand, in cases in which strong suspicions of the existence of acute miliary tuberculosis are entertained, a careful search for tubercles in the choroid, and tubercle bacilli in the blood and sputum (if there be any), is to be carried forward. C. Loeb[1] has recently emphasized the value of ophthalmic examinations in the differential diagnosis between typhoid fever and acute miliary tuberculosis. The personal history is often most helpful. In doubtful cases an attempt should be made to cultivate the typhoid bacilli from any suspicious eruption that may be present. There are not a few cases in which a positive diagnosis, however, must be withheld, for lack of discriminating features.

DISTRIBUTION OF THE ULCERS IN TYPHOID FEVER.

By Joseph Louis Baer, S.M.,
of Chicago.

(From the Pathological Laboratory of the University of Chicago and Rush Medical College.)

The occurrence of two cases of typhoid fever with an unusual distribution of the ulcers suggested the desirability of a general investigation of the distribution of ulcers in this disease. The two cases are presented in detail, and are followed by an analysis of a series of 89 cases, and by a review and discussion of the literature on the subject.

The first case showed ulcers in the œsophagus and colon, and in no other part of the alimentary tract:

Case I.—This series 33; Rush Medical series 945. A. B., male, aged twenty-four years; died January 31, 1901.

Clinical Diagnosis. Typhoid fever; tonsillitis; pharyngitis; laryngitis; pleuritis; probable pneumonia.

Anatomical Diagnosis (Dr. H. G. Wells). Typhoid fever (colotyphoid); ulcerative colitis; follicular enteritis; swelling of mesenteric lymph glands and spleen; follicular pharyngitis; œsophageal ulcers; acute serofibrinous pleuritis; bronchopneumonia; fibrous perisplenitis and perihepatitis; healed pulmonary tuberculosis.

Tongue. Lymphoid follicles prominent.

Pharynx and Epiglottis. Covered by mucopus.

Œsophagus. Covered by thin mucopus. There are prominent follicular swellings. At a point 1 cm. below the cricoid cartilage is

[1] Archives of Ophthalmology, New York, 1903, vol. xxxii. pp. 453–469.

a superficial ulcer 5 mm. in its long diameter, which is parallel to the axis of the œsophagus. Near this are three smaller ulcers; floor smooth, margins sharp, outline oval, long axis vertical.

Larynx and Trachea. Covered by thin mucopus. No ulcers.

Stomach. No ulcers.

Small Intestines. There is a slight hyperplasia of the solitary lymph follicles, especially in the lower part. Peyer's patches are normal. There is some hyperæmia. No ulcers.

Large Intestine. Beginning at a point 30 cm. below the ileocæcal valve and extending 70 cm. are twenty-five ulcers, 2 mm. to 6 mm. in diameter, with swollen, elevated edges. None have perforated. There is some hyperæmia and hyperplasia of the lymph follicles.

Bacteriology. The typhoid bacillus was isolated from the heart's blood and kidney.

In the second case the ulcers were limited strictly to the ascending and transverse colon, the sigmoid flexure, and rectum.

Case II.—This series 45; St. Luke's Hospital 38. E. T., male, aged twenty years; died and examined February 24, 1903.

Clinical Diagnosis. Typhoid fever; hypostatic pulmonary congestion; pseudohypertrophic muscular atrophy.

Anatomical Diagnosis (Dr. H. G. Wells). Typhoid ulceration of the colon; hypertrophic pulmonary emphysema; purulent bronchitis; bronchopneumonia, and left hypostatic pneumonia; œdema of the right lower lobe; acute lymphadenitis, peribronchial and mesenteric; hypoplasia of the aorta; hypertrophy of the left ventricle; parenchymatous degeneration of the liver and kidneys; fibrous pericholecystitis; atrophy of vermiform appendix; hyperplasia of the spleen; calcification of the peripancreatic and mesenteric lymph nodes; chronic diffuse nephritis; decubitus; hypoplasia of the testicles; fibrous increase in the thyroid; atrophy of the muscles of the lower extremities, with replacement by fatty fibrous tissue; contractures of the feet.

Œsophagus. The lymphoid nodules are prominent, but none are ulcerated.

Stomach. The mucous membrane is contracted, but the folds can be pulled out. No ulceration.

Duodenum. Lymphoid structures are prominent.

Lower Small Intestine. The last Peyer's patches are slightly swollen. A few irregular pigmented spots are found above the swollen Peyer's patches.

Large Intestine. Immediately below the ileocæcal valve is an ulcer 1 cm. in diameter. In the upper 30 cm. of the large bowel are five ulcers, the largest 2 cm. in diameter. There are also a few pigmented spots. 50 cm. below the valve are two ulcers, 1.5 cm. in diameter; 20 cm. farther another ulcer is found, 1 cm. in diameter; 35 cm. above the anus is an ulcer, 5 mm. in diameter; 10 cm. above the anus three ulcers are present, placed parallel, 3 cm., 2 cm., and 1 cm. in diameter, and transverse to the long axis of the bowel.

The series of 89 cases whose analysis is presented here was obtained from two sources, 44 cases from the Cook County Hospital, June, 1897, to June, 1903, and 45 cases from the Presbyterian Hospital, August, 1895, to July, 1902.

The distribution of the ulcers is as follows:

	Cases.	Percentage.
Mouth	0	0
Larynx	3	3.4
Trachea	1	1.1
Pharynx	0	0
Œsophagus	1	1.1
Stomach	2	2.2
Duodenum	0	0
Jejunum	1	1.1
Ileum	67	75.3
Ileum, lower half	32	35.9
Ileum alone	29	32.6
Meckel's diverticulum	1	1.1
Small intestine (not specific)	12	13.5
Total cases of involvement of small intestine	77	86.5
Ileocæcal valve	1	1.1
Vermiform appendix	1	1.1
Cæcum	15	16.9
Ascending colon	13	14.4
Transverse "	12	13.5
Descending "	5	5.6
Colon (not specific)	12	13.5
Sigmoid flexure	3	3.4
Rectum	3	3.4
Large intestine (not specific)	9	10.1
Large intestine alone	5	5.6
Cæcum alone	2	
Cæcum and ascending colon	1	
Cæcum and appendix	1	
Ascending colon, transverse colon, sigmoid flexure, and rectum	1	
Total cases of involvement of large intestine	45	50.6
No ulcers (with bacteriology)	2	2.2

Comparison of the percentages of distribution of the ulcers derived from this series with those derived from the general statistics in the literature, and which are presented later, reveals a close correspondence, except in two important items: In this series the percentage of involvement of the small intestine (in any part), 86.5 per cent., and of the ileum, 75.3 per cent., is markedly lower than the figures obtained from the older statistics, 99.4 per cent. and 89.9 per cent., respectively; while, on the other hand, the involvement of the large intestine in this series, 50.6 per cent., is more than double the percentage derived from other statistics—*i. e.*, 22.7 per cent.

This difference seems to me to indicate careful examination at the autopsies in this series, rather than variations that are the result of chance, and this explanation is further borne out by the fact that the same differences, though in less degree, exist between the earlier and the more recent statistics in the literature.

The bacteriology has been recorded in 37 of the 89 cases.[1] The typhoid bacillus, with or without other organisms, was found in 31 cases. Other organisms only were recovered in 6 cases.

Perforations were found in 14 cases (15.7 per cent.), distributed as follows: ileum, 9 cases (10.1 per cent.); cæcum, transverse colon, and large intestine, each 1 case (1.1 per cent.); and "vague," 2 cases. As is well known, the number of ulcers in typhoid fever varies considerably, and in this connection it is interesting to note that in one of these cases of perforation of the ileum the bowel presented but one ulcer, 30 cm. above the ileocæcal valve, and this solitary ulcer perforated, causing death by peritonitis.

Indeed, in recent years a large number of cases of typhoid fever entirely without ulceration has been reported. In this series there occur two such cases, and in both the bacteriology was carefully worked out, the typhoid bacillus being recovered and identified from the kidney, spleen, liver, and mesenteric lymph glands in one case, and from the kidney, spleen, and gall-bladder in the other case. This subject of typhoid fever without ulceration has been reviewed recently by Picchi, Bryant, Flexner and Harris, McPhedran and Ophüls. I have collected 26 cases, which, with the 2 cases in this series, make a total of 28 cases that seem to me to be valid on bacteriological grounds.[2] Search through the literature has yielded abundant data on the distribution of the ulcers in typhoid fever.

The material has been grouped in two divisions: first, a series of 83 individual cases, each involving unusual distribution of the ulcers; and second, a series of statistical analyses.

The 83 individual cases have been dissected below, in order to show the relative frequency of ulcerations in unusual sites:

		Cases.[3]	
Involvement of	larynx	17	
" "	pharynx	16	
" "	œsophagus	10	(4 are strictures)
" "	trachea	1	
" "	stomach	10	
" "	jejunum	3	
" "	Meckel's diverticulum	1	
" "	appendix	5	
" "	ileocæcal valve	3	
" "	cæcum	12	
" "	ascending colon	6	
" "	transverse "	5	
" "	descending "	4	
" "	sigmoid flexure	3	
" "	rectum	4	
" "	skin at anus	1	
" "	ileum and colon	12	(total 29)
" "	small and large intestine (not specific)	17	
" "	large intestine (alone)	6	

[1] Sex: males, 66; females, 22; not given, 1. Age: twenty-one to thirty-five, 42; before twenty-one, 12; after thirty-five, 16; not given, 19 cases.

[2] Nine cases have been omitted because of a questionable bacteriology: 3 by Karlinski; 2 by Goodall; and 1 each by Banti, Thue, Guarnieri, and Dogliotti.

[3] In the appended bibliography all articles marked with an asterisk (*) contain one or more of these cases.

The general statistics from the literature have been dissected and rearranged on an anatomical basis, rather than a classification based on authorship, thus affording a more intelligible arrangement for comparative purposes. Under each anatomical division the average obtained from the data presented by the various authors is given first, followed by the result of the analysis of my series of 89 cases, and finally an average of the two totals, where both are given:

	Literature. Total cases.	Literature. Per ct.	My series of 89 cases. Per ct.	Average. Per ct.
Ulcers of mouth	......	.....	....	none mentioned.
" larynx	1020	21.3	3.4	19.9
" trachea	439	0.2	1.1	0.38
" pharynx	648	2.5	...	2.2
" œsophagus	134	6.7	1.1	4.5
" stomach	1019	1.9	2.2	1.98
" duodenum	891	0.3	...	0.30
" jejunum	1269	6.1	1.1	5.9
" ileum	1334	89.9	75.3	89.0
" ileum (lower half)	316	37.0	35.9	36.8
" ileum (alone)	245	60.8	32.6	58.3
" Meckel's diverticulum	.....	......	1.1	1.1
" common bile-duct	439	0.23	....	0.23
" small intestine (in any part)	534	99.4	86.5	97.5
" ileocæcal valve	....	......	6.7	6.7
" vermiform appendix	352	2.8	1.1	2.5
" cæcum	1307	31.3	16.9	30.3
" ascending colon	532	9.6	14.4	10.3
" transverse "	532	3.2	13.5	4.5
" descending "	532	2.1	5.6	2.6
" colon (not specific)	1092	29.1	....	29.1
" sigmoid flexure	12	33.3	3.4	6.9
" rectum	967	2.2	3.4	2.4
" large intestine	1084	22.7	50.6	33.3
" large intestine (alone)	......	......	5.6	5.6
No ulcers (with a bacteriology)	......	......	2.2	2.2

In reviewing the results obtained from a study of the literature, several facts worth noting are brought into prominence. Probably most striking among these is the wide distribution of the typhoid ulcers. They are found in every division of the alimentary tract, excepting the mouth, and they are found also in the larynx and trachea. One case has been reported by Mitchell, in which the observer speaks of a "loss of substance on each side of the tongue." No other mention of buccal involvement has been found.

Ulceration of the larynx in typhoid fever has been the occasion of much dispute, the point at issue being whether the lesion was due to typhoid bacillus or to fresh infections with pyogenic organisms (Kanthak and Drysdale, G. Duffy). Williams, in 1894, recovered the typhoid bacillus from the laryngeal ulcers in 2 cases, and since then the tendency has grown to regard these ulcers as primarily typhoidal. As long ago as 1829 Louis said: "The rarity of ulceration of the larynx is the more remarkable since ulcerations are frequently met with around that organ at the epiglottis, pharynx, and œsophagus. If laryngeal ulcers are found on a body dead of an acute disease, they will establish with nearly perfect certainty, and without going any farther, that the affection was typhoid fever."

Ouskow has analyzed the time of appearance of the ulcers in the larynx with these results: ulcers in the first week, none; in the second week, 79 cases; in the third week, 144 cases; in the fourth week, 89 cases.

The site of the ulcers, as determined by Lüning, in a series of 165 cases, was: supraglottic in 50 cases, infraglottic in 36 cases, and in the glottis in 18 cases. The author states that the process begins in the arytenoid cartilages and extends to the cricoid cartilages.

Ulceration of the trachea, while extremely rare, occurred in 3 cases in these statistics (Ouskow, Greffier, and this series).

Pharyngeal ulcers have been noted by many observers, and I have found 32 cases.[1]

Ulceration of the œsophagus, though found repeatedly by the earlier observers, Louis, Jenner, and Chomel, later became a rarity, as is strikingly shown by Packard's review of 5000 cases, none of which showed œsophageal ulceration. To a certain extent this negative result should be regarded as due to too brief a scrutiny or complete oversight on the part of the observer, for recently Mitchell, Riesman, and Pyle have presented a total of 10 cases (4 of which were strictures with recovery) and in this series there is another case (Case I.), which is given in detail because of the unique distribution of the ulcers, they being found only in the œsophagus and colon.

Gastric ulceration, though very unusual, is now regarded as quite possible in typhoid fever and may serve to explain some cases of hæmatemesis. In one of the 2 cases of gastric ulceration in this series the entire stomach has been preserved. Sections showed the ulcers to be fairly typically typhoidal, with numerous endothelioid phagocytic cells. In addition to 20 cases found in statistics,[2] a total of 10 individual cases is presented by Chauffard, Dignat, Perignon, and Keen.

The duodenum is the second rarest site for typhoid ulcers, only 3 cases being found. Two are by Louis and the third by Andral.

The low percentage of ulcers in the jejunum, 5.9 per cent., calculated from a total of 1358 cases, confirms the general impression as to the infrequency of jejunal involvement.

Involvement of the ileum is found in 89 per cent. of the cases; of the lower half of the ileum in 36.8 per cent., and of the ileum alone in 53.3 per cent. That typhoid ulcers elsewhere than in the ileum are found more commonly than has been supposed is demonstrated by the last percentage given, especially when this is viewed in connection with the high percentage of colonic involvement about to be presented.

[1] Murchison, Moore, Osler, Ouskow, Roque, Derignac, Riesman.
[2] Murchison, Moore, Hawkins, and Andral.

Ulceration of the small intestine in any part has been recorded in 97.5 per cent. of 623 cases. Ulceration of Meckel's diverticulum has been noted twice, once in this series and once by J. Sailer.

Ulceration of the common bile-duct has been reported once by Ouskow in a series of 439 cases. This is the rarest site for typhoid ulcers. However, not only here but throughout all the statistics there is an element of doubt in the diagnoses. Perhaps it would be well to regard the ulcers as typhoidal only after recovery of the typhoid bacillus from the affected area and satisfactory demonstration of the histological picture shown by typhoid ulcers. The abrupt termination of the ulcer zone at the ileocæcal valve is well shown by the low percentage of involvement of the valve itself, 6.7 per cent.

The distribution of the ulcers in the large intestine has been considered under various captions. Involvement of the large intestine (without specification of locality) in 33.3 per cent. of 1173 cases, and of the colon in 29.1 per cent. of 1092 cases, only 65 of which are duplicates of the former number, is convincing evidence of the comparative frequency of ulceration in those sites. The division of the large intestine most frequently involved is the cæcum, 30.3 per cent. Next in order of frequency come: ascending colon, 10.3 per cent.; sigmoid flexure, 6.9 per cent.; transverse colon, 4.5 per cent.; descending colon, 2.6 per cent.; vermiform appendix, 2.5 per cent.; and rectum, 2.4 per cent.

Involvement of the large intestine alone was not found in any statistics in the literature. In this series, however, 5 cases (5.6 per cent.) were found. One of these is presented in detail (Case II.).

Chantemesse, Rendu, Hodenpyl, and Laveran describe single cases of ulceration of the large intestine alone. It may be mentioned here that Chantemesse[1] states that the typhoid ulcers may be absent throughout, except in the appendix, but he gives no details.

The distribution of the ulcers in typhoid fever having been elaborated in the foregoing statistics, the question naturally arises as to what determines this distribution, usually so typical and yet frequently so bizarre.

The answer has not yet been attained in its entirety. It is obvious that one important factor in determining the seat of the lesions is the extent and character of the lymphatic apparatus in the part. Yet the frequent occurrence of pharyngeal and laryngeal involvement, and the occurrence of such atypical cases as the two presented in this paper, indicate that accidental lodgement of the typhoid bacilli is another factor of considerable importance.

Moreover, the many authentic cases of typhoid fever without ulceration point to the existence of other possible factors, such as a lowered resistance of the gastrointestinal mucosa, which in these cases without ulcerations has reached its lowest ebb.

[1] Traité de Médecine, p. 744.

In conclusion, I desire to thank Prof. L. Hektoen and Dr. H. G. Wells for much valuable advice and criticism.

BIBLIOGRAPHY.

*Allen. Australasian Medical Journal, Melbourne, 1884, n. s., vol. vi. p. 217.

*Allyn, H. B. Pennsylvania Medical Journal, 1902. vol. v. p. 486.

Andral. Tweedie's Cyclop. of Med. Also under Hawkins, F.

*Arkle, C. Trans. Path. Soc. Lond., 1894, vol. xlvi. p. 63.

Arnaud. Arch. de méd. et pharm. mil., Paris, 1893, vol. xxii. p. 529.

*Barth, M. Progrès méd., Paris, 1884, vol. xii. p. 703.

Bryant, M. British Med. Journ., London, 1899, vol. i. p. 776.

*Carter, W. S Proc. Path. Soc. Philadelphia, 1898, vol. xviii. p. 38.

*Chantemesse. Semaine méd., 1890.

Chantemesse. Traité de méd., p. 744.

*Chuffard, A. Determinations gastriques. Paris, 1882, J. B. Baillière.

Chomel. (See under Riesman.)

*Cockle. Med. Times and Gaz., London, 1883, vol. i. p. 92.

Coupland, S. Clinical Journal, London, 1895–96, vol. vii. pp. 45–51.

*Curnow, J. Trans. Path. Soc. London, 1882, vol. xxxiv. p. 116.

Curshman. Deutsche med. Wochenschr., 1888, vol. xxi. p. 421; also Nothnagel, iii. i. p. 85.

*Derignac, P. Thèses de Paris, Le Mans, 1883, No. 111.

*Dignat, P. Journ. de méd. de Bordeaux, 1884-85, vol. xiv 297.

*Druon, E. Journ. de Sc. méd. de Lille, 1897, vol. i. p. 299.

*Duffy, G. Dublin Journ. Med. Sci., 1898, 3d s., vol. cv. p. 185.

Flexner and Harris. Johns Hopkins Hospital Bulletin, 1897, vol. viii. p. 259.

Flexner, S. Johns Hopkins Hospital Reports, 1899–1900, vol. viii. p. 241.

Goodall. Trans. Clin. Soc. London, 1896–97, vol. xxx. p. 120.

*Greenhow, E. H. Trans. Path. Soc., London, 1872, vol. xxiv. p. 110.

*Greffier, L. Progrès méd., Paris, 1882, vol. x. p. 1028.

Griesinger, Wil. Handbch. d. Path. u. Therap., Virchow, 1864, vol. vi. p. 173.

Hawkins, F. Lancet, London, 1893, vol. ii. p. 245.

*Hodenpyl. British Med. Journ., London, 1897, vol. ii. p. 1850.

Hoffman, C. E. E Untersuchungen über die path. anat. Veränderungen beim Abdomtyphus. Leipzig, 1869.

Jenner. (See under Murchison.)

Kanthak and Drysdale. New York Med. Journ., 1896, vol. lxiii. p. 533.

*Keen, W. W. Surgical Complications of Typhoid, 1898.

Lartigau. New York Med. Journ., 1899, vol. lxx. p. 158.

*Laveran. Le bull. méd., Paris, July 23, 1893.

*Le Wald. Medical Record, New York, 1898, vol. liv p. 891.

Louis. (See under Murchison.)

Luning. (See under Keen, W. W.)

*Lyons. Dublin Journ. Med. Sci., 1868, vol. xlvi. p. 228.

*MacKenzie. Trans. Path. Soc. London, 1882, vol. xxxiii. p. 161.

McPhedran, A. Canada Journ. Med. and Surg., Toronto, 1899, vol. vi. p. 251.

*Mercier, J. A. Thèse de Paris, 1888, No. 349.

*Mitchell, J. F. Johns Hopkins Hospital Reports, 1900, vol. viii. p. 295.

Moore. Trans. Path. Soc. London, 1882, vol. xxxiii. p. 150.

Murchison. Fevers, 1873.

Ophüls, W. New York Med. Journ., 1900, vol. lxxi. p. 728.

Opie and Bassett. Johns Hopkins Hospital Bulletin, 1901, vol xii. p. 198.

*Orton, J. British Med. Journ., London, 1899, vol. ii. p. 142.

*Osler, W. Canada Journ. Med. and Surg., Montreal, 1885, vol. xiv. p. 7.

Osler, W. Johns Hopkins Hospital Reports, 1895, vol. iv. p. 12.

Ouskow, N. W. Arch. d. Sc. biol., 1892, vol. ii. p. 3; also Annual Univ. Med. Sci., 1894, vol. i. p. 23.

Packard. (See under Riesman.)

*Perignon. Journ. de Sc. méd. de Lille, 1890, pp. 2, 11, 14.

Picchi, L. Lo Sperimetale, 1899, p. 299.

*Pyle, John S. Philadelphia Med. Journ., 1900, vol. v. p. 303.

*Reichal, B. Inaug. Dis., Erlang, 1892; also under Hodenpyl.

*Rendu. Le bull. méd., Paris, July 23, 1893.

*Riesman, D. Philadelphia Med. Journ., 1899, vol. iv. p. 578.
*Roque. Provence méd., Lyon, 1891, vol. v. pp. 3-15.
*Sailer, J. Proc. Path. Soc. Philadelphia, 1897-98, n. s., vol. i. p. 304.
Sailer, J. Ibid., 1899, n. s., vol. ii. p. 151.
Sorel, F. Gaz hebd. de méd., Paris, 1889, 2d s., vol. xxvi. p. 416.
Vanzetti Journ. de phys. et path. gén., 1902, vol. iv. p. 575.
*West, S. Trans. Path. Soc. London, 1882, vol. xxxiv. p. 114.
Williams, P. W. British Med. Journ., London, 1894, vol. ii. p. 1353; also under Duffy, G.

TYPHOIDAL PERFORATION:

WITH A REPORT OF EIGHT CASES SUBJECTED TO OPERATION; TWO RECOVERIES.*

By Francis T. Stewart, M.D.,

PROFESSOR OF SURGERY, PHILADELPHIA POLYCLINIC; SURGEON, GERMANTOWN HOSPITAL; ASSISTANT SURGEON, JEFFERSON HOSPITAL; OUT-PATIENT SURGEON, PENNSYLVANIA HOSPITAL.

In 1884 Leyden first suggested and Mikulicz first practised suture of a perforated typhoid ulcer. In 1885 James C. Wilson brought the subject before the profession of America, and more recently (1898) interest was aroused in this subject by the brochure of Keen. That operation is still too seldom resorted to is evident when we recall that probably over 16,000 cases perish from perforation annually in the United States,[1] and that in 1903 Harte[2] was able to collect from the literature the records of only 339 cases subjected to operation.

The mortality of typhoid fever is probably about 10 per cent., and it is said that one-third of the fatalities are due to perforation of the intestine.

Perforation usually occurs during the third, fourth, or fifth week, but may happen at any stage of the disease. Males are more frequently affected than females, and the catastrophe is more liable to take place in adolescence than in infancy or old age. When the intestinal wall becomes thinned by the process of sloughing the immediate cause of perforation may be the pressure of hardened feces, straining at stool, excessive gaseous distention of the bowel, or sudden change in posture; in a number of cases ascarides have been found in the peritoneal cavity. Perforation is usually acute and followed by marked symptoms; occasionally it is chronic and the symptoms are insidious, the peritoneal cavity being protected for some time by previous adhesions.

In approaching a case for diagnosis the age, sex, previous condition of the bowels, previous presence or absence of hemorrhage, previous severity or mildness of the disease, and the period of the

* Read before the Germantown Medical Society, October 12, 1903.

disease may be disregarded entirely. Pain is a reliable and constant symptom, occasionally violent, usually severe, and rarely mild in character. As a rule, the pain is sudden in onset, begins in the right lower quadrant of the abdomen, quickly becomes generalized, and persists, despite the hebetude of the patient. Le Conte suggests that in view of the great sensibility of the parietal peritoneum the character of pain may be influenced by the proximity of the perforation to the abdominal wall. In a few instances the pain is reflected to the rectum and is accompanied by a frequent desire but inability to defecate. Frequency of micturition, with vesical pain, has also been noted.

Tenderness is most marked in the region of perforation, usually in the right iliac region, to which area it is limited in the beginning. Rectal or vaginal examination reveals tenderness on the right side at the onset, and later on both sides. Tenderness is of more value than pain. Rigidity of the abdominal muscles is the most valuable sign of perforation of the intestine; it is at first localized over the area of perforation, thence becoming general with the spread of infection. In uncomplicated cases of typhoid, pain is a frequent symptom; tenderness is common over the ileum, and slight rigidity may be present, but the association of these three features is an indication for exploration, and with a fair degree of accuracy indicate, by their character and extent, the intensity and area of peritonitis. The hardening of the belly-wall, due to meteorism, to emaciation, to the application of cold water, or to associated pulmonary disease, must not mislead the surgeon, who should be familiar with the feel of the abdomen in all stages of the disease.

Distention of the abdomen is often present throughout the disease, and is not an important sign, although it becomes more pronounced after perforation. The vital point is to determine whether the gas is within the bowel or in the peritoneal cavity outside the bowel. Partial absence of liver dulness may be produced by tympanitic distention of the intestine, but total obliteration of liver dulness not associated with distention of the abdomen is due to gas outside the bowel and indicates perforation of the alimentary canal. It has been suggested that in cases in which gas is free in the peritoneal cavity the chest sounds may be distinctly heard over the abdomen, but this is equally true when the intestine is distended with gas without perforation. Tschunowsky[3] claims to have heard an amphoric murmur, synchronous with respiration, over the point of perforation; he attributed the sound to the exit and entrance of air through the opening in the intestine. "In pneumatosis of the abdominal cavity one sometimes gets a peculiar quality of sound on deep percussion which resembles the cracked-pot sound."[4]

As the result of experiments on animals, Connell[5] believes that perforation may be diagnosticated by tapping the abdomen, injecting air or salt solution, and, after regaining the injected material, testing it for hydrogen sulphide. It seems to us that exploratory incision would be more certain and less dangerous.

It has been advised in cases of suspected intestinal perforation to inject air, hydrogen, or ether into the rectum; if there be no perforation the gas will pass through the intestine and out of the mouth; if an opening into the peritoneal cavity exists the gas will pass through the perforation, increase the distention of the abdomen, and obliterate the liver dulness. This method increases the extravasation of intestinal contents and is not to be employed.

Dulness in the flanks, as indicative of fluid in the peritoneal cavity, is a fallacious sign, as it is sometimes present in the absence of perforation and often absent in cases in which perforation has occurred and in which there is a large quantity of fluid in the peritoneal cavity.

Localized impairment of resonance is of little value as a sign, as it is seldom found, even when there is an attempt at walling off the peritoneal cavity.

Immobility of the abdomen and thoracic respiration accompany rigidity, and are important signs.

Auscultation rarely reveals a friction sound, but may elicit the presence or absence of peristalsis, which is of more value from the standpoint of prognosis than of diagnosis.

Nausea and vomiting occur in less than 25 per cent. of the cases and are often present without perforation. A chill at the onset of perforation is not common. The classical symptoms of shock do not ensue as often as is generally believed. In many cases the temperature remains unchanged, and in some it rises. Sweating is a frequent symptom. The respirations are increased in frequency and thoracic in character; the pulse is accelerated and the blood pressure, as determined by the Riva Rocci sphygmomanometer, is distinctly raised.[6] The facial expression is altered and characteristic in many cases, and is a feature on which much stress is laid. A leukocytosis is only of value when corroborative of other signs.

Typhoidal perforation may be confounded with almost any other lesion producing a peritonitis, but as treatment in these cases would usually demand exploration a failure to differentiate would not be productive of harm. The most difficult differential diagnosis to make is that between intestinal hemorrhage and perforation, as the symptoms are sometimes identical and the differentiation is of the greatest importance, for to mistake hemorrhage for perforation means an unnecessary operation at a very critical period, and to mistake perforation for hemorrhage means death. The appearance of blood in the stools is not conclusive, as the two conditions may coexist. A reduction in the number of red cells and in the hæmoglobin would point toward hemorrhage, whereas an excess in the number of white cells would incline toward perforation. It is of the utmost importance to withhold opium in cases of hemorrhage in which perforation is suspected, because of the danger of clouding the symptoms.

With Osler we may say: "That time-honored picture of perforation with the Hippocratic facies; the feeble, running pulse; the profuse sweat; the distended, motionless abdomen must be erased as not a picture of perforation, but of peritonitis, or, better still, a rough draught of death. What we need more than anything at present is a fuller knowledge of the symptoms of perforation, particularly of its onset, apart from those of the consecutive peritonitis."[7] But, unfortunately, there is nothing in the perforation itself which will enable one to suspect it; the signs and symptoms that are elicited are due to peritoneal infection, the very onset of which we should make an effort to recognize. Obliteration of liver dulness in a flat belly or resonance over the postérior and lateral area of hepatic dulness in a distended abdomen and cellular emphysema are the only pathognomonic signs of an opening into the intestine. The former, however, is a late sign, and the latter does not occur in typhoidal perforations.

The only safe rule is to have every typhoid watched most carefully, to examine thoroughly at the onset of any of the above symptoms, and to open the abdomen if the evidence gathered leave a doubt as to perforation. If there be doubt, exploration may be conducted under local anæsthesia; but if the diagnosis be positive or if exploration reveals perforation, ether should be employed, as the operation may be performed more quickly, the abdominal cavity may be cleansed more thoroughly, and the patient is not subjected to the deleterious effects of fright and struggling. Operation should be done at the earliest possible period. Some authors advise waiting for the subsidence of shock, but if shock is present the danger of delay far outweighs the danger of a rapid operation, in which the ether and the flushing of the abdominal cavity with hot salt solution tend to combat rather than aggravate the symptoms of shock. All cases should be operated upon, no matter how ill they are, as some remarkable recoveries have been reported. The incision is made in the right iliac region, as from 85 per cent. to 90 per cent. of all perforations are found in the last twenty or thirty inches of the ileum or in the cæcum or appendix. If the perforation be not found in the ileum and there are evidences of peritonitis, the sigmoid, the colon, and the remainder of the small intestine should be explored in the order mentioned, making a median incision if necessary. If the ileum be intact and there are no evidences of peritonitis, a mistake in diagnosis has probably been made, but the incision should not be closed without further exploration. Ross[8] reports a case of suspected perforation in which exploration revealed a normal peritoneum and an intact ileum; an intussusception was found in the jejunum. The perforation may be sutured with a double row of continuous Lembert sutures of silk. The continuous suture is more rapid than the interrupted suture and just as safe. It is not necessary to excise the ulcer. A large perforation should be sutured obliquely, so as not to interfere with the fecal current. Search for a second perforation should always be made, for in 17 or 18 per cent. the openings are multiple. All suspicious spots are invaginated with a continuous silk suture. In some cases suture is impossible because of the size of the opening, because of the number of openings in a segment of the bowel, or because a piece of the bowel is gangrenous. Resection would be the ideal treatment in these cases, but as it consumes so much time surgeons have been afraid to try it. Plugging the hole with omentum or fastening the omentum over the perforation may succeed in some instances, but is a hazardous procedure. Isolating the affected portion of bowel by gauze packing has been advocated and may be employed in certain cases. The safest plan is to anchor the intestinal loop outside the abdominal cavity; this not only makes the isolation more complete, but relieves threatening symptoms of distention, and allows the local application of medicaments to the interior of the bowel for the treatment of the remaining typhoid ulcers.

After dealing with the perforation the abdomen should be flushed with gallons of hot salt solution, unless the infection be distinctly limited, in which case the affected coils should be drawn from the abdomen and thoroughly washed extraperitoneally, as a general peritoneal lavage in these cases would disseminate the infection. The abdomen is usually drained by gauze, one strip of which is pushed down into the pelvic cavity. The after-treatment is that of other abdominal cases, excepting that the patient must be carefully watched for symptoms of secondary perforation.

The prognosis is more favorable when the perforation occurs early in the disease, when the diagnosis is made quickly after the onset, and when the surgeon possesses skill and good judgment. According to Harte,[2] the mortality in 277 cases in successive intervals was as follows: 1884 to 1889, 10 cases, 90 per cent.; 1890 to 1893, 16 cases, 87.5 per cent.; 1894 to 1898, 110 cases, 74.5 per cent.; 1899 to 1902, 141 cases, 66.6 per cent.

The following is an abstract of eight cases operated upon.

Case I.—Male, aged ten years; operated upon July 28, 1901, at the Pennsylvania Hospital, twelve hours after perforation, which occurred on the thirteenth day of the disease. Pain during the entire disease, worse at the time of operation, but not severe. Tenderness all over the abdomen, but most marked in the right iliac region. No vomiting. Obliteration of liver dulness, movable dulness in the right flank, rigidity of the right rectus, thoracic breathing, distention, fall of temperature from 103° F. to normal, leukocytes 4000. Incision in the right semilunar line; liquid feces in the abdominal cavity. In the ileum, six inches from the cæcum, was a large indurated area, with a pinhole perforation in the centre. Double row of continuous Lembert sutures. Peritoneum injected. Death in sixty hours. Post-mortem revealed a closed perforation, the lumen of the bowel constricted one-third, and a general peritonitis.

CASE II.—Female, aged twenty-three years; operated upon December 15, 1901, at the Pennsylvania Hospital, forty-eight hours after perforation, which occurred during the fifth week of the disease. This patient walked about until the time of perforation, which was inaugurated with violent pain in the region of the appendix. Admitted to the hospital immediately before operation. Vomiting, Hippocratic facies, swollen belly, obliteration of liver dulness, no dulness in the flanks, belly immobile, moderate tenderness in the right iliac region. Temperature 103° F., pulse scarcely perceptible; anæsthetic 1 per cent. cocaine solution; incision right semilunar line; large quantity of yellow fluid mixed with flakes of lymph; perforation in ileum three inches from the cæcum, one-eighth of an inch in diameter. Patient died one-half hour after operation.

CASE III.—Male, aged nineteen years; operated upon August 25, 1902, at the Polyclinic Hospital during the third week of the disease, fourteen hours after perforation. Sudden severe pain, distention, tenderness and rigidity on the right side, tympanitic over liver, leukocytes 10,000. Previous diarrhœa. No vomiting, no dulness in the flanks, thoracic respiration, temperature unchanged. Perforation in ileum five inches from the cæcum, size of a lead-pencil; liquid feces in the peritoneal cavity; gauze drain through the primary incision and rubber tube through the loin. Vomited once after operation, distention less, pain absent, fever persistent, diarrhœa continued, death third day. Post-mortem revealed closed perforation, dry peritoneal cavity, and a few adhesions. Cause of death typhoid(?).

CASE IV.—Male, aged twenty-three years; operated upon February 4, 1902, at the Jefferson Hospital, during the third week of the disease and twelve hours after perforation. Admitted to hospital just before operation. Pain, tenderness, and rigidity in the right iliac region. Temperature 104° F., pulse 120, respirations thoracic; severe pain, reflected to the rectum and associated with tenesmus; distention, liver dulness obliterated one-half, no dulness in the flanks, no vomiting, leukocytes 7200. Perforation in ileum six inches from the cæcum, size one-quarter of an inch; yellow feces and gas in the peritoneal cavity; gauze drain. Pulse and temperature fell to normal after operation, later rose to 103° F., and remained elevated. There were no further abdominal symptoms, but the patient died on the eighth day, apparently from typhoid. No post-mortem.

CASE V.—Male, aged thirty years; operated upon June 6, 1903, at the Pennsylvania Hospital, immediately after admission. No satisfactory history could be obtained, as the patient was a Pole who understood no English. Dulness and rales over the bases of both lungs; pinched expression. Temperature 100° F., respirations

40, pulse 140, sweating; retracted, rigid belly; absence of liver dulness; costal respiration. Diagnosis perforative peritonitis; median incision; perforation in ileum eighteen inches from the cæcum, one-half inch in diameter; a smaller perforation was found one-half inch above the first perforation. Abdominal cavity filled with feces and pus. Death one hour later.

CASE VI.—Male, aged forty-two years; operated upon June 7, 1903, at the Pennsylvania Hospital, immediately after admission. No history obtainable, as the patient was a Pole who could understand no English. Temperature 100° F., pulse 100, respirations 30. Great pain in the abdomen and right shoulder; tenderness all over the abdomen, and especially marked over the site of a left inguinal hernia; belly immobile and rigid, dulness in the flanks, liver dulness decreased one-half, vomitus nigra. Diagnosis perforative peritonitis; median incision; liquid feces and pus in the abdominal cavity; mesentery glands enlarged; perforation in the ileum one-half inch in diameter, three feet from the cæcum. Closure of perforation with a double row of Lembert sutures, lavage with hot salt solution, gauze drainage. Uneventful recovery. Widal reaction positive.

CASE VII.—Female,* aged nine years; operated upon June 24, 1903, at the Jefferson Hospital, on the thirteenth day of the disease, three hours after perforation. The temperature had been running along at about 104° F., the pulse 120, and the respirations 20. She complained of severe pain in the right iliac region; this lasted for a short time, and the patient complained no more, even when questioned. The temperature, pulse, and respirations remained unchanged. No vomiting, slight tenderness and rigidity in the right iliac region, movable dulness in the right flank, liver dulness one finger's breadth above the costal margin, abdominal respiration. Two bowel movements between the time of perforation and operation. Tenderness on the right side per rectum, leukocytes 18,000. Incision in the right semilunar line; clear fluid in the belly, no feces or pus; peritoneum normal; perforation in ileum the size of the lead in a lead-pencil, ten inches from the cæcum and midway between the mesentery and the free border of the bowel. The perforation was closed by a small, yellowish slough, which became dislodged as the bowel was pulled through the wound. Continuous Lembert suture, flush with salt solution, and closure of the abdomen without drainage. The patient continued with the typhoid symptoms, and made a good recovery.

CASE VIII.—Male, aged forty-one years; operated upon July 8, 1903, at the Jefferson Hospital, two weeks after the beginning of the

* This patient developed a small hernia at the site of incision, for which a second operation was performed four months after the suturing of the intestinal perforation. There were no adhesions in the peritoneal cavity, the mesenteric glands were still enlarged, and the site of the perforation was marked by a small grayish patch which was perfectly smooth and slightly indurated. There was no constriction of the intestine.

symptoms of typhoid and nineteen hours after perforation. The patient had been walking about up until nineteen hours before the operation, when he was seized with a sudden severe pain in the lower part of the abdomen. He was admitted to the hospital immediately before the operation. Temperature 101° F., pulse 140, respirations 30. Typical picture of a general peritonitis, liver dulness undiminished, no dulness in the flanks. Diagnosis perforative peritonitis; median incision; fecal matter and pus in the peritoneal cavity; perforation in ileum three-eighths inch in diameter, one foot from the cæcum. Death in thirty hours from peritonitis.

Analyses of cases operated upon: Sex, 6 males, 2 females. Ages nine, ten, nineteen, twenty-three, twenty-three, thirty, forty-one, and forty-two years. Day of disease on which perforation occurred: 2 on thirteenth day, 1 during second week, 2 during the third week, and 1 during the fifth week; in 2 cases no satisfactory history could be obtained, the patients being unable to understand English. Number of hours elapsing between the time of perforation and operation: three hours in 1 case (recovered), twelve hours in 2 cases, fourteen hours in 1 case, nineteen hours in 1 case, and forty-eight hours in 1 case. In 2 cases, 1 of whom recovered, the time elapsing between perforation and operation could not be determined. Pain during the entire course of the disease in 2, absence of pain previous to perforation in 4, unknown in 2. Location of pain in right iliac region in 5, general in 3. In 1 case the pain was reflected to the right shoulder, and in 1 case the pain extended to the rectum and was associated with tenesmus and a frequent desire but inability to defecate. The pain was violent in 1 case, severe in 6, and moderate in 1; in 1 case in which the pain was severe at the onset it disappeared soon after its appearance and remained absent up until the time of operation. The facial appearance was altered in all except the 2 that recovered. Mental hebetude was present in all. Previous bleeding from the bowel was absent in 6 and unknown in 2. Vomiting was absent in 5 and present in 3. Constipation had been present in 2, diarrhœa in 4, and 2 unknown. A chill was not noted in any of the 6 cases from whom a history could be obtained. In 1 case the temperature fell 3 degrees to normal, in 5 the temperature remained unchanged, and in 2 the temperature at the time of perforation could not be obtained. The pulse and respirations were accelerated in all. Localized impairment of resonance was not noted in any of the cases. Sweating was present in 6 and absent in 2. Distention was absent in 2 only. Immobility of the abdomen and thoracic respiration were present in 7 and absent in 1 case. Friction sound was not heard in any of the cases. Peristalsis was heard in 1 case, in which the bowels moved twice after perforation and in which recovery ensued. The liver dulness was totally absent in 4, partly absent in 2, and present in 2. Dulness in the flanks was present in 2 cases only. Rigidity was present in all. Tenderness was general in 5 cases and limited to the lower right abdomen in 3. Rectal examination revealed tenderness in the 7 cases in which it was made. The leukocytes in 4 cases were 4000, 7200, 10,000, and 18,000. The diagnosis was made in 5 cases, and the incision was made in the right iliac region; in 3 cases a diagnosis of perforative peritonitis was made and the abdomen opened in the middle line. The perforations were situated in the ileum within three feet of the cæcum in all cases, and varied in size from a pinhole up to one-half inch in diameter. In 1 case there were two perforations. Fecal matter was present in the peritoneal cavity in all except 1 case, in which the fluid was clear and in which recovery ensued. The peritoneum was inflamed in all but 1 case, in which recovery ensued. Mesenteric glands were enlarged in all. In only 1 case was it necessary to tear through adhesions to find the perforation. In all cases a double row of continuous Lembert suture of silk was employed. All were drained with gauze, surrounded by a rubber dam, except 1 (recovered); in 1 case (died) in addition to the gauze drainage in the primary incision a rubber tube was brought out through the loin. Ether was used as an anæsthetic in all cases except 1, in which the operation was performed under cocaine. 5 of the cases were admitted to the hospital immediately before operation, and 2 walked about until the time of perforation. 2 recovered, 2 died of typhoid (?), and 4 died of peritonitis.

References.

1. H. M. Taylor. New York Medical Journal, February 1, 1903.
2. R. H. Harte. Annals of Surgery, July, 1903.
3. Berliner klin. Wochenschrift, 1869, Nos. 20, 21.
4. Liebermeister. Ziemssen's Cyclopedia.
5. Connell. Journal American Medical Association, March 28, 1903.
6. Crile. Ibid., May 9, 1903.
7. Osler. Proceedings Philadelphia County Medical Society, January, 1901.
8. G. G. Ross. Transactions of the Philadelphia Academy of Surgery, 1903.

PAROTITIS COMPLICATING APPENDICITIS.[1]

By F. E. Bunts, M.D.,

of Cleveland, Ohio.

The first reported instance of parotitis as a postoperative complication of appendectomy is that reported by Barlow, in 1886, who, in a male aged twenty years, reports the occurrence of a parotid bubo, "which did not suppurate." In the operation, collections of fetid pus around the cæcum had been found. The appendix vermiformis was noted to have been much thickened, but apparently it was not re-

[1] Read before the Academy of Medicine of Toledo, Ohio, October 23, 1903.

moved. Elder and Thomas next, as recently as 1901, each mentions the occurrence of parotitis as a sequel to appendicitis. In Elder's case, a male aged twenty years had a sudden onset of pain in the right iliac region. The operation revealed pericæcal abscess. Three days after the operation the temperature began to rise, and a stiffness and swelling in the right parotid region, with intense pain, appeared. "The swelling rapidly increased for about ten hours, when the pain subsided. At this time the whole parotid region and the upper part of the neck were enormously swollen, the swelling coming forward over the cheek and involving the eyelids, especially the under one. Thirty-six hours after the left parotid began to swell in the same way, while the right parotid began slowly to decrease. The left parotid attained almost exactly the same size as the right, and the temperature reached 103° F. The swellings were very painful to pressure, but there was no indication of suppuration in either of them. The second parotid reached its maximum in about twelve hours after it showed symptoms of enlarging." Both parotids gradually subsided, and recovery followed. As a probable etiological cause in this instance, infection is suggested.

In Thomas' case, that of a young woman aged twenty-two years, the appendix was found adherent to the pelvic bottom, but no suppuration was present. Six days after the operation a parotitis developed on the right side, which was extremely painful and persisted for ten days, then subsiding without suppuration.

In these three instances of postoperative parotitis following appendectomy are to be found the only records of this complication subsequent to this operation. As noted, in two, suppuration occurred, while in one of these a septic condition was presumably not present. To these three cases I wish to add three others which have come under my own observation.

Case I.—Male, aged twenty-nine years, entered Charity Hospital May 12, 1902, with severe attack of appendicitis. Patient refused operation, and a large mass formed in the right side. All food was withheld from the stomach, and feeding was carried on exclusively by the rectum. In about seven days, when the general symptoms were improving, though the tongue remained dry and hard, he developed a tenderness over the right parotid. Ichthyol and hot fomentations were applied, suppuration occurred, and the abscess was opened May 24th. The left parotid up to this time had not been involved, but in a few days became inflamed, suppurated, and was opened May 28th. The pus was at first very thick and white, but later it became thin, the drainage was better, and they slowly healed. The mass entirely disappeared, and the patient was discharged June 27th, entirely recovered. He was seen at the expiration of one year and had had no recurrence of the trouble.

Case II.—Male, aged twenty-nine years, entered Charity Hospital January 28, 1903, with an attack of acute appendicitis, this being the fifth attack within the past year. At this time the patient had a mass in the right side, and vomited severely, apparently obstruction of the bowels. Immediate operation revealed abscess cavity and gangrenous appendix, peritoneal cavity well walled off. Appendix was removed and wound drained. No movement of the bowels was obtained until the second day. He suffered from great pain and extreme distention of the abdomen, and was allowed nothing by mouth but hot water and occasionally a little beef broth. About February 6th he developed a right parotitis, which slowly went on to suppuration, and was opened. In two or three days the left parotid became involved, and though greatly swollen and very painful, never had to be opened, but was treated with local applications of ichthyol and moist heat. The bacteriological examination showed a pure culture of bacillus coli communis from the appendiceal abscess and staphylococcus pyogenes aureus from the parotid abscess. Patient discharged cured March 25th. At no time did the parotid inflammation appear to threaten the life of the patient, and in the one which suppurated, recovery followed fairly rapidly upon its evacuation.

Case III.—Female, aged sixty-two years, admitted to Mt. Sinai Hospital July 16, 1903, had been sick for one week, suffering intense pain in abdomen, especially in the right iliac region, had severe diarrhœa, brought on by purging, vomited frequently, abdomen markedly distended, large mass in the right iliac region. Diagnosis, appendicitis. No operation was performed; patient was allowed only water by the mouth, and was fed by the rectum, and ice-bags applied to the abdomen. Under this treatment the fever gradually declined until July 22d, when it reached normal, and remained, with slight variation, at that point till July 26th, when it rose to 100.4° F. Coincidently there was a beginning tenderness of the left parotid, which increased greatly in size, the swelling extending back of the ear and well down on the neck. On account of the pain and swelling she could only separate her jaws about one-quarter of an inch. The tongue was very dry and hard. Five days later, under local anæsthesia, the parotid was opened and a small amount of very thick pus escaped. The pus was so thick that for several days the flow was much impeded. By July 30th the temperature was again normal, but August 2d it rose to 100° F., and a beginning parotitis of the right side was discovered. This was treated as was the first, by local applications of ichthyol and hot fomentations. The tongue remained dry and harsh, the jaws almost entirely closed, but the inflammation gradually subsided without evidence of suppuration, and the patient's general condition improved very markedly till August 9th, when she complained of some pain and discomfort in the right iliac region. The mass had disappeared after a week's confinement to rectal feeding, and was not again present, but the temperature rose to 101.4 F., and then gradually resumed the normal, remaining there for several days prior to her death on August 21st. No autopsy was permitted, so that the exact cause of death was not known. Both parotids had, however, entirely recovered. There was no evidence of metastatic processes, but the condition seemed to be rather one of low sepsis and exhaustion.

The records of these cases, especially the bacteriological findings, are unfortunately incomplete, but in the second case, or the only one in which an operation was performed and an opportunity given to compare the bacteriological cause of the appendicitis and also of the parotitis, the examination showed colon bacilli in the one and staphylococci in the other, thus showing the improbability of its being metastatic in its origin, and in all three cases both parotids became entirely well and no metastasis developed, and aside from the additional debility or exhaustion which ensued, the parotitis did not seem to be *per se* a serious complication.

Since the completion of this paper the following report of a case of parotitis complicating appendicitis has been kindly given me by my colleague, Dr. C. A. Hamann:

E. R., aged twenty years; operation on November 23, 1901. Three weeks before operation was attacked with usual symptoms of acute appendicitis. Condition at time of operation: Large tender mass in median line of abdomen, below and to left of the umbilicus, plainly to be felt per rectum; fluctuation not to be determined, temperature, 101° F.; pulse, 92; leukocytosis, 27,000. Incision in median line. Abscess cavity contained about one pint of pus, walled off. Pus had a fecal odor. Bacillus coli communis found. Appendix could not be found. On November 28th the left parotid region was greatly swollen; œdema over gland; pain; temperature, 102° F. November 29th, incision; no pus evacuated. December 4th, another incision; much pus; About this time the right parotid became enlarged. Soon pus appeared in the external auditory canal. December 7th, incised right parotid; much pus; bacillus coli communis and staphylococci found in pus from parotids. Patient progressed gradually to complete recovery. Discharged from the hospital January 4, 1902.

It will be noted that in this case the colon bacillus, as well as staphylococci, were found in the examination of the pus obtained from the parotid, but no other evidence of metastatic infection appeared, and the patient eventually made a favorable recovery.

The occurrence of parotitis as a sequel or complication of various operations and diseases, though known and described by many clinicians, is still of interest and of importance, and while the object of this paper is to emphasize the possibility of its occurrence in appendicitis, it is also my desire to refer as briefly as possible to a number of cases which have been from time to time reported and the theories which have been advanced to account for them.

Parotitis as occurring subsequent to abdominal sections has been most frequently noted in relation to ovariotomy. Goodell, in a series of 153 ovariotomies, noted its occurrence in 4 cases, in only 1 of which did suppuration occur. Moricke, in 200 ovariotomies, observed 5 cases, 4 of which suppurated. Paget, in a collection of 101 cases of parotitis, the result of injury, either traumatic or operative, to the abdomen or pelvis, reports that in 27 it was the sequel to ovariotomy or oöphorectomy. In 90 of these cases both parotids were attacked, and in 3 the submaxillary and sublingual glands were also involved. Brunne, in a report of 17 cases of parotitis supervening upon ovariotomy, reports that in 4 cases it was bilateral, while in 9 cases suppuration occurred.

From this great preponderance of parotitis subsequent to ovariotomy it was at one time assumed that it occurred only in this operation to the exclusion of all others. Moricke asserted that he had never observed this complication in any other laparotomy excepting that involving an ovariotomy. This statement was, however, soon contradicted by more accurate observations, and other operations followed by this complication were soon reported.

According to McDonald, parotitis was not an unusual or uncommon complication in the early history of abdominal surgery, it being regarded by some surgeons as invariably fatal. This statement regarding the fatality of postoperative parotitis was seemingly substantiated by Moricke, who also regarded the parotitis following ovariotomy as a severe complication, stating that in 2 cases it was seemingly the sole cause of death, and in 2 cases it at least contributed to the fatal issue.

As to the etiology of postoperative parotitis, the theory which was primarily advanced assumed the sympathetic relation between the generative organs and these glands. This theory, which gained some corroboration from the frequent occurrence of orchitis or mastitis following the so-termed mumps of childhood, was apparently even more strongly verified by some peculiar instances of parotitis following injuries or operations on these organs.

In the male sex parotitis had been observed secondary to injury of the testicle (Billroth, Hutchison), after the passage of the catheter (O'Conner, Crimm, Paget), as also subsequent to cystitis (Paget). In the female sex, however, parotitis had been even more frequently observed in the various affections of the generative organs. Peter, in a woman with irregular menstruation, speaks of the substitution of the menses by parotitis of either one side or the other, most frequently the left. Hawkins mentions the instance of a woman who, during six successive pregnancies, had an enlargement of the left parotid, which increased with the advance of gestation, and totally disappeared after delivery. He states that "she had learned to recognize this as one of the first indications of her condition." Cribb, in connection with the interrelation of parotitis and the sexual organs, speaks of an instance in which parotitis followed the insertion of a pessary in the vagina. Parotitis following delivery, abortion, and the menopause, has also been mentioned by other observers, also as a sequence to operative procedures on the generative tract, as has been observed after the excision of the cervix, uterus (Goodell), the repair of a lacerated cervix (Emmet), the repair of a vesicovaginal fistula (Emmet), abdominal hysterectomy (Krussen, Ross, Baldwin, McDonald), salpingectomy (Ricketts), perineorrhaphy (Auld), myoenucleation of the uterus (Gotschauer).

In the frequent observance of parotitis as resulting from disease, injuries, or operations upon the sexual organs, the sympathetic bond between these respective organs seemed assured, even although a more or less direct anatomical connection could not be determined. Trousseau already referred to it in a vague manner. Brunn advanced the explanation that stimuli were transferred from one organ to the other by means of certain nerve channels. In this way irritation in operations on the ovary was said to cause vasomotor disturbances in the parotid gland, from which an inflammation soon followed, which at the onset was assumed to be simple. If suppuration subsequently occurred, this was supposed to be the result of micro-organisms, whose portal of entrance was through Stenson's duct, the partial suspension or inhibition of the salivary secretion being considered a most favorable and influential factor for the admission of the micro-organism.

Paget similarly assumed a nervous relation, although he, too, could advance no more definite statement as to the nature of the relation. The assumption of Paget was largely based on instances of persistent alteration of the parotid gland of both a physiological and clinical nature. In the dog, for instance, the action of the gustatory nerve is known to suffer inhibition when a loop of intestine is drawn from the abdominal cavity, and the secretion of saliva is thereby diminished or totally arrested until the loop of the intestine is replaced. Clinically, he states, arrest of saliva has also been observed during gastritis, as also during menstruation, while in pregnancy salivation is a common occurrence.

This influence of the nervous system on the salivary glands is said to be both direct and reflex. In all of these assumptions a clear elucidation of the exact anatomical and physiological interrelationship of these organs to either the nervous system or to the parotid gland seemed lacking, so that they presented but little which could logically commend itself. With more accurate observations on this form of parotitis it was also found that the affection was not entirely limited to operations upon the sexual tract, but occurred after other cœliotomies and operations. In the report of such instances it had been noted as a sequel to gastrectomy (Clark), gastrostomy (Paget), enterostomy (Dunkworth), colostomy (Dashwood, Rosenbach), laparotomy for peritonitis (Goode, Addenbrook), partial removal of the omentum and retroperitoneal tumor (Paget), operation for gastric ulcer (Hawkins and Herbert), as well as after a division of a rectal stricture and excision of hemorrhoids (Paget, Auld), and after an amputation of the leg (McDonald), so that the statement that parotitis following operation is confined exclusively to operations upon the generative tract is no longer valid, and the theories which had been advanced were changed to include all interference upon the peritoneal cavity. A definite relation identical to that which had been theoretically applied to the ovaries was, however, assumed to exist between the peritoneum and the parotid gland.

In this connection Brunn mentioned that in the cases of parotitis following ovariotomy which he had observed this seemed to be most frequent when multiple adhesions between the viscera were encountered. To explain the occurrence of parotitis subsequent to laparotomy or operative interference in the peritoneal cavity in general, a new theory, however, soon came in, viz., that of direct metastasis. As has been frequently stated, parotitis was more apt to result if purulent foci were encountered in the course of the operation subsequent to peritonitis, pyæmia, appendicular abscess, etc., than after non-septic cœliotomies.

Pozzi regarded the occurrence of parotitis after cœliotomy as strong evidence of the fact that a certain degree of septicæmia was present. In general, however, the theory of metastasis where no purulent affections and septicæmic processes were present could not be regarded favorably. Among later writers this theory too has been discarded, as it could not logically be assumed that septic metastasis should involve the parotid gland to the exclusion of all other organs. The more rational view that parotitis was to be associated with an ascending infection from the mouth along Stenson's duct began to prevail, and the clinical facts, when carefully considered, in part if not wholly, served to substantiate this view. Certain predisposing factors favoring the ascending infection along the course of Stenson's duct were soon determined to be present in the instances in which parotitis supervened. Among the most influential of these is the dryness of the mouth, which may supervene after operations and in conditions of enjoined rest of the patient. Contributory causes are the stagnation of the saliva and the injury to the duct in the course of the operation. That dryness of the mouth predisposes to a parotitis has been attested by clinical observations of various writers.

In the affection termed erostomia the occurrence of repeated attacks of parotitis has not been infrequently noted (Hutchison, Harris, and Battle). Gee, in the consideration of the inflammation of the parotid as complicating the various fevers, regards it as being caused by the dryness of the mouth, the irritation being assumed to extend from the mouth along Stenson's duct to the gland. Next to the dryness of the mouth the stagnation of the saliva may be said to constitute the most favorable factor for an ascending infection along Stenson's duct.

The conditions under which a patient is placed subsequent to the operation may well be considered as powerful contributory factors in the causation of parotitis. The feverish condition often following operations, by reducing the quantity of secretion, leads to a still further stagnation of the saliva within the glands and ducts. The failure to clean the teeth in the first few days following the operation may also act as a contributory cause. Thus in 2 cases reported by Malcolm the opening of Stenson's duct was visibly inflamed when attention was first directed to the gland, and in both cases carious teeth were situated opposite the opening of Stenson's duct. Hawthorne noted this early infection of the duct, stating that from the very earliest appearance of parotitis, pressure over the duct would cause the expulsion of a drop of pus from its orifice.

The histological investigation of Hannau in several fatal cases complicated by parotitis also bears out this view that an ascending infection from the mouth is the primary and direct cause of this affection. Paget at once refuted this theory, advancing as the most patent argument against it that the socia parotidis were never inflamed before the main body of the gland. This objection seems, however, not to be of great value, as clinically it must be difficult to establish an inflammation of such a small portion of the gland. Its attendant enlargement can be but slight, and the pain upon palpation cannot probably be so accurately localized as to enable us to say whether it is in this part or the anterior portion of the gland proper. Moreover, as has been determined histologically and clinically, inflammation of Stenson's duct precedes that of the parotid gland, so that the refutation of Paget may be considered as resting on insufficient or faulty observations.

One of the possible contributory causes not heretofore mentioned is the injury to the gland or duct, which may occur during the administration of anæsthesia. In the various manipulations of the face, as in the forward action of the mandible, the traction of the tongue or the removal of the accumulated secretion of the mouth, the duct may be easily compressed. A somewhat severe compression might at times result in slight injury, such as contusion of Stenson's duct, a locus minoris resistentiæ be thereby established, which, either singly or in conjunction with the dryness of the mouth and stagnation of saliva, would prepare a favorable field for a parotid infection. Occlusion of the duct at its most constricted portion, the papilla, which is situated opposite to the second upper molar tooth, would, similarly, be at times the result of this manipulation in the course of the anæsthesia. That these injuries of the duct favor the development of a parotitis is maintained in the cases reported by Johnson, in which the only cause that could be ascertained was an inflammation of the duct, with stagnation of the salivary secretion. Similar cases have been reported by Choppell, Battle, Kussmaul, and others. In several of these cases it was noted that pressure over the duct or gland relieved the swelling, and it was found that the pressure caused the expulsion of a plug of thick, turbid mucus from the duct, thus relieving the obstruction to the escape of saliva.

The various theories which have been advanced to explain the occurrence of postoperative parotitis may be stated as follows:

1. A sympathetic or nervous connection between certain viscera, notably the ovary and the parotid gland.
2. Metastasis.
3. Direct infection of the gland by way of Stenson's duct.

The theory of a sympathetic relation is not only entirely hypothetical, but extremely improbable. It is based for the greater part on a collection of facts having little apparent relation to each other, except that in all the parotid gland is involved, and there seems to be no relation other than that indefinite one termed reflex, which may not only take place after operations and injuries of various organs, but as the result of psychical emotions. Similar or identical reflex disturbances are also encountered in other gland structures, and are not, therefore, confined to the parotids. It is known, for instance, that in the emotion of fear the secretion of the parotid gland is inhibited, and in surgical shock also the flow of saliva is in part arrested. In neither of these, however, is the parotid gland alone involved. If shock is of any duration all glandular structures are said to be similarly involved. The increased salivation of pregnancy cannot be directly attributed to the uterus. It is more likely the consequence of the general condition. The statement that in camels the parotid glands enlarge during the breeding season may be included under this explanation. The functional alterations in the parotid secretions after operations, if it occur, is of temporary duration, so that it is doubtful whether as such it could favor inflammation.

The clinical observations of the occurrence of orchitis following mumps might possibly be explained by the theory that the causative agent was transferred accidentally by the hand from the mouth to the urethera, thence to the vas deferens, and finally involving the testicle. The occurrence of parotitis following catheterization attended by pain and fear might be due to the psychical effect which temporarily inhibited the secretion of saliva, and thus favored infection, but it could scarcely be more than a contributing agent, and, therefore, the role of sympathy in the production of inflammation of the parotid should be excluded.

That metastasis may and sometimes does occur in the parotid gland cannot be denied, especially in pyæmic or septicæmic cases, but it seems hardly probable that the parotid alone should be involved, while all the other organs of the body and more frequent sites of metastatic deposits should escape. So that while in single instances this metastasis may be assumed to have occurred, we cannot insist upon this being the universal or even common cause.

Direct infection, in the light of modern pathology and from the clinical study of many cases, would seem to be the only tenable theory, and while no doubt a large percentage of these infections occur primarily in Stenson's duct, the known fact that many pathogenic bacteria are cast off through the salivary glands make it not improbable that the locus minoris resistentiæ having been prepared by the dryness of the mouth, the stagnation of saliva, the inactivity of the masticatory muscles from the enforced liquid diet, or from possible injury to the duct or gland in operation, the bacteria may develop directly in the parotid, even while the duct is the site of an inflammation derived from bacteria within the buccal cavity.

PROGNOSIS. So far as may be judged from the few reported cases of parotitis following appendicitis, this complication is not to be considered a serious one or one likely to lead to any grave results, obviously very different from those rare cases of pyæmia, with coincident involvement of the parotid.

TREATMENT. The treatment must be regarded as (1) prophylactic and (2) surgical. The prophylactic treatment consists in attention to the buccal cavity, frequent cleansing of the teeth, washing out the mouth with a mild antiseptic, such as boric-acid solution, freeing the tongue so far as possible from the foul deposit which so often accumulates upon it, and in the cases in which stomach-feeding has been interdicted, giving the patient something to chew, so as to bring into action the masticatory muscles, and not only help in this manner to evacuate Stenson's duct of the accumulated mucus, but in a mild way stimulate the salivary secretion. Where not objectionable to the patient, chewing-gum might prove the most suitable agent. It might be proper, again, to call attention to the possibility of injuring the duct or gland by external manipulation, especially during the administration of an anæsthetic.

The surgical treatment consists in the application of heat or cold in the hope of checking the inflammation, but where pus is obviously present, nothing remains but to evacuate and drain, and a satisfactory recovery may be confidently anticipated.

BIBLIOGRAPHY.

Paget, P. J. Clinical Lecture and Essays. Lecture I., p. 364.
McDonald, A. Edinburgh Med. Journ., 1885, vol. xxx. p. 1020.
Hawthorne, C. O. Glasgow Med. Journ., vol. xliv. p. 17.
Malcolm, J. D. British Med. Journ., 1899, vol. ii. p. 1671.
Addenbrooke, B. Lancet, 1900, vol. ii. p. 1873.
Jellet, H. Cent. f. Gyn., 1897, vol. xxi. p. 975.
Frederick, C. C. Amer. Journ. Obstet., 1895, vol. xxxiii. p. 772.
Keith, S. Edinburgh Med. Journ., 1886, vol. xxxii. p. 306.
Reference Handbook of Medical Science, vol. vi. p. 51?.
Hawkins, H. P. British Med. Journ., 1897, vol. i. p. 914.
Transactions of the Amer. Gyn Society, 1885, vol. x. p. 211.
Everke. Deut. med. Wochensch., 1895, vol. xxi. p. 319.
International Encyclopædia of Surgery, Ashhurst, vol. v. p. 614.
Hulke. Lancet, 1886, vol. i. p. 735.
Elder, W. Ibid., 1901, vol i. p. 176.

British Med. Journ., January to June, 1887, pp. 612, 676, 828.
Addinsell. Lancet, 1898, vol. ii. p. 1260.
Barker, A. E. Ibid., 1886, vol. i. p. 734.
Dashwood. Ibid.
Cyclopædia of the Practice of Medicine, Ziemssen, vol. v. p. 122.
Brewis, N. T. Edinburgh Med Journ., 1894, vol. xxxix. p. 423.
British Med. Journ., July to December, 1887, p. 1396.
Ahern, M. J. Amer. Journ. Obstet., 1896, vol. xxxiii. p. 232.
Trousseau's Clinical Med., Lecture XI., vol. ii.
Clarke, W. B. Lancet, 1886, vol. i. p. 734.
The Lancet, January to June, 1886, vol. i. pp. 86, 130, 227, 335, 374, 732.

NASAL SYPHILITIC TUMORS.

By Max Toeplitz, M.D.,
of New York.

The tertiary manifestations of syphilis, in the nose the most frequent, are often seen very early—a few months to one year after the first infection, but, as a rule, much later. The tertiary lesions of hereditary lues are the same as those of the acquired, and occur either soon after birth or during puberty.

The anatomical lesion is a gummous infiltration of the mucous membrane, independent affection of cartilage, periosteum and bone, and simple infiltration, with softening, ulceration, either from without inward or inversely. The favorite seat of the infiltration is the septum, particularly on the boundary line between the quadrilateral cartilage and the perpendicular lamina of the ethmoid, bilaterally, often as the only sign; but it also occurs on other places of the septum, rarely on the lateral nasal wall, the turbinates first, but most frequently on the septum and nasal floor.

The tumors are either extremely large gummata or so-called granulomata. Such a syphiloma occurred in a woman, aged twenty-six years, an inmate of the Montefiore Home, who suffered from obstruction of the left nostril, formation of thick crusts, loss of sense of smell, and severe epistaxis. In the right nostril the most anterior portion of the lower turbinate covered with fibrinous deposits was seen only, owing to a deviation of the septum. The left nostril was obstructed by a gray, reddish, movable, smooth tumor, which was removed piecemeal with the cold snare, with much hemorrhage. It sprang from the upper portion of the bony septum, viz., from the upper raised boundary of a perforation, through which the tumor disappeared into the right nostril. The interior of the nose was covered with thick, foul-smelling, green-gray, adhesive crusts. The middle turbinate was atrophied. The histological examination, made by Dr. Henry Kreuder, revealed the body of the growth to consist of loose fibrous connective tissue covered in places by epithelium of the stratified columnar variety. The epithelium dipped down into the tumor and formed small retention cysts, which were lined with stratified columnar epithelium and were filled with mucus. Throughout the connective tissue many large bloodvessels with thin walls were seen and areas of inflammatory round-celled infiltration. Besides, there were areas of larger cells, almost round, with large nuclei, which were suspicious of sarcoma. When the patient entered the Home, on June 20, 1902, she was considered tubercular. Bacilli resembling tubercle bacilli were twice found in the urine. She was removed to the tubercular ward, but as the sputum was always negative she was transferred to another ward. Iodide of potassium was first given on March 3, 1903, in doses of 20 gr., t.i.d., which were increased to 50 gr., and continued till September 20, 1903. Two courses of mercury rubbings, each lasting six weeks, were applied between April 1st and July 23, 1903. Iodide of potassium (10 gr.) and Fowler's solution (3 minims), t. i. d., were given for one month. On February 1, 1904, began hypodermic injections of bichloride of mercury, $\frac{1}{10}$ gr. daily. The antisyphilitic treatment was continued for other than nasal lesions; an annular stricture of the rectum, causing obstruction, which was relieved by cutting through the ring, but along which a syphilitic neoplasm still remained.

An analogous case is reported by Kuhn, in which a mother of four healthy children presented in the vestibule of the left nostril a soft, slightly bleeding tumor, the size of a walnut, covered with smeary pus, and connected, through a perforation the size of a quarter in the cartilaginous septum, with a similar, somewhat smaller tumor in the right nostril, both of which obstructed the nasal cavities completely. Microscopically the tumor consisted of cellular tissue of moderate vascularity, mostly round cells and young connective-tissue cells. Besides, it contained a large number of partly rounded, partly elongated giant cells, with numerous processes and marginal nuclei, and at some places firmer tracts of connective tissue.

Another such case with perforation of the septum is given by Kuttner, who holds that a gummous growth originating from the periosteum had broken down, causing a carious destruction of the septum. The syphiloma or granulation tumor had grown alongside of it. Another explanation is this: The decay of the gumma produced an inflammatory irritation of the surrounding tissue, giving rise to granulation.

These tumors obstruct the nose when large enough, and discharge fibrinous, smeary, and purulent secretions. They cause pain in the head, face, shoulder, and paralytic-like weakness in the arm. They are of variable size, and are implanted upon the mucous membrane with a broad or pedunculated base. Their favorite seat is the anterior lower portion of the septum, occasionally, also, the nasal floor. They are red, reddish-gray, not quite smooth, show frequent erosions, but rarely ulcerations. They are covered with fibrinous, purulent, firmly adherent exudations, in some cases with thin, fluid, mucopurulent secretion. The tissue is boggy, brittle, still without tendency to decay, its main distinction from gumma.

Von Esmarch has warned against superfluous and harmful operations which are carried out for these syphilitic tumors when their nature is not recognized.

In Knight's case the appearance of manifest specific signs prevented the operation. A girl, aged fifteen years, had suffered from epiphora through a stenosis of the nasal duct due to an enormous enlargement of the right inferior turbinated body, which blocked up the nostril completely and was adherent to the septum. The mass was removed, but in two weeks had resumed its original proportions. Another recurrence took place after removal, and microscopically a small round-celled sarcoma was diagnosed. A general surgeon advised excision of the upper jaw. Ten days later a sensitive swelling of the left chin and a semifluctuating tumor of the size of a hen's egg appeared over the crest of the tibia. Under mercury and iodide of potassium in rapidly increasing doses the tumors of the nose, chin, and tibia disappeared within two weeks.

Many such histories could be related in which the microscopic examination revealed apparently a sarcoma, which disappeared under antisyphilitic treatment.

In several of Kuhn's cases the tumor was due to direct infection, while in a girl, aged eight years, numerous syphilomata had appeared in the nose as late manifestations of congenital syphilis.

I have seen a number of cases of multiple tumors under and along the lower turbinate which resembled a papillomatous growth and recurred as rapidly as they were removed, but were cured with mercury and iodide of potassium.

Theisen reports three cases: The first in a child, aged seven years, with tumors of the septum, of the size of small cherries, pedunculated, like papilloma, which contained spindle cells, recurred after removal and disappeared under iodide of potassium. The second case in a man, aged thirty-six years, was a tumor, of the size of a walnut, and was attached to the septum. It contained tubercle bacilli and giant cells. The third case was a large tumor in a man, aged fifty-eight years, springing from the inferior turbinate, which also showed a swelling of the right cheek.

The diagnosis of these tumors is difficult if the patients do not exhibit other syphilitic signs and the history does not furnish any support. Microscopic examination does not give any positive results as to the specific nature.

The new formations are true tumors, pure connective-tissue growths originating from the submucous connective tissue. The giant cells, which resemble the tuberculous giant cells of Langhans, are proliferations of endothelia from the walls of small veins, and the leukocytes also take part in their production.

The fibrous connective-tissue stroma is the distinguishing feature between these tumors and the round-celled and spindle-celled sarcoma, in which the fundamental substance is sparse and more homogeneous or slightly granular.

The granulomata or syphilomata are not to be confounded with the frequently occurring nasal gummata, which are an inflammatory infiltration into the mucous membrane along its prominent surface, and which soon decay and ulcerate. The syphilomata, however, originate from a small circumscribed place of the mucous membrane, develop to a considerable size, and do not exhibit any tendency to decay.

The clinical proofs are the history and other syphilitic lesions. Perforations of the nasal septum are not always specific; they may be due to congenital or developmental influences, traumatic (operations), contiguous pathological conditions, and influences engendered by constitutional diseases, local inflammations, and allied processes. I have found the greater majority of workingmen in a Paris green factory with perforations of the nasal cartilaginous septum.

The best criterion for the diagnosis is the success of the antisyphilitic treatment. Kuttner had in one case given iodide of potassium without success, and, therefore, had considered the growth as non-specific, but when he later combined it with mercury he succeeded in curing the case.

The antisyphilitic treatment shows the best results with nasal syphilomata.

Bibliography.

Kuhn. Verhandlungen d. Deutsch. Otol. Gesellsch. 1895, No. 4; Deutsche mediz. Woch., 1896; Vereinsbeilage, No. 5.

Frank, Th. Ueber syphiliche Tumoren, Dissertation, Strasburg, 1894.

Manasse. Virchow's Archiv, 1897, vol. cxlvii.

Kuttner. Archiv für Laryngologie, No. 7.

Von Esmarch. Verhandlungen d. Deutschen Chirurgen-Congresses, 1893.

Knight, C. H. The Sequelæ of Syphilis and Their Treatment. Nasal Sequelæ, New York Medical Journal, September 19, 1903.

Ripault. Annales des maladies de l'oreille, 1895.

Locoarret. Ibid.

ICTERUS IN SECONDARY SYPHILIS.

By W. J. Calvert, M.D.,
MISSOURI STATE UNIVERSITY.

C. D., aged twenty-seven years, male, American, white, was admitted to the Post Hospital, Fort McHenry, Md., on June 6, 1902, with intense jaundice. Family history was negative; personal history includes ordinary diseases of childhood; no recent sickness.

Present illness began six weeks ago, when a hard chancre developed on the right side of the glans penis. About three days ago, June 3, patient thinks he had a very slight fever (doubtful), when he also noticed his jaundiced condition. All duties pertaining to his profession were performed until the day previous to entering the hospital. Physical examination on admission revealed an intense general icterus; hard, indurated chancre with one enlarged, hard, right inguinal gland; slight general glandular enlargement; no fever; no pain; no skin lesions; thorax and abdomen negative. Liver was normal in size and not sensitive to pressure. Urine showed bile pigments, no albumin. Feces were not totally decolorized. Three days after admission the first appearance of a general macular eruption was noted.

On admission calomel and soda were given and patient put on bichloride $\frac{1}{16}$ grain and potassium iodide 10 grains t. i. d. On January 25th all secondary symptoms and jaundice had disappeared and patient was discharged from the hospital with the usual instructions.

During his stay in hospital no fever or digestive disturbances were noted, appetite and general condition good. Patient at no time complained of pain. Diagnosis was icterus associated with secondary syphilis.

While icterus in secondary syphilis has long been known, the literature on this subject is comparatively limited.

Extracts from literature: Paracelsus, in 1510, speaks of icterus associated with syphilis, and in 1555 noted the frequency of liver affections in hereditary syphilis. In 1740 Astuc pointed out that icterus followed obstruction and congestion of the liver, as was later mentioned by von Swieten, in 1743, and Fabre, in 1765. Rosen de Rosenstein, in 1764, admitted the co-existence of icterus and syphilis, but thought the icterus was due to the mercurial treatment. Portal, in 1812, admits that icterus is associated with secondary and tertiary syphilis. Guebler, in 1852, reported 5 cases; and Luton, in 1856, first pointed out the difference between icterus in secondary syphilis and that in catarrhal conditions. Three cases were reported, in 1864, by Lancereaux. Lacombe, in 1874, and Morelard, in 1879, report new cases; while Schroeder, in 1887, reported 7 cases. Engel-Reimers, 1887, recorded a case of acute yellow atrophy in secondary syphilis terminating fatally. More recently, Lasch, in 1894, reported 3 of his cases and 46 from the literature; Neumann, in 1895, records 14 cases; Lowenstein, 1. From the records in Allgemeinen Krankenhause in Hamburg, Werner reports 57 new cases of icterus in secondary syphilis out of a total of 15,799 cases, or 0.37 per cent. Aschner, in 1896, reports 3 cases; and Jaumenne, in 1899, 2 cases.

It is difficult to ascertain the exact number of cases as the literature at my disposal often says that some new cases were reported.

Starting with Lasch, who reports 46 cases from literature and 3 of his own, we have, Neumann 14, Lowenstein 1, Werner, 57, Aschner 3, Jaumenne 2, Calvert 1, or a total of 127.

Naturally the etiology of this manifestation is obscure, consequently it has given rise to numerous speculations, no one of which covers all the cases.

Lancereaux, Engel-Reimers, Quincke, and others think the icterus is caused by enlarged glands pressing on the bile-ducts.

Senator, Hutchinson, and Chapotot agree with Guebler, who thinks the secondary eruptions in the intestines cause an obstruction in the flow of bile.

Maurice thinks the hyperæmia of the bile capillaries, due to inflammation of the liver, is sufficient cause. Schroeder believes general catarrhal condition, similar to the infectious diseases, exists. While Quadillac holds that the changes in the blood due to syphilis produce icterus. Several French writers think the general condition of the nervous system plays a role; sò use the term "jaunisse émotive," while others use "meta-syphilitique."

Neumann considers changes in the vessels a sufficient cause; Eichhorst and others favor the chemicotoxic theory; and Liebermeister advocates Menkowsky's idea of acatactic or diffusions icterus.

It is perhaps safe to say that one or more of these causes may be present in the same case. Two types occur—benign and grave.

In benign cases icterus develops rapidly without the usual digestive symptoms of catarrhal jaundice, as was first pointed out by Luton. In 75 per cent. of the cases jaundice develops simultaneously with the secondary symptoms; in the remaining percentage of cases either before or after the onset of secondary manifestations. The character of the secondary lesions is unimportant. In degree, the jaundice varies from a light tinge to a deep discoloration. Its course runs parallel with the secondary symptoms and, like them, may recur. In duration icterus exists from a few days to two months, and if treatment is neglected may become chronic. Occasionally, varying degrees of sensitiveness is present in the hypochondriac regions. Two of Werner's cases presented enlarged livers. Spleen is normal in size. Urine shows ordinary findings. Feces more or less decolorized. Pruritus seldom. Werner noted xanthopsia three times.

In the grave cases icterus develops as above recorded, but on the fifth or sixth day, delirium, hemorrhage, purpura, or coma, often followed by death, may develop in a remarkably short time.

The diagnosis of this manifestation is usually easy. There is a history and evident signs of syphilis. The secondary eruption may be present when the patient is first examined. The following points are most distinctive:

1. Appears in secondary stages of syphilis.

2. Simultaneous appearance with secondary lesions.
3. Influenced by specific treatment.
4. May vary in degree as the secondary eruption varies in intensity during the course of the disease, and, like the eruptions, may recur.
5. Rapid appearance without digestive disturbances.

Even the grave cases if properly treated are rarely fatal. Treatment consists in ordinary treatment for syphilis in this stage.

LITERATURE.

Total literature is too voluminous to republish in toto. See the following articles, where may be found the majority of citations:

Goujon. Sur l'Ictere de la periode secondaire de la syphilis acquise, Paris Thèse, 1896.
Laubry. L'Ictere syphilitique secondaire, La tribune médicale, 1901, vol. xxxiii. p. 1027.
Werner. Beiträge zur Pathologie des Ikterus syphiliticus, Münch. med. Wochensch., 1897 Bd. xliv. p. 736.
Index Catalogue of the Library of the Surgeon-General's Office.

BRIEF REPORT OF A CASE OF SPRING CONJUNCTIVITIS RESEMBLING MALIGNANT GROWTH OF THE CORNEAL LIMBUS.[1]

BY C. A. VEASEY, A.M., M.D.
OF PHILADELPHIA,
ASSISTANT OPHTHALMIC SURGEON AND CHIEF OF EYE CLINIC, JEFFERSON MEDICAL COLLEGE HOSPITAL; OPHTHALMIC SURGEON, METHODIST EPISCOPAL HOSPITAL; CONSULTING OPHTHALMOLOGIST, PHILADELPHIA LYING-IN CHARITY, ETC.

EARLY in October, 1902, H. H., a male, aged twenty-four years, native of Virginia, was brought to me by one of my clinic assistants for the purpose of having a growth removed from the corneal limbus of the right eye. This growth had been observed first about two years before as a small elevation 2 mm. to the temporal side of the limbus in the centre of a small, circumscribed patch of conjunctival injection, and had increased in size until at the time of my examination it was 5 mm. by 7 mm. in breadth and encroaching upon the cornea. It presented an angry, bluish-red appearance, and, though apparently situated in the conjunctiva, was firmly adherent to the underlying episcleral tissue. The patient complained of the disfiguring appearance, sensation of a foreign body, slight burning, and some conjunctival discharge. Further examination of the eyes and lids revealed nothing abnormal, excepting a moderate refractive error, and the patient was confident that the condition had been uninfluenced by the seasons and that the growth had been gradually increasing in size for two years. No family history of tumors of any kind could be obtained.

[1] Read before the Section on Ophthalmology of the College of Physicians of Philadelphia, March 15, 1904.

The growth was excised under cocaine anæsthesia, the site thoroughly curetted, and healing was prompt, with amelioration of all the symptoms.

The specimen was hardened in a 5 per cent. solution of formalin and sections prepared for microscopic study by Dr. E. A. Shumway. Considering the clinical history just referred to, the condition at the time of examination, and the fact that in the tumor were found small, round mononuclear cells, some pigment, and an alveolar arrangement, together with a tendency of the thickened surface epithelium to proliferate inward, it was thought that we were probably dealing with an alveolar sarcoma, which had developed from a pigmented nævus of the conjunctiva.

In May, 1903, nearly eight months after the operation had been performed, the patient was again seen, and examination showed a marked recurrence on the former site, which, according to the patient's statement, had first been observed two months before, or nearly six months after removal. The appearance of the recurrent growth was not red and angry-looking, as was the original, but of a much paler hue—in fact, markedly resembling a lump of paraffin covered by the delicately tinted conjunctiva.

Expectant treatment was employed, and a few weeks later somewhat similar but smaller patches appeared at the nasal and temporal margins of the left eye, together with three isolated enlarged papillæ of the conjunctiva of the upper lid, the latter now presenting a bluish-white appearance, as if covered by a thin layer of well-diluted milk.

Further study of the microscopic specimens of the original growth at this time, considering the clinical history in its later aspects, proved, beyond doubt, that the condition was spring conjunctivitis and not sarcoma. The subsequent history of the case has confirmed this opinion.

Dr. Shumway's report of the histological conditions is as follows:

The sections of the tissue measure 5 mm. by 2.5 mm. The greater portion of the growth is composed of a loose-meshed, fibrous connective tissue, which contains a moderate number of bloodvessels. It is covered by a thick layer of epithelial cells, which have a tendency to send inward processes of cells beneath the surface. Directly below the epithelial layer the mass is densely infiltrated with mononuclear round cells, and the bloodvessels contain a few polymorphonuclear cells. In places there are, in addition, larger, flat cells, which are arranged in nests and have the appearance of proliferated endothelial cells, such as are found in beginning alveolar sarcoma of the conjunctiva. Scattered between them is a small amount of light-yellow pigment. The majority of the cells, however, are small and represent ordinary lymphocytes, whose presence is due to irritation of the tissue. Some of them are broken down, their nuclei are fragmented, and the neighboring connective-tissue bundles have an œdematous appearance. The mass is evidently a new-growth, simulating a fibroma, with a decided inflammatory infiltration. The presence of the proliferated endothelial cells and the pigment is suggestive of commencing alveolar sarcoma. Similar cells, however, were described in a case of vernal conjunctivitis reported by de Schweinitz and myself, published in the *University Medical Bulletin*, and, in view of the clinical appearance and history, this portion of the growth should be considered of minor importance, and the diagnosis made of growth at the corneal limbus due to spring catarrh.

The chief points of interest in the case are:

1. The clinical and microscopic appearances of the growth so greatly resembling sarcoma.
2. The confinement of the ocular variety of spring conjunctivitis to one eye for nearly three years before it made its appearance in the other.
3. The fact that spring conjunctivitis was present in one eye for two years and eight months before the symptoms became sufficiently characteristic to permit a positive diagnosis to be made.
4. That the clinical history must always be given consideration in the establishment of a diagnosis from the study of a microscopic specimen.

INVESTIGATIONS OF THE NEWER METHODS FOR DIAGNOSING UNILATERAL KIDNEY LESIONS.

BY M. KROTOSZYNER, M.D.,

AND

W. P. WILLARD, M.D.,

OF SAN FRANCISCO, CAL.

CYSTOSCOPY at last seems to have gained its well-earned place among the reliable and scientific diagnostic methods. Even strong opponents to its use, as James Israel, are now converted into ardent advocates of its diagnostic value, but the same is not yet true of ureteral catheterization. It seems as if the opposition is generally headed by those unfamiliar with its technique; to them ureteral catheterization appears to be a procedure of unsurpassable difficulty. They admit the desirability of obtaining urine from either kidney separately, but claim this end may be obtained with less danger and inconvenience to the patient and with the same accuracy for examining purposes by one of the many clever devices known as urinary segregators. Whoever has worked with these instruments will admit that they are more bulky and their introduction therefore more painful and dangerous to the patient than any of the ureteral cystoscopes in use. I. Cohn,[1] who conducted at Posner's clinic a number of experiments with nearly all urinary segregators brought to the knowledge of the profession, found that in some instances the instruments had to be withdrawn from the bladder on account of their causing severe pain to the patient while *in situ.* Whenever methylene blue or milk under low pressure was injected through one side of the separator, the fluid coming from the other side was soon afterward noticeably colored. Admitted that injection of a fluid under the lowest possible pressure may enter one of the bladder chambers, separated from the other merely by a very thin rubber wall, under different conditions from those where the urine emerges drop by drop from the ureter, still, these experiments prove conclusively that an accurate separation of fluids by these devices cannot be accomplished.

Lichtenstern,[2] who principally experimented with the two segregators devised by French authors (Luys and Cathelin), concluded that the thin and easily movable rubber membrane cannot always produce an accurate separation of the bladder in two parts.

Kummell[3] reports a case of a woman, where nephrectomy had been performed on the right side, in which, by the use of Luys' segregator, urine was obtained only from the right side. He concludes from the fact that, as very often, on cystoscopy, the ureteral openings are seen to be very close to each other or in abnormal location, results from the use of segregators must be inaccurate. His strongest argument against the promiscuous use of these instruments is that the urine is obtained indirectly and is mixed with material that may be in the bladder.

Our experience with the different segregators coincides with these statements. Urinary segregators should be restricted to the very few cases in which cystoscopy is impossible (bladders of children or those that cannot be cleansed for cystoscopical purposes). In ureteral catheterization we have a method easy of execution in most cases and not very painful to the patient if dexterously performed, while the results obtained are absolutely reliable. The term "dexterously performed" does not imply a more than ordinary skill. Here, as elsewhere, it is true that practice makes perfect. On the other hand, it may be stated that, once familiar with the method, one becomes an enthusiastic adherer to it, on account of the accurate, faultless, and quick diagnostic results obtained. In our experience, as in that of many others, ureteral catheterization can be successfully done in almost every case, provided that the examinations are carried out with the necessary patience and perseverance. One of our cases (Case X.) required many painstaking and tedious sittings before we succeeded in clearing the diagnosis, which only could have been accomplished by ureteral catheterization. We will show later that examinations with one of the segregators would have led to unreliable and faulty conclusions.

The cystoscopes for catheterization of the ureters, in use by the majority of workers in this field, are those designed by Albarran, Casper, and Nitze, all three being modelled after the same design, the idea of which belongs to Casper. In Nitze's and Albarran's instruments the movements of the ureteral catheter in the bladder can be directed at different angles by a knee mechanism attached to the distal end, which is controlled by a screw at the ocular end of the cystoscope. The French instrument unites in itself three different cystoscopical types, viz., the ordinary examining, the irrigating, and the catheterizing. The vesical end of the ureteral catheter can be easily moved into an angle of 180 degrees; the only disadvantages are its small field of vision and low illuminating intensity.

Nitze's cystoscope combines the cystoscopical types of irrigation and ureteral catheterization; but it has two advantages over Albarran's instrument, viz., its larger field of vision and its excellent light.

In Casper's ureteral cystoscope the movements of the vesical end of the catheter to different angles are accomplished by the fact that the catheter lies in a canal the upper wall of which is formed by a movable cover. The farther this cover is pushed toward the bladder, the narrower becomes the slit from which the catheter emerges and the greater becomes its curvature, and *vice versa*. This instrument has one great advantage over the two cystoscopes previously mentioned, viz., after having catheterized one ureter, a second catheter can be introduced through the instrument while it is *in situ*, with which the other ureter can be catheterized. The removal of the instrument after catheterizing is more easily accomplished than in the other instruments, as the tension on the catheter is avoided by the removal of the cover. Lately Casper has constructed a double-barrelled cystoscope for catheterizing both ureters.

Bierhoff[4] has devised a cystoscope carrying two catheters, which are under separate control. This instrument is of small calibre (23 F.), but only a catheter of a small diameter can be used. It also having two cannulæ, a double-current irrigation can be employed for changing the fluid in the bladder while the instrument is *in situ*.

Kelly's cystoscope is not described here, as its use is limited to females. To our knowledge, one more catheterizing cystoscope is in use in this country, that devised by Bransford-Lewis. We regret to say that our attempts at cystoscopy with this instrument have been unsatisfactory.

Our own work was mostly done with Nitze's cystoscope, preferably on account of its illuminating properties.

We do not wish to dwell here on the technique of ureteral catheterization, but desire to point out a few facts that proved to be valuable in our work. The bladder was, in some instances, so sensitive and its capacity so small that the first attempts at cystoscopy failed entirely. Whenever, after innumerable washings, the fluid seemed to return from the bladder fairly clear, it had become very cloudy by the time the cystoscope was introduced. In Case X., where this difficulty was experienced, the bladder could not be filled with more than 60 c.c. to 90 c.c. of fluid under local anæsthesia. We succeeded, though, under spinal anæsthesia with 0.05 tropacocaine, in filling the bladder with about 150 c.c. of fluid, which remained fairly clear for a few minutes, so that the regions of the ureteral openings could be inspected. Only the left opening was recognized as such, and fluid was seen to escape from it. The other ureter was apparently buried in a patch of ulcerated tissue. After repeated examinations we learned to locate the presumable site of the ureter by taking our bearings from the left ureter and describing with the cystoscope an angle of 45 degrees along the sphincter, where, under normal conditions, the ureteral opening should be located. To this point the vesical end of the catheter was pressed under a rather sharp angle and thus introduced into the ureter. Four or five times in this manner the right ureter was catheterized, but never could the catheter be pushed farther than about four or five inches above the vesical opening. The catheter was repeatedly left a whole hour *in situ* without obtaining a drop of any liquid. Even aspiration with a large hand-syringe did not produce anything. Meanwhile, the left ureter had been successfully catheterized and the urine obtained from it subjected to the usual tests. Through a catheter passed to the bladder, while the ureteral catheter was in the left side, a few drops of pus and blood were obtained, too small a quantity for examining purposes. Finally, after many futile attempts, the catheter was passed to the pelvis of the right kidney, and, after waiting some time for fluid to appear, we aspirated again with a hand-syringe, which was readily filled with several drachms of pure pus.

If we in this case would have relied upon segregation, which, on account of the great irritability of the patient's bladder, probably never could have been accomplished, we certainly would have concluded that blood or pus appearing on the right side was due to the tubercular foci seen in the bladder. This case shows conclusively that a correct diagnosis was only possible by ureteral catheterization, which, if possible here, can be carried out in the vast majority of cases.

It is very important, after the catheter has entered the ureter, to push it forward under the control of the eye; it may otherwise be caught in its progress and fold up in the bladder unnoticed by the operator. This may be overcome by drawing back the catheter and giving its ureteral end another angle by means of the extravesical screw.

In the majority of cases the bladder was anæsthetized by 30 c.c. of a 4 per cent. cocaine solution, but in many instances no local anæsthetic was used, save a few cubic centimetres of the cocaine solution in the posterior urethra. The passing of the catheter in the ureter was always found to be absolutely painless.

Much has been said against ureteral catheterization, on account of the danger of infection to healthy kidneys. If such a danger exists it must certainly be a very remote one or only occur very rarely. Margulies,[5] who reports on 200 ureteral catheterizations, has never seen any bad results, and particularly states that never after ureteral catheterization was a rise of temperature observed in patients whose temperature was normal before the examination. The same has been experienced by Casper, Albarran, and others. In our material once a chill followed by some increase of temperature was observed in Case IX., most decidedly caused by the more than usually severe instrumentation, for, in order to catheterize both ureters with Nitze's instrument, it had to be withdrawn and introduced again into the bladder with one catheter *in situ.*

For the verification of certain doubtful points in the diagnosis of renal functional capacity, we examined the blood and urines obtained by ureteral catheterization of a number of patients with presumably healthy kidneys.

The value of cryoscopy of blood, as well as of urine, for determining the function of the kidneys appears to be a mooted question, from the mere fact that the firm molecules in urine continually change in number with the varying blood pressure. The cryoscopical point of the urine of a patient examined soon after drinking large quantities of water will, of necessity, differ from that determined in the same patient under usual dietary conditions. This fact was demonstrated to us in Case IX., where an examination was made after the patient had taken a large amount of mineral water. Here were found low cryoscopical urine points, —0.63 and —0.83 against —1.1 and —1.2, when liquids only had been taken in quantities to which the patient had ordinarily been accustomed. We deduced from this the important fact that one cryoscopical determination is of little value, and that by repeated tests only, done under various physical conditions of the patient, can a somewhat safe conclusion be arrived at.

Little has been published in this country upon cryoscopy, but the few publications at hand unanimously state that this method permits of reasonable accuracy in diagnosing renal insufficiency and the type of renal lesion present,[6] and that one may solely rely upon cryoscopy to determine the condition of the kidneys, provided it is possible to obtain specimens by catheterizing both ureters.[7] These statements must be considered, from our experience, as being too radical. The real value, in our opinion, lies in the comparison of the points of either side.

From our limited material we learned that wherever, in unilateral kidney lesions, the cryoscopical urine-point was very low, as compared with that of the presumably healthy side, it could be concluded that one kidney was diseased. A striking illustration of this fact is given in Case VIII., where the right kidney gave —0.4, while the left side showed —1.2, which certainly could be only interpreted as an impaired function of the side with the low cryoscopical point.

Less conclusive are our results with the determination of cryoscopy of blood. Casper and Kummell, who have the widest experience on this point, state that molecular concentration of blood only varies where a bilateral renal affection is present. In unilateral kidney diseases, where one healthy kidney does the work of both, the blood-point was found in almost all cases to be a stable one, between —0 56 and —0.58. We have only obtained blood for our investigations in a small number of patients, and our results do not coincide with those of the authorities just mentioned. We are satisfied, though, that this is due to the inaccuracy of Beckmann's cryoscope, and possibly also to certain faults in our methods.

The phloridzin test was found to be equally as valuable in regard to comparative results in our few pathological cases. The statements of one of us upon the value of this test made in a previous paper[8] were found to be verified by subsequent larger experience with the method. Phloridzin is perfectly harmless. The separation of sugar from phloridzin takes place in the epithelial structure of the glomeruli and tubules of the renal cortex and nowhere else in the human organism. Watson and Baily,[9] in their report upon experiments with phloridzin on patients with normal and diseased kidneys, conclude that the phloridzin test gives accurate indications of the condition of renal function and of the existence of renal disease; but they also found the reverse to be true in a series of observations.

Our experience with the phloridzin test is that no absolute conclusion can be drawn from it upon the function of the kidneys, but that the value of the test lies in comparing results on both sides from urines obtained by ureteral catheterization. We are certain that the quantity of sugar excretion does not afford a safe guide as to the condition of the kidney. Neither are we prepared to claim any particular pathognostic value for the retarded appearance of sugar after the injection of the usual dose of phloridzin.

Israel, of Berlin, reports observations in which, after phloridzin injection, no sugar appeared in the urine. Barth,[10] in his report, mentions a case in which, without any plausible reason, no phloridzin reaction occurred where in a former examination the same dose of phloridzin had given a prompt positive result. We are, from our experience, inclined to think that the solution used in these instances was not fresh. Wherever we used fresh solutions of phloridzin we found sugar present in the urines one-half hour after the injection. In those cases where we got negative results, we injected the next day the same quantity of a new solution, and our results were positive for sugar.

As for urine cryoscopy, Case VIII. is also for the phloridzin test a striking example of its comparative value. Here we found on the diseased side 0.25 per cent. sugar, while the healthy side showed 1.28 per cent. This is such a striking difference that, other tests being equally conclusive, positive conclusions could be drawn from it.

Equally important seems to be the comparative study of quantitative values of urea excretion in urines separately obtained by ureteral catheterization. Unfortunately, our pathological material was too small to afford us sufficient proof for the verification of results obtained by others. (Kummell, Barth.) In our cases with normal kidneys the quantitative value of urea appeared to be almost equal.

Our microscopic findings of both urines were not without an element of grave error, caused by the fact that we only catheterized one ureter in almost all our cases, taking the bladder urine as representing the secretion of the other kidney for microscopic examination. This resulted in showing, in a majority of the cases, red blood cells, certainly caused by a mechanical lesion of the bladder wall, through the introduction of the cystoscope.

For the following reports the urine was obtained by catheterizing one ureter, removing the cystoscope, and passing a soft-rubber catheter to the bladder, care being taken that the bladder was empty before collecting specimens. The urine passing through the bladder usually contains blood, as above stated. A few red cells from the catheterized side may be also present, due to the passage of the catheter, it being withdrawn a short distance in taking out the cystoscope. This method does not alter the cryoscopical, urea, or phloridzin findings, but does not give accurate microscopic results, for the urine passing through the bladder may, besides blood, contain elements from that organ (pus, epithelial cells, etc.).

The cryoscopical examinations were made with a Beckmann's cryoscope, the thermometer being corrected often by testing with distilled water. We adopted the plan of placing the inner tube directly in the freezing mixture until the mercury dropped below zero before placing in the air chamber; by this procedure the time of freezing is shortened about one-half. For the blood cryoscopy we obtained from the median basilic vein about 20 c.c., allowing the blood to flow directly into the small tube of the cryoscope and agitating with the mixture wire, then proceeding immediately as with the urine. Although the points obtained by this instrument cannot be considered absolutely reliable, still, we found them to be sufficiently accurate for comparison. The amount of urea was estimated by the Doremus ureometer, and the findings given in milligrams per cubic centimetre. Just before catheterizing 20 minims of a ½ per cent. phloridzin solution was given hypodermically. The phloridzin must be thoroughly dissolved and only a fresh solution used, for in some of the cases no sugar was found after injecting an old solution. It is also well to add an equal quantity of Na_2Co_3 to keep the phloridzin in solution.

We found, as did Baily and Watson, that the most sugar is excreted during the first half-hour, and most of our estimations were made with this urine. We used Lohnstein's new saccharometers and found them very accurate for comparison, being able to detect a difference of $\frac{1}{100}$ per cent. Three instruments were used, one for the urine of each kidney and the third for a control of distilled water, so that the results might be obtained under the same conditions.

CASE I.—*July 2d.* Blood cryoscopy, —0.61; left ureter catheterized. Cryoscopy: Left kidney, —1.6; sugar, 0.77. Cryoscopy: Right kidney, —1.5; sugar, 0.85 (one hour after injection of phloridzin).

21st. Right ureter catheterized. Cryoscopy: Right kidney, —1.5; urea, 0.016; sugar, 0.35. Cryoscopy: Left kidney, —1.62; urea, 0.018; sugar, 0.3 (two hours after injection of phloridzin). Microscopic: Right kidney, few red cells, leukocytes, calcium-oxalate crystals, conical epithelium, bacteria. Left kidney, numerous red cells.

CASE II.—*July 14th.* Blood cryoscopy, —0.58.

16th. Right ureter catheterized. Cryoscopy: Right kidney, —1.8; urea, 0.012. Cryoscopy: Left kidney, —1.57; urea, 0.013 (sugar not present one, two, and three hours after injection of phloridzin, which had been in solution about ten days. Next day fresh solution gave positive results). Microscopic: Right kidney, few red cells, numerous round and conical epithelial cells; hyaline casts. Left kidney, numerous red cells, flat epithelial cells.

23d. Cryoscopy: Right kidney, —1.42; urea, 0.011. Cryoscopy: Left kidney, —1.75; urea, 0.013; sugar, not present. Phloridzin solution, old. (Next day fresh solution showed sugar.) Microscopic: Right kidney, red cells, calcium-oxalate crystals, flat epithelium. Left kidney, few red cells, round and conical epithelium, granular cast, bacteria.

CASE IV.—*July 28th.* Left ureter catheterized. Cryoscopy: Right kidney, —1.54; urea, 0.012; sugar, 1.32. Cryoscopy: Left kidney, —1.49; urea, 0.011; sugar, 1.3. Microscopic: Right kidney, red cells; flat, conical, and round epithelium; bacteria. Left kidney, few red cells, round epithelium, leukocytes, bacteria.

August 5th. Blood cryoscopy, —0.46.

CASE V.—*August 26th.* Right ureter catheterized. Cryoscopy: Right kidney, —1.44; urea, 0.015; sugar, 1.4. Cryoscopy: Left kidney, —1.22; urea, 0.0145; sugar, 1.1. Microscopic: Right kidney, round and conical epithelial cells. Left kidney, flat, round and conical epithelial cells; red cells.

The above sugar percentages were determined with urine passed during the first half-hour after phloridzin injection. The urine passed during the second half-hour showed 0.3 per cent. of sugar.

Case VI.—*March 7th.* Left ureter catheterized. Cryoscopy: Right kidney, —1.33; urea, 0.0095; sugar, 0.45. Cryoscopy: Left kidney, —1.38; urea, 0.01; sugar, 0.6. Microscopic: Right kidney, pus cells, red cells, uric-acid crystals. Left kidney, red cells, uric-acid crystals.

The following cases are of pathological note and are, therefore, reported at length:

Case VII.—J. F., aged thirty-five years. Family history: father died of pneumonia, uncle on father's side of tuberculosis. Previous history: typhoid fever six years ago; gonorrhœa several times, last attack eight years ago; orchitis five years ago.

Present illness began one year ago with œdema of lower limbs and some ascites, which disappeared after three weeks' treatment. Urine at this time showed albumin, hyaline and granular casts, round cells, pus cells, and red cells. Has been dropsical off and on since.

May 28, 1903. First saw patient; temperature, 96° F.; pulse, feeble; nausea; vomiting; diarrhœa. *Examination.* Patient emaciated, having lost twenty-five pounds in last year; heart and lungs negative; kidneys not palpable, but some tenderness on deep pressure over the right. Urine showed 0.2 per cent. albumin; numerous pus cells and tubercle bacilli. Pigs injected with this sediment gave negative results. Cystoscopic examination showed on the bladder-wall numerous patches of ulcerations.

July 11th. Right ureter catheterized. Cryoscopy: Right kidney, —0.95; urea, 0.0045; sugar, 0.25. Cryoscopy: Left kidney, —1.4; urea, 0.004; sugar, 0.2. Microscopic: Right kidney, pus, few red cells, round and conical epithelium, no tubercle bacilli. Left kidney, red cells, few pus cells, no tubercle bacilli. Patient's condition at this time not permitting further examination he was sent to the country, where he died three months later of uræmia. No autopsy.

Case VIII.—A. H., aged fifty-five years; brewer. Family history negative. Has been a heavy beer-drinker. Previous history unimportant. Present illness began one year ago, when he passed bloody urine; this again occurred one month later. Six months ago, December, 1902, was confined to bed for three months, during which time the urine contained a large amount of blood; bladder became irritable, patient urinating every hour. Pain at the end of the penis. Chills, fever, and sweats at this time.

June 1st. Again passing blood; no pain; feels weak; constipation, alternating with diarrhœa. Has lost forty-five pounds. *Examination.* Poorly nourished; skin pigmented on right side of face and left thigh. Heart and lungs negative. Tumor palpable on the right side of the abdomen, about the size of an orange, smooth and slightly movable. No pain or tenderness on palpation.

July 10th. Right ureter catheterized. Cryoscopy: Right kidney, —0.4; sugar, 0.25. Cryoscopy: Left kidney, —1.2; sugar, 1.28.

Microscopic: Right kidney, numerous red cells and round epithelia. Left kidney, red cells, pus cells, and round epithelia.

16th. Right ureter catheterized; cryoscopy, —0.3.

18th. Left ureter catheterized; cryoscopy, —1.5.

21st. Blood cryoscopy, —0.55.

22d. Right kidney removed by Dr. Weil; about twice the normal size, irregularly contracted. Examination proved it to be a Grawitz tumor.

23d. Passed 560 c.c. of urine in first twenty-four hours.

24th. 800 c.c.; cryoscopy, —1.63.

This man made a good recovery, but his urine two months after operation still contained some red cells, which were thought by Dr. Jellinek, his attending physician, to be from the remaining right ureter. Further cystoscopic examinations were not permitted.

CASE IX. (By courtesy of Dr. L. Gross).—M., Japanese merchant; father has pulmonary tuberculosis. Previous history: malaria ten years ago; typhoid fever two years ago. Three months ago patient first passed blood, mixed with urine; no clots. This continued for a month intermittently, bloody for a few days, then clear. Urine remained clear if patient stayed in bed. Has had no pain, chills, or fever; appetite good, and general health not impaired. Passed urine about ten times during the day and twice at night. No blood within the last two months (since first catheterization of the left ureter, September 1st). Before examination patient passed about ten ounces of very bloody urine. After catheterization a great amount of urine was passed, the patient having taken a large amount of liquid during the day; this fact is mentioned in order to account for the low cryoscopic points.

Left ureter catheterized. Cryoscopy: Right kidney, —0.62; urea, 0.007; sugar, 1.05. Cryoscopy: Left kidney, —0.83; urea, 0.01; sugar, 1.5. Microscopic: Right kidney, pus cells, few red cells, flat and round epithelial cells. Left kidney: numerous red cells, round epithelia, and casts.

September 14th. Blood cryoscopy, —0.51.

Sept. 23d. Both ureters catheterized. Cryoscopy: Right kidney, —1.1; urea, 0.0075; sugar, 0.6. Cryoscopy: Left kidney, —1.2; urea, 0.0095; sugar, 0.5. Microscopic: Right kidney, few red cells, crystals of uric acid; sediment, small amount. Left kidney, numerous red cells.

Both examinations did not prove satisfactorily the presence of any pathological condition. Whether the hæmaturia was due to a kidney or ureteral condition we cannot say, but the findings of the second examination show conclusively that the renal function was not at fault. Operative procedure was advised against, and at the present time, two months and a half after examination, the patient has had no return of his hæmaturia and is in excellent health.

CASE X. (By courtesy of Dr. Jellinek).—J. M., aged thirty-nine years; farmer. Mother and one brother died of pulmonary tuberculosis. Nineteen years ago took care of tubercular brother, after which he became ill and was told he had pulmonary tuberculosis; since then until the present trouble has lived an out-of-door life and has been in good health. One year ago noticed some trouble on urination; passed blood two or three times in one day. Health became impaired, but had no urinary symptoms, with the exception of a little pain in the region of the bladder, until four months ago. Then had pain on urinating, which occurred about every hour, day and night. Urine became very foul-smelling. Condition on admission to the German Hospital, about two months ago: poorly nourished, nervous, unable to sleep, night-sweats, irregular temperature, continuous pain in bladder region, more marked at the end of urination. Heart negative; tubercular involvement of apex of right lung; appetite fair; no trouble with digestion; passes urine about every hour, which contains abundance of pus and tubercle bacilli. Pigs injected with this sediment died of tuberculosis.

September 25th. Cystoscopy: numerous ulcerated patches over bladder-wall; left ureter catheterized; a good quantity of urine obtained, but nothing came from the bladder catheter that could be utilized. Cryoscopy: Left kidney, —0.9; sugar, 0.4. Microscopic: Some pus, round epithelia, few uric-acid crystals, bacteria, no tubercle bacilli.

October 24th. Right ureter catheterized, and over an ounce of greenish-yellow pus obtained, which contained tubercle bacilli.

26th. Urine cryoscopy: bladder urine, —1.08.

November 4th. Operation (by Dr. Weil). Right kidney about twice normal size, lower portion fluctuating; about eight ounces of greenish-yellow pus removed; kidney drained.

8th. Passed thirty-eight ounces of urine in last twenty-four hours; large amount of pus; cryoscopy, —1.12.

CASE XI.—S. S.; previous history unimportant.

March 18th. Attack of severe pain on left side, which necessitated giving morphine (¼ grain) for relief; complete anuria for twenty-four hours. From the symptoms a diagnosis of renal calculus was made. The first urine passed showed a trace of albumin, numerous red cells, leukocytes, and uric-acid crystals. Condition gradually improved, so that on March 25th normal amount of urine was passed.

August 18th. Another attack of pain, but less severe; slight chill, urine diminished to twelve ounces, contained trace of albumin, amorphous urates. After four or five days the patient was able to get about again, and has remained in good health since.

30th. Left ureter catheterized. Met with resistance about five inches from the bladder, beyond which point the catheter could not be passed. Cryoscopy: Right kidney, —1.31; urea, 0.0085; sugar, 2.8. Cryoscopy: Left kidney, —1.47; urea, 0.008; sugar, 2.8.

Microscopic: Right kidney, flat epithelium, uric-acid crystals, red cells. Left kidney, round epithelium, uric-acid crystals, numerous red cells.

We have presented this rather small material because we believe that in the diagnosis of unilateral kidney lesions any contribution is of value. As we have stated above, none of the methods fŏr determining the functional capacity of the kidneys enable us to arrive at a conclusion upon the actual function of both kidneys or either organ. In other words, none of these methods alone are sufficiently accurate to decide upon the basis of one of them the question whether a kidney should be removed or not. The real value of the methods worked out in our material lies in the comparative results and in the coincidence of the methods. A "conditio sine qua non" for the application of these methods is ureteral catheterization, and wherever feasible, catheterization of both ureters. If both urines obtained in this way are subjected to cryoscopy, phloridzin test, urea examination, and microscopic examinations, we are certainly enabled to get a fair idea upon the functional value of either kidney and to arrive at safe conclusions from our findings as to intended operative procedures.

BIBLIOGRAPHY.

1. I. Cohn. Kann der Harnleiterkatheterismus durch Harnsegregatoren ersetzt worden? Berliner klin. Wochenschr., 1903, No. 16.
2. Lichtenstern. Ueber Harnsegregatoren, Wien med. Presse, 1903, No. 13.
3 Kummell. Die neuerem Untersuchungs-methoden u. die operativen Erfolge bei Nierenkrankh., Thirty-second Congress of German Surgeons, 1903.
4. F. Bierhoff. A New Cystoscope for Simultaneous Catheterization of Ureters, etc., Medical News, March 8, 1902.
5. Michael Margulies. 200 Faelle von Katheterismus der Ureteren, Monatsber f. Urologie, 1903, No. 8.
6. S. Grim. Cryoscopy, Philadelphia Medical Journal, March 21, 1903.
7. M. Tinker. Cryoscopy, Bulletin of the Johns Hopkins Hospital, June, 1903.
8. M. Krotoszyner. Determination of the Functional Capacity of the Kidneys, etc., Occidental Medical Times, May, 1903.
9. F. S Watson and W. T Baily. Some Observations upon the Value of the Phloridzin Test, etc., Boston Medical and Surgical Journal, December 4, 1902.
10. Barth. Ueber funkt. Nierendiagnostik, Arch. f. klin. Chir., vol. lxxi. p 3.

THE PRODUCTS OF GLYCOLYSIS IN BLOOD AND OTHER ANIMAL FLUIDS.

BY A. E. AUSTIN, M.D.,
OF BOSTON.

(From the Medical Chemistry Laboratory of Tufts College.)

IT is a well-known fact that normal blood of almost all species of animals when freed fresh from its albumins shows a reducing body which is unquestionably largely made up of dextrose. When, however, the blood is allowed to stand some time, even when kept free from bacterial decomposition by antiseptics (thymol), this reducing body disappears, and only a substance which is able to hold copper in solution in an alkaline medium is found, but no reduction takes place. Biernocki, Pavy, and Lepine have shown further that if dextrose be added to blood under similar conditions, not only is the blood-sugar destroyed, but also a large proportion of that which has been added. To this process they give the name of glycolysis. My attention had been directed to the fact, and efforts had already been made by me to determine what became of the sugar thus destroyed, when, in 1901, P. Mayer[1] demonstrated that ox blood contained paired glycuronic acid, one of the oxidative products of dextrose, and very closely allied to it, and Mayer[2] further showed that if glycuronie acid be given to an animal and oxidation be experimentally restricted, saccharic acid is eliminated. It has also been demonstrated by the same author that if glycuronic acid or even dextrose be given in great excess, an increase of oxalic acid is found in the urine, and also that the liver is found to be surcharged with the same acid, from which he deduces the principle that if there is present an actual or relatively diminished oxidation (overwhelming the organism with carbohydrate) these partially oxidized products will appear in the urine. Based upon these facts, my efforts were directed toward determining whether the products of the so-called glycolysis of the blood might be any of these substances, viz., glycuronic, saccharic, oxalic, or carbonic acid, the final product of oxidation; of these the three last do not reduce Fehling's solution, which would account for the loss of the blood sugar in blood which is allowed to stand.

Experiment 1.—570 c.c. hydrocele fluid which had been kept two weeks on ice, was precipitated by twice its volume of 95 per cent. alcohol, filtered and washed, the alcohol driven off, acidified with acetic acid, boiled, and filtered. The resulting fluid did not show any immediate reduction with Fehling's solution, such as would be expected of dextrose. For the purpose of isolating the supposed carbohydrate body, the method of Salkowski, for obtaining xylon[3] was used, but the resulting product was a blue syrupy fluid which could not be made to crystallize, but which, when again dissolved in sodium hydrate, reduced promptly upon warming. The peculiarities of this substance suggested that it was glycuronic acid, but it was not proven. The copper suboxide formed (0.148 grams) showed 0.0667 gram of reducing body reckoned as dextrose.

Experiment 2.—500 c.c. fresh ox blood was precipitated by alcohol as before, and an effort made to isolate the reducing body by the same means as before, but ineffectually, since no precipitate could be obtained.

Experiment 3.—(*a*) 100 c.c. fresh ox blood as control for the following was precipitated with alcohol, the resulting filtrate freed

[1] Zeit. f. phys. Chemie, vol. xxxi.

[2] Berlin. klin. Wochenschr., 1899, pp. 27, 28.

[3] Zeit. f. phys. Chemie, vol. xxxiv. p. 162.

from alcohol and warmed with 40 c.c. Fehling's solution. There was no immediate precipitate, but twenty-four hours afterward a whitish-yellow precipitate had formed, but it was too small in amount to furnish identification.

(*b*) 500 c.c. of the same ox blood as above was charged with 5 grams of dextrose and allowed to remain in the same brood-oven at a temperature of 38° C. for forty-five hours, decomposition being avoided by the addition of toluol. By that time it had acquired a deep purple color; and after the toluol had been driven off over the water-bath, it was freed from albumin by alcohol, the precipitate again rubbed up with alcohol in a mortar, the alcoholic extracts united, and the alcohol removed by distillation. After establishing the volume at 1000 c.c., 50 c.c. of this clear fluid was cooked with Fehling's solution, but no reduction took place, nor was there any reaction with phloroglucin or orcin. This liquid was then allowed to stand several weeks in the refrigerator, whereupon it was filtered from the slight precipitate formed, reduced to 500 c.c. by evaporation, and then treated with subacetate of lead and ammonia; the precipitate removed, washed, suspended in water, acidified with acetic acid, and the lead removed by sulphuretted hydrogen, and the fluid reduced to 50 c.c. at 40° C. This had no reducing power, did not modify the light in the polariscope, and the remaining 40 c.c. when distilled with an equal amount of hydrochloric acid gave no furfurol with phloroglucin in the distillate; from this it is safe to say that while the dextrose was wholly converted it must have passed beyond the stage of glycuronic acid, either into a volatile substance like CO_2, or into the less readily identified carbohydrate acids.

Experiment 4.—(*a*) In order to determine whether the blood-sugar or added dextrose was converted into carbon dioxide, the final product of oxidation, as well as of yeast fermentation, 1 litre of fresh ox blood to which toluol has been added, and in a stoppered flask from which a tube led into a flask containing barium hydrate solution, which was protected from the outer air by a drying tube containing sodium hydrate, was allowed to remain in the brood-oven for twenty-four hours. When removed some insoluble barium carbonate had been formed in the adjoining flask, which was tightly stoppered and placed on ice until opportunity offered for the determination of the carbon dioxide. The blood was freed from albumin by the method of Abeles (zinc acetate and absolute alcohol), the zinc removed and the solution concentrated to 250 c.c. at 40° C. The solution had a left-turning power of 0.05 per cent. reckoned as dextrose, and gave a faint phloroglucin and orcin reaction, but no lines in the spectroscope, even when shaken out with amyl alcohol. It was now precipitated with lead and ammonia, and, after removal of the lead, concentrated to 50 c.c. Its turning power was now lost; it gave still a weak orcin and phloroglucin reaction, but no spectroscopic lines, and an osazone which was largely soluble in absolute alcohol. The barium carbonate which was formed in the barium hydrate solution was removed and the carbon dioxide determined according to Fresenius (*Quantitative Analysis*, vol. i. page 439). It amounted to 0.1054 gram in the litre of blood.

(*b*) 5 grams dextrose were added to 1 litre of the same blood as above and under the same conditions, the mixture was allowed to remain in the brood-oven the same length of time. It was then removed and treated in the same way. The resulting fluid, which was free from albumin, gave a weak phloroglucin and orcin reaction, did not reduce, but kept copper in solution in alkaline medium, and had no turning power. It was then treated as before, with lead and ammonia, and the resulting fluid concentrated to 50 c.c. It now gave a much stronger Tollens reaction, but no spectroscopic lines, and still had no turning power. The amount of carbon dioxide, determined in the same way, which had been given off was 0.1163 gram. In this case we see that 5 grams dextrose had utterly disappeared, and yet it could not have been converted into carbon dioxide, for the amount of this in the latter instance was but a trifle more than in the former, or 0.1163 gram as compared with 0.1054 gram, and in both cases it may have come from the blood itself, since Ludwig, Pfleuger, and others have found as much as 40 per cent. in dog's arterial blood.

Experiment 5.—(*a*) 5 grams dextrose were added to 250 c.c. fresh hydrocele fluid—obtained through the courtesy of Dr. Gardner W. Allen—connected with a carbon-dioxide apparatus, and the whole placed in the brood-oven for eighteen hours. It was then removed, and, without disconnecting from the apparatus, air was drawn through the blood for thirty minutes. It was then poured into an equal amount of a solution, saturated when warm with both sodium chloride and mercuric chloride, allowed to stand overnight, filtered, washed, and the filtrate and wash water freed from mercury reduced to 250 c.c. It now gave a marked phloroglucin reaction, with a line in green in the spectroscope, had a right-turning power equal to 0.5 per cent. as dextrose, and a reducing power which was equivalent to 0.66 per cent. dextrose, determined according to Allihin. Its carbon dioxide equalled 0.0804 gram.

(*b*) 10 c.c. of the same fluid taken as control and immediately precipitated, had a slight reducing power, gave no Tollens reaction, had a slight dextrorotatory power, and gave a fine, yellow, needle-like osazone, which was mostly soluble in absolute alcohol. As can readily be seen, 3.35 grams of the dextrose added to this fluid disappeared, forming no carbon dioxide, for this amount of sugar by fermentation would produce, theoretically (43.3 per cent.), 1.45 grams carbon dioxide, instead of the 0.0804 gram found, but glycuronic acid presumably, since, when paired, being a left-turner, it reduced the actual amount of carbohydrate 0.66 per cent. to 0.5 per cent. in the polariscope and gives a marked Tollens reaction.

EXPERIMENT 6.—(*a*) 1 litre fresh beef blood was placed in a flask connected with a carbon-dioxide apparatus, toluol added, and the whole placed in the brood-oven for twenty-two hours, air drawn through for thirty minutes, and then freed from albumin by sodium and mercuric chloride, and the latter removed. The resulting clear fluid was then reduced to 50 c.c., which had no turning power, but a reducing power equal to 0.0586 gram of dextrose, or 11 per cent. The remainder was then cooked in an autoclave with 1 per cent. sulphuric acid for one hour and neutralized, whereupon it acquired a dextrorotatory power of less than 0.1 per cent. It formed an osazone of lemon-colored needle-like crystals mixed with globules of a darker hue, which were almost entirely soluble in absolute alcohol. The original blood emitted 0.1878 gram carbon dioxide.

(*b*) To another litre of the same blood 5 grams dextrose were added in a flask which was connected with the carbon-dioxide apparatus, and the whole placed in the brood-oven as before for the same time. It was then freed from albumin and reduced to 50 c.c. It was levogyr to 0.1 per cent., and had a reducing power equivalent to 0.0591 gram, or 0.118 per cent. as dextrose. The remainder was now cooked with sulphuric acid, but it remained a left-turner and gave a marked phloroglucin and orcin reaction without spectroscopic lines. It gave an osazone consisting of a few crystals (needles), but chiefly of globules, which were soluble in absolute alcohol. Its carbon dioxide amounted to 0.9564 gram.

(*c*) 1 litre of the same blood was precipitated at once and reduced to 50 c.c. It then had a turning power of +0.1 per cent. and a reducing power of 0.0403 gram as dextrose, or 0.08 per cent. It formed an osazone soluble in alcohol, consisting of irregular, feathery masses.

In both (*a*) and (*b*) the fact that the rotatory power was less than the reducing power and that (*a*) was converted to a dextrogyr body and that (*b*)'s levogyr power was very much lessened by splitting with sulphuric acid shows that at least a portion of the reducing substance was in the form of glycuronic acid, a fact still further emphasized by the marked orcin and phloroglucin reaction in (*b*), which, based upon its reducing power and compared with the control (*c*), had lost all of the dextrose added. A part of this may have been converted to carbon dioxide, since there was a marked increase in this over (*a*), to which no dextrose was added. As is well known, the paired glycuronic acid being a left-turner, diminishes or obliterates the dextrogyr power of dextrose.

EXPERIMENT 7.—(*a*) 1 litre of a pleuritic exudate, obtained through the courtesy of Dr. Mackechnie, guarded against decomposition by toluol, was placed in the brood-oven for twenty hours, removed, freed from albumin by the mercury process, and reduced to 200 c.c. The rotatory power was now +0.1 per cent. and the reducing 0.23 per cent. as dextrose. There was no Tollens reaction.

The fluid was then cooked with sulphuric acid, after which it still retained a rotatory power of +0.1 per cent.; Tollens weak. In producing the osazone in this and all the following experiments a strict proportion between the phenylhydrazin added and the amount of reducing body, as determined by the polariscope after splitting, was maintained, so that one molecule of the reagent was added to one molecule of the suspected glycuronic acid, which, according to their molecular weights, gave 0.55 gram of the reagent to 1 gram of the substance sought, or as my reagent was in the form of the chloride, 0.735 gram was used. Another improvement which was suggested by Neuberg was to place the substance and reagent in a brood-oven for twelve to fourteen hours instead of boiling it, and this proved very satisfactory in increasing the product and avoiding tenacious masses, which would form on the edges of the flask in the old way. This limited addition of phenylhydrazin is supposed to cause the glycuronic acid to form an osazone to the exclusion of dextrose, or, if the latter does form, it can be separated by washing with hot water and absolute alcohol. It is true that Neuberg and Mayer use bromphenylhydrazin, but I think I have demonstrated that the ordinary reagent can be used in the same way.

(*b*) 10 grams of dextrose were added to 1 litre of the same exudate and the whole placed in the brood-oven for the same time as before, then freed from albumin and reduced to 200 c.c. Polariscope showed +0.7 per cent. and reduction 1.201 per cent., while there was no phloroglucin and no orcin reaction. After cooking with sulphuric acid, rotatory power 0.75 per cent. as dextrose, both orcin and phloroglucin positive, and osazone of well-formed globules of dark color.

(*c*) 400 c.c. same exudate freed at once from albumin and reduced to 50 c.c. Polariscope showed +0.2 per cent. and reduction 0.35 per cent. After splitting polariscope showed +0.25 per cent., but there was no Tollens reaction. Attention must be called here to these general features repeated in the other experiments; the reduction is greater than the polariscopic reading in (*a*) and (*b*); the Tollens reaction is brought out strongly by the splitting with sulphuric acid, as is also an increase in the polariscopic reading. It becomes evident, also, that during the process of evaporation, even if the reaction is kept slightly acid, as was the custom, a partial splitting of the paired acids takes place, else we should much oftener come across levogyr bodies. The separation of the glucosazone from the combination of glycuronic acid and other acids with phenylhydrazin could be accomplished with repeated washings with hot water and after drying with absolute alcohol upon the filter paper. The wash water and alcohol upon cooling would often cause a precipitation of a crystalline nature, which consisted almost entirely of glucosazone, and its needles are very different from the globules which the other compounds form. The demonstration of the nature of the precipitate, which is insoluble in hot water and absolute alcohol, was most difficult. Since the glucosazon is soluble in absolute alcohol, presumably the residue which was left was an hydrazin of glycuronic or saccharic acid, but no solvent could be found which would enable one to determine its power in the polariscope. Mayer and Neuberg use a mixture of absolute alcohol and pyridine, and its left-turning power is so great (0.2 gram in 10 c.c. of the mixture gives a reading of —7° 25′) that it can be easily distinguished from all other osazones or hydrazins, but the pyridine could not be procured, and after various attempts to find a solvent in mixtures of glacial acetic acid, acetone and absolute alcohol, the attempt to identify the substance in this way was abandoned. It suffices to say, however, that the insoluble portion had all the characteristics of the hydrazin of glycuronic acid described by Mayer.[1]

Another fact worth mentioning is that the product obtained with phenylhydrazin from the normal blood was perfectly soluble in hot water and alcohol, while that from both bloods subjected to the brood-oven temperature was only partially so. In no case was there sufficient evidence that more than an infinitesimal amount of the lost dextrose was converted to the carbohydrate acids, and we must fall back upon the suggestion made that the dextrose may combine with the albumin of the blood and be removed with that.

The next point to establish was whether the dextrose could have been converted to oxalic acid by the process of glycolysis, as is assumed by Mayer, in the animal when oxidation is impaired. For this purpose four portions of fresh ox blood were taken and treated in the following manner:

(*a*) 1 litre was precipitated at once by mercuric and sodium chlorides, the mercury removed, and, keeping the steadily increasing acid reaction in check by sodium carbonate, the whole was reduced to 200 c.c. It was then shaken three times with ether, no hydrochloric acid having been added on account of that present from the mercuric chloride removed, and an effort made to determine the oxalic acid, if present, according to the method of Salkowski; but only the merest traces of this substance were found too small for estimation. The remaining watery solution was freed from ether and reduced to 50 c.c., when its turning power was found to be +0.2 per cent., while by the method of Allihin there was found to to be 0.199 per cent., or practically the same as shown by the polariscope. It gave no reaction with phloroglucin. It was then split with 1 per cent. sulphuric acid in a closed flask, and the volume having been re-established, with due calculation for the amount used in the reduction determination, it now gave a turning power of +0.15 per cent., and afforded, dried at 110° C., 0.0888 gram of an osazone which dissolved in 3.5 c.c. glacial acetic acid, gave a turning power of —0.2

[1] Zeit. f. Physiol. Chemie, 29, 67.

per cent. reckoned as dextrose. From all the evidence found here probably nothing but dextrose existed in the blood.

(*b*) 1 litre of blood, to which 10 grams of dextrose were added, was attached to a water-pump, after having been treated with toluol, in hopes of at least partially preventing decomposition, and air was drawn through it for twenty-four hours. It was then freed from albumin in the same way, reduced to 200 c.c., and shaken three times with ether, in order to extract the oxalic acid, but only traces were found. The ether was driven off from the watery solution, and the whole reduced to 50 c.c. Its turning power was now +1.875 per cent., and it gave the phloroglucin but not the orcin test. By the Allihin method with copper it showed 1.54 per cent. of a reducing body; a peculiarity in the reduction was noticed which is suggestive of glycuronic acid, as well as other substances apart from dextrose. The Fehling solution became at first greenish when boiled, and a yellowish precipitate was thrown down, in which were seen particles of the red suboxide of copper. Owing to the fact that on evaporation a large amount of salts had been thrown out of solution and the possibility that some dextrose was mechanically held by this mass from which it had been filtered, these were extracted with water until the last water showed no reduction. The volume had now risen to 225 c.c., giving a polariscopic reading of +0.51 per cent., which was cooked in a closed stone flask for eight hours with 1 per cent. sulphuric acid. This solution, when neutralized, possessed a turning power of +0.425 per cent. and both the phloroglucin and orcin reactions, but no lines. It also gave, dried at 110° C., 1.244 grams of an osazone or hydrazin, consisting of microscopic rosettes and globules, which was insoluble in hot water and absolute alcohol, whose optical properties could not be determined, as before stated, for want of a suitable solvent. In this, as in previous instances, an attempt was made to determine the nitrogen by Kjeldahl, but, though the destruction of the substance by the acid seemed complete, no ammonia could be distilled over; yet it is not safe to judge from this that no nitrogen existed in the compound.

(*c*) This litre of blood, treated with toluol, was allowed to remain at brood-oven temperature for twenty-four hours without the addition of dextrose, freed from albumin, reduced to 200 c.c., an almost neutral reaction having been maintained, shaken out with ether, freed from the same, concentrated to 50 c.c., and tested for reducing bodies. No oxalic acid was found beyond the mere traces mentioned in the other samples. It showed no reduction, no turning power and phloroglucin test, hence no further attempts were made to isolate an osazone. It simply proves what has been so often established, that a blood loses its native dextrose, even when by strong antiseptics the possibility of fermentation is practically excluded, without leaving any traces of discoverable oxidative or glycolytic products of the dextrose which has disappeared.

(*d*) 1 litre of blood, to which was added 10 grams of dextrose and sufficient toluol to cover surface of the fluid, was placed in a brood-oven for twenty-four hours and treated as before. No oxalic acid was found, but it gave a marked phloroglucin reaction. The polariscope showed, in 100 c.c. of fluid, 0.503 per cent., while by reduction of copper and weighing, 0.5 per cent. was found. The remainder after these tests was diluted again to 100 c.c., showing a turning power of +0.15 per cent., and after splitting with 1 per cent. sulphuric acid, +0.2 per cent. It also gave marked phloroglucin and orcin reactions, as also 0.370 gram of an hydrazin, insoluble in hot water and absolute alcohol. Here we have no decided increase of reduction over polariscopic reading, as would be present were the levogyr paired glycuronic acid present to any extent, nor do we find a marked increase of turning power after splitting with acid, as would be expected under the same conditions. We do, however, find an insoluble hydrazin and Tollens reaction, particularly after splitting, in both cases where dextrose has been added. Taken all in all, there is evidence that paired glycuronic acid exists in ox blood, as demonstrated by Mayer, and human serum, but none to substantiate the conversion of dextrose into that substance by means of any glycolytic ferment existing in the blood. We think that we have also demonstrated that the large amount of dextrose failing to reappear in these experiments is not converted into carbonic acid or oxalic acid. Where this change takes place, if it does, as insisted upon by Mayer, we do not know. One thing is evident to everyone who has worked with blood: that our means of separating the albumin are crude, and that the enormous coagulum or precipitate formed by the albumin must of necessity carry with it a considerable portion of the blood-sugar which cannot be separated from it. The problem of what becomes of the sugar in glycolysis still remains to be solved.

The methods of isolating the rarer forms of the oxidative products of dextrose, like glycuronic and saccharic acids, are still so crude that they offer but little hope of success in this direction. A glycolytic enzyme undoubtedly exists in the liver, but its action has been demonstrated on glycogen only, and can probably have nothing to do with the oxidation of dextrose. Croftan also claimed to have found an enzyme in the leukocytes which would destroy dextrose, but, beyond demonstrating that the sugar disappeared, nothing further was proved. Salkowski suggests that the oxidase which is found in the tissues may be the active agent, but, as far as I can learn, this agent has only been able to oxidize the more highly oxidizable bodies, like benzaldehyde and salicyldehyde, but never dextrose. The proof of the former action has been established by the detection of benzoic and salicylic acids; but, as far as can be learned, never of the latter by the detection of glycuronic, glycuric, saccharic acids, etc., the oxidative products of dextrose.

THE BACTERIAL EXAMINATION OF 104 SAMPLES OF WATER:

TOGETHER WITH A DETAILED STUDY OF THE COLON BACILLUS.[1]

By William G. Bissell, M.D.,
BACTERIOLOGIST, DEPARTMENT OF HEALTH, BUFFALO, N. Y.

There does not appear to be a subject at the present time that is shrouded with a greater uncertainty than the sanitary interpretation of the presence of bacilli coli in a water supply. This uncertainty has been largely augmented by the fact that many reliable observers have found colon bacilli in waters which, presumably, were not polluted with fecal material.

At the meeting of the American Public Health Association at New Orleans, La., after considerable consultation between many of the laboratory workers, it was decided that several should conduct, independently, an investigation along the following lines:

1. The consideration of what should constitute a colon bacillus.
2. The amount of water most advisable to test in order to arrive at some conservative conclusion as indicating the presence or absence of fecal pollution.
3. The length of life of the colon bacillus in water under its natural environment.
4. The degree of frequency with which colon bacilli can be found in different amounts of water known to contain sewage.
5. To ascertain, if possible, the relative degree of frequency with which colon bacilli can be detected in water presumably not polluted with sewage.

After considering the subject, it appeared to the writer that his residential district was most fortunate, in that it afforded a favorable field for an investigation of this character, and, after obtaining the co-operation of an able laboratory assistant who could devote his entire time to the work, an investigation was started.

During the progress of the work many difficulties were experienced, and particularly was this true in considering the fifth division of the work, for the reason that, although many wells were found which, upon inspection, did not reveal the probable access of fecal pollution, it was impossible to locate but one body of water (Lake Hemlock, near Rochester) where sewage pollution could presumably be eliminated.

The first division of the work, as to what constitutes a colon bacillus, was conducted along the following lines:

[1] Read at Washington, D. C., October 26, 1903, before the Laboratory Section of the American Public Health Association.

1. An organism responding to the full colon test was isolated from fifteen different samples of human feces. These organisms were cultured in all the common media and in different lots of the same media, and the comparative results checked. It was found that the same organism in the same class of media, but of different generations (and particularly was this true in regard to the use of the Smith fermentation tube), would frequently differ as to the amount of gas produced during a definite interval. In two instances organisms giving indol and odor reactions in older generations would fail in different lots of the same class of media in earlier generations. It was the writer's endeavor by this procedure to ascertain as near as possible the actual degree of uniformity of results that it was possible to obtain with the present colon test.

2. In ascertaining what constitutes a colon bacillus was the study of certain lactic-acid producing organisms and their comparison with known colon bacilli. Many of the members of this section will recall that Prescott has pointed out a great similarity between certain lactic-acid organisms found upon grain and the colon organism.

The writer at the meeting of the American Public Health Association at New Orleans, La., exhibited cultures showing the similarity in the cultural manifestations between the bacillus acidi lactici of Hoeppe and the colon bacillus. The work in this connection was conducted as follows:

Fifteen different laboratories were communicated with and cultures purporting to be lactic-acid bacilli were received. After thorough cultural investigation it was impossible, by any of the usual methods, to demonstrate a constant difference between ten of the cultures received and the colon bacillus. These results at first puzzled the investigators, for it suggested the possibility of the lactic-acid organism not being a distinct species of the bacteria. It is now the writer's belief that such cultures were none other than colon bacilli mistaken for the lactic-acid organism, for the reason that the remaining five cultures contained an organism absolutely non-motile; nor was it possible, under different modes of procedure, to cause these organisms to develop motility, and they in that manner differed from the colon bacillus. It is the writer's opinion that such cultures were true lactic-acid bacilli, and this has been recently strengthened by the positive demonstration of spores in four of the five cultures.

3. The next step as to what should constitute a colon bacillus was devoted to the use of presumptive tests. This work was carried on to ascertain to what degree it was necessary to carry on confirmative work in order to arrive at a positive diagnosis where a presumptive test was most marked. The organisms tested were two common to most waters, namely, the bacillus fluorescens liquefaciens and the bacillus fluorescens putridus. All results were checked with cultures of colon bacilli.

The presumptive test included the use of three fermentation tubes containing 2 per cent. of dextrose bouillon and the subsequent testing of gas formulæ after forty-eight hours, the production of acidity, the coagulation of milk, the production of indol, and the production of a disagreeable odor. It was found that the organisms mentioned gave results that could be easily mistaken for colon bacilli, if no greater time than forty-eight hours be allowed and the exact morphology of the organisms not determined.

The result of this division's work seems to justify the following conclusions:

(*a*) That the factors liable to great variation in tests for colon bacilli are those pertaining to the amount of gas produced, the production of indol, and the production of a putrefactive odor.

(*b*) That it is necessary, in order to arrive at a positive diagnosis of colon in water, to completely culture the organism, and the results obtained include the following:

1. A motile organism.
2. Slender rods without spores.
3. An acid-producing organism.
4. One that will coagulate milk within forty-eight hours without a redigestion of the casein.
5. An organism producing marked turbidity in broth within twenty-four hours.
6. An organism capable of fermenting 2 per cent. of dextrose bouillon in a Smith fermenting tube giving 25 per cent. to 75 per cent. gas production within forty-eight hours, the gas having an approximate formulæ of two parts hydrogen to one part carbon dioxide.
7. The production of indol.
8. The reduction of nitrates to nitrites.
9. The production of a putrefactive odor.
10. An organism that will ferment lactose and saccharose as well as dextrose.

(*c*) That there are other organisms common to water which may be easily mistaken for colon bacilli if presumptive tests are alone considered.

The second division of the work, as to the amount of water advisable to test in order to indicate the presence or absence of fecal pollution, was conducted as follows:

Buffalo, a city of 400,000 inhabitants, is situated at the head of the Niagara River. This river has an average velocity of nine miles per hour, and, although a rapidly running stream, is not of excessively great volume. The sewage of Buffalo is emptied into this river, and, in consequence of its being a turbulent stream, becomes mixed with the water of the river in a very short distance. It appeared to the writer that examination of different amounts of the water at distances of twelve and twenty-two miles down the stream would be productive of much valuable information as regards the amount of water advisable to test, as this river certainly received a tremendous amount of direct sewage pollution.

The investigation covered an examination of 104 samples. Fifty-two of these samples were collected twelve miles below Buffalo and the remaining fifty-two samples ten miles below this point, or twenty-two miles down stream. All samples were examined in quantities ranging from $\frac{1}{10}$ of a c.c. to 1 litre.

The results obtained were as follows: From the samples collected twelve miles down stream colon bacilli were present in:

21	per cent. when the amount examined was	1/10 c.c.
29	" " " " "	½ "
52	" " " " "	1 "
59	" " " " "	5 "
69	" " " " "	10 "
80	" " " " "	50 "
87	" " " " "	100 "
90	" " " " "	500 "
91	" " " " "	1 litre.

Of the samples collected twenty-two miles down stream the results were as follows:

19	per cent. when the amount examined was	1/10 c.c.
21	" " " " "	½ "
34	" " " " "	1 "
39	" " " " "	5 "
41	" " " " "	10 "
47	" " " " "	50 "
51	" " " " "	100 "
53	" " " " "	500 "
59	" " " " "	1 litre.

There were several doubtful results during the progress of the work, and all such results were recorded as being positive.

In several instances, if the presumptive test mentioned in Division No. 1 was alone considered as being conclusive evidence of the presence of colon bacilli, many errors would have resulted, and a much larger percentage of positive results recorded. As it is, the result of this work does not correspond with similar work conducted by Winslow and Miss Hunnewell, as recorded in a statement issued by Prescott, in that the percentage of 1 c.c. of samples examined revealing positive evidence of colon bacilli are much larger than in their investigation. This may be accounted for by the fact that it is the writer's belief that the relative frequency of colon bacilli in a given quantity of water is largely dependent upon the amount of dilution that the raw sewage or fecal material undergoes. It will be noted that the results at twelve and twenty-two miles show a considerable variance in favor of colon bacilli being less frequently found in the same amounts of water at the greater distance. The cause of this decrease does not seem easy of explanation, for the reason that the natural influences which tend to produce disintegration of organisms as worked out and recorded by Jordan do not seem to be present in this clear, shallow, rapidly running stream, having a bed largely composed of rock.

Agitation would not seem accountable for the result, for the reason that samples collected immediately above and below Niagara Falls failed to reveal any difference in the number of organisms present. It would seem to the writer that sunlight is the only remaining natural factor that could possibly be considered, and the reduction may be due to this cause. The land on either side of the Niagara River is subject to constant cultivation, and, as many of these samples were taken during and following heavy rainfalls, it would seem, if the cultivation of lands in the near vicinity supplies any great amount of colon bacilli to a stream of this character, that the relative numbers of coli would have been materially increased at such times. As a matter of fact, this was not the investigator's experience. The number of coli present in the amount of water was materially lessened following rainfalls. This, of course, might be due to the great dilution produced by the rainfall. As judged by the investigators, the relative amount of colon supplied, if any, must have been extremely small to permit of the reductions noted. As a recapitulation of the results of the second division's work, the following conclusions would seem justifiable:

1. The presence of colon bacilli in the majority of 10 c.c. lots of a sample should be looked upon as suspicious.

2. When found in the majority of 5 c.c. lots of a sample it should be looked upon as decidedly suspicious.

3. When found in 50 per cent. of 1 c.c. lots of a sample it can be considered as evidence of direct fecal pollution.

4. That whereas cultivated lands bordering on water supplies may furnish sufficient quantities of colon bacilli during certain periods to permit of their being detected when large quantities of water are examined, it does not appear that in the examination of 1 c.c. amounts of samples that colon bacilli coming from this source will be present in sufficient numbers to permit of their detection in the majority of the 1 c.c. examinations.

The third division of the work, the length of life of the colon bacillus in water under natural environment, was conducted as follows:

Three wells were found, which, after thorough inspection of the surrounding territory and careful bacterial examination, did not reveal colon bacilli. There was placed in each well one quart of excrement, the source of same being as follows:

Human in Well A, cow in Well B, and horse in Well C.

After ten days all wells were examined and colon bacilli were found in abundance, the exact number being in the neighborhood of: Well A, 500 to 800 per c.c.; Well B, over 3000 per c.c.; Well C, over 1000 per c.c.

After thirty days the number of colon in Well A were approximately the same; in Well B the colon had greatly decreased; in Well C the colon had decreased 10 per cent. After ninety days the number of colon bacilli in Well A had decreased over 11 per cent.; in Well B could be found only occasionally in c.c. quantities, and in Well C there was but an average of four colonies of colon bacilli to the c.c., counting four plates. It was impossible at this time to continue the investigation of Wells B and C, but an examination of Well A one hundred and ninety days after the introduction of excrement revealed five colonies of colon bacilli per c.c., averaging three lactose litmus agar plate. From these tests it would seem that the length of life of colon bacillus in well water under natural conditions varies with the variety. It was impossible to conduct an investigation relative to the length of life of colon bacilli in stream water. The following recapitulation of results would seem justifiable:

1. The resistance of the colon bacillus in water is influenced by the animal source of the material.

2. That there is a gradual decrease in the number of organisms where there is no additional pollution.

3. That colon bacilli in human excrement is capable of surviving at least one hundred and ninety days in well water.

The fourth division of the work, that of considering the degree of frequency with which colon bacilli can be found in water known to be polluted with sewage, is covered under the results reported in the work of the second division.

The fifth division of the work, the degree of frequency with which colon bacilli can be found in waters not presumably contaminated with fecal material, was conducted as follows:

The work of this division was mostly confined to the examination of well waters, for the reason that after a most diligent search the investigators were unable to locate in the near vicinity to Buffalo a single stream, and but one lake (Hemlock, near Rochester) from which the presence of sewage could be presumably eliminated. The source of this lake is said to be springs, and it is not immediately connected with any other great body of water. The great distance of this lake from the point where the work was conducted rendered it impossible to obtain any great number of samples for investigation. Seven samples were examined, all being collected upon the same day, at different locations in the lake, and, fortunately, at a time following a forty-eight-hour rainfall. The land surrounding Lake Hemlock for a considerable number of feet is controlled by the city of Rochester, and is protected as a water-shed to this lake. The remaining adjacent lands are used for farming purposes.

After many attempts, using 1 c.c., 3 c.c., 5 c.c., and 10 c.c. lots from each of the seven samples, it was impossible to detect the presence of colon bacilli. The well-water tests included, on an

average, four examinations of two different samples from thirty-one different wells. 5 c.c. was the amount selected in each instance. None of the examinations revealed the presence of colon bacilli.

A recapitulation of the results of the five divisions of the work seems to justify the following conclusions:

1. That there is a difference between the bacillus acidi lactici of Hoeppe and the colon bacillus.
2. That presumptive tests, although of unquestionable value as primary procedures, and serviceable for prolonged routine test of a supply, where the analyst is familiar with all conditions and can ascertain at a glance any variable feature, must not be relied upon in arriving at a positive definite diagnosis of the colon bacillus.
3. That the colon bacillus cannot be constantly detected in c.c. amounts of water from the same source, although it may be heavily polluted with sewage.
4. That the presence of colon bacilli in 50 per cent. of c.c. amounts of water is strongly indicative of sewage pollution.
5. That the ordinary cultivation of farm lands, although it may be the source of some colon bacilli to a water supply, does not seem to play any great role as such, and that this source need hardly be considered when the majority of 1 c.c. samples reveal the organism.
6. That agitation has little or no destructive influence upon colon bacilli in water, and that light appears to exert a destructive influence.
7. That the positive detection of the presence of true colon bacilli in waters not presumably receiving sewage is rare.
8. That it is possible there have been organisms mistaken for colon bacilli, probably through too great reliance upon presumptive tests.

OBSERVATIONS UPON THE CHROMATIC VARIATIONS IN THE PRECIPITATED AND SEDIMENTED CHLORIDES, SULPHATES, AND PHOSPHATES OF URINE.[1]

BY EDWARD F. WELLS, M.D.,

AND

JOHN C. WARBRICK, M.D.,

OF CHICAGO.

IN making quantitative analyses of urine for chlorides, sulphates, and phosphates by the volumetric method, using the centrifuge for the purpose of throwing down the precipitate, certain chromatic variations in the sediment have long attracted our attention. Although

[1] Read before the Chicago Medical Society, January 6, 1904.

such variations in color were particularly noted by one of us in the earliest days of centrifugal analysis, yet no systematic record of these was made until about eighteen months ago, since which time an accurate notation covering this point has been made in every urinary analysis made in our laboratories. These examinations, numbering more than 2000, have been sufficiently numerous to warrant an analysis of the results of our observations, and these are herewith presented, in the form of a preliminary report.

The urines analyzed were from healthy persons, mainly beyond middle age, who presented themselves, as a routine, for physical examination, and from invalids of all ages and affected with a great variety of ailments. In the latter class were included cases of the acute infections, tuberculosis, carcinoma, diabetes, nephritis, anæmias, circulatory disturbances, etc. Various foods and medicaments were ingested, and these were noted. In nearly every case the twenty-four hours' urine was employed and the examinations were repeated daily or at longer intervals.

The analyses were made in the ordinary manner and included information upon the nature of the specimen, quantity in twenty-four hours, transparency, sediment, color, reaction, specific gravity, total solids, urea, chlorides, phosphates, sulphates, albumin, sugar, diazo reaction, indican, bile, hæmoglobin, casts, blood elements, epithelium, crystals, amorphous sediment, etc. The chlorides were precipitated by a 10 per cent. solution of nitrate of silver, the phosphates by the alkaline magnesium solution and the sulphates by the standard acidulated chloride of barium solution. For the purpose of estimating the color the sediment was compared with a standard chromatic scale.

The chlorides showed the greatest variations in color, and for the sake of brevity our remarks will be confined mainly to this phase of the subject.

The colors assumed by the chloride sediment varied from the purest white, through innumerable shades of yellow, orange, green, and red to black, as shown in the drawings. It is worthy of note that no two specimens were exactly alike. Thus, if two specimens, either of which would be designated as pure white, were compared, noticeable differences in shade could be readily detected.

The white sediments were more numerous than any other. These varied infinitely in shade, through pure white; white with a more or less distinct yellowish or, and oftenest, a pinkish tinge; white with a slight bluish tinge; grayish and dirty white. These in turn ran, by insensible gradations, into the drabs and slates. The yellow sediments rose up from the yellowish-white and passed on through the various shades of light yellow, canary yellow, ochre and deep yellow, losing themselves in the oranges, salmon colors, old-gold and green sediments. The reds began with the most delicate shades of pink, pale reds, yellowish reds, rose tints, wine colors to dark reds; light, dark, yellowish, and seal browns to blacks. In two specimens a beautiful light lilac-purple color was developed. In numerous instances the colors were strikingly pure and beautiful. If the test-tube were not well shaken after the addition of the nitrate of silver solution a marbled or mottled appearance was likely to be produced.

In some instances the chromatic bodies were soluble and imparted to the supernatant liquid a coloring more or less nearly approximating that of the sediment—usually of a lighter shade. In others the supernatant liquid was colored some shade other than that of the sediment—*e. g.*, pink with a white sediment. In yet others more or less of the coloring matter was abstracted from the urine, leaving it distinctly lighter. In a small proportion of cases the supernatant liquid was unchanged in color.

The variously colored chloride sediments were compared with the color, reaction, specific gravity, total solids, total urea, diazo reaction, indican, sugar, albumin, phosphate, and sulphate sediments of the urine; with exposure of the sediment to light; with the medication, etc., without observing any constancy of relation.

For example: Although the white sediments were usually obtained from yellow urines, yet such sediments were also seen in red and even brown urines. The same applied to the yellow sediments. The peculiar and beautiful old-gold sediments were found in light yellow, yellow, yellowish-red, and red urines. The pale-green, bright-green, and dark-green sediments were observed only in yellow urines. Olive sediments were noted in variously colored urines, but were almost uniformly present in those which were bile-stained. Orange sediments were found only in red urines. Pink, light-red, and yellowish-red sediments were seen in yellow, amber, red, and brown urines. Rose-tinted and wine-colored sediments were noted in yellow, amber, and red urines. A single lilac sediment was encountered in an amber urine. The variously shaded brown sediments were usually observed in red urines, but in a few instances were seen in yellow urines. The brownish-black and black sediments were usually met with in light-yellow and yellow urines, rarely in amber and red urines.

In one notable case of chronic interstitial nephritis, in which the urine has been habitually a very light yellow, the sediment was, for several years, regularly dark brown or black. Recently, without recognizable cause, it has changed to a dirty white or gray color.

In comparing the colors of the chloride sediment with the specific gravity of the urine it was noticeable that the average specific gravity diminished as the colors darkened, but very low and very high densities were observed in every group of color shades. The opposite, with like exceptions, applied to the lighter shades of color and the moderate and higher ranges of specific gravity. Similar statements may be made regarding the relations existing between the urea and color of the sediments.

The presence in the urine of albumin, of sugar, of indican, of the diazo reaction, etc., were without apparent influence, and this could be said of the medication observed, especially with reference to salol, guaiacol, acetanilid, salicylic acid, morphine, iron, mercury, iodide of potassium, etc.

The bulk percentage of the chloride sediment, which varied from a mere trace to 50 per cent., appeared to have no bearing upon the color. It is true, however, that in some groups of colors—*e. g.*, the wine-colored sediments, the percentages were uniformly low, while in others, as note the pink sediments, they were as uniformly high.

The color of the chloride sediment was independent of the action of light upon the precipitate, before and after sedimentation. When exposed to light it underwent, upon the surface, the changes which are usual with solutions of nitrate of silver in the presence of organic matters, but this had no connection with the phenomena which we observed.

The colors of the phosphate and sulphate sediments bore no close relation to those of the chlorides. They were usually some shade of white or fawn color. We might say that the phosphates were oftenest of a pure white color, or of a delicate fawn or buff color, while the sulphates were oftener of a dirty white or buff color. It rarely occurred that these were of any other color where the chlorides were white or light in color. On the other hand, the chloride sediment might have shown any of the darker colors, even black, while the phosphates and sulphates remained white or light in color.

In many instances these sediments appeared in a variety of colors —*e. g.*, pinks, light browns, yellows, drabs, etc., rarely in the darker colors. In some cases striking colorations were noted. In one specimen the chlorides were black, the phosphates yellow, and the sulphates orange. In another the chlorides were seal brown, the phosphates orange, and the sulphates green. In yet another the chlorides were dirty white, the phosphates a beautiful pink, and the sulphates a bright, deep yellow.

In conclusion we will say that no reasonable explanation is offered or known to us for the phenomena observed. We have been unable, as yet, to find the key to the situation. That these chromatic variations in the sedimented chlorides, phosphates, and sulphates depend upon more or less important vital processes, most probably in the intestines, and of a fermentative or putrefactive nature, we believe to be true. We are of the opinion, also, that a clear understanding of this subject would probably be of diagnostic importance. For this reason we have thought it best to present our observations at the present time, with the hope that by attracting attention to the subject the solution of the problem may be expedited.

EXPERIMENTAL STUDIES ON THE ETIOLOGY OF ACUTE PNEUMONITIS.*

BY AUGUSTUS WADSWORTH, M.D.,

ALUMNI FELLOW IN PATHOLOGY; ASSISTANT IN BACTERIOLOGY AND HYGIENE, DEPARTMENT OF PATHOLOGY, COLLEGE OF PHYSICIANS AND SURGEONS, COLUMBIA UNIVERSITY, N. Y.

INTRODUCTION.

ACUTE exudative inflammation of the lungs may develop as a metastatic lesion secondary to disease processes in other parts of the body, or it may accompany acute interstitial processes arising usually from the pleura, or it may arise as a primary infection of the lung forming patchy bronchopneumonic or diffuse lobar lesions. The bacterial incitants of acute primary infectious processes in the lung are now well known. Our knowledge of the essential conditions which determine the extent and nature of the disease processes in the lung and elsewhere, however, lacks the precision which can come only from exact experimental data. This may be attained only when it is possible to reproduce at will the various disease processes in animals. With pneumococcus pneumonia this has not heretofore been satisfactorily accomplished. As a result of a long series of experiments, I have finally determined a method by which the diffuse lesions of pneumococcus pneumonia may readily be incited in the rabbit. This method it is the purpose of this paper to record; but the failures and successes of others have in such large measure contributed to my final results that they may with advantage be briefly considered. The significance of this previous work, however, may not be fully appreciated without summing up our knowledge of the distribution and disposal of bacteria in general in the respiratory apparatus, of the bacterial incitants of pneumonia, and of the paths of infection.

BACTERIA OF THE NORMAL RESPIRATORY APPARATUS. Inspired foreign particles and bacteria, as shown by the researches of Arnold[3] and many others, are deposited chiefly on the moist surfaces of the upper respiratory passages, although they may occasionally be carried to the alveoli of the lung. For most bacteria the healthy mucous membrane is an unfavorable environment, yet this varies greatly in different parts of the tract and with different species of bacteria. In the *mouth* and *nares* bacteria are being constantly deposited on the mucous membranes. As indicated by the researches of Thomson and Hewlett,[178] Wright,[197] Nenninger,[131] Müller,[126] and Laschtschenko,[109] some of them disappear very rapidly; others may develop and exist as harmless parasites. These secretions thus contain

* Read in abstract before the American Association of Pathologists and Bacteriologists, April, 1903.

many different species of micro-organisms, among which the bacteria commonly associated with pneumonia—the pneumococcus, streptococcus, staphylococcus, and the bacillus of Friedländer—have often been found. Suffice it to note that the pneumococcus was present in a large proportion of Sternberg's cases,[173] 20 per cent. of Fraenkel's cases,[67] 17 per cent. of Besser's cases,[17] 20 per cent. of Wolf's cases,[196] 30 per cent. of Bein's cases,[15] 55 per cent. of Miller's cases,[123] 4 per cent. of Neumann's normal cases,[136] and in 100 per cent. of the forty tonsils examined by Bezancon and Griffon.[20] Netter[132] divided his cases into those with and those without a history of pneumonia, and found the pneumococcus in four out of five and in one out of five cases, respectively, and he also claims to have found the organisms virulent five, ten, or more years after a pneumonic infection. Furthermore, it is significant to note that it has been experimentally shown by Guarnieri,[80] by Bordonni-Uffredozzi,[24] by Grawitz and Steffen,[77] by Spolverini,[170] and by Ottolenghi[138] that the pneumococcus in sputum may remain alive and virulent for two to four months.

In the *trachea* bacteria are also deposited on the mucous membranes,* but under normal conditions these are comparatively few in number and are rapidly disposed of by the cilia, and also by the action of the mucus, which, in the researches of Wurtz and Lemoyez[198] with sputum, of Walthard,[187] of Stroganoff,[175] and of Morisani[124] with the uterine secretions, and more recently of Arloing[2] with pure mucus, has shown marked bactericidal qualities.† Examination of the human trachea at autopsy, as in the studies of Baumgarten,[10] Hoffmann,[91] v. Besser,[19] Ritchie,[152] Claisse,[38] and Durck,[45] has revealed the presence of micro-organisms in a considerable proportion of the cases, but the trachea and lung at autopsy, although of normal appearance, may not be considered to be under normal conditions. Normal conditions, it is evident, are more closely approximated in the researches conducted on animals, as in the studies of Hildebrandt,[89] Klipstein,[102] Gobell,[74] Rosenthal,[154] Beco,[12] Buttersack,[30] Boni,[23] Barthel,[9] and Calamida and Bertarelli.[31] In these examinations of the trachea of animals, bacteria have not often been found, and the lower portions of the trachea and the bronchi have thus been considered to be practically sterile.‡

* As suggested by the researches of Slawjansky[157] and of Kuttner[107] with the injection of foreign substances, and of Pernici and Scagliosi[143] with the injection of bacteria into the general circulation, the possibility of bacteria being carried to and through the mucous membrane from the circulating blood may also be considered.

† In the experiments of Grawitz,[77] Steffen,[77 171] and also of Hopkins[92] this action of mucus was not detected in sputum sterilized by heat.

‡ In the course of my experiments, examination of the lower portion of the trachea clearly indicated that in the rabbit, at least, this portion of the respiratory tract is normally free from micro-organisms; but that contaminations, attributed very largely to the death agony, readily occur; and that the bacteria of such contaminations may grow so that, unless the animal be examined immediately after death, considerable numbers of bacteria may be found. Furthermore, animals dying of disease, when compared with those killed, frequently showed the presence of contaminating bacteria in this portion of the respiratory apparatus, although the entire tract was apparently normal.

In the normal *lung* bacteria do not, so far as is known, exist as harmless parasites. The researches of Prudden and Northrup,[144] Tschistovitch,[180 181] Grammatschikoff,[75] Silfast,[165] and others show that pathogenic as well as non-pathogenic bacteria in the air spaces degenerate: some are taken up by the phagocytes and carried into the lymph channels; others are destroyed by the body fluids. By these processes considerable numbers of bacteria may be disposed of in a comparatively short time.

BACTERIAL INCITANTS OF PNEUMONIA. The infectious nature of pneumonia was first definitely established by the researches of Friedländer,[71] Talamon,[176] and Fraenkel.[67] The various studies of the pneumonic lung at autopsy in long series of cases by many subsequent observers, notably, Weichselbaum,[190] Wolf,[196] Finkler,[62] Prudden and Northrup,[144] Kreibach,[105] Netter,[133 135] Pearce,[141] Durck,[44] and Howard,[93] have served to indicate the etiological importance of the different bacterial incitants. The pneumococcus is now considered as practically the sole incitant of the diffuse lobar lesions. Netter believes the disease to be specific; others concede a small percentage of the lesions to the bacillus of Friedländer. In bronchopneumonia the more recent researches indicate that the pneumococcus rather than the streptococcus is more frequently the incitant, yet in the secondary lesions following certain of the exanthemata the streptococcus is still considered the more important.

Although the inflammatory reactions induced by the pneumococcus, streptococcus, staphylococcus, and pneumobacillus are somewhat similar, they differ in many respects, so that there are certain types of lesion more commonly associated with one species than with others. The pneumococcus lesions are in general more diffuse, œdematous, fibrinous, hemorrhagic, and less necrotic than those induced by either the streptococcus or pneumobacillus. In pneumococcus lesions gangrene rarely develops, except as the result of secondary infection; on the other hand, the pneumobacillus is not infrequently associated with such a condition. The pneumococcus and streptococcus are, on the whole, more similar in their pathogenic effects than any of the others; but in the lung the streptococcus rarely if ever gives rise to the lobar form of pneumonia. The staphylococcus processes are less variable, almost always circumscribed, rarely diffuse or fibrinous, as compared with those of the other three species.

These broad differences, to some extent dependent upon the virulence of the bacterial species, may be modified by many conditions, such as the age or susceptibility of the individual, and more particularly by the susceptibility of the race or species of animal infected. In respect to infection with the pneumococcus, Behring and Nissen,[14] Fraenkel,[67] Gamaleia,[72] Kruse and Pansini,[106] and many others have determined that mice and rabbits are the most susceptible; guinea-pigs, rats, squirrels, cats, dogs, sheep, horses, and man are in varying degrees less susceptible; and fowls more or less immune.

PATHS OF INFECTION IN PNEUMONIA. Infection through the air-passages is undoubtedly the rule in bronchopneumonia; but certain secondary pneumonias arising by hæmatogenous infection may so closely simulate bronchopneumonia that the rule must either be excepted for these cases or they must be classified with the metastatic pneumonias. Most observers believe that lobar pneumonia also develops from an infection through the air-passages; but regarding the universality of this there is some question, doubtless arising from the unsatisfactory results that have attended tracheal inoculations in animals and other similar experimental attempts to induce the lobar lesion. Two other paths of infection, the hæmatogenous and the lymphatic, have therefore been considered by some theoretically possible. As supporting hæmatogenous infection, the results of the blood examinations of pneumonia patients have been cited. Careful scrutiny of these, however,* reveals the fact that while bacteriæmia develops early as well as late in the disease, there is no indication that this is other than secondary to the local lesion. The occurrence of pneumonia in the foetus offers the clearest example of hæmatogenous infection. Cases of such infection have been reported by Strachan,[174] Marchand,[117] Thorner,[179] Netter,[134] Viti,[184] Czmetscha,[41] and Delestre.[42] These reports, however, are in many respects inadequate; in some histological examinations of the lesions were not made, in others infection by the air-passages after birth could not be excluded. They, therefore, fail to establish the occurrence of lobar pneumonia from placental infection. Experimental support of hæmatogenous infection in lobar pneumonia is certainly very meagre, uncorroborated, and relatively insignificant. Finally, suffice it to note that, clinically as well as experimentally, pneumonic lesions of the lobar type are uncommon in races or individuals very susceptible to systemic pneumococcus infection and more common in resistant individuals or species in which systemic infections are less usual.

There are few facts to support a theory of lymphatic infection. Grober's[79] interesting work on the tonsil and its lymphatic connections is extremely significant as applied to tuberculous and pleural infections, but the plague bacillus is the only species which is definitely known to reach the lung through the cervical lymphatics and give rise to an acute exudative pneumonitis. These plague pneumonias, however, are of a peculiar metastatic lymphatic type, quite different from the lobar lesions.

In view of these facts and in the absence of reliable positive data,

* Witness, for example, the studies of Guarnieri,[80] Fraenkel,[61] Banti,[8] Belfanti,[16] Sittmann,[166] Sello,[164] James and Tuttle,[96] Prochaská,[145] White,[193] Baduel,[7] Pane,[139] and Wandel,[189] many of which, and others not cited, have been reviewed recently by Ewing.[60]

the possibility of lobar pneumonia arising by hæmatogenous or lymphatic infection must be considered as not yet established.*

PREVIOUS RESEARCHES ON EXPERIMENTAL PNEUMONIA.

The earliest attempts to induce pneumonia in animals, which were made when the disease was attributed to exposure or fatigue and before its infectious nature was determined, are now chiefly of historic interest. The first significant experiments comprised the inoculation of animals with the exudates and autopsy material from pneumonia cases. After the infectious nature of the disease had thus been established and the several bacteria concerned isolated and differentiated, greater scope and precision of experimentation became possible, pure cultures replaced the exudates, etc.; or if the exudates were used the bacteria contained in the exudates were previously determined, and special methods of inoculation were adopted. At first the lungs were inoculated through the chest-wall, then this rather crude method was discarded and the animals were forced by various contrivances to inhale the infectious material. Finally, tracheal injections of the infectious material were used. Although infection of the normal lung of various animal species were not infrequently secured by certain of these methods, typical diffuse pneumonic lesions rarely developed. Attention was therefore directed to the animal and attempts were made through injury to render the lung more susceptible to infection. The results of these experiments as regards the development of circumscribed bronchopneumonic types of lesions were more satisfactory and uniform; but as regards the development of diffuse lobar types of lesion were uncertain and far from satisfactory.

The experiments of former observers may, therefore, be divided into two main classes: those on normal and those on artificially predisposed animals.

PREVIOUS ATTEMPTS TO INDUCE PNEUMONIA BY INFECTION OF THE UNINJURED OR NORMAL LUNG. *Intravenous*, *subcutaneous*, *infraocular* inoculations—in short, all methods giving rise to a primary general infection, whether practised in the ordinary laboratory routine or in the hope of securing pneumonic lesions—have, with a few uncorroborated exceptions,† uniformly failed to give rise to the

* This, however, does not exclude the possibility of a metastatic pneumonia, as has been exceptionally noted, simulating the diffuse lobar processes. In fact, between the more typical processes of all forms of acute exudative pneumonitis intermediate lesions occur which histologically are distinguished with difficulty.

† Schultz[103] reports pneumonic lesions in eight out of fourteen rabbits inoculated intravenously with pneumococci. Apparently the collapsed lungs were examined, and certainly the lesions found were inaccurately described as typically exudative. Klipstein[101] reports one instance of a diffuse pneumonia being found after subcutaneous inoculation with a colon bacillus, and Fraenkel[43] noted the exceptional development of pneumonic lesions after subcutaneous inoculation of the thorax with the pneumococcus. An early observer, Klebs,[100]

definite lesions of either bronchopneumonia or lobar pneumonia. *Intraperitoneal* inoculation has similarly failed, the few exceptional lesions being of the pleuropneumonic type.

With *intrathoracic* inoculation the needle may or may not penetrate the lung; if the lung tissues are entered a local injury, with more or less hemorrhagic extravasation, results; if not, the pleural cavity only is inoculated and the infection of the lung is secondary, thus pleuropneumonia is incited. By intrathoracic inoculation of pneumococci, Talamon,[178]* in eight out of twenty rabbits, Weichselbaum[190] rarely, Gamaleia,[72] in dogs and sheep always, obtained pneumonic lesions, some of which were described as diffuse and lobar in type. With the pneumobacillus, Friedländer,[71]† in thirty-two mice and in one out of four dogs, Weichselbaum,[190] occasionally in mice and rabbits, obtained pneumonic lesions. In other similar experiments of these and many other observers, notably Kruse and Pansini,[106] Fraenkel,[67] Salvioli,[157 158] Foa and Rattone,[66] Klein,[101] Sternberg,[172] v. Besser,[19] and Silfast,[165] with pneumococci, streptococci, staphylococci, and the pneumobacillus, conducted on mice, rabbits, guinea-pigs, dogs, and horses, the inoculation failed to give rise to pneumonic lesions, although in the very susceptible animals a general systemic infection often ensued.

The *inhalation* of infectious material has been used chiefly as a test of the permeability of the normal lung to bacteria; but owing very largely to changes occurring in the virulence of the bacteria as a result of cultivation or the drying and pulverizing, and to the uncertainty as to how much if any of the infectious material ever reaches the air spaces, inhalation has proved a most uncertain method of infecting the lung. Pneumonic lesions usually circumscribed have, nevertheless, in exceptional instances, been noted, as in the researches of Buchner, Merkel, and Endelen,[29 64] Eppinger,[55] and Grammatschikoff,[75] with anthrax; of Friedländer,[71] Emmerich,[51]‡ and Chester,[36] with the pneumobacillus; and of Silfast,[165] with streptococci. Weichselbaum[190] failed to secure pneumonic lesions in his experiments with inhalation. The inhalation of the plague bacillus, as in the experiments of Batzaroff[11] and others, doubtless owing to the extreme virulence of this organism and the susceptibility of the animals used, has been remarkably successful in giving rise to the different types of plague pneumonia.

reports the development of pneumonic lesions after intraocular inoculations with exudates which were not obtained in Veraguth's[188] similar experiments. In the course of my experiments, I have occasionally found at autopsy extensive consolidations of the lung, in which no bacteria or bacteria other than those inoculated were present, and which could only be attributed to chance or an intercurrent infection. A similar undetected infection may account for some of these unusual findings, especially in the early researches.

* Exudates were used for inoculation.

† Identity of cultures used is somewhat doubtful.

‡ Emmerich[52 53] claims to have invariably secured typical diffuse lesions in animals which had inhaled virulent pneumococci. His observations have never been corroborated; in fact, such inhalations have usually proved harmless.

By *tracheal injection* of the infectious material greater precision was given to the experiments and more definite results were thereby attained; but the virulence of the different bacteria in these experiments, as in those with inhalation, was a most important and variable factor. With pneumococci introduced in this way, Fraenkel[67]* rarely, Salvioli[159] in one rabbit and in two of four guinea-pigs, Kruse and Pansini[106] in possibly one of twenty-eight dogs, Tschistovitch[181] in seven of nineteen cats, and exceptionally in rabbits, obtained diffuse pneumonic lesions. Similar experiments of these and other observers, notably, Gamaleia,[72] Klein,[101] Guarnieri,[80] Griffiini and Cambria,[78] Talamon,[176] Lipari,[112] Welch,[191] Arustamow,[4] Müller,[125] Aufrecht,[5] Durck,[46] Coco and Drago,[39] and Carnot and Fournier,[33] with pneumococci, conducted on rabbits, guinea-pigs, cats, dogs, and sheep, failed to give rise to typical lesions, the inoculation proving either harmless or, as in very susceptible animals, giving rise to systemic infection, usually without, but in some instances, with small circumscribed lung lesions.

Patchy or circumscribed lesions have been occasionally induced by the tracheal injection of other bacteria, as in the experiments of Prudden and Northrup,[144] Orloff,[137] Fleck,[65] Laehr,[108] Durck,[46] Silfast,[165] and Beco,[13] with streptococci and staphylococci; of Lépine and Lyomet[111] with the typhoid bacillus; of Gamaleia[72] and of Tschistovitch[180] with the chicken cholera bacillus; and of Tschistovitch[180] with the bacillus of rouget du porc. Diffuse lesions following endotracheal inoculations have been reported by Gamaleia[72] with the bacilli of anthrax and chicken cholera, and by Bosc and Galavielle[25] with the micrococcus tetragenus. Finally, the various forms of plague pneumonia have been frequently induced by this method of inoculation. These are often hemorrhagic, usually bronchopneumonic, sometimes confluent and diffuse.

Experiments on the normal animal having given unsatisfactory results, attempts were made to render the lung more susceptible to infection by means of predisposants, which may be considered as acting chiefly upon the lung locally or upon the system at large. Many conditions, such as the inspiration of irritating substances, exposure to cold, trauma, fatigue, and disease, have long been recognized clinically as favoring the development of pneumonia in man. These and other conditions used as experimental substitutes for them have been extensively studied as to their effect *per se* on the animal and when combined with inoculation.

PREVIOUS ATTEMPTS TO INDUCE PNEUMONIA IN THE LOCALLY PREDISPOSED ANIMAL. The early researches of Heidenhain,[84] Arnold,[3] and Massalongo,[119] and the more recent work of Klipstein[102] and Beco,[13] in which the lungs of animals were exposed by inhalation or injection to various noxious substances in gaseous, liquid, or

* More often with attenuated than with virulent cultures.[69]

solid state, suffice to show that a series of changes largely desquamative, but often exudative, are effected in the tissues of the lung by these irritants.* That the changes thus induced in the lung tissue favor infection and the formation of lesions is well shown by the numerous experiments in which the injured lung has been directly inoculated through the trachea or the predisposed animal has been forced to inhale the infectious material. Such are the experiments of Buchner, Merkel and Enderlen,[29] and Muskatbluth[127] with anthrax; and of Prudden and Northrup,[144] Silfast,[165] and Beco[13] with streptococci and staphylococci; but the lesions in these experiments were usually circumscribed and bronchopneumonic in type. Typical diffuse lesions, however, Gamaleia[72] claims were always obtained when the injured lungs of resistant animals, such as the dog and sheep, were inoculated through the trachea with virulent pneumococci; in the normal lungs of these resistant animals the inoculation proved harmless, in the more susceptible animals this injury merely favored the development of fatal bacteriæmia without lung lesions.

As a result of *trauma* the lung tissues may be injured and thus predisposed to infection. If the integrity of the thorax is destroyed and the lung thereby exposed to external contamination, a wound infection accompanied by various disease processes of the lung, as well as of other tissues, may develop. If, on the other hand, the thorax remains intact, the trauma, acting purely as a predisposant, may give rise to changes in the lung, such as have been noted experimentally by Reineboth[146, 148] and others,† which may favor the development of infectious material carried to the lung by the usual channels. In experimental pneumonia trauma is obviously a constant and possibly a determining factor.

Exposure to *cold*, long considered an all-important factor in the development of pneumonia, is now classed with trauma as a predisposant,‡ which, only in certain cases, may be a determining factor.§ Experimentally the effect of exposure to cold has been extensively studied. The changes brought about in the animal tissues have been attributed to the retention of deleterious products

* Extensive lesions closely resembling those of acute exudative pneumonitis have been secured by such treatment without bacterial agency, but this is exceptional and the reports are confined to a few of the earlier observers.

† Traumatic pneumonia has also been extensively studied by Litten,[113] Meunier,[121] Reynaud,[160] Souques,[168] Gauthier,[73] and Schild.[161]

‡ Witness, for example, the table compiled by Comby:[40]

Bouilland	attributed to cold	75	per cent.
Grisolle	" "	20	"
Ziemssen	" "	9	"
Jurgenson	" "	4	
Griesinger	" "	2	"
Massalongo	" "	0	"

§ Ruhemann,[155] however, considers the exposure to cold the exciting factor, and the presence of the bacteria the predisposing factor in the etiology of pneumonia.

of the body metabolism from diminished excretion (Eisenmann[50]), to reflex nervous action (Heymann[83]), and to the direct action of the cold on the tissues (Rosenthal[155]). These are very largely dependent upon the nature and extent of the exposure, upon the animal species used, and as shown by the researches of Nasaroff,[129] Durig,[47] and Lode,[115] upon the nutritive condition of the individual exposed. As a result of exposure the body temperature may be greatly influenced, as in the experiments of Eve,[59] who found that the experimental extremes compatible with recovery approximate those clinically observed in man, viz., 45° C. (113° F.) and 25 C. (77° F.). The marked fluctuations in blood pressure following exposure to either heat or cold, as in the experiments of Hegglin,[83] Grawitz,[76] Hermann,[87] Hadl,[81] and others, may give rise to hyperæmia, congestion, transudation, or even hemorrhage. Marked anæmia,* with reduction of both cells and hæmoglobin and with hæmoglobinuria, may develop, as in the studies of Chvostek,[37] Erhlich,[48] Grawitz,[79] Ebstein,[49] Fischl,[64] and Rheinboth and Kohlhardt.[149] Other cells of the body may undergo parenchymatous degeneration, as was noted by Lassar[110] and many others since his time. That these changes in the tissues resulting from exposure to cold predispose to many infections has been established by a great variety of researches, notably the early observers, Pasteur,[140] Wagner,[185] Ernst,[56] and Sawtschenko,[160] and the more recent writers, Chelmonski,[35] Lode,[114] Dieudonne,[43] Silfast,[165] Sanarelli,[159] Kisskalt,[99] and Reineboth and Kohlhardt.[149]

Owing to the anatomical structure of the lung these circulatory disturbances and the changes dependent upon them are especially well marked in this organ. Thus, in exposed animals, extensive lesions of the lungs were noted as early as 1862 by Walther,[188] and in 1870 by Wertheim,[192] and also recently by Durck.[45] The development of pneumonic infection in animals exposed to cold has been studied by means of the tracheal injection or the inhalation of infectious material, as in the experiments of Lode[114] and of Platania,[142] with the pneumobacillus and staphylococcus; of Silfast,[166] with streptococci; of Beco,[13] with staphylococci; of Carrière,[32] with attenuated pneumococci; and of Lipari,[112] with virulent pneumococci. In these experiments infection developed, and lesions, usually circumscribed or bronchopneumonic, were obtained more frequently than in normal animals. Lipari[112] alone reports definite results. Diffuse lobar pneumonia was obtained in all the exposed, but in none of the normal, rabbits of his experiments.

Circulatory changes, whether purely reflex and evanescent or associated with definite lesions and damage to the tissues, have been considered determining factors of local predisposition in the lung

* The stimulating effect of mild exposure to cold has long been recognized, and the blood as well as other tissues may be greatly benefited by such exposure, as in the studies of v. Breitenstein,[26] Thayer,[177] Winternitz,[196] and of Speck.[169]

as in other organs and tissues. Attempts to demonstrate this experimentally have not been satisfactory: thus, Buchner[28] concluded that arterial hyperæmia was salutary; Kisskalt,[98 99] that arterial hyperæmia favored infection, but that stasis hyperæmia, as in tuberculosis, may act differently; Frenkel,[70] that sensory paralysis increased the susceptibility, while vasomotor paralysis increased the immunity, but neither had any effect in determining the general infection. Other observers, notably, Hermann,[86] Kasparek,[97] Meltzer,[120] Nekam,[130] Charrin and Ruffer,[34] and Roger,[153] have obtained results which suggested that innervation of a part favored the development of infection. These uncertain results are obviously to be attributed to many variable and indeterminate conditions, relating chiefly to the susceptibility of the animal, on the one hand, and to the nature and virulence of the bacteria on the other.*

The normal lung, however, as compared with the other tissues and fluids of the body, is such an unfavorable environment for bacterial growth that a hyperæmia, with transudation by creating a more favorable soil, may be theoretically considered to favor infection in this organ. For experimental support of this, suffice it to refer to the above-noted predisposing action of irritation and trauma and of exposure to cold, the effects of which in the lung are largely due to circulatory changes.

The so-called *vagus pneumonias* have been studied by many of the early investigators, by Schou,[162] and recently by Müller[125] and by Esser.[58] Section of the vagus nerve, on one or both sides, has been frequently followed by the development of pneumonia, which has usually been of the patchy, bronchopneumonic type, though occasionally diffuse. The paralysis of the larynx, which facilitates infection of the lung by bacteria contained in the secretions of the upper respiratory passages and the circulatory changes set up in the lung, are the main factors in these experimental pneumonias. The results of these experiments prove that the method is uncertain, and, as compared with the direct inoculation of the lung with pure cultures of accurately determined bacterial species, such procedures are obviously crude.

Clinically, *previous disease processes*, especially those of the respiratory apparatus, are said to precede the development of pneumonia, and experience has shown that such inflammatory processes not only impair the protective resources of the parts, but afford favorable conditions for an increase of virulence in the bacteria present in the secretions. In Esser's[57] experiments the permanent changes left by healed inflammatory processes also favored the development of infection, and Aufrecht[6] cites statistics to show that the primary pneumonia predisposes to subsequent pneumonic infec-

* If the circulating blood is a favorable environment for the growth of the bacteria, a hyperæmia obviously favors infection; if unfavorable, retards infection. The experiments in this field have thus as yet added but little to our general theoretical knowledge.

tions. The predisposition effected by disease processes in other parts of the body, except possibly the heart, is obviously the result of an increased general susceptibility of the individual.

Previous Attempts to Induce Pneumonia in the Systemically Predisposed Animal. Many conditions influencing the system at large are well-known predisposants to infection. Some of these are clinically known to favor the development of pneumonia, and certain of the substances or conditions used as local predisposants undoubtedly act to some extent on the general system. Special methods of securing a systemic predisposition, however, have not been used in the experimental study of the etiology of pneumonia, except indirectly by Kaminer,[96] in his work on fibrin formation in the lung. Kaminer obtained pathological changes in the lungs of rabbits poisoned by phenylhydrazin in small repeated subcutaneous doses. In one animal a diffuse fibrinous lesion was found in the lung at autopsy. Bacterial examination failed to reveal micro-organisms.

Summary of the Results of Previous Researches on Experimental Pneumonia. General systemic infection of the animal by intravenous or by subcutaneous inoculation, whether practised on the normal or on the predisposed animal, has uniformly failed to give rise to pneumonic processes. Local infection of the lung from the inhalation of infectious material or by inoculation with virulent bacteria through the chest-wall, or, preferably, through the trachea, has, in some instances, been followed by the development of pneumonia. Practically all the various forms of primary acute exudative pneumonitis have thus been occasionally induced in predisposed and even in normal animals by many different kinds of bacteria. Of the different forms of pneumonia the bronchopneumonic or patchy has been most commonly incited; the typical diffuse lobar lesions have been secured with great difficulty and exceptionally.

It is evident and was early recognized that the nature and virulence of the bacteria inoculated were extremely important factors in each experiment; but it does not alone suffice to secure infection of the lung by means of highly virulent cultures, for this may, and does, as a rule, in susceptible animals, lead to a general fatal bacteriæma, which in nowise contributes to the development of local processes. A precise experimental control of subtle relationships between the virulence of the micro-organism, on the one hand, and the susceptibility of the animal, on the other, should therefore be sought. The virulence of the micro-organisms may be, and has been in many previous experiments, controlled by passing the cultures through animals of the species to be experimented upon. The susceptibility of the animal, however, has not been so definitely kept in hand. The various grades or conditions of susceptibility were not accurately determined and cannot be precisely compared, however suggestive in theory they may be.

THE WRITER'S RESEARCHES ON EXPERIMENTAL PNEUMONIA.

My studies were undertaken with a view of determining accurately the effect of increasing or diminishing the virulence of the incitant upon the development of pneumonic infection in normal animals and in animals whose susceptibility, local and systemic, was definitely increased. By using one micro-organism, the pneumococcus, and carefully controlling its virulence, and one animal species, the rabbit, whose susceptibility to pneumococcus infection was well known, it was hoped that comparison of the results obtained in a series of systematic researches would lead to more precise methods, and thus to more uniform and certain results.

TECHNIQUE. The media used for growing the pneumococci were made from meat infusion and were brought to a final reaction of less than 1 per cent. acid,* phenolphthalein being the indicator. Although glucose proved a valuable addition to the media, it was rarely used, as these cultures were very short-lived, probably on account of the acid developed. Ascites fluid was, in some instances, added to the broth. In tubes of pleuritic fluid, heated until semi-solid, although still transparent, the pneumococcus stock cultures were kept at a temperature of about 10° in an accessible form, alive and virulent for several (eight or more) months. By this means the changes in the biological state of the micro-organism that usually attend repeated transfers were largely eliminated. It was, therefore, possible to work with the same unmodified races of pneumococci in all the experiments.†

Two races of pneumococci were used, one of low, the other of high virulence for rabbits. The first (A) was isolated from a fatal case of lobar pneumonia. The virulence of this organism may be approximately suggested by the fact that intravenously inoculated, 1 c.c. of a twenty-four-hour broth culture proved fatal; injected through the trachea this dose was harmless; subcutaneously inoculated, 0.5 c.c. of a twenty-four-hour broth culture induced an abscess at site of inoculation in two rabbits, and fatal septicæmia in two others inoculated from the same culture tube. The second (B) was obtained, through the kindness of Dr. Alexander Lambert, from the laboratory of the New York Health Department, where, by repeated serial inoculation in rabbits, it had been brought to a high virulence, 0.00001 c.c. of a twenty-four-hour serum broth culture at one time proving fatal to the average rabbit. This culture had, however, lost some of its virulence, for I found that although 0.1 c.c. of a twenty-four-hour broth culture intravenously inoculated excited severe reactions in rabbits, these were not always fatal. Owing to

* A reaction of 0.5 per cent. acid, which Dr. T. C. Janeway in some unpublished experiments has found to be an optimum, was in most instances used.

† For a more complete account of this method and media, see the Proceedings of the New York Pathological Society, April, 1903.

the previous adaptation of this race to rabbits, the potential strength of the culture was perhaps greater than was represented by my figures.

The inoculations were made with a Koch syringe into the ear vein or through the soft parts between the tracheal rings into the lumen of the trachea, which had previously been exposed by an incision through the skin and fasciæ. By careful technique in operating infection of the wound was avoided. The culture fluid was directed to the left lung by elevating and tilting the animal, but forced inspirations of the fluid carried it, in some instances, to the right as well as to the left lung. At the autopsies cultures and smears were usually made from the heart blood, trachea, and liver; in addition, the pleuræ were often, the spleen and kidney sometimes, examined. The smears were stained by the Welch[191] method for staining the capsules and also by the newer methods recommended by Hiss.[90] The lungs were distended with alcohol and all the specimens were hardened in this fluid. Sections of the lung, liver, spleen, and kidney were stained and examined for bacteria by the Gram-Weigert method. Other methods were also used in special instances, and by some of these, as yet not carefully determined, capsules could be demonstrated on the pneumococci in the sections of the lesions.

Scope of the Experiments on Normal and Predisposed Animals. Intravenous, subcutaneous, and intrathoracic inoculations with pneumococci of varying grades of virulence were made in normal and in predisposed animals, with a view of retesting and corroborating the results similar methods had given in other hands. A number of tracheal injections with pneumococci of varying degrees of virulence were made in normal animals with the same object in view. The series of researches on predisposed animals with tracheal injections were thus accurately controlled. The predisposition was secured in three ways: the systemic susceptibility was increased by a chronic phenylhydrazin poisoning; the lung was locally injured by exposure to severe cold; and finally, by combining the two methods, a predisposition both local and systemic was obtained. In sets* of parallel experiments the effect of these forms of predisposition upon the development of pneumonic infection was studied by the tracheal injection of pneumococci of low and of high virulence.

Attempts to Induce Pneumonia in the Uninjured or Normal Rabbit. *Subcutaneous, intravenous,* and *intrathoracic*† inoculation of normal animals with pneumococci of varying grades of virulence failed to give rise to exudative pneumonia. *Tracheal injection* of

* Each set comprised three rabbits, not including the controls.

† Of fifteen normal rabbits, four cats, and one guinea-pig, inoculated through the right chest-wall, one cat developed a typical but small area of diffuse pneumonitis. The lungs of the other animals were comparatively free from lesions, although all the rabbits and the guinea-pig died, and local processes were found in the pleura and pericardium.

these organisms, however, yielded variable results. Pneumococci of low virulence when injected through the trachea had practically no effect on the lung and were rapidly disposed of. More virulent organisms incited varying, but for the most part small, central areas of exudative pneumonitis: of seven animals inoculated by the trachea, four died, and in two of these typical and extensive lesions of diffuse pneumonitis were found at autopsy. Pneumococci of still greater virulence injected through the trachea of five normal rabbits incited fatal bacteriæmic infections, with small areas of central bronchopneumonitis in but two. Thus in my experiments on normal animals, as in those of other observers, the diffuse lesions of exudative pneumonitis were rarely incited, and only when pneumococci of just the requisite grade of virulence were injected through the trachea; higher grades inducing fatal bacteriæmias, lower grades proving harmless.

Attempts to Induce Pneumonia in the Poisoned or Systemically Predisposed Rabbit. In order to determine the effect of increasing the rabbit's systemic susceptibility upon the development of pneumonic infection, studies were made with intravenous inoculation and with tracheal injection of pneumococci of high and of low virulence on animals previously poisoned with phenylhydrazin hydrochlorate. As brought out by many researches, notably those of Heinz,[85] Kaminer,[96] Mya and Sanarelli,[128] and Lubarsch,[116] this drug in rabbits, besides many interesting but for the present purposes unimportant structural changes in the blood elements, gives rise to severe grades of anæmia of a secondary pernicious type with hæmoglobinæmia, hæmoglobinuria, and albuminuria. Various stages of parenchymatous degeneration and an œdematous condition of the tissues are also to be found in such animals.

Six rabbits previously poisoned by the repeated subcutaneous administration of phenylhydrazin in small doses were divided into two sets and injected through the trachea with pneumococci of low and of high virulence, respectively. All died in from twelve to fifty-six hours of a general bacteriæmic infection, and the only pneumonic lesion found was a small patch of exudative pneumonitis in the rabbit which lived fifty-six hours. The development of rapidly fatal general infections with little or no lung lesion in these poisoned animals, whether inoculated in the ear vein or through the trachea, and whether cultures of high virulence or of low virulence were used, shows that such rabbits are even less favorable subjects for the experimental incitement of diffuse lesions than the normal animal. The studies were then directed to the effect of increasing the local susceptibility of the lung.

Attempts to Induce Pneumonia in the Injured Lung or Locally Predisposed Rabbit. An increase in the susceptibility of the lung without much disturbance of the system at large is obviously best accomplished by means of local irritation. Such methods have been so exhaustively studied by others and have proved, in the rabbit at least, so consistently unsatisfactory as a means of obtaining diffuse lesions that exposure to cold—another method of rendering the lung more susceptible—was adopted.

The animals were tied to trays and placed in ice baths at temperatures of 7° C. to 12° C. for five minutes. Immediately after the bath the animals were taken from the trays and wiped with towels. After these exposures various changes were noted. In the lungs large and small areas of hyperæmia and congestion, occasionally small hemorrhagic extravasations were found. The rectal temperature fell for a period of five, ten, or even twenty minutes after the bath; the lowest observed in animals which recovered was 26.5° C.

A general bacteriæmic infection without lung lesions followed the intravenous inoculation of these animals with pneumococci of varying degrees of virulence, and the exposure of normal rabbits to cold when combined with the tracheal injection of pneumococci also proved an inadequate means of securing definite pneumonic lesions. A study of the effect of combining these methods was therefore made.

Attempts to Induce Pneumonia in the Systemically and Locally Predisposed Rabbit. Intravenous inoculation as heretofore failed to give rise to local processes in the lung and similarly the tracheal injection of the more virulent pneumococci incited but little reaction* in the lungs of these animals, all three of which died of a general infection. With pneumococci of comparatively slight virulence the tracheal injection of these emaciated and exposed rabbits gave rise to extensive and diffuse lung reactions, which were considered typical and comparable to the lobar pneumonias of man in two of the three animals of the experiment.

Of these three rabbits: one died in twenty hours and developed slight bronchial reactions similar to those found in the animals injected with the more virulent organisms; another died in thirty hours, and diffuse lesions in an early stage involved the upper portion of the lower and the lower portion of the upper left lobes; the third lived four and one-half days, and at autopsy typical red and gray hepatization, macroscopically and microscopically, were found in the upper left lobe.

Summary of the Researches on Normal and Predisposed Animals. It was thus finally possible to approximate at least the balance of conditions as to the virulence of the bacteria on the one hand and on the other the special degrees of local and systemic susceptibility of the animal necessary for the development of typical diffuse lesions of the lung. With an increased susceptibility of the animal pneumococci of low virulence only could be used. More-

* One rabbit of the set of three lived sixty hours and showed more marked lesions than the others which died in twenty-four and thirty-six hours. None of the lesions were typical.

over, both the local and systemic susceptibility of the animal in varying degrees must be increased. Such a fine balance of conditions, it is obvious, might not always be easily obtained, and the practical solution of the problem had to be sought along other lines.

Heretofore, in the experiments of others and in my own described above, the predisposition was secured by methods which increased the susceptibility of the animal to infection. In the lungs of such animals organisms of sufficient virulence to incite extensive lesions gave rise to a rapidly fatal bacteriæmia, and the reaction of the body tissues was thereby generalized or inhibited, so that the local processes failed to develop. The attempts of others to obviate this early development of a bacteriæmic infection by selecting less susceptible animals for experimentation having proved uncertain and as yet impracticable, I sought a method of rendering the rabbit less susceptible to such infection. As this could easily be accomplished by immunization, my studies were directed to this field of experimentation.

Attempts to Induce Pneumonia in the Immunized Rabbit.

Preliminary Experiments. Two animals were immunized by the inoculation of non-virulent cultures of pneumococci. Their blood serum failed to agglutinate pneumococcus cultures in dilution of 1:1, and they died from the virulent tracheal injection in twelve and eighty hours. Two other rabbits were immunized by the subcutaneous inoculation of virulent pneumococci, which induced serious but not fatal local disease processes. Their blood sera agglutinated the pneumococcus cultures in dilution of 1:1, and they survived the tracheal injection. In the rabbit which died twelve hours after the tracheal injection, an early stage of an exudative pneumonitis involving the whole left lung was found at autopsy. Similarly extensive and diffuse lesions of a later stage were present in the animal which lived eighty hours. The other two rabbits recovered from the effects of the tracheal injection and were killed on the third day. Lesions of a resolving diffuse exudative pneumonia involving large areas in one animal and small, more circumscribed areas in the other were found in the lungs.

Additional researches were divided into three sets of experiments, respectively, comprising: five immunized and two normal rabbits, four immunized and three normal rabbits, four immunized and two normal rabbits. Of the thirteen immunized rabbits injected through the trachea, but one died of the infection, and of the seven normal animals three recovered from the inoculation. Diffuse and typical lesions were incited in a considerable proportion of the animals, and the processes were more marked and more frequently found in the immunized than in the normal control animals; but the difference was not sufficiently definite, and it was evident that there were certain errors in the methods used. Obviously either the virulence of the pneumococci inoculated or the degree of immunization attained by the animals was at fault.

At first the immunization of the animals was thought to have been inadequate, but the fallacy in this was apparent on recalling the fact that many animals had died in the process of immunization, and the survivors used for the experiment, though often greatly emaciated, withstood the virulent tracheal injection. By means of a specially devised technique insuring accurate results* the blood sera of these animals was tested as to its agglutinative action on pneumococcus cells, and the results were compared with those obtained with other blood sera of better-known strength. Thus it was determined that the rabbits had attained an extremely high degree of immunization.

The cultures used for inoculation were of pneumococci grown in exudates taken from animals dying of pneumococcus infection and diluted with broth in about equal proportions. Inoculation with such cultures often failed to kill the normal rabbit, whereas cultures of this pneumococcus in broth or in normal sera by tracheal injection or by intravenous inoculation in much smaller doses ($\frac{1}{400}$ c.c.) invariably proved fatal. A similar loss of virulence in organisms grown in immune sera was noted by Metschnikoff,[122] and that this loss in virulence is only apparent, not real, was determined by the researches of Metschnikoff's pupils, Isaeff[94] and Arkharow,[1] and also by the recent studies of Walker.[186] The lack of virulence in the tracheal injections of my experiments was therefore attributed to the presence, in the exudates used for culture media, of protective substances, which, in the lungs of the immunized or even of the fresh normal rabbit, became active. In this way an effect was obtained comparable to a lack of virulence not actually existing in the pneumococci.

It thus became evident that in these researches, as compared with the first preliminary experiments, the conditions essential to the development of pneumonic processes in the rabbit had unwittingly been altered by the above-noted errors in technique; so much so in fact that the necessary balance for the formation of typical diffuse lesions was present in a majority but not in all of the immunized animals.

Final Experiments. By avoiding what in the previous experiments seemed to be the chief faults, namely, a too high degree of immunization in the animal, and a neutralization of the virulent inoculation, more complete results were expected and obtained in a final experiment on eleven immunized† and five normal rabbits.

* Fully described in a paper published in the Journal of Medical Research, 1903, vol. x., No. 2.

† Eight normal rabbits in the process of immunization received: *March* 6, 1903. 1.5 c.c of a salt solution suspension of pneumococcus cells dissolved by normal rabbit bile: subcutaneous. *10th.* 5 c.c. sterilized broth culture of pneumococci: intravenous. *12th.* 2 c.c. of the bile solu-

March 6, 1903. The eleven immunized and five normal control rabbits were tracheally injected with 1 c.c. of a culture of the extremely virulent pneumococci grown in normal rabbits' serum diluted with broth.

Of the five control animals, three died in forty-eight hours without lung lesions; a fourth lived four days, and a small area of exudative pneumonitis was found at autopsy. The fifth was dying on the fifth day, when it was killed, and a similar lesion of the lung was found in this animal.

Of the eleven immunized animals none died; but a few were seriously ill for twenty-four to thirty-six hours. The first set of eight were killed on the third day; the second set of three on the fourth day after the tracheal injection. The various lesions of acute diffuse pneumonitis involving considerable areas of the left lung were present at autopsy. The smallest lesion found in any of these rabbits comprised at least a quarter of the lower lobe. In one animal, however, the entire left lung, with the exception of the lowermost tip, was solid. Cross-section showed the granular appearance seen more markedly in the human lung.

SUMMARY OF THE EXPERIMENTS ON IMMUNIZED ANIMALS. It is evident from these experiments that in the lungs of immunized rabbits virulent pneumococci do not give rise to an early general infection, but are confined to the lung, where, if the animal be not too highly immunized, they develop, inducing disease processes comparable to the lobar pneumonia of man. In the experimental control of these conditions under which diffuse lesions may be obtained, there are but two chief variable factors to be considered—the virulence of the micro-organism on the one hand, and the degree of immunization on the other—both easily and accurately determined by the ordinary routine methods of the modern laboratory.

GENERAL CONSIDERATIONS.

THE HISTOLOGY OF THE EXPERIMENTAL PNEUMONIAS. The type of inflammation in all the experimental lesions obtained with the pneumococcus was purely exudative and diffuse, usually with abundant formation of fibrin. All stages in the development of the reactions were present in the different lesions, and it was impossible to draw any sharp lines of distinction between the simple bronchitis and the bronchopneumonic reactions, or between the bronchopneumonias and the diffuse lobar lesions. The one merged gradually into that of the other, although the types were easily distinguished.

The leukocytes were usually numerous and particularly prominent

tion of pneumococcus cells: subcutaneous. *26th*. 1.5 c.c. of clear salt solution extract of pneumococcus cells: intravenous.

Three normal rabbits in the process of immunization received: *March* 2, 1903. 3 c.c. of a salt solution suspension of sediment from pneumococcus growth in glucose broth; intravenous. *3d*. 3 c.c. subcutaneous.

in the early stages of the lesion. The exfoliation of epithelium also occurred early in the process, but the desquamated cells were relatively more numerous in the later stages. Few fibrin fibrils could be found in the very early stages, but granules were often abundant. As has been noted by Kohn,[103] Hauser,[82] Bezzola,[21] and others, the fibrin developed and was more abundant in the early stages along the walls of the air spaces, and in places the fibrils could be traced from one alveolus to another. In the more advanced lesions the fibrin formation was most marked in the centre of the exudate, a clearer zone lying next the alveolar wall.*

The pneumococci were present, often in large numbers, in all the early stages of the lesions. The cocci were for the most part outside the cells. In resolving lesions the bacteria were often absent, even though large portions of the lung were involved. This was particularly noticeable in the lesions which were found in the immunized animals. Areas of irregular development gave to the lobar lesions during the early stages a patchy appearance. These areas may or may not correspond with the lobule of the lung; certainly they were not as distinct as the lobular patches present in human lobar pneumonia, nor could the intralobular structure described by Bezzola[21] and Ribbert[151] be definitely made out. The lung of the rabbit doubtless offers certain differences in the anatomical structure or arrangement of its lobules which may possibly explain these slight discrepancies. Furthermore, the posture of the animal doubtless influences the absorption and accumulation of exudates in the lung and thus, to some extent, the character of the lesion.

The Development of Experimental Pneumonia. It is obvious that the development of localized disease processes in the lung, as elsewhere, is determined by conditions referable either to the infecting micro-organism or to the animal infected. The infecting micro-organisms are extremely susceptible to environmental influences and thus exhibit considerable biological variation of both species and race. The biological character of the bacterial species as regards the peculiarities of growth and the elaboration of toxins and the special adaptation of the individual or race to the animal infected, commonly though inadequately expressed by the term virulence, are thus essential determining, but extremely variable factors in the development of all infections. On the other hand, the animals infected, within certain variable limits, afford favorable or unfavorable environments for the incitants of infection; in short, the animals are in varying degrees susceptible of infection.† This

* In distended or inflated lungs an artefact is often produced which should not be confused with these appearances.

† An important and co-operating factor intimately associated with the susceptibility of the animal is the chemotaxis. In animals very susceptible to certain infections it has been shown experimentally that, with extremely virulent cultures of the incitants, the chemotaxis is negative. In less susceptible animals or in immunized animals or with less virulent incitants the chemotaxis is in varying degrees positive.

susceptibility may be local as affecting certain tissues or parts of the animal or it may be systemic. When the bacterial incitant is extremely virulent or the animal very susceptible a systemic infection is induced, but when the bacterial incitant is less virulent or the animal only partially susceptible, a local infection is induced.

The morphological character of the disease processes depends in part upon the grades of susceptibility in the animal tissues, but chiefly upon the nature and virulence of the bacterial incitants, which, as noted above, are extremely variable. Different races of the same bacterial species thus often give rise to very different types of lesion in different or even in the same species of animal. Similarly, according to the degree of specialization necessary in the bacterial incitant, the different types of lesion may each be induced by a large or a small number of bacterial species or even by only one species, as in the so-called specific lesions. For example, in the lung, many different kinds of bacteria give rise to bronchopneumonia, but few to diffuse lobar pneumonia, and only one, the tubercle bacillus, to a specific productive necrotic process called tuberculosis.

Owing to the special anatomical arrangement of the epithelial, vascular, and lymphatic tissues of the lung, and to the physiological or pathological adaptation of these tissues, the lung surface acts, to some extent, similarly to the skin and mucous membrane as a barrier to infection, yet is peculiarly fitted not only for the rapid absorption and elimination of toxic material, but for the rapid diffusion of such material and the accumulation of exudates. The problem of infection in the lung is thus obviously complicated, and the relationship between the above-cited essential factors of infection more subtle than in other parts of the body. For most bacteria the normal lung is unfavorable, and similarly for the bacteria commonly found in pneumonic lesions the lung, as compared with other tissues, is, in most animals, a less favorable environment; thus for infection of the lung special adaptation or virulence of the bacterial excitant is essential. If this virulence be too great, the micro-organisms gain early access to and develop more rapidly in the other more favorable tissues of the susceptible animals. If this virulence be moderate, localized processes are incited in the lung, the surface of which, acting as a barrier to infection, prevents the invasion of the more susceptible tissues until the animal becomes, in a measure, immunized or the organisms acquire the requisite virulence for systemic infection. For the development of extensive diffuse lesions of the lung a relatively extreme adaptation or virulence of the incitant is obviously essential; thus these lesions rarely develop in animals very susceptible to the infection. Furthermore, bacteriæmias, whether temporary or terminal, are apt to complicate such disease processes. A relative systemic insusceptibility, whether natural to the animal species or acquired by the individual,* is, therefore, an extremely important factor in the development of lobar pneumonia. For the formation of circumscribed or patchy lesions of the lungs less specialization or virulence of the incitant is required; thus the protective mechanism of the lung is usually an efficient barrier shielding the more susceptible tissues from infection, and bacteriæmias are comparatively rare. Occasionally, however, as in susceptible animals infected with incitants which possess or quickly attain a high virulence, a systemic infection supersedes the localized pneumonic lesion. Plague pneumonia is an apt illustration of the development of bronchopneumonia under these conditions, which, except for the lack of systemic insusceptibility, are the same as give rise to lobar pneumonia. Thus it is that in bronchopneumonia and in lobar pneumonia similar etiological conditions in slightly varying relationship give rise to slightly varying lesions differing only in type.

THE PNEUMONIC PROCESS IN MAN IN THE LIGHT OF THESE EXPERIMENTAL RESEARCHES ON ANIMALS. All grades of reaction from the idiopathic lung congestions (Maladie de Woillez) to the diffuse lobar pneumonic lesions may be induced by pneumococci in the lung of man. In these the different races of pneumococci exhibit wide variations in virulence. Carrière[32] found attenuated pneumococci in the lung congestions, whereas it is well known that those isolated from lobar lesions are usually extremely virulent. Eyre and Washbourn[61] tested four stocks of pneumococci: one from the sputum of a healthy person, three from pneumonia cases. The pneumonia cultures became excessively virulent by passing them through from eight to eleven rabbits, 0.00001 loop proving fatal in rabbits. The sputum culture was passed through forty-three rabbits before 0.001 loop was fatal, and fifty-three before 0.00001 loop proved fatal. The subsequent observations of these authors confirm the above-noted results.

It is well known that, relative to other species, man is more resistant† to pneumococcus infection. However, the resistance offered by different races of men varies greatly. Billings,[22] from the census report, found that the negro is markedly susceptible to pneumonic infection. Marchoux[118] reports an epidemic of pneumococcus infection of a bacteriæmic type occurring in a body of French colonial negro troops. Although disseminated lesions were present, well-

* This systemic insusceptibility may be acquired by individuals normally susceptible, in the early stages of the infection which may for a time be confined to the air spaces where the exudates collect: thus lobar pneumonia is occasionally induced in very susceptible animals. Such a fine balance of conditions is for the present at least beyond experimental control.

† The presence of the pneumococcus in the sputum of health and in many of the disease processes of the nose, throat, and ear suggests that more or less specific resistance may be developed at times in some if not in many individuals. By means of a special technique I have obtained agglutinin and precipitin reactions with the blood serum from certain animal species not usually susceptible to pneumococcus infection, and with the normal human sera, tests these reactions were more marked and developed in higher dilutions. (Journal of Medical Research, 1903, No. 2, vol. x.)

developed pneumonias were comparatively rare. Kolle[104] noted a similar epidemic among the negroes of South Africa, but lesions were found in the lungs of some of these cases. Brodie, Rogers, and Hamilton[27] studied two epidemics of severe general pneumococcus infection, characterized by rhinitis and gastrointestinal disturbances, occurring in the Kaffirs. Pneumonic lesions were rare. Tostivant and Remlinger[182] describe the marked susceptibility of certain Arab tribes to pneumococcus infection and the difference in the lesions induced.

Aside from racial susceptibility, the individual at different ages and under different conditions offers striking analogies, in some instances to the susceptible, in others to the resistant, animal. In general, the newborn and the infant are remarkably susceptible to infection. At this age lobar pneumonias are rare; infection of the lungs with pathogenic bacteria gives rise to the bronchopneumonic type of lesion. Here, then, is a direct analogy to the susceptible animal. In the adult, as in the resistant or immunized animal, lobar lesions are more commonly found in the primary pneumonias; but, on the other hand, the adult may be rendered in varying degrees susceptible by other disease processes, and exudative pneumonitis developing under these conditions, the so-called secondary pneumonia, is more apt to be of the bronchopneumonic type.

It has long been recognized clinically that in the lobar pneumonias of man there is no definite relation between the extent of the lesion and the gravity of the infection upon which a prognosis may be safely based. This is even more pronounced in the experimental pneumonias in animals, and, as shown by the researches on animals, is due to the fact that extensive lesions may be incited by virulent infections when confined to the lung without seriously endangering the life of the individual; whereas less extensive lesions are often followed by general infections which terminate fatally. Thus the lesions in the fatal lobar pneumonias of old people are often small, sometimes unrecognized; whereas the lungs of a robust individual with good protective resources may be extensively involved, and yet recovery take place. As suggested by the researches on animals, the generalization of the infection is the real danger. Upon the determination of this only can a prognosis be safely based.

It is therefore evident that the various phenomena of pneumococcus infection observed in animal inoculation also occur in man. The rule of one is, however, the exception of the other; thus, general infections, except as transitory or terminal conditions complicating the local processes are comparatively rare in man, but common in the ordinary laboratory animal.

Summary and Conclusions.

As a result of the numerous and varied researches of other observers it has been determined that the bronchi and lung under normal conditions are practically free from micro-organisms; that the secretions of the upper respiratory tract in both health and disease often harbor the bacteria commonly found in pneumonia, namely, the pneumococcus, the streptococcus, the staphylococcus, and the pneumobacillus; that the incitants of pneumonia may be carried to the lung by the lymph channels, inducing an interstitial pleuropneumonitis; or by the bloodvessels, giving rise to secondary metastatic processes; or, as is usual, by the air-passages, inciting the various lesions of exudative pneumonitis, of which two main types, the bronchopneumonic and the diffuse lobar, are recognized; and, finally, that the bronchopneumonic lesions, whether arising in man or induced experimentally in animals, may be incited by a great variety of bacteria, most frequently by the pneumococcus or the streptococcus; whereas, comparatively few species of bacteria give rise to diffuse lesions in animals, and in man practically but one species, the pneumococcus, ever attains the necessary specialization for the incitement of lobar pneumonia.

In the researches of others patchy or circumscribed lesions comparable to the bronchopneumonia of man, have been induced experimentally with comparatively little difficulty. Previous attempts to induce diffuse lobar lesions in animals, though successful in a few exceptional instances, have failed to determine the exact conditions under which the lesion develops and offer no reliable method of securing typical pneumonic processes.

By means of accurately controlled series of experiments which allowed of precise comparison, it was possible in my researches to determine the effect of increasing or diminishing the virulence of the incitant, the pneumococcus, in systemically predisposed, in locally predisposed, and in both systemically and locally predisposed animals. These experiments show that the incitement of diffuse lesions in the normal rabbit is extremely uncertain, and only possible in the predisposed rabbit when both the general and local susceptibility are increased and when organisms of comparatively low virulence are used. Thus, and owing chiefly to the fact that the lung surface acts as a barrier to infection, the development of acute exudative pneumonitis offers an especially clear example of the nice balancing of the essential conditions determining infection. These conditions are, on the one hand, the specialization or virulence of the incitant, and, on the other hand, the animal susceptibility, both local and systemic. Organisms of low virulence induce evanescent bronchial reactions; more virulent organisms by a local infection, give rise to the more typical bronchopneumonic lesions; while organisms of still greater virulence, if confined to the lung, incite diffuse processes of the lobar type, but if not so confined and bacteriæmic infection occurs, the lung lesions are less marked and of the bronchopneumonic type. The extremely fine balance of these conditions essential to the formation of lobar lesions in normal as well as in predisposed animals is as yet for practical purposes beyond experimental control.

Finally, as a result of these systematic researches on normal and predisposed animals, an entirely new procedure was adopted: the preliminary immunization of the rabbits, so that extremely virulent cultures of pneumococci can be used without giving rise to bacteriæmic infection. The experiments with this procedure showed that diffuse exudative lesions comparable to the lobar pneumonia of man may be incited experimentally in the immunized rabbit; and that in securing this result there are but two chief variable factors, the virulence of the incitant and the immunization of the animal; both easily and accurately controlled by the routine technique of the modern laboratory.

I am deeply indebted to Professor T. Mitchell Prudden and to Professor Philip Hanson Hiss, Jr., for their suggestions and criticism.

BIBLIOGRAPHY.

1. Arkharow. Archiv. de méd. exp., 1892, p. 498.
2. Arloing. Journ. de physiol. et de path. gén., 1902, p. 291. Bibliog.
3. Arnold. Untersuchungen über Staubinhalation u. Staubmetastase, Leipzig, 1885.
4. Arustamow. Woenno-Medicinskij, 1889, Hft. 2–4. Baumgarten Jahrbrt., 1889, p. 61.
5. Aufrecht. Nothnagel specielle Path. u. Therapie, 1899, part ii. vol. xiv. pp. 1–63. Bib.
6. Aufrecht. Ibid., pp. 55, 56.
7. Baduel. Riforma Medica, 1899, No. 15, p. 170.
8. Banti. Lo Sperimentale, 1890, vols. lxv.–lxvi. pp. 349, 461, 573.
9. Barthel. Centralblatt f. Bakt., 1898, vol. xxiv. pp. 401, 433, 574–577.
10. Baumgarten. Mycologie, 1889, vol. ii. p. 602.
11. Batzaroff. Annales de l'Institut Pasteur, 1899, p. 385.
12. Beco. Archiv. de médecine expér., 1899, p. 317.
13. Beco. Ibid., 1901, p. 51. Bibliog
14. Behring and Nissen. Zeitschrift f. Hygiene, 1890, vol. viii. p. 412
15. Bein. Charité Annalen, 1895, vol. xx. Bibliog.
16. Belfanti. La Riforma Med., 1890, vol. i. p. 338.
17. v. Besser. Ziegler's Beiträge, 1889, vol. vi. p. 333.
18. v. Besser. Ibid., p. 339.
19. v. Besser. Ibid., pp. 351–362.
20. Bezancon and Griffon. Soc. méd. des hôpitaux, April 15, 1898.
21. Bezzola. Virchow's Archiv, 1894, vol. cxxxvi. p. 345.
22. Billings. Census Report, 1890
23. Boni. Deutsches Arch. f. klin. Med., 1901, vol. lxix. p. 542. Bibliog.
24. Bordonni-Uffredozzi. Centralblatt f. Bakt., 1891, p. 305.
25. Bosc aud Galavielle. Soc. de biol., 1898, p. 981.
26. v. Breitenstein. Archiv f. exper. Path. u. Pharm., 1896, vol. xxxvii. p. 253. Bibliog.
27. Brodie, Rogers, and Hamilton. Lancet, 1898, p. 1045.
28. Buchner. Munchener med. Wochenschrift, 1899, pp. 1261 and 1301.
29. Buchner, Merkel, and Enderlen. Archiv f. Hygiene, 1888, vol. viii.
30. Buttersack. Zeitschr. f. klin. Med., vol. xix. p. 411. Bibliog.
31. Calamida and Bertarelli. Centralblatt f. Bakt., 1902, vol. xxxii. p. 428.
32. Carrière. Revue de méd., 1898, pp. 765 and 951. Ibid., 1899, p. 54. Presse méd., Jan. 27, 1898.
33 Carnot and Fournier. Archiv. de méd. exper., 1900, vol. xii. pp. 367–369.
34. Charrin and Ruffer. Compt.-rend. de la Soc. de la biol., 1889, p. 208.
35. Chelmonski. Deutsches Archiv f. klin. Med., 1897, vol. lix. p. 140.
36. Chester. Report of Delaware Agricultural Experimental Station, 1899–1900.
37. Chvostek. Ueber das Wesen der Hemoglobinurie, Leipzig u. Wien, 1894. Bibliog.
38. Claisse. Les infectiones bronchique, Paris, 1893. La semaine méd., 1893, No. 38, pp. 297–300.

39. Coco and Drago. Gazzetta degli ospitali, 1899, p. 104.
40. Comby. Traité de mal. de l'enfance, 1898, vol. iv. p. 56.
41. Czmetscha. Prager med. Wochenschr., 1894, vol. xix. p. 233.
42. Delestre. Compt.-rend. de la Soc. de biol., 1898, p. 150.
43. Dieudonne. Arbeit. a. d. kaiserl. Gesundheitsamte, 1894, vol. ix. p. 492.
44. Durck. Deutsches Archiv f. klin. Med., 1897, vol. lviii. pp. 368–415.
45. Durck. Ibid., pp. 418–429.
46. Durck. Ibid., pp. 435–444. Bibliog.
47. Durig and Lode. Archiv f. Hygiene, 1901, vol. xxxix. p. 46. Bibliog.
48. Ehrlich. Zeitschrift f. klin. Med., 1881, vol. iii. p. 383.
49. Ebstein. Arch. f. exper. Path., vol. ii.
50. Eisenmann. Archiv f. Wissensch. Heilk., 1862, vol. vi. p. 325.
51. Emmerich. Fortschritte der Med., vol. ii. p. 153.
52. Emmerich. Seventh International Congress of Hygiene, London, 1891. British Medical Journal, 1891, pp. 379, 380.
53. Emmerich. Münchener med. Wochenschr., 1891, p. 554.
54. Enderlen. Deutsch. Zeitsch. f. klin. Med., vol. xv. p. 50.
55. Eppinger. Die Hadenkrankheit., Lubarsch and Ostertag, 1896.
56. Ernst. Ziegler's Beiträge, 1890, vol. viii. p. 203.
57. Esser. Centralblatt f. d. gesammte Med., January 26, 1901.
58. Esser. Arch. f. exper. Path. u. Pharm., 1903, vol. xlix. p. 200. Bibliog.
59. Eve. Journal of Physiology, 1900, vol. xxvi. p. 119.
60. Ewing. Clinical Pathology of the Blood, 1903. p. 289.
61. Eyre and Washbourn. Lancet, 1899, vol. i, p. 19.
62. Finkler. Die Acuten Lungenentzundungen, 1891.
63. Finkler. Thesis, 1895, Bonn, Baumgarten Jahrbt., 1895.
64. Fischl. Zeitschrift f. Heilk., vol. xviii. p. 321. Prager med. Wochenschr., 1897, p. 49.
65. Fleck. Diss., Bonn, 1886.
66. Foa and Rattone. Gazzetta degli ospitali, 1885, No. 12, p. 94.
67. Fraenkel. Zeitschrift f. klin. Med., vol. x. p. 401; vol. xi. p. 437. Bibliog.
68. Fraenkel. Ibid., pp. 417, 418.
69. Fraenkel. Ibid., p. 423.
70. Frenkel. Achiv. de méd. exper., 1892, p. 638.
71. Friedländer. Virchow's Archiv, 1882, vol. lxxxvii. p. 319. Fortschr. der Med., 1883, vol. vii. p. 715.
72. Gamaleia. Annales de l'Institut Pasteur, 1888, p. 440.
73. Gauthier. Lyon méd., 1900, vol. xcv. pp. 329, 372.
74. Gobell. Diss., 1897, Marburg.
75. Grammatschikoff. Arb. a d. Geb. de path. anat., Inst. zu Tübingen, 1891, p. 450.
76. Grawatz. Zeitschrift f. klin. Med., 1892, vol. xxi. p. 459. Centralbl. f. inn. Med., 1894, vol. xv. p. 33.
77. Grawitz and Steffen. Berl. klin. Wochenschr., 1894.
78. Griffini and Cambria. Giornales internazionale de sc. méd., 1882, vol. iv. p. 353. Archiv. ital. de biol., 1883, vol. iii. p. 189.
79. Grober. Deutsches Archiv f. klin. Med., vol. lxviii. p. 296.
80. Guarnieri. Atti d. e. accad. med. di Roma, 1888, Ser. 2, vol. iv. p. 97.
81. Hadl. Inaug. Diss., Würzburg, 1896.
Hauser. Münch. med. Wochenschr., 1893, p. 155.
. Hegglin. Zeitschr. f. klin. Med., 1894, vol. xxvi.
. Heidenhain. Virchow's Archiv, 1877, vol. lxx. p. 441.
Heinz. Ziegler's Beiträge, 1901, vol. xxix. p. 299.
Hermann. Annales de l'Institut Pasteur, 1891, p. 243.
Hermann, L. Pflüger's Archiv, 1870, vol. iii. p. 8.
Heymann. Berliner klin. Wochenschr., 1872, p. 447.
82. Hildebrandt. Ziegler's Beiträge, 1888, vol. ii. p. 411.
[illegible] Hiss. Centralblatt f. Bact., vol. xxxi. p. 302.
91. Hoffmann. Nothnagel's Specielle Pathologie, 1896, vol. xiii. (Th. iii. abth. i.).
92. Hopkins. International Dental Journal, August, 1903.
93. Howard. Cleveland Journal of Medicine, 1900, vol. v. p. 450.
94. Isaeff. Annales de l'Institut Pasteur, vol. vii. p. 260.
95. James and Tuttle. Presbyterian Hospital Reports (New York), vol. iii.
96. Kaminer. Zeitschr. f. klin. Med., 1900, vol. xli. p. 91.
97. Kasparek. Wiener klin. Wochenschr., 1895, pp. 570, 593.
98. Klaskalt. Münchener med. Wochenschr., 1900, p. 110.

99. Kisskalt. Archiv f. Hygiene, 1900, vol. xxxix. p. 142. Bibliog.
100. Klebs. Archiv f. exper. Path., vol. iv. p. 420.
101. Klein. Centralblatt f. d. med. Wiss., 1884, No. 30.
102. Klipstein. Zeitschr. f. klin. Med., 1898, vol. xxxiv. p. 191.
103. Kohn. Münch. med. Wochenschr., 1898, p. 42.
104. Kolle. Deutsches med. Wochenschr., 1898, p. 425.
105. Kreibach. Breiträge zur klin. Med. u. Chir., 1896, Heft 13, p. 1.
106. Kruse and Pansini. Zeitschr. f. Hygiene, 1892' vol. xi. pp. 337–355.
107. Kuttner. Centralblatt f. die med, Wissensch., 1875.
108. Laehr. Diss., Bonn, 1887.
109. Laschtschenko. Zeitschrift f. Hygiene, vol. xxx. p. 125.
110. Lassar. Virchow's Archiv, vol. lxxix. p. 168.
111. Lépine and Lyomet. Soc. de biol., 1899, p. 583. Compt.-rend. de la Acad. sc., Feb. 13, 1899.
112. Lipari. Il Morgagni, 1888, pp. 523, 575, 651.
113. Litten. Zeitschr. f. klin. Med., 1882, vol. v. p. 26.
114. Lode, Alois. Archiv f. Hygiene, 1897, vol. xxviii. p. 344. Bibliog.
115. Lode, A., and Durig, A. Münchener med. Wochenschr., 1900, p. 109.
116. Lubarsch. Geschwulsten u. Infectionskrankheiten, 1899, p. 144.
117. Marchand. Arch. f. path. Anat., 1887, vol. 109, p. 86.
118. Marchoux. Annales de l'Institut Pasteur, 1899, p. 198.
119. Massalongo. Archiv. de Physiol., 1885, 3d ser., T. vi.
120. Meltzer and C. Meltzer. Journal of Medical Research, 1903, No. 1, vol. x.
121. Meunier. Du rôle du systeme nerveux dans l'infection de l'appareil broncho-pulmonaire, Paris, 1896.
122. Metschnikoff. Annales de l'Institut Pasteur, 1887, vol. i. p. 42. Ibid., 1892, vol. vi. p. 297.
123. Miller. Dental Cosmos, 1891, vol. xxxiii.
124. Morisani. Arch. di Ost. e Ginec., 1897, vol. iv, p. 133.
125. Müller, W. Deutsches Archiv f. klin. Med., 1901, vol. lxxi, p. 513; and 1902, vol. lxxii. p. 80. Bibliog.
126. Müller, F. Münch. med. Wocenschr., 1897, No, 49, p. 1382. Bibliog.
127. Muskatbluth. Centralblatt f. Bakt., 1887, vol. i. p. 321.
128. Mya and Sanarelli. Vide Lubarsch.
129. Nassaroff. Virchow's Archiv, vol. xc. p. 482.
130. Nekam. Centralblatt f. Bakt., 1894, vol. xvi. p. 932.
131. Nenninger. Zeitschr. f. Hygiene, 1901, vol. xxxviii.
132. Netter. Soc. de biol., November 29, 1887; Traité de médecine (Bouchard-Brissaud), 1901, vol. vi. pp. 485, 486.
133. Netter. Ibid., pp. 475, 476.
134. Netter. Bulletin de la Soc. anat., April 9, 1886.
135. Netter. Traité de médecine (Bouchard-Brissaud), 1901, vol. vi. p. 506.
136. Neumann, R. Zeitschrift f. Hygiene, 1902, vol. xl. p. 33.
137. Orloff. Wratsch, 1887, pp. 385 and 401.
138. Ottolenghi. Arch. f. le Sc. Med., vol. xxii. p. 425.
139. Pane. Riforma medica, 1899, vol. iii. p. 376.
140. Pasteur. Bulletin de l'Acad. méd., 1878, vol. vii. p. 253.
141. Pearce. Boston Medical and Surgical Journal, No. 23, vol. cxxxvii. Bibliog.
142. Platania. Giornale internaz. delle sc. med., 1889, p. 344. Bibliog.
143. Pernici and Scagliosi. Riforma medica, 1892, pp. 97, 98.
144. Prudden and Northrup. THE AMERICAN JOURNAL OF THE MEDICAL SCIENCES, 1889.
145. Prochaska. Archiv f. klin. Med. vol. lxx. p. 559.
146. Reineboth. Münch. med. Wochenschr., 1898, p. 1170.
147. Reineboth. Deutsches Archiv f. klin. Med., 1899, vol. lxii. p. 63.
148. Reineboth. Ibid., 1900, vol. lxix. p. 144.
149. Reineboth and Kohlhardt. Ibid., vol. lxv. p. 192.
150. Reynaud Bulletin médicale, July 1, 1899. Bibliog.
151. Ribbert. Fortschritte der Med., 1894, p. 371; Virchow's Archiv, 1894, vol. cxxxvi. p. 359.
152. Ritchie. Journal of Pathology and Bacteriology, 1901, p. 13. Bibliog.
153. Roger. Compt.-rend. de la Soc. de biol., 1896.
154. Rosenthal. Inaug. Diss., Erlangen, 1893.
155. Rosenthal, J. Berliner klin. Wochenschr, 1872, p. 453.
156. Ruhemann. Thèse, Leipzig, 1898. Zeitschrift f. Krankenpflege, 1898.
157. Salvioli. Arch. per le sc. méd., 1884' No. 7, vol. 8.
158. Salvioli and Zaslein. Centralblatt d. med. Wiss., 1883, p. 721.

159. Sanarelli. Centralblatt f. Bact., 1891, vol. x. p. 817.
160. Sawtschenko. Ibid., vol. ix. p. 473.
161. Schild. München. med. Wochenschr., 1902, vol. xlix. p. 1569.
162. Schou. Fortschritte der Med., 1885, No. 15.
163. Schultz. Arch. de sc. de biologie, St. Petersburg, 1901, vol. viii. p. 1.
164. Sello. Zeitschrift f. klin. Med., vol. xxxvi. p. 112.
165. Silfast. Ziegler's Beiträge, 1899, vol. xxv.
166. Sittmann. Deutsches Arch. f. klin. Med., 1894, vol. liii. p. 323.
167. Slawjanski. Virchow's Archiv, 1869, vol. xlviii.
168. Souques. Presse médicale, 1900, p. 109. Bibliog.
169. Speck. Zeitschr. f. klin. Med., 1901, vol. xliii. p. 377.
170. Spolverini. Annali d'igiene sperim., 1899, p. 202.
171. Steffen. Centralblatt f. Bakt., 1895, vol. xviii. p. 464.
172. Sternberg. THE AMERICAN JOURNAL OF THE MEDICAL SCIENCES, 1885, vol xc. p. 117.
173. Sternberg. Text-Book of Bacteriology, 1893, p. 298.
174. Strachan. British Medical Journal, 1886.
175. Stroganoff. Centralblatt f. Gynäk., 1893, No. 40.
176. Talamon. Progrès méd., 1883, pp. 281, 301, and 1030.
177. Thayer. Johns Hopkins Hospital Bulletin, 1893, p. 37.
178. Thomson and Hewlett. Medical and Surgical Transactions, 1895, p. 239. British Medical Journal, 1896. vol. i. p. 137.
179. Thorner. Thèse, Munich, 1888. Cited by Netter.
180. Tschistovitch. Annales de l'Institut Pasteur, 1889, p. 337.
181. Tschistovitch. Ibid., 1890, vol iv. p. 285.
182. Tostivant and Remlinger. Archiv. de méd. et pharm. mil., 1901, vol. xxxviii. p. 107.
183. Veraguth. Virchow's Archiv, 1880, vol. lxxxiii. p. 238. Bibliog.
184. Viti. Arch. ital. di pediatris, 1890.
185. Wagner. Annales de l'Institut Pasteur, 1890, vol. iv. p. 570.
186. Walker. Journal Pathology and Bacteriology, 1902, vol, viii. p. 34.
187. Walthard. Centralblatt f. Bakt., 1895, vol. xvii. p. 311; Arch. f. Gynäk, vol. xlviii. pp. 233-244.
188. Walther. Virchow's Archiv, 1862, vol. xxv.
189. Wandel. Deutsches Archiv f. klin. Med., 1903, vol. lxxviii. p. 1.
190. Weichselbaum. Wiener med. Wochenschr., 1886, Nos. 39, 40, and 41.
191. Welch. Johns Hopkins Hospital Bulletin, 1892, p. 125.
192. Wertheim. Wiener med. Wochenschr., 1870.
193. White. Journal Experimental Medicine, vol. iv. p. 425.
194. Widal and Bezancon. Revue trimens. suisse d'odontolog., 1894, p. 185.
195. Winternitz. Centralblatt f. klin. Med., 1893, vol. xiv. p. 1017.
196. Wolf. Wiener med. Blätter, 1887, Nos. 10. 11, 12, 13, and 14.
197. Wright. New York Medical Journal, July 27, 1889.
198. Wurtz and Lemoyez. Compt.-rend. de la Soc. de biol., 1894.

HEREDITARY ŒDEMA.

BY ARTHUR WILLARD FAIRBANKS, M.D.,
OF BOSTON,
VISITING PHYSICIAN TO THE BOSTON FLOATING HOSPITAL FOR CHILDREN; PHYSICIAN TO THE BOSTON DISPENSARY.

ALTHOUGH the influence of heredity as a factor in the production of certain forms of œdema, not of cardiac or renal origin, was mentioned by Quincke in 1882, it was not until 1888, when Osler published the details of a case, that the subject attracted general notice in this country. This was probably due, first, to the eminent position held by the latter writer in the medical world, and, second, to the exceptionally favorable circumstances that enabled him to obtain a full and accurate history of the patient's antecedents. Too often, in our attempt to learn the family history of any given case, are we met by absolute ignorance on our patient's part of facts concerning even his immediate progenitors, or receive information possessing the authenticity of tradition.

Rarely are we permitted to look back, with reasonably accurate vision, four, five, or even six generations into our patient's past. Cases have, however, been reported of the affection we are considering in which we are afforded such privilege.

Dinkelacker,[1] a pupil of Quincke, wrote a dissertation in 1882 on acute œdema, using as the basis of the essay cases referred to later by Quincke.[2] Among these was a case of a watchmaker, who had for years been afflicted with periodical attacks of acute œdema, whose son, a child of one year, had suffered from his third month with the same affection.

In 1885 Valentin,[3] who had occasion to see this family after the appearance of the papers of these two observers, adds the interesting information that another son, then two years old, not born when the above observations were made, was also afflicted with similar attacks from the first week of life. Another child, a daughter, had shown no sign of the affection up to the time of observation.

In 1885 Strübing[4] reports a case in a man, aged seventy years, who for forty-five years had had attacks of acute œdema of the face, throat, pharynx, and larynx, the latter so severe that extreme dyspnœa ensued. This would last a few hours and then subside. Between his sixty-third and sixty-eighth year he was entirely free from the throat attacks; then without any evident cause he felt pain on swallowing, with beginning inspiratory dyspnœa. This increased rapidly until in fifteen minutes it had attained such a degree that tracheotomy seemed unavoidable. Respiration was attended with the highest degree of orthopnœa, with action of all the accessory muscles. This condition lasted for a few minutes, then gradually subsided, until six hours later no sign of the distress remained. Now, however, œdema of the face and genitals developed. Four days later all disturbance had disappeared. More frequently than the attacks of œdema have occurred since his twenty-sixth year, at intervals of four to six weeks, attacks of severe vomiting, preceded by a slight sensation of abdominal pain, increasing in intensity up to the culmination in the vomiting. These attacks were attended by marked prostration and followed by sleep, out of which he awoke feeling well. At times the attack was ended in three or four hours, after vomiting four or five times. On other occasions it lasted twenty-four hours, with twenty to thirty repetitions of the emesis.

His sixteen-year-old son suffered from his third year with similar attacks, except that œdema was not so marked a feature. Much more frequent were the attacks of vomiting, in which a large quantity of fluid was ejected. A daughter also suffered from attacks similar to those of her father.

Falcone[5] reports a case of acute recurrent œdema in a child, aged seven years, whose grandfather was afflicted with similar attacks.

Osler,[6] in 1888, reported a case of great interest in which, through the fortuitous recollections of some of the members of the family, and especially the unimpaired memory of a great-grandfather, aged ninety-two years, who had himself been afflicted for seventy-four years, a history of the affection extending through five generations, and involving twenty-two members, was obtained.

The characteristics of the affection in this family noted by Osler were: the occurrence of local swellings in various parts of the body; the almost invariable association of gastrointestinal disturbance, —colic, nausea, vomiting, and sometimes diarrhœa; the strongly marked hereditary disposition:

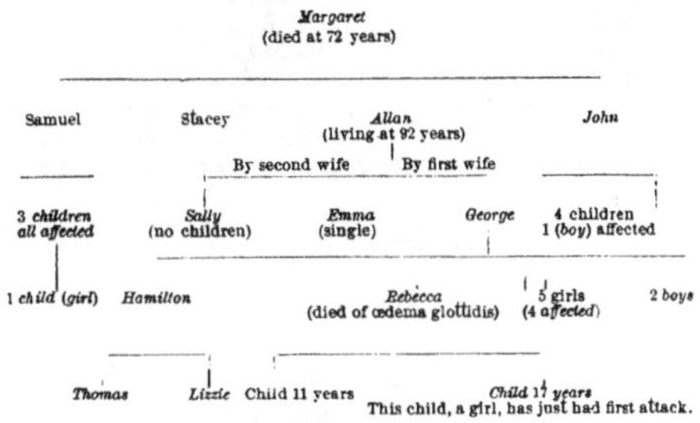

Krieger[7] cites a case in a man, aged twenty-five years, whose mother was also affected.

In one of Smith's[8] cases, that of a young woman, subject to recurrent attacks of œdema, the mother was similarly affected.

Fritz[9] gives the history of a man, aged twenty-three years, who fell and struck on the right temple. Shortly after the left eyelid began to swell, until the eye became completely closed. The swelling extended to cheek, lip, and neck. On entrance to the hospital there were cyanosis, dyspnœa, almost entire aphonia, and frothy expectoration. Examination showed the uvula swollen, the left tonsil, the left pillar of fauces, and the left side of the glottis very œdematous. During the night the swelling appeared in the right side of the face, subsiding in the places where it had first made its appearance. On the following day it entirely left the face, but appeared in the right foot and ankle. Lungs and heart normal. Urine 900 c.c., 1022, acid. Urea, 28.8 grams. No albumin or sugar. He was otherwise well and had always been so, except that after drinking on an empty stomach, overeating, or after slight injuries, swelling, usually in extremities and eyelids, would ensue. These attacks had occurred since he was four years old. His paternal grandmother died of œdema of the glottis. One aunt had recurrent attacks of œdema. Two cousins, children of this aunt, died of œdema of the glottis. One of his sisters is also affected with attacks of glottic œdema. Both of his brothers died with the same form of œdema. Eight members in all were affected in this family.

Roy[10] mentions cases of acute circumscribed œdema in a mother and her daughter.

Ricochon[11] reports three generations of acute œdema, accompanied by colic, vomiting, meteorism, fever, and malaise. His cases show a close symptomatic resemblance to the cases of Strübing, already mentioned, and to those of Yarian,[12] which follow. This patient was a woman, aged fifty-four years, who since childhood had acute attacks, commencing with general malaise, followed by swelling of some part of the body, usually the face or extremities, sometimes the shoulders or chest. One or two days later she is taken with very severe sharp pain in the region of the epigastrium, occasionally elsewhere over the abdomen, with marked prostration. This is soon followed by nausea and vomiting, with severe retching. Mental emotion is capable of precipitating an attack with great suddenness.

At times with the œdema, or just as it is subsiding, there have appeared "purple rings" on the chest, neck, arms, and hypogastrium. After free vomiting the pain and œdema disappear, and such an attack in the forenoon does not incapacitate her for work in the afternoon. The attacks appear on an average of every two weeks, nine weeks being the longest period during which she has been free from its occurrence. Her mother had identical attacks from childhood, and died at the age of sixty-three years, "from dropsy." After the menopause she also had attacks of purpura. Her uncle on her mother's side had similar attacks, and died at the age of forty-two years, from œdema of the glottis. This uncle left a child, a girl, who suffers from periodical œdema without the gastralgia and vomiting. A brother of this child, now dead, also had attacks. Her maternal grandfather and some of his brothers had similar attacks, but without the pain and vomiting. Her maternal great-grandfather also suffered with the affliction, but he, too, never had the pain or vomiting. This is as far back as the affection can be traced. Her two children, both girls, while of irritable disposition, never showed signs of her trouble. One died of tuberculosis when twenty-one years of age. The other is living at twenty-five years of age and married. Her grandchild by this daughter has thus far shown no evidence of the affection.

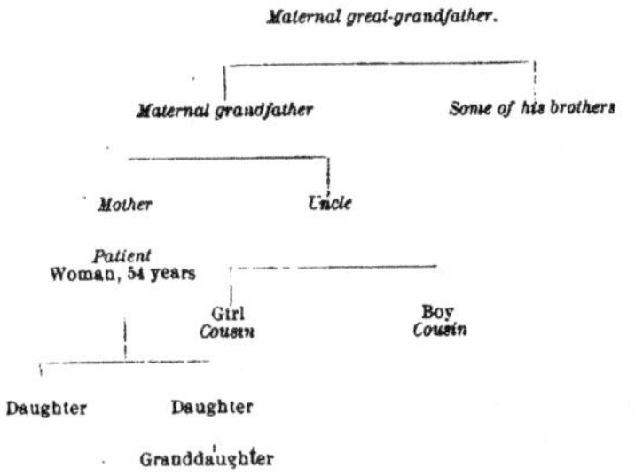

Schlesinger[13] cites an instance in which the affection appeared in four generations. The patient, a man, aged forty-four years, has been subject for twenty-two years to the following attacks:

Commencing with a subjective feeling of irritation or depression, an exanthem appears on some part of the body. After six or eight hours this disappears, then on some portion of the body a rapidly developing swelling occurs, usually attended by pain in the epigastrium. This swelling develops with great rapidity, reaching its maximum in a few moments, lasts from one to three days, and then disappears. In the earlier years it occurred every half-year, later on at intervals of every ten or eleven days.

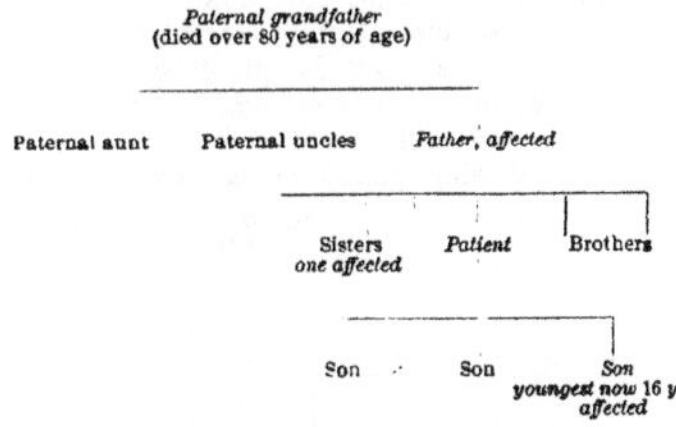

T. Wardrop Griffith,[14] of Leeds, reports a case of an adult woman, aged twenty-three years, who from infancy had been subject to attacks of localized œdema involving the hands, feet, shoulders, genitals, and throat. At the age of twenty-three years death occurred suddenly from laryngeal obstruction. Her father had been subject to similar attacks from earliest infancy. At the age of twenty-one years he had a laryngeal attack; a few years later another; and at the age of twenty-nine years a third attack caused his death. Examination of the larynx of the woman showed, in cross-sections, that the œdema involved not merely the mucous membrane, but also the deeper connective tissue, and even the substance of the muscles themselves, which condition Griffith thinks would prevent the abductors from enlarging the aperture during inspiration, and so lead to death.

These instances leave no doubt of the influence of heredity in some of these cases of acute œdema. The characteristics of this affection are recurrent attacks of acute œdema in varying portions of the body, usually of rapid development and brief duration, and often associated with disturbances of the gastrointestinal tract.

We now come to the consideration of a form of œdema with quite different characteristics. This variety is as slow in its development and as sluggish in its course as the form we have just described is acute and transient.

Higier[15] says, in speaking of œdema not of organic origin, but occurring in connection with some neurotic condition: "It may appear and disappear in some hours or some days, but it may also last the life long. It is not rarely hereditary." This would seem to indicate that this author regards these two forms as in close relationship. It is questionable, however, whether we are justified in so considering them, on the basis of their clinical characteristics.

Heredity is as strongly indicated in some of these chronic cases as in the above-cited acute forms. The features peculiar to this chronic form of œdema are swelling in one or more extremities or parts of an extremity, of gradual onset, and usually life-long course, unattended by pain or disturbance of the general health. Some slight exceptions to this definition may be found in individual cases; such as transient pain, or the presence of some coincident affection, usually of the nervous system; but they are so seldom as to but emphasize the rule.

The following remarkable cases are reported by Milroy:[16]

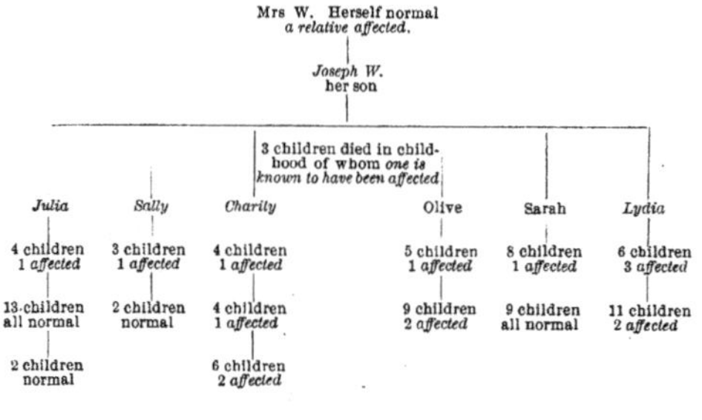

Of six generations, comprising ninety-seven individuals, over 22 per cent. were affected. In the third generation there were nine individuals, all children of one father. Of these, three died in childhood of unknown cause. Of the remaining six, four lived to be over seventy years of age, and two were eighty and eighty-two years, respectively, at time of death. The other two died at the ages of sixty-six and thirty-eight years. This indicates in a striking way how absolutely harmless this form of œdema appears to be. We shall see that it is, in this respect, in sharp contrast to the form we have previously considered.

Jopson[17] reports two cases of marked subcutaneous œdema of the lower extremities of congenital origin in children, aged four years and one and one-half years, respectively, whose father, during his childhood, had a similar condition, which disappeared as he became older. The swelling in both cases pitted on pressure. In the older child the foreskin at birth was also involved.

In 1899 Meige[18] reported cases of a similar affection occurring in eight members of one family through four generations. The reader is referred to his excellent article for photographs of the condition.

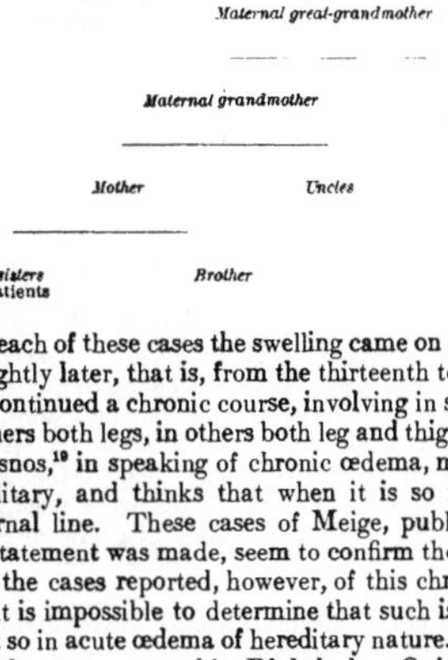

In each of these cases the swelling came on at the period of puberty or slightly later, that is, from the thirteenth to the twenty-third year, and continued a chronic course, involving in some cases only one leg, in others both legs, in others both leg and thigh.

Desnos,[19] in speaking of chronic œdema, mentions that it may be hereditary, and thinks that when it is so it is usually down the maternal line. These cases of Meige, published eight years after this statement was made, seem to confirm the opinion. So few have been the cases reported, however, of this chronic hereditary œdema that it is impossible to determine that such is the case. It certainly is not so in acute œdema of hereditary nature.

In the cases reported by Dinkelacker, Quincke, and Valentin, and in the instances cited by Strübing, it was transmitted from a father to a son.

In Osler's cases this repeatedly occurs. In one instance the disposition can be traced through the male line for four generations;

great-grandfather, grandfather, father, and son each being subject to the attacks. This is strikingly exemplified in Schlesinger's cases, where also four generations in the paternal succession were affected. In Yarian's patient the maternal element is somewhat more evident, but even here we see that among her ancestors and relatives a father transmitted the disposition to several of his sons, and through one of these, not alone to a granddaughter, but to a grandson and great-grandson.

There have been many endeavors to solve the problem of the production of œdema. One of the earliest attempts at the solution of the question was that of Lower,[20] in 1669. Lower ligatured the inferior cava and claimed to have thereby obtained œdema of the lower extremities and ascites, as the result of the venous stasis, the blood serum passing through the vessel walls as through a filter. This was the mechanical filtration theory. Wherein the error in his experiment lay does not now appear. At all events, this was the prevailing view for two hundred years up to 1869.

Virchow,[21] in his *Handbook of Special Pathology and Therapy*, published in 1854, says: "I have never been able to convince myself that in mechanical dropsy the fluid passes through the walls of the veins. The location of the transudation is mainly the capillaries. With a certain degree of lateral pressure the capillary wall may be permeable for watery fluid."

This is a practical acceptance of the mechanical filtration theory for certain forms of œdema, but he says further: "Exceedingly difficult is finally the question of the primary essential or idiopathic, and the secondary, consecutive, or symptomatic dropsies. One may assume that these primary and essential dropsies are brought about by an arterial fluxion in parts whose blood and lymph vessels are in a state of disturbed nutrition."

In 1869 Ranvier[22] took up Lower's experiments and utterly failed to obtain œdema in that way. All the signs of venous stasis appeared, but œdema was not one of them. When, however, he cut the sciatic nerve on one side, on that side he obtained œdema, while on the other side no transudation from the vessels occurred. To the writer the most interesting result of Ranvier's experiments is the following: Œdema was only obtained when the sciatic nerve itself, outside of the spinal canal, was cut. When its roots of origin inside the canal before the accession of many sympathetic fibres were severed no dropsy resulted.

In 1877 Cohnheim and Lichtheim[23] published the results of numerous experiments. They concluded that a hydræmic condition of the blood in itself alone cannot cause œdema. For its production there must exist coincidently some injury to the vessel walls. They show that transfusion of salt solution, even to the extent of 64 per cent. of a dog's weight, is not followed by œdema of the skin. Such injury to the vessel walls may, however, be brought about in time by a hydræmic condition itself. "The normal function of the vessel walls is dependent upon the continuation of normal circulation in the vessels. . . . It is hardly to be doubted that not alone the oxygen, but other constituents of the blood are equally important factors for the maintenance of the normal function of the vessels."

Sotnischewsky[24] thought that œdema could be produced by simple constriction of the veins, provided the total venous outflow of the limb was cut off, while every opportunity for the afflux of blood to the part was afforded. He found, however, that when he also cut the nerve supplying a vein, œdema occurred, even if the total venous outflow was not restricted.

Cohnheim[25] again, in 1882, emphasizes the greater facility with which œdema occurs in hydræmia from the poorly nourished and permeable vessels. He cites the experiment of Ostroumoff, in the course of his remarks. Ostroumoff irritated the peripheral end of cut lingual nerve with an induced current of gradually increasing intensity. He obtained a primary hyperæmia, followed in ten minutes by œdema, which, ten minutes later, had reached marked proportions. In 1884 some exceedingly interesting experiments were carried out by Landerer[26] to determine the part played by the elastic tissue in transudation. He found tissues subject to dropsy markedly deficient in elasticity, and concluded that this factor was one of great influence on the circulation of the blood and lymph. He considers œdema and inflammation also, an impairment of "the elastic equilibrium of the circulating fluids of the body." This subject was mentioned by Monro previous to 1777, for in the German translation of his work on dropsy of that date, on page 11, is the following: "Es giebt viele und mancherlei Ursachen von der Wassersucht. Die vornehmsten davon sind folgende. . . . Eine Erschlappung und Schwäche der Fasern. Diese Ursache fällt öfters vor."[27]

Gaertner,[28] repeating the experiments of Cohnheim and Lichtheim, thought that their injection of the salt solution was too rapid, and that œdema ensued when the fluid was more slowly introduced.

Gergens[29] found that in frogs the vessels allowed much more fluid to pass through when the medulla was destroyed.

Of much interest are the experiments of Salvioli.[30] He found that an excess of artificial hydræmia did not cause transudation into the subcutaneous tissue, but did to a certain extent produce œdema of some of the internal organs. When, however, he ligatured the renal and inferior mesenteric vessels, fluid did collect in the subdermal spaces of the abdomen, thorax, and thighs. From this he concluded that some vessels are naturally more permeable than others, and that when these vessels are cut off from the circulation, in this state of artificial hydræmia, those next in order of permeability permit transudation to take place. He regards the different organs as possessing different degrees of permeability, and thinks that the location of such transudation may be varied by suppressing the vessels that under usual conditions most readily allow filtration.

Jankowski[31] says that œdema from hydræmia in itself alone does not exist, but that in such condition where the vessel walls are injured even slight disturbances of circulation suffice to produce transudation.

Recklinghausen[32] considered œdema the product of increased filtration of blood plasma, dependent on abnormal pressure in blood- and lymph-vessels or on chemical change in the blood plasma.

Heidenhain[33] and, at about the same time, Hamburger,[34] of Utrecht, advanced the theory that the capillary endothelium possesses powers of secretion, and is not merely a filtering agent.

Horsley and Boyce[35] saw the results of Ranvier's experiments confirmed in nine out of twelve cases, and, in an enumeration of the various factors in the production of œdema, quote the paper of Tigerstedt and Santesson[36] (which was not available to me) as disposing once and for all of physical theories, and of the dependence of transudation on mere variation in pressure on the two sides of a permeable membrane.

Hamburger,[37] in a paper on the regulation of the "osmotic tension" of fluids in the peritoneal and pericardial cavities, considers as factors in transudation, venous hyperæmia, increased permeability of vessel walls, and irritation of the capillary endothelium by some substance produced by disease, and later adds,[38] as a fourth factor, "retardation of absorption."

Lazarus-Barlow,[39] in a most valuable contribution to the subject, concludes that œdema is not caused by merely mechanical means, even in the cardiac variety; that there is no evidence of any damage to the bloodvessels, other than that caused by starvation of the same; and that anæmia, being in fact a starvation, in conjunction with non-removal of waste products, is an important cause of œdema.

The non-removal of waste products introduces the element of poisoning, which, he thinks, is a more important factor than mere anæmia.

Senator[40] believes that dropsy does not necessarily depend on disease of the kidneys, but upon a coincident injury to and consequent increased permeability of the blood- and lymph-vessels of the skin, and of the serous and mucous membranes.

Boddaert[41] says: "It is the general scientific opinion that obstruction of the lymphatics plays no part in the development of œdema by constriction," but concludes from his researches that œdema by constriction *is*, at first, at least, essentially lymphatic.

He considers, as a result of direct experiment, that the œdema produced in one extremity by ligature of the lymphatics alone is identical in kind with that produced in the other limb by constriction of its entire circumference (in the upper part of the thigh). His researches were conducted on rabbits.

Opitz[42] presented, in 1899, an excellent general consideration of the whole subject of œdema.

He thinks that the filtration theory received a hard blow from the experiments of Cohnheim and Lichtheim, whose work he considers the starting-point for the modern theory of œdema.

Howell[43] classes œdema as follows: Œdema of engorgement, œdema of inflammatory origin, that of hydræmic or cachectic nature, and that of angioneurotic character. Changes in the vessel walls of nutritive character, qualitative changes in the blood and toxæmias resulting in malnutrition and nerve irritation, are all causative factors. Instances of such blood conditions are seen in anæmia, chlorosis, scurvy, slow starvation, chronic discharges, etc., and all debilitating influences resulting in hydræmia.

Funck,[44] in an exceedingly interesting paper on the physiology and pathology of dropsy, says that it has been experimentally shown that, within moderate limits, as in ordinary disease, neither a diminution of albumin nor an excess of water in the blood is sufficient to cause œdema. To produce œdema, something more is required than more facility of filtration of watery blood, in fact, malnutrition of the vessel wall, lessened elasticity from vasomotor paralysis, rendering the vessels more permeable for fluid.

Albu[45] believes that a watery condition of the blood, with loss of albumin, favors the transudation of serum from the vessels; that a "hydræmic plethora," with lessened outflow of fluid, tends to the same condition; while the *sine qua non* is an increased permeability of the vessel walls. These three theories are practically those of Bright, Bartels, and Cohnheim, respectively, combined.

Among the latest works on the causation of œdema known to the writer, and which practically brings the subject up to date, is the interesting work of Jacques Loeb,[46] of Chicago. Loeb considers the filtration theory utterly erroneous. He says: "I consider that the power for the movement of fluid in the tissues in cases of œdema (as in all other cases) is essentially to be sought for in osmotic force, and that the œdematous conditions, that is to say, the penetration of fluids into the tissues, occur when the osmotic force in the tissues is higher than that of the blood and lymph. In other words, the œdema must have as its basis such causes as raise the osmotic force of the tissue or lessen the osmotic force of the blood and lymph." This may be a change in the tissues of chemical nature that increases its osmotic force. Loeb produced such a change in a muscle by totally shutting off its circulation, and suggests that it may have been due to lack of oxygen. He shows that the osmotic pressure may be 300 times the degree of intravascular pressure that has been thought sufficient to produce the highest degree of œdema of the lungs.

Many experiments with frogs showed that a given muscle in a limb, when the circulation to the limb was totally restricted, absorbed fluid to from 1 per cent. to 3 per cent. of its weight in eighteen hours,

15 per cent. in forty-eight hours, 25 per cent. to 40 per cent. in seven days. A similar result ensued when the muscle was removed and placed in salt solution.

This chemical change in the muscle, which increases its osmotic force, and is apparently due, he thinks, to lack of oxygen, is accompanied by acid formation. Osmotic force may be increased in the tissues by alkalies, acids, and loss of water.

"The occurrence of œdema is brought about by chemical changes in the tissues. These chemical changes influence first the osmotic force in the sense that in the tissues that are œdematous it is higher than in the blood and lymph. Second, these chemical changes may also bring about morphological changes."

As Sewall[47] pointed out some years ago, there can be no question but that osmosis in living animal tissue is a different problem than it is in dead membrane. The endothelial walls of the capillaries are composed of living cells engaged in active vital process, vital, at least, as regards their own existence, if in no other way. That this living cell membrane allows the fluid of the blood or tissues to pass through it, subject only to the law of diffusion, as applicable to dead inert membrane, seems to the writer extremely problematical, although, perhaps, possible. Another source of error is the assumption that deductions drawn from experiments on lower animals are, without further qualification, applicable to physiological or pathological processes in the human being.

Not alone do different animals vary greatly in the degree to which a physiological or pathological process may be carried out, but also corresponding organs in the different species may possess functions differing greatly in degree, if not in kind. This is, perhaps, nowhere more evident than in the cutaneous covering of the various animals. Thus the skin of man is an organ of excretion of the utmost importance, while in the dog this is, by comparison, a function of infinitely less value. In the rabbit and guinea-pig such is also the case, while in some animals scarcely any analogy exists. The dog, and occasionally the rabbit, have, as a rule, been the animals employed in the attempt to solve this question. It would seem that such marked variation in the function of an organ, in man of the greatest importance, in the animals experimented upon of relatively little importance, in the elimination or retention of the watery constituents of the body, must have its influence on the results of these experiments, and should be considered in the deductions drawn therefrom for application to similar processes in the human being.

However, the actual process of transudation may take place, we know, beyond all reasonable doubt, that the *exciting* factor in this process may be, in numerous cases, of neurotic nature. It is not necessary to go beyond the limits of the human species to find convincing evidence of this fact.

The occurrence of œdema in traumatic or surgical injury to a nerve or in other nerve disturbance has frequently been seen.

The œdema following nerve section; the transudation occurring in the area of distribution of a nerve which has been the seat of neuralgic pain; the œdema occasionally met with in neuritis; that of paralyses, and that sometimes seen in tetany are all instances in which the neurotic factor is apparently direct. Further evidence is found in the occasional occurrence of not only a circumscribed but a unilateral œdema, of which a case will be noted among these here reported. (Fritz.) These cases are somewhat analogous to those of unilateral hyperhidrosis or hemidiaphoresis sometimes seen. The occurrence, simultaneous with the transudation, of symptoms of undoubted nervous origin, or the occurrence of the same at other times, or occasionally in alternation with the œdema, furnishes also strong presumptive evidence of its neurotic character. The extremely rapid onset, development, and disappearance of the acute attacks can hardly be accounted for on any other than a neurotic basis.

Finally, the heredity itself in the cases above mentioned strongly suggests a neurosis.

Of interest in this connection are the cases of periodical vomiting described by Leyden,[48] who cites their analogy to the "gastric crises" of Charcot. These attacks closely resemble those of Strübing's and Yarian's cases, apart from the œdema. They were, as in the case of Strübing's younger patient, accompanied by the vomiting of large amounts of watery fluid. In none of these cases did œdema ever appear, but the gastric symptoms are practically identical with those seen so frequently in these cases of acute œdema.

The neurotic element in the chronic cases is not evident, although Meige is inclined to consider them analogous to the trophic disturbances seen in lesions of the cord.

No more curiously interesting affection exists than this recurrent acute œdema. Here we have in one family a man living in unimpaired vigor of mind and body at ninety-two years, having suffered with the affection for seventy-four years, while in his family a child died of the affliction in early life, and an adult woman forfeited her life to the same disease. That death may be narrowly escaped is illustrated by the fact that his mother at one time nearly died of "shortness of breath," but, nevertheless, lived to be seventy-two years old.

That death may come with great suddenness and without warning is shown by Griffith's case. This woman was playing on the floor with her baby, apparently in perfect health, when she was seen to suddenly put her hand to her throat as if she felt trouble there and immediately fell over dead.

This affection has occasionally been regarded as one of little seriousness to life. It is, however, a condition of serious import, and, once occurring, renders the patient's future always insecure.

Krieger's case was found dead in bed, and autopsy showed that death was due to œdema glottidis. Five of the eight members of the family cited by Fritz died of glottic œdema, including both of the patient's brothers.

Griffith's case died at twenty-three years and her father at twenty-nine years, both of œdema of the glottis.

These cases are only those occurring in the families where the affection manifested some hereditary tendency. Many fatal cases have been recorded in instances of acute recurrent œdema where heredity was not manifested, and which, therefore, are not included among those we are considering. But if we consider the mortality in these hereditary cases alone, we shall see that the affection shows a death rate of about 16 per cent.; while of the remaining cases, 6 per cent. had had attacks in which death was imminent.

This is a mortality in strong contrast to the prognosis given by some writers for acute recurrent œdema; and it will at once be evident why this is so, when we consider that cases of this affection are rarely under the observation of any one observer for any prolonged period of time.

The full life history of the individual is, therefore, not obtained.

In a somewhat extensive review of the general subject of acute œdema previous to the study of the hereditary cases, it was evident to the writer that the mortality was much greater than was generally considered, but no conception of as high rate as the above percentage indicates was obtained. It would seem, however, that we must be nearer the truth in deduction based on these hereditary instances, for here we know the life history of many of the individuals, and further knowledge of the ultimate fate of those still living would tend not to diminish but to rather increase the death rate.

In the fatal cases death was due, almost without exception, to œdema of the glottis.

If in the adult death may occur with the extreme suddenness seen in so many of these instances from obstructive œdema of the throat, it might well be thought that in the child this would be much more likely to occur.

Curiously enough, however, the majority of the deaths in the cases here reported occurred in adult life, notwithstanding the fact that many of the individuals had been afflicted with the affection in childhood.

Another singular fact is that while in almost every family there were many cases that began in childhood, there were a number in which the affection did not appear until after this period; and in one family, in four generations, no case occurred until adult life was attained.

Direct exciting cause seems often to be present in the individual attacks. In a number of instances trauma appeared responsible for the onset; in others exposure to extremes of temperature or emotional excitement were apparent factors. These can but be regarded as merely the sparks that induce the explosion of nerve force, already in a state of hereditary unstable equilibrium.

Of the ultimate neurotic nature of the affection, it would seem that there could be no serious doubt.

References.

1. Dinkelacker. Inaugural Dissertation, Kiel, 1882.
2. Quincke. Monatshefte f. practische Dermatologie, 1882, vol. i. p. 129. Ref. in Archiv f. Dermatologie und Syphilis, 1882, p. 544.
3. Valentin. Berliner klinische Wochenschrift, 1885, p. 150.
4. Strübing. Zeitschrift f. klinische Medicin, 1885, vol. ix. p. 381.
5. Falcone. Gazzetta degli Ospedali, 1886, vol. vii. p. 125; also Rivista veneta di scienz. med., Venezia, 1887, vol. vii. p. 251.
6. Osler. The American Journal of the Medical Sciences, 1888, vol. xcv. p. 362.
7. Krieger. Meditzinskvie Obozrenie, 1889.
8. Smith. Medical News, 1889, vol. liv. p. 320.
9. Fritz. Buffalo Medical and Surgical Journal, 1893–94, p. 286.
10. Roy. Medical Record, 1894, vol. xlvi. p. 42.
11. Ricochon. La semaine médicale, 1895, p. 365.
12. Yarian. Medical News, 1896, vol. lxix. p. 238.
13. Schlesinger. Wiener klinische Wochenschrift, 1898, p. 335.
14. Griffith, T. W. British Medical Journal, 1902, vol. i. p. 1470.
15. Higier. St. Petersburger medicinische Wochenschrift, 1894, vol. iv. p. 50.
16. Milroy. New York Medical Journal, 1892, vol lvi. p. 505; and Omaha Clinics, 1892–1893, vol. v. p. 101.
17. Jopson. Pediatrics, 1898, p. 69.
18. Meige. Nouvelle Iconographie de la Salpêtrière, 1899, vol. xii. p. 453.
19. Desnos. Société méd. des hôpitaux de Paris, February 13, 1891.
20. Lower. Tractatus de corde, London, 1669, chap. ii. Quoted by Virchow (21).
21. Virchow. Die Wassersucht. Handbuch der speciellen Pathologie und Therapie, 1854, vol. i. pp. 182 and 209.
22. Ranvier, Lazarus-Barlow. The Pathology of Œdema. British Medical Journal, 1895, vol. i. p. 634.
23. Cohnheim and Lichtheim. Virchow's Archiv, 1877, vol. lxix. p. 106.
24. Sotnischewsky. Ibid., 1879, vol. lxxvii. p. 85.
25. Cohnheim. Vorlesungen über allgemeine Pathologie, Berlin, 1882, vol. i. pp. 135, 445, and 492; and vol. ii. p. 438.
26. Landerer. Die Gewebspannung in ihrem Einfluss auf die örtliche Blut und Lymphbewegung. Leipzig, 1884.
27. Monro. Wagner. Deutsches Archiv f. klinische Medicin, 1887, vol xli. p. 509.
28. Gaertner. Wiener medicinische Presse, 1883, Nos. 20–21.
29. Gergens. Pflüger's Archiv, 1876, vol. xiii. p. 591.
30. Salvioli. Archivio per le Scienze Mediche, 1884–1885, vol. viii. p. 421; also Adams, London Medical Record, 1885, p. 315.
31. Jankowski. Virchow's Archiv, 1883, vol. xciii. p. 259.
32. Recklinghausen. Allgemeine Pathologie des Kreislaufs und der Ernährung, Stuttgart, 1883, p. 96.
33. Heidenhain. Pflüger's Archiv, 1891, vol. xlix. pp. 209, 222, and 223.
34. Hamburger. Zeitschrift f. Biologie, 1890, vol. xxvii. p. 259.
35. Horsley and Boyce. British Medical Journal, 1893, vol. i. p. 111.
36. Tigerstedt and Santesson. Bihang vid. k. Svenska Set Akad. Handlingar, vol. ii.; and Mittheilung vom Physiolog. Laborat. des Carol. Med. Chir. Inst. in Stockholm, 1886.
37. Hamburger. Du Bois-Reymond's Archiv, 1895, p. 281.
38. Hamburger. Virchow's Archiv, 1895, vol. cxli. p. 398.
39. Lazarus-Barlow. British Medical Journal, 1895, vol. i. p. 634.
40. Senator. Die Erkrankungen der Nieren, Vienna, 1896, p. 176.
41. Boddaert. Étude expérimentale de la pathogénie de l'œdème par constriction. Bull. l'Acad roy de méd. de Belg., 1898, vol. xii. p. 422; and Bull. Soc. de méd. de Gand, 1898, vol. lxv. p. 178; also La presse médicale Belge, 1898, vol. l. p. 194.
42. Opitz. Journal of the American Medical Association, 1899, vol. xxxii. p. 51.
43. Howell. Buffalo Medical Journal, 1899–1900, vol. xxxix. p. 176.
44. Funck. Cincinnati Lancet-Clinic, 1900, vol. xlv. p. 73.
45. Albu. Virchow's Archiv, 1901, vol. clxvi. p. 87.
46. Jacques Loeb. Pflüger's Archiv, 1898, vol. lxxi, p. 467.
47. Sewall. The Denver Medical Times, 1893, p. 174.
48. Leyden. Zeitschrift f. klinische Medicin, 1882, vol. iv. p. 605.

REVIEWS.

A Treatise on Orthopedic Surgery. By Royal Whitman, M.D., Instructor in Orthopedic Surgery in the College of Physicians and Surgeons of Columbia University, New York; Associate Surgeon to the Hospital for Ruptured and Crippled; Orthopedic Surgeon to the Hospital of St. John's Guild; Chief of the Orthopedic Department of the Vanderbilt Clinic; Member of the Royal College of Surgeons of England; Member and some time President of the American Orthopedic Association; Corresponding Member of the British Orthopedic Society; Member of the New York Surgical Society, etc. Second edition, revised and enlarged. Illustrated with 507 engravings. Philadelphia and New York: Lea Brothers & Co., 1903.

The second edition of this book triply applauds its author. The first edition, profusely illustrated by line and half-tone prints, completely and concisely presented the best and latest thought of to-day in orthopedic surgery. The prompt exhaustion of this edition is but a merited acknowledgment of the appreciation of the medical bookbuyer. The bookmaker's tribute to the writer follows and will be welcomed by the booklover, since it accords a more generous, fitting, and attractive publication to the second edition. In the latter, contrasted with its predecessor, suitably selected paper has vastly improved the printing of the half-tones, while the judicious leading of a smaller printed page, framed with wider margins, and marked by a freer use of boldface headings, has much increased the ease of reading and reference and materially enhanced the beauty as well as the number of the new book's pages. Not resting on the double laurels won by the first edition, the author has proceeded to deserve a third variety on account of new features introduced in text and illustration in the second edition. Not only has the work been brought abreast of the moment by a number of valuable additions, but the matter of the first edition has been revised and in a couple of instances reclassified.

The Lorenz refinement of the Pravaz and Paci manipulative articulation by "bloodless method" of congenitally unarticulated hip-joints is described in minute detail, and step by step illustrated through each stage of operation, fixation, and after-treatment. This supplement to what in the first edition was rather a comprehensive chapter will doubtless be scrutinized first and with ungrudging approval by each reader of the new volume. Congenitally malformed hips, however, are comparatively rare deformities, and the greater usefulness of this book lies in the excellent chapters, with which we are familiar, dealing with the more prevalent tubercular lesions of spine and hip, with rachitic deformities, with scoliosis, with paralyses, and the congenital and other distortions of the feet, including the practically universal ones due to conventional shoeing, and not forgetting the newly inserted method of correcting hallux valgus by Sampson's ingenious toe-post. One cannot glance at these chapters, in either edition, without admiration for their illustrative demonstration—clear beyond mistake—of the most modern orthopedic methods and apparatus.

The topical division of subjects with subclassifications on a pathological basis has been preserved, and doubtless will be of practical assistance in reference for physicians not devoted to this specialty. On the other hand, both scientifically and for the instruction of students, it would seem preferable to group the subjects according to their pathological origin and subdivide them in reference to their anatomical distribution. J. M. S.

Radium and Other Radioactive Substances: Polonium, Actinium, and Thorium. With a consideration of Phosphorescent and Fluorescent Substances, the Properties and Applications of Selenium, and the Treatment of Disease by the Ultraviolet Light. By William J. Hammer, Consulting Electrical Engineer. New York: D. Van Nostrand Co., 1903.

Coming at this time, when the attention of students of both pure and applied science is focused on the extraordinary phenomena manifested by radium, polonium, and their allies, this little work is singularly opportune. Within the brief compass of 72 pages the author presents clearly and concisely a great deal of very interesting and instructive matter.

To the physician the subject has a double interest: he follows with appreciation the work of the physicists in their investigations into those activities, the manifestations of which have so changed our views of matter; he seeks for therapeutic possibilities in the practical application of this radioaction against disease.

The first part is devoted to a consideration of phosphorescent and fluorescent substances, which the author aptly likens to "step-down transformers," in that they lower the vibration frequency of ultraviolet rays to such a number that the human eye can appreciate them. The fact that many of these substances respond to the stimulation of radioaction and emit light makes their study one of importance. As an example of this is given the fact that a diamond will phosphoresce from stimulation by radium, thus differentiating it from an imitation diamond.

Briefly and clearly the author gives the history of radioactive substances from their extraction from the common source, pitchblend, through the record of observed facts and ingenious hypotheses. The author discusses the substances in the order of their activity, taking uranium as a standard; the emanating rays are classified according to their power of penetration and susceptibility to deflection by a magnet, and, further, their properties are compared with those of *x*-rays. Several interesting radiographs are shown, giving the photographic record of the power of penetration of the emanations from the radioactive substances through materials of varying resistance. In conclusion, we are given a short though entertaining account of the Finsen Light Institution and the method of treatment employed there, some of the results in cases of lupus vulgaris being shown by photographic plates. H. M. W.

INFECTION AND IMMUNITY, WITH SPECIAL REFERENCE TO THE PREVENTION OF INFECTIOUS DISEASES. By GEORGE M. STERNBERG, M.D., LL.D., Surgeon-General, U. S. Army (retired). New York and London: Putnam & Sons.

To present the subjects of infection and immunity as these phenomena are now interpreted in a form which is intelligible to the non-medical reader is indeed a difficult problem. Owing to the new technical terms which the investigations upon antitoxins, agglutinins, precipitins, and bacteriolysins have brought into use, and to the complexity of Ehrlich's side-chain theory, these subjects have been practically omitted as being unsuitable for popular treatment. The volume therefore narrows down to discussions upon the general subjects of "susceptibility to infection," "disinfection," "immunity," and a series of chapters upon the various infectious diseases which form the second and major part of the volume. Bubonic plague, Asiatic cholera, typhoid fever, etc., are all discussed separately. Each disease is considered from an historical, etiological, and epidemiological standpoint, while special regard is paid to prophylaxis and measures of prevention. Technical terms are avoided as much as possible and the main facts regarding each form of infection are given in a concise, clear, and interesting manner. The chapters on yellow fever and malaria are particularly good.

Perhaps the title of the book is somewhat misleading, but the text is none the less interesting. W. T. L.

Die Fermente und Ihre Wirkungen. Von Carl Oppenheimer, Dr. Phil. et Med.; Assistent am Thierphysiol. Inst. d. Landwirth. Hochsch, Berlin, Zweite Neubearbeitete Auflage. Leipzig: F. C. W. Vogel, 1903.

The general subject of Ferments has assumed so much importance within the last few years that without a proper knowledge of their action one is at a loss to explain many of the processes concerned in physiology or pathology. A book such as this is particularly acceptable, and it is really impossible to overestimate its value. The subject is treated in a purely scientific manner and each chapter contains such a wealth of information that it may be read many times without exhausting the benefits to be derived from it, so carefully has the material been collected and so concisely put forth. The first and minor portion of the book deals with the subject in general terms, while in the second portion the various ferments are grouped together in sections, but discussed fully in separate chapters. Cytolysins, agglutinins, and precipitins receive recognition and are classed as substances related in a way to the true ferments. The book has both subject and author indices. One realizes the great care and precision with which the book has been prepared when he finds over 1500 references to literature. The book numbers 439 pages in all. W. T. L.

Surgical Diseases of the Abdomen, with Special Reference to Diagnosis. By Richard Douglas, M.D., Formerly Professor of Gynecology and Abdominal Surgery, Medical Department, Vanderbilt University, Nashville, Tenn.; ex-President of Southern Surgical and Gynecological Association, etc. Illustrated, 883 pp. Philadelphia: P. Blakiston's Son & Co., 1903.

Surgeons both in their journal articles and text-books have, we feel, paid undue attention to operative technique to the neglect of the important question of diagnosis. It is therefore with pleasure that we review this book on *Surgical Diseases of the Abdomen*, which deals almost entirely with the diagnosis of these conditions and which is yet written by a practical surgeon. A book dealing with the diagnosis of abdominal diseases from the surgical point of view has been a want felt by all surgeons, and the present volume bids fair to supply that want very satisfactorily. Abdominal surgery has become a wide field and has extended its boundaries far into the territory formerly considered entirely the domain of the medical man. Consequently the question of diagnosis in this field of surgery is of as much, if not more, importance to the surgeon than to the physician.

The book before us presents each of the subjects under discussion in a most extensive and satisfactory manner. At the close of each chapter is a list of references which will be found of great value to the reader who desires to further investigate any particular subject. The illustrations are not profuse, but supply every want.

It is impossible in a review of this kind to comment upon each portion of the book, but nevertheless certain comments may not be out of place.

The first chapter is an excellent one on Peritonitis, in which the symptoms and diagnosis are presented in a most comprehensive manner. Instead of describing extensively the steps of the surgical treatment, the author briefly presents the surgical indications. Although we agree with him that drainage is too constantly employed in pelvic work, we are not prepared to say the same, as he does, of appendiceal work. He heartily approves the postural drainage, suggested by Fowler, which has proved so very satisfactory in cases of peritonitis. The diagnosis and surgical indications of typhoid perforation are carefully considered, but in our judgment the author does not urge with sufficient energy immediate operation as soon as symptoms indicate perforation. It is now practically agreed by all having experience in this condition that it is a mistake to delay operation for the recovery from shock, but that the sooner the abdomen is opened and properly treated the better will be the result.

We fully concur with Douglas in his attitude toward the exploring needle as a diagnostic measure in liver abscess. He states that the needle should not be employed unless the surgeon is prepared to operate at once in case pus is found.

The portions of the book dealing with diseases of the kidney and with abdominal injuries meet with our particular approval. The latter portion of the volume is devoted to surgery of the female pelvis, and is not proportionately as extensive as other parts. One criticism that might be offered is that the diseases of the ureter have not been considered.

This book is one which every surgeon and every physician can read with profit, and it will undoubtedly take its place as a most satisfactory book of reference. J. H. G.

Cancer and Precancerous Changes, Their Origin and Treatment. By G. H. Fink, M.R.C.S., L.S.A. Lond., Major Indian Medical Service (retired). London: H. K. Lewis, 1903.

This pamphlet is a highly speculative and often vague discussion upon the changes in the animal organism as well as in the surrounding hygienic conditions which may lead to the development of

cancer. An analogy is drawn between the life-cycle of the malarial parasite and the life-history of cancer, while great importance is given to the hypothetical "materies morbi" of new-growths. Much of the dissertation is far from lucid, owing both to the abstruse nature of the problems dealt with and to the faulty English used. To some persons the book may prove interesting, but scarcely instructive.
W. T. L.

A Text-book of Obstetrics. By J. Clarence Webster, M.D., F.R.C.P.E., F.R.S.E. Philadelphia, New York, and London: W. B. Saunders & Co., 1903.

This is a thoroughly good work. Not only is the practical side of the subject well handled, but, in addition, the scientific receives its required consideration Throughout the author has shown a nice sense of proportion, and seems to us to have succeeded in his endeavor to make a book suitable both for the needs of the active practitioner and the scientific student.

As might be expected, his section upon Placentation is especially good, as are the chapters on Ectopic Pregnancy and Eclampsia.

His chapter upon Pelvimetry is up to date in every way, even to the figuring of Ehrenfest's pelvigraph and kliseometer.

Throughout the volume his advice as regards treatment is marked with most satisfactory conservatism.

The consideration of the subject of "Puerperal Infection" is, in our opinion, one of the most valuable portions of the whole book. In this chapter the subject is considered in a thoroughly scientific manner, and the treatment is in accord with the views which receive the adherence of most experienced men.

In a word, the author has produced a very satisfactory volume which, undoubtedly, will receive the commendations of the profession.
W. R. N.

A Text-book of Obstetrics. By Barton Cooke Hirst, M.D. Philadelphia, New York, and London: W. B. Saunders & Co., 1903.

Four editions since first issued, in 1898, is a record which makes the formal review of this work a rather useless procedure.

To be a satisfactory subject for review a volume should have some rather glaring faults either of omission or commission, thus enabling the one who criticises to express his opinion without being compelled to make a very searching examination. Unfortunately, this volume is not satisfactory from the reviewer's standpoint, as a rather intimate knowledge of the earlier editions and an examination of the changes and added material in the present one have not enabled us to find any points about which one can write adversely. We are, therefore, compelled to consider the good points of the book, a study which, while not as exciting to us, is, nevertheless, in the present instance, one which affords us decided satisfaction, as we believe this to be one of the best books on obstetrics published up to the present time for the use of both the undergraduate student and the man engaged in active practice.

As samples of the general excellence, we would refer to the chapters upon the Pathology of the Puerperium, the Pathology of the Newborn Infant, and the section devoted to the Major Obstetrical Operations. The chapter on Puerperal Sepsis is also particularly complete, and we are glad to note that while the use of the Döderlein or Menge tube is described and advocated as an aid to diagnosis, its limitations and the possible factors of inaccuracy in its use are clearly defined.

The book is even more profusely illustrated than the previous editions.

W. R. N.

ROLE DES POISON DU BACILLE DE KOCH DANS LA MENINGITE TUBERCULEUSE ET LA TUBERCULOSE DES CENTRES NERVEUX. Par DR. P. F. ARMAND-DELILLE. Paris: G. Steinheil, editeur.

THIS monograph is a study upon the effect which different poisons isolated from the tubercle bacillus may produce upon the central nervous system. The research is divided into three parts. The first part deals with the experimental aspect of the subject; the second with the histological lesions, and the third gives the conclusions which the author draws from his work and the theories which may be deduced therefrom. From the experimental investigations it was found that the tubercle bacillus is capable of producing two varieties of poisons which act in different ways upon the meninges and brain. One group has a local action. It causes more especially caseation of the tissue, and through the mechanical action of these lesions vascular alterations follow in the surrounding tissue, resulting in degenerative changes of the nervous elements. The second group of poisons is of a diffusible nature and gives rise to phenomena of nerve-cell intoxication without evident histological modifications in either the nerve cells or meninges.

Tuberculosis of the meninges, studied from the histological standpoint, was never complicated by actual inflammatory lesions of the elements of the nervous tissue; but important degenerative alterations were found in the nervous centres immediately surrounding the diseased meninges and were ascribed to the changes in the blood-vessels.

The author, from these observations, formulates a conception of the pathological physiology of tuberculous meningitis. Three periods may be distinguished in the genesis of clinical symptoms. The first period, the stage of excitation, is explained by the circulatory disturbances in the cortex, and in a small measure by the toxic phenomena; the second period is characterized by symptoms of paralysis of the cortex, which seem to be produced by the toxic phenomena, and the third period ends in death, caused by paralysis of the spinal cord and medulla from intoxication by the diffusible poisons of the tubercle bacillus. W. T. L.

A SYSTEM OF PHYSIOLOGIC THERAPEUTICS. Edited by SOLOMON SOLIS COHEN, A.M., M.D., Senior Assistant Professor of Clinical Medicine in Jefferson Medical College, etc. Philadelphia: P. Blakiston's Son & Co., 1903.

VOLUME VIII. REST, MENTAL THERAPEUTICS, AND SUGGESTION. By FRANCIS X. DERCUM, M.D., PH.D., Professor of Nervous and Mental Diseases in the Jefferson Medical College of Philadelphia, etc. Pp. 318.

VOLUME X. PNEUMOTHERAPY, INCLUDING AEROTHERAPY AND INHALATION METHODS AND THERAPY. By DR. PAUL LOUIS TISSIER, one time Interne of the Paris Hospitals; Assistant Consulting Physician to Laennec and Lariboisière Hospitals, etc. Pp. 479.

VOLUME VIII. presents much that has been the subject of other volumes in times gone past and also much that is of more recent date. If the author had merely given us a modern presentation of "Rest and Pain," as Hilton taught us, we would have been only grateful for the opportunity of again reviewing a book which made a deep impression upon us in our earlier career. But he has done more, for he has traced the connection farther than our fathers and added to it the best of Mitchell and of those who have introduced modifications of more or less importance. In pointing out how far this is applicable to the treatment of hysteria and the symptom-complex of neurasthenia we find the field enlarged, and conditions more or less allied to the latter subjects offered for discussion. Hypochondria, according to the author, becomes a "readily differentiated clinical entity," and with this view we will agree so far as concerns the plan upon which he bases his hopes for relieving those troublesome patients of their symptoms. At any rate he makes them a class by themselves, and in that differentiation we are more hopeful both for the neurasthenics and hysterics. In the sixth chapter, on the application of rest in chorea and other functional nervous diseases and in organic nervous diseases, we find a curious assemblage of symptoms and diseases, although we are not disposed to be critical, for the practical points abound and the large experience of the author is well in evidence. The therapeutics of mental diseases is well presented in two chapters comprising eighty pages. To those who believe that the subject cannot be summed up in mechanical and chemical restraint we commend this section of the work. So thorough has the writer been that we are of the opinion that those whose especial work lies in the treatment of these unfortunates will find much to learn, while those in the broader field can find much that the physician should know and apply in the way of prevention. Finally we come to suggestion for which, as is pointed out, there is a legitimate field and, as we all know, one that should be understood only to condemn. For those who have gone over the dreary wastes of speculation or read pages of invective these chapters are refreshing.

In Vol. X. we have a book of a different type—an effort to assemble together practically all that can be said in favor of the method, and in this compilation an *ex parte* argument is presented with the resultant lack of perspective. Granted that this method has been neglected, its presentation need not include the antiquated and the obsolete, which obscure the present. Completeness may suggest that all be presented, but in every-day and practical work they are unnecessary. Air as a therapeutic agent is presented from all viewpoints—composition, density, temperature. The therapeutic applications follow closely upon the physical and chemical facts. The special therapeutic indications are not the subject of separate chapters, but are included in the broader statements, but, however, with sufficient differentiation of particular interest, as in the chapter on "General and Respiratory Gymnastics and Mechanical Pressure Methods," which, however, should be read in connection with Vol. VII. of this series. In the second part "Inhalation Methods and Therapy" will doubtless prove to be of greater interest to the physician. Dealing with gases, fumes, and vapors in general, the author takes up the medicaments suitable for use (vapors, atomization of liquids, insufflation of powders) in satisfactory detail. If any matter of importance has been omitted we have failed to note its absence. In this portion the literature is full, the directions precise, and the indications fully set forth. How much can be accomplished by these methods only one who has intelligently practised them can believe. As one lays down this volume he must admit that it contains a mass of information of real value; that it has reconciled many hitherto disputed points; that theory has been modified to the point of furnishing a working basis for practice, and that all methods and matters are readily accessible. If, as in other volumes of the series pharmacology is in evidence to a greater extent than the plan of the work would seem to indicate, we must remember that no complete scheme of therapeutics can be built on any one or on all physical agencies combined, and that physiological properties are possessed by matters other than those presumably here presented. Excluding what has seemed to us as unnecessary in a book which is to appeal to the practising physician, we believe that this volume represents the present state of our knowledge upon this subject, and that its information is in a presentable form, for which the reviewer and reader will congratulate Drs. Eshner, Brickner, and Goepp for their skilful and painstaking translation. R. W. W.

A Thesaurus of Medical Words and Phrases. By Wilfred M. Barton, M.D., and Walter A. Wells, M.D. Philadelphia, New York, and London: W. B. Saunders & Co., 1903.

The most striking feature of this work is its entire originality both of conception and execution. There is no other book just like it, and it has been so carefully compiled and covers the ground so thoroughly that we doubt if there will be room for a similar publication for years to come. The method of its use is explained in a well-written introduction. It is intended to play for medical literature the part which Roget's *Thesaurus of English Words and Phrases* has long done for general literature. It is not a medical dictionary because it does not furnish definitions, but merely synonyms, and in fact reverses the ordinary dictionary method, as instead of supplying a meaning or idea for a given word, the Thesaurus supplies the word necessary to express the idea which we have in our mind. The persons to whom it will prove especially useful will undoubtedly be those who, while deficient in medical education, are employed at work in medical literature. Thus, as its authors claim, it will possess great value to stenographers engaged in transcribing the proceedings of medical societies or reporting medicolegal testimony. It will also be of great value to translators of medical works.

Although the authors suggest its value to lawyers, journalists, or novelists who are dealing with subjects requiring the employment of technical medical terms, nevertheless, we take leave to express the opinion that it would be most unfortunate should these three classes of laymen attempt to write technical descriptions from its pages. We could imagine the ridiculous effect produced in their writings by the choice of some of the synonyms which are given for words in ordinary use, and as there is no guide to the definition of the various synonyms, the *Thesaurus* would leave them at perfect liberty to choose anything they might desire; and when it is remembered that medical men no longer talk the ridiculous jargon which amuses us so much from the lips of Dr. Slop in *Tristam Shandy,* we can but conclude that it is much safer for a layman not to provide himself with a *Thesaurus,* but to write in the ordinary vernacular. To all those engaged in medical literary work, this book will prove invaluable. Its thoroughness, accuracy, and the skilfulness with which the subject-matter has been arranged leaves nothing to be desired in it as a work of reference. F. R. P.

DIE KRANKHEITEN DER OBEREN LUFTWEGE. Aus der Praxis für die Praxis. Von PROF. DR. MORITZ SCHMIDT. Dritte sehr verbesserte Auflage. Berlin: Verlag von Julius Springer, 1903.

THIS valuable work of Prof. Schmidt, which has long been a standard text-book in Germany, deserves to be much more widely known and consulted in America than is the case. It is probably too advanced and thorough to be of much service to the ordinary American medical student as a college text-book, but as a work for consultation and reference, it should be in the library of every physician who is engaged in doing special work in diseases of the nose, throat, and ear. One is especially struck with the author's breadth of view in regard to the connection between disorders of the nose and throat, and constitutional diseases or conditions, which is manifest throughout the entire work. The author is thoroughly conversant with all of the most recent methods of diagnosis and treatment, and, what is probably more remarkable in a German, he is thoroughly familiar not only with Teutonic medical literature, but with the work being done by physicians belonging to other nationalities. It is to be hoped that a translation of this invaluable work will at some time be available for the use of the American physician. F. R. P.

PATOLOGIA E TERAPIA DELLA ORECCHIO E DELLE PRIME VIE ÆERE (OTOLOGIA, RHINOLOGIA, LARINGOLOGIA). DR. GIUSEPPE GRADENIGO. Torino: S. Lattes & Co., Librai Editori, 1903.

THIS large volume presents in the form of lectures the teachings of Gradenigo, the distinguished professor of laryngology at the University of Turin. Although intended primarily for the use of students, it is written with almost Germanic thoroughness, and consequently possesses value for the more advanced workers in laryngology and otology. Scientific medicine has in recent years been greatly benefited by the activity of the Italian profession.

The present work conveys the teachings of the most prominent Italian authority on laryngology and otology. The marginal notations which are to be found on every page are of great service as guides, especially to the reader who is not a fluent Italian student.

Although, as stated before, the book is of a more or less elementary character, it would nevertheless be of value to all workers in this special field if for nothing else because of the originality of many of the author's views upon important subjects. The great tendency in the American medical profession is to confine their researches in medical literature to works published in English, German, and occasionally French. Of course, this is owing to the fact that but few American physicians are sufficiently familiar with the Latin tongues to acquaint themselves with publications in Italian or Spanish. The converse of this proposition is, however, not true in the book at present under discussion, the references in which are of the most polyglot character, the author evincing familiarity with the medical literature of all tongues. F. R. P.

THE CARE OF THE BABY. A Manual for Mothers and Nurses. By J. P. CROZER GRIFFITH, M.D., Clinical Professor of Diseases of Children in the Hospital of the University of Pennsylvania. Third edition, thoroughly revised. Philadelphia, New York, and London: W. B. Saunders & Co., 1903.

THE appearance of a third edition of Dr. Griffith's well-known manual is a satisfactory indication of the favor with which the earlier editions have been received. In its present form it has been submitted to a thorough revision, a large number of illustrations have been added, and a few to which objection had been raised have been omitted.

While primarily intended as a popular book for the guidance of mothers and nurses, it contains a large amount of material that should be a part of the equipment of every physician whose work brings him into frequent contact with childish patients. It therefore offers an excellent primer for the student, inasmuch as every young practitioner is early brought face to face with baby patients; and it behooves him to be well prepared to face with confidence the discriminating criticism of the experienced mother and her gossipy friends.

Throughout the whole work the author aims to discourage over-confidence in the mother, and seeks to teach her what not to do for her child in case of illness rather than to assume responsibilities which should properly be relegated to the physician. It is therefore a safe book to put into the hands of mothers and nurses, and should prove a valuable adjunct to the nursery. T. S. W.

SERUM THERAPY. By R. T. HEWLETT, M.D., D.P.H. LOND. Philadelphia: P. Blakiston's Son & Co.

THIS small work of two hundred and fifty pages contains a concise account of the treatment of disease by antitoxins and antisera, with a brief description of the preparation and administration of these materials, the way in which they are supposed to act as curative agents, etc. Ehrlich's side-chain theory is clearly set forth and a chapter is devoted to transfusion of animal blood, saline solutions, and artificial sera. Those interested in this subject will find the book useful and quite complete for its size. T. A. C.

THE MEDICAL EPITOME SERIES. AN EPITOME OF INORGANIC CHEMISTRY AND PHYSICS. By A. MCGLANNAN, M.D., of the College of Physicians and Surgeons, Baltimore. Series edited by V. C. Pedersen, M.D. Philadelphia and New York: Lea Brothers & Co.

THIS small volume contains an excellent epitome of the most important facts in physics and inorganic chemistry. It will prove of special value to undergraduate students of those subjects, but will be a most serviceable companion to more advanced scholars who desire a résumé for handy consultation. To the medical man a book of this kind is a most useful little work of reference for consultation in some of the points which come up so frequently in his practice in relation to the sciences with which it deals. The plan upon which the matter is arranged is most practical. It is a pity that in the proof-reading a number of errors have been overlooked. They are not, however, of great importance, and do not in any way mar the accuracy of the scientific facts set forth.

E. A. C.

THE MEDICAL EPITOME SERIES. NORMAL HISTOLOGY. A MANUAL FOR STUDENTS AND PRACTITIONERS. By JOHN R. WATHEN, M.D. Philadelphia and New York: Lea Brothers & Co.

THE qualities that distinguish the Medical Epitome Series and which have made it justly popular are conspicuous in the present member of the group. It presents the same judicious arrangement of subject-matter, clear and concise language in the letter-press, with an adequate number of engravings selected from authoritative text-books, and the same continuity in the text in place of the fragmentary method of questions and answers of the older "quiz compends." The manual is as compact as it could be made without sacrificing comprehensiveness, and is especially adapted to the needs of those for whom it is designed—students and practitioners confronted with the necessity of "getting up" knowledge on short notice when time is an important factor. R. M. G.

THE MEDICAL ANNALS OF MARYLAND, 1799–1899. Prepared for the Centennial of the Medical and Chirurgical Faculty. By EUGENE FAUNTLEROY CORDELL, M.D. Baltimore, 1903.

THIS volume, which was published as a commemoration of the Centennial of the Medical and Chirurgical Faculty of the State of Maryland, is a contribution of the greatest importance to the history of American medicine. Its author has long been distinguished for his labors in the field of American medical history. Had it not been for his zeal for research the immensely important part played by the profession of Maryland in the development of medical science in this country would hardly have been appreciated. There are indeed few States which can boast of a prouder record in this respect than Maryland. In this volume its claims are well presented. The work is divided into three sections, namely, an historical, a biographical, and a chronological section, the first portion being devoted to a history of the Medical and Chirurgical Faculty, the second to biographical sketches of its members, and the third to a chronological record of events of importance in the medical history of Maryland. The Medical and Chirurgical Faculty of Maryland for many years occupied a peculiarly important position in the fact that until the year 1859 physicians desiring to practise within the limits of Maryland were obliged to have a license from it. In that year this power was taken from it by legislative enactment.

In the chronological record we would note that in all probability the autopsy stated as having been made in that colony in 1637 is the earliest recorded in America, and in addition there are also a number mentioned subsequently, all of which were performed prior to the autopsy performed in Massachusetts in 1674, and very generally supposed to have been the first.

Another "first event" is noted in the year 1768, when John Archer, of Maryland, received the first medical diploma, "M.B." from the University of Pennsylvania, ever granted after attendance in America. In more recent times, the first annual meeting of the American Medical Association was held in Baltimore in 1848. Many other interesting facts might be quoted from this well-compiled record did space allow.

Among the biographical sketches are several of the greatest interest and value, dealing with the early celebrities in the profession, many of whom have not so far been brought adequately before the public. Among these may be mentioned those of Upton Scott, John Archer, John Crawford, and Horatio Gates Jameson.

Dr. Cordell's book is one of the greatest interest not only to the physicians of Maryland, but to those of the whole United States. It is an excellent example of what should be done in various localities to gather up as much of the local medical history as possible, and preserve it before it is irretrievably lost. F. R. P.

A TEXT-BOOK OF THE PRACTICE OF MEDICINE. By JAMES M. ANDERS, M.D., PH.D., LL.D. Sixth edition, thoroughly revised. Philadelphia, New York, and London: W. B. Saunders & Co., 1903.

THE appearance of the sixth edition of this work in six years in itself attests its popularity among students and practitioners. The work has been revised and brought up to date, as has become necessary in those diseases where information is rapidly accumulating. In addition new diseases or symptom groups have been introduced.

The author has made use—as in former editions—of a tabular parallel in differential diagnosis of diseases which present like symptoms. Many of these tables are original with the author. Of the new subjects introduced are paragraphs on paratyphoid fever, the fourth disease; trypanosomiasis, orthostatic albuminuria, transcortical aphasia, adiposis dolorosa, and amaurotic family idiocy.

In a work of such general excellence it is difficult to pick out any particular portion as deserving of special notice. The chapters on Tuberculosis, Diseases of the Heart, Anæmias, Malaria are very complete reflections of our present knowledge of these subjects, and the same statement applies to the book *in toto*. The author has a very clear method of expressing himself and does not overload us with facts in support of theories already proven and accepted. Also, in discussing diseases of unknown or disputed etiology and pathology, both sides of the question at issue are given and not too much weight placed on an individual opinion. As an illustration of this method of treatment, the chapter on Diabetes may be cited.

Dr. Anders has been aided by others in revising the parts on the Nervous System and some of the section on Children's Diseases, and this work has been done in the same thorough way. The combination of careful methodical work, of studying and making use of current medical literature, with the author's own wide experience, has made this a standard text-book second to none.

J. N. H.

PROGRESS

OF

MEDICAL SCIENCE.

MEDICINE.

UNDER THE CHARGE OF

WILLIAM OSLER, M.D.,

PROFESSOR OF MEDICINE, JOHNS HOPKINS UNIVERSITY, BALTIMORE, MARYLAND.

AND

W. S. THAYER, M.D.,

ASSOCIATE PROFESSOR OF MEDICINE, JOHNS HOPKINS UNIVERSITY, BALTIMORE, MARYLAND.

The Measurement of the Pressure in the Right Auricle (a New Clinical Method).—GUSTAV GAERTNER (*Münchener med. Wochenschrift*, 1903, No. 47). Gaertner's method depends upon the well-known fact that when the arm hangs by one's side the veins fill with blood, which empties out when the arm is raised. This Gaertner calls the "vein phenomenon." It occurs normally when the vein to be tested in the arm is raised to the level of the costal insertion of the third, fourth, or fifth rib. Gaertner argues that the occurrence of the "vein phenomenon" is dependent upon the pressure in the right auricle. The veins form manometers, which, although not transparent, indicate the position of the blood column. A slight positive pressure suffices to distend their walls, while they collapse if the pressure is zero or negative.

He recognizes two limits: 1. The elevation of the arm at which emptying of the veins just occurs. 2. The elevation of the arm at which the veins just do not collapse. Of these only the first is important. The pressure in the right auricle is measured by determining the vertical distance between the level of the right auricle and the level of the vein examined. The pressure in the right auricle is subject to rhythmical variations. It rises during systole and sinks during diastole, and varies with inspiration and expiration. The veins of the arm constitute, as it were, a "minimum manometer."

By adjusting the arm at the proper height, Gaertner observed pulsation in the veins in cases of mitral disease, and in cases of dyspnœa. A voluntary increase of pressure in the right auricle can be produced by forced expiration when one holds the nose (Valsalva experiment).

He found that the pressure in the veins is not identical with the pressure in the thorax. By increasing the pressure in the thorax artificially to the equivalent of 10 cm. of water, the pressure in the auricle rose only about 6 cm. With an increase of 15 cm. in the thorax the auricular pressure rose only about 11 cm. He noticed the curious fact that negative pressure in the thorax produced no diminution, but actually an increase of pressure in the auricle.

Gaertner had an opportunity to test the pressure in a number of patients in Prof. Neusser's clinic.

His experiments showed that in all cases, without exeeption, in which there was congestion of the right heart he was able to demonstrate by his method an increased auricular pressure. The difference from the normal was naturally dependent upon the nature of the case. In almost all cases it was so material a difference as to be readily recognized. Usually in healthy people the veins collapse when the hand is at or below the level of the shoulder; some cases when it is raised to the level of the eye or top of the head. He designates the auricular pressure as V. D. (Vorhofsdruck). He took as his standard the upper border of the fifth rib. He found that the pressure varied from 9 cm. to 23 cm. In the case of pericarditis about 20 cm., in lung emphysema about 18 cm., in lobar pneumonia 29 cm. He found also increase of pressure in tuberculosis, pleural exudation, and so on. The highest pressure was 37 cm. in an individual with beginning infiltration of the apices of the lungs. In this last case a satisfactory explanation of the pressure was not found.

He records the varying changes of pressure in the infarct of the lungs that was observed very early.

At times the increased auricular pressure was the only objective symptom that indicated damaged circulation. In one case the pressure was 20 cm. in a woman, aged about forty years, in whom the investigation of the heart and lungs gave no signs of disease. Clinical history, however, showed that there was cardiac insufficiency.

In describing his method, Gaertner suggests that changes may be required after further experiences. The determination is best made with the patient sitting upright. The back should be supported in order to prevent alterations of the position during the determination. With fat people or with those with abdominal tumors, ascites, etc., the feet should rest on the ground, since when sitting in bed the abdominal pressure produces circulatory changes. Thin patients could be measured even while sitting in bed. The anterior plane of the thorax should be as upright as possible. In semirecumbent position the determination is more difficult. The chief difficulty occurs when one attempts to determine what point must be selected as the normal zero point. At first he was inclined to select the upper limit of heart dulness; but he later concluded to select a point on the skeleton, and chose the sternal insertion of the upper border of the fifth rib. This is easily demonstrable, and there can be no question of its position, while there might be controversy about the limits of cardiac dulness. Furthermore, this point corresponds in healthy human beings to the level of the tricuspid valve. Finally, the horizontal plane that passes through this point is to be regarded, according to his observations, as the lowest limit at which the vein phenomenon occurs. In all cases, then, one will obtain a positive value for V. D., while if a higher point be selected the value for V. D. may be either positive or negative. It may be said that the auricle in diastole forms a space 6 cm. to 8 cm. in vertical measurement, so that in the auricle itself there must be differences of pressure according as the measurement is at the top or bottom of the auricle, and by selecting the lowest point of the auricle, that is, the tricuspid valve, as his zero point, he always obtains a positive value for his auricular pressure.

Having determined that one will select the lowest plane of the auricle for the measurements, it remains to determine where this lowest point falls. It would be simple to determine this matter by means of

Roentgen-ray pictures, but this is a complicated procedure. For practical diagnostic purposes such exactness is superfluous, for in pathological cases the extent of the pressure is so far from the normal that it is readily perceived by less exact means.

Of the veins that may be selected for examination, those of the back of the hand and the radial surface of the forearm are the most suitable. At times these are not available, and any vein that presents must be selected, such as the median basilic. It is rare in adults that no vein occurs available for this determination, though this is common among well-nourished children.

Under the action of cold the veins become invisible; the use of warmth in any form, however, quickly restores the circulation to the skin and brings out the veins. One must select a vein that collapses readily. On the backs of the hands of old people it is not uncommon to find thickened varicose veins which do not collapse. Exceptionally, such veins occur also on the forearm and upper arm. The collapse of even the most delicate vein is sufficient for the determination. A good illumination and a suitable position of the observer are essential for this. If the eye of the observer is a little bit higher than the vein and if the light comes over the shoulder of the observer, one can see the shadows cast by the rising vein over the congested skin and can determine the moment of collapse by the disappearance of the shadow. Of course, one must be careful that articles of clothing do not interfere with the circulation and must be sure that the handling of the arm does not occlude any of the veins. The person examined must not hold his breath; the arm examined must not be too sharply bent at the elbow, at the most about 120 degrees; nor should the arm be everted from the shoulder.

Before beginning the final determination, let the arm hang vertically and wait until the blood column accumulates to the shoulder after two or three minutes. Then bend the arm, held in adduction to an angle of 120 degrees at the elbow and pronated. The forearm must be raised from the shoulder so that the whole forearm stays horizontal. In this case the collapse occurs simultaneously in the whole extent of the forearm. The movements must be executed by the physician with care not to compress the vein. The muscles of the person examined must be as relaxed as possible. Several determinations must be made, preferably using both left and right arms. Often the first determinations are higher than the later ones, as the patients are frequently somewhat excited by the examination. Once Gaertner observed a very great increase of pressure after only very slight muscular exertion in the case of a patient with mitral disease. The determination of the difference of level between the auricle and the observed vein can be either approximate or accurate. According to the first method, one roughly measures the height of the vein at the point of emptying and projects it upon the median plane of the body, and in this way finds how much above the given zero point the collapse occurs. It is much more accurate to measure this pressure in centimetres, which Gaertner does with a simple apparatus that he describes.

The first objection that may be raised is that he is obtaining hydrodynamic relations and not hydrostatic, and second that the pressure in the peripheral vein is modified by a suction action where the small vein empties into the jugular. Third, that the elasticity of the vein walls modifies the result.

He also made determinations using the veins in the foot and leg

He thinks that a comparison of the results given on the upper and lower extremities gives us a means of determining intra-abdominal pressure. His conclusions are as follows:

1. An observation of the "vein phenomenon" puts us in a position to determine the pressure in the right auricle in a manner beyond objection, as far as the laws of physics are concerned.

2. By means of the method here described we can recognize the presence of congestion in the right heart not only with certainty, but actually can measure the degree of injury and follow the course of alterations. We will be able to follow very accurately the limits of therapeutic measures.

3. The method is so simple, the appearance is so unmistakable that its application will recommend itself for diseases of the circulation and respiratory organs.

OSKAR PRYM (*Münchener med. Wochenschrift*, 1904, No. 2, p. 60) raises several objections to Gaertner's method which was recently proposed. Having tried this method repeatedly in the clinic at Bonn, he finds: 1. The vein phenomenon occurs in the same individual at unequal heights in different veins; the difference amounted to 6 cm. or 8 cm. or more. 2. There was often a rapid change in the height at which the vein phenomenon occurred, which depended apparently upon the rapidity with which the arm was raised. With more rapid raising of the arm the vein phenomenon occurred at a greater height. 3. On account of the influence of varying pressure and varying volume of blood passing through the veins, and on account of the varying tonus of the veins, he concludes that the vein phenomenon does not always indicate either the lowest pressure in the right auricle nor the highest pressure. The vein phenomenon may indicate either too high or too low a pressure. He thinks it not allowable to regard the veins as simple manometers, for the height at which the vein empties is dependent not only upon the pressure in the right auricle, but also upon the amount of flowing blood, upon the resistance to the outflow, and upon the tonus of the vein. He thinks that Gaertner's method may be of use clinically if these factors are borne in mind.

SURGERY.

UNDER THE CHARGE OF

J. WILLIAM WHITE, M.D.,

JOHN RHEA BARTON PROFESSOR OF SURGERY IN THE UNIVERSITY OF PENNSYLVANIA; SURGEON TO THE UNIVERSITY HOSPITAL,

AND

F. D. PATTERSON, M.D.,

SURGEON TO THE X-RAY DEPARTMENT OF THE HOWARD HOSPITAL; CLINICAL ASSISTANT TO THE OUT-PATIENT SURGICAL DEPARTMENT OF THE JEFFERSON HOSPITAL.

The Treatment of the Congenital Dislocation of the Hip.—REINER (*Centralblatt f. Chir.*, 1904, No. 2) considers this subject under two separate headings: first, radical treatment in relation to the age of the patient, and, second, the after-treatment. The method of Schlesinger, of Dresden, consists in reduction followed immediately by immobilization in a plaster cast, but we must remember that he states that three years is the age limit for this procedure. Reiner has found, however, that this method may be tried up to the twelfth year where both sides are involved, and to fifteen years in the single variety. In patients of this age the idea should be not to accomplish complete reduction at the first sitting, but instead to merely bring the head of the femur near the articular surface of the acetabulum. The reduction should then be completed in from eight to fourteen days, and in 12 cases the method was successful. In regard to the after-treatment, active and passive motion are essential, care being taken to see that reduction is absolute at the end of the movement.

Intracapsular Resection of the Prostate for Hypertrophy.—RYDYGIER (*Centralblatt f. Chir.*, 1904, No. 1) states that there have lately appeared three articles on the subject of the treatment of prostatic hypertrophy by Riedel, Zuckerkandl, and Völcker; Riedel not only goes into the technique, but also into the operative indications, and his conclusions are in the same line with those of Rydygier, who, however, does not agree with Zuckerkandl and Völcker. The author notes that in 1900 he fully described partial perineal prostatectomy and also in 1901 and 1902 the intracapsular operation as related to resection, but Zuckerkandl evidently did not come across these references, for at one place in his article he notes his priority in this field of work. The author's method differs from those of Alexander, Nicoll, Jabulay, Freyer, and others; also from Czerny, which Völcker describes, and from Zuckerkandl. As this condition usually exists only in men who are senile, the author's idea is to make the operative interference as slight as possible so as to avoid shock. The technique consists in making an incision in the raphé of the perineum, then separating the capsule to one side about 1 to 2 cm. from the median line in a longitudinal direction. The urethra should not be opened as Zuckerkandl advises, as no advantage is gained by doing so. Total extirpation is certainly not necessary in every case and it is far more dangerous than a partial reduction. Care, too, should be taken not to injure the rectum as happened in several of Zuckerkandl's cases, and also not to injure the ejaculatory ducts. That recurrence is more common after resection than after other methods does not seem probable; the operation should be performed in the early stages of the disease, and it is one that is but very slightly dangerous and which should not be followed by disagreeable sequelæ.

Some Practical Points Associated with Appendicitis.—SPANTON (*British Medical Journal*, February 6, 1904) states that the early symptoms are often not only obscure but positively misleading, and the typical signs the books describe so mathematically are often represented by a cipher. The author then reports 10 cases in detail and remarks that the ordinary symptoms of simple appendicitis are sufficiently familiar and so need not be detailed here. But there are some to which undue importance is attached, while there are others which may readily be mistaken for those of other morbid conditions. Pain, for example, is relied upon by some as essential, but in several of the cases the pain was so slight as to be hardly mentioned by the patient.

The locality of the pain, too, is very misleading. In a large proportion of the worst cases the pain is referred to the epigastrium or along the course of the colon. Epigastric pain is almost invariably associated with peritonitis and is one of the most valuable indications of its presence and the need for operation in these cases. Tenderness on pressure and referred pain should be kept distinct. Tenderness is usually over the seat of the appendix, but it must be borne in mind that the appendix may be fixed in one of the hernial openings (it occupied the obturator foramen in one case) or, on the other hand, it may be free and move its position considerably; hence the location of the tenderness may vary greatly. In women it is liable to be confounded with ovarian tenderness, and it is not an uncommon thing for the appendix and ovary to be adherent—both inflamed—and the author has elsewhere pointed out the comparative frequency of appendicitis in young women occurring at the catamenial periods. The presence of a lump is again very misleading, for a good proportion of such cases without very marked constitutional symptoms do well and recover without operation, while, on the other hand, the absence of such a swelling indicates little, for the appendix may be gangrenous, may be hidden away down in the pelvis, or may be doubled down behind the ileum, in which cases no lump would be perceptible.

But when we come to abdominal tension, especially with rigidity of the right abdominal muscles, we have an indication of a more definite character, almost always denoting formation of pus or circumscribed peritonitis, which in conjunction with constitutional symptoms, especially persistent sickness, is almost pathognomonic. In such cases operation is demanded. Constipation is no doubt usually present, but, on the other hand, spurious diarrhœa is not uncommon. There is frequently a history of more or less habitual constipation, with some unusual meal followed by sickness and diarrhœa, which may persist even as the graver symptoms increase. Temperature counts for little, except when a sudden rise gives indication of grave mischief, which is ordinarily apparent enough already. The same as to pulse; it is often quiet and even slow when the necessity for operation is clear enough. The necessity for operation must be judged on the merits of each individual case, but it is far safer to operate too soon than to defer it a minute too long. A certain proportion of patients will get well with ordinary care and treatment, especially strict recumbency; but in all cases of doubt it is far safer for the patient and more to the credit of surgery to act soon, and make practically certain of saving the patient's life. No one ought to be allowed to die unopened unless practically moribund, and some most desperate cases do get well.

Notes on the Ineffectual Treatment of Cancer.—Power (*British Medical Journal*, February 6, 1904) states that in cancer, with its apparently increasing mortality, it is only right that a fair trial be given to every method of treatment which promises to give relief, provided that the method can be adopted without ill consequences to the patient. With this end in view, three cases were treated by the injection of the Schmidt serum; one, a woman, from whom had recently been removed a part of the breast for a scirrhous carcinoma; a man, the half of whose tongue had been removed for epithelioma, and a patient from whose neck had been removed a malignant growth the origin of which was not clear. After noting in great detail the progress of each of these cases the author states in conclusion: 1. In regard to the reaction. There is no doubt that a reaction takes place after the injection of Schmidt's serum. The temperature rises and with it the pulse, but the respirations as a rule are not affected. In this rise of temperature there was nothing peculiar, for it follows the injection of serum which admittedly contains toxins and in all probability any similar serum would produce a similar result if it were active. It cannot therefore be said with accuracy that the reaction is specific, and this is proved by the fact that the first case showed the most typical reaction, yet subsequent examination of her tissues failed to detect any malignant disease. 2. The local effect upon the tumor was shown in each case, for the breast in the first case and the malignant masses in the other two cases became inflamed and reddened as the result of the injection. Yet here again one could not see that the serum acted by selection upon malignant tissues only. It seemed to intensify any pre-existing inflammation. This was effectually shown in the first case, where the lymphatic glands in the right axilla became enlarged in addition to those in the left armpit, the original seat of cancer being the left breast. For here again subsequent examination showed that none of the glands which had thus become enlarged after the injections of the culture were affected with cancer. 3. The treatment is certainly painful apart from the succession of hypodermic injections.

Lastly, malignant disease progresses even to a fatal issue while the injections are being given, as happened in the second case. The author believes that this method is of no service at present, either from a prophylactic, diagnostic, or curative standpoint, but it may fairly be argued tha this trial has been insufficient and that further observations are desirable.

THERAPEUTICS.

UNDER THE CHARGE OF

REYNOLD WEBB WILCOX, M.D., LL.D.,

PROFESSOR OF MEDICINE AND THERAPEUTICS AT THE NEW YORK POST-GRADUATE MEDICAL SCHOOL AND HOSPITAL; VISITING PHYSICIAN TO ST. MARK'S HOSPITAL.

Mineralization and Hypochloruration in the Bromide Treatment of Epilepsy.—M. Toulouse considers that hypochloruration aids materially the action of the bromides in the treatment of epilepsy, but it causes a demineralization of the patient, who is thus rendered more liable to infection, especially that of tuberculosis. To remedy this, sodium chloride is replaced by sodium phosphate. Five patients were treated by the administration of 75 to 150 grains of sodium phosphate per day. No crises occurred. It seems rational to admit that sodium phosphate does not interfere with the absorption of the bromides. A diet rich in chlorides seems to create, on the part of the tissues, a desire for homologous salts, such as the bromides. The author's experiences confirm the theory of modifying the nutrition in order to augment the action of drugs.—*La presse médicale*, 1904, No. 11, p. 86.

Radium in Certain Nervous Affections.—M. A. Darier has succeeded in two cases in terminating neurotic convulsive attacks which had in one patient been accustomed to occur every day, and in the other three or four times a week, by applying tubes containing radium to the temples. Also in a case of neurasthenic pseudo-ataxia and in a case of recent facial paralysis, cure resulted after a day's application of the radium. The activity of the radium employed varied from 10,000 to 7000 units, and the feeble intensities were applied for three or four days or even up to fifteen days, pain appearing a short time after the cessation of the application. With intensities of from 1000 to 7000 units the duration of the sittings was from two to six hours per day.—*La semaine médicale*, 1904, No. 7, p. 51.

Solanum Carolinense in Epilepsy.—Dr. Trusch, after a study of this drug, has arrived at the following conclusions: 1. That solanum carolinense possesses great value in the treatment of idiopathic, non-hereditary *grand mal*, especially when the disease begins after childhood. 2. That it is also very useful in hystero-epilepsy with convulsions; in *petit mal* its effect is less marked. 3. In advanced epilepsy, where cell degeneration in the brain seems to have been established, the drug seems to have an almost specific action, but its effect does not last so long as does that of the bromides. 4. The author's observations show that the vegetable depressomotors possess real advantages over the mineral salts employed to produce this effect. With solanum the bad effects of the continued use of the bromides are avoided, especially the dermatoses and the influence upon the mind. 5. The fluid extract of the drug seems to be the preparation to be preferred.—*Journal de médecine de Paris*, 1904, No. 8, p. 74.

Intravenous Collargolum Injections in Septic Affections.—Dr. George Tucker Harrison reports a case of pyæmia following criminal abortion which, when first seen, had a weak pulse, remittent temperature, effusion in the right knee-joint, and a gluteal abscess. After the first injection of collargolum in twenty-four hours the pulse and temperature were nearer to the normal and the general condition was much better. Two more injections were given during the following three weeks, but the fever continued because of an abscess which developed in the right thigh. This was incised, drained, irrigated, and dressed. On the following day not a drop of pus was present, and recovery rapidly ensued. The author remarks this as being unusual in such cases, and reports a case of puerperal sepsis, and, in conclusion, states that he has seen no such brilliant recoveries as those following the use of collargolum.—*Virginia Medical Semi-monthly*, 1904, No. 20, p. 477.

Epidural Injections in Genito-urinary Diseases.—Dr. Artur Strauss reports his results in 18 cases of various genito-urinary disorders. Of 10 cases of enuresis, 1 was cured by an operation for phimosis rather than by the injections, in 2 the enuresis by day was cured, while that of the night was improved; 5 others were also improved, while 3 passed out of observation. Two cases of incontinence were cured. Of 7 cases of pollution all were cured, while of 3 of spermatorrhœa 2 recovered, while the third was unimproved. One case of prostatorrhœa and 2 out of 3 cases of impotence were cured, while of 2 cases of neurasthenia sexualis 1 was improved, while the other remained *in statu quo*. The author used for injection at first 0.2 per cent. sodium chloride to each 10 c.c. of which 2 drops of 5 per cent. carbolic acid had been added; later Schleich's solution was used. From 10 c.c. to 35 c.c. were injected into the lumbar sacral region of the cord at each sitting, and, in the author's opinion, the operation, when done under strict asepsis, is not in the least dangerous. The indications for its performance seem to be: infantile eneuresis, incontinence without mechanical obstruction, emissions, impotence, spermatorrhœa, and neuropathic polyuria.—*Therapeutische Monatshefte*, 1903, No. 2, p. 74.

Treatment of Tuberculous Meningitis by Lumbar Puncture.—DR. H. SERAFIDI has treated three patients suffering from this affection by lumbar puncture with the following results: The first patient, aged nine years, when seen was in the position of opisthotonos, with photophobia, frequent emesis, etc., and a pulse of 160 per minute. On the fourth day of the disease 10 c.c. of fluid were drawn off by lumbar puncture, and amelioration began at once. In three days recovery was assured. The second patient, aged fifteen years, exhibited practically the same symptoms as the first. On the eighth and ninth day of the disease lumbar puncture was performed. The patient's condition rapidly improved and a few days later he was entirely well. The third patient, aged one and a half years, presented classical symptoms of the disease, and upon the fourth day of the illness 10 c.c. of clear fluid were drawn from the spinal canal. Slight improvement followed, and two days later 34 c.c. of fluid more were withdrawn. Recovery followed without event. The author states that if any conclusion can be drawn from these three cases it is that the cure of tuberculous meningitis is not absolutely impossible. He considers these recoveries permanent, since considerable time has elapsed.—*Revue de thérapeutique*, 1903, No. 3, p. 80.

Secretine.—M. ED. ENRIQUEZ, who has made extensive experiments with this substance (which is an acid extract prepared by macerating the duodenal mucous membrane), has demonstrated that it is not exclusively an excitant of the pancreatic secretion, but that it increases also the flow of bile, and that the result of introducing an acid substance into the duodenum and that following the injection of secretine into the circulation are identical. Seven patients in whom the dominant symptom was habitual constipation were treated by the author, with the result that the motor and secretory functions of the intestine were stimulated and regular evacuations of the bowel were obtained. Of five cases in which the constipation was accompanied by the symptoms of mucomembranous colitis, such as painful abdominal crises and passages of mucus, four were relieved of the constipation, and at the same time the other symptoms were rendered much less distressing. Of four patients in whom the constipation was associated with lack of motility of the stomach, delayed digestion, and general lassitude, all were favorably and rapidly affected by the treatment. In conclusion, the author states that the acid duodenal medication has an undoubted stimulant action upon secretion, and since it increases the quantity of bile and pancreatic juice and also excites the motility of the intestine, it should prove of considerable value in intestinal dyspepsias.—*La presse médicale*, 1903, No. 14, p. 106.

PEDIATRICS.

UNDER THE CHARGE OF

LOUIS STARR, M.D.,
OF PHILADELPHIA,

AND

THOMPSON S. WESTCOTT, M.D.,
OF PHILADELPHIA.

A Simple Method for Obtaining Sputum in Children.—LEONARD FINDLAY, of Glasgow (*Archives of Pediatrics*, February, 1904, p. 126), referring to the difficulty experienced in obtaining specimens of sputum from young children, describes a method which has been in use for years in the French hospitals, but which he has not found described in any English work. It consists in irritating the pharynx and especially the epiglottis with the forefinger wrapped with a piece of gauze; cough is thus excited, and any expectoration that is coughed up is swept out of the mouth by the finger before it has time to be swallowed. The quantity thus obtained varies, but, as a rule, is sufficient for bacteriological examination. Several attempts may be required, but even in children as young as six months sufficient has been obtained on which to found a diagnosis. This method he has practised as a routine measure for nine months in the Royal Hospital for Sick Children, Glasgow, and with very gratifying results. Many cases of not very well-marked tuberculosis of the lungs were diagnosticated early, even on the day of admission to the hospital, and, with only one exception, no case of pulmonary tuberculosis went to post-mortem examination without the tubercle bacillus having been found in the sputum at some time. In cases of meningitis, also, supervening upon local pulmonary disease, in which there was a doubt as to its being tuberculous or pneumococcic in origin, the finding of the tubercle bacillus in the expectoration removed in the manner described cleared up the diagnosis.

Impetigo and Ecthyma Showing the Diphtheria Bacillus.—RAOUL LABBE and DEMARQUE, of Paris (*Revue mensuelle des maladies de l'enfance*, February, 1904, p. 49), report two cases in young children exhibiting extensive lesions of impetigo and ecthyma, in which were found, besides staphylococci in one case and staphylococci and streptococci in the other, various forms of Klebs-Loeffler bacillus. The same organisms were found in the throats of the patients, and both received injections of Roux's serum (20 c.c.), although no clinical symptoms of faucial diphtheria were observed, and no history of previous sore throat could be elicited in either case. The cutaneous lesions resembled those of a staphylococcic infection, but differed in their slow and chronic evolution. Without doubt, such cases are not exceptional, but the authors have failed to find reference to similar observations in the literature. They advise recourse to bacteriological examination of all cases of impetigo or ecthyma with multiple localizations in children, and that serum should not be neglected as one of the culture media. In such cases serotherapy should be employed early, but local treatment should not be neglected, and here, probably, the method of topical application of antidiphtheritic serum recently suggested by L. Martin (*Comptes-rendus soc. de biologie*, May 16, 1903) may find an appropriate field.

The Open-air Treatment of Bronchopneumonia Complicating Whooping-cough.—KER (*Scottish Medical and Surgical Journal*, January, 1904) gives the results obtained in the treatment of the complicating bronchopneumonia of whooping-cough by the open-air method, as practised at the Edinburgh City Hospital.

The writer calls attention to the high death rate from this disease, especially among the lower classes and in children living in institutions, and to our helplessness in its treatment.

Although much can be done to secure the patient rest and to maintain his strength, the practical point is some method of successfully treating the bronchopneumonia, which is the cause of death in the vast majority of cases.

The records of the Edinburgh Hospital show a death rate of 71 per cent. for the cases with bronchopneumonia, and statistics from other hospitals give about the same results.

The fact that many of the whooping-cough patients developed bronchopneumonia after admission, evidently from ward infection, influenced the writer to try the open-air treatment. At least any method, however heroic, could hardly increase the death rate.

Many writers have recommended that children suffering from pertussis be allowed out in the open air, but the occurrence of a pulmonary complication is usually said to be a contraindication of this treatment.

The first cases were selected from the worst in the wards, and many of them were regarded as hopeless. They were carried out and left in the open air for about six hours daily, provided it did not rain. No bad results were noted, and there was a very marked improvement in some of them. The children were warmly covered, and the chest was protected with cotton. The main effects of the treatment were as follows: The whoops were unaffected in number or severity. The patients took their food ravenously, and their general strength was improved. They also slept better, and the whole nervous tone of the children was improved. Another practical advantage was the complete rest given the wards for a period of from one to seven hours daily. While one case, which was admitted uncomplicated, developed bronchopneumonia and several had relapses in convalescence, it may be said that under this treatment bronchopneumonia of hospital origin became extinct. As regards the severity of the cases treated there is no doubt at all. Many were admitted cyanosed, with temperatures of 103° F. or 104° F., respirations of 60 to 80, and pulse running from 140 to 170. Even in the favorable cases these symptoms continued for a long time, though the pulse and respiration rate slowly decreased and the cyanosis disappeared.

The writer gives tables of various groups of cases treated over certain periods, the results of which are briefly stated as follows: Treated indoors entirely: cases, 74; deaths, 51; death rate, 66.9 per cent. Treated outdoors partly or entirely: cases, 76; deaths, 24; death rate, 31.5 per cent.

Pyelitis Due to the Bacillus Coli Communis.—McCay (*Indian Medical Gazette*, December, 1903) reports a case of pyelitis in a child, aged seven years, the true nature of the infection not being discovered until the patient had been under treatment for several weeks. The child was taken ill suddenly with pain in the left side extending down the leg. There was tenderness over the left lumbar region, coated tongue, constipation, and a temperature of 101° F. A week after the onset the temperature had risen as high as 105° F., with marked remissions. Pus was suspected, but could not be localized. The urine at this time was acid, with a trace of albumin. There was some abdominal distention, and constipation was a prominent symptom. The case was then thought to be possibly atypical typhoid fever. The patient continned to have high, irregular fever, accompanied by chills and vomiting, and when seen by the writer for the first time was extremely weak, anæmic, and much emaciated. There was œdema of the forehead and below the eyelids.

The blood examination gave a negative Widal reaction, while the urine showed a moderately large quantity of pus and abundant lively colon bacilli. The patient was given citrate of potassium in large doses, which had the effect of rendering the urine alkaline and of diminishing the amount of pus, but had no influence upon the bacilli. They grew rapidly on the various media and were very mobile. Urotropin was then given, and at once the bacilli, to a certain extent, lost their motility, and the number of colonies were fewer. After a few days they had entirely disappeared from the urine. The patient made a rapid recovery.

GYNECOLOGY.

UNDER THE CHARGE OF

HENRY C. COE, M.D.,

OF NEW YORK.

ASSISTED BY

WILLIAM E. STUDDIFORD, M.D.

Changes in the Endometrium in Ectopic Gestations.—Cazeaux (*Annales de gyn. et d'obstétrique*, Feb., 1904) arrives at the following conclusions: The expulsion of a complete membranous cast of the uterine cavity in ectopic gestation is not constant, nor does it imply the death of the fœtus. It has not been proved that this occurrence signifies some disturbance at the site of the ovum. This cast is formed by the superficial layer of the mucous membrane of the uterus, and the line of separation is never beyond the limits of the ampulla.

Function of the Corpus Luteum.—Labusquiere (*Annales de gyn. et d'obstétrique*, Feb., 1904) concludes from a study of Fraenkel's work and from his own observations that the corpus luteum is a true ovarian gland which is renewed regularly and affects the nutrition of the uterus and the periods of puberty and the menopause. It is not the pressure upon the nerves of the ovary by the growing follicles that excites the menstrual flow, but the activity of the corpus luteum, since the latter presides over the periodical hyperæmia of the uterus which terminates in either menstruation or pregnancy.

Direct Illumination in Gynecology.—D. de Ott (abstract of monograph in *Annales de gyn. et d'obstétrique*, Feb., 1904) advocates the general application of electric illumination in gynecological examinations and operations, using a number of simple appliances which are clearly figured and explained in his original *brochure*. A suitable head mirror is worn by the operator during abdominal and vaginal cœliotomies, the patient being in the exaggerated Trendelenburg posture on a special table.

Examinations of the rectum and bladder are similarly conducted, the interior of the latter viscus being exposed by separating the opposing surfaces of the urethral and vesical sphincter by means of small retractors, instead of with an endoscope. One blade of the retractor carries an electric light.

(The French editor properly calls attention to the fact that the advantages of extreme pelvic elevation during examination of the bladder were long ago recognized by American gynecologists, and that there is nothing new about the method of illumination.)

Torsion of the Pedicle.—Hammer (Inaugural Dissertation; abstract in *Zentralblatt f. Gynäkologie*, No. 5, 1904) analyzes 43 cases of torsion of the pedicle noted in 248 ovariotomies at the Würzburg clinic. In 7 per cent. there were sudden colicky pains; in 60.5 per cent. several minor attacks were noted; 32.5 per cent. were unattended with symptoms, the condition being found at the time of operation. Torsion occurred in 32 cystoadenomata, 4 dermoids, 3 parovarian cysts, 1 fibroma, and 1 cystosarcoma. Twenty-three torsions were from left to right and 18 in the opposite direction.

The writer agrees with Hofmeier that unsymmetrical development of the neoplasm is the direct cause of the accident, pregnancy having little influence upon it. All the patients recovered but two, who were in collapse when admitted.

Late Recurrence of Mammary Cancer.—Marggraff (Würzburg Inaugural; abstracted in *Zentralblatt f. Gynäkologie*, No. 5, 1904), in reporting a case of recurrence eight years after amputation of the breast for scirrhus, analyzes 860 cases in which the disease reappeared in 430 (50 per cent.). The longest period of immunity was eleven years.

(We have recently removed a recurrent cancerous nodule thirteen years after the primary operation.—H. C. C.)

Pathology of Uterine Fibroids.—Watt-Keen (abstract of Inaugural Dissertation in *Zentralblatt f. Gynäkologie*, No. 5, 1904) in 417 cases from Hofmeier's clinic notes the following complications: ovarian cyst, 27; diseased tubes, 19; hernia, 7; uterine displacements, 14; carcinoma and sarcoma of the corpus uteri, 9. Myxomatous degeneration of the fibroid was present in 8 and necrosis in 8. Twenty per cent. of the married women were sterile.

Myomectomy (abdominal) was performed 123 times, supravaginal amputation 44, total extirpation 15. Forty-five vaginal myomectomies and 43 total hysterectomies were performed. The total mortality after all operations was only 6.48 per cent.

Tuberculosis of the Tubes.—Fellenberg (*Zentralblatt f. Gynäkologie*, No. 5, 1904) reports 10 cases from the Bern clinic in which the diagnosis was confirmed microscopically. All the patients were nulliparæ; in none were there any characteristic symptoms, and no ulcerations were present on the vagina or cervix. The peritoneum was affected in two cases and the ovary only once, the uterus being free from disease in every instance.

The writer regards the prognosis after salpingectomy as generally favorable. In this respect he differs from those who advocate extirpation of the uterus and adnexa in every case of tuberculosis of the tubes.

Pruritus Vulvæ.—Lorand (*La policlinique*, vol. xii., No. 6) believes that diabetes is the etiological factor in the majority of the cases, and that it is frequently overlooked because the urine is not carefully and repeatedly examined, especially after giving test meals.

Three conditions may favor the development of pruritus in diabetes, viz.: 1. The toxic influence of the blood. 2. Direct irritation from the urine, which is rich in uric acid, as well as sugar. 3. Local hyperæsthesia of nervous origin. As regards treatment, the writer states that in addition to regulation of the diet he has obtained good results from the use of ointments containing 10 per cent. naphthalin and anæsthesin.

Torsion of the Omentum.—Vignard and Girandeau (*La policlinique*, vol. xii., No. 6) add 2 new cases to the 18 already reported. In both the symptoms warranted the diagnosis of appendicitis, the true condition being found only at the time of the operation. Of the 20 recorded cases 15 occurred in men and 5 in women. In all a hernia existed, so that this condition is evidently the principal etiological factor. The diagnosis is obscure and can seldom be made before operation. The treatment consists in resection of the affected portion of omentum above the point of torsion.

Deciduoma Malignum after the Menopause.—McCann (*British Obstet. and Gyn. Journal*, No. 3, 1903) reports the case of a woman, aged fifty-three years, who had borne ten children, the last nine years before. Menstruation had ceased a year and a half before she came under observation, complaining of profuse metrorrhagia of four weeks' duration. The patient succumbed on the sixth day after hysterectomy. Examination of the uterus showed the presence of a deciduoma malignum.

Vaccinia of the Female Genitals.—Löwenbach (*Monatshefte f. prakt. Dermatologie*, Band xxxvi.) states that he has observed four cases in which healthy women were infected on the genitals from individuals who had been recently vaccinated. He was able to find only one other similar recorded case. Infection took place through the medium of clothes, by direct contact, scratching, and in one instance because a physician who had dressed a vaccination sore on a child's arm made a vaginal examination of the mother without washing his hands. In the early stage the vesicle must be differentiated from pemphigus, eczema, and herpes, in the later stage from the syphilides.

OBSTETRICS.

UNDER THE CHARGE OF

EDWARD P. DAVIS, A.M., M.D.,

PROFESSOR OF OBSTETRICS IN THE JEFFERSON MEDICAL COLLEGE; PROFESSOR OF OBSTETRICS AND DISEASES OF INFANCY IN THE PHILADELPHIA POLYCLINIC; CLINICAL PROFESSOR OF DISEASES OF CHILDREN IN THE WOMAN'S MEDICAL COLLEGE; VISITING OBSTETRICIAN TO THE PHILADELPHIA HOSPITAL, ETC.

Diabetes Mellitus and Metritis.—LEIPMANN (*Archiv für Gynäkologie*, Band lxx., Heft 2, 1903) reports the case of a patient, aged thirty years, in her sixth pregnancy. The abdomen was more enlarged than the gestation warranted, heart sounds could not be heard, fetal movements could not be felt, and the patient suffered from dyspnœa. There was a history of diminution in the quantity of urine voided; the feet were swollen; the urine contained large quantities of sugar with a trace of albumin, with leukocytes, but no casts and kidney epithelia in the sediment. The membranes were ruptured and about eleven pints of amniotic liquid allowed to escape. The head of the child could be felt freely movable above the pelvic brim. A quarter of an hour later a large blood clot was expelled, followed by free hemorrhage. Version was at once performed, but the patient suffered severe shock. Extraction of the child was followed by the discharge of a very large quantity of dark blood and the placenta had partially separated. It was at once removed, the uterus douched and packed with gauze. The patient's condition was desperate, but she rallied under stimulation. There was at first no sugar found in the urine immediately after labor. When the gauze was removed from the uterus, streptococci were found upon microscopic examination. Antistreptococcus serum was injected and sugar appeared in considerable quantity in the urine. The patient became actively delirious and abundant acetone appeared in the urine. The temperature fell; the patient shortly afterward died in coma. Upon autopsy the cortex of the kidneys was found in fatty degeneration, there was ulcer of the stomach, arteriosclerosis of the aorta, and hyperæmia and œdema of the lungs. There was dissecting metritis.

This case presented polyhydramnios and diabetes as coexisting conditions. The immediately complicating circumstance which led to the patient's death was severe hemorrhage. Upon examining the uterus, the connective tissue was found necrotic, while the muscle fibre was intact. The lamellated structure of the uterine muscle could still be discerned, although the nuclei could not be seen. Abundant bacteria were present in the vessels.

Leukocytosis in the Complications of Pregnancy and the Puerperal State.—CARMICHAEL, in a recent paper before the Edinburgh Obstetrical Society (*British Medical Journal*, December 5, 1903), found that leukocytosis was an unsafe gui[illegible] as a symptom unless taken in connection with other well-defined conditions. In some severe cases of puerperal septic infection there was no leukocytosis. In eclampsia an increase in leukocytosis often accompanied a diminution in the severity of the attacks. No leukocyte count was of much value in determining the necessity for puerperal hysterectomy.

A Clinical Comparison of Pelvis and Fœtus.—LANE (*Lancet*, September 26, 1903) has made a clinical study of the development of Indian children and of the size of the pelvis in the mother.

In measuring the pelvis, advantage was taken of the relaxed condition of the abdominal walls after labor, and the conjugate was measured by pressing the tip of the middle finger strongly against the promontory of the sacrum and depressing the end until its radial edge came in contact with the anterior edge of the symphysis. This manipulation is successful when the uterus has undergone sufficient involution to descend into the pelvic cavity. It was observed that when the dark and white races mixed the result seemed to be the lessening in the pelvic diameters of the white individual. The average conjugate diameter among Indian natives was 4.008 inches, the average measurement between the spines 7.818 inches, and the average measurement between the crests 9.607 inches. In European women the average conjugate measurement was 4.411 inches, the interspinous diameter 8.24 inches, and the intercristal 10.367 inches. In Indian women the average proportion of the interspinous to the intercristal was 81.828 per cent. In European women this percentage was 79.477.

It was found that there existed a distinct ratio between the size of the child and the conjugate diameter. As the weight of the child increased so did the size of the conjugate diameter. The writer believes that in most cases the moulding of the head is largely due to the soft parts. When the head fits tightly in the pelvic brim it may be compressed by the pelvis during labor and subsequently expanded during its passage through the remainder of the birth canal. He concludes that except in the case of small pelves, a parallelism of the biparietal diameter of the head and the conjugate diameter of the pelvis is the result of natural growth and not of pressure. His conclusions are summed up in the statement that the child grows in utero in such a manner that its size is proportional to that of the mother's pelvis.

OTOLOGY.

UNDER THE CHARGE OF

CLARENCE J. BLAKE, M.D.,

OF BOSTON, MASS.,

PROFESSOR OF OTOLOGY, HARVARD UNIVERSITY.

ASSISTED BY

W. A. LECOMPTE, M.D., E. D. WALES, M.D., AND D. H. WALKER, M.D.

On Lumbar Puncture in Endocranial Complications of Otitis.—CHAVASSE and MAHU (*Annales du maladies de l'oreille, du larynx,* etc., pp. 384–479) state that lumbar puncture was introduced in December, 1890, by Quincke, of Kiel, who first employed it with a therapeutic aim to lower the abnormal pressure in the cerebral ventricles, but afterward as a means to diagnose, recognize, and measure the elevation of this pressure in certain pathological cases. It soon passed into the domain of general medicine and there was not much delay in acknowledging it as an efficacious proceeding of direct investigation of the central nervous system. It is supposed that even as the effusion in the pleural cavity reflects quite exactly the state of the serous membrane which contains it, so the composition of the cerebrospinal fluid undergoes special modification produced by the alterations of the meninges or perhaps of the nervous system itself. It is then, especially in this direction, that researches have been directed, for it is well known that the therapeutic value of lumbar puncture is limited. Empirically in the beginning, lumbar puncture has become a scientific means of exploration. Abroad, especially in Germany, where puncture is done commonly through manometric pressure, the clinical and bacteriological characteristics and the therapeutic value of the cerebrospinal fluid has been studied. In France the study of the cells in the cerebrospinal fluid by Widal, Ravant and Sicard has given a new impetus to this means of diagnosis.

Subject is divided into the following chapters:

I. Technique of Lumbar Puncture, Accidents and Dangers.
II. Technique of the Examination of the Cerebrospinal Fluid.
III. Diagnostic Value of Lumbar Puncture.
IV. Therapeutic Value of Lumbar Puncture.

Chapter I. Under the Technique of Lumbar Puncture, Accidents and Dangers, the anatomy of the lumbar region is first reviewed. In the adult, puncture between the fourth and fifth lumbar vertebræ, that is, in the fourth interlaminar space. In the child, puncture in the third or even in the second space. (Quincke.) In certain cases and especially in elderly people, where the cartilages have ossified, if nothing is obtained in the fourth interspace, repeat it in the third space. The needle is very simple, hollow with short head, made of platinum-iridium, and of sufficient resistance to penetrate without bending or breaking. Outside diameter of $1\frac{1}{2}$ mm., inner diameter of $\frac{8}{10}$ mm. to 1 mm., and a length of 10 cm. for adults; 4 to 5 cm. is sufficient length for infants. The end of the needle should have a shoulder to which a short rubber tube can be fastened to regulate the flow of the liquid. Quincke uses a trocar to which a V-manometer tube filled with water is fastened to measure the pressure. A piece of silver or platinum wire to keep the needle open. Strict asepsis of the instrument and the region to be punctured; also, the hands of the operator. In the faint-hearted an injection of cocaine or a jet of ethyl-chloride may be necessary. The penetration of the deep tissues is almost painless. The position of the patient varied, according to the method of the operator. Some place the patient near the edge of the bed, the back strongly bent, head between the hands, elbows touching the thighs. This is a good position for the operator, but cannot always be taken by the patient, and then again the position causes increased intraspinal pressure which may cause the fluid to flow too rapidly. The patient may take a lateral, or a slightly lateroventral position on the right or left side, the head slightly raised by a pillow. Pressure on the abdomen prevents unseasonable movements on the part of the patient, especially when the needle is suddenly thrust in. In frightened patients and especially those with meningitis, several assistants may be necessary to get sufficient immobility. This is not easily accomplished in the lateral position.

The point of puncture in the fourth interlaminar space is carried out according to Jacoby's line described in 1895. The liquid falls drop by drop and is best gathered in a sterile centrifugal tube. The needle is withdrawn quickly and the wound stopped by a drop of antiseptic collodion or by a light application of tincture of iodine. There is practically no danger in doing lumbar puncture. Of the difficulties, a dry tap is rarely made. The needle may be too short; strike the vertebræ, or the needle may plug up, or there may be a gelatinous exudate. Again there may be abnormal position of the interspaces, deformity or ossification of the ligaments.

Among the possible accidents, the needle may break, bleeding from a rachidian vein, and, in infants, the aorta could be punctured. It is also possible to injure the filaments of the chorda and cause spasmodic movements of the thighs; these passed away in twenty-four hours. If the fluid is collected too rapidly it may cause pain in the head, vertigo, tinnitus, and irregularity of the pulse. If this occurs, stop the flow and lower the head. Never let the pressure fall below 40 mm. After lumbar puncture there may be nausea or vomiting; a tendency to faint if the flow is too rapid or pressure falls below 40 mm. Often there is headache next day; sleep is impossible. These symptoms increase to the third day and then lessen till the sixth or seventh day.

Death may result, especially in cerebral tumor or uræmia. Cases of death have occurred after aspiration and after chloroform. Death nearly always results by paralysis of respiration. The respiration is first intermittent (Cheyne-Stokes) and then stops. Artificial respiration is of no benefit.

Accidents may be avoided by—

1. Puncture without aspiration even without a Pravaz syringe.
2. Place the patient in a prone position.
3. Never give ether or chloroform.
4. Avoid gathering the fluid too fast or too much.
5. Do not drain off more than 20 c.c. of fluid.
6. Avoid puncture in cases of cerebral tumor and be prudent in uræmic cases.

Chapter II. Technique of the Examination of the Cerebrospinal Fluid. It is important to know—

1. The pressure under which the fluid escapes.
2. Its color diagnosis.
3. The bacteriological investigation.
4. The cytological diagnosis.
5. Its chemical characteristics and its "cryoscopic."

In its normal state the cerebrospinal fluid is clear, transparent, and of a density varying from 1003 to 1004. Its quantity varies from 60 to 150 grams, but can be 300 grams and even 400 grams in old people. In pathological states its color is often altered and its density varies from 1002 to 1009

I. *Pressure.* About 125 mm. of water. In tubercular meningitis and tumors of the brain, 80 to 600 mm.

II. *Color.* Compare a tube filled with sterilized water of the same size as the tube in which the fluid is collected.

III. *Bacteriological Examination.*

1. *Direct examination the quickest:* Inoculation can only be performed in chronic cases and in tubercular meningitis. Among the bacteria found are staphylococci, streptococci, pneumococci of Fraenkel and Weichselbaum, meningococci of Weichselbaum, bacillus of Eberth, bacterium coli, streptococcus of Bonome, bacillus of Koch, etc.

2. *Transplantation and cultures:* Colonies only appear at about the end of fifteen days to three weeks, so that this method is inapplicable. A positive result is of extreme value; a negative result is of no use whatever.

3. *Inoculation of animals:* This method takes at least three weeks.

IV. *Cell Diagnosis.* Normal cerebrospinal fluid contains one or two lymphocytes in each field. If the meninges are irritated or inflamed the elements vary according to the intensity and nature of the process; a qualitative and quantitative reaction at the same time. Three or four cubic centimetres of fluid should be collected, best in a centrifugal tube and placed in the centrifuge ten minutes.

The cells contained in diseased states of cerebrospinal fluid are:

1. Mononuclear lymphocytes with small round nuclei. If they are increased in number or predominate, we call it lymphocytosis.

2. Polymorphonuclear leukocytes.

3. Large mononuclear lymphocytes, which are impossible or very difficult to differentiate in this liquid from the single endothelial cells.

1. Lymphocytosis of the cerebrospinal fluid only signifies the existence of an irritation of the meninges and does not give us any indication of the irritative process. They are observed especially in chronic meningitis (tabes, syphilis) and in tubercular meningitis.

2. The presence of polymorphonuclear leukocytes indicates a severe and acute irritation. Observed in acute meningitis, non-tubercular form, with pneumococcus, staphylococcus, and meningococcus, etc. In the first days of the disease the polynuclear leukocytes are very numerous and diminish as convalescence is established; the lymphocytes take their place and, having predominated, disappear as recovery takes place.

3. The cerebrospinal fluid remains normal when there is no anatomical lesion of the meninges. This is the case in cerebral tumor, hysteria, "meningisme" neurasthenia, thrombophlebitis of the sinus, cerebral abscess without complications, etc. The leukocytic formula of a meningitic exudate is in relation to the anatomical reaction which has caused it.

V. *Chemical Properties.* These researches have not been of much practical value.

VI. *Cryoscopy and Hæmatology.* Normally the point of coagulation of serum is about 0.56. That of cerebrospinal fluid is lower; it varies between 0.72 and 0.78. In diseased conditions it varies between 0.56 and 0.74, and in the large majority of cases between 0.60 and 0.65. The hæmatology is of less value than the point of coagulation. The results have little practical bearing as yet.

Chapter III. The Diagnostic Value of Lumbar Puncture. Diagnosis of the endocranial complications of otitis, especially in the early stage, when a judicious intervention could save the life of the patient, often presents great difficulties, sometimes even insurmountable. It is often necessary to ask, in cases with cerebral phenomena well accentuated but poorly defined, whether a true complication exists, and what, a sinus thrombophlebitis, abscess, meningitis especially in children, or an affection with localized meningitis, cerebrospinal meningitis, tubercnlar meningitis, or whether a simple reflex phenomenon. Is it "meningisme" hysteria or neurasthenia? The importance of deciding what to do in these difficult cases is such that the specialist is under obligations to try all means of exploration which general medicine provides to solve these hard problems. It is not indifferent in effect to go on an error of diagnosis, open the skull, explore the meninges, and puncture the brain to find an abscess which does not exist, or inversely to do nothing, believing a diffuse bacterial meningitis or tuberculosis when a thrombophlebitis or a brain abscess exists.

Lumbar puncture which permits the examination of the fluid in direct contact with the meninges, the brain, and the spinal cord, gives us knowledge of the actual state, the means of establishing with certainty the presence of an otitic complication, or of revealing the existence of an intercurrent meningeal affeetion. The study of these questions is the object of this chapter, which is the most important of our report.

I. *Thrombophlebitis of the Sinus, Particularly of the Lateral Sinus.* The cerebrospinal fluid is of normal composition, but its quantity, according to the Halle Clinic, shows an important increase. This fact has not been verified by French observers in cases of thrombosis without complications.

II. *Abscess of the Cerebrum and Cerebellum.* When the abscess is not complicated by other endocranial affection, sinus thrombophlebitis, diffuse or circumscribed meningitis, the liquid is as a rule normal, clear, without micro-organisms, and does not coagulate.

III. *Bacterial Meningitis.* Sicard has divided bacterial meningitis into three groups:

1. Bacterial meningitis caused by pneumococcus, staphylococcus, streptococcus, bacillum of Eberth, colon bacillus, bacillus of Pfeiffer, bacillus pyocyaneus and tetragenus.

2. Epidermic cerebrospinal meningitis due to the meningococcus of Weichselbaum.

3. Serous meningitis which represents the first stage of meningeal infection, the inflammatory exudate remaining serous without terminating in pus, and in which one finds pneumococcus, staphylococcus, bacillus of Pfeiffer and of Eberth, that is, nearly all the bacilli of the first group. Among the meningeal inflammations diffuse suppurative meningitis, caused by bacteria of different kinds, is most frequently observed as a complication of suppurative otitis.

Diffuse Suppurative Leptomeningitis. The suppuration in the majority of cases is in the meshes of the subarachnoid space, exceptionally in the subdural space. Thus, as a rule, suppurative meningitis occurs as a sole complication of an aural affection or accompanies at the same time a sinus thrombosis or a brain abscess. The cerebrospinal fluid obtained by lumbar puncture shows changes in its composition. It shows a varying disturbance, from greenish-yellow to true purulence, and contains a marked quantity, or predominating quantity, of polynuclear leukocytes and very often micro-organisms of different kinds. The pressure under which it is collected is variable, on an average somewhat increased. The predominance of polynuclear leukocytes here plays an important part and indicates the existence of a meningitis or a meningeal irritation. There are exceptions to this rule where the brain has been found covered with pus and the cerebrospinal fluid clear, normal, or without polynuclear lenkocytes.

IV. *Circumscribed Suppurative Meningitis.* Here we may have the same symptoms as in a diffuse meningitis. The puncture is not always demonstrative and can show a normal fluid. In all negative lumbar punctures in the course of symptoms of otitic meningitis there is the possibility of a circumscribed meningitis.

V. *Extradural Suppuration; Internal Suppurative Pachymeningitis; Intradural Abscess.* In these suppurative inflammations the cerebrospinal fluid is normal in composition

VI. *Serous Meningitis.* Serous meningitis is still poorly defined. We find described under this class bacterial meningitis not yet come to suppuration; meningitis from absorption of toxins, from suppurative ears, the temporal bone or the brain. Then the serous meningitis of Quincke. Serous meningitis is observed almost exclusively in infancy or youth and sometimes shows true meningeal symptoms; it takes most frequently a subacute course with tendency to dropsy of the ventricles, giving rise to symptoms of cerebral pressure, clinically like a cerebral abscess, with which it is frequently confused.

Merkens, Brieger and Körner believe that the great majority of cases of serous meningitis are due to the absorption of toxins from a suppurative seat producing a serotoxic inflammation of the meninges leading to an internal hydrocephalus. A sufficient number of observations of the cerebrospinal fluid has not been made to draw conclusions, though it is generally clear and under pressure.

VII. *Cerebrospinal Meningitis.* Due to the meningococcus of Weichselbaum. The cerebrospinal fluid is generally of a greenish tint and sligh ly cloudy. It can be purulent. Councilman has found it mostly tclear. Dr. Councilman observed the diplococcus of Weichselbaum thirty-eight times in fifty-five cases.

VIII. *Tuberculous Meningitis.* Most common in infants, caused by an otitic, or concomitant with, a general tuberculosis. Rarely it has been confounded with an ordinary meningitis or even with a brain abscess. The fluid obtained by puncture is most often clear, limpid, sometimes greenish-yellow, or tinted with blood. It is collected generally under increased pressure. The coagulum which forms is white, dull or gray, hard. The bacillus of Koch is found in about 50 per cent. of cases and always in small numbers. The lymphocytes predominate. The accuracy of information derived by lumbar puncture has put aside all ideas of intervention.

IX. "*Meningisme.*" *Pseudomeningitis of Bouchut.* A simulation more or less perfect of meningitis by a process independent of all cortico-meningeal lesions. Cases where no inflammatory lesion can be suspected. It should be distinctly separated from serous meningitis. Sometimes observed in suppurative otitis and to be diagnosed from simple or tubercular meningitis or cerebral abscess. Occurs in youth and also in the adult. Attributed to hysterical neurasthenic meningitis, non-bacterial intoxication, or toxins from pneumococcus, or reflex symptoms from suppurative labyrinthitis.

X. "*Labyrinthisme.*"

XI. *Traumatic Lesions of the Labyrinth and of the Base of the Skull.* Two cases cited by Moure. Numerous blood globules in the cerebrospinal fluid.

XII. *Influences Exercised by Certain Diseases on the Cerebrospinal Fluid.* 1. Syphilis. 2. General paralysis. Tabes. 3. Chronic alcoholic meningitis. 4. Mental aberration, senile dementia. 5. Hysteria and neurasthenia.

Discussion on the Diagnostic Value of Lumbar Puncture. The following conclusions are generally true, but not constant:

1. Clear liquid, normal, non-coagulable; thrombophlebitis of the sinus, brain abscess supra and subdural, serous meningitis so-called simple; "meningisme," hysteria, sometimes circumscribed meningitis. If the fluid gathers in a stream under pressure, very great probability of a sinus thrombophlebitis, serous meningitis or sometimes abscess of the brain.

2. Clear liquid, without bacteria or cells forming a coagulum; meningitis probable, perhaps by toxins (?), sometimes tuberculous.

3. Clear liquid or yellowish or slightly cloudy with lymphocytosis predominating, or the bacillus of Koch: tubercular meningitis (climinate clinically the causes of lymphocytosis if the bacillus of Koch is not found).

4. Fluid opalescent or purulent, forming coagulum with polynuclear leukocytes predominating, and eventually micro-organisms of different kinds; acute suppurative diffuse meningitis or non-suppurative cerebrospinal meningitis if there is the meningococcus of Weichselbaum and if the puncture is early, sometimes circumscribed meningitis. This is quite exceptional in brain abscess.

Then for differential diagnosis of the different kinds of meningitis and meningitis and brain abscess, simple serous meningitis, "meningisme" and sinus thrombophlebitis, lumbar puncture with its color, bacterial and cell diagnosis of the cerebrospinal fluid, does not give us an absolute diagnosis but one of great importance, especially if we are aided by clinical observation.

Chapter IV. Therapeutic Value of Lumbar Puncture. In practical otology, in meningeal complications, lumbar puncture seems as if it could be therapeutically of a certain utility, at least as a means to suppress the initial seat of suppuration. If one decides to use it for this effect one must, following the advice of Netter and Sicard, withdraw each time 20 to 30 c.c. of fluid and repeat the lumbar puncture as many times as one deems it necessary.

CONCLUSIONS. 1. Lumbar puncture is a valuable means of diagnosis in intracranial complications of aural suppuration on condition that an examination of the cerebrospinal fluid is made as to its color, bacteriology, and cytology. Lumbar puncture without aspiration, without general anæsthesia, and with the patient lying down is almost always without danger.

2. Positive as well as negative results should be considered, also the clinical status and the exact stage in which the puncture is made. The influence of certain general diseases on the condition of the cerebrospinal fluid must not be overlooked.

3. The existence of a bacterial meningitis is indicated in the great majority of cases, if the liquid is turbid or even clear after centrifugalization and contains bacteria or polynuclear leukocytes or both. A clear

liquid or one slightly turbid, containing mononuclear lymphocytes in abundance, indicates as a rule tubercular meningitis, positively, if it contains the bacillus of Koch. Lymphocytosis is also seen in other chronic meningeal affections and in the convalescence from acute meningitis, especially in cerebrospinal meningitis.

4. In extradural and subdural suppuration the cerebrospinal fluid remains normal so long as the arachnoid membrane is free from all irritation.

5. Lumbar puncture in circumscribed meningitis up to the present has not given much satisfaction as an aid to diagnosis of these affections.

6. In brain abscess, in thrombophlebitis of the lateral sinus, and in the serous non-bacterial meningitis the fluid is clear and normal, often increased in quantity and under increased tension, more in the last two complications.

7. The fluid is normal in "labyrinthisme" and "meningisme."

8. After traumatic lesions of the labyrinth or base of the skull with ear symptoms, red blood corpuscles are often found in the cerebrospinal fluid.

9. The condition found in the fluid should never stop surgical intervention; on the contrary, the operator should be more exact in his purpose, starting effectively.

10. Till now the therapeutic value of lumbar puncture has been doubtful; nevertheless, considering the results obtained in general medicine and in some cases of meningitis of otitic origin, lumbar puncture may be performed, together with surgical intervention, so long as the situation does not appear hopeless clinically.

11. Lumbar puncture has demonstrated curability of certain cases of meningitis.

12. Examination of the cerebrospinal fluid, particularly as to its cellular characteristics, makes a great step forward in the diagnosis of intracranial complications of otitis, and we think it ought to be generally employed.

DERMATOLOGY.

UNDER THE CHARGE OF

LOUIS A. DUHRING, M.D.,

PROFESSOR OF DERMATOLOGY IN THE UNIVERSITY OF PENNSYLVANIA,

AND

MILTON B. HARTZELL, M.D.,

INSTRUCTOR IN DERMATOLOGY IN THE UNIVERSITY OF PENNSYLVANIA.

A Tuberous Iodide of Potash Eruption Simulating, Histologically, Epithelioma.—D. W. MONTGOMERY (*Journal of Cutaneous Diseases*, February, 1904) reports the following case: A man, aged fifty-two years, who, fifteen years previously had had a sore upon the penis followed by a generalized scaly eruption, presented an eruption of tumor-like and papillary elevations scattered over the scalp, face, trunk, and extremities after taking considerable doses of iodide of potassium. The eruption was accompanied by some elevation of temperature and evidences of renal insufficiency. One of the most characteristic lesions, situated on the forehead over the left eye, was a quarter-dollar-sized, soft, rounded tumor with a broad, constricted base and ulcerating summit. A portion of this tumor examined microscopically showed a structure closely resembling epithelioma, there being the same connective-tissue *loculi* filled with atypical epithelial cells. The author calls attention to the ease with which mistakes in the microscopic diagnosis of such lesions may be made.

Sublamine in Parasitic Diseases of the Scalp.—W. S. Gottheil (*Medical News*, October 17, 1903) found this drug valuable in an epidemic of tinea tonsurans in New York, where out of 900 children in an orphan asylum, 450 were affected. A solution of 1:1000 proved less irritating than corrosive sublimate and was found to cause less inflammatory reaction, and cures were quicker with the new remedy than with the old. The author states that a fungus not to be distinguished from the trichophyton could be cultivated from the scalps of persons who seemed to have no disease.

The Varieties of Lineæ Albicantes.—W. Osler (*Medical News*, November 7, 1903) divides lesions of the kind into three groups: first, those due to distention of the skin, as observed in ascites and pregnancy; secondly, post-febrile instances, especially such cases as are met with after scarlet and typhoid fever; and thirdly, the idiopathic form. The author gives the notes of a case of an adult in whom after typhoid fever transverse scar-like lines developed in the sacral region. Some cases are difficult of explanation.

Periodical Shedding of the Hair.—H. Ledermann (*Journal of Cutaneous Diseases*, January, 1904, p. 53) describes the case of a woman, aged twenty-two years, whose hair was shed every winter and grew in again in the summer. Last winter she became entirely bald, and this summer her hair did not grow in again. Absence of hair existed on the general surface, which began in circular patches when she was twelve years old.

A Case of Systemic Blastomycosis, with Multiple Cutaneous and Subcutaneous Lesions.—Ormsby and Miller (*Journal of Cutaneous Diseases*, March, 1903) report a case of systemic blastomycosis—the third on record—accompanied by numerous cutaneous lesions. The patient, a Swede, fifty-six years old, ten years before his death exhibited symptoms of pulmonary disease accompanied by fever, weakness, and emaciation. Two months after the beginning of this illness cutaneous lesions appeared which consisted of cutaneous and subcutaneous nodules and abscesses, and open and crusted ulcers extensively distributed over the entire body, but most abundant upon the head, face, and extremities. Pure cultures of blastomycetes were obtained from the abscesses ante-mortem and from various tissues and organs postmortem. Microscopic examination of the various lesions failed to show any tubercle bacilli, but revealed great numbers of blastomycetes. No reaction to tuberculin was obtained, and experiments upon animals were likewise negative as to tuberculosis. At the autopsy the lungs were found to contain great numbers of abscesses and tubercle-like lesions; the pleura was studded with nodules, and the liver and kidneys contained many miliary abscesses and nodules. The spleen was extensively diseased, portions of it being practically destroyed. The mesentery contained many nodules. Blastomycetes were demonstrated microscopically and culturally in all these situations, but no tubercle bacilli. While the early pulmonary and other symptoms and the patient's family history suggested tuberculosis, the failure to demonstrate the tubercle bacillus by any of the methods employed for this purpose, the absence of the histological features characteristic of tubercular tissue, the extraordinary number and rapid evolution of the cutaneous lesions, and the great numbers of blastomycetes in every lesion, in the opinion of the authors, exclude tuberculosis.

Pemphigus Neonatorum in the Light of Recent Research.—H. G. Adamson (*ibid.*) concludes from his investigations that it is generally admitted that pemphigus of the newborn is an infantile form of impetigo contagiosa, and that it is due to streptococcic infection. It would seem therefore reasonable to suppose that observers who have described the staphylococcus pyogenes aureus as the infective agent in pemphigus of the newborn have been concerned with a secondary infection, and that investigation by special culture methods will discover the streptococcus pyogenes as the primary cause.

Tinea Versicolor of the Finger Nails.—Campana, of Rome (*Journal of Cutaneous Diseases*, January, 1904), cites a case in which the fingers and finger nails were affected. For a long time prior to the appearance of the disease on the fingers the nails had been thickened. The microscope showed the presence of the mycelian and sporon of the microsporon furfur.

Pityriasis Rosea.—Weiss (*Journal of the American Medical Association*, July 4, 1903), in a paper read at the Fifty-fourth Annual Session of the American Medical Association in the Section on Cutaneous Medicine and Surgery, reports the results of his study of this affection. He believes the disease to be of internal origin, due to some pathogenic substance circulating in the blood. Microscopic examination of scales and sections and culture experiments failed to reveal any fungus in the cases which he has studied. The microscopic picture presented by the malady is that of a mild subacute exudative inflammation affecting the cutis chiefly.

Acute Contagious Pemphigus in the Newly Born.—G. J. Maguire, of London (*British Journal of Dermatology*, December, 1903), presents an interesting paper on a subject about which there is not much definite knowledge. A series of 18 cases is given, illustrating an epidemic of this disease. The author summarizes his experience as follows: That his cases, occurring epidemically, belonged to the group designated pemphigus acutus neonatorum. The disease was due to a pathogenic micro-organism, the staphylococcus pyogenes aureus, conveyed from case to case by a certain midwife. While occurring chiefly in the newly born, and only fatal to these, it also attacked older children and adults.

It was characterized by a bullous eruption on the skin, variable in distribution and extent, the specific organism being found in the contents of the blebs. In many of the cases no symptoms other than the skin eruption were manifested, but a certain group of cases showed grave symptoms of a general infection, and invariably ended fatally. The point at which the systemic invasion arose in these fatal cases was the unhealed umbilical scar. The treatment had little or no effect upon the course and duration of the disease, whatever the result.

Influence of the Becquerel Rays upon the Skin.—HALKIN (*Archiv für Dermatologie und Syphilis*, Bd. lxv., Heft 2), experimenting with radium-barium bromide upon the skin of young pigs, found that effects very similar to those produced by the Roentgen ray were produced. After exposures of varying length, the portions of skin exposed were excised and examined microscopically. It was found that the Becquerel rays acted upon the vessels, the epithelium, and the connective-tissue cells much in the same way as the Roentgen rays. Experiments were then made to determine whether these rays might be employed therapeutically, lupus vulgaris being the disease selected for the experiments. Exposures of moderate duration were apparently without effect. After exposures lasting from two to four hours, repeated daily for from fourteen to nineteen days, ulceration followed; but even in these cases the most careful microscopic examination failed to show any effect upon the deeper portions of the lupus deposit.

Six Cases of the Miliary Perifollicular Syphiloderm Resembling Lichen Scrofulosorum and Lichen Pilaris.—JONITESCU (*Annales de Derm. et de Syph.*, June, 1903) describes the pathological anatomy of five cases which consisted of a perifollicular cellular deposit of plasma cells, with here and there giant cells, such as are commonly met with in the papular syphilodermata, the peculiarity being that they were perifollicular.

A Case of Chronic Purpuric Erythema (Eight Years' Duration), with Pigmentation of Skin and Enlargement of Liver and Spleen.—OSLER (*Journal of Cutaneous Diseases*, July, 1903) reports the following unusual and interesting case: A man thirty-three years old was admitted to the Johns Hopkins Hospital, complaining of an extensive cutaneous eruption and soreness of the wrists, ankles, and knees. The illness had begun seven years before with red spots about the ankles, and from that time the legs had never been free from eruption, which gradually grew worse, spreading slowly up the legs. Some years later spots appeared upon the arms. The face remained free. The eruption was not accompanied by itching. For a year past there was a good deal of pain in the joints, chiefly pain on motion, but no swelling nor redness. When admitted to the hospital the legs presented an almost uniform, deep brownish pigmentation with here and there lighter areas; wide-spread areas of hemorrhagic infiltration into the skin; localized and distinctly raised areas of hyperæmia and hemorrhage resembling purpura urticans, and lastly a general scaliness. The condition extended to the groins in front and to the sacral region behind. The skin was hard and brawny to the touch. The greater part of the back was free, but there were a few spots above the sacral region and in the left interscapular area. Upon the left arm along the posterior axillary fold were linear ecchymoses, and a few spots of hemorrhage and infiltration over the biceps. The spleen and liver were both enlarged. The patient improved decidedly during his stay in the hospital. The continuous warm bath was used, the patient remaining seventeen or eighteen hours in the tub. The skin improved very much, but fresh hemorrhages occurred at intervals. Examination of the skin excised from the leg showed much iron-containing pigment in the connective tissue of the corium, and an increase in the small mononuclear elements. Six months later the condition of the skin had changed very little. About one year after the last examination the patient died of pernicious malaria.

PATHOLOGY AND BACTERIOLOGY.

UNDER THE CHARGE OF

SIMON FLEXNER, M.D.,

DIRECTOR OF THE ROCKEFELLER INSTITUTE FOR MEDICAL RESEARCH, NEW YORK.

ASSISTED BY

WARFIELD T. LONGCOPE, M.D.,

RESIDENT PATHOLOGIST, PENNSYLVANIA HOSPITAL, PHILADELPHIA.

Report of Investigation of Spotted Fever.—WILSON and CHOWNING (*First Biennial Report of the Montana State Board of Health*). The disease known in Montana as "spotted fever" has been recognized as a distinct clinical entity by physicians of the Bitter Root Valley for fifteen to twenty years. It is confined to the eastern foot-hills of the Bitter Root Mountains in a valley on the western side of the Bitter Root River, but outside of this comparatively small area the disease is rarely if ever seen. Sp[illegible] fever is met with only in the spring months, appearing between March and July. Persons who are constantly out-of-doors upon the foot-hills and mountains are the ones oftenest attacked, and apparently for this reason the disease is more common in males than in females. The mortality is very high; 70 per cent. to 80 per cent. of the cases end fatally. Death usually occurs between the sixth and eleventh days of the disease, but should the termination be favorable the attack is prolonged, and convalescence is slow. An initial chill usually marks the onset of the disease, while the early symptoms are headache, backache and joint pains. The general appearance is much like that of typhoid fever. After the initial chill the temperature rises to 103° or 104° F., and in five to seven days may reach 105° or 107° F. If the patient recovers the temperature usually falls by lysis. The eruption, which has given the name to the disease, makes its appearance from the second to the fifth day after the chill, spreading from the wrists, ankles and back over the entire body. At first the rash is macular, of a rose-red hue, and disappears on pressure; but later the spots become permanent, much larger, and assume a deep purple hue. Purplish petechiæ may be present. The skin ordinarily shows some jaundice, and the vessels of the conjunctivæ are injected. Superficial gangrene, pneumonia, and articular rheumatism may arise as complications. At autopsy no specific lesions are found. All the organs are congested and show the evidences of an acute infection.

In the red blood cells of the circulating blood the authors found an organism which they believe is a hitherto undescribed hæmatozoon. In a fresh drop of blood from the patient's ear the parasites are not very numerous, though they may be found with careful search during the entire course of the disease. As far as may be determined, two stages can be recognized in the life-cycle of this parasite. In the first phase the organisms appear as small hyaline oval bodies, 1 micron in thickness by 1½ microns in length. Two of these bodies may occur in the same corpuscle. Motility has not been observed. In the second stage oval or irregular solitary bodies are seen within the red blood corpuscles. This form measures from 2 to 3 microns in breadth and 5 microns in length; it is actively amœboid, and constantly throws out and draws in small pseudopodia, thus changing its shape with gı a rapidity. The parasites are readily stained by methylene blue, Nocht-Romanowsky, hæmatoxylin and Jenner's mixture. While the organisms are scarce in the circulating blood, they may be found in abundance within the red blood cells of the internal organs. In sections and smears from the heart muscle, spleen, liver, and kidneys great numbers of red blood corpuscles are seen containing parasites, and frequently many phagocytes are observed which have absorbed one to eight infected red blood cells.

By means of subcutaneous inoculations of spleen and heart's blood from autopsy cases the disease can be transmitted in a mild form to rabbits, and for many days the red blood corpuscles of these animals are found to harbor parasites. The mode of infection is believed to be through tick bites, although direct proof of this means of transference is not yet established. The tick is not suspected, however, of carrying the parasite from man to man, but is considered to act as an intermediate host and to receive the parasite from the "gray gopher" or "ground squirrel." This rodent is plentiful in the infected district, and, moreover, its geographical and seasonal distribution bears a close relationship to the situation and occurrence of "spotted fever." Several "gray gophers" were captured, and in the blood of many of these animals parasites were found which were similar in all respects to those seen in the red blood corpuscles of the blood from cases of spotted fever.

The interesting fact was also noted that only the gophers from the west side of the river harbored parasites, while those from the east side, where spotted fever does not occur, were entirely free from the infection. The authors in concluding suggest that many points will have to be investigated before the study of the disease or its mode of transmission can be completed.

On a Dysentery Antitoxin.—Charles Todd (*Brit. Med. Jour.*, 1903, vol. ii. p. 1457) concludes from his work upon dysentery antitoxins that by growing the dysentery bacillus in a somewhat highly alkaline broth a soluble toxin is obtained. Certain animals, notably the horse and rabbit, are highly susceptible to this toxin. The toxin is fairly stable, and though destroyed by an exposure to a temperature of 80° C.

for an hour, it is not altered by exposure to a temperature of 70° C. for the same period. When injected into suitable animals, for example the horse, the toxin gives rise to a powerful antitoxin. The combination of the toxin and antitoxin "in vitro" does not take place immediately, but requires a certain time, and the rate of combination varies with the temperature.

Bacteriological and Anatomical Studies of Scarlet Fever, with Special Reference to Blood Examinations.—JOCHMANN (*Deut. Arch. f. klin. Med.*, Bd. lxxviii. p. 209) contributes an interesting article upon this subject. In 161 cases of scarlet fever streptococci were found in the blood twenty-five times during life, pneumococci twice, and paratyphoid bacilli once. Streptococci were never isolated from the blood duing the first two days of the disease, nor from the blood of any of the fulminating cases. Their presence was always coincident with some secondary infection, usually a tonsillitis. All the cases from which positive cultures were obtained ended fatally, death occurring within one or two days. The bacteriological examination of 70 autopsy cases showed that in a very large proportion streptococci were present not only in the heart's blood, but in the spleen, bone-marrow, and less frequently in the kidney. This streptococcic infection appeared as a secondary event in the course of the disease. The usual portal of entry was the tonsils. In all but one of the cases showing streptococci in the blood during life, microscopic examinations of the tonsils after death revealed very definite lesions with accumulations of streptococci in the bloodvessels and lymphatics of the surrounding tissues. The one exception was a case of otitis media with mastoid infection. The author concludes that streptococcic infection plays an exceedingly important role in scarlet fever, although the condition has no etiological significance and must be considered as a secondary event.

The Pathological Anatomy of Whooping-cough and the Presence of the Whooping-cough Bacillus in the Organs.—ARNHEIM (Virchow's *Archiv*, 1903, Bd. clxxiv. p. 530) concludes, from a study of eight fatal cases of whooping-cough, that the disease is an infectious catarrh of the mucous membrane of the respiratory tract, affecting particularly the trachea. In the secretion of the air-passages and in their mucous membranes it is possible to demonstrate the characteristic polar-staining bacillus, which has been described by Czaplewski as the exciting cause of the áffection. The bacilli often occur in colonies. A desquamative catarrh is usually present. Great numbers of bacteria are found in the bronchopneumonic patches in the lungs. The onset of the characteristic coughing spells is caused by the presence of bacterial colonies in the typical "cough areas," the situation of which Nothnagel and Kohts have described. The coughing spells should thus be considered as a healing process, since with the expectorated sputum innumerable bacteria are carried away. The secretion is viscid. Healing follows with *restitutio ad integram* after the expulsion of the colonies of bacteria from the mucous membrane.

Periarteritis Nodosa.—VESZPREMI and JONCSO (*Ziegler's Beit.*, 1903, Bd. xxxiv. p. 1) say this affection was first described by Kussmaul and Maier in 1866, but it is of such rare occurrence that the authors have only been able to collect eight authentic cases reported since that time. The case under discussion was that of a boy, aged fourteen years, who for six months before death had had occasional choreiform attacks and a petechial eruption over parts of the body. He was admitted to the hospital with symptoms of cerebral hemorrhage. At autopsy a large hemorrhage was found over the cortex of the cerebrum. Multiple miliary aneurisms were discovered in the coronary arteries and in the lesser arteries of the stomach and intestines, besides which there were small nodules situated above the vessels and occasional thromboses, giving rise in the heart to disseminated areas of necrosis. Histological examination of the aneurisms and periarteritic nodules showed that the earliest change consisted in an invasion of the adventitia of the smallest vessels by great numbers of leucocytes, while in a later stage the process extended to the media and produced grave defects in that coat. Owing to these alterations the vessel walls appeared unable to withstand the blood pressure, and therefore the coats were stretched and thinned, or the elastica torn into short fibres. In the more advanced lesions the infiltration of leucocytes had subsided, and connective tissue cells made their way from the adventitia through the media and elastica into the intima, overgrowing and replacing the leucocytes. The hyaline-like band described by Meyer, Graf, Müller, and Freund which lies between the thickened intima and the atrophied media was formed by a coagulation necrosis of the exudate in the vessel walls. The authors conclude, in reviewing the cases so far recorded, that the symptomatology of the disease is so varied and confusing that one can scarcely recognize the affection clinically as an entity. They emphasize particularly the fact that the changes in the vessels and thickening of the intima especially are dependent upon a process which originates in the adventitia of the arteries.

Lesions of the Red Bone-marrow in Typhoid Fever with Special Reference to the Vertebræ.—E. Fraenkel (*Mit. aus den Grenzgeb. der Med. u. Chir.*, 1903, Bd. x. p. 1) says that in 1894 Quincke made the announcement that he had found typhoid bacilli in the bone-marrow of eight out of nine cases of typhoid fever. Since then his observations have been confirmed by other authors. Fraenkel investigated thirteen cases of typhoid, and in every instance recovered typhoid bacilli in great numbers from the marrow of the vertebræ. The presence of the bacilli in the bone-marrow bore no relation to their numbers in the blood; in the former situation they were found as late as the sixth week of the disease. Sections from the bone-marrow of the femur and vertebræ showed definite histological lesions. Besides hemorrhages, accumulations of small round cells, and diffuse areas of degeneration, changes which may occur in other varieties of acute infections, and were not considered specific, certain other lesions which the author believes are peculiar to typhoid fever were found with great constancy. These lesions consisted in small areas of focal necrosis infiltrated with a delicate network of fibrin threads, but not surrounded by a zone of reaction. They are probably produced by a slow action of the typhoid toxin upon the bone-marrow cells and upon the lymphatics, in the latter case causing rupture of the wall of the lymph vessel and an escape of lymph, thereby giving rise to the mesh of fibrin lying between and about the necrotic cells. Typhoid bacilli were not necessarily associated with the lesions. The condition is not known to occur in diphtheria, scarlet fever, erysipelas, pneumonia or peritonitis, but in variola Chiari has described somewhat similar areas. The author believes these areas of focal necrosis are as characteristic of typhoid fever as any of the histological lesions found in the other organs, and suggests the name of "osteomyelitis typhosa" to describe the condition.

The Dysentery Bacillus in a Series of Cases of Infantile Diarrhœa.—WOLLSTEIN (*Journal of Med. Research*, 1903 vol. x. p. 10) during the past winter examined the stools in one hundred and fourteen cases of infantile diarrhœa occurring in New York. In thirty-nine instances she was able to isolate the B. dysenteriæ (Shiga). The clinical picture of dysentery associated with frequent bloody and mucous stools was present in most of the positive cases; but in some stools, though mucus was noted, there was no blood. For early diagnostic purposes the serum reaction could not be relied upon, since it rarely occurred during the first week, and frequently was not positive for two weeks. The isolation of the B. dysenteriæ from the stools was the only positive evidence of infection during life. The bacilli were found in the stools for a period of two to three weeks, and they occasionally remained for a longer time.

A Study of the Proteolytic Enzymes and of the So-called Hæmolysins of Some of the Common Saprophytic Bacteria.—ABBOTT and GILDERSLEEVE (*Journal of Med. Research*, 1903, vol. x. p. 42) conclude from their experiments made with the filtered products of the growths of B. prodigiosus, B. proteus vulgaris, B. subtilis, etc., in gelatin, bouillon, and other media that the destiny of these non-toxic but otherwise physiologically characteristic products of bacterial life in the body is determined by the presence of a specific neutralizing substance that can be demonstrated in the circulating blood. By the customary methods of artificial immunization the amount of such antidotal substances in the blood may be increased, though only to a slight degree; and through the use of sera from animals immunized from the non-toxic bacterial products it is possible to distinguish the proteolytic enzymes resulting from the growth of different bacterial species from one another as well as from certain physiologically analogous enzymes of animal origin such as trypsin.

The proteolytic enzymes elaborated by certain bacteria in the course of their growth are much more resistant to high temperatures than is generally supposed, some being capable of exhibiting their characteristic function after exposure in the moist state to a temperature of 100° C. for fifteen to thirty minutes. The so-called hæmolysins of bacterial origin, are at least in some cases proteolytic enzymes. The authors believe that it is possible by experimental means to contribute material support to the doctrine of Welch concerning the origin of bacteriogenic cytotoxins.

Experimental Researches in the Inoculation of Syphilis in the Monkey ("Bonnet Chinois").—NICOLLE (*Ann. de l'Instit. Past.*, 1903, T. xvii. p. 636) reports three experiments which were made before Metschnikoff's and Roux's communication, but which have hitherto remained unpublished. The cutaneous inoculation of three monkeys with the products of chancre resulted in the development, after fifteen to nineteen days' incubation, of certain local lesions. Papules appeared at the site of inoculation in two cases and in one case a hard indurated nodule, together with swelling of the adjacent lymph glands. The local lesions soon disappeared and no further symptoms suggestive of syphilis made their appearance.

Protozoa in a Case of Tropical Ulcer (Delhi Sore).—WRIGHT (*Jour. of Med. Research.* 1903, vol. x., p. 472), while studying a case of tropical ulcer, found certain peculiar bodies in both smear preparations and stained sections which he believes are protozoa and the cause of the condition. For the staining of these bodies in smear preparations the best results were obtained by using the methylene-blue-eosin mixture which the author has previously described. The bodies are generally round, sharply defined, and from 2 to 4 micromillimetres in diameter. A large part of the periphery stains a robin's egg blue, while the central portions are unstained or white. A prominent feature is a small lilac-colored mass which always appears near the periphery. The bodies are found in great numbers and often occur within cells. In sections the cortical portion stains faintly with nuclear stains, while the peripheral mass, considered to be the nucleus, stains deeply with methylene blue or gentian violet. It is possible that these same cells have been described before by Cunningham and Firth. All efforts to reproduce the lesions in rabbits by subcutaneous injections of material obtained from the ulcer were attended with negative results. It was also impossible to cultivate the organisms upon fresh human blood or other media. Wright suggests the name of *helcosoma tropicum* for this newly described parasite.

Pale Cells in the Human Liver.—ADLER (*Ziegler's Beit.*, 1903, Bd. xxxv. p. 127) has found that in the liver of the human fœtus two different varieties of liver cells can be distinguished. Besides the ordinary polygonal cells large, rounded, pale cells are seen, which, from their small fat and pigment content and the presence of mitotic figures must be regarded as young liver cells. Between this cell and the ordinary liver cells all grades of transition may be observed. In certain pathological conditions the livers of adults show the presence of pale cells which bear some resemblance to those in the fetal livers. When part of the liver parenchyma has been destroyed and there is a tendency to cell regeneration, as in cirrhosis, red atrophy, primary carcinoma, etc., these pale cells are numerous in the atypical portions of the parenchyma and appear exactly like those in the fetal livers. It is thus possible by histological examination to recognize those portions of the liver where regenerative processes are in progress.

Notice to Contributors.—All communications intended for insertion in the Original Department of this Journal are received only *with the distinct understanding that they are contributed exclusively to this Journal.*

Contributions from abroad written in a foreign language, if on examination they are found desirable for this Journal, will be translated at its expense.

A limited number of reprints in pamphlet form will, if desired, be furnished to authors, *provided the request for them be written on the manuscript.*

All communications should be addressed to—

DR. FRANCIS R. PACKARD, 1831 Chestnut Street, Philadelphia, U. S. A.

CONTENTS.

ORIGINAL COMMUNICATIONS.

REVIEWS.

PROGRESS OF MEDICAL SCIENCE.

MEDICINE.

UNDER THE CHARGE OF

WILLIAM OSLER, M.D.,

AND

W. S. THAYER, M.D.

SURGERY.

UNDER THE CHARGE OF

J. WILLIAM WHITE, M.D.,

AND

F. D. PATTERSON, M.D.

THERAPEUTICS.

UNDER THE CHARGE OF

REYNOLD WEBB WILCOX, M.D., LL.D.

OBSTETRICS.

UNDER THE CHARGE OF

EDWARD P. DAVIS, A.M., M.D.

GYNECOLOGY.

UNDER THE CHARGE OF

HENRY C. COE, M.D.,

ASSISTED BY

WILLIAM E. STUDDIFORD, M.D.

OPHTHALMOLOGY.

UNDER THE CHARGE OF

EDWARD JACKSON, A.M., M.D.,

AND

T. B. SCHNEIDEMAN, A.M., M.D.

DISEASES OF THE LARYNX AND CONTIGUOUS STRUCTURES.

UNDER THE CHARGE OF

J. SOLIS-COHEN, M.D.

HYGIENE AND PUBLIC HEALTH.

UNDER THE CHARGE OF

CHARLES HARRINGTON, M.D.

PATHOLOGY AND BACTERIOLOGY.

UNDER THE CHARGE OF

SIMON FLEXNER, M.D.,

ASSISTED BY

WARFIELD T. LONGCOPE, M.D.

THE

AMERICAN JOURNAL

OF THE MEDICAL SCIENCES.

JUNE, 1904.

RETROPERITONEAL SARCOMA.

BY J. DUTTON STEELE, M.D.,

ASSOCIATE IN MEDICINE, UNIVERSITY OF PENNSYLVANIA; PHYSICIAN IN THE MEDICAL DISPENSARY, UNIVERSITY HOSPITAL.

IN a paper that appeared in this JOURNAL[1] for March, 1900, the writer published a series of conclusions based upon the study of 61 cases of sarcoma originating in the retroperitoneal space. Since then I have had the opportunity of observing 3 new cases of retroperitoneal sarcoma, and have collected a supplementary series of 32 cases, making a grand total of 96 cases.

The reports of my own cases are as follows:

CASE I.—*Female, white, aged eighty years; abdominal tumor in the upper central region that was thought to be an enlargement of the liver due to passive congestion; no cachexia; course fifteen months; death from acute bronchitis. Autopsy. Pathological diagnosis: spindle-cell sarcoma of the retroperitoneal space growing from the connective tissue around the cœliac axis. The colon lay upon the anterior surface of the tumor, and the stomach was displaced forward to the left.*

The patient was a woman, aged eighty years, who had been bedridden for some twenty years on account of an intracapsular fracture of the femur. She was a private patient of Dr. Musser, with whom I had the privilege of attending her. There were the usual arterial changes due to age. Her heart was considerably enlarged, both to the right and left, and there was evidently some degeneration of the myocardium.

[1] "A Critical Summary of the Literature of Retroperitoneal Sarcoma," THE AMERICAN JOURNAL OF THE MEDICAL SCIENCES, March, 1900.

About eighteen months before her death we noted that apparently her liver was enlarged. The interval of rapid enlargement was about three months, and at the end of this time the mass in her abdomen, that we took to be the liver, was as large as it was at any time during the fifteen months that intervened before her death. The abdominal mass very closely resembled the liver, and we considered it to be an hepatic enlargement due to passive congestion. The mass did not move freely on respiration, but we explained this by the fact that her respirations were very shallow, and were probably not sufficiently strong to move the enlarged liver up and down.

For over a year we examined the mass at very frequent intervals and never noticed anything that caused us to doubt our diagnosis.

The patient was not cachectic, and the presence of the abdominal tumor did not seem to have any effect upon her general health. It caused her some slight discomfort and pain, but that was all. If the idea of malignant growth had occurred to us we would probably have excluded it on account of the absence of wasting and cachexia.

A note made six months before her death upon the size and position of the liver is as follows:

"The liver is much enlarged and extends to the level of the umbilicus in the midclavicular line. The right lobe extends almost to the crest of the ilium, and there is very little if any movement of the lower edge in respiration. The breathing is very shallow, and there is hardly any movement of the diaphragm. The upper dulness of the liver commences at the seventh rib. The surface is hard and a little rough on the right side. The left lobe apparently extends to a point just below the umbilicus."

The patient had a goitre of moderate dimensions. She died eighteen months after the abdominal growth was first noticed, of an acute capillary bronchitis.

An autopsy was performed twelve hours after death. There was much arterial sclerosis involving the coronary arteries and considerable degenerative change in the myocardium.

The notes upon the abdomen were as follows.

There was a tumor as large as a child's head, eight inches in diameter, originating behind the peritoneum in the upper central portion of the abdomen. It grew just back of the lesser curvature of the stomach. The left lobe of the liver lay flattened out along the upper border of the mass. The pressure that this part of the liver had undergone had caused some atrophy, and the edge of the organ was considerably thinned. The right lobe of the liver was thickened and elongated and extended to the crest of the ilium. Its surface was rough and typically hobnailed.

Microscopic examination of the growth showed that it was a compact spindle-cell sarcoma. The tumor had a well-marked capsule, which sent trabeculæ of fibrous tissue in various directions to the growth. The bloodvessel supply was not profuse. There was considerable hemorrhage in various areas of the tumor, and in many places there were the usual blood channels without walls characteristic of sarcoma.

The liver showed an extreme degree of interlobar cirrhosis with atrophy of the liver cells, and proliferation of the bile-ducts. In the lappet of the liver, which was flattened against the tumor, the liver substance was almost entirely destroyed, and the anterior edge of the organ had been converted into fibrous tissue rich in round cells, with here and there a bloodvessel and proliferated bile-ducts.

The stomach lay against the lower and anterior edge of the tumor and was carried forward, downward, and to the left by the growth of the tumor behind it. The small intestines were pushed downward. The hepatic flexure of the colon was displaced downward, while the splenic flexure remained in approximately its normal condition, so that the transverse colon ran diagonally upward across the abdomen and lay against the lower anterior surface of the tumor somewhat overlapping the stomach. The tumor appeared to spring from near the sheath of the great vessels above the cœliac axis and adherent to them. It lay just above the pancreas, but did not involve it.

The kidneys and adrenals had no connection with the tumor. The retroperitoneal lymph glands above and below the tumor were not affected. The tumor was freely movable, and might easily have been moved on respiration if the breathing had been strong enough. It was covered by peritoneum, which was somewhat thick and shining. It was nearly round and was encapsulated. On section it was white and hard, except for a small area in the centre which had softened. In several places it was distinctly lobulated. The lower border extended to within one inch of the umbilicus. The tumor's close connection with and its adherence to the left lobe of the liver, together with the enlargement of the right lobe of that organ, gave the whole mass of the tumor and the liver taken together a shape that approximated the general shape of an enlarged liver.

The lack of respiratory movement was explained by the weakness of breathing and absence of the movement of the diaphragm.

The case illustrates well several points in the diagnosis of retroperitoneal sarcoma. The position of the colon and stomach was very characteristic. The transverse colon lay upon the anterior and lower surface of the growth, and was pushed forward and downward. The stomach was pushed outward and slightly upward. The onset was very insidious and without objective symptoms. The tumor was elastic and resembled the liver very closely in its physical characteristics, so that the physical examination entirely misled us. It is probable that if the patient had been stronger and had taken a more liberal diet, she would have experienced some disturbance of digestion on account of the interference with the functions of the stomach and colon.

It is probable also that if the patient had been able to take a long breath the movement of the diaphragm would have imparted some motion to the tumor, since the growth was not as firmly fixed as retroperitoneal growths usually are. Indeed, the tumor was quite easily movable at the autopsy.

The tumor differed from other retroperitoneal sarcomata in its protracted course, in the absence of areas of softening and degeneration, which could be detected by physical examination, and in the small effect that it had upon nutrition. The advanced age of

FIG. 1.

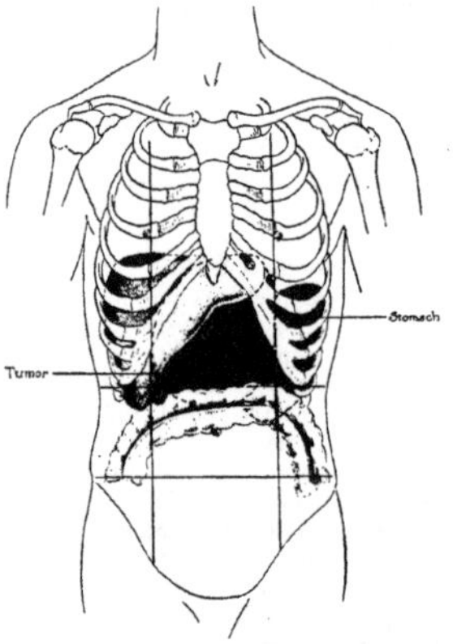

CASE I.—Retroperitoneal sarcoma. The transverse colon is pushed forward and crosses the anterior and lower half of the tumor. The stomach is pushed forward and to the left. Compare Fig. 4.

the patient may explain two of these points of difference, since the tissue changes of advanced age are necessarily slower than in youth, and if cell metabolism had been more active there would probably have been wasting and cachexia enough to have caused the death of the patient from exhaustion in a much shorter time than fifteen months.

As far as we could determine the presence of the tumor had very little effect upon the length of life.

CASE II.—*A white girl, aged four years. Six months after a fall which caused a hard blow upon the upper portion of the abdomen, there was enlargement of the left side of the abdomen accompanied by loss of weight and cachexia. Tumor and left kidney removed by* **operation;** *death in several months; metastasis to skin of the thorax.* ***Pathological diagnosis:*** *Spindle-cell sarcoma, which sprang from the capsule of the left kidney. Tumor was centrally degenerated.*

Case II. has already been reported before the Pathological Society of Philadelphia as an "Endothelioma of the Retroperitoneal Space." Further study of the case convinces me that I was mistaken in my first diagnosis, and that the growth was a round-cell and spindle-cell sarcoma.

The patient was four years old. She had always been quite well and active. One year before admission she fell from a considerable height across a rail fence, striking the rail with her abdomen. Six months after this enlargement of the left side of the abdomen was noticed. This increased steadily and caused a marked protrusion. Her general health began to fail, and she rapidly lost weight. Examination on admission to the hospital showed a large, firm, and smooth mass occupying the entire left side of the abdomen and extending about one inch to the right of the median line. The day after admission Dr. Willard operated and removed the tumor, which occupied the whole left half of the abdomen and lay behind the peritoneum. The left kidney was adherent to the mass and was removed with it. The child was much shocked, but recovered from the effect of the operation.

The patient went home and for a time was perfectly well. The growth, however, soon recurred. The physician in attendance reported metastasis in the skin of the thorax near the heart, but from the rapid loss of strength of the patient it is probable that there was some visceral involvement as well. She died three months after the operation. There was no autopsy.

The tumor removed at operation was a large oval mass measuring 15 cm. at its largest diameter, 7 cm. in its transverse diameter, and 22 cm. in its greatest circumference. The surface was smooth and firm. The tumor appeared to be made up of a number of spherical masses, averaging 3.5 cm. in diameter. These spheres around the edge of the mass were firm and hard, and on section they were pinkish-white in color. There was a well-defined framework of connective tissue surrounding these bodies and separating them from each other. The centre of the mass was much degenerated, and the central cavity was filled with a cheesy semifluid material. There did not appear to have been any extensive hemorrhage, although the undegenerated portions were studded here and there with small hemorrhagic spots.

The tumor was closely adherent to the left kidney and lay anterior to it and below it. The kidney was compressed and flattened from front to back. On section it was pale and somewhat light in color. Sections of the cortex of the kidney immediately adjacent to the tumor showed that the organ was considerably affected by the pressure of the growth. The capsule of the kidney was also much thickened and merged into the capsule of the tumor. In no place was there evidence that the neoplastic process had invaded the kidney or its capsule. The capsule of the tumor was about 2 mm. thick and sent trabeculæ between the tumor cells, so as to give the section a distinctly alveolar arrangement. The blood supply of the capsule was very abundant, while that of the tumor itself was fairly so.

Some of the bloodvessels in the tumor had the lack of true walls characteristic of sarcoma. Others had fairly perfect walls and carried with them a very delicate framework of fibrous tissue. The portion of the tumor nearest the kidney was traversed by bands of fibrous tissue and by collection of cells which had a distinctly columnar appearance. These cells were of varying shapes. Some forms had a deeply staining and large nucleus, while others had a distinctly oval nucleus. There was a very fine intracellular cement substance which was homogeneous and stained faintly with eosin.

The mass of the tumor was made up of round cells and spindle cells and was evidently a sarcoma of mixed type. There was considerable connective-tissue stroma dividing the growth into alveoli, but the fibrils of connective tissue did not run between the cells. The diagnosis of endothelioma was based upon the presence of columns of cells which were apparently endothelial in type and that ran through the tumor, suggesting lymph spaces. Further study, however, has convinced me that these columns were small bloodvessels with proliferation of their lining endothelium. Well-formed bloodvessels were very few in number and the greater part of the blood supply was furnished by blood channels with endothelial lining, but without true walls. The growth was evidently a sarcoma of mixed type, and apparently sprang from the capsule of the kidney or the fibrous tissue immediately adjacent to it. Apparently it had included a number of lymphatic glands.

The case is of interest, because the history of injury seems to bear a quite distinct relation to the beginning of the growth. The pathological anatomy agrees very closely with that found in most of the reported cases.

It is to be regretted that no record was kept of the physical examination or of the relation of the tumor to the mass. Its course was very rapid, though not more so than in a great many of these retroperitoneal sarcomata.

CASE III.—*White man, aged sixty-three years. Attacks of colic-like pains in the epigastrium commencing ten years before and becoming more frequent and severe until they resembled gastric crises. Six months before a tumor had appeared under the costal margin upon the right side. This grew rapidly until at the time of examination it was as large as a child's head. Œdema of the right ankle and leg;*

emaciation and cachexia. The tumor was immovable, hard, and nodular, with one spot of softening. The colon lay on the anterior upper surface of the tumor and separated it from the liver. Urine negative; no jaundice.

The third case was seen at the University Hospital through the courtesy of Dr. Musser. The diagnosis was not verified by operation or autopsy, but the history and the result of the physical examination presented a typical picture of what the study of the reported cases has taught one to expect. The case is reported with a tentative diagnosis.

FIG. 2.

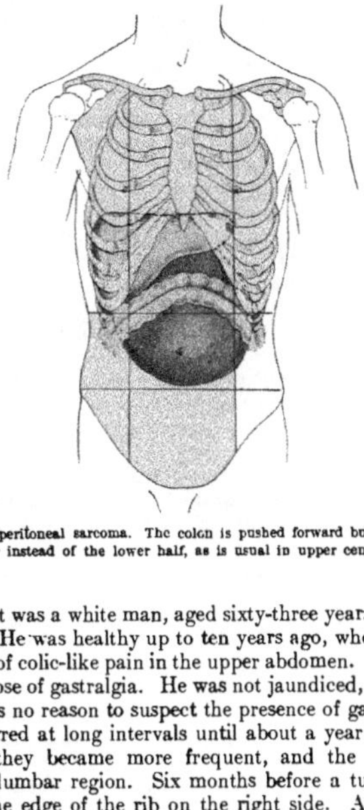

CASE III.—Retroperitoneal sarcoma. The colon is pushed forward but crosses the upper half of the tumor instead of the lower half, as is usual in upper central retroperitoneal tumors.

The patient was a white man, aged sixty-three years, and a native of Virginia. He was healthy up to ten years ago, when he began to have attacks of colic-like pain in the upper abdomen. These attacks resembled those of gastralgia. He was not jaundiced, did not vomit, and there was no reason to suspect the presence of gallstones. The attacks occurred at long intervals until about a year before admission, when they became more frequent, and the pain radiated through the lumbar region. Six months before a tumor appeared just under the edge of the rib on the right side. About this time there was œdema of the right leg and ankle, which lasted about four weeks. There was no pain in either leg. The patient had very frequent attacks of sharp pain over the tumor. There was no nausea or vomiting. He was much emaciated and cachectic, and suffered from constipation. The tumor was the size of a child's head and lay in the upper central portion of the abdomen. It extended slightly farther to the right than to the left. It was generally hard and nodular, although in the lower half there was a spot of softening with obscure fluctuation. The tumor was firmly fixed and immovable. The colon was full of gas and could be seen as well as mapped out by percussion. It ran over the upper anterior surface of the tumor, between it and the liver. The edge of the liver could be plainly felt just above the colon (Fig. 2). The patient refused operation and passed out of observation. Examination of the urine showed that the specific gravity was 10.16. It contained no albumin and no sugar, and it was negative microscopically.

The position of the colon showed quite clearly that the tumor was retroperitoneal. The fact that the colon lay between the tumor and the liver indicated that it had no connection with that organ. The absence of jaundice was against tumor of the head of the pancreas, and the hardness and solidity of the tumor excluded cyst of that organ or of any other structure. The growth was apparently a solid malignant retroperitoneal growth, and the diagnosis would seem to lie between a retroperitoneal tumor proper and a tumor originating in the adrenals or kidneys.

The result of urinary examination was against a growth of the kidney, but did not exclude it. The fact that the tumor was beginning to degenerate and soften was in favor of its being retroperitoneal sarcoma. The diagnosis must be a tentative one, but the picture that the case presented is very much in accord with that of a typical case of retroperitoneal sarcoma.

The notes of the following cases were given me by Dr. Howard J. Williams, of Macon, Georgia. I wish to express my very deep obligation to Dr. Williams for the privilege of recording these cases, which are as yet unpublished, and for the help and suggestions that he has given me in our correspondence during the past few months. This makes six cases that Dr. Williams has had under his observation.

CASE IV.—*Female, aged forty-four years. Six months before operation a small tumor was discovered in the left upper quadrant of the abdomen. The subjective symptoms were those of indefinite intestinal disturbance and constipation. The tumor was fixed and did not move on respiration. The omentum overlay the growth, but the intestines were not carried forward on the anterior surface of the tumor. Operation showed the tumor originated in the retroperitoneal space, just below the splenic flexure of the colon. Death six months after.*

Female; white; aged forty-four years. The family history and her past history are both good. She is the mother of nine children.

She was somewhat spare of build, but her general health had been perfect. In June, 1903, she began to suffer from some flatulence after eating, and constipation. Her family physician was called in and discovered a small lump or mass to the left and above the umbilicus. The mass rapidly grew and interfered decidedly with the functions of the bowels, producing obstinate constipation. The tumor prevented her from standing erect. She had never had pain, nausea, or vomiting, and practically no loss of flesh or strength. A physical examination made upon November 11, 1903, revealed a tumor as large as a croquet ball, which could be easily outlined through the thin abdominal wall. The tumor was fixed and was uninfluenced by respiration. There was no evidence that any portion of the intestines lay between the tumor and the abdominal wall.

An exploratory operation upon November 13, 1903, revealed a tumor adhering to the omentum and through it to the anterior abdominal wall. When the adhesions were broken it was found that the descending colon lay to the left of the growth and the small intestines to the right. There were many large veins on the surface of the tumor.

The tumor sprang from the retroperitoneal space to the left of the point where the transverse colon with its mesocolon crosses the duodenum. The mesocolon was not involved.

The situation of the tumor and the condition of the patient were such that the extirpation of the tumor could not be undertaken. The patient recovered from the operation and returned home in two weeks. She died six months after the tumor was first noticed.

Although there was no microscopic examination of the tumor, there can be do doubt that the growth was primary in the retroperitoneal space, and that it was malignant in character. These two facts render it almost certain that the growth was sarcoma.

The case is interesting because the tumor originated in such a position that it did not dissect up the layers of the mesocolon and carry the bowels forward on its anterior surface. It grew in such a manner that the omentum was the only structure pushed forward by its growth. In its insidious onset, in the production of indefinite digestive disturbances, and in its quick course and absence of cachexia until the growth was large enough to seriously interfere with the abdominal organs, the tumor closely follows the type of retroperitoneal sarcomata of the upper left quadrant.

If Dr. Williams had not operated so promptly, it is probable that in due time the tumor would have dissected up the mesocolon and carried the colon forward on its anterior surface. It is probable that this did occur before death, but as there was no autopsy no information can be given upon this point.

CASE V.—*Female, aged three years. History of constipation and vomiting for several months; decided cachexia; examination showed a large tumor occupying the left side of the abdomen; enlargement of the abdominal veins and œdema of the left leg. The mass was immovable on palpation and upon respiration. It was flat upon percussion, except for an area of tympany over the right edge, which was shown on operation to be the colon. Operation: The tumor sprang from the anterior surface of the left kidney and pushed the descending colon over to the right; extensive central colloid degeneration; death in twenty hours after operation.*

R. P., female, aged three years. Family history was very good. The child had never been strong. For several months there had been digestive disturbance, constipation, vomiting, loss of weight, and inability to walk. The child received no regular medical attention until the end of January, 1904. Examination at that date showed the presence of a large tumor occupying the left side of the abdomen, from the costal border to the iliac crest and extending to the right of the umbilicus. The veins on the surface of the abdomen were enlarged and the left leg was œdematous. On palpation the mass was firm and appeared to be solid. It was flat upon percussion, except over the right edge, where there was tympany. The growth was immovable upon palpation, and did not move during respiration. The child was anæmic and cachectic. Examination of the urine showed a specific gravity of 10.20, no albumin, no sugar, and no blood.

Dr. Williams operated at once, and I quote the description of the operation from his report:

"An incision was made on the left semilunar line five inches long. The omentum was not adherent and there were no adhesions. The peritoneum could be moved over the growth, which was the size of a small child's head. The descending colon was pushed over to the right, and the mesocolon rested upon the mass and was loosely adherent to it. The peritoneum over the presenting surface of the tumor was incised and stripped up. There were enlarged veins over the surface of the growth. On palpating the exposed portion of the tumor a sense of softness was obtained, and an exploring trocar was thrust into the growth and drew off some drops of gelatinous fluid. The incision was enlarged and a quantity of grumous colloid material escaped. The interior of the tumor was broken down with the finger, and this greatly reduced the size of the growth and made the further steps of the operation easier. The tumor was now enucleated by blunt dissection. The tumor was in this way separated from the colon and mesocolon and then from the left abdominal walls. Its base was found to be adherent to the capsule of the left kidney on its anterior surface, and it was necessary to remove the kidney with the tumor. The spleen, pancreas, and stomach were free. The tumor was not adherent to the posterior abdominal wall.

"Hemorrhage was checked by the free use of ligatures. The circulation of the descending colon was not disturbed, which was satisfactorily demonstrated after completing enucleation. Deep drainage was provided and the abdomen closed. Dissection of the mass showed that the tumor was attached to the capsule of the kidney. The kidney was easily shelled out of its capsule, and the renal tissues were not involved, except in one small area, the size of a hazelnut. The suprarenal body was not involved."

The child stood the shock of the operation fairly well and quickly recovered from the anæsthetic. She showed symptoms of shock during the following night. Pulmonary œdema developed, and the patient died twenty hours after leaving the operating table. A microscopic examination of the tumor made by Dr. H. F. Harris, of Atlanta, showed that it was a spindle-cell sarcoma with colloid degeneration. No kidney tissue was found.

During the four years that have elapsed since my first review of the literature of retroperitoneal sarcoma nothing new has been contributed to the diagnosis and symptomatology. However, many new cases of great interest have been recorded in current literature. These cases have been studied with greater care than was formerly the custom to give to such tumors, especially with regard to the physical signs and the relation of the colon, small intestines, and stomach to the growth. Witzel's observations upon the relation of the hollow viscera to tumors originating in the retroperitoneal space have been accepted as one of the most important diagnostic signs of this condition.

In general, it may be said that the attention given to such tumors is beginning to assume the importance that they deserve, and the physical signs and symptomatology are recognized as forming a definite symptom-complex.

Rudolf Goebell has contributed, perhaps, the most important article of the past four years upon solid tumors of the retroperitoneal space. He considers the subject of lateral retroperitoneal tumors of all varieties, and includes in his list 30 cases of sarcomata. His series contains 10 cases, to which I did not have access. The remaining 20 were included in my first series. He does not report any new instances of the condition, nor do his conclusions add anything new to the diagnosis or symptomatology. His paper is classical in its thoroughness, but is confined to the consideration of lateral tumors and is consequently limited in its scope.

M. L. Harris and M. Herzog have contributed an excellent article upon the tumors of the mesentery proper, that is, those that grow in or around the lymphatic glands situated between the layers of the mesentery. Such tumors have little in common with solid tumors of the retroperitoneal space, and none of the 57 cases which they have collected are available for my list.

Howard J. Williams reports 3 new cases of retroperitoneal sarcoma, which are included in my second series. He states that he has collected 11 new cases, but on referring to the authorities given, it was discovered that 9 of these were tumors originating in the mesenteric glands, and, therefore, cannot be considered retroperitoneal, as the term is generally used. The tenth case (reported by R. C. Smith) was included in my second series, and the eleventh case to which he refers could not be found in the reference given. Dr. Williams gives an exceedingly interesting review of the subject, especially the operative treatment of the condition. He has seen more cases of retroperitoneal sarcoma than have been reported by any one American observer. I wish again to express my deep obligation to him for the privilege of reporting Nos. 4 and 5 of the new cases recorded here for the first time.

Otto Hartman reports a new case of upper central retroperitoneal sarcoma, which is referred to at length as Case 69 of the new series.

R. Douglas reports 1 new case and gives a short excellent review of the symptomatology and diagnosis of such tumors.

In addition, new cases have been reported by W. E. Hughes, John McLachlan, R. C. Smith, and J. M. Withrow.

My first series contained 61 cases. The second series contain those that have been recorded in current literature since January, 1900, and those that were overlooked or to which I had no access at the time of writing my first paper, and amount to 30 in all.

The first series together with the second series and the 5 new cases amount in all to 96 cases, upon which the following conclusions are based:

AGE. The combined table of 96 cases show that retroperitoneal sarcoma is more frequent in the first, fourth, and sixth decades. 71 per cent. occurred in the third, fourth, fifth, and sixth decades. The oldest case was a woman of eighty years (Case II. of my own series), the youngest was a baby under a year, reported by C. A. Martin (Case 38).

Age.		Age.	
0 to 10 years	14	51 to 60 years	21
11 " 20 "	4	61 " 70 "	5
21 " 30 "	11	71 " 80 "	4
31 " 40 "	15	Not given	5
41 " 50 "	16		

SEX does not appear to be a predisposing cause. The combined tables show 44 males and 46 females. In 6 the age was not recorded.

POSITION. The whole list of cases have been reclassified as to their position, with rather more elaboration than in the original report. The table is as follows:

Central	19	Left lumbar region	12
Upper central	6	Left iliac region	5
Pelvic	6	Left central region	1
Right lumbar region	18	Lumbar region, side not given	1
Right iliac region	12	Whole abdomen	1
Right central region	6	Not given	8

Total central tumors	31
Total lateral tumors	56
Total right-sided tumors	36
Total left-sided tumors	19

MULTIPLE TUMORS.

2 tumors, both left upper region	1	2 tumors, left upper and pelvic	1
2 tumors, left upper and right lower	1	3 tumors, in region of kidney	1

ORIGIN. It is very hard to determine the point of origin with any degree of confidence. It is perhaps fair to assume that a tumor composed of round, fairly separate nodules, and consisting of small, round cells, had its origin in the lymphatic glands. On the other hand, spindle-cell sarcomata probably spring from fibrous tissue.

In some instances it is fairly easy to determine the point of origin, as when the tumor grows from the periosteum the capsule of the kidneys or the sheath of the great vessels. The following table is more condensed and simpler than the one in the original paper, and the number of cases classified as doubtful is much larger:

Lymphatic glands about spine	5	Periosteum of ilium	1
" root of mesentery	6	Connective tissue of retroperitoneal space	6
" root of mesocolon	4	Sheath of great vessels	2
" on promontory of sacrum	1	Wall of retroperitoneal abscess	1
Capsule of kidney	10	Connective tissue of pelvis	1
Periosteum of spine	7	Uncertain	52

Naumann suggests that the tumor in his case originated in the Neben-Körper of Zuckerkandl.

MORBID ANATOMY. The physical characteristics of the tumors in the new cases accord very closely with the description of the gross morbid anatomy of the retroperitoneal sarcoma given in my original paper. In the early stages the tumor is hard or elastic, usually round, and very often nodular. It is well encapsulated and white and glistening. The tumor is very prone to degeneration. This degenerative process usually commences in the centre and often progresses to such a stage that the tumor becomes cystic. The degeneration does not always commence in the centre of the growth, but may occur at any point in the periphery, giving rise to softer areas that may be distinctly felt through the abdominal wall. The combined list shows that in 29 cases the tumor was so degenerated as to form a cyst. In almost every one of the remaining cases there were areas of softening in some part of the tumor. Usually there is considerable hemorrhage in the tissue of the growth, and the fluid of the cyst is often described as brown and sanguineous.

The combined tables of the variety of sarcoma in 64 cases are as follows:

Small round cell	13	Myxosarcoma	1
Large round cell	2	Angiosarcoma	1
Polymorphic	9	Myxosarcoma cavernosus	1
Spindle cell	21	Giant-cell sarcoma	1
Lymphosarcoma	6	Alveolar sarcoma	2
Fibrosarcoma	3	Variety not stated	4

In the second of my own cases and in those of McGraw (Case 28) and McLachlan (Case 75) microscopic examination showed that the tumor contained unstriped muscle fibre. This is easily explained by the fact that bands of unstriped muscles traverse the retroperitoneal space, and are, therefore, easily included in tumors arising in this region.

Metastasis occurred in 31 cases, and the following table gives the different localities of the secondary growths:

Liver	11	Lungs	8
Spleen	3	Skin	8
Kidneys	3		

Lymphatic glands, scrotum, adrenals, muscle, mesentery, mesocolon, pleura, heart, bone, cord, dura, neck, 1 each.

SYMPTOMATOLOGY. The onset of retroperitoneal sarcoma is insidious, and the symptoms are not characteristic until the tumor has become large enough to be detected by physical examination. The growth generally manifests itself first by signs of pressure upon some of the structures in the peritoneal cavity or retroperitoneal space. The character of these symptoms can best be described by considering the results of pressure produced in the different regions of the abdomen.

In tumors developing in the *upper central region* the most common symptoms are those of gastric disturbance. In the early stages these are usually indefinite in character and consist of discomfort after eating, vague pain, and nausea. As the tumor enlarges pain is more severe and vomiting occurs.

In 3 of the cases (Cases 65, 68, and No. III. of my own series) there were crises of abdominal pain with vomiting much resembling cholelithiasis, but without tenderness over the gall-bladder, jaundice or other symptom of gallstones. The tumor in every case was in the upper central region and displaced the stomach downward and backward.

In Case 69 the sarcoma grew behind the lesser curvature and cardiac end of the stomach and by its pressure diminished the capacity of that organ, so that the patient experienced a feeling of satisfaction and loss of appetite after taking a very small quantity of food. He had dysphagia due to pressure upon the cardiac end of the œsophagus. The hydrochloric acid of the gastric contents was diminished, and this fact, combined with the presence of a mass, led to the diagnosis of gastric cancer, and to the operation which revealed a retroperitoneal sarcoma growing behind the stomach.

When the tumor originates in the *right or left upper quadrant* pressure symptoms are not pronounced, and consist chiefly of digestive disturbances of the indefinite character already mentioned, nausea, vomiting, and vague abdominal pain.

The growths in the *lower half of the abdomen* give earlier signs of their presence and produce pressure symptoms which are more severe and more easily localized.

In tumor of the *lower right or left quadrant*, the result of interference with the veins and nerves of the iliac fossæ, are œdema and neuralgic pains in the foot and leg of the same side. Occasionally this pain is very much localized, especially in the early stages of the growth.

In Rogowski's case (Case 78) the first symptom was pain in the right foot, most marked in the heel and gradually spreading over the whole leg. The tumor grew from the right iliac fossa. Keresztszeghy's case in the first series (Case 21) was strikingly similar. The tumor was in the left iliac fossa and the pain was at first very severe and localized in the left foot, and gradually spread over the leg.

In Case 80 of the second series there was contraction of the adductor and flexor muscles in the leg on the same side, accompanied by severe pain. The tumor grew from the right iliac fossa.

Ellis (Case 11) reports the case of a boy, aged seven years, who had œdema of the left lung and of the left side of the face. The tumor surrounded the left kidney, but did not involve it.

In Osler's case (No. 44) there was polyuria without sugar, and the tumor grew in the median position. It seems probable that the symptoms in both of these cases were due to pressure upon the sympathetic system of the abdomen.

Femoral phlebitis occurred three times.

In Lunier's case (No. 27) blood was passed from the urethra, and on one occasion a piece of tissue was discharged through the same channel. Microscopic examination showed that this was from a lymph gland, and a diagnosis of tumor of a retroperitoneal lymph gland was made. Autopsy revealed a retroperitoneal sarcoma that had perforated the bladder.

Ascites may occur, but is not frequent. Hydronephrosis is also rare, and occurred in but 3 cases.

Tumors of the *pelvis and lower central abdomen* produce early and definite pressure symptoms, as would be naturally supposed. Difficult micturition is one of the earliest and most common manifestations of retroperitoneal sarcoma in this region. It varies from frequent urination in the early stages to the complete obstruction of the neck of the bladder in the later stages.

Pelvic tumors usually produce constipation, which may amount to intestinal obstruction. Other cases, especially in the earlier stages, have persistent diarrhœa.

If the tumor encroaches upon both iliac veins, there will be œdema of the genitalia and both legs.

Occasionally, if the tumor originates in such a position that it does not press upon any of the structures of the peritoneal cavity and retroperitoneal space, there are no pressure symptoms, properly speaking, but merely evidences of interference with the function of the digestive tract. In such cases pain and œdema and the other signs of pressure appear later in the course of the condition after the tumor has attained sufficient size to encroach upon the neighboring structures.

PHYSICAL EXAMINATION. In the early stages the physical signs of retroperitoneal growths are those of a deep-seated abdominal tumor, concerning which little can be determined by palpation. Such tumors are rarely observed in their early stages, since their symptoms are so vague at the onset that medical advice is not sought until the tumor has grown to such a size that it is plainly perceptible to the patient himself.

The insidious onset of retroperitoneal sarcoma is a real source of danger, since by the time that the tumor is discovered it has grown to such a size that an operation is exceedingly difficult or impossible, and this is probably the reason why the results of operative treatment are decidedly unsatisfactory.

As the tumor enlarges, its retroperitoneal position can usually be determined by the signs that are becoming definitely recognized as peculiar to growths originating in the retroperitoneal space.

The relation of the colon and other hollow viscera to the tumor is by far the most important part of the examination in determining whether or not the growth originated behind the peritoneum. Since Witzel first called attention to the characteristic relation of the stomach and bowel to retroperitoneal tumors, many writers have verified his statements.

The conclusion of my first paper as to the relations of the colon to retroperitoneal tumors proper agreed substantially with those of Witzel, except that several of the collected cases demonstrated conclusively that the transverse colon may be displaced forward by retroperitoneal tumors in the median position, although Witzel claimed that this could not be the case. Two cases reported here for the first time illustrate the importance of careful study of the relation of hollow viscera in the diagnosis of retroperitoneal tumors.

The most important systematic observations that have as yet been made upon the relation of the colon to abdominal growths are those given in the recent classical paper by W. L. Harris entitled "The Relation of the Colon to Intra-abdominal Tumors."[1] Dr. Harris confirms the conclusions of my first paper, but has carried the subject farther, and has included in his observations tumors that are not of retroperitoneal origin.

If the colon is carried forward upon the anterior surface of the tumor, it is proven almost beyond doubt that the tumor originates in the retroperitoneal space.

[1] Journal of the American Medical Association, February 18, 1899.

The stomach is displaced outward and to the left by upper central tumors, and coils of small intestines may be found upon the anterior surface of tumors that sprung from the root of the mesentery and grew up between its layers. However, the relation the stomach and small intestines bear to retroperitoneal tumors is not as characteristic as the displacement of the colon to which reference has just been made.

The following is a classification of the relation of the colon to tumors originating in the various regions of the retroperitoneal space:

1. *Upper central* or *median tumors* sooner or later dissect up the peritoneum until they reach the transverse mesocolon, and then, as they enlarge and grow between its leaflets, the colon is carried forward upon the anterior surface of the mass. The bowel usually runs across the anterior and lower surface and curves slightly downward, with the convex of the curve toward the umbilicus. But it may run along the anterior and upper surface, as in Case III., where the transverse colon occupied the sulcus between the tumor and the liver (Fig. 2).

If the tumor is not exactly in the median position, but grows a little to one side or the other of the median line, the transverse colon may cross the anterior surface of the growth diagonally. (See Fig. 1.)

2. *Lateral tumors* carry the ascending or descending colon forward upon their anterior and inner surface in the same manner. Then the colon curves slightly inward with the convex portion of the curve toward the umbilicus. Here, also, under some conditions depending upon the direction of the tumor's development, the colon may cross it diagonally. The important fact is that the tumor has grown between the layer of the mesocolon and has carried the large bowel forward on its anterior surface. This cannot occur with tumors originating within the peritoneal cavity.

This relation of the colon to retroperitoneal growths is not characteristic of retroperitoneal tumors proper in the accepted sense of the term, as was insisted upon in my first paper. It is seen in tumors developing in the kidneys (Fig. 3), in the adrenals or in the accessory adrenals, in the remains of the Wolffian ducts, in pancreatic cysts, in abdominal aneurism (Fig. 4), and, in fact, in any growth originating in the retroperitoneal space, using the term in its broadest sense.

Harris states that in 95 per cent. of 34 cases of pancreatic cysts the colon was carried forward and downward, but the relation of the colon to pancreatic cysts is not as characteristic as its relation to retroperitoneal growths developing farther down, since the pancreas lies almost entirely above the transverse colon; consequently the colon will not cross a pancreatic cyst as far up upon the surface of the tumor as it would in the case of a retroperitoneal tumor originating in the middle of the retroperitoneal space.

A true retroperitoneal tumor may be so situated as not to affect the colon. In the growths originating in the upper central or upper left portion of the retroperitoneal space, the stomach and not the colon is displaced. In such cases the stomach is pushed forward and to the left.

In tumors growing from the attachment of the mesentery and separating its layers, the small bowel surrounds the growth like a crown and may even cover it completely, so that there is tympany in front of the mass, and as the tumor extends laterally and reaches the abdominal wall in the flank, there will be dulness in this region with the tympany in front, so that the whole picture suggests abdominal effusion. In several of such cases attempts have been made to draw fluid with the aspirator.

The presence of the colon between the tumor and the anterior abdominal wall can best be demonstrated by inflating the bowel with air through the rectum.

In the early stages the tumor is firm in its consistency and is often nodulated or knotty, especially when it originates in the retroperitoneal lymph glands. The tumor may be very hard, but the term elastic is used with striking unanimity by the various observers in describing its physical characteristics.

In Case I. the large and firm spindle-cell sarcoma originated in the upper central region, possessed this peculiar elastic consistency, and resembled the liver so closely on palpation that the growth was supposed to be the liver enlarged from passive-congestion.

In Case III. the tumor was distinctly elastic without fluctuation, except in one small area.

In the case reported by Jacoby (No. 15) a thrill was felt over the mass resembling that often observed in an echinococcus cyst. The autopsy shows a sarcoma with multiple area of degeneration.

Although in the earlier stages the tumor of retroperitoneal sarcoma is hard or elastic, there is a distinct tendency to degeneration, which occurs rather earlier in the course of retroperitoneal sarcoma than other solid tumors of the abdomen. This tendency to softening is distinctly characteristic of retroperitoneal sarcoma, and is practically the only point in the diagnosis by which it can be distinguished from other solid malignant tumors of the retroperitoneal space.

The degeneration is usually described as hemorrhagic, and, unless the growth is removed in its first stage by the surgeon, the autopsy reveals, in a majority of cases, a central cavity filled with a cheesy, brownish fluid containing old blood pigments, or the evidences of recent hemorrhages.

In 30 of 96 cases the tumor was so-degenerated that it had become practically a cyst, of which the walls were formed by the remains of the tumor mass, and the centre was filled with the fluid contents described above.

In 12 of the cases fluctuation of the mass as a whole was obtained before death, and in many more small softened areas were observed, although the rest of the tumor remained firm and hard.

The tumor is usually immovable, owing to its deep position and broad attachment. However, in 15 cases the tumor could be moved on palpation, and in 6 it moved on deep inspiration. When the mass was affected by the movement of the diaphragm, the growth was most often in the right lumbar region, and the movement is probably explained by attachments to the liver or the pressure of that organ upon it. But there may be movability synchronous with respiration in tumors which originate in other localities. Stiller reports such an instance in which the mass was in the upper left quadrant of the abdomen. In Witzel's case the tumor moved with deep respiration and sprung from around the lumbar vertebræ. R. Johnson reports a tumor that sprung from the left lumbar region, which moved on respiration. In a case reported by S. W. Morton there were two tumors, one in the lower right quadrant and one in the splenic region, that were influenced by respiration, probably on account of adhesions between them and the abdominal wall. Wilutski reports a sarcoma occupying the left side of the abdomen, which sprang from the periosteum of the spine, which was freely movable, and Lossen records an instance of a sarcoma springing from the capsule of the right kidney, which was extraordinarily movable on palpation.

The growth of the tumor is decidedly rapid. In 58 cases in which the duration could be definitely determined, the average length of the time from the beginning of subjective symptoms to operation or death was eight and a half months. The shortest case reported by Chassagne ran thirty-two days. McGraw reports a case of a man who had had a slowly developing tumor in the abdomen for five years, but in which the increase in size was very rapid in the last six months of life. It seems possible that the period of rapid growth in this case represented the true duration of malignancy. In Case I. we noticed no change in the tumor during the last fifteen months of life, although its development before this time had been rapid and occupied a space of about two months. Case I. is also remarkable for the lack of cachexia, and for the very slight influence that the sarcoma had upon the patient's general health and strength. Indeed, her death was due to other causes than malignant tumor. It is probable that the patient's advanced age prevented the rapid tissue changes that would have occurred in a similar growth in a younger person.

TERMINATION. The termination is usually death from exhaustion, unless there is surgical interference.

Case 49 died in collapse from rupture into the stomach of a sarcoma that had become cystic from central degeneration.

In Case 81, the tumor ruptured into the small intestines.

Case 88 died from rupture of an enlarged vein upon the surface of the tumor.

In three instances death resulted from the rupture of the softened tumor in the peritoneal cavity.

Tapping was resorted to in 5 cases. Case 65 gave a few drops of blood. Case 80 gave yellow fluid, with pigmented round cells and spindle cells. The tumor was a round-cell sarcoma that sprang from the periosteum of the spine. Case 90 was tapped three times, and each time gave a small amount of clear serous fluid. Case 39 gave viscid blood. Aspiration offers some aid in differentiation between cysts and solid retroperitoneal tumors, but it is questionable whether the measure is justifiable, in view of the fact that running a needle through the peritoneum into the tumor must be attended with some risk, and that the only hope of recovery in any malignant retroperitoneal tumor lies in operation.

In a certain number of cases wasting and anæmia appeared slowly and comparatively late in the course of the tumor's development, but, taken as a whole, cases of retroperitoneal sarcoma present the same degree of emaciation and cachexia that are characteristic of other malignant tumors.

Diagnosis. The differential diagnosis between solid malignant tumors of the retroperitoneal space and other tumors in the abdominal cavity which might be confused with them, has been fully discussed in my previous paper, and a study of the cases here reported for the first time, and of the additional cases collected from literature, only emphasizes the fact that a positive diagnosis as to the origin of solid malignant retroperitoneal tumors is practically impossible without exploratory incision.

Tumors of the kidneys and pancreas may manifest themselves by the urinary and digestive disturbances peculiar to these organs. New-growths in the adrenals may give more or less definite symptoms of Addison's disease. However, tumors may develop in any of these three organs without characteristic clinical symptoms.

The following case illustrates very well the difficulty of distinguishing between a solid tumor of the kidney and the so-called retroperitoneal tumor proper. The case was one of carcinoma of the kidney, and is clinically identical with a typical case of malignant retroperitoneal growth.

Case VI.—*Woman, aged fifty-five years; rapid loss of flesh and strength for three months and severe pain in the epigastrium; œdema in both legs; a large tumor occupying the right and lower portion of the abdomen; the tumor was hard and slightly movable; the transverse colon ran across the upper anterior surface; death from exhaustion. Autopsy. Large carcinoma originating in the right kidney.*

The patient was a woman, aged fifty-five years, who had been failing rapidly in strength for three months previous to applying for treatment. The only subjective symptom that she complained of was a severe pain in the epigastrium. There had been no pain in the legs and very little in the lumbar region. About a week before death there was considerable swelling of both legs below the knees. There was no diminution in the amount of urine, which was passed involuntarily and could not be examined. Her bowels were open and there was no symptom of intestinal obstruction.

Physical examination showed a tumor occupying the lower portion of the abdomen. Its upper border was at the umbilicus, the left border extended 9 cm. to the right of the median line. Lower border extended within 2 cm. of the umbilicus, and its right border ran

FIG. 3.

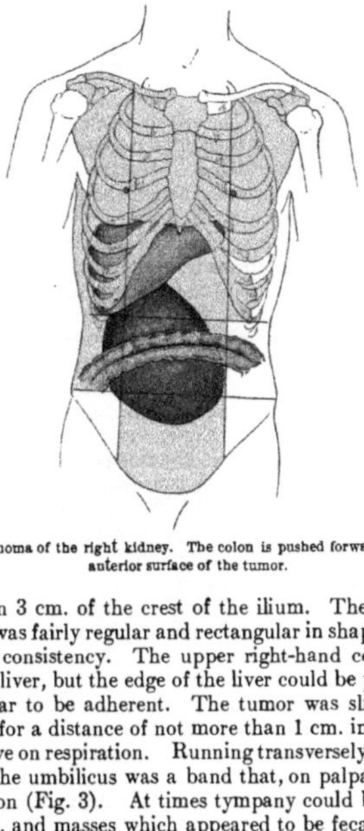

CASE VI.—Carcinoma of the right kidney. The colon is pushed forward and crosses the anterior surface of the tumor.

over to within 3 cm. of the crest of the ilium. The lower portion of the tumor was fairly regular and rectangular in shape. The tumor was hard in consistency. The upper right-hand corner extended up under the liver, but the edge of the liver could be plainly felt and did not appear to be adherent. The tumor was slightly movable on palpation for a distance of not more than 1 cm. in any direction. It did not move on respiration. Running transversely across it about 2 cm. below the umbilicus was a band that, on palpation, appeared to be the colon (Fig. 3). At times tympany could be elicited over this structure, and masses which appeared to be fecal masses, from their consistency and changeability of position, were plainly felt in.

it. On the right and left edge of the tumor could be felt vertical bands that were thought to be the ascending and descending colons. At a point a little below and to the right of the umbilicus was a point where indistinct fluctuation could be obtained. The liver was slightly enlarged, extending from the fifth rib 4 cm. below the mid-clavicular line. Several nodules were felt upon its surface, which appeared to be about the size of a cherry; otherwise the surface of the liver was smooth. With the exception of the structure supposed to be the colon, there was nothing between the tumor and the anterior abdominal wall. The flanks were full, but palpation did not give the impression that the right flank contained more than the left.

I am indebted to Dr. W. B. Stanton for the notes upon the autopsy, which was limited to the abdomen.

There was a large tumor originating in the right kidney and extending from the ilium to the costal arch. The abdominal cavity was smooth and contained almost no fluid. The descending colon lay upon its anterior surface. The spleen was not enlarged. The liver was not enlarged, but its right lobe contained one yellow nodule about the size of a quarter-dollar. The stomach and intestines were healthy. The microscopic examination showed that the tumor was carcinoma of the kidney.

The immovability of the tumor and the position of the colon rendered a diagnosis of retroperitoneal growth easy. The fact that a specimen of the urine could not be obtained made it difficult to tell anything of the condition of the kidneys, although it is quite possible that the urine might not have furnished any information. The case was seen only for the last three days of life, and the autopsy was limited and hurried, so that the report is not very thorough, but the case illustrates very well the relation of the colon to tumors of the kidney.

Retroperitoneal lipomata and the rare retroperitoneal congenital cysts may usually be distinguished by their physical characteristics, and tapping would be conclusive. Various rare, solid, non-malignant tumors of the retroperitoneal space have been reported, such as myofibromata and osteoenchondromata. The distinction between them and retroperitoneal sarcomata should be made by the history and course.

Tubercular enlargement of the retroperitoneal lymph glands should offer no difficulty in diagnosis. For a more detailed consideration of this subject, see my previous paper.

Mesenteric cysts present a fluctuating tumor, which lies at first laterally, but which enlarges and comes to occupy the middle of the abdomen, points toward the umbilicus, is freely movable, especially transversely, and rotates upon its axis. It is surrounded by a zone of tympany and has a zone of tympany passing over it.[1]

[1] Moynihan, Annals of Surgery, July, 1897.

Solid tumors originating in the mesentery are very movable, and are distinguishable by this characteristic from the retroperitoneal tumors originating at the base of the mesentery and growing up between its leaflets. In other respects, namely, the arrangement of the small bowel in front of the tumor and the dulness in the flanks simulating abdominal effusion, the two tumors are very similar.

Aneurysm of the abdominal aorta may very closely simulate a solid retroperitoneal growth. When the physical signs characteristic of aneurysm are well marked, such a mistake could hardly be made, but when the aneurysmal sac has reached a great size and has been so nearly filled with organized clots that the usual thrill, bruit, and pulsation are much lessened or entirely gone, such an error may readily occur.

Parker Syms reports a case of aneurysm of the aorta that so closely simulated a solid tumor that an exploratory operation was undertaken.

In the case reported by Phillipson (No. 46), a retroperitoneal sarcoma in the right lumbar region showed a distinct up-and-down pulsation.

One of the best demonstrations that such a mistake might occur is furnished by the following case that occurred in the service of Dr. Musser and under the care of Dr. A. O. J. Kelly, in the medical wards of the University Hospital during the past winter. These gentlemen will, no doubt, publish the case in detail in the future. I will merely refer to the points in the history of the physical examination, which show how closely a large aneurysm of the abdominal aorta may simulate a solid retroperitoneal tumor. I am much indebted to them both for the privilege of publishing the following summary of the history and physical signs:

Case VII.—*White man; aged sixty years. Pain in the whole of the right side referred to the spine and right hip; a large tumor in the centre and right of the abdomen, which was smooth and elastic; the transverse colon overlaid the tumor, and the stomach was pushed out into the left. At this stage the tumor resembled a solid retroperitoneal growth. Later expansile pulsation and bruit developed. Sudden death by hemorrhage from the lungs. Autopsy showed a large abdominal aneurysm, eroding the spine and rupturing through the diaphragm into the lungs.*

The patient was a man aged sixty years. During the past thirty years he had had occasional attacks of pain in the right hip, which had grown worse within the past two years, and had extended over the whole of the right side. Two months previously a prominence was noticed in the epigastrium, which subsequently began to enlarge. The tumor was large and smooth and somewhat elastic. The relation of the tumor to the liver, colon, and stomach is shown in Fig. 4.

When the colon was inflated it overlay the lower portion of the tumor. Inflation showed that the stomach was pushed up and to the left. The growth could not be differentiated from the liver by palpation or ordinary percussion, but auscultatory percussion rendered it very easy to demonstrate the lower border of the liver. Pulsation was occasionally noticed over the mass in front, but this was not expansile in character, and there was no bruit or thrill. The pulsation was considered to be transmitted from the aorta, and at this period of observation the diagnosis was thought to lie between pancreatic cyst, solid tumor of the retroperitoneal space, or a similar tumor originating in the kidneys. Gradually pulsation spread over the whole area of the mass and was very marked posteriorly in the

Fig. 4.

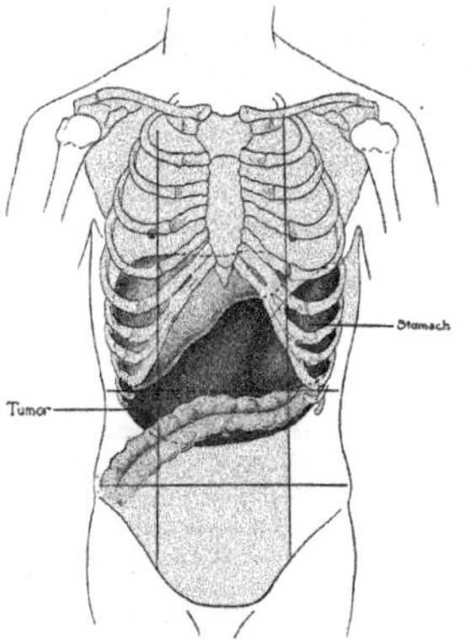

Case VII.—Aneurysm of the abdominal aorta. The colon is pushed forward and crosses the anterior and lower half of the tumor. The stomach is pushed forward and to the left. Compare Fig. 1.

right flank, and a bruit developed over the whole tumor, thus forming a very characteristic picture of aneurysm.

The man died suddenly, and the autopsy showed a large aneurysm of the abdominal aorta that had ruptured into the lung.

The case is mentioned because in its earlier stages the growth resembled a solid tumor of the retroperitoneal space so closely that at one time an exploratory operation was seriously considered. The fact that an aneurysm is a retroperitoneal tumor explains the displacement of the colon and stomach that is so characteristic of any growth originating in the retroperitoneal space.

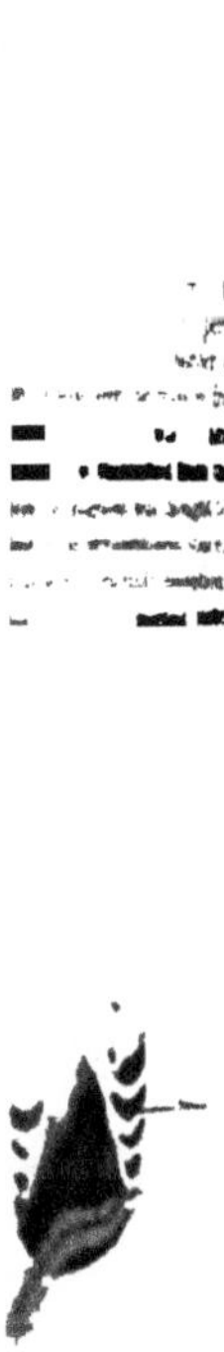

TREATMENT. The only hope for the patient lies in surgical interference and removal of the tumor. Naturally, the earlier in the course of the affection that this is done the better the prognosis. Consequently, the responsibility of making as early a diagnosis as possible lies with the medical man, and hence the importance of including retroperitoneal sarcoma in the list of possibilities when a case is under examination that shows indefinite abdominal symptoms with loss of weight. It is probable that physical examination in deep narcosis after thorough emptying of the bowel might often reveal a retroperitoneal tumor at a much earlier stage than such tumors are generally discovered.

It is not my intention to enter into a discussion of the surgery of retroperitoneal sarcoma. It is sufficient to say, that the only hope of recovery lies in the earliest possible diagnosis and removal of the tumor.

In the 96 cases here reported operation was undertaken 29 times, with 18 deaths and 11 recoveries.

The survival of the patient for two months after operation has been arbitrarily considered a recovery.

CONCLUSIONS. *Frequency.* Sarcoma of the retroperitoneal space is not so very uncommon. In the past few years it has become recognized that the development of such tumors has a definite symptom-complex, and more reference is being made to the condition in current medical literature, with a relatively larger number of reports of cases.

Etiology. The condition is more frequent in the first, fourth, fifth, and sixth decades; 53 per cent. occurred in the interval from the thirtieth to the sixtieth years.

Sex is not a predisposing cause. In 90 cases there were 44 males and 46 females.

In 4 cases there seemed to be a direct relation between an abdominal injury and the development of the tumor.

In 1 case the tumor grew from the wall of a retroperitoneal abscess.

Course. The development of the tumor is very quick. The average interval from the time the growth was first detected to operation or death in 58 cases was eight and a half months.

Position and Morbid Anatomy. The most common point of origin of these tumors is in the lumbar region (30 cases, or 32 per cent.), and the right side is oftenest affected. The next most frequent point of origin is the centre of the retroperitoneal space (19 cases, or 20 per cent.). Next comes the iliac region (17 cases, or 18 per cent.). In 6 cases the tumor grew in the pelvis, and in 4 cases it originated in the upper central region above the level of the umbilicus. The tumor was lateral in a majority of cases (56, or 60 per cent.), and two-thirds of the lateral tumors were upon the right side. The tumor is almost always single. It is usually lobulated and encapsulated, and is hard and firm in the earlier stages, but is very prone to degeneration. The degenerative process is oftenest hemorrhagic in character, but may be puriform or myxomatous. In a third of the cases degeneration progressed to such a degree that the growth assumed a cystic character.

Metastasis occurred in one-third of the cases. The secondary growths are most often found in the liver and lungs. In many of the cases the new-growth involves the intestines, and in 5 cases a cystic tumor ruptured into the gastrointestinal tract or the peritoneal cavity.

Symptomatology and Diagnosis. Emphasis must be placed upon the fact that the symptoms and signs vary so greatly in accordance with the position of the tumor that a very comprehensive classification cannot be made. The signs most characteristic of sarcoma of the retroperitoneal space may be stated as follows:

The earliest manifestation is the presence of a hard or elastic nodular tumor usually quite immovable, growing deep in the abdominal cavity and giving rise to rather indefinite digestive disturbances. If the mass is placed so as to interfere with the important structures of the abdomen or retroperitoneal space, there may be characteristic pressure symptoms, such as pain and œdema in the legs or genitalia, or obstruction of the urethra or the large or small bowel. As the tumor enlarges, the symptoms of interference with the abdominal viscera are aggravated, and there may be constipation, sometimes amounting to intestinal obstruction, difficult micturition, violent vomiting, or signs of perforation of the bladder, stomach, or bowel.

The point of most value in the physical diagnosis is the relation of the colon and intestines to central and lateral growths, and the relation of the stomach to upper central tumors. The determination of the position of the stomach or the colon in most cases should decide whether or not the tumor is retroperitoneal. When this has been done, the diagnosis is narrowed to tumors of the kidney, adrenals, accessory adrenals, remnants of the Wolffian ducts, tumors of the pancreas, cysts of the pancreas, aneurysms, and solid retroperitoneal tumors in the restricted use of the term.

Perhaps the only sign that is at all characteristic of retroperitoneal sarcoma, and that can be used in distinguishing between sarcomata and other solid tumors of the retroperitoneal space, is the tendency of retroperitoneal sarcomata to degenerate early in their course. When a tumor that is evidently retroperitoneal and that was at first hard and nodular rapidly softens and shows spots of fluctuation, the evidence is strongly in favor of its being a sarcoma springing from the retroperitoneal glands or connective tissue.

An exploratory incision is the only certain means of determining the origin of solid malignant tumors of the retroperitoneal space, and surgical interference offers the only hope of prolonging the patient's life.

The prognosis of the condition is distinctly unfavorable. The chief danger lies in the insidious development and lack of characteristic signs and symptoms in the early stages of the growth of the tumor. An early diagnosis is imperative, if any benefit is to be derived from surgical interference. It is important, therefore, to recognize that such tumors are not excessively rare and that their development presents a somewhat obscure but still characteristic symptom-complex. Hence it is important to include retroperitoneal sarcoma in the list of possibilities in the examination of cases with indefinite disturbance of digestion and loss of weight, especially if there are signs of pressure upon any of the structures included in the retroperitoneal space.

BIBLIOGRAPHY.

The following list of references includes the cases of the first and second series.

CASES OF FIRST SERIES.

1. H. Arnott. Proceedings of the Pathological Society of London, 1886.
2. Arnstein. Inaugural Dissertation, Berlin, 1883.
3. Bardeleben. Charité-Annalen, 1887, p. 439.
4. Bellevue Hospital Reports, 1879.
5. H. M. Biggs. New York Medical Record, July 29, 1893.
6. A B. Buchanan. Glasgow Medical Journal, 1864, p. 52.
7. J. R. Chadwick. Boston Medical and Surgical Journal, 1884.
8. A. Chassagne. Gaz. méd. de Paris, May 8, 1886.
9. Czerny. Archiv für klinische Chirurgie, 1888, p. 878.
10. G. F. Elliot. Proceedings of the Pathological Society of London, 1879.
11. E. Ellis. Lancet, January 20, 1866.
12. M. H. Fussell. Proceedings of the Pathological Society of Philadelphia, vol. xvii. p. 272.
13. Heidelberg klin. Annal., 1832.
14. W. E. Hughes. Proceedings of the Pathological Society of Philadelphia, vol. xvi. p. 230.
15. A. Jacoby. Transactions of the New York Pathological Society, 1877, p. 205.
16. R. Johnson. Proceedings of the Pathological Society of London, 1889.
17. Kapuscinski. Inaugural Dissertation, Berlin, 1873.
18. Howard Kelly. Text-book of Gynecology.
19–20. Kelsch and Wannebourge. Progrès médicale, 1881, p. 728.
21–22. Keresztaszeghy. Beiträge zur path. Anat. und zur allg. Path., 1893, vol. xii.
23. J. B. Knapp. Transactions of the New York Pathological Society, 1877, p 203.
24. Kohler. Charité-Annalen, 1887, p. 542.
25–26. C. B. Lockwood. Transactions of the Medical Society of London, 1895, vol. xviii.
27. N. Lunier. Wratsch, 1888, No. 3; Jahrbuch für kinderheilkunde, 1897, vol. xxix. p. 89.
28. T. A. McGraw. Detroit Medical Age, 1887.
29. E. Mairinger. Jahrbuch der Wiener k. k. kranken Anstalt, 1896, vol. ii. p. 354.
30–36. Middlesex Hospital Reports, 1883, p. 164; 1886, p. 104; 1888, p. 275; 1890, p. 122; 1895, p. 102; 1895, p. 110.
37. E. Monnier. Bulletin de la Soc. anat. de Paris, 1897, p. 88.
38. C. A. Martin. British Medical Journal, October 17, 1896.
39. S. W. Morton. University Medical Magazine, 1890, p. 713.
40. D. Nasse. Virchow's Archiv, vol. xciv. p. 473.
41. Nicolaysen. Centralblatt für Chirurgie, vol. xiii. p. 496.
42. W. Netzel. Centralblatt für Gynakologie, vol. viii. p. 127.
43. E. Neumann. Archiv für Heilkunde, vol. x. p. 421.
44. W. Osler. Proceedings of the Pathological Society of Philadelphia, vol. xiii. p. 211.
45. Pilliet and Vean. Bulletin de la Soc. anat. de Paris, 1896, p. 719.
46. Phillipson. Lancet, May 23, 1885.
47. Pitres. Bulletin de la Soc. anat. de Paris, 1874, p. 25.
48. J. Ransohoff. Medical News, November 24, 1883.
49–50. B. Stiller. Wiener med. Presse, 1890, 50 and 51.
51. H. Storser. Wiener medicinische Wochenschrift, 1888, 4 and 5.
52–53. B. Stort. Das Sarcom und Seine Metastases, Berlin, 1877.
54. J. Tyson. Proceedings of the Pathological Society of Philadelphia, vol. xii. p. 253.

55. R. Van Santrood. New York Medical Record, 1887.
56–57. Virchow. Geschwulste, 1856, p. 566.
58–59. C. A. Weber. Chirurgische Erfahrungen und Untersuchungen, 1859, p. 364.
60. O. Witzel. Deutsches Archiv für klinische Chirurgie, 1886, p. 326.
61. Zahn. Virchow's Archiv, vol. cxv. p. 60.

CASES OF SECOND SERIES.

62. Bardenheuer. Extraperitoneal Explorativ Schnitt, Stuttgart, 1897.
63. Cecil F. Beadles. Transactions of the Pathological Society of London, 1899, vol. i. p. 239.
64. Bergh. Hygeia, 1897, p. 550.
65. W. H. Day. Proceedings of the Pathological Society of London, 1881, vol. xxxii. p. 142.
66. Dorn. Inaugural Dissertation, Würzburg, 1894.
67. R. Douglas. Annals of Surgery, March, 1903, p. 372.
68. R. B. Hall. Journal of the American Medical Association, October 14, 1899.
69. Otto Hartman. Deutsches Zeitschrift für Chirurgie, 1902, vol. lxv. p. 75.
70. Henoch. Beiträge zur Kinderheilkunde, 1863.
71. Heyder. Archiv fur Gynäkologie, 1890, vol. xxxviii. p. 301.
72. W. E. Hughes. Proceedings of the Pathological Society of Philadelphia, N. S., vol. ii. p. 260.
73. Raymond Johnson. Proceedings of the Pathological Society of London, 1889, vol. xl. p. 295.
74. Lossen. Deutsches Zeitschrift für Chirurgie, 1879, Bd. xiii. p. 199.
75. John McLachlan. Lancet, November 7, 1903.
76. Middlesex Hospital Reports, 1898, p. 194.
77. Naumann. Nordskt. mediciniskt Arkiv, 1902, Bd. xxv., Heft 3.
78. Rogowski. Inaugural Dissertation, Freiburg, 1899.
79. J. W. Ross, from service of William Osler. Canada Medical and Surgical Journal, 1880, vol. ix. p. 161.
80. Ruge. Inaugural Dissertation, Greifswald, 1892.
81. H. Sainsbury. Proceedings of the Pathological Society of London, 1885, vol. xxxv. p. 343.
82. R. C. Smith. Journal of the American Medical Association, September 7, 1901.
83. Stande. Geburthielfliche Gesellschaft zu Hamburg, October 12, 1897.
84. J. K. Thornton. Proceedings of the Pathological Society of London, 1882, vol. xxxiv. p. 141.
85. Wiesinger. Münch. med. Woch., August 15, 1899.
86–88. Howard J. Williams. THE AMERICAN JOURNAL OF THE MEDICAL SCIENCES, August, 1903.
89. Willutski. Inaugural Dissertation, Königsberg, 1891.
90. F. Winckel. Deutsches Archiv für klin. Medicin, 1893, vol. lv. p. 289.
91. J. M. Withrow. Cincinnati Lancet-Clinic, September 12, 1903.

TRAUMATIC INTESTINAL RUPTURE, WITH SPECIAL REFERENCE TO INDIRECT APPLIED FORCE.[1]

BY EMANUEL J. SENN, M.D.,
OF CHICAGO, ILL.,
ASSISTANT PROFESSOR OF SURGERY, RUSH MEDICAL COLLEGE, UNIVERSITY OF CHICAGO; ASSISTANT SURGEON, PRESBYTERIAN HOSPITAL, CHICAGO.

THIS subject merits much more conscientious consideration than is usually given to it by surgical authors. I have reference to internal injuries with no manifest external lesions. The degree of injury is no criterion whatever as to the future aspect of the case. Frequently a slight abdominal contusion is followed by great damage to the underlying viscera; while, conversely, a crushing injury to the

[1] Read before the Chicago Medical Society, January 6, 1904.

abdominal parietes, severe enough to cause fracture of neighboring bony structures, will not have interfered with the integrity of the abdominal organs. I wish to lay stress on the importance of the absolute necessity of examining carefully all patients suffering from abdominal contusions, and of cautious observation for a requisite period after the time of injury to preclude the possibility of having made a diagnosis of simple abdominal contusion. Then, having assured the patient and his friends of a quick recovery, only to hear later that the patient became suddenly very ill, and in all probability died from a perforative peritonitis.

Relatively speaking, how often we hear of a fracture of the skull or severe injury to the cranial contents having been diagnosticated by the first surgeon in charge as a simple scalp contusion.

Frequency of Segment of Intestine Involved. These injuries are found most often in men and young adults, by reason of their greater exposure to injury. In a study of the statistics of the relative frequency of rupture of the different portions of the intestinal tract, no mention is made in many instances of the exact anatomical location of the lesion.

Jalaguier claims that in all contusions of the abdominal wall, in which the viscera are injured, the digestive tube is involved in one-eleventh of the cases. These statistics are based upon those of Thomas Morton, 234, and those of Coull Mackenzie, 111, making a total of 345, of which 31 concerned the gastrointestinal tract. Chavasse found the ileum and jejunum injured 106 times, large intestine 19, duodenum 7, small and large intestine together 7, and the rectum 1. Curtis, in 113 cases, found the large intestine injured only 4 times. Bryant, in a series of cases, gives the duodenum 2, jejunum 7, and the ileum 10. Croft, in 10 cases, collected between 1873 and 1890, states there were 7 of the ileum and 3 of the jejunum. Maylard recorded 10 cases, of which 6 were injuries of the ileum and 4 of the jejunum. Poland discovered 5 cases of rupture of the large bowel out of 64 injuries to some portion of the intestinal tract. In 40 cases of rupture of the small intestine, only 4 occurred in the duodenum. It will be seen that while the duodenum is firmly fixed in its position, it is, comparatively speaking, rarely injured. It is protected by its thick walls and also by its deep position.

As we proceed in a downward direction to the ileocæcal valve, traumatic rupture becomes correspondingly more frequent. This condition is explained by the greater exposure, especially of the ileum; the mobility of the intestinal coils, and by the gradual attenuation of the tunics of the small intestine. The large bowel is protected in the loin and hypochondriac region. Its contents, which are usually of a semisolid or solid consistency, militate against injury; while we know that the fluid contents in the small intestine play an important role in rupture.

The stomach is rarely injured, on account of its protected position.

Coull Mackenzie, in 111 cases, found the stomach injured only once, and then there was an accompanying injury of the spleen, showing that great force had been exercised.

MECHANISM OF INJURY. Speaking in a general sense, blows directed above the level of the umbilicus are unlikely to cause intestinal injuries. There are certain injuries which should invite suspicion of rupture. Thomas Bryant has well said: "When an individual has been run over, the wheel passing over the abdomen or back, had a kick from a horse, a fall from a height or a crush between two obtuse bodies, there is a great probability of injury to some solid viscus or laceration of the intestine." The usual nature of injuries which produce rupture is shown by the 149 cases of gastro-intestinal involvement collected by Chavasse: 36 were due to kick of a horse; 13 were due to kick of man, blows by clubs, etc.; 23 were due to crushing of wagon wheels. It is obvious that we must first consider the force applied in consideration of the mechanism of the injury. We may classify such force into first, direct; second, indirect.

By direct force I mean that the vulnerating body has been applied in the nearest line to the exposed intestines—that is, against the abdominal parietes. By indirect force, I wish to call attention to an impulse conveyed to the intestines by an impact directed upon the buttocks or the lumbar region. Again, we can classify such injuries in regard to the nature of the applied force into (1) percussion and (2) compression. Strictly speaking, the great majority of cases of traumatic rupture of the intestine are due to compression, although there is only one vulnerating body. A blow is administered upon the abdominal wall; but the rupture is due to the compression between two solid bodies; that is, the vulnerating force and the vertebral column behind or the bony pelvis. This is substantiated by Makin's observation, that intestinal ruptures are found most often in that portion of the intestine which is low in the pelvis. There are undoubtedly ruptures produced in the true sense of percussion—that is, the impulse of the blow might cause violent momentary vibrations in a coil of intestine overdistended with fluid contents, and thus cause a rupture. This supposition is supported by the fact that in the great majority of cases the rent in the bowel is at the convex surface, diametrically opposite the mesenteric border. All cases of rupture produced by indirect force would be effected in this manner.

In a careful search of the literature, I have found only 2 well-authenticated cases of rupture produced in this manner, both of which were published in 1902.

Dr. J. F. Bottomly reports a case where the patient was struck in the back below the left shoulder-blade by an approaching wagon. Operation showed a perforation of the first portion of the jejunum. Westbrook describes a case where a wagon-pole struck a man in the lumbar region. Autopsy revealed a rupture at the junction of the duodenum and jejunum large enough to admit two fingers.

I wish to report the following case as illustrative of an injury to the intestine, which was produced in a unique way, and shows the possibility of a force of small degree directed upon the buttocks, capable of producing intra-abdominal laceration.

Mrs. J. F. O., aged twenty-six years, married; previous health good; on July 17th, at 6 P.M., while hurrying into her house to escape a thunder-storm, slipped and fell, striking the ground upon the right buttock. She had just partaken of a hearty supper. No immediate alarming symptoms were noticed, and the patient retired as usual. At midnight she awoke with severe abdominal pains; vomited once. The following day she was seen by her physician, Dr. G. F. Berger, who prescribed opiates and turpentine stupes. The pains increased and the patient rapidly grew worse. I was called in consultation on the morning of the 19th. The appearance of the patient was critical. She had an anxious expression, and complained bitterly of abdominal pains. Temperature, 104.3° F. (rectal); pulse, 140. Manual palpation revealed diffuse abdominal tenderness. There was marked tympany, most noticeable over a limited area in the region of the appendix. Without the history of the injury a diagnosis of appendicitis would have been the most probable. A provisional diagnosis of perforative peritonitis was made, and the patient advised to undergo immediate operation. She was transferred to the German Hospital. Stimulation with strychnine and salt solution enemata.

Operation. Anæsthetic, ether, by the open method. Median incision, four inches long, below the umbilicus. Upon opening the peritoneal cavity there was an escape of cloudy fluid, but no gas. Spider-web adhesions of the great omentum, which were separated, followed by a gush of fluid heavily loaded with fibrinous flakes. Small intestine was greatly distended and of a bluish-black color, and covered with a fibrinous exudate. No collapsed bowel seen. The intestine was now grasped at a fixed point by an assistant, and a search for the perforation made. After a long exploration a sudden escape of gas was noticed deep down in the pelvis. Further examination revealed feces in the peritoneal cavity, and a small perforation, about the size of the little finger-nail, was discovered on the convex surface of what appeared to be the lower portion of the jejunum. The patient was now nearly pulseless, and she was given a subcutaneous injection of salt solution. The abdominal cavity was next thoroughly cleansed by dry sponging, and the perforation in the intestine sutured into the abdominal wound. The lower angle of the incision was left open, and four large gauze drains were placed into the abdominal cavity, two in the direction of the pelvis, and two well up toward the diaphragm. This drainage was supplemented by a tubular drain. The patient was returned to her room in a very weak condition. She was stimulated with strychnine, camphorated oil, and salt enemata; each administered every three hours, but given at such intervals that the patient had one of these stimulants every hour. The patient rallied, and on the second day was in a fair condition. She recovered entirely from the operation, but the fistula persisted, and the adjacent surface was aroused into a severe dermatitis due to the digestive action of intestinal fluids. I saw her one week after the operation, and she was in good condition. I did not see her again until October 3, 1903, she in the mean time having been treated by Dr. Berger. I found her very much emaciated, literally having starved to death. She had been nourished for eleven weeks per rectum. Food taken by the mouth greatly increased the discharge, and appeared undigested at the opening. The fistula was still patent, in spite of the repeated cauterization with the Paquelin cautery. During the last two days she had two sinking spells. I advised immediate operation as the only means of saving her life; although the wound was unfavorable for operation, on account of the dermatitis.

A second operation was performed October 4, 1903. Two curvilinear incisions around the fistula were made; then a layer of gauze with an opening in the centre was sutured to the wound margins. The opening in the gauze exposed the field of operation and the layer of gauze protected the wound from the surrounding infected skin. The loop of intestine was dissected loose from the abdominal wall. The general peritoneal cavity was next packed off with compresses. The margins of the fistula were trimmed and closed by transverse suturing with two rows of continuous sutures. The first row was passed through all the intestinal coats, the second being Lembert sutures. The line of suture was covered with an omental graft, and the repaired intestine dropped into the abdominal cavity. The external wound was closed without drainage. The patient bore the operation well. The following day she was given peptonoids, two ounces every four hours per rectum. October 6th, peptonoids were given by mouth, and then, October 9th, white of an egg; October 10th, milk; October 11th, oatmeal; October 12th, soft-boiled eggs and bread; October 14th, steak. Her recovery was perfect, and she left the hospital October 23, 1903. I heard from her November 19th. She had gained twenty-five pounds, weighing more than ever before in her life.

Remarks. The history of the cause of the injury was reliable, and that the fall was not severe I can vouch for, as she complained of no soreness in the region of the buttock, nor was there any bruise visible. I did the enterostomy for two reasons, and believe it was the means of saving the patient's life. First, on account of the collapsed state of the patient, requiring rapidity of execution, and, second, because of the paralytic state of the intestine, overdistended with gas, allowing its evacuation as the bowel regained its tone.

The state of the abdominal muscles at the time of injury plays an important role in intestinal injuries. A blow delivered upon a rigid abdomen loses considerable of its force; while an impact directed against the same structure in a relaxed state is transmitted directly to the underlying intestinal coils, and enhances the liability of a rupture. This assertion has been demonstrated beyond a doubt by the beautiful experiments of Eichel.

He first made a series of experiments upon dogs profoundly etherized. The animals were placed upon the back, the extremities being tied and extended. A forcible blow was struck upon the abdomen with a heavy club. The experiments were all negative, laparotomy showing the intestines intact and only slight extravasation in the tissues of the abdominal wall. The same experiments were performed on dogs which had been overfed for two days in advance, but the results were also negative. In another series of experiments the hind-legs were loosened before the stroke. In the first experiment the blow was delivered too high, producing a rupture of the liver. The stomach wall was also the seat of suggillation. In other experiments a hammer was used instead of a stick to produce the trauma, and rupture of the intestine was almost invariably produced. Experiments were also made by striking the lumbar region, the intestines having previously been insufflated with air through the rectum, but no rupture of the intestines was produced. Chauveau maintains that the reverse is the rule. He claims that contraction of the abdominal muscles diminishes the abdominal cavity, and also immobilizes the intestinal coils, and thus favors rupture. This argument, however, should bear no weight, as it stands simply as a personal conviction, or rather an hypothesis, while Eichel's opinion rests upon the firm basis of experimental research. Other conditions may predispose to injury, such as adhesions, alteration of intestinal walls, old reducible hernia, in which the intestinal walls have been weakened by pressure. There has been much discussion as regards gaseous distention facilitating rupture. Longuet, in 1875, claimed that the elasticity of the gas was unfavorable to rupture, while liquid distention favored it. This theory was accepted by Mugnier. The hydrostatic pressure of intestinal fluids is evidently the cause of rupture in those cases produced by indirect force. That gaseous distention would act as an elastic cushion seems plausible.

PATHOLOGY. From a pathological standpoint, we can divide these injuries into (1) contusions; (2) rupture: incomplete, complete.

Contusions may be of all degrees, either a simple interstitial ecchymosis or a submucous infiltration; or else there may be an infiltration through the entire thickness of the intestinal coats. The contused surface is more or less rounded or oval, and the long diameter is usually in the long axis of the bowel. The color of the ecchymotic area depends upon the amount of infiltration, and is usually white or yellow. The surface is denuded and covered by an exudate. Sometimes different areas of contusion are found in the same intestinal loop, or in different loops in the same region. Contusion probably is often produced and causes no untoward symptoms. However, there are cases on record where, after an injury, the patient progressed well for days or even weeks, when there arose suddenly symptoms of a perforative peritonitis, and the autopsy revealed a perforation. At the time of the accident there was a contusion produced, which in time became the seat of an infection; or else, by reason of an interfered-with circulation, a necrosis resulted, which compromised the integrity of the intestine. Thomas Bryant reports 2 cases of delayed rupture. One progressed favorably after the accident until the nineteenth day, when the patient died. Necropsy showed perforation of the duodenum, and an ulcer on the posterior wall of the stomach. In the other case there was a perforation on the fifth day. Autopsy demonstrated a perforation of the ileum four inches above the cæcum. Incomplete ruptures, when one or two of the tunics are torn, in all probability are frequent; however, as far as pathological investigation can be pursued, they are supposed to be rare. In a case observed by Jobert, in 1825, ecchymotic spots were found in the small intestine, and a rupture of the longitudinal fibres of the colon discovered. Poland reports 2 cases of such ruptures in the stomach; in 1 the mucous coat was torn, and in the other the peritoneal coat.

Complete ruptures, when all the tunics are ruptured, are more often brought to view on the operating table and in the post-mortem room. Chavasse, in 149 cases, found this condition 14 times; duodenum, 1; junction of duodenum and jejunum, 3; jejunum and ileum, 10.

Complete ruptures are usually single, but may be multiple, especially following the kick of a horse. Moty claims that there are often two perforations corresponding to the two lateral extremities of the horseshoe. It is a marvellous fact that a contusion of sufficient intensity to cause a complete rupture does not often injure other viscera; for Coull Mackenzie, in 111 cases, only found 2 with accompanying injury to the spleen and liver. The rent in the intestine always occupies the point diametrically opposite the point of the mesenteric insertion. It is sometimes a clean-cut wound, and sometimes the border is ragged and irregular. Leakage after rupture is hindered and even entirely prevented through two factors. We must remember there is no abdominal cavity in reality, the whole of the visceral contents being so closely and equably brought into contact by the pressure of the abdominal muscles and the diaphragm that considerable force is required of the intestinal contents to overcome this. The influence of the pressure of the abdominal muscles upon the intestinal contents is well known clinically; because if an injured coil of intestine protrudes from the abdomen devoid of the intra-abdominal influence, extravasation takes place much more readily. The intrinsic contractility of the intestinal tunics is another inhibitory agent against extravasation. Travers long ago pointed out that in a puncture of the gut, or even an incision two or three lines in length, an eversion or prolapsus of the mucous membrane takes place, and hermetically seals the opening. If the aperture is more than four lines in extent the protuberant mucous membrane is incapable of protecting the perforation. The protrusion of mucous membrane is due to the retraction of the longitudinal fibres. There is also contraction of the circular muscular fibres around the protruded mucous membrane, according to Jobert; thus, temporarily at least, preventing extravasation. Even in extensive complete rupture there is little likelihood of visible fecal extravasation, for Makins, in an exhaustive report of 20 cases, in St. Thomas' Hospital, London, found no appreciable escape of fecal matter.

SYMPTOMS. As this pathological condition is usually the consequence of a severe trauma in the neighborhood of the sympathetic centres, we usually find the classical symptoms of shock. The more serious symptoms soon pass away, unless there is injury of the abdominal viscera or internal hemorrhage, which is denoted by long-continued shock. If there is intestinal rupture, with fecal extravasation, the symptoms of shock merge into those of a general perforative peritonitis. It is difficult to tell where shock ends and peritonitis begins. In an injury produced by a sharp blow, the resulting shock appears more marked than that which follows a severe compression of the abdomen. In cases of contusion or incomplete rupture of the intestine, after the symptoms of shock have subsided, there is some temperature on account of local peritonitis, but not much variation in the pulse. Constipation or diarrhœa may be present and possible blood-stained stools. There is slight pain and abdominal tenderness upon pressure. Such cases, as a rule, follow a favorable course, but may terminate disastrously by reason of secondary perforation internally, or favorably by rupture externally, causing a fecal fistula. In those cases where the contusion is followed by immediate extravasation of the intestinal contents into the general peritoneal cavity, an entirely different picture confronts the surgeon. There is immediate excruciating localized pain. The face is pale, the pupils dilated, respiration superficial, the pulse small, and the temperature subnormal. This complexus of symptoms is soon followed by vomiting. The abdominal muscles are at first fixed and contracted, which is gradually followed by a ballooned abdomen; while respiration becomes of a costal nature. The symptoms now progress rapidly from bad to worse; shallow costal respiration gradually merges into dyspnœa; the anxiety of the patient becomes intense; the eyes are sunken; the pulse thready; the extremities cold and cyanosed, and the patient dies in collapse. These symptoms are the usual outcome in cases of complete rupture. However, the gravity depends upon the condition of the intestine, whether empty or distended, and also upon the virulence of the infective bacteria. Violent visceral injuries may cause no immediate symptoms. Michaux, out of 100 cases of grave contusions, had 10 cases where patients followed their vocations long after injury, in some of which there was complete laceration. Rioblanc reports 2 similar cases. Poland mentions a case of a child, aged thirteen years, struck upon the abdomen, who walked a mile after the injury, and died thirteen hours later. There was a complete rupture of the duodenum. Holland mentions a girl, aged eleven years, who fell down a flight of stairs. She vomited and then had no symptoms for twenty-four hours, when she died. Autopsy showed rupture of one-half of the jejunum. Chavasse speaks of an injury by kick of a horse at 3 A.M. Patient had severe pain and then felt well until the following night, when he vomited and died in collapse. Post-mortem revealed a complete rupture of the jejunum.

I wish to call attention to retroperitoneal emphysema as an indication which signifies injury to the duodenum or the colon. The loss of liver dulness is an orthodox symptom in many text-books on surgery. This diagnostic resource is by no means infallible, especially if the laceration is limited. While fecal matter is less prone to escape than gas, the latter may escape in very small quantities. Again, we should remember that these injuries usually lie toward the pelvis and the upper quadrant of the abdomen may be isolated by omental adhesions. It is obvious that where a great quantity of gas was liberated in the general peritoneal cavity, the liver would fall away from the abdominal wall, so that a resonant note would be heard but not always, as a highly distended bowel may encroach upon the liver dulness.

Vomiting is considered of great diagnostic importance by many. Trendelenburg and Berndt consider it almost a positive sign of rupture. Berndt claims that in contusion of the abdominal wall without rupture, there may be slight vomiting, it being entirely a reflex process, but in complete rupture peristalsis forces the intestinal contents into the opening, and thus irritation of the cut end of the nerves causes vomiting. While continued interrupted vomiting is by no means absolute evidence of rupture, great weight should be placed on its presence in connection with other corroborative symptoms. The abdominal rigidity soon after injury is ominous. Hartmann, in 37 cases, found rigidity 17 times. He treated such patients by laparotomy, and found visceral injury in each. In the 20 other contusions there was no rigidity; the patients were treated expectantly, and all recovered. Kirstein also dwells upon the importance of this symptom.

PROGNOSIS. The prognosis depends upon certain conditions. An injury soon after a hearty meal, while there is a copious physiological secretion of intestinal juices, would, of course, facilitate extravasation. The prognosis of wounds which are inflicted in the duodenojejunal region is relatively bad, because they are near the source of secretions and because of the difficulty in dealing surgically with this anatomical region. Horse-kicks upon the abdomen have usually an especially bad prognosis. However, Pech reported 67 cases during the years 1890 to 1897 at the garrison of Luneville, France, with only 2 deaths, treated upon the conservative plan. These statistics seem improbable. Dubujadoux observed 8 coutusions from horse-kick, and found intestinal lesions 8 times. The mortality of these injuries in the past has been shocking, and it is only due to the great advance of surgery in the last decade that statistics give a more cheerful aspect.

In 1896 Petry collected 160 cases of rupture of the intestine treated expectantly, of which 149, or 93 per cent., died, and 11, or 7 per cent., recovered. He also collected 42 cases of rupture of the stomach and intestine which had been operated upon; 14, or 33.6 per cent., recovered, and 28, or 66.7 per cent., died. Kirstein collected 18 cases operated upon from the German literature since the publication of Petry's paper, of which 44.5 per cent. recovered and 55.5 per cent. died. D. N. Eisendrath collected statistics of 40 cases of which 19, or 47.5 per cent., recovered, and 21, or 52.5 per cent., died. The prognosis of the future will rest upon an early diagnosis. Immediate operation will reduce the mortality to a minimum. The statistics of Siegel, which I consider of the greatest scientific importance, bearing upon this subject, are as follows: In 532 cases treated expectantly, the mortality was 55.2 per cent.; in 376 cases operated upon there was a mortality of 51.6 per cent. An analysis of these statistics proves that the high mortality is due to late operation, when a general peritonitis had already developed. When the time of operation is taken into consideration, the true status of early aggressive surgery can be conceived, as is proven in a further study of Siegel's statistics.

Cases operated upon first four hours, mortality	15.2 per ct.
" " " " five to eight hours, mortality . . .	44.4 "
" " " " nine to twelve hours, mortality . . .	63.6 "
" " " later	70.0 "

TREATMENT. In all cases of abdominal contusions the prognosis should be guarded, and the patients ought to be kept under careful observation. Upon the least suspicion of rupture immediate laparotomy is the only course to be followed. The statistics of Siegel place this argument beyond question. The surgical treatment of perforating wounds of the abdomen has been decided for all time to come, and a plea for equally decisive measures is made for this pathological condition.

The first laparotomy for rupture of the intestine was performed by Bouilly in 1883, but the case terminated fatally. Moty, in 1889, was successful in the first case on record. The incision should be made through the linea alba below the umbilicus, notwithstanding the advice of F. Spaeth to make the incision at the point of greatest tenderness. This incision will give a better survey of the abdomen. Usually the injured intestine will lie in close proximity, and if there are concomitant injuries of other organs, they can be most easily reached through such an incision. Upon opening the peritoneum there may be an escape of gas, also exudate containing albuminous flakes. The bowel should be examined methodically from a fixed point until the injured segment is found. I wish again to call attention to the great possibility of multiple rupture, especially in cases due to horse-kick. Small rents should be sutured transversely to the long axis of the bowel. Large lacerations should be dealt with by resection, provided the patient is in good condition. In all cases when there are alarming symptoms, the injured bowel should be anchored in the abdominal wound. Personally, I believe this is a good practice to follow in the great majority of cases. Intestinal drainage is of prime importance where the bowel is paretic and distended. Again, in such injuries, especially if operation is delayed, there is a zone of infection which cannot be rendered sterile by secondary disinfection; hence the great danger of tearing through of the stitches and a resultant secondary peritonitis. In the case I reported in this paper, there was a permanent fistula as a result of the operation, but the patient was in such a desperate condition and time was of such moment that the intestine was sutured to the tissues too near the skin. The proper course to follow, when possible, is to unite the bowel, but leave a small fistula and anchor the segment to the abdominal wall. This procedure has been practised by Bouilly. Verneuil, Farquhar Curtis, Treves, Thomson, and Smith have advised an artificial anus after resection of the bowel. I believe this is unnecessary, as it always insures a secondary operation, while the principles are fulfilled equally well by the procedure of Bouilly, and the fistula will close spontaneously in the great majority of cases. When it is deemed advisable to drop the repaired intestine back into the abdomen, the line of suture should always be re-enforced by an omental graft, as advised by N. Senn. When an expectant course is followed in simple contusion or in cases of ruptured intestine, when for some reason operation cannot be performed, the patient should be placed at rest, with an ice-bag on the abdomen. Feeding by mouth should be prohibited, and nourishment given by rectal enemata. Opium is indicated to diminish peristaltic action of the bowels, and thus inhibit extravasation.

BIBLIOGRAPHY.

1. Croft. Transactions of Clinical Society of London, 1890, vol. xxiii.
2. Poland. Guy's Hospital Reports, 3d series, vol. iv. p. 142.
3. Cahier, L. Revue de Chirurgie, Paris, 1902, vol. xxii.
4. Makins. Annals of Surgery, 1899, vol. xxx. pp. 137–170.
5. Spaeth, F. Berliner klin. Woch., 1887, vol. xxiv. p. 883.

6. Klistein. Deut. Zeit. f. Chir., Leipzig, 1900, vol. lvii.
7. Von Angerer. Verhand. der Deut. Gesellschaft f. Chir., Berlin, 1900, vol. xxix.; pp. 475–492.
8. Eichel. Beiträge z. klin. Chir., 1898, vol. xxii. pp. 219–242.
9. Eisendrath. Journal of the American Medical Association, October 25, 1902.
10. Westbrook. Brooklyn Medical Journal, 1902, p. 417.
11. Duplay and Reclus. Traité de Chirurgie.
12. Schönwerth. München. med. Woch., 1899, No. 4.
13. Siegel. Beiträge z. klin. Chir., 1899, Bd. xxi.
14 Bryant, T. The Lancet, December 7, 1895.
15. Battle, W. H. Ibid., December 10, 1898.
16. Curtis. International Journal of the Medical Sciences, 1887, p. 329.
17. Berndt, F. Deut. Zeit. f. Chir., vol. xxxix. pp. 516–521.
18. Bottomly, J. F. Boston City Hospital Reports, 1902.
19. Maylard. Surgery of the Alimentary Canal.
20. Ashhurst. Erichsen's Science and Art of Surgery.

CASTRATION FOR TUBERCULOSIS OF THE TESTICLE.[1]

By Charles Greene Cumston, M.D.,

of Boston Mass.

Not many years ago it was generally admitted that a radical operation for extensive tuberculosis of the testicle and epididymis was indicated when only the genital apparatus was affected by the disease, the remaining organs of the body being free. In the *Deutsche Chirurgie*, edited by Billroth and Luecke, will be found Kocher's classical article on the subject. In this he says that the reason for this procedure is the chance of a radical cure, although he admits the possibility of a spontaneous recovery, but which is, in most cases, accompanied by the functional loss of the organ involved. He also points out that a cure without operation is only a possibility, and if the organ with its disease is left intact, with the hope that the affection will finally disappear, the patient is exposed to all the dangers attendant upon suppuration. In other instances the condition demands a radical treatment. In a patient having tuberculosis of one testicle which is left untreated, it is always to be expected that within a short time its fellow will also become invaded by the process. This not only applies to the other testicle, but to the whole organism as well, and if the tuberculous testicle is not removed a metastasis of the process will take place in other parts of the body, usually in the form of a general miliary tuberculosis. From this it would appear that castration is absolutely indicated, and although the prostate and seminal vesicle were enlarged and other subjective symptoms of tuberculous infection of the genital organs were manifest, Kocher noted that these symptoms disappeared in a relatively short time after castration had been done. He even found that suppuration of the spermatic cord and abscesses of the prostate would

[1] Read by title at the French Urological Society, Paris, October 22 to 24, 1903.

oftentimes heal after incision if the diseased testicle were removed at the same time.

König also confirms Kocher's views, and, in his opinion, infection of the prostate and urinary organs is no contraindication to castration, for the reason that the removal of the tuberculous testicle has a favorable action on the disease when located in other parts of the genito-urinary system, as well as upon the general condition of the patient. Southam, Simon, and others are also in accord on this point.

Various are the methods of performing castration, but in most instances, as there is only evidence of the disease involving the testicle and epididymis, the operation has usually been thought sufficient when the organ was simply removed. The technique employed simply consists in a longitudinal incision starting above the spermatic cord and extending down to the lower pole of the testicle. When one or more fistulæ exist, or if the skin should be adherent to the organ, the incision is carried round on both sides, so that an elliptical portion, including the fistulous openings in the scrotum, is removed along with the testicle. After peeling off the scrotal integument the spermatic cord is dissected out from its various coverings and then the arteries, veins, and vas deferens are ligated and the cord is cut through. The ligatures should be left long in order to keep the cut end of the cord from slipping up into the inguinal canal.

The testicle is then dissected out from above downward, and when it is adherent to the scrotal tissues this usually occurs in the neighborhood of its lower pole. When the organ has been removed all hemorrhage should be carefully controlled, the wound irrigated, and, after a final inspection of the stump of the cord, the threads are cut and it is allowed to slide up into the inguinal canal. A gauze wick should be inserted, the parts sutured, and the usual dressings applied.

Von Bungner has pointed out a fact which is well known, that the spermatic cord is often diseased without presenting much evident infection at the time of operation. From this arises the danger that the diseased parts which are left behind in the cord will act as disseminating foci for further tuberculous infection, and, in order to avoid this danger, he recommended a new method which he termed castration with evulsion of the spermatic cord. As in castration, the spermatic cord is separated from the vessels and its surrounding coverings, the vessels are tied off below the external inguinal ring, and then the isolated vas deferens is slowly but steadily pulled upon until it breaks. The piece of vas is removed along with the diseased testicle and epididymis. In his operations, von Bungner was able to extract about four-fifths of the spermatic cord by his method of evulsion, and, according to his statistics, he obtained a cure in 50 per cent. of his cases.

It is quite evident that removal of the vas deferens should be undertaken as far as possible in every case of castration, especially when it is evidently diseased, but the method of evulsion is certainly not devoid of danger. Lauenstein and Helferich pointed out the danger of hemorrhage occurring in the pelvic tissue from the traction exercised on the vessels accompanying the spermatic cord. The first-mentioned authority performed castration with evulsion of the vas in thirteen cases, and in several succeeded in removing quite large portions of the cord with much benefit to the patient, but in two instances such severe hemorrhage arose that it was extremely difficult to control it. Since this time Lauenstein only removes as much of the vas deferens as can be pulled down without exercising traction upon it.

A point which should not be forgotten is that in the method of evulsion the peritoneum can be easily torn, and with the raw surface of the cord the peritoneal cavity might easily become infected. Consequently, the method of evulsion is certainly not devoid of danger, and it also should be remembered that in all probability the diseased spermatic cord will rupture at a point where it is infected by the tuberculous process on account of lesser resistance. If this be true, and there is every apparent reason that it should be so, it would naturally scatter tuberculous material, which would be the starting point for a new dissemination of the disease. For these reasons Shede employs a technique similar to that described by Lauenstein, dissecting the spermatic cord up as high as possible and then ligating it at a point where it appears to be healthy, and, for this purpose, it may be necessary to dissect the peritoneum off the cord to a certain extent. It is evident that in this operation, as in others, the spermatic cord is not always removed beyond the point of disease, and, consequently, the affection still remains in the intra-abdominal portion of the vas which is left behind.

The length of the spermatic cord has been estimated as 32 cm. by König, who also resects the vas deferens under the control of the eye, and he has been able to remove as much as 25 cm.; von Bungner removed four-fifths of its entire length, which means practically about 25 cm., thus leaving from 7 cm. to 8 cm. of the cord, which in all probability was diseased.

Now, supposing the seminal vesicle or the prostate is affected by the disease, if it cannot be denied that the removal of the testicle has a favorable influence on the process, it must also be said that it certainly is insecure as regards the prognosis, especially when the tuberculous process within the organ is advanced, and, therefore, simple castration also must be considered insufficient. The involvement of the other genito-urinary organs in a case of tuberculosis of the testicle should always be admitted as more than probable, even when the spermatic cord appears so be perfectly intact; and von Bungner, in his paper, laid stress upon the fact that tuberculosis of the urogenital apparatus does not extend in continuity, and that occasionally the orifice of the vas deferens may be diseased, yet at its middle it may be healthy.

König has reported a case in which he found a spindle-shaped thickening at the external inguinal ring extending up the inguinal canal, which proved to be a tuberculous infection, although the spermatic cord seemed to be quite healthy. He points out the fact that the points of election for the development of the tuberculous process are where bends or curves take place in the canal.

The removal or direct local treatment of the infected seminal vesicles or prostate is most advisable, but these organs, unfortunately, are most difficult of access, and that to reach them is a most arduous undertaking is demonstrated by the numerous techniques that have been described.

The procedure described by Zuckerkandl is too severe to combine at the same time with castration, and resection of the vas deferens had better be done at a later date, when the patient has recovered from the operation of removal of the testicle.

The diseased parts are reached by the perineal route, a curved incision being made between the scrotum and anus. The posterior wall of the bladder is exposed and the prostate and seminal vesicles are reached after the connective tissue covering the latter has been opened. As numerous bloodvessels are to be found here, the hemorrhage must be controlled before proceeding, although this is very often a most difficult thing to do, on account of the depth of the parts in which one is working.

The question of hemorrhage has deterred many surgeons from selecting the perineal route, and even so great an authority as König advises against its use, suggesting another technique, which avoids this difficulty, using the sacral route, according to the method of Kraske, for resection of the rectum. The operation is preceded by several days' preparatory treatment of the patient, principally to thoroughly empty the intestine. The patient receives only liquid diet and the bowels are thoroughly emptied daily by castor oil and enemas.

The technique of the operation consists in making two longitudinal incisions, beginning on each side, 2 cm. from the median line at the highest point of the anterior border of the anus, the patient being in the lithotomy position, and carried downward midway between the anus and tuber ischii to the fourth or fifth sacral vertebra. After control of the hemorrhage, the incisions are deepened until the fascia pelvis parietales is reached. The space between the anus and tuber ischii is filled with cellular tissue, in which the inferior hemorrhoidal veins pass, supplying the external sphincter of the anus. There are, however, sufficient anastomoses present, so that there is no danger in cutting and ligating these vessels. The pelvic fascia being exposed, a third incision is made transversely over the sacrum down to the bone, which connects the two lower ends of the incision. The sacrum is then separated between the fourth and fifth vertebra, which is at about the level of the seminal vesicle.

In order to accomplish this a chain saw is passed through the fourth sacral foramen and the bone sawed through. At this point of the operation it should be remembered that severe hemorrhage may take place on account of section of the middle sacral artery and vein, consequently they should immediately be ligated before the operation is proceeded with.

A flap containing the soft parts and bone has now been formed and is then turned upward and the pelvic fascia is incised on the left side of the rectum, the gut being pushed over to the right. When this has been accomplished the structures to be reached are exposed and the posterior part of the bladder and prostate can be seen. On each side of the latter organ the vasa deferentia may be found, running downward to the point where the seminal vesicles are situated.

Each seminal vesicle is covered by a capsule of a fibromuscular nature, deprived almost completely of any blood supply on its posterior aspect, and, consequently, the capsule may be incised and the seminal vesicle peeled out without any danger of hemorrhage.

It is quite impossible to injure the bladder or the urethra at this point, and it is also fairly easy to remove the entire remaining part of the vas deferens up to the point where it enters the prostate. If thought necessary, the seminal vesicle on the other side may be removed, and should the prostate be found diseased the cheesy foci can be cleaned out with the curette. The parts are then plugged with iodoform gauze and the wound can be closed, only one long tampon being left protruding through the incision, which may be removed on the fourth day. The wound may also be left open for the purpose of local iodoform treatment, but a secondary suture does not give such brilliant results.

As to the after-treatment, it consists in confining the bowels for four or five days and the internal administration of tincture opii in sufficient quantity is indicated during this time, after which the bowels may be opened.

In a way this operation presents evident advantages, principally from the fact that the field of operation is easily reached and all the steps are under the control of the eye. The structures to be attained are not very deeply seated when this method is employed, severe hemorrhage is avoided, and the parts easily drained. The two methods just described are probably the best, but there are many others, principally those of Roux, Villeneuve, Guelliot, Rydygier, and others, that I should like to discuss were the limits of this paper sufficient to permit of it.

Unless the patient is in fairly good constitutional condition, such prolonged operation can hardly be advisable, and that this has also been so considered by other surgeons is well demonstrated from the fact that attempts have been made to treat the diseased parts by means of iodoform-glycerin injections. Von Bungner experimentally investigated upon the cadaver to what extent injections made directly into the lumen of the vas deferens might be pushed. He injected iodoform-glycerin into the lumen of the spermatic cord after section in both directions, and found that the entire genital tract from the epididymis to the urethral orifice was filled with the solution. Some of it ran out through the urethra. The seminal vesicles were filled, but contained a certain amount of the injected fluid. The liquid came in contact with those parts of the vas deferens which are usually involved in the tuberculous process, as well as the intra-canalicular parts and the mucous membrane, both of which become involved during the progress of the process.

It was thought that by this method a cure might result without operation in those parts remaining after castration, but the iodoform treatment might also be employed without having done castration in cases where the tuberculous process is so far advanced that it cannot be eliminated, even by the removal of the entire urogenital tract. Under these circumstances this treatment will relieve the suffering in the later stages of the disease, and it also may be indicated in the very early stages of tuberculosis of the genital organs when a radical operation does not seem to be imminently necessary. It may also be employed where only a suspicion of tuberculosis exists.

Von Bungner's results are uncertain, because the method has only been employed for a short time, but it would appear to me that nevertheless a surgical operation should in the first place be undertaken, because the hopes of the instigator of the iodoform-injection method do not appear to me to be at all certain. Recently, however, a number of operators have appeared to give up the radical measures and adopted the milder ones, even going so far as to institute an expectant treatment. Some uphold that in most cases the epididymis is alone the seat of the disease, and that consequently destruction of the tuberculous foci seated within it is quite sufficient, and that castration is too radical, and should only be reserved for extreme cases. Senn claims good results by the sclerogenous method, but does not appear to be a strong advocate of its use.

Platon believes that the removal of one testicle in no way prevents the occurrence of the disease in the remaining organ, and should this arise it is hard to persuade a patient to lose his remaining seminal gland. Albert believes that he has also seen the disease appear in the remaining testicle and also the development of a general tuberculosis after castration has been done on one side, and for this reason he favors conservative treatment. Other authorities of late also oppose radical measures and deem that destruction of the diseased parts or ultimately an incision of the epididymis will be sufficient.

Among the conservative operations may be mentioned the experiments of Mauclaire, who endeavored to bring about atrophy of the testicle by ligation and section of the elements of the spermatic cord. It appeared to him that the best method was section of the entire spermatic cord, with the exception of the vas deferens and its accompanying vessels. Upon the appearance of the atrophic process, the tuberculous foci disappeared and a hard lump remained, which led the patient to believe that he still possessed his testicle.

It would appear to me, however, that the work done in this direction by Mauclaire has not been sufficiently controlled, and more recently there has been a tendency, not only to preserve the testicle itself, but also its functions as well, which, with the other methods described, were always lost.

Rasumowski, in an article which appeared in 1902, states that Bardenheuer tried to attain this end by endeavoring to give an exit to the semen by the formation of an anastomosis between the spermatic cord and the capsule of the testicle. To accomplish this the diseased epididymis was peeled out of its capsule and then the stump of the spermatic cord was sutured to the capsule, with the hope that the seminal fluid escaping from the rete testis would find its way into the space left by the excision of the epididymis and from there into the vas deferens, but this method naturally could never amount to anything. To form an anastomosis of any duration a simple mechanical union of the parts is not sufficient, for the reason that both mucosæ, covered with their epithelium, must be united in intimate relation to each other in the entire circumference of the anastomosis.

Rasumowski claims that he developed the same idea independently of Bardenheuer. He devised two methods of operation which would accomplish the same end; in one the indications for its use are when the entire epididymis has to be resected and a reunion of the vas deferens must be made with parts of the coni vasculosi. In the second operation the spermatic cord is united to the remainder of the epididymis when the tail and the part of the body of the latter have been removed. The technique of the first operation consists in resection of the epididymis, taking care that the vessels passing at the inner border of the epididymis to the testicle are carefully preserved. The cut end of the healthy part of the vas deferens is split up to the extent of about 1 cm., and, thus enlarged, it is stitched with fine catgut near to the rete testis, at a point where the epididymis was in close relation to the testicle. The sutures should only include the external connective tissue and muscular layers of the vas, while at the testicle the connective tissue of the corpus Highmorii is used. By this method the mucosa of both organs is supposed to be uninjured.

Now, in a certain sense, one is working in the substance of the testicle, and the connective tissue of the corpus Highmorii and that of the albuginea should be securely sutured in a manner similar to that employed for the fixation of the drainage-tube in the wall of the stomach in Witzel's method of gastrostomy. These sutures are then buried by pulling over the remainder of the covering of the testicle and suturing them. A small drain is inserted and the scrotum closed.

In the second method of anastomosis of the vas and epididymis the diseased parts are first resected, the end of the vas is split, and then a canal is formed in the cut surface of the epididymis; this canal should be about 1 cm. deep. Fine catgut sutures are inserted in the external layers of the stump of the spermatic cord, both ends of the sutures being threaded on needles. The stump is then introduced into the canal, the sutures are drawn through to the surface of the epididymis, and are tied in such a manner that the spermatic cord is fixed into the substance of the epididymis. By this method the borders of the mucous layer come into close apposition with the coils of the cut epididymis, and in order to bring about a more perfect apposition the borders of the transverse section of the epididymis can be brought together around the inserted vas. The wound is then closed with drainage.

Should the case require the resection of a large amount of the spermatic cord, so that its insertion within the epididymis would cause considerable tension, or should the testicle be pulled upward too much in order to obtain approximation, the body of the epididymis should be separated from the testicle and by turning it upward the parts can be approximated. Rasumowski states that in cases where a portion of the testicle has already been removed on account of tuberculous infection, the last-mentioned technique can be employed by making anastomosis with the tubuli contorti and recti.

That by such means anastomosis can in reality be established is proven by experimental work, and Skaduto was able to demonstrate microscopically that the sexual gland could by this means preserve its functional relations; but whether or not this histological demonstration would be the same in man, and whether or not sexual activity can be continued without impediment, Rasumowski does not say. This modern method has been as yet insufficiently experimented with for any conclusion to be made, and, although it is most ingenious, I do not believe that practically it will ever be of any real value.

In opposition to those who believe in simple resection of the diseased parts and who are opponents to the radical treatment, there are other surgeons who believe that an operation cannot be too radical, because other parts of the urogenital apparatus are first involved, while the testicle is invaded by the tuberculous process only secondarily, consequently being involved in a descending extension. For this reason removal of the entire testicle is insufficient. The tuberculous process continues to spread and the immediate good effect of the operation sooner or later proves to be an illusion.

In Germany a descending extension of urogenital tuberculosis is admitted by a large number of surgeons, and so eminent an authority as König believes that the testicle becomes involved by descending tuberculous process seated in the prostate or bladder, and that a primary infection of the seminal gland, without the disease being present in any other part of the body, is an exception. It was Gussenbauer's opinion that the testicle was involved secondarily by a descending infection of the disease. These authorities considered castration of one testicle as absurd, and they look upon double castration as practically useless, for the reason that if the affection involves one gland the disease already exists in the prostate and seminal vesicle. In their opinion another factor should also be taken into consideration, which would be decidedly against the entire removal of the testicle, namely, the mental effect of the operation. It has been shown by a number of writers that the internal secretions of the testicle play an important part in metabolism. These recent discoveries in physiology have worked riot among a number of surgeons, but we would consider attentively the ideas emitted by von Bruns, because of their importance and also for the light they throw upon the subject. In Kocher's writings, already mentioned, the idea is expressed that partial resection means only accomplishing half the necessary work, and it is also stated that the seminal gland is more involved than can clinically be detected, and that consequently recurrences are practically certain. Von Bruns emits the same opinion, and gives statistics showing that in 40 per cent. of his cases, six months after anything was noticed, the testicle was diseased, as proven at the time of operation. If the duration was over six months, it was present in 60 per cent. of the cases. Now, taking into consideration that the process often proceeds without any evident clinical changes, it can readily be conceived how little partial excision of the parts apparently involved can help the patient in the majority of cases, and how seldom a durable success can be recorded unless the entire seminal gland is removed.

Still another argument speaks against limited excision of the testicle, namely, that in about 50 per cent. of all cases of tuberculosis of the organ the disease at a later period develops in the other gland, and, according to the statistics of von Bruns, 23 per cent. of cases in which castration was performed on one side developed the disease in the remaining testicle. From this it may be concluded that prevention of the development of the disease in the apparently healthy testicle is to be found in early castration of the one afflicted. It stands to reason that the partisans of partial resection are baffled, and their various methods of interference have no significance whatever. The opponents of radical treatment declare castration superfluous, while others uphold that the operation is most disadvantageons to the patient, because the primary focus is left behind in the body. Of course, it is here understood that, according to their views, tuberculosis of the testicle is due to a descending infection from the prostate and seminal vesicle, consequently a secondary process.

Baumgarten has thrown much light on this subject, for he has experimentally demonstrated on rabbits that tuberculosis of the bladder, in the pars prostatica urethræ, and in the prostate, could be produced by injecting cultures of very virulent tubercle bacilli, but he was never able to demonstrate tuberculosis of the spermatic cord or testicle. He observed the animals for a long period of time, and the process did not extend upward along the ureters. On the other hand, by experimentally infecting the testicle, he was able to demonstrate an ascending infection along the spermatic cord. In this case he injected the bacillus directly into the epididymis and the spermatic cord, and in order to avoid the objection that the virus might have attained the deeply seated part of the vas deferens he ligated it. It was also proven that none of the inoculation fluid entered the spermatic cord when injected into the epididymis, as no swelling of the cord near the epididymis could ever be found, and, microscopically, no tuberculous lesions could be demonstrated.

In all these experiments a rapid ascending extension of the process took place, but the testicle on the other side never became involved. Von Baumgarten rightly concludes, I believe, that the tuberculous process always follows either the current of secretions or the lymph, and never in an opposite direction. He believes that the explanation of this fact is to be found in the mode of living of the tubercle bacillus; this organism, being devoid of motion and being obliged to rely on passive transportation, must naturally follow the circulating currents. Beside this, they are unable to develop and grow in secretions, and for this reason they are powerless to resist the secretory currents unless retained by some obstruction.

Pathologically and clinically these experiments seem to be correct, and certainly coincide with facts, namely, that tuberculosis of the testicle often occurs when the other parts of the urogenital apparatus are intact. It would also go to show that descending infection by the bacillus of tuberculosis is impossible and that castration performed when the disease is still of short standing and not advanced will bring about a complete recovery, because it prevents the possibility of an ascending infection from taking place.

Von Bruns gives quite an imposing number of complete recoveries after castration of one testicle, namely, 46 per cent., and what makes it particularly valuable is that the observation of his cases continued over a period of thirty-four years.

If, however, one finds frequently other portions of the urogenital tract involved, it is only in very advanced stages of the process, especially where the prostate and bladder become infected secondarily from the testicle or by a descending infection from the kidneys. Only 12 per cent. died, according to von Bruns, from tuberculosis of the urogenital apparatus after castration had been performed on one side, and in almost all of the fatal cases the patient presented the picture of tuberculosis of the urinary apparatus before the operation was undertaken. The same may be said regarding the cases of double castration, of which 15 per cent. died from tuberculosis of the urogenital apparatus, but the majority recovered, thanks to the operation. The ultimate duration of cure in double-sided castration amounted to 56 per cent., and the time over which the cases were observed was thirty years.

The great number of recoveries in which unilateral castration was done would seem to refute the statement that an extension of the process from one testicle to another takes place.

Equally favorable results have been reported by Simon, who, during the space of twenty-two years, had operated on 107 cases of tuberculosis of the testicle; the lapse of time during which they were followed varied from ten to twenty years. Out of 92 cases, 59 were alive, 54 of whom were free from any evidence of tuberculosis. Of the 33 who died, 26 succumbed to the tubercle bacillus and 7 from an intercurrent disease. 61 cases had remained free from tuberculosis after the operation, which gives us 66.3 per cent. recoveries. Simon learned the ultimate outcome in 29 out of 34 cases in which bilateral castration had been done, with the astonishing result that only 8 of them had died.

Regarding the question of psychical changes occurring after bilateral castration, it would appear to me that they have been considerably exaggerated, and where mental disturbances occur they usually only amount to a decrease in sexual desire.

The conclusions that may be deduced from what has been put forward in this paper, as well as from some little personal experience, would be that radical treatment should not be allowed to become obsolete, that castration has an exceedingly low mortality, considered as an operation, and that if performed at an early period of the disease there is a good chance of preventing further infection from the bacillus of tuberculosis from taking place. Castration certainly complies with one of the most urgent demands of modern therapeutics, namely, the eradication of the soil breeding the disease, when, of course, the affection has not been present for too long a period and has not extended to other parts of the body. Conservative surgery applied to the testicle is practically useless when the organ is affected by tuberculosis, and it allows the dangerous consequences to arise which the radical treatment directly tends to avoid.

THE RELATION OF CELLS WITH EOSINOPHILE GRANULATION TO BACTERIAL INFECTION.[1]

By Eugene L. Opie, M.D.,

ASSOCIATE IN PATHOLOGY IN JOHNS HOPKINS UNIVERSITY; FELLOW OF THE ROCKEFELLER INSTITUTE FOR MEDICAL RESEARCH.

(From the Pathological Laboratory of the Johns Hopkins University and Hospital.)

In a preceding article I have described the behavior of the eosinophile cells during the course of experimental infection with a parasite belonging to the animal kingdom, namely, trichina spiralis. Both the polynuclear leukocytes with fine granulation and the coarsely granular eosinophile leukocytes of the blood are increased in number; but increase of eosinophlie cells constitutes the predominant feature of the local and hæmal leukocytosis which results. Infection with a large variety of bacteria, on the contrary, causes migration of finely granular leukocytes into tissues where bacteria or their products have accumulated, and, in addition, hæmal leukocytosis occurs. The behavior of the leukocytes with eosinophile granulation in the presence of bacterial infection, though repeatedly the subject of investigation, has not been clearly defined.

That the eosinophile cells have a part in resisting bacteria which have entered the body was first suggested by Hankin,[2] who maintained that the bactericidal substances of the blood serum are derived from the leukocytes with eosinophile granulation. Answering a critical review of this theory by Metschnikoff,[3] Hankin[4] subsequently stated that his observations made upon rabbits had reference to the amphophile or pseudoeosinophile cells of Ehrlich, and not to the coarsely granular cells which correspond to the eosinophile leukocytes of human blood.

Kanthack and Hardy,[5] following the suggestion of Hankin's hypothesis, studied in the frog the behavior of the eosinophile leukocytes in the presence of micro-organisms. If bacillus anthracis were injected below the skin of a frog, eosinophile cells, they found, accumulated in large numbers during the first three or four hours and collected in masses about the bacilli. Large cells with non-granular protoplasm and large nuclei, called by Kanthack and Hardy hyaline cells, then made their appearance, entered the masses of eosinophile cells, and finally ingested the bacteria. The micro-organism became the prey of the hyaline cell only after it had been

[1] The present investigation has been conducted with the aid of a grant from the Rockefeller Institute for Medical Research.

[2] Cent. f. Bakt., 1892, vol. xii. pp. 777, 809

[3] Ann. de l'Inst. Pasteur, 1893, vol. vii. p. 50.

[4] Cent. f. Bakt., 1893, vol. xiv. p. 852.

[5] Philosophical Transactions of the Royal Society of London, 1894, vol. clxxxv., B., part i. p. 279; and Proceedings of the Royal Society, 1894, vol. lii. p. 267.

subjected to the influence of eosinophile cells. Such influence, according to Kanthack and Hardy, is exerted by the granules of these cells. In hanging drops they saw the granules stream toward that side of the cell which happened to be in contact with the micro-organism and then gradually disappear.

Hardy and Wesbrook[1] have shown that when fresh cultures of the bacillus of anthrax or of the spirillum cholera are injected into the intestines of frogs, eosinophile cells migrate through the epithelium into the lumen, so that they finally disappear from the intestinal wall.

Mesnil,[2] studying the means by which lower vertebrates resist bacterial infection, has repeated many of the experiments of Kanthack and Hardy, but has not obtained the same results. Within two and a half hours after injection of bacillus anthracis into the dorsal lymph sac of the frog non-granular leukocytes with round or lobed nuclei begin to accumulate and immediately approach and ingest the bacteria. Leukocytes with eosinophile granulation may congregate at the point of inoculation, but their number is inconstant, and, while in some instances they constitute even 50 per cent. to 80 per cent. of the leukocytes at the site of inoculation, they are often, particularly in rana esculenta, not 1 per cent. of those present. That cells with eosinophile granulation in lower vertebrates do not play an essential part in resisting bacterial invasion is, Mesnil believes, further shown by the fact that the perch (perca fluviatilis), which is not susceptible to bacillus anthracis, possesses no granular leukocytes; injected anthrax bacilli, as in the frog, are engulfed by non-granular leukocytes possessing irregularly round or lobed nuclei. In accordance with the view held by Metschnikoff and himself, Mesnil believes that the eosinophile granules represent transformed material previously ingested by the leukocyte; such old phagocytes filled with reserve material still possess some remains of their phagocytic power. Mesnil states that he has observed these cells in the frog ingest bacteria, rarely after subcutaneous inoculation, but more frequently after the injection of bacteria into the circulation.

In a previous paper[3] I have reviewed the evidence which demonstrates, I believe, that the eosinophile cells of mammals are not derived from the polynuclear leukocytes with finer granulation, but exclusively from eosinophile cells in the bone-marrow. These cells of the marrow, which may be designated eosinophile myelocytes, are analogous to the myelocytes with finer granulation, the parent cells of the finely granular leukocytes. In lower vertebrates the relation of the various granular leukocytes to one another and to those of higher mammals are less clearly understood. In birds, for

[1] Journal of Physiology, 1895, vol. xviii. p. 490.

[2] Ann. de l'Inst. Pasteur, 1895, vol. ix. p. 301.

[3] The American Journal of the Medical Sciences, 1904, vol. cxxvii. p. 217.

example, the more common polynuclear leukocytes are provided with large spindle-shaped granules, which, like the less numerous coarsely granular leukocytes of mammals, have a strong affinity for eosin. Hence, conclusions reached by a study of lower vertebrates, some of which apparently possess no granular leukocytes, even were they in accord, are not with our present knowledge applicable to mammals.

In the article just mentioned I have considered certain facts which indicate that the polynuclear leukocytes with fine and with coarse granules in different mammalian species bear corresponding relations to one another. A second series of experiments performed by Kanthack and Hardy[1] on rabbits, guinea-pigs, and rats has, therefore, a more direct bearing upon the activities of the eosinophile cells in man and in other higher mammals. In mammals, as in lower vertebrates, according to Kanthack and Hardy, those wandering cells which are first attracted by micro-organisms and a variety of other irritant substances are coarsely granular oxyphile (eosinophile) cells, which have their origin in the neighboring connective tissue. This conclusion has been based upon a series of experiments in which various bacteria and a variety of substances, such as nitrate of silver, turpentine, and filtrates from bacterial cultures have been introduced into the peritoneal cavity or into the subcutaneous tissue of the animals just named.

If Ziegler's chambers containing cultures of bacillus anthracis or of the spirillum of cholera are introduced into the peritoneal cavity of the rabbit, at the end of seven hours only coarsely granular eosinophile cells have succeeded in entering. When a less virulent organism, such as bacillus ramosus, is employed, large non-granular cells with round or indented nuclei ("hyaline cells") have accumulated in large numbers at the end of two and a half hours. The more virulent bacteria, according to Kanthack and Hardy, cause rapid destruction of these non-granular cells, while the less virulent organism allows them to accumulate. In another series of experiments Kanthack and Hardy have injected bacillus anthracis, bacillus pyocyaneus, or the spirillum of cholera in small amount into the peritoneal cavity of the guinea-pig or of the rat. The primary result has been disappearance of the cells present in the cavity, and as fragments of eosinophile cells are to be found in the peritoneal fluid, they are believed to have been destroyed in part at least. The injected bacteria are quickly attacked by the coarsely granular cells, and even within five minutes after the inoculation of bacillus anthracis into the rat 40 per cent. of the eosinophile cells found are applied to bacilli. These cells do not ingest bacteria, but their granules, Kanthack and Hardy have maintained, exhibit the phenomenon noted in the frog. Bacteria are engulfed by the "hyaline" cells, the

[1] Journal of Physiology, 1894, vol. xvii. p. 81.

process beginning within ten minutes after inoculation. Destruction and removal of bacteria, they conclude, is due to the combined activity of two kinds of cells, the coarsely granular oxyphile (eosinophile) and the "hyaline" cell.

Durham[1] has studied the local reaction which occurs when various bacteria are injected into the peritoneal cavity of guinea-pigs. He has failed to observe the preliminary attack of eosinophile cells described by Kanthack and Hardy, and reaches the conclusion that these cells have no important part in the destruction of bacteria. Durham says, however, that in animals which die within thirty hours after inoculation, the only cells in the peritoneal fluid at the time of death are finely granular polynuclear leukocytes in abundance, together with a variable number of coarsely granular leukocytes. At times only one coarsely granular cell is seen in ten fields of the $\frac{1}{12}$ objective, while in other instances one may be found in almost every field. Judged by their relative numbers, the eosinophile cells at this stage, Durham believes, can have but a small share in the work of destroying bacteria.

Noesske[2] has performed experiments with the tubercle bacillus which have a bearing upon the present subject. Studying this organism under conditions which cause it to assume a radiate formation suggesting actinomycosis bovis, he found at an early stage of infection, about such colonies of the bacillus, free granules, which, he thought, were derived from eosinophile cells. He supported his views by demonstrating that the granules react to stains like eosinophile granules and are similarly affected by digestive ferments, but does not bring more conclusive evidence of their nature. Introduction of tubercle bacilli into the muscle of rabbits showed more clearly that eosinophile cells accumulate at the seat of infection. Colonies of bacillus tuberculosis were placed within an incision made into the muscle of the back, and at the end of four days the surrounding tissue was removed. In immediate contact with the implanted colonies the tissue was necrotic; polynuclear leukocytes were numerous, and eosinophile cells were few. Near-by, however, eosinophile leukocytes were present in great number within degenerate muscle fibres, among which were scattered tubercle bacilli. A similar result was produced in rabbits with tubercle bacilli killed with steam. Noesske, moreover, obtained an accumulation of eosinophile cells in the subcutaneous tissue of a human subject by injecting the dead bacilli. He reaches the conclusion that these cells are always abundant during the first stage of tuberculous infection. Pyogenic bacteria, on the contrary, Noesske found caused no accumulation of eosinophile cells.

Ehrlich[3] found that with acute leukocytosis only the mononuclear

[1] Journal of Pathology and Bacteriology, 1897, vol. iv. p. 338.
[2] Deutsche Zeitsch. f. Chirurgie, 1900, vol. lv. p. 211.
[3] Zeit. f. klin. Med., vol. i. part iii.

and neutrophile polynuclear forms of the blood are increased, while the eosinophile cells exhibit an apparent diminution. Subsequent observers have noted a well-marked diminution of the eosinophile leukocytes during various infectious diseases caused by bacteria. Müller and Rieder[1] have found that eosinophile cells are diminished during typhoid fever. Rieder[2] noted their diminution or complete absence from the blood in cases of pneumonia, while Canon[3] noted a diminution in association with septic processes. Zappert[4] has carefully studied the behavior of the eosinophile leukocytes during the course of various infectious diseases, and reaches the conclusion that fever is associated with such constant diminution of the absolute number of these cells that this diminution may be regarded as one of the manifestations of febrile intoxication. With pneumonia, typhoid fever. erysipelas, and certain pyogenic infections eosinophile cells are diminished so long as fever persists, but after its subsidence return to normal or, in a certain proportion of cases, undergo a more or less well-marked increase above their normal number. Zappert quotes observations of Ehrlich[5] upon the destruction of leukocytes in the spleen during febrile processes, and reaches the conclusion that eosinophile cells are diminished because the normal transformation of leukocytes with neutrophile granulation into eosinophile leukocytes is prevented.

Observations similar to those of Zappert have been made by Türk[6] and others in cases of pneumonia, typhoid fever, diphtheria, and with various suppurative processes. It is, however, noteworthy that in certain diseases not due to bacterial infection, such as scarlet fever (Kotschetkoff[7]) and smallpox (Ferguson[8]), there is a moderate increase of eosinophile cells.

In hardened tissues which have been the seat of a variety of inflammatory processess several observers have noted the presence of eosinophile cells, occasionally in considerable number. Numerous observations have shown that eosinophile cells are often abundant in carcinomata of the cervix uteri, in nasal polyps, and in a variety of other benign and malignant tumors. From a study of tissue obtained at autopsy and from the operating table, Noesske[9] reached the conclusion that tumors of mucous membranes, particularly when they are exposed to injury, are rich in eosinophile cells; immense numbers are not infrequently found in epitheliomata of the lip or of the tongue, in carcinomata of the cervix uteri, and in laryngeal

[1] Deutsches Arch. f. klin. Med., 1891, vol. xlviii. p. 47.

[2] Beiträge zur Kenntniss der Leukocytoses. Leipzig, 1892.

[3] Deutsche med. Woch., 1892, vol. xviii. p. 206.

[4] Zeit. f. klin. Med., 1893, vol. xxiii. p. 227.

[5] Zur Kenntniss des acuten Milztumors, Charité-Ann., 9 Jahr.

[6] Klinische Untersuchungen über das Verhalten des Blutes bei Infectionskrankheiten, Wien und Leipzig, 1898.

[7] Ref., Cent. f. allg. Path. u. path. Anat., 1892, No. 11.

[8] Journal of Pathology and Bacteriology, 1903, vol. viii. p. 411.

[9] Loc. cit.

tumors. Tumors situated below the skin contain eosinophile cells when the overlying epithelium is lost and ulceration is beginning. When benign or malignant tumors are situated in internal organs where they are protected from infection, eosinophile cells are scant or absent. Noesske thinks that these cells have a part in protecting the tissue from bacterial infection. Where, however, the tumor tissue is the seat of an advanced inflammation, and, indeed, in the lesions of various pyogenic or other inflammatory processes, such as erysipelas, osteomyelitis, and pneumonia, eosinophile cells are present in small number or are completely absent. Eosinophile cells, at times in very large number, have been found by Howard and Perkins[1] in the lesion of appendicitis, salpingitis, oöphoritis, and perioöphoritis, acute interstitial and suppurative nephritis, enteritis, and of a variety of other inflammatory processes. Their association with such lesions has not been found constant, and in some instances they are normally present in the affected tissue.

In an article to which reference has already been made, I have collected evidence to show that the bone-marrow is the seat of origin of the eosinophile leukocytes, and the vascular system the path by which they are distributed to various tissues of the body. Changes in the blood being subject to observation during the entire course of an experimental infection, it is possible to determine if the eosinophile cells of the blood exhibit a characteristic reaction to bacterial invasion.

METHODS. In counting the relative and absolute number of eosinophile leukocytes in the blood, I have used the methods previously described.[2] For the purpose of these experiments the guinea-pig has been found particularly suitable, since the blood of apparently healthy full-grown animals usually contains from 5 per cent. to 10 per cent. of eosinophile leukocytes. Hence the effect of conditions which cause a diminution of these cells can be far more accurately determined than in animals possessing only a very small proportion of such cells. In order to test the behavior of the eosinophile cells, I have employed a variety of bacteria, including bacillus tuberculosis, bacillus anthracis, bacillus choleræ suis, and bacillus mucosus capsulatus (of Friedländer), all of which are pathogenic in small quantity for guinea-pigs. Bacillus pyocyaneus has been selected as a convenient means of studying the effect of a relatively severe infection from which the animal is capable of recovering. Bouillon cultures incubated from twenty-four to forty-eight hours have been employed in varying amount. The injection of as much as 3 c.c. of sterile bouillon into the peritoneal cavity has caused no noteworthy change in the number of eosinophile cells nor in the weight of the animal.

[1] Johns Hopkins Hospital Reports, 1902, vol. x. p. 249.
[2] Loc. cit.

Behavior of the Eosinophile Leukocytes during the Course of Fatal Bacterial Infection.

Infection of guinea-pigs with a moderate number of trichinæ, I have shown,[1] causes a gradual increase of the eosinophile leukocytes, but death is preceded by rapid diminution. The administration of a very large number of parasites is more quickly fatal; the eosinophile cells diminish in number and completely disappear from the blood. The effect of fatal bacterial infection is similar, though the eosinophile cells may disappear from the circulating blood more gradually.

CHART I.

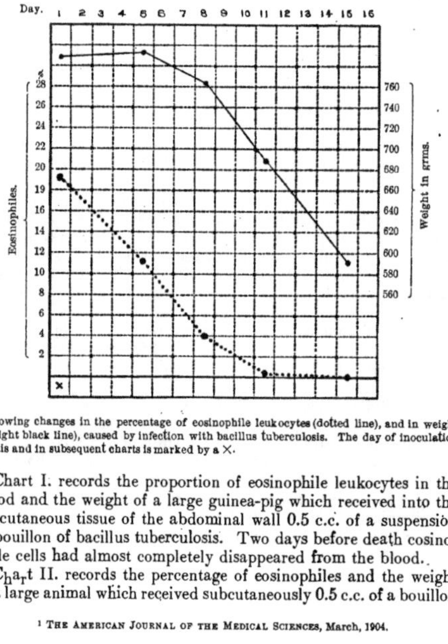

Showing changes in the percentage of eosinophile leukocytes (dotted line), and in weight (straight black line), caused by infection with bacillus tuberculosis. The day of inoculation in this and in subsequent charts is marked by a ×.

Chart I. records the proportion of eosinophile leukocytes in the blood and the weight of a large guinea-pig which received into the subcutaneous tissue of the abdominal wall 0.5 c.c. of a suspension in bouillon of bacillus tuberculosis. Two days before death cosinophile cells had almost completely disappeared from the blood.

Chart II. records the percentage of eosinophiles and the weight of a large animal which received subcutaneously 0.5 c.c. of a bouillon

[1] THE AMERICAN JOURNAL OF THE MEDICAL SCIENCES, March, 1904.

culture of bacillus choleræ suis incubated twenty-four hours. Death did not occur until the ninth day, but the eosinophile leukocytes, which at the beginning of the experiment constituted 15 per cent. of the white blood corpuscles, had almost completely disappeared on the fifth day.

In both experiments the tissues from the animals were hardened in Zenker's fluid and stained, after embedding in paraffin, with hæmatoxylin and eosin, so that eosinophile cells might be identified. The paucity of eosinophile cells in the tissues in both experiments is in harmony with their disappearance from the blood. In the spleen, where the number of eosinophile cells normally present corresponds

CHART II.

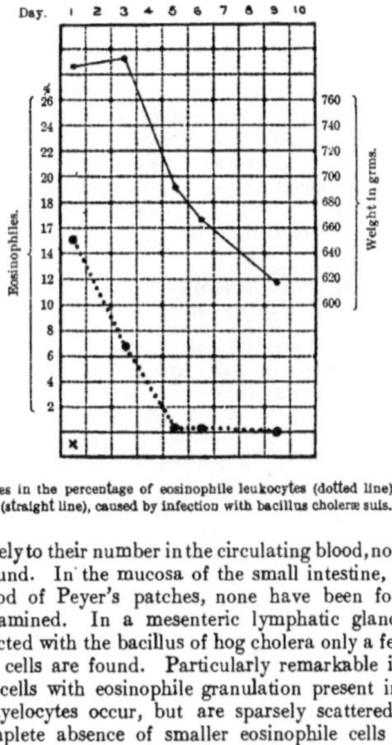

Showing changes in the percentage of eosinophile leukocytes (dotted line) and in weight (straight line), caused by infection with bacillus choleræ suis.

approximately to their number in the circulating blood, no eosinophile cells are found. In the mucosa of the small intestine, even in the neighborhood of Peyer's patches, none have been found in the sections examined. In a mesenteric lymphatic gland from the animal injected with the bacillus of hog cholera only a few scattered eosinophile cells are found. Particularly remarkable is the small number of cells with eosinophile granulation present in the bone-marrow; myelocytes occur, but are sparsely scattered, while the almost complete absence of smaller eosinophile cells with lobed nuclei is noteworthy. In the bone-marrow from both animals occur very small eosinophile cells, with a diameter approximately two-thirds that of an eosinophile leukocyte. These dwarfed cells have nuclei which are round or only slightly indented, resembling in the latter case intermediate stages between the nucleus of the myelocyte and the typically lobed nucleus of the mature eosinophile leukocyte.

With bacterial infections which are more acute than those just described, eosinophile leukocytes disappear much more quickly from the circulating blood; indeed, none may be found in specimens examined at the end of a few hours. Injection of 1 c.c. of a bouillon culture of bacillus pyocyaneus, which had been incubated four days, into the peritoneal cavity of a guinea-pig possessing 5.7 per cent. of eosinophile leukocytes, caused their disappearance within twenty-four hours; death occurred at the end of forty hours. Subcutaneous inoculation of 0.5 c.c. of a twenty-hour culture of the same organism caused the percentage of eosinophile leukocytes to fall from 9.7 to 0.5 in eight hours. Bacillus mucosus capsulatus (0.3 c.c. of a forty-eight-hour-old bouillon culture injected into the peritoneal cavity) caused the eosinophile leukocytes to diminish during four hours from 20.7 per cent. to 7.3 per cent. of the number of white blood corpuscles. The injection of streptococcus pyogenes into the peritoneal cavity had a similar effect; 1 c.c. of a culture four days old caused the eosinophiles of a guinea-pig possessing 5.7 per cent. to diminish to such an extent that none were found in a specimen examined at the end of four hours.

Behavior of Eosinophile Leukocytes during the Course of Non-fatal Bacterial Infection.

The disappearance of eosinophile leukocytes under the influence of severe, usually fatal infections has suggested the desirability of studying their behavior during the course of acute infections from which the animal is capable of recovery. For this purpose bacillus pyocyaneus has been selected and has been injected into the peritoneal cavity in order to avoid the prolonged effect of a localized abscess. The injection of 0.5 c.c. to 1 c.c. of a culture in bouillon incubated at 37° C. during twenty-four hours causes an acute general peritonitis, from which the animal usually recovers. The well-known effect of such inoculation upon the blood being an increase of the polynuclear leukocytes with fine granulation, I have limited my attention to the behavior of the eosinophile cells.

Chart III. records the effect of the intraperitoneal inoculation of 0.7 c.c. of a bouillon culture of bacillus pyocyaneus upon a large guinea-pig of which the eosinophile leukocytes constituted 7.3 per cent. of the white corpuscles.

At the end of twenty-four hours after inoculation eosinophile leukocytes had diminished to such extent that none were found in the specimens of blood examined. The proportion gradually rose and reached a maximum on the sixth day, when it exceeded that originally present; on the eighth day the percentage count agreed approximately with that before inoculation. The absolute number of eosinophile cells has been estimated from the total number of leukocytes, counted daily by the same Thoma-Zeiss apparatus, and the changes which it undergoes are found to correspond with those of the percentage count. The weight of the animal has been recorded, since it gives an indication of the effect of infection upon the general metabolism of the animal.

CHART III.

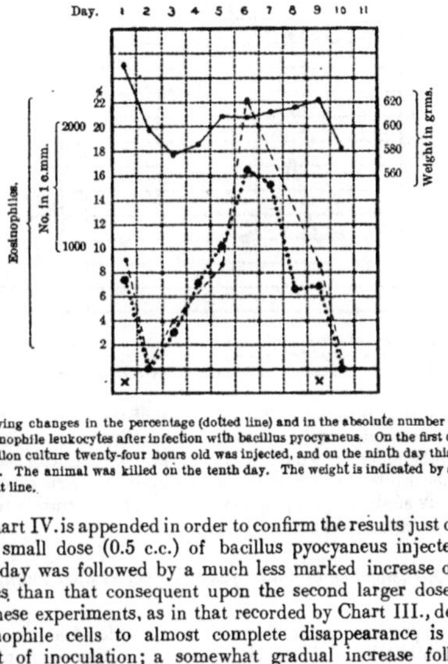

Showing changes in the percentage (dotted line) and in the absolute number (broken line) of eosinophile leukocytes after infection with bacillus pyocyaneus. On the first day 0.7 c.c. of a bouillon culture twenty-four hours old was injected, and on the ninth day this dose was repeated. The animal was killed on the tenth day. The weight is indicated by an unbroken straight line.

Chart IV. is appended in order to confirm the results just described. The small dose (0.5 c.c.) of bacillus pyocyaneus injected on the first day was followed by a much less marked increase of eosinophiles than that consequent upon the second larger dose (1 c.c.). In these experiments, as in that recorded by Chart III., decrease of eosinophile cells to almost complete disappearance is the first effect of inoculation; a somewhat gradual increase follows and reaches a maximum on the fifth or sixth day, when, after inoculating 0.7 c.c. or 1 c.c. of the culture, the number of eosinophile cells in 1 c.mm. of blood is more than twice the original number. A return to normal then follows. Such changes in the blood suggest that destruction of eosinophile cells has been followed by regeneration causing an accumulation in excess of the normal. In order to obtain an explanation of this phenomenon it is essential to know the cause of their temporary disappearance during what may be termed the stage of eosinophile leucopenia.

In order to determine the fate of the eosinophile leukocytes which have disappeared from the peripheral circulation during the early stages of acute bacterial infection attention has been directed

CHART IV.

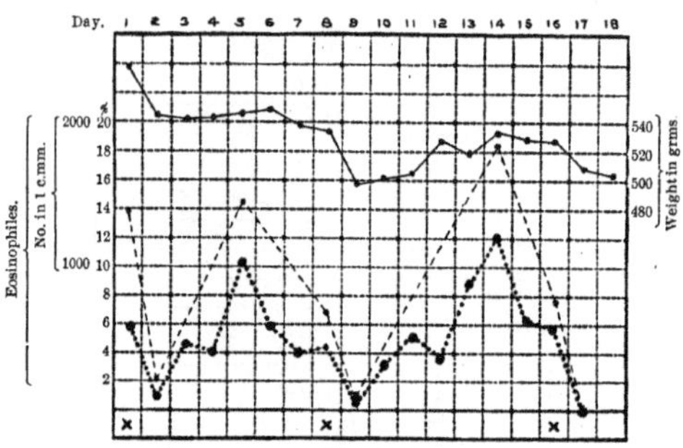

Showing the effect of infection with bacillus pyocyaneus. On the first day 0.5 c.c., on the eighth day 1 c.c. of a culture twenty-four hours old was injected; on the sixteenth day the animal received 1 c.c. of a culture four days old, and death occurred on the eighteenth day.

to the seat of infection. For the study of the local changes which follow inoculation the peritoneal cavity offers obvious advantages. The inflammatory exudates which accumulate can be readily obtained while the phenomena occurring in the tissues can be conveniently studied in preparations made from the transparent tissue of the omentum and mesentery.

Local Accumulation of Eosinophile Leukocytes after Intraperitoneal Inoculation of Bacteria.

Since previous studies have shown that local accumulation of eosinophile cells is the result of their migration from the blood-vessels, it has been considered desirable to study with especial care the contents of the vessels at the site of inoculation and to note perhaps the occurrence of migration. For this purpose the following method has been employed: At the end of a variable time after inoculation the animal is etherized and, while breathing still continues, the peritoneal cavity is opened in the midline. After specimens of the peritoneal exudate have been prepared, Zenker's fluid (containing 5 per cent. of acetic acid) warmed to a temperature of 40° C. is poured into the cavity. The omentum and mesentery, together with the peritoneum elsewhere, are thus quickly hardened. The tissues to be preserved are removed and kept in Zenker's fluid about twenty-four hours, after which they are treated in the usual way. Small pieces of the omentum and mesentery are stained without embedding. Treatment of these membranes, previously stained with hæmatoxylin, with 0.5 per cent. aqueous solution of eosin has served to demonstrate so clearly the granules of the eosinophile leukocytes that these cells are readily distinguishable from the more numerous polymorphonuclear leukocytes with fine granulation; at the same time they are recognizable within the blood-vessels. The amœboid shape of the leukocytes is often well preserved and not infrequently they are fixed in process of migration from the vessels. Methylene blue used with eosin has the advantage of staining bacteria.

The peritoneal cavity contains normally a small amount of clear fluid in which are suspended a considerable number of cells. The character of these wandering cells has been the subject of special study by Kanthack and Hardy, who found the following varieties: 1. Polymorphonuclear cells with coarse eosinophile granules forming in guinea-pigs from 30 per cent. to 50 per cent. of the total number of cells. 2. Cells with basophile granulation occurring in small number. 3. Small cells, identical with the lymphocytes of the blood, possessing a single round nucleus surrounded by a narrow rim of protoplasm. 4. Larger mononuclear cells with round or indented nuclei and fairly abundant non-granular protoplasm. The latter Kanthack and Hardy designate "hyaline cells." Both Durham and Beattie have found in the peritoneal cavity of guinea-pigs three types of wandering cells described by Kanthack and Hardy, but have not noted the presence of cells with basophile granulation. The "hyaline cells" of these authors in part at least are the macrophages of Metschnikoff.

Before describing my observations upon the behavior of the eosinophile cells in the presence of bacterial infection I will briefly define the reaction which occurs when bacteria are injected into the peritoneal cavity. These changes have been studied by Issaeff,[1] Metschnikoff,[2] Durham,[3] and Beattie.[4] The first effect of intraperitoneal inoculation is the partial disappearance of cellular elements normally present, so that in the guinea-pig, according to Durham, five or six minutes after injection almost all cells save lymphocytes have disappeared.

[1] Zeit. f. Hygiene, 1894, vol. xvi. p. 287.
[2] Ann. de l'Inst. Pasteur, 1895, vol. ix. p. 369.
[3] Journal of Pathology and Bacteriology, 1896. vol. iv. p. 338.
[4] Ibid., 1903, vol. viii. p. 129.

This stage of leucopenia persists about one hour (Durham), during which time the amount of peritoneal fluid increases. Metschnikoff has maintained that the disappearance of leukocytes is the result of their destruction by the toxic products introduced with the micro-organisms. Durham has brought forward evidence to support a different explanation. At the end of only two minutes after injection he has noted that "hyaline" and eosinophile cells begin to adhere in clumps, the lymphocytes being exempt. At first these groups are small, but later large masses containing many cells may be found. Such masses tend to adhere to the peritoneal surfaces, but especially to the omentum, so that at the end of about twenty minutes (Durham) "hyaline" and eosinophile cells are here present in considerable number. At the end of about an hour polynuclear leukocytes with fine granulation make their appearance and subsequently accumulate so that about fifteen hours after inoculation they are present in enormous number. They are actively phagocytic and ingest bacteria. If, however, infection is caused by a large dose of a virulent organism, few polynuclear leukocytes may be found and the stage of leucopenia may persist until death. With a relatively mild infection which has caused the accumulation of polynuclear cells in great number, cells of another type appear at the end of about fifteen hours. They are larger than polynuclear leukocytes and have a large round, oval, or indented nucleus. These cells, which are the macrophages of Metschnikoff, are actively phagocytic and ingest not only bacteria but polynuclear leukocytes as well, so that frequently several of the latter are seen within one macrophage. Upon the fourth, fifth, or sixth day after infection, the peritoneal fluid has assumed its normal characters, disappearance of the polynuclear leukocytes being followed by that of the macrophages.

Observers who have studied the foregoing phenomena have not failed to note the presence of eosinophile cells in the exudate which accumulates. Such cells, however, exist in the normal peritoneal cavity, and the difficulty of determining whether they are increased or diminished is considerable. The divergent conclusions reached by observers who have studied the effect of intraperitoneal inoculation have already been cited.

Study of the blood has shown that eosinophile cells partially or completely disappear from the peripheral circulation within a few hours after intraperitoneal inoculation. Study of the membranes which are contained within the peritoneal cavity has explained this phenomenon. Eosinophile cells constitute a considerable proportion of the immense number of leukocytes which within several hours are attracted to the bloodvessels which abut upon the infected peritoneal surface. Their migration and accumulation within the peritoneal cavity are demonstrable. These facts may be best illustrated by a series of experiments performed with *bacillus pyo-*

cyaneus. The following observations have been made upon fourteen animals inoculated intraperitoneally and killed after intervals varying from a few minutes to twenty-four hours:

Within a few minutes after the injection of one cubic centimetre of a bouillon culture of bacillus pyocyaneus incubated twenty-four hours large mononuclear and eosinophile cells disappear from the peritoneal cavity, so that in animals killed at the end of eight and fifteen minutes after inoculation only one or two eosinophile lenkocytes have been encountered while counting several hundred cells, almost exclusively lymphocytes. Examination of the omentum fixed and stained confirms the statements of Durham. Large mononuclear cells form compact clumps, often containing a hundred or more cells, among which are eosinophile cells in varying number. Altered or fragmented eosinophile cells were not seen, and evidence that these cells had undergone destruction was not obtained. In animals killed at the end of eight, fifteen, or thirty minutes after inoculation the number of leukocytes within the bloodvessels of the omentum and mesentery has undergone no change. Within small veins having a diameter equal or twice that of a polynuclear leukocyte, white corpuscles are scattered among the red corpuscles at such long intervals that the labor of counting them is considerable. In the tissue of the mesentery eosinophile cells occur in considerable number, but are not more numerous than in the normal animal.

At the end of one hour the number of cells in the peritoneal exudate is still small, though polynuclear leukocytes with fine granulation have made their appearance. Eosinophile cells are also present in small number. In the tissue of the mesentery a few polynuclear leukocytes are found about many of the bloodvessels. Within the lumen of the vessels leukocytes are much more numerous than before and are in large part finely granular polynuclear leukocytes, some of which are flattened out upon the endothelial surface of the vessel, while others are in process of migration.

At the end of two hours the same changes are more advanced. In the peritoneal exudate cells are not numerous and about one-half of those present are polynuclear forms with fine granulation; eosinophile cells are fairly numerous and constitute about 10 per cent. Leukocytes have accumulated in the bloodvessels of the mesentery and are often found in fair number about them, while cells in process of migration are numerous. Eosinophile cells are present both in the tissue and within the bloodvessels, but their proportion does not differ notably from that in the peripheral circulation before inoculation. In an animal (weight 553 grams), of which the eosinophile leukocytes numbered 5.7 per cent. before inoculation, 4 per cent. were counted in small veins in diameter about twice that of a polynuclear leukocyte. Since, however, the total number of leukocytes within these vessels has been enormously increased, such percentage indicates that many eosinophile cells have been held in the vessels of the inflamed region. Eosinophile cells are occasionally found in process of migration.

At the end of four hours the influence of bacterial infection upon the eosinophile leukocytes is more clearly demonstrable. The omentum is now covered by purulent exudate and, as Durham has described it, is rolled into a compact mass lying in contact with the stomach. In the peritoneal cavity is a considerable amount of turbid fluid containing an immense number of cells which are almost wholly polynuclear leukocytes. Eosinophile cells are present, but in small number, so that one or two are encountered while counting successive hundreds of cells. In the tissue of the mesentery polynuclear leukocytes are numerous and eosinophile cells are present in smaller proportion. In the bloodvessels leukocytes are closely crowded and eosinophile cells are very numerous. In blood from the ear of a guinea-pig weighing 604 grams the eosinophile leukocytes which had constituted 8.3 per cent. of the white corpuscles before inoculation had fallen at the end of four hours to 1.3 per cent. The animal was killed within the next half-hour.. In small veins of the mesentery with a diameter from three to four times that of a polynuclear leukocyte, 21, 26, 20, and 23 eosinophile leukocytes were counted in successive hundreds of white corpuscles, which are here present in very large numbers. In smaller vessels with a diameter approximately half as great, leukocytes are less numerous and a smaller number of eosinophile cells are present, the count in two successive hundreds being 11 and 13. Where eosinophile cells are so numerous the process of migration is readily demonstrable. Some cells with eosinophile granulation are flattened and closely applied to the inner surface of the vessel; others have been fixed while making their way through the wall of the vessel, part of the cell being still within the lumen, while a part has penetrated the intima and projects upon the outer surface of the small vein which is formed by little more than a layer of endothelial cells. That part of the leukocyte which projects from the vessel wall is occasionally connected with the remainder, still in the lumen of the vessel, by a strand of protoplasm drawn out into a narrow thread. Upon the surface of the omentum polynuclear leukocytes are present in great number and are usually collected to form compact clumps. Within and about such masses eosinophile leukocytes are numerous. In the bloodvessels of the omentum, polynuclear leukocytes, both with fine and with coarse granulation, are abundant.

At the end of eight hours polynuclear leukocytes are present in the peritoneal exudate in immense number and are in large part collected into masses held together by a network of fibrin. From 1 to 2 per cent. of eosinophile cells can be counted in the fresh exudate. The masses of leukocytes just mentioned are particularly numerous upon the surface of the retracted omentum. In specimens of the omentum stained with eosin and methylene blue eosinophile cells are clearly demonstrable even though embedded in masses of finely granular leukocytes, and are particularly numerous within the clumps of leukocytes already mentioned. From such specimens one obtains convincing evidence that eosinophile cells in number far greater than that originally present have found their way into the peritoneal cavity.

Eosinophile leukocytes upon the surface of the omentum are in part normal in appearance and are provided with lobed nuclei which stain most deeply at the periphery. Eosinophile cells exhibiting degenerative changes are however, readily found. Though the eosinophile granules are still well preserved, the nucleus of the cell is contracted into one or more small round masses which stain deeply and homogeneously. While the finely granular leukocytes almost uniformly contain many ingested bacteria, the bodies of the eosinophile cells are free from such inclusions.

Examination of the mesentery demonstrates that leukocytes are less numerous in the small bloodvessels than at an earlier period. Though polynuclear leukocytes and eosinophile cells are still abundant, migration is less active and at the end of sixteen hours has apparently ceased completely.

At the end of sixteen hours eosinophile leukocytes still form a conspicuous feature of the exudate upon the surface of the omentum and to less extent upon the surface of the mesentery. Many are still well preserved, but a considerable proportion exhibit degenerative changes, the nucleus being contracted into one or more small masses of chromatin which stain deeply and homogeneously. Occasionally a clear vacuole is situated within the otherwise compact globule of chromatin. In some instances, on the contrary, the lobed nucleus of the eosinophile cell is swollen and stains poorly. Changes of a similar nature affect the nuclei of the finely granular polynuclear leukocytes. At this stage large mononuclear cells have made their appearance.

At the end of twenty-four hours large mononuclear cells have become numerous. Eosinophile leukocytes form a small proportion of the great number of cells present in the exudate. Ingestion of polynuclear cells by the large mononuclear phagocytes has begun. In this process the eosinophile and finely granular leukocytes are equally concerned, and within a macrophage may be found a round clump of coarse eosinophile granules from which the nucleus has completely disappeared.

In order to confirm the preceding observations, repeating the experiments, I have employed, instead of bacillus pyocyaneus, bacillus mucosus capsulatus (of Friedländer), an organism far more pathogenic for guinea-pigs.

Experiment A (Bacillus Mucosus Capsulatus). An animal weighing 492 grams received 0.3 c.c. of a bouillon culture twenty-four hours old. The eosinophile leukocytes before inoculation constituted 3.3 per cent. of the white blood corpuscles. In the peritoneal exudate at the end of three hours free bacteria are present in large number; polynuclear leukocytes, lymphocytes, and eosinophile cells are present, the latter forming 35.3 per cent. In the tissue of the mesentery leukocytes occur in moderate number. In the small veins leukocytes are very numerous, and in four successive hundreds of white corpuscles the proportion of eosinophile leukocytes was 14, 17, 13, and 17 per cent. Eosinophile cells are found fixed in process of migration.

Experiment B (*Bacillus Mucosus Capsulatus*). An animal weighing 625 grams received intraperitoneally 0.3 c.c. of a culture of bacillus mucosus capsulatus forty-eight hours old. The eosinophile leukocytes in the peripheral circulation which before inoculation numbered 24.3 per cent. fell at the end of four hours to 7.3 per cent. The animal was killed at the end of four and a half hours. Cells are fairly numerous in the peritoneal exudate and are almost wholly polymorphonuclear leukocytes and eosinophile cells, the latter constituting 7.7 per cent. In the mesentery polynuclear leukocytes and eosinophile cells occur in considerable number, particularly in the neighborhood of the bloodvessels. In the vessels leukocytes are usually accumulated in such number that the lumen is closely packed with cells of which eosinophile leukocytes constitute considerably more than half. To obtain an approximate estimation of their relative number they were counted in small vessels with a diameter from one and a half to twice that of an eosinophile cell; the percentage count was 65 per cent. Many of these cells are found flattened and closely applied to the endothelial surface of the vessel, while others are found in process of migration; a small process containing part of the nucleus may project between the endothelial cells, the remainder of the leukocytes being within the lumen. Sections of the mesentery embedded in paraffin confirmed the observations just described. In the lumen of one comparatively small vein differential count showed the presence of 73 per cent. of eosinophile leukocytes.

Experiment C (*Bacillus Mucosus Capsulatus*). A guinea-pig weighing 597 grams, with eosinophile leukocytes numbering 20.3 per cent., received intraperitoneally 0.5 c.c. of a bouillon culture of bacillus mucosus capsulatus. The animal died at the end of twenty hours, and the peritoneal cavity was found to contain about 3 c.c. of turbid fluid in which polynuclear leukocytes numbered 69 per cent., eosinophile cells 29 per cent., and large mononuclear cells 2 per cent.

The phenomena which occur after inoculation with bacillus pyocyaneus are reproduced by infection with bacillus mucosus capsulatus. The experiments with the two organisms are not wholly comparable, since the number of eosinophile leukocytes in the circulating blood before inoculation in different animals has differed considerably. Nevertheless, with the more virulent bacillus mucosus capsulatus migration of eosinophile cells appears to be much more active, so that at the end of a given time the proportion of eosinophile leukocytes in the peritoneal exudate is much greater than with bacillus pyocyaneus. The chemotactic influence which virulent bacteria exert upon the eosinophile cells is further shown by study of the bloodvessels in the mesentery. In two of the experiments just described eosinophile leukocytes constituted respectively 65 per cent. and 15.2 per cent. of the total number of white corpuscles in these vessels, though their proportion in the peripheral circulation before inoculation had been only 24.3 per cent. and 3.3 per cent. Doubtless the earlier migration of polynuclear leukocytes with fine granulation explains in part the large proportion of eosinophile leukocytes present in the vessels three or four hours after inoculation. The experiments demonstrate that both types of polymorphonuclear leukocyte are attracted to the inflamed region.

Results of a similar nature have been obtained with *bacillus anthracis.*

Experiment A (Bacillus Anthracis). A guinea-pig weighing 533 grams, with eosinophile leukocytes numbering 27.3 per cent., received into the peritoneal cavity 0.5 c.c. of a bouillon culture of bacillus anthracis forty-eight hours old. At the end of four hours the animal was killed. The peritoneal exudate is found to contain polynuclear leukocytes in great number, together with eosinophiles, constituting 7 per cent. of the cells present. In the tissue of the mesentery eosinophile cells are numerous. The small bloodvessels are closely packed with leukocytes, among which those with eosinophile granulation, counted in small veins with a diameter approximately one and one-half that of a leukocyte, constitute in three successive hundreds 23, 21, and 20 per cent.

In the foregoing experiment it is evident that a large number of eosinophile leukocytes have been held in the inflamed area, even though it be recalled that their proportion in the peripheral circulation before inoculation slightly exceeded that found in the vessels of the mesentery four hours later, for they then constituted one-fifth of the immense number of leukocytes which are crowded together in the vessels of the inflamed membrane. With bacillus anthracis, as with bacillus pyocyaneus (see Chart IV.), a small dose of the micro-organism has a less marked influence upon the eosinophile cells.

Experiment B (Bacillus Anthracis). A guinea-pig weighing 560 grams, with eosinophile leukocytes in the peripheral circulation numbering 2.3 per cent., was inoculated with 0.1 c.c. of a twenty-four-hour-old culture of bacillus anthracis. At the end of four hours the peritoneal exudate contained polynuclear leukocytes in great number, together with eosinophiles, constituting 2.2 per cent. of the cells present. Of the leukocytes which are closely packed together in the bloodvessels of the mesentery 1 per cent. are cells with eosinophile granulation.

Accumulation of Eosinophile Myelocytes in the Spleen.

Study of the spleen during the first few hours which follow bacterial inoculation of the peritoneal cavity has afforded further evidence of a profound disturbance of the eosinophile cells. In the venous sinuses of the spleen four hours after inoculation are found both finely granular and coarsely granular or eosinophile myelocytes, together with a small number of giant cells identical in structure with the so-called megakaryocytes of the bone-marrow.

When a rabbit is repeatedly bled the spleen undergoes what has been designated by Dominici[1] "myeloid transformation." Cells which are characteristic of the bone-marrow make their appearance in the organ. During the course of prolonged infection with the bacillus of typhoid fever, Dominici has observed a similar phenomenon, but all the cells peculiar to the marrow are not represented, megakaryocytes and eosinophile cells being rare or absent. In the spleen of three guinea-pigs killed eighteen weeks after inoculation with bacillus tuberculosis, Dominici[2] found myelocytes both with fine and with coarse (eosinophile) granulation and megakaryocytes. Dominici believes that new formation of myeloid tissue occurs in the spleen, so that the organ again takes on the hæmatopoietic activity which it normally possesses only during embryonic life.

Muir, moreover, has found myelocytes in the spleen of rabbits subjected to repeated infection with staphylococcus pyogenes aureus. He has not attempted to distinguish forms with fine and coarse granulation. He has observed similar cells in the circulating blood and thinks that it is a function of the spleen to remove such abnormal elements from the blood.

In the spleen of individuals dead with scarlet fever, diphtheria, erysipelas, septicæmia, pneumonia, peritonitis, purulent meningitis, and phthisis Hirschfeld[3] has found both neutrophile and eosinophile myelocytes. Since, he says, myelocytes have been found (Engel,[4] Türk[5]) in the blood in association with the hyperleukocytosis of infectious diseases, it may be suspected that those in the spleen are derived from the bone-marrow. Against this view is the occurrence in the spleen of eosinophile myelocytes which have never been observed in the blood with hyperleukocytosis. Hirschfeld maintains that he has found transitions between the non-granular

[1] Arch. de médecine expérimentale, 1901, vol. xiii. p. 1.
[2] Compt. rend. Soc. de biol., 1900, p. 851.
[3] Berliner klin. Woch., 1902, vol. xxxix. p. 701.
[4] Deutsche med. Woch., 1897, Nos. 8 and 9.
[5] Loc. cit.

lymphoid elements of the spleen and the granular myelocytes, which can thus, he thinks, be formed within the organ.

I have observed the occurrence of eosinophile myelocytes in the spleen after inoculation with bacillus pyocyaneus, bacillus anthracis, and bacillus mucosus capsulatus. For control the spleens from six apparently healthy guinea-pigs have been carefully studied. Eosinophile leukocytes in the circulating blood of these animals just before death varied in different animals from 0.3 to 17.2 per cent. Eosinophile cells which are identical with those of the blood are readily recognizable, both in the sinuses of the spleen and in the intervening pulp, and are particularly numerous when the proportion of eosinophile leukocytes in the blood has been large. Eosinophile myelocytes have not been found. The spleens from two animals which had been killed respectively during the third and fourth week after infection with trichina spiralis were also examined. In one instance the proportion of eosinophile leukocytes in the peripheral circulation had increased from 5.7 to 17.3 per cent., in the other from 6.7 to 17.7 per cent., the latter figures being noted just before death. Eosinophile leukocytes were present in large number in the spleen, both in the sinuses and in the pulp, but eosinophile myelocytes were entirely absent. Megakaryocytes not improbably occur occasionally in the spleen of apparently healthy rodents, but none were found in the spleens of the eight guinea-pigs examined for control.

The accumulation of eosinophile myelocytes in association with other elements which are characteristic of the bone-marrow has been studied in the previously mentioned series of animals killed at varying intervals after inoculation with bacillus pyocyaneus. At the end of one-half and of one hour after inoculation no myelocytes are found. In the spleen of an animal killed at the end of two hours after inoculation an occasional myelocyte with eosinophile granulation is present in the venous sinuses. Two cells with a diameter from three to four times that of a polynuclear leukocyte are identified by their lobed or budding nuclei as megakaryocytes.

At the end of four hours the sinuses of the spleen exhibit a characteristic appearance. Within the lumen of the larger sinuses are often found ten or more cells with a diameter almost twice that of an eosinophile leukocyte; the coarse granules which stain deeply with eosin and with acid fuchsin (of the Biondi-Heidenhain mixture) are identical with those of the eosinophile leukocytes, but the nucleus of the cell is large, round or oval, and of vesicular type; one or more well-defined nucleoli are present. Similar cells undergoing karyokinetic division are found with little difficulty. The chromatin stains deeply and homogeneously and exhibits the variations characteristic of different stages of indirect division, ranging from the so-called skein formation to the diaster stage. Myelocytes with fine granulation appear to be less numerous than eosinophile myelocytes, but are present in considerable number and at times have been fixed while undergoing indirect division. Megakaryocytes are found in the sinuses and are usually somewhat larger than those seen at an earlier stage. Polynuclear leukocytes occur in very great number, while eosinophile leukocytes with polymorphous nuclei are sparsely scattered in the tissue.

At the end of eight hours eosinophile myelocytes are present, but are much less numerous than in the spleen just described. Eosinophile leukocytes are rarely found. Megakaryocytes are present. After sixteen hours eosinophile cells have almost completely disappeared from the spleen; after twenty-four hours a small number are still present, but only one or two may be found in a single section. At this time megakaryocytes are found in considerable number.

Four hours after inoculation, at a time when eosinophile leukocytes are migrating into the peritoneal cavity and eosinophile myelocytes are numerous in the spleen, the latter may be found occasionally in the bloodvessels elsewhere. In hardened sections eosinophile myelocytes are numerous in the splenic vein and in several instances have been fixed while undergoing karyokinetic division. In a small vein of the mesentery was found one typical myelocyte.

In order to confirm the preceding observations I have studied the spleen from animals killed after infection with bacillus mucosus capsulatus and bacillus anthracis. Four hours after the injection of 0.3 c.c. of a bouillon culture of bacillus mucosus capsulatus typical eosinophile myelocytes have been found in the spleen, several not infrequently occurring in the sectioned lumen of a large sinus. Small polynuclear eosinophile leukocytes are also present in moderate number. Myelocytes with fine granulation in two instances have been found undergoing karyokinetic division, and one megakaryocyte of relatively small size has been seen.

Four hours after intraperitoneal inoculation with 0.5 c.c. of a bouillon culture of bacillus anthracis fine and coarsely granular myelocytes have been abundant in the venous sinuses of the spleen. One eosinophile myelocyte undergoing karyokinetic division has been found. Megakaryocytes are particularly numerous and vary much in size.

The occurrence of myelocytes together with megakaryocytes in the spleen a few hours after bacterial inoculation, and at a time when leukocytes both with fine and with coarse granulation are attracted in immense number to the seat of inflammation, demonstrates, I believe, that these cells have their origin in the bone-marrow and are temporarily held in the spleen. They occur in smaller number in the circulating blood. It appears probable that bacterial poisons which, Werigo and Jegunow[1] have shown, exert within from twenty minutes to an hour after inoculation a chemotactic

[1] Pflüger's Arch. f. Phys., 1901, vol. lxxxiv. p. 451.

influence upon the finely granular leukocytes of the bone-marrow, are in less degree effective in attracting from the marrow cells which are usually fixed within its substance. Myelocytes with both fine and coarse eosinophile granulation, finding their way to the spleen, are still capable of karyokinetic division, so that in the spleen and in the portal circulation multiplication of polynuclear leukocytes occurs temporarily. Eosinophile cells, both myelocytes and forms with polymorphous nuclei, have within about sixteen hours almost completely disappeared from the spleen, but megakaryocytes are still present.

CONCLUSIONS. Certain bacteria (bacillus tuberculosis, bacillus choleræ suis) producing somewhat chronic, fatal infection in guinea-pigs cause the eosinophile leukocytes to gradually disappear from the circulating blood. After death few eosinophile cells can be found in those tissues in which they are usually present in abundance. Hence the study of tissues removed at autopsy gives little indication of the behavior of the eosinophile leukocytes during the course of bacterial infections. During more acute infections produced by inoculating bacteria into the peritoneal cavity (bacillus mucosus capsulatus of Friedländer, streptococcus pyogenes) eosinophile leukocytes rapidly disappear almost completely from the peripheral circulation within a few hours.

After the inoculation of an organism (bacillus pyocyaneus), producing an infection from which the animal is capable of recovering, eosinophile leukocytes disappear from the peripheral circulation, so that their proportion may fall from 5 or 10 per cent. to less than 1 per cent. The number of eosinophile leukocytes then increases, and at the end of four or five days both the relative and absolute number of these cells may considerably exceed that present in the peripheral circulation before inoculation. At the end of six or seven days the number of eosinophile leukocytes is again normal.

When bacteria (bacillus pyocyaneus, bacillus mucosus capsulatus, bacillus anthracis) are introduced into the peritoneal cavity of the guinea-pig the large mononuclear and eosinophile cells contained in the peritoneal fluid form compact clumps which adhere in great part to the surface of the omentum, so that for a time eosinophile cells have almost completely disappeared from this fluid. At the end of about an hour they have again made their appearance. Some of the eosinophile cells normally present in the tissues of the mesentery and omentum doubtless make their way into the cavity, but soon eosinophile cells begin to accumulate in the bloodvessels of both membranes, but particularly in those of the mesentery. These cells adhere to the wall of the small veins and migrate into the surrounding tissue. This process begins about one hour after inoculation, reaches its maximum several hours later, and is more marked the larger the quantity of bacteria introduced and the more virulent the organism employed. At the end of about four hours, when the number of eosinophile leukocytes in the peripheral circulation has undergone well-marked diminution, the same cells have accumulated in great number in the vessels of the inflamed mesentery and omentum. Similar changes are less marked below the peritoneum of the abdominal wall and below the serosa of the viscera. Though eosinophile cells are migrating from the bloodvessels into the peritoneal cavity, their relative number in the peritoneal exudate diminishes, and at the end of four hours is only 1 or 2 per cent. Polynuclear leukocytes at this time have accumulated in such immense number that they constitute an overwhelming proportion of the cells present.

Eosinophile cells are present in the cavity at the time of inoculation, but only after a period of about an hour do they begin to accumulate in increasing numbers. A primary attack of eosinophile cells such as that described by Kanthack and Hardy has not been observed. Polynuclear leukocytes with fine granulation accumulate in great quantity upon the surface of the omentum and form compact clumps held together by a network of fibrin; eosinophile leukocytes in large number penetrate into these masses of cells. Unlike the polynuclear leukocytes eosinophile cells rarely if ever, acting as phagocytes, ingest bacteria.

Eosinophile leukocytes upon the surface of the omentum, doubtless under the influence of the bacterial poisons, undergo degenerative changes of which nuclear fragmentation is the most characteristic. In such cells the eosinophile granules are still preserved. Evidence that the cells discharge these granules has not been obtained. At a somewhat later period eosinophile leukocytes are ingested by large mononuclear cells (macrophages).

Under the influence of severe bacterial infection eosinophile myelocytes together with other elements, usually regarded as characteristic of the bone-marrow, accumulate in the spleen and may be found in the circulating blood. The occurrence of this phenomenon within from two to four hours after inoculation demonstrates that these elements are derived from the bone-marrow and are not formed in the spleen. Myelocytes both with fine and with coarse (eosinophile) granulation, which have found their way to the spleen, here multiply by karyokinetic division.

Bacteria exert a chemotactic influence upon cells with eosinophile granulation, attracting them from the circulating blood to the site of inoculation and from the bone-marrow into the blood. Eosinophile leukocytes, like the finely granular polynuclear leukocytes, accumulate in the neighborhood of bacteria injected into the body and, though they rarely act as phagocytes, have a part in the series of changes which follow bacterial invasion.

THE ENVELOPE OF THE RED CORPUSCLE AND ITS ROLE IN HÆMOLYSIS AND AGGLUTINATION.

By S. Peskind, B.S., M.D.,
of Cleveland, Ohio.

One of the most important fields of medical research at present is that which relates to hæmolysis. The brilliant theories of Ehrlich have served to explain a large number of facts bearing on the subjects of hæmolysis and immunity. But Ehrlich's work, while it concerns itself almost exclusively with the various properties and modes of action of the biological lakers, does not sufficiently take into account the chemical, physical, and histological changes which take place in the corpuscles themselves, when these are subjected to the action of hæmolytic agents. The importance of determining as far as possible these alterations is very clear, and it is evident that only after we have an intimate knowledge of the structure of the blood corpuscles can the nature of these changes be understood.

Two theories have been advanced concerning the structure of the red blood corpuscle. According to Schäfer and others, the corpuscle is merely a vesicle and consists of an envelope which contains a fluid mass. The other—proposed by Rollet and modified by Hamburger—assumes that the corpuscles consist of a network or stroma in whose meshes are found a fluid or semifluid mass composed of hæmoglobin and electrolytes.[1]

The first hypothesis is held by very few at the present date, while the latter—which has the support of many experimental facts—is endorsed by the majority of hæmatologists. Hamburger ably discusses the latter theory and gives good reasons for its acceptance. One argument which seems particularly convincing may be quoted here: "Osmotic experiments have shown that the amount of water which a corpuscle can imbibe and give out—*i. e.*, the amount of swelling and shrinkage which it is capable of— is less than would be the case if the corpuscle were simply a vesicle. Therefore, the interior of the corpuscle must be filled up with some protoplasmic substance—a stroma or network in whose meshes is contained the water-attracting fluid of the corpuscle."[2]

As Dr. G. N. Stewart has pointed out, the presence of an envelope or limiting layer about the corpuscles seems an almost necessary assumption.[3] It is well known that there is a constant interchange of substances between the corpuscles and surrounding medium; while the metabolic products and salts within the corpuscles make their way out, these are replaced by the requisite serum constituents.

[1] Hamburger, Osmotischer, Druck und Ionenlehre, p. 171.
[2] Ibid.
[3] Journal of Physiology, 1899, vol. xxiv. p. 211.

On the other hand the corpuscles keep out bodies inimical to themselves. Both of these processes which are continually going on together, and which require a selective ability on the part of the corpuscles, could hardly take place were they not provided with envelopes which permit of the entrance of some substances and the exclusion of others.

It is the principal object of this paper to adduce evidence of the existence of such an envelope and to point out the role which it plays in hæmolysis and agglutination.

The presence of an envelope may be demonstrated by histological, chemical, and physical methods.

Histological Proof. The most obvious way of demonstrating the limiting membrane of a cell is by means of differential staining, but this has proved itself to be an especially difficult method in the case of blood corpuscles. I have been able to find in the literature only one reference to a staining reaction, whereby an envelope is said to be made visible in the red blood corpuscles.

H. Deetjen[1] stains corpuscles dried on a slide and heated to a certain temperature, with gentian violet; the envelopes, according to him, are thus easily made apparent.

Dr. G. N. Stewart has published some histological plates in which is given convincing evidence of the presence of an envelope in the necturus corpuscle.[2]

In the case of some cells the envelope may be clearly seen if it be mechanically separated from the underlying intracellular substance. By this method, for instance, the sarcolemma of a muscle fibre is rendered visible.

Through a peculiar reaction which takes place when hydroxylamine hydrochlorate is added to blood, I think it is possible to produce the above-mentioned separation of envelope and cell contents in the case of mammalian red corpuscles.[3]

In this reaction bubbles of nitrogen gas are formed at the periphery of the corpuscles. These bubbles are lined externally by a delicate, apparently hæmoglobin-free membrane (Fig. 1, *a*), and internally by hæmoglobin (*b*).

The membrane is hardly stained by any of those dyes which stain the hæmoglobin in the rest of the corpuscles very deeply. This indicates that it does not contain hæmoglobin. It appears colorless in the unstained corpuscle. This might be because the color of a very thin layer of hæmoglobin might escape detection. Only by observing the corpuscles during the formative stage of the bubbles is it possible to make out that they are not formed within the hæmoglobin at all, but that the latter merely forms their inner boundary.

[1] Virchow's Archiv f. experimentelle Pathologie, 1901, vol. clxv. p. 232.
[2] American Journal of Physiology, 1902, vol. viii. p. 103.
[3] Peskind. Ibid., 1903, vol. viii. p. 424.

About ten minutes after the reagent and blood are mixed, the first sign of the intracorpuscular bubble formation becomes evident; it consists in a flattening or depression of the hæmoglobin on the periphery of a corpuscle, the outer lining of the bubble being too close to the hæmoglobin at this stage to be visible (Fig. 2).

The next stage is represented by Fig. 3, and shows some separation between the surface layer of the corpuscle (*a*) and the hæmoglobin.

The completed bubble appears in Fig. 4, the outer lining (*a*) often projecting considerably above the surface.

The most striking part of the reaction lies in the depression of the hæmoglobin from the surface of the corpuscle in the first stage. It demonstrates that the accumulation of gas takes place between an enveloping layer and the hæmoglobin, causing the repulsion of

FIG. 1.

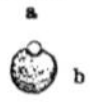

FIG. 2.

FIG. 3.

FIG. 4.

FIG. 5.

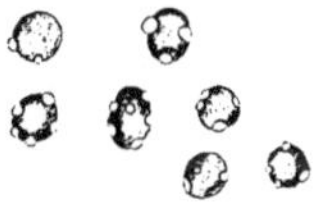

FIG. 6.

FIG 7.

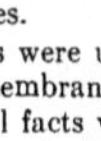

FIG. 8.

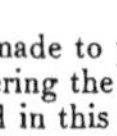

FIG. 9.

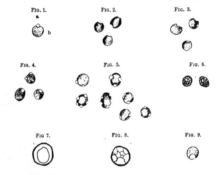

the latter from the surface of the corpuscle toward the centre and, at the same time, separating the envelope from the hæmoglobin underneath.

Although gas is formed immediately on mixing the blood and reagent, yet about ten minutes elapse before bubbles are formed inside the corpuscles. This could be explained on the hypothesis that the envelope must be hardened to a certain extent before it will be sufficiently unyielding to retain the bubbles within the corpuscles.

Efforts were unsuccessfully made to produce a differential stain of the membrane-like film covering the bubbles.

Several facts will be observed in this reaction:

1. That the bubbles are lined by a delicate and very thin membrane. This, together with the observations made on the evolution

of the bubbles, renders it almost certain that the membrane lining the bubbles is the envelope of the corpuscles.

2. That the bubbles are all of small size and sharply circumscribed. This speaks very strongly for the presence of a stroma whose meshes are continuous with trabeculæ derived from the envelope; for, if the envelope were a differentiated membrane and not connected to the intracellular substance, then we would expect that the gas formed in the reaction as it collects at the periphery of the corpuscles would produce a diffuse and extensive stripping of the envelope from the contents underneath, and would not form localized accumulations or bubbles. (See Fig. 7.)

But if the envelope is part of the stroma which forms the boundary of the corpuscles, then we can readily understand how the gas accumulation would be limited to the space between the trabeculæ, thus giving rise to bubble formation. (See Fig. 8.)

CHEMICAL EVIDENCE. We come next to the consideration of such chemical facts as point to the presence of an envelope.

In a recent paper I have described a reaction between blood corpuscles on the one hand, and acids and acid salts on the other.[1] When a mere trace of most acids and acid salts is added to a suspension of blood corpuscles, the latter are immediately agglutinated and precipitated. If the corpuscles be laked, then the stromata are precipitated by the same reagents. This reaction is apparently due to the combination of the nucleoproteid of the surface layer of the corpuscles with the reagents. The reasons for this view are given elsewhere.[2]

An interesting observation in connection with this reaction throws light on the subject under consideration.

We know that all the precipitating agents—*i. e.*, acids and acid salts in dilute solution—convert oxyhæmoglobin first into methæmoglobin and then into acid hæmatin. Now if the hæmoglobin in the intact corpuscles were present in the surface layer, then we should expect it to be rapidly altered by the precipitating agents into methæmoglobin. But it was found that the hæmoglobin contained in the corpuscles was not altered in the least if the exact amount of reagent necessary to precipitate the latter was employed. Even if a moderate excess of reagent were employed in precipitating the corpuscles no methæmoglobin band appeared for five or ten minutes. However, if we lake the corpuscles first—*e. g.*, by sapotoxin or water—and then add the same amount of reagent, it will be observed that part of the hæmoglobin is instantly converted into methæmoglobin and this conversion proceeds rapidly until complete.

What is it that temporarily shields the hæmoglobin in the intact corpuscles from the action of the reagents?

[1] American Journal of Physiology, 1903, vol. viii. p. 404.
[2] Ibid., p. 420.

Is this protection due to the fact that an intervening layer on the periphery of the corpuscle must be penetrated before the hæmoglobin can be reached, or is this conversion delayed by some chemical constituent of the corpuscles which combines with the reagent as rapidly as it enters? Such a chemical protection could be afforded to the hæmoglobin by the alkali of the corpuscles, by the stroma substance, or through the firm combination of the hæmoglobin with the stroma.

It can be shown that neither the alkali nor the stroma substance shields the hæmoglobin from the action of the reagents, since after laking the presence of stromata and liberated alkalies protects the oxyhæmoglobin but slightly and not at all if excess of reagent be present.[1]

Moreover there are many facts which suggest that the hæmoglobin compound within the corpuscle is a weak one and is easily split up.

Seeing that the temporary immunity of the hæmoglobin cannot be explained on chemical grounds, we are forced to adopt the view that there is something in the *structure* of the corpuscles, some mechanical or physicochemical barrier, which shields the hæmoglobin from the immediate action of the reagents. In other words, the hæmoglobin is protected by an envelope.

The laking of blood corpuscles by ether affords additional evidence of the existence of an envelope. It has been generally assumed that ether laking is due to the removal from the corpuscles of some or all of their cholesterin and lecithin.

This I have attempted to prove along the following lines:[2] First I determined how much ether is necessary to exactly lake 5 c.c. of blood. Then I extracted the corpuscles derived from 5 c.c. of blood with ether. The extract consisting of cholesterin and lecithin was suspended in 5 c.c. of serum or saline. Then ether was added cautiously to this suspension until the cholesterin and lecithin were perfectly dissolved and the amount of ether used noted.

It was found that the amount of ether necessary to dissolve the cholesterin and lecithin contained in the corpuscles of 5 c.c. of blood and suspended in 5 c.c. of saline or serum was about one-half again as much as was required to lake 5 c.c. of blood. So that the amount of ether required to lake blood bears a definite relation to the quantity of ether necessary to dissolve the cholesterin and lecithin of its corpuscles.

It appears from the above experiments that only a certain proportion of the cholesterin and lecithin is dissolved in ether laking,

[1] American Journal of Physiology, 1903, vol. iii. p. 422.

[2] These experiments will be published elsewhere in detail. Here I assume, in accordance with the general view, that cholesterin and lecithin are the only bodies dissolved out of blood corpuscles by ether. If, as some investigators believe, other ether-soluble substances exist, then my experiment shows that laking can be caused by the removal of other substances than cholesterin.

and this is probably the part that exists in the peripheral layer of the corpuscle. The cholesterin and the lecithin which remains undissolved during the laking in all probability remains in the interior of the corpuscle—*i. e.*, the stroma.

That the removal of lecithin alone from the envelope gives rise to laking can, I think, be readily demonstrated by the use of ether saturated with cholesterin.

If, as we have reason to believe, the cholesterin in the blood corpuscles has the same properties as the ordinary commercial cholesterin (Merck's was used in my experiments), then it would not be dissolved out from the corpuscles by ether which has been saturated with the commercial cholesterin. I found by experiment that a given amount of blood was laked by practically the same quantity of cholesterin-saturated ether as of pure ether, and, moreover, that the time required in the laking was the same in both instances.

The ether which was saturated with cholesterin laked blood just as though no cholesterin were dissolved in it. Here, I believe, we have good evidence to show that the removal of lecithin alone is capable of producing laking of the corpuscles.

Physical Proof. Dr. G. N. Stewart has made an extensive research on the conductivity of blood corpuscles. As was mentioned previously, the necessity for assuming the presence of an envelope in all animal cells became clear to him early in his experiments, and realizing this he set about to determine what changes could be produced in the envelope of the red blood corpuscles by various laking agents, using them as convenient test-objects. Unfixed corpuscles being unsuitable for various reasons, he employed formaldehyde-hardened corpuscles. Sapotoxin and sodium taurocholate when added to a suspension of formaldehyde-hardened corpuscles produced the surprising effect of greatly increasing the conductivity of the latter.

"Unhardened blood corpuscles or formaldehyde-hardened corpuscles not treated with saponin or sapotoxin permit NH_4Cl to pass much more readily into them than NaCl, and there is evidence that some of the NH_4Cl is bound by substances in the corpuscles or at any rate does not pass as freely out of them as it passes into them. After the formaldehyde-hardened corpuscles have been acted on by sapotoxin they seem to exhibit little if any power of binding either NH_4Cl or NaCl, and the ions both of NaCl and NH_4Cl wander easily through the corpuscles."[1]

It will be seen from the above that there is beyond doubt a great change in the surface layer or envelope of the corpuscles after they are acted upon by the sapotoxin.

For the purpose of determining what constituents of the formalde-

[1] G. N. Stewart, Journal of Medical Research, No. 1, vol. viii. p. 270.

hyde-hardened corpuscles are acted upon by sapotoxin the corpuscles were extracted with ether. The solvent took up a considerable quantity of cholesterin and lecithin. The ether-extracted corpuscles were carefully washed many times with salt solution and then suspended in a known volume of salt solution. For this suspension, Dr. Stewart found "the conductivity markedly greater than for a suspension of the unextracted formaldehyde corpuscles containing approximately the same proportions of corpuscles and salt solution. Sapotoxin caused no change in the conductivity of the extracted corpuscles. This renders it highly probable that sapotoxin increases the permeability of the formaldehyde corpuscles by action on the substance soluble in ether."

It can readily be shown that when a suspension of cholesterin is shaken up with sapotoxin the latter is removed by the cholesterin or rendered inert so that the liquid obtained after filtering off the cholesterin has no laking power. Apparently a definite amount of cholesterin neutralizes a certain amount of sapotoxin. I found, moreover, that formaldehyde-hardened corpuscles will also remove sapotoxin completely from a solution in twenty-four hours. So that changes in permeability produced by adding sapotoxin to formaldehyde-hardened corpuscles is clearly due to a combination of the sapotoxin with the cholesterin contained in the surface layers of the corpuscles.

While it seemed most likely to Dr. Stewart that sapotoxin exerted an action on unfixed corpuscles similar to that produced on formaldehyde corpuscles—and he gave evidence to that effect—he was unable at the time of the first research to prove this. The difficulty lay in the rapidity with which the sapotoxin causes laking. During the course of some experiments on hæmolytic agents, I made the observation that cold retards sapotoxin laking for a considerable period. This provided the means of proving the above-mentioned surmise, and to this effect a series of experiments, in some of which I assisted, were carried out. The conclusion drawn from the research are taken from Dr. Stewart's paper.[1]

1. At 0° C. the laking action of sapotoxin is much retarded, and it can be shown that before any hæmoglobin has been liberated the conductivity of the blood is increased, and presumably owing to the increase in the permeability of the corpuscles to electrolytes. At this stage sapotoxin has been fixed by the corpuscles.

2. Both at 0° C. and at ordinary temperature a dose of sapotoxin just sufficient to cause liberation of the hæmoglobin causes the discharge of a small proportion of the electrolytes of the corpuscles; when the dose is increased the electrolytes are discharged.

3. It seems permissible to divide the action on the corpuscles in three stages:

[1] American Journal of Physiology, No. 2, vol. ix. p. 96.

(*a*) An action on the envelope, which does not necessarily nor immediately lead to the liberation of the hæmoglobin.

(*b*) An action on the hæmoglobin or the stroma which causes a discharge of the pigment.

(*c*) An action on the stroma leading to the setting free of electrolytes.

RESISTANCE OF BLOOD CORPUSCLES. The so-called "resistance of blood corpuscles" affords good evidence of the existence of an envelope. "It is well known that in certain physiological states and in disease laking begins to take place in a more concentrated salt solution than is required to lake normal corpuscles. This could be due to one of several causes—either that the stroma contents of the corpuscles in disease have a greater power of absorbing water or that they possess a greater volume—or that the envelope of the corpuscles has been so altered by the disease that, when it is stretched to a certain degree, it is less able to prevent the escape of bæmoglobin than would the envelope of a normal corpuscle. That the latter is in all probability the correct explanation may be seen from the action of hæmolytic and certain bacterial toxins on blood corpuscles.

"These poisons, in very small doses, alter the corpuscles in such a manner that they cannot bear such small salt concentrations as in the normal state. This change is found to be due neither to a modification of the water-absorbing power of the corpuscular contents nor to an increase of the intraglobular volume. So that we are forced to the assumption that the hæmolytic sera give rise to a diminished resistance of the protoplasmic envelope, thus favoring the escape of the hæmoglobin when a degree of internal tension has been reached which would still leave the normal corpuscle intact."[1]

BIOLOGICAL HÆMOLYSIS. Granting that the toxins of disease do cause a diminished resistance of the envelope, it is of interest to inquire whether at the same time an increased permeability of the envelope is produced. And if so, whether the corpuscle becomes more permeable to ions or to the hæmolytic agents only. It will be remembered that sapotoxin causes a primary increase in the permeability of the envelope, and by analogy one might reason that the intermediary body necessary to biological hæmolysis acts by making the envelope more permeable to the complement. In a conjoint experiment performed by Dr. Stewart and myself no evidence was obtained that dogs' serum can produce any change in the conductivity of the rabbit blood before liberation of hæmoglobin takes place.[2] This is also in agreement with the fact that the permeability of the formaldehyde-fixed corpuscles of the rabbit is

[1] Hamburger, Osmotischer, Druck und Ioneulehre, p. 391.
[2] American Journal of Physiology, No. 2, vol. ix. p. 81.

not affected by dogs' serum. Since the envelope is not made more permeable to ions by the intermediary body, it is likely that the function of the latter is to effect such changes that the complement will be able to penetrate to the interior of the corpuscle, where it can exert its specific action.

PROPERTIES OF THE ENVELOPE. The foregoing will, I think, be considered satisfactory evidence of an envelope in the red corpuscles, and we shall proceed to discuss the role that the envelope plays in hæmolysis and agglutination.

It will be appropriate at the outset to review what is known regarding the chemical and physical properties of the envelope. That it is hæmoglobin-free we have demonstrated by the action of hydroxylamine hydrochlorate and also by experiments with acid salts. (See previous pages.) That the envelope contains nucleoproteid as well as lecithin and cholesterin is shown respectively by the agglutination reaction with acids and acid salts and by the ether-laking experiments quoted previously. Alkalies must be present in combination with the nucleoproteid,[1] and salts, which always exist in protoplasm, must be contained in the envelope.

PHYSICAL PROPERTIES. The envelope of the red corpuscle appears to be smooth. That it also possesses a certain glaze I would infer from the crisp and sparkling reflex seen in fresh blood, and from the fact that the circulating corpuscles do not agglutinate with each other. This property of the envelope may subserve some defensive purpose. We can readily imagine that a corpuscle having a smooth surface will not offer so good a foothold—if the expression may be allowed—to any toxin, as would a corpuscle having a sticky envelope such as is produced by the action of an agglutinin. In support of this view we find that, as a rule, hæmolysis is preceded by agglutination. This is especially true of biological laking. In nature, wherever a biological hæmolysin occurs, there is usually also present an agglutinin in the same medium, and it seems as though the two bear a co-operative relation similar to that found between a complement and its intermediate body—which likewise are usually coexistent in nature.

When blood corpuscles are exposed to the simultaneous action of a hæmolysin and an agglutinin, the result varies with the relative strengths of the two. If the toxin be relatively weak, and the agglutinin strong, then we get primarily a powerful agglutination of the corpuscles followed by their gradual hæmolysis. If the toxin be very powerful and the agglutinin comparatively weak, then agglutination may not occur, especially if any swelling of the corpuscles is produced by the toxin. It seems that swelling of the corpuscles is inimical to agglutination.[2]

[1] Compare Hammaesten, Physiolog. Chemie, p. 80.
[2] Peskind, American Journal of Physiology, No. 5, vol. viii. p. 416.

The envelope is distensible and elastic. It is this elasticity of the envelope which permits of the expansion and shrinkage of the corpuscle brought about by osmosis. Most hardening agents do not affect the elasticity of the envelope to any degree, since after the corpuscles are fixed by these reagents they still may be caused to swell.

The envelope being protoplasmic, and therefore semifluid, must exhibit the phenomenon of surface tension. This surface tension is one of the forces which co-operate to give the corpuscles their biconcave shape. During equilibrium the intraglobular pressure must be equal to the sum of the surface tension and the pressure exerted by the liquid about the corpuscle. If for any reason the surface tension be lessened, then the intraglobular pressure could assert itself and would tend to produce a greater distention of the envelope.

Such a diminution of the surface tension in blood corpuscles is brought about, I believe, by the emulsifiers, sapotoxin and sodium taurocholate, which are known for their ability to lessen the surface tension of liquids.[1] Reasons for this view will be advanced in the discussion of the permeability of blood corpuscles.

Permeability of Envelope. A very important property of the envelope is the selective permeability with which it is endowed. A great deal of investigation has been bestowed upon this complex subject, but it still rests upon a rather unsatisfactory basis. One fact has been pretty well established, namely, that the envelope is not permeable to salt molecules but to ions only. Not all ions, however, can penetrate the corpuscles; for the most part it is the electronegative ions, the halogens and acid radicals, which have this power. The envelope is permeable for NH_4 and to free acids and alkalies, but not for Ba, Str, Ca, Mg, and in all probability it is impermeable to Na and K, although this is still under some dispute.

Of the non-electrolytes there are a considerable number which can enter the corpuscles, among which may be mentioned alcohols, aldehydes, ketone, ether, antipyrin, urea, urethane. The corpuscles are impermeable to the various sugars, but allow bile acids and salts to penetrate.[2]

One can readily imagine that the size of certain molecules may be a cause of their inability to pass through the envelope. But if the intermolecular spaces of the envelope be enlarged—as must occur when the corpuscle swells and the envelope becomes distended—then it is conceivable that some large-sized molecules could enter which, under normal circumstances, would be unable to penetrate the corpuscles.

[1] Hay's test for bile salts in urine is founded on the fact that these salts lower the surface tension of the urine.

[2] Hamburger, Osmotischer, Druck und Ioneulehre, p. 260.

Causing the corpuscle to swell is one way of enlarging the spaces which exist between the molecules of the envelope. Another method consists in removing some of the molecules which compose the envelope—*e. g.*, the cholesterin and lecithin. When these substances are extracted by ether the envelope is left in a porous condition, which makes it very permeable. This has been well shown in the experiment quoted above, in which formaldehyde corpuscles were extracted with ether. The conductivity of the corpuscles was found to be much increased by this procedure.

The suggestion may be ventured at this point that the action of sapotoxin consists partly in widening the intermolecular spaces of the envelope, making the latter more permeable to the sapotoxin molecules, which are presumably of large size. I conceive the mechanism of the process to be as follows:

First, as Ransom has shown, sapotoxin is taken up by the cholesterin of the envelope. The cholesterin and lecithin molecules are bound to the other molecules of the envelope merely by cohesion and not by firm chemical ties, since they may be dissolved out mechanically by ether. Now sapotoxin is an emulsifier; and, being such, lessens the cohesive power of fatty particles. Therefore, sapotoxin, once it has gained a foothold in the envelope, lessens the cohesion between the cholesterin-lecithin group and the other molecules which compose the protoplasm. Since surface tension is the result of the force of cohesion exerted between molecules of the surface layer, it follows that sapotoxin, in lessening the cohesion of these molecules, also lessens the surface tension of the corpuscles.

As soon as the surface tension becomes diminished the intra-globular pressure exerts itself and distends the envelope. Ions and water must now enter and the corpuscle swells.

This theoretical description corresponds very well to the actual first stage of sapotoxin laking. The corpuscles are seen to lose their biconcave shapes, become globular, and swell, showing that a great change in the surface tension has taken place, and that water and ions have entered.

At the same time it can be demonstrated that a great increase in the electric conductivity has taken place, which is probably due to the enlargement of the intermolecular spaces which accompanies the distention of the envelope.[1] The size of these interspaces being increased, the large-sized sapotoxin molecules can enter the corpuscles and split up the hæmoglobin-stroma compound, thus giving rise to laking.

DETERIORATION OF THE ENVELOPE. The red corpuscles, like other cells of the body, are often exposed to pathological influences and suffer changes which may seriously affect their value to the

[1] It may be noted here that sodium taurocholate causes laking without any notable previous swelling of the corpuscles; the increase in the permeability produced by this reagent is also much less than that produced by sapotoxin.—G. N. Stewart.

organism. Some of these alterations are without doubt due to a deterioration of the envelope and stroma, and it will be of interest in this connection to consider under what conditions the envelope of the red corpuscles will become damaged.

The following agents may be cited as producing deleterious changes in the envelope:

1. Toxins produced in disease.
2. Chemicals—*e. g.*, acids and alkalies.
3. Drying of corpuscles.
4. Fixing blood by throwing it into boiling saline.
5. Freezing and thawing.
6. Agglutinins.
7. Aging of corpuscles.

We shall discuss these in the order mentioned.

1. *Action of Toxins Produced in Disease.* The change in the resistance of the envelope produced by hæmolysins has been considered elsewhere. A diminished resistance of the corpuscles in typhoid, pneumonia, and other diseases has been constantly observed and is in all probability due to a deterioration of the envelope caused by the specific toxins formed during the course of these diseases. Some evidence to this effect may be derived from experiments that I recently made on the sera and corpuscles of various affections.[1]

An observation, which I have made on the blood of some severe cases of anæmia and several cancer cases may be mentioned here. On exposing a drop of blood to pressure between cover-slip and slide the hæmoglobin escapes quite readily from the corpuscles. (A similar phenomenon is observed in the case of corpuscles precipitated by ammonioferrous sulphate or other acid salts.)

Hamburger[2] has shown that pressure has no effect on the resistance of normal corpuscles, so that the above observation tends to show that the resistance of the envelope had been lowered by some product of the disease.

Vacuolization. I should like to suggest here that the condition known as "vacuolization of the hæmoglobin" might be due to a localized deterioration of the envelope. Let us imagine that a very small part of the circumference of a corpuscle were injured; this would allow the very gradual escape of hæmoglobin at this point and at the same time would permit water and ions to enter so that a seeming vacuole would be produced. (See Fig. 9.)

According to this view "vacuolization of the hæmoglobin" may be considered as a localized laking of the corpuscle.

2. *Action of Chemicals.* Acids and alkalies both effect the resistance of the envelope. Corpuscles acted upon by acids give up their hæmoglobin in a weaker NaCl solution than the normal corpuscles,

[1] American Medicine, No. 23, vol. v. p. 919.

[2] Ioneulehre, p. 175.

while the contrary is the case with blood corpuscles acted upon by alkalies.[1]

3. *Drying of Corpuscles.* The effect produced on the envelopes of red corpuscles by allowing the latter to dry in air has been carefully studied by Dr. Guthrie.[2] He made the interesting observation that chickens, and human red blood corpuscles, allowed to dry in the air at room temperature, are readily laked by 0.9 per cent. NaCl solution.

It has been shown that fixing washed corpuscles by pouring them into boiling salt solution greatly increases their permeability to ions. Dr. Guthrie reasons "that a similar effect is produced by drying at a temperature below that necessary for fixation, so that the permeability of the corpuscles for diffusible substances is greatly increased, while it allows of the escape of hæmoglobin when enough water to dissolve it is present."

I have observed that when a drop of blood or of a washed suspension of corpuscles is placed on a slide and covered with a slip, those corpuscles which are at the edge of the drop—*i. e.*, where a gradual drying out occurs—become markedly swelled. And it may be demonstrated that there is also extensive laking at the edge of the drop, even in the case of corpuscles which at the moment of laking are floating in the liquid.

Dr. Guthrie in mentioning these experiments explains them very satisfactorily on the hypothesis "that the drying of a portion of the circumference of a corpuscle at the edge of the drop—or the action on it of the concentrated salt solution produced by evaporation —may render the rest of the circumference more freely permeable to the salts of the solution or to the water, and thus give rise to water laking."

4. Throwing blood corpuscles into boiling salt solution greatly increases their permeability to ions.[3]

5. Freezing and thawing causes laking, and while I have no proof to offer that this is due to an injury to the envelope, yet such an assumption seems very reasonable. The alternate contraction and expansion produced by freezing and thawing could very well have a disintegrating effect on a protoplasmic envelope consisting of heterogeneous molecules but loosely combined.

6. Agglutinins cause marked changes in the properties of the envelope, and that it also diminishes the resistance of the latter may be seen from the fact that an agglutinated mass of corpuscles loses hæmoglobin if exposed to slight pressure between slide and coverslip. Normal corpuscles cannot be laked in this manner.

7. *Aging of Corpuscles.* Old corpuscles may be distinguished in the circulating blood by the fact that they have lost a large part of

[1] Ioneulehre, p. 322.
[2] American Journal of Physiology, No. 5, vol. viii. p. 444.
[3] G. N. Stewart.

their hæmoglobin. This is most likely due to the deterioration of the envelope effected by the wear and tear to which the corpuscles are exposed.

Soon after blood is shed from an artery its permeability to NH_4Cl is greatly increased.[1] This indicates that there is a difference between corpuscles within the blood stream and those *in vitro*. It may be shown, moreover, that the envelopes of corpuscles which have been removed from the body deteriorate after a certain length of time. The behavior of corpuscles to hydroxylamine hydrochlorate may be cited as proof of this. Fresh blood, and blood less than three days old, when treated with this reagent, show bubble-formation within the corpuscles (see above). Blood that has stood for about three days will not show any bubbles with the reagent, but the corpuscles have a perforated appearance as though gas bubbles had escaped from their interior. This may be explained as follows:

Hydroxylamine hydrochlorate has a double action; not only does it permeate the corpuscles and produce gas bubbles within them, but it hardens them at the same time. If the envelope be intact, then the reagent penetrates but slowly and thus has time to harden the envelope before much of the salt enters the corpuscle. The evolution of gas produced by the reagent is thus very gradual and, as the bubbles are formed at the periphery of the corpuscle, they are retained by the partly hardened envelope. When the blood becomes old, however, the envelope deteriorates, in consequence of which the hydroxylamine hydrochlorate penetrates very rapidly, before the envelope is hardened sufficiently to be able to retain the bubbles. The result is that the reagent which enters the corpuscles in large quantities gives rise to an immediate and copious evolution of gas bubbles whose escape cannot be hindered by the weakened and only slightly hardened envelope.

The rents in the envelope produced by the escaping bubbles remain open and give rise to the perforated appearance above mentioned.

This observation shows strikingly how the envelope deteriorates with the aging of the blood corpuscles.

Hardening of Envelope. The effects of various hardening agents on the envelope and stroma are of considerable importance and merit some mention here. Among the principal hardening and fixing agents may be mentioned $HgCl_2$ (Hayem's solution), formaldehyde, osmic acid, hydroxylamine hydrochlorate, alcohol, ether, chromic acid.

In another part of the paper was brought out the fact that the distensibility and elasticity of the envelope and stroma were practically unaltered by most hardening agents, since the hardened corpuscles may still be caused to swell by suitable means.

[1] G. N. Stewart.

Agglutination of corpuscles hardened by formaldehyde, osmic acid, and ether, may still be brought about by certain means. But after fixation with $HgCl_2$ I was unable to produce agglutination. Chromic acid and picric acid agglutinate while they harden the corpuscles.

The envelopes of corpuscles hardened by formaldehyde and those hardened by $HgCl_2$ show a dissimilarity in their behavior toward sapotoxin; whereas the electric conductivity of formaldehyde-hardened corpuscles is greatly increased by sapotoxin, corpuscles hardened by $HgCl_2$ show no such effect, presumably owing to the more complete hardening produced by the latter reagent.

A peculiar effect is produced by acid salts when added to blood just shed from an artery. If to a definite amount of blood taken from the carotid and diluted with saline is added just enough ferric chloride to precipitate all the corpuscles, it will be found that the supernatant serum, after the corpuscles have settled, will not clot even after three days. This serum is neutral in reaction. The ferric chloride, combining as it does with the envelopes of the corpuscles, probably prevents the exit of the fibrin ferment, but possibly the neutralization of the alkali in the serum by the ferric chloride is the cause of its not clotting. The former mode of action is the most likely, since the addition of alkali to the serum did not produce real clotting. Further experiment must decide this point.[1]

RESUME. Various facts of a histological, chemical, and physical character show that the red blood corpuscles possess an envelope.

From the action of hydroxylamine hydrochlorate, which produces sharply circumscribed accumulations of nitrogen gas—*i. e.*, bubbles —on the periphery of blood corpuscles and not an extensive separation of the envelope from the contents underneath, it appears most probable that the envelope is not a differentiated membrane, but a part of the stroma which is condensed to form the surface layer of the corpuscle.

The envelope is hæmoglobin-free and consists of nucleoproteid, cholesterin, lecithin, and mineral constituents.

It is elastic, smooth, and apparently possesses a certain glaze which prevents the agglutination of normal corpuscles with each other and makes the corpuscles less accessible to the action of toxins.

Agglutination of blood corpuscles is due to an effect on the envelope produced by various biological products and chemical reagents whereby the envelope is made sticky.

Agglutinins, by modifying the envelope, probably lower the resistance of blood corpuscles toward toxins and other agents. From the fact that in nature they almost always occur in company with a hæmolysin, the suggestion is offered that the agglutinins

[1] American Journal of Physiology, 1903, vol. viii. p. 412.

bear some co-operative relation to the hæmolysins similar to that existing between the intermediary body and the complement, which likewise are usually coexistent in nature.

The "resistance" of blood corpuscles depends in large part upon the condition of the envelope. The latter may be caused to deteriorate by various agents principal among which are the toxins of disease. Deterioration of the envelope may be complete or partial —*i. e.*, involving the whole circumference or only a small part of the same.

So-called "vacuolization of the hæmoglobin" can be explained very satisfactorily on the assumption of a minute lesion in the envelope which allows the surrounding fluid to enter and thus permits of a localized laking at this point.

The function of the envelope is in part to make possible various metabolic processes, principal among which is the complex process known as internal respiration. This is accomplished through the medium of a selective permeability.

Another important use of the envelope is to protect the corpuscles from the action of various substances deleterious to the latter. But the very chemical constitution of the envelope may at times serve for the undoing of the corpuscles, since it has been well shown by Ransom, Kyes, Sachs, and others that the cholesterin and lecithin of the envelope fix certain toxins and thus act as intermediary bodies.

HÆMOLYSINS IN HUMAN URINE.*

By Roger S. Morris, A.B., M.D.,
INSTRUCTOR IN MEDICINE, UNIVERSITY OF MICHIGAN, ANN ARBOR, MICH.
(From the Clinical Laboratory of the Johns Hopkins Hospital.)

Since the epoch-making experiments of Bordet,[1] such a vast amount of work has been done upon hæmolysis and allied subjects that a review of the literature seems superfluous. For present purposes, it is only necessary to refer to some of those instances in which specific bodies have been shown to pass from the blood into the secretions or excretions.

Ehrlich and Brieger[2] showed, in the case of a goat immunized against tetanus toxin, that the specific antibody could be demonstrated in the milk. By Kassel and Mann[3] it was shown that the milk of a woman suffering from typhoid fever possessed the power of agglutinating typhoid bacilli.

Friedberger[4] was the first to demonstrate the passage of agglutinins and hæmolysins from the blood into the urine. For this purpose

* Read at the meeting of the American Association of Pathologists and Bacteriologists at New York, April 1 and 2, 1904.

he immunized a rabbit to defibrinated pigeons' blood. In conducting his experiments upon hæmolysis, he used 1 c.c. of urine from the immunized rabbit, to which were added 1 c.c. of a solution of pigeons' blood in physiological salt solution and a few drops of normal pigeons' serum. In a second experiment 1 c.c. of urine of the immunized rabbit was added to 1 c.c. of pigeons' blood in physiological salt solution, *no serum* being added. Microscopically and macroscopically merely agglutination was observed in each case. After the lapse of several hours, the cells having collected at the bottom of the test-tubes, leaving a clear fluid above, it was found that in the first experiment, to which a few drops of normal pigeons' serum had been added, the supernatant fluid was stained red, while that in the second experiment remained plainly yellow. In experiments carried out in the same manner with the urine of normal rabbits, no red staining of the fluid was obtained. Friedberger concluded from his researches that the intermediary body passed into the urine, but that the complement either did not pass into the urine or was destroyed in the urine.

Camus and Pagniez[5] are, I believe, the first to have studied the "globulicidal action" of human urine. They pointed out that the red blood cells may be destroyed in a urine (1) by virtue of its being hypotonic and (2) by the action of certain substances which isotonic or hypertonic urines may contain. Under the second group are included specific hæmolysins and other substances. They found that a normal urine, hypertonic, was at times capable of producing hæmolysis in the red blood cells of a rabbit; and this was seen to be the case only when the urine possessed a marked acid reaction. The acidity of the urine is due to the acid phosphates for the most part, to uric and hippuric acids to a smaller degree. The monobasic acid phosphate of soda in an isotonic NaCl solution gave no diffusion of hæmoglobin. Uric acid, because of its slight solubility, was not used. Hippuric acid, they say, gave positive results; after neutralization, no hæmolysis resulted. They then report pathological urines, in which the reaction was neutral or weakly alkaline, which caused hæmolysis in the erythrocytes of the rabbit; two of these were cases of chronic nephritis, the remaining two being cases of pneumonia during the period of defervescence.

Sabrazès and Fauquet[6] showed that urines, in which laking of blood did not occur, when made poor in chlorides by a rigid milk diet attained the power of laking. When the chlorides were raised to 7 grams per litre no diffusion of hæmoglobin resulted. Laking was also obtained when using the first urine of newborn infants shown to be poor in chlorides. In their experiments they added 20 c.mm. of blood to 1 c.c. of urine.

Pugnat,[7] examining urines from cases of croupous pneumonia during the febrile period, when the chlorides are greatly reduced in amount, failed to obtain laking. In each of his eight cases he found the freezing point of the urines greater than that of the blood, and concluded that the degree of molecular concentration of a urine, as determined by the cryoscope, indicates the action which the urine will have upon the red corpuscles, laking being produced only in urines hypotonic to the blood.

The hæmolytic theory of pernicious anæmia has been ably set forth by Hunter.[8] Warthin[9] has added to it in his observations upon the hæmolymph glands in pernicious anæmia. It was with a view to determining whether hæmolysins are present in the urine in cases of this disease that the present work was undertaken. As a working hypothesis, it was assumed that pernicious anæmia is essentially the result of increased hæmolysis, which arises from the absorption of bacterial hæmolysins from the alimentary canal, the latter appearing in the urine as an excretion.

In the first place, it becomes necessary, if possible, to exclude the hypotonicity of the urines examined. To this end the cryoscope would appear at first thought to be well suited. The freezing point, however, is no criterion of the tonic strength of a urine, for the following reason: Gryns[10] has shown that solutions of urea have an action upon red blood cells similar to that of distilled water—*i. e.*, laking takes place; but urea is an influencing factor in the determination of the freezing point. A method both accurate and requiring not too much time was not obtained. Still, the estimation of the percentage of sodium chloride, the inorganic salt which is present in the urine in largest amount, will often give valuable information in cases where hæmolysis does occur. For example, if the percentage of NaCl in the urine is 0.9, one can be certain, when working with rabbits' corpuscles, that a hæmolytic action is not due to hypotonicity of the urine. In fact, percentages lower than this may be obtained, the urine still being isotonic or hypertonic, for one must not lose sight of the remaining solid constituents other than urea. The freezing point was obtained in the majority of instances, as it was often of definite aid in showing that a urine was hypotonic.

The urines examined were obtained from patients suffering with various diseases in the wards of Dr. Osler, together with urines from two obstetrical cases, for which I am indebted to Dr. Slemons, and from individuals in good health. Freshly voided samples of urine were used. For testing the urines a 5 per cent. solution of the red blood corpuscles of a rabbit was used. The blood was drawn from a vein of the ear, defibrinated, centrifugalized, and the serum was drawn off. A solution of sodium chloride, 0.9 per cent., was added. This was again centrifugalized. In all, the corpuscles were washed three times in the salt solution. A 5 per cent. solution of the rabbits' corpuscles was then made in a 0.9 per cent. solution of the NaCl. The percentage of sodium chloride in the urines was obtained by the method of Lütke-Martius.[11]

No. of case.	Diagnosis.	Hæmolysis.	Reaction of urine.
1	Typhoid fever.	—	Acid.
2	Typhoid fever (convalescent).	—	Alkaline.
3	" " "	—	Acid.
4	" " "	—	"
5	" " "	—	"
6	" " "	—	Alkaline.
7	" " "	—	Acid.
8	" "	—	Alkaline.
9	" "	+ (hypotonic).	Neutral.
10	" "	—	Acid.
11	" "	+ (hypotonic).	Alkaline.
12	" "	—	Acid.
13	" "	—	Neutral.
14	" "	—	Acid.
15	" "	—	Neutral.
16	" "	—	Acid.
17	Typhoid periostitis.	—	"
18	Croupous pneumonia (febrile).	+ (hypotonic).	Alkaline.
19	" "	+ (hypotonic).	Acid.
20	" "	—	"
21	" "	—	"
22	" "	—	"
23	Tuberculosis (lung).	—	"
24	" "	—	"
25	" "	—	"
26	" "	—	"
27	Tuberculosis (brain).	—	"
28	Tuberculosis (peritoneum).	—	Alkaline.
29	" "	—	Acid.
30	Tuberculosis (intestines) (atrophic cirrhosis of liver).	—	Neutral.
31	Bronchial asthma.	—	Acid.
32	Influenza.	—	"
33	Pleurisy with serous effusion.	—	Neutral.
34	" " " "	—	Acid.
35	Pleurisy.	—	"
36	Amœbic dysentery.	—	Neutral.
37	" "	—	Acid.
38	Dysentery (bacillary ?).	—	"
39	Catarrhal jaundice.	—	Alkaline.
40	" "	—	Acid.
41	Obstructive jaundice (gallstones).	—	"
42	" gallstones.	—	Neutral.
43	Chronic jaundice (cause ?).	—	Acid.
44	Hypertrophic liver cirrhosis.	—	Neutral.
45	Acute rheumatic endocarditis.	—	"
46	" " "	—	"
47	Chronic endocarditis.	—	Alkaline.
48	" "	—	"
49	Myocarditis.	—	Acid.
50	" and arteriosclerosis.	—	"
51	" and angina pectoris.	—	"
52	Mitral insufficiency and stenosis.	—	Neutral.
53	Aortic " neurasthenia.	—	Alkaline.
54	" " aneurysm.	—	Acid.
55	" "	—	Alkaline.
56	" "	—	Acid.
57	Thoracic aneurysm.	—	"
58	Pericarditis with effusion.	—	"
59	Acute articular rheumatism.	—	Neutral.
60	Gon rrhœal arthritis.	—	Acid.
61	Arthritis deformans.	—	"
62	"Still's disease."	—	"
63	Spondylitis.	—	"
64	Transverse myelitis (acute).	—	Alkaline.
65	Syphilis.	—	Acid.
66	" aneurysm.	—	"
67	" (congenital).	—	"
68	Basedow's disease.	—	Alkaline.
69	Neurasthenia.	—	Neutral.
70	"	—	Acid.
71	"	—	Neutral.
72	"	—	Alkaline.
73	"	—	Acid.
74	Anorexia nervosa.	—	"
75	Chronic interstitial nephritis.	—	"
76	" " "	+ (hypotonic).	Neutral.
77	" " "	+ (hypotonic).	Acid.
78	" " "	—	"
79	Chronic interstitial and parenchymatous nephritis.	—	Alkaline.

No. of case.	Diagnosis.	Hæmolysis.	Reaction of urine.
80	Hæmatoma of kidney.	—	Acid.
81	Diabetes mellitus.	—	Alkaline.
82	" "	—	Acid.
83	" "	—	"
84	Uncinariasis.	—	"
85	Splenomyelogenous leukæmia.	—	"
87	Henoch's purpura.	—	"
88	Polycythæmia.	—	"
89	Pernicious anæmia I.		
	Examination *a*.	+ ($\Delta = -1^\circ.805$)	"
	" *b*.	—	"
	" *c*.	—	"
90	Pernicious anæmia II.		
	Examination *a*.	+ (NaCl = 0.7605 %)	"
	" *b*.	+ (NaCl = 0.6903 %)	"
	" *c*.	+ (NaCl = 0.6318 %)	"
	" *d*.	—	"
	" *e*.	—	"
91	Pernicious anæmia III.		
	Examination *a*.	+ (NaCl = 0.5031 %)	"
	" *b*.	—	"
	" *c*.	+ ($\Delta = -0^\circ.61$)	"
	" *d*.	—	"
	" *e*.	—	"
	" *f*.	+ (NaCl = 0.74 %)	"
	" *g*.	—	"
92	Pernicious anæmia IV.		
	Examination *a*.	+ ($\Delta = -0^\circ.916$)	"
	" *b*.	—	Alkaline.
	" *c*.	—	"
	" *d*.	—	"
93	Pregnancy.	—	Acid.
94	Puerperal eclampsia (6 examin.)	—	"
95	Healthy individual.	—	"
96	" "	—	"
97	" "	—	"
98	" "	—	Alkaline.
99	" "	—	Acid.
100	" "	—	Alkaline.
101	" "	—	Acid.
102	" "	—	"
103	" "	—	Neutral.
104	" "	—	Alkaline.
105	" "	—	Acid.
106	" "	—	"

The above table will serve to show partially the results obtained. The sign + denotes hæmolysis, the sign — its absence.

The experiments were conducted in small test-tubes, after Friedberger, in the following manner:

Experiment A. Ten drops of urine; ten drops of a 5 per cent. solution of rabbits' corpuscles; three to four drops of normal rabbits' serum.

Experiment B. Ten drops of urine; ten drops of a 5 per cent. solution of rabbits' corpuscles.

The test-tubes, after having been filled, as above, were placed in an incubator at 37° C. for two hours. They were then placed in a temperature of 0° C. for about twenty hours. The tubes were then examined macroscopically and spectroscopically. In all cases where sedimentation was not satisfactory, the contents of the test-tubes were centrifugalized. The supernatant fluid was in each instance examined with the spectroscope for the bands of oxyhæmoglobin.

From the foregoing table it is seen that in no instance, except in cases of pernicious anæmia, was hæmolysis obtained where hypotonicity could be excluded. The results in the cases of pernicious anæmia require further explanation.

Solutions of sodium chloride of various strengths were prepared in which rabbits' corpuscles were suspended. The solutions were placed in test-tubes which were put in the incubator, and later in the refrigerator; in fact, treated exactly as in the experiments described above. A 0.66 per cent. solution of sodium chloride showed no diffusion of hæmoglobin from the rabbit's corpuscles, while hæmoglobin was present in the supernatant fluid in a 0.64 per cent. solution. Thus it is seen that in case No. 90, examinations *a* and *b* and in Case No. 91, examination *f*, the positive result may not be explained on the ground of hypotonicity. Again, it must be kept in mind that in the experiments ten drops of urine were added to ten drops of a 0.9 per cent. solution of NaCl; so that in each case where percentage of NaCl is recorded the resulting strength in sodium chloride is above 0.7 per cent. None of the pernicious anæmia urines showed the bands of oxyhæmoglobin on examination previous to the addition of the solution of rabbits' corpuscles.

In all cases where hypotonicity could be proven to exist, the supernatant fluid took on a deep-red color soon after the addition of the rabbits' red blood cells. This was the case in none of the pernicious anæmia urines. In no instance did the supernatant fluid show a marked pink color in this disease. On the contrary, only the suggestion of a pink color was to be seen. But in each case recorded as positive, the bands of oxyhæmoglobin were present on spectroscopic examination. In each of the examinations designated as positive, the fluid in experiment A was perceptibly darker than that in experiment B, and, in the former, the spectroscopic bands of oxyhæmoglobin were darker. In no case was this observed in any of the hypotonic urines. This fact convinces me that coloring of the fluid was not due to hypotonicity of the urine. If this were the case, why should twenty drops of a hypotonic solution, to which three drops of normal rabbits' serum has been added, show greater diffusion of hæmoglobin than twenty drops of the same solution to which no serum was added? The darker coloring in the tube to which normal serum was added coincides with Frieberger's results, although it seems that some complement is present in the urine.

No results were obtained comparable to those of Camus and Pagniez in working with normal urines. In every instance where diffusion of hæmoglobin took place, excepting the cases of pernicious anæmia, hypotonicity was proven to exist. It is to be regretted that details of their experiments are so meagre. In the cases of pneumonia, in which they report hæmolysis to have been present, neither freezing point nor percentage of chlorides is given, so that one cannot judge of the tonic strength of the urines.

The presence of hæmolysis in the urines of the pernicious anæmia cases has, so far as can be seen, no definite relationship to a rising or falling number of red blood cells. The observations extended over too short a space of time, however, to answer this point satisfactorily.

The fact that hæmolysis was not found constantly in the urines, that it was present at one examination, absent in the next, would seem to support Warthin's[9] theory as to the cyclical or intermittent nature of the hæmolysis in this disease, though one cannot deny that this may be due wholly to temporary changes in the excretory power of the kidneys irrespective of other changes in the organism.

The possibility of pernicious anæmia being due to the absorption of bacterial toxins is clearly set forth by Hunter.[8] Elders[12] reports a case treated successfully by antistreptococcus serum which supports Hunter's view. Welch[13] mentions the possibility of "certain obscure anæmias" being due to the absorption of toxins of bacteria. It is possible that the hæmolysis found in the urines of pernicious anæmia is due to bacterial hæmolysins which have been absorbed, though hæmolysins from other sources cannot be excluded.

It is my pleasure to thank Professor Osler for his kindness in facilitating the work; also Dr. Emerson, the director of the clinical laboratory.

BIBLIOGRAPHY.

1. Ann. de l'Inst. Pasteur, 1898.
2. Deutsche med. Woch., 1892.
3. Münch. med. Woch., 1899.
4. Berlin. klin. Woch., 1900.
5. Journ. de Physiol. et de Path. Gén., 1901.
6. Comptes-rendus de la Soc. de Biologie, 1901.
7. Ibid.
8. Pernicious Anæmia, London, 1901.
9. THE AMERICAN JOURNAL OF THE MEDICAL SCIENCES, 1902.
10. Pflüger's Archiv, 1896.
11. Sahli. Klin. Untersuchungs-Methoden.
12. Lancet, 1900.
13. Bulletin of the Johns Hopkins Hospital, December, 1902.

MENTAL SYMPTOMS ASSOCIATED WITH PERNICIOUS ANÆMIA.

BY WILLIAM PICKETT, A.M., M.D.,
INSTRUCTOR IN NEUROPATHOLOGY AND INSANITY, JEFFERSON MEDICAL COLLEGE; EXAMINER OF THE INSANE, PHILADELPHIA HOSPITAL.

THE spinal cord lesions and symptoms of pernicious anæmia, through the work of Lichtheim, C. W. Burr, and others, have become an old story, of which the sequel, written by Putnam and

Taylor, and others, reveals the probable role of anæmias and cachexias in a large group of combined degenerations of the cord.

Mental symptoms of the character of delirium and confusion in pernicious anæmia were early recognized. "The mind occasionally wanders," said Addison, in his classic portrayal of idiopathic anæmia,[1] and subsequent writers have, in similar comments, noticed mental disturbance as a terminal incident in this grave blood disease. A Swedish observer, Henry Marcus, in the *Neurologisches Centralblatt*, May 16, 1903, describes a psychosis resembling expansive paresis, but associated with anæmia which he designates as "pernicious," although the lowest blood estimation was 2,400,000 red cells and 27 per cent. hæmoglobin; while no differential count of leukocytes is published and no mention is made of nucleated red cells. The mental symptoms in Marcus' case subsided in the course of six months with very little improvement in the blood state, and had not returned two years later, which I think is the strongest support for his claim that this was a true pernicious anæmia—psychosis.

Yet, I have seen the wildest delusions of grandeur fade in a few weeks, giving place to a remission of four years' duration, apparently, and as the late D. E. Hughes believed, through the correction of a simple anæmia; and I have seen paretic symptoms lighted up by alcoholic debauches at three periods about a year apart, to fade again as the alcoholic influence was eliminated in the first and second accesses, but apparently to become established in the third access, the patient appearing then as a confirmed paretic. It would seem that these toxic states belong in the category of exciting causes of paresis along with trauma and the puerperium; and so it is possible that Marcus' patient is a paretic after all.

Secondary anæmias are found in association with various mental states. About two years ago it occurred to me that cases of paresis in which the cord succumbs to the disease first might show a peculiar blood state as compared with those in which mental symptoms usher in the disease; and I made blood examinations of 7 cases of paresis of the spinal type in order to compare them with the ordinary cases which might be called, in view of the studies of Storch and of Schaffer, the *forebrain* type.

Assuming that the cases studied by Capps in 1896[2] and by Jelliffe in 1897[3] belong mainly to the latter or ordinary type, the comparison of the two types appears as follows:

[1] Osler, in his Practice, quotes all that Addison said of the disease.
[2] The American Journal of the Medical Sciences, June, 1903.
[3] New York State Hospital Bulletin, July, 1903.

Name.	Station and gait.	Knee-jerks.	Pupils.	Light reaction.	Accommodation.	Red corpuscles.	White corpuscles.	Hæmoglobin.	Polymorphonuclear	Lymphocyte.	L. mononuclear.	Eosinophiles.
9	....	....	....	....	....	3,700,000	21,066	65 %	69 %	19 %	5 %	7 %
W. M.	Very poor, paraplegia.	Absent.	Large; right larger.	Both good.	Good; nystagmus.	3,260,000	25,400	50 %	53 %	12 %	29 %	6 %
J. F. B.	Moderate ataxia; weakness.	Very quick.	Right larger.	Absent.	Poor; horizontal nystagmus.	3,380,000	14,400	70 %	54 %	40 %	4 %	2 %
G. R.	Moderate ataxia; weakness.	Absent.	Fairly large; right slightly larger.	Absent.	Good.	2,820,000	24,000	80 %	95 %	4 %	1 %	0 %
H. D.	Poor station; ataxic gait.	Absent.	Small; right larger.	Both slight.	Better than light.	3,800,000	22,983	65 %	58 %	35 %	12 %	0 %
H. M. D.	Ataxic gait.	Plus; ankle clonus.	Large; left larger.	Left none; right good.	Both good.	4,240,000	32,588	72 %	68 %	24 %	7 %	1 %
C. H.	Ataxic gait.	Plus.	Pinpoint; left larger.	Both slight.	Sluggish.	3,580,000	36,266	60 %	69 %	20 %	8 %	8 %
	Spinal type (averages of above)					3,516,000	25,922	66 1/6 %	65 1/3 %	22 1/2 %	10 1/6 %	2 %
	Ordinary type (averages in 19 cases reported by Capps)					4,789,774	12,288	84 9/10 %	75 1/3 %	14 3/4 %	7 7/8 %	2 3/5 %
	" " (In Jelliffe's 18 cases)					5,714,333	7,106	83 %	78 2/3 %	16 2/3 %	7 1/3 %	1 4/5 %

If we may draw a conclusion from this small series of cases, it is this: When the spinal cord bears the brunt of the disease process in paresis, a simple anæmia with leukocytosis is found; when mental symptoms alone appear, the blood state is not characteristic. Perhaps anæmias or the toxins of anæmias are a factor in the cord lesions even of paresis.

My cases were, mentally, early ones, yet the blood counts resemble those obtained by Diefendorf[1] in the last stage of ordinary paresis; so it may be that simple anæmia with leukocytosis is merely a consequence of advanced paretic degeneration, whether this be spinal as in my cases, or cerebral as in Diefendorf's.

The frequency of spinal-cord involvement in pernicious anæmia is evidently great; diffuse degenerations occur even when spinal symptoms are not apparent; tract degenerations have been traced by Spiller and others into the brain stem; but of cerebral lesions from pernicious anæmia nothing of value is known. I hope to report upon this point later, as I have two brains from cases in which the blood state was extreme, and mental symptoms prominent; and Professor Coplin has a third brain from a case in which I have been interested medicolegally, since the individual's testamentary capacity was called in question by reason of mental disturbance that arose in the last month of his life.

Dr. E. Q. Thornton has furnished me with notes of this case: A merchant, aged fifty-five years, consulted Dr. Thornton on November 12, 1902, complaining chiefly of languor, but appearing of such a bad color that he was sent for a blood examination at once to Dr. Rosenberger, who reported the following: red corpuscles, 1,500,000; white corpuscles, 7500; hæmoglobin, 35 per cent. Poikilocytosis; large and small nucleated red cells.

On January 25, 1903, the man took part in an interview that agitated him; the next day his temperature rose to 103° F. and he became delusional, declaring that his wife was trying to poison him; that she was unfaithful and that the nurses and doctors were in a conspiracy with her to get his property; he exhibited his hands from which "poison" was exuding; described disagreeable odors of poisonous gases, and attempted to escape by the windows repeatedly. He disinherited her by tearing up a will made in her favor long before. Yet he was not much disoriented and could talk clearly of other matters. Death occurred on February 18, 1903.

Lena P. was an inmate of the Insane Department, Philadelphia Hospital, for twelve years; she had pernicious anæmia on admission in 1890; a blood count made by Dr. Gilmore at that time showed red corpuscles, 590,000. She died of the disease in 1902. The blood count four days before death was: red corpuscles, 1,107,000; white

[1] The American Journal of the Medical Sciences, December, 1903.

corpuscles, 9166; hæmoglobin, 18 per cent. Macrocytes, microcytes, gigantoblasts, and normoblasts.

She had the color and other evidences of the disease throughout the entire period, and was mildly demented; but she was subject to exacerbations of the blood disease—in a number of which blood counts were recorded—and at the same time of her mental symptoms becoming dreamily confused.

Catharine McB. was brought to the Philadelphia Hospital from the House of Correction, in a state of confusion with excitement—a mild delirium. Examination of the blood revealed the following: red corpuscles, 690,000; white corpuscles, 12,000; hæmoglobin, 15 per cent. Marked poikilocytosis, many macrocytes and microcytes, normoblasts and gigantoblasts.

Michael F. was sent to the Philadelphia Hospital by Dr. J. O. W. Kelly, on account of a hallucinatory confusional state, of three months' duration. The patient's color and weakness suggested to the late Dr. Hughes a blood disease, which was found: red corpuscles, 2,990,000; white corpuscles, 11,466; hæmoglobin, 38 per cent. The man cleared mentally and left the hospital after five weeks of treatment, although he was still anæmic.

Bessie M. is at present under treatment at the Philadelphia Hospital Insane Department. The blood count is: red corpuscles, 3,230,000; white corpuscles, 28,133; hæmoglobin, 55 per cent. Normoblasts and gigantoblasts are abundant. The mental state, as much as the color of the skin, suggested pernicious anæmia in her case.

A composite picture of the mental disturbance in these cases presents a shallow confusion with impairment of the ideas of time and place (disorientation), more marked on awakening from sleep. The patient fabricates, relating imaginary experiences of "yesterday" in a circumstantial way.

Illusions, particularly of identity, are common. Hallucinations appear at times, pertaining to any of the senses.

Based upon these illusions and hallucinations, persecutory delusions arise. These are usually transient, causing episodes of fear and agitation, but they may persist for considerable periods and be thus somewhat fixed; they may be even systematized, as in Dr. Thornton's case.

The pernicious anæmia psychosis is mainly an abeyance of mind; it rarely presents that spontaneous excitement by which some types of confusion seem to merge into true mania; so that the term amentia, in Meynert's sense, seems appropriate for it. Of Meynert's two groups, *idiopathic* and *symptomatic* amentia, the latter, of course, would embrace the pernicious anæmia psychosis. Korsakoff's disease and folie Brightique resemble it closely.

CLINICAL AND HISTOLOGIC STUDY OF THE OPHTHALMIC CONDITIONS IN A CASE OF CEREBELLAR NEOPLASM OCCURRING IN A SUBJECT WITH RENAL DISEASE.[1]

By Charles A. Oliver, A.M., M.D.,
of Philadelphia.

In the month of February, 1898, A. C. T., a white woman, aged forty-eight years, married, and the mother of one living child, came under the care of Dr. J. Hendrie Lloyd in the Wards for Nervous Diseases at the Philadelphia Hospital. Dr. Lloyd's most careful notes of the case state that the principal complaints of the patient upon her admission into the hospital were double vision "with incomplete loss of vision in the left eye," and weakness in the legs and lumbar region. The patient's family history showed that both her father, a man aged seventy-nine years, and her mother, a woman aged sixty-nine years, were living. The patient was one of thirteen children, of whom four brothers and four sisters were living; of the remaining four children, all brothers, two died during infancy; the third in adult life (from hypertrophic cirrhosis of the liver), and the fourth from some unknown cause.

The patient had had "all of the diseases of childhood." She first menstruated at twelve years of age, and had been "regular" up to her forty-sixth year of age, the epochs usually lasting for three or four days' time. The flow was always moderate in quantity, and the crisis was never painful. Menopause had been slowly though undisturbingly establishing itself for the past two years. She had one living healthy child. She never had any miscarriages. Seven years before admission she had suffered from an attack of acute articular rheumatism, followed four years later by inflammation of the lungs. She reported that she had never had venereal disease, and she had never had any gross accidents or operative interference. She had never used alcohol or tobacco.

She said that following her recovery from the pneumonia she suffered from occipito-vertical pains and vomiting at each premenstrual period, the headache having ceased during the last eight attacks, but the vomiting being preceded by gross exacerbations of nausea. She stated that she had been unable to walk without assistance for three years' time. For two years she had had "weakness in the lower part of the back." There was frequent desire with difficulty in micturition, the patient not always being able to urinate. There had never been any retention or incontinence of

[1] Read before the March, 1904, meeting of the Section on Ophthalmology of the College of Physicians of Philadelphia.

urine. Her bowels had been constipated much of the time for fully a year.

Four weeks before she was seen she had experienced a severe attack of nausea and vomiting which had lasted for three days' time. Just previous to this attack she had had so much dizziness as to cause her to fall from a chair. After this accident she noticed that objects appeared double and that she was told at times that her eyes seemed crossed. At this time vision with the left eye began to fail. These symptoms were almost immediately followed by loss of vision in the left eye. The vertiginous seizures persisted, though to a much less degree, while the patient was placed in a prone position.

Upon admission to the hospital, the patient appeared to be well nourished. Her radial pulse was 100, small and compressible. Her heart sounds were rapid, the second beat being accentuated. The tongue was protruded straight, and there was not any marked tremor. There was not any trembling of the lips. The masseter, the temporal, and the pterygoid muscles acted well. Neither the sensory nor the motor portions of the fifth nerve seemed involved. A slight trembling of the hands and arms upon extension was noticeable. Hand grip was equally good on both sides. Sensation and localization were good in both arms. The biceps jerks were apparent. The patellar tendon reflex was exaggerated on the right side, and ankle clonus was absent on both sides. The plantar reflex was increased, while sensation in the legs was somewhat greater than normal. Pressure upon the sacral region gave rise to tenderness. Station was poor, while gait was slightly ataxic in character. There was marked inco-ordination. Examination of the urine gave a low specific gravity, a minor amount of albumin, and the presence of a few granular and hyaline casts.[1]

The pupil of the right eye was 1 mm. larger than that of the left, which was 4 mm. wide in the horizontal meridian. Iris reactions to light stimuli were very feeble, and were not so good in the left eye as in the right one when gross attempts at accommodative efforts were made. A medium degree of paresis of the left external rectus muscle, together with a slight paresis of the corresponding orbicularis muscle, could be determined both objectively and subjectively. There was imperfect action of the muscles which were supplied by the left oculomotor and pathetic nerves.

The ophthalmoscope showed that there was a marked degree of neuroretinitis, the swollen tissues of the left optic nerve-head being denser and more extensive than those of the right eye (seven dioptres as compared with six dioptres for the right optic nerve-head swelling). There were numerous superficial and deeply seated hemorrhages in both the neural and retinal tissues, particularly along the

[1] For a most interesting and instructive difference between these findings and those of the urine which had been examined eight years previously, see later notes in report of this case.

larger temporal vessels. Great numbers of commencing degeneration areas could be seen in both papillomacular regions, though more pronounced in the left eye.

Uncorrected vision with the right eye equalled one-third of the normal, this being improved to one-half of normal by having the patient gaze through a pinhole. Vision with the left eye was one-sixth of normal, being brought to one-fifth by use of the pinhole. The visual fields were lessened somewhat concentrically with the presence of great numbers of mutable relative and absolute scotomatous areas with fixed enlargements of the physiological blind

Fig. 1.

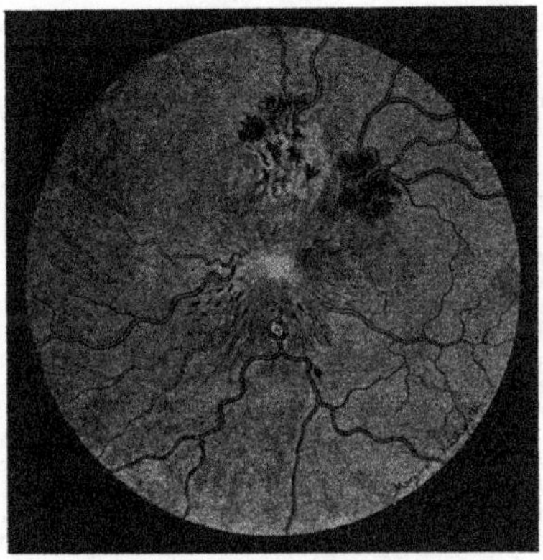

Ophthalmoscopic appearance of left eye-ground.

spots. There was not any accommodative play, the one-half dioptre type being clearly and fixedly defined at 30 cm. when looked at through a convex spherical lens of four dioptres' strength with the right eye, and the three-quarters of a dioptre type being seen clearly at 25 cm. distance with the same correcting lens. Intraocular tension in each eye was normal.

The ticking of a watch, which could be heard at 30 cm. distance from the right ear, was not audible even when the watch was held close to the left ear.

Upon re-examination of the ocular conditions eleven days later it was found that the patient was unable to make use of the lower fibres of the left orbicularis muscles, the upper fibres, and partienlarly those in the unstriated series at the inner angle, being but slightly contractile, with compensatory movement of the globe, given in order to place the cornea beneath the upper lid.

Ophthalmoscopic examination of both eye-grounds as pictured in the accompanying sketch (Fig. 1) of the left eye-ground, made by Miss Margaretta Washington, of this city, showed fresh hemorrhages, both superficial and deep, in the retinal tissues. The swelling of the optic disks had subsided to about two dioptres, and the tissues of the nerve-heads had become much thickened. The retinal plaques and patches noted in the previous study still existed.

In the lower part of the superficial layers of the left cornea there was a large saturated and markedly anæsthetic ulcerous area, which was rapidly extending into the corneal layers, giving rise to an extreme irritability of the eyeball. The conjunctival membrane, particularly that portion of it which was situated in the neighborhood of the ulcerous spot, was proliferating its external squamous cells, and there was a corresponding desquamation of the neighboring epithelium. The previous convergence was now noted as having become bilateral, this being produced by a paresis of the right external rectus muscle, though to a lesser degree than that of the left eye.

At this time the patiênt voluntarily gave the information that for the first time she had experienced attacks of irritation phosphenes in the shape of golden rain, which was situated directly in front of the right eye. The visual fields both for form and color were lessened irregularly to a greater degree than they had been at the earlier examination. Intraocular tension had become slightly diminished in the inflamed eye. Vision with this eye had decreased to an uncorrectable one-thirtieth of normal.

From this time on vision in both eyes steadily failed until she became practically blind; postneuritic changes set in; muscle palsies of the most bizarre types appeared; and the general condition gradually weakened until in some six weeks' time after she had been first studied she died from apparent uræmic poisoning.

A most careful autopsy was made. The scalp and the calvaria did not present anything abnormal. The dura mater was not especially adherent. There was not any excess of fluid in the subarachnoid spaces. The small vessels of the pia mater were injected, and the large ones were distended. The membrane itself was almost transparent.

Springing from the left lobe of the cerebellum was a cone-shaped mass which proved to be sarcomatous in character. The apex of the growth was nipple-shaped and projected forward to a point which was situated slightly anterior to the middle line of the pons varolii and reached to within $1\frac{1}{2}$ cm. of the origin of the left crus cerebri. The base of the tumor was found to be placed somewhat anterior to the middle of the left cerebellar hemisphere. The tumor-mass was 3 cm. broad at its base; its total length was 55 mm., and its greatest width was 33 mm. Laterally, toward the median line, the growth pressed upon the medulla oblongata, while on the left side it rested upon the posterior part of the pons varolii. The medulla, which was flattened laterally, was twisted on its longitudinal axis in such a manner that it was directed at an angle of forty-five degrees away from the median line, causing its normally placed left lateral surface to be turned obliquely upward. The growth was sharply circumscribed and could be readily removed from the cerebellum. Its posterior aspect was covered by pia mater, while its anterior face was possibly similarly conditioned.

The mass, which was firm in consistency, had an irregularly convoluted surface, resembling that of brain tissue. Upon section, it was yellowish-red in color and exhibited a few distended vessels and small free hemorrhages.

The seventh and eighth nerve trunks on the right side appeared to be in good condition, while the corresponding left ones were swollen and indistinct. There was a marked softening of the pons varolii in the position where the neoplasm pressed upon it. This softening extended to about 2 cm. in advance of the growth. The tumor was adherent to the base of the skull.

After removal of the brain it was found that the posterior part of the petrous portion of the temporal bone was deeply eroded. The cavity made by the growth was 2 cm. long, 14 mm. wide, and 1 cm. deep. The central part of this excavation corresponded in position to that of the internal meatus. The bone surface in the excavated area was rough and was crossed by a series of serrated elevations. The cavity was filled with soft tumor-like masses of reddish tint.

The body was emaciated. The cæcum and ascending colon were distended with gas. The appendix was bound to the cæcum and the ascending colon by adhesions. The pleuræ were free. Both the right and left lower lobes of the lungs were somewhat congested, while the upper lobes were slightly emphysematous. There were a few adhesions between the lobes of the left side. The pericardium showed a great deal of fatty infiltration. The heart muscles were some 18 mm. thick. Both the aortic and the pulmonary valves were normal; the tricuspids were thickened. The mitral valve exhibited a few yellowish opaque spots. The liver was small, its right lobe being 19 cm. long and its left lobe 16 cm. long; its average thickness was $4\frac{3}{4}$ cm. The gall-bladder projected for some 5 cm. beyond the surface of the liver. There was a slight increase of connective tissue between the lobules of the organ. The interior of the aorta was both roughened and thickened. The spleen was small, very dark in tint, and quite soft. The pancreas did not present anything abnormal. The left suprarenal capsule showed fatty degeneration in its cortex. The capsules of both kidneys could be stripped with difficulty. The organs themselves were somewhat smaller in size than normal. Their cortices, which were red in tint, were reduced in thickness. The pyramids were fibroid in character. The pelvic membranes were injected, those of the left kidney being infiltrated with pus. The bladder was contracted; its walls were greatly thickend, and its cavity was filled with pus.

The posterior halves of the eyes, together with the orbital portions of the optic nerves, were removed and placed in formalin.

Some few months later, while inspecting some notes in my clinical service at Wills Hospital, I unexpectedly came across a carefully prepared record of this patient who had visited my out-patient service in December, 1890. The symptoms complained of at that time were typically those of renal disease. The ophthalmic examination, which was most complete, showed the presence of some faint star-like degeneration radii in both macular regions, with a few superficial and deeply seated hemorrhages in the papillomacular areas, in association with a small mosaic of pigment aggregations with intervening fatty degenerations, slightly down and out from the left optic nerve-head, and extending into the macular region. Vision with the right eye was reduced to four-fifths of normal and to two-thirds of normal with the left eye. The visual fields were large. They presented proper color sequences and were well shaped; small but negative central scotomas being present. Examination of the urine at that time revealed a fluid of good specific gravity, but containing a faint trace of albumin and some granular casts. The patient, who was ordered an appropriate regimen and was given a prescription for Basham's mixture, failed to return after the third visit.

Through the kindness of Dr. Edward A. Shumway of this city, the left eyeball was embedded in celloidin, and sections were made through the optic nerve and neighboring ocular tunics.

Macroscopically, the optic nerve was much thinner than ordinary, and its intraocular extremity showed decided swelling.

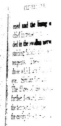

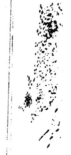

Microscopically, the optic nerve-head was found to be swollen, the result of the swelling being $\frac{87}{100}$ mm. above the level of the lamina vitrea of the chorioid. The tissues were infiltrated with a great number of cells which had assumed spindle-like forms; these cells being particularly numerous around the vessels, forming complete mantles in places. (*Vide* sketch by Dr. Ellen C. Potter, Resident Physician at the Woman's Hospital of Philadelphia). In those sections which were stained by the Van Gieson method, the intercellular substance stained with fuchsin, and appeared to be composed of fine connective-tissue fibres (by the contraction of which the optic nerve fibres had become atrophic, as no trace of them could be found). The vessel walls were very much thick-

ened and the lining endothelial cells were proliferated, but the chief increase in thickness was situated in the adventitia. Embedded in the swollen nerve-head were several irregularly round bodies, staining faintly pink with eosin, and light red with the Van Gieson reagents. These bodies were without structure, and resembled those which are found in the nerve-head in senile conditions of the eye. Similar formations were also found in the intervaginal space. The fibres of the lamina cribrosa were thickened and extended further forward than usual. Posterior to the lamina cribrosa, on the temporal side, the intervaginal space was widely distended, and the cavity thus formed, which extended backward for a distance of

FIG. 2.

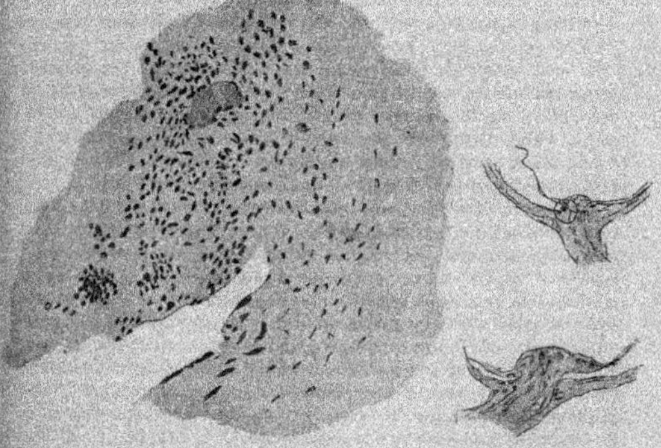

Spindle-like cells around vessels in swollen optic nerve-head.

1 mm., was filled with a loosely coagulated fluid and crossed by swollen connective-tissue processes. Everywhere else the space between the dural and pial sheaths was filled with a mass of proliferating cells. These cells were similar in type to the endothelial cells that line the processes of the arachnoid. In consequence of these changes, no lymph space existed around the optic nerve. The connective-tissue septa within the optic nerve were normal in thickness and were moderately infiltrated with lymphoid cells —particularly around the central vessels. The decrease in the diameter of the nerve was due to an almost complete atrophy of the nerve fibres. With the Weigert sheath stain only an occasional

tenuous thread, continuing for a short distance to end in a minute globule, could be seen.

The retina exhibited circumpapillary inflammation and œdema. The changes were situated chiefly in the outer layers, and consisted in hypertrophy of the supporting elements, their separation by fluid, and the formation of cystic cavities.

In one place (the macular region) there was a mesh-like deposit of fibrin, such as is common in retinitis albuminurica. Swollen, fatty cells were occasionally seen, but no hemorrhages could be found. The rods and cones were degenerated, their outer ends being converted into irregularly shaped masses. The fibre layer of the retina showed œdema and hypertrophy of the supporting fibres, but there were not any large cavities. The nervous elements in this layer had apparently disappeared, no fibres could be determined, and but a few of the cells present could be isolated as highly degenerated ganglion cells. The vessels showed the same changes as those in the optic nerve-head. The so-called retinal pigment cells were decidedly proliferated, and the surface of the chorioid presented several masses of partially organized exudate to which some of the cells of the outer retinal layer remained adherent.

The chorioidal vessels were widely distended with blood, which contained numerous polymorphonuclear leukocytes; the stroma being moderately infiltrated with mononuclear round cells.

Remarks. The case is of interest from several standpoints: the formation of a cerebellar tumor of sarcomatous type in a subject with previous renal disease; the existence of a low grade macular chorioretinitis in both eyes, with the characteristic ophthalmoscopic phenomena of a true retinitis albuminurica without any coarse signs of endarteritis or perivasculitis eight years before the gross type of neuroretinitis, which is so peculiar to increased intracranial pressure, and particularly to that which is found in subtentorial neoplasms, appeared; the masking of the primary changes in the macular regions by the later gross ones of neuroretinitis with their post-mortem exposure by the microscope (*i. e.*, the finding of the solitary remnant of the previous localized retinal and chorioidal inflammation from disturbance in the vascular network—the mesh-like deposit of fibrin); the final rapid loss of vision in so brief a period of time (three months) (the reason for which was so well shown post-mortem by the almost, if not quite complete, atrophy of the nervous elements of the retina and the optic nerve); the disappearance of the negative scotomas with the subsequent irregular peripheral contraction, with remaining star-like sectors, of the rapidly lessening visual fields; the progressive types of exterior and interior ocular pareses and palsies, which were always more marked in the groups of the left side; the occurrence of trophic disturbances in the corneal membrane of the left eye (the eye which was always the one which was the more greatly involved); the enormous lengthening of the fibres of Müller—especially in the nuclear layers of the retina—giving rise to irregular elevations on the outer surface of the retina, and the gross hyperæmia and moderate degree of inflammatory infiltration of the chorioid.

A CASE OF FIBROADENOMA OF THE TRACHEA:*

WITH REMARKS ON TUMORS OF THE TRACHEAL IN GENERAL.

By Sylvan Rosenheim, M.D.,

and

Mactier Warfield, M.D.,

ASSISTANT AND INSTRUCTOR IN LARYNGOLOGY, JOHNS HOPKINS MEDICAL SCHOOL.

(From the Clinic of Professor Mackenzie, Johns Hopkins Hospital.)

Tumors of the trachea are exceedingly rare. Among 3120 tumors of the upper respiratory tract seen by Moritz Schmidt (1903) there were 7 tracheal new-growths. This is less than 1 per cent. of their frequency in the larynx. This is due to the passive role played by the trachea as compared with the larynx. The lack of susceptibility of the trachea is strikingly shown by Schroetter's statistics. Among 3639 cases of disease of the upper respiratory organs, there were only 26 cases of pure catarrh of the trachea. The description of these growths is usually dismissed in a few words in the text-books. Owing to their almost certain fatality if not recognized and removed, the report of a case is not only of unusual interest, but also serves to keep the subject fresh in our mind.

The following will consist of a report of our case and a review of the literature on new-growths of the trachea. We wish to thank Dr. Mackenzie for his permission to report the case and for his supervision of our work. Our thanks are also extended to Dr. C. W. Potter for his beautiful photomicrographs illustrating the microscopic specimens.

History of Case. Mrs. J. L., aged twenty-three years, white. Was admitted to the Johns Hopkins Hospital February 2, 1903, complaining of difficulty in breathing.

Family History. Negative.

Past History. Always well and strong. Before the present trouble, no cough. Married at the age of twenty-one years; has one child living aged five months. Is now pregnant, at the beginning of the third month.

Present Illness. Nine months ago the patient noticed a slight heaviness and a feeling of choking at night. She began to cough, and there was soon some expectoration. She thought there was something wrong with the lungs or with the heart. The difficulty in breathing has gradually grown greater, and now there is a marked shortness of breath on exertion and a constant feeling of lack of air. There is no expectoration and only a slight, hacking cough.

Physical Examination. Well-nourished woman; mucous membrane slightly pale; the teeth show a lack of enamel and a slight notching of the cutting edge. The glands of the neck are not enlarged. The lungs, heart, and the abdomen are negative.

Larynx. The vocal cords and larynx are normal. A short distance below the vocal cords one sees a tumor mass, apparently about the size of a small marble, almost hemispherical, surface smooth, mucous membrane covering it very red. It almost fills up the lumen of the trachea, and does not move on respiration or on phonation.

The patient was operated on several days after admission by Professor Halsted under chloroform anæsthesia. A preliminary tracheotomy was first performed, and then the trachea was opened above the tracheotomy wound. The growth was seen to be on the posterior wall opposite the cricoid cartilage and upper tracheal rings. At this stage of the operation the patient suddenly stopped breathing, necessitating artificial respiration. Natural respiration was established again by means of dilatation of the rectum and the growth was excised. The tracheal cannula was left in place for several days and then removed. Convalescence was uninterrupted. Dr. Mackenzie saw the patient six months later, when there was no sign of a return of the growth.

Macroscopic Description of the Tumor. The specimen is 1.5 cm. in diameter, definitely circumscribed and encapsulated. It is quite firm and elastic, with a somewhat softer area to one side. This softer area corresponds to a hemorrhagic zone. The cut surface of the tumor shows a definite capsule. On one side there is a firm tissue with a distinct fibrous network, between the meshes of which are translucent-looking areas. On pressure drops of a pure mucoid fluid are expressed, apparently from these areas. From this firm area strands and trabeculæ extend through the rest of the specimen. Between the trabeculæ are spaces of various sizes, the largest near the colloid material. Scattered through them are numerous pinpoint to pinhead size, tawny yellow, open spots.

Gross Diagnosis. Colloid adenoma. The tissue was fixed in alcohol, embedded in celloidin, and the sections were stained in hæmatoxylin and eosin, hæmatoxylin and Van Gieson's stain, and thionin.

Microscopic Description of the Tumor. The greater mass of the tumor is made up of fibrous connective tissue, which partly surrounds it as a capsule. It occurs in long, wavy masses. Intermixed with this connective tissue is a fair amount of cellular structure. The latter occurs in two forms: first as acini, secondly as cell nests without any definite arrangement. The acini are lined by a single layer of cells, some columnar, some irregularly shaped. The nucleus of the cells is large, fairly well stained, and contains a small nucleolus. The protoplasm takes no stain and has a reticulated appearance.

The cell nests consist of round and polygonal cells between strands of connective tissue. The nuclei stain deeply, and the protoplasm is a faintly stained, homogeneous matter.

Treated with thionin, the contents of the acini take on a deep-blue stain. With Van Gieson's stain they are of a brownish color.

The fibrous tissue is present in very large amount, forming more than half of the growth. It occurs in long, wavy masses. In the section stained with thionin, numerous "mast-cells" are seen in the fibrous tissue.

The tumor is poorly supplied with bloodvessels. These consist of large blood spaces lined by a single endothelial layer.

These details are very well seen in the accompanying photographs.

The tumor is a mixture of fibrous and glandular tissue, the former predominating, and the name fibroadenoma is therefore proper.

The staining characteristics of the contents of the acini make one think of the thyroid tumors, which are described as occurring in the trachea, but the cells are certainly not thyroid gland cells and they are not arranged as in the thyroid gland tumors.

Clinically there is but little difference between new-growths of the trachea. They can be conveniently studied, however, in the following classes: 1. Neoplasms. 2. Infectious granulomata. 3. Granulations following tracheotomy and other wounds of the trachea. 4. Intratracheal thyroid growths.

1. *Neoplasms.* The following classification covers all the growths seen in the trachea:

1. Non-malignant	Papilloma. Fibroma. Lipoma. Enchondroma and chondro-osteoma. Adenoma. Lymphoma. Amyloid growths.
2. Malignant	Carcinoma. Sarcoma.

Previous to the clinical use of the laryngoscope by Türck and Czermak, growths in this region were discovered only at autopsy. Türck, in 1861, first saw a growth in the trachea in the living person. Despite the diligent use of the laryngoscope since that time, there are on record but a comparatively few cases of intratracheal tumors.

Cohen had collected, in 1889, 57 cases, all he was able to find in literature. He included in this list one case of tuberculous tumor. Lemoine, in an inaugural dissertation in 1889, added 44 new cases. As, however, 11 of these were vegetations following tracheotomy and one a syphilitic tumor, they must be excluded. Bruns, in Heymann's *Handbuch*, has made an exhaustive analysis of the literature up to

1898. He found 95 benign and 45 malignant growths, including in the latter only primary carcinoma and sarcoma of the trachea. These tumors were divided as follows: Non-malignant—fibroma, 23; papilloma, 33; lipoma, 3; chondroma and osteoma, 29; adenoma, 5; and lymphoma, 2. Malignant—carcinoma, 31; sarcoma, 14. Since that work has appeared we have been able to collect the following: papilloma, 1; chondro-osteoma, 1; carcinoma, 2; sarcoma, 8; amyloid tumors, 8; 1 case of multiple fibromyxoma of ours not yet reported, and the present reported case.

Adding these cases to those enumerated by Bruns, we have the following table, which comprises all the growths of the trachea on record:

Non-malignant	Papilloma	34	
	Chondroma and chondro-osteoma	30	
	Fibroma	23	
	Adenoma	5	
	Lipoma	3	
	Lymphoma	2	
	Fibroadenoma	1	
	Multiple fibromyxoma	1	
	Amyloid tumors	5	
			104
Malignant	Carcinoma	33	
	Sarcoma	22	
			55
			159

This makes a total of 159 tracheal tumors described up to the present date.

As in the larynx, the greater proportion of these growths belong to the papilloma and fibroma groups. They occur most frequently in the upper part of the trachea, next in the lowest part, and least frequently in the middle portion. Exceptionally they run the entire length of the trachea. They are most often found on the posterior wall.

2. *Infectious Granulomata.* In this class tuberculosis and syphilis are represented. Chronic tuberculosis gives rise to subepithelial cellular infiltrations, which break down and form ulcers of various sizes. They may extend deep, laying bare the rings, and by perichondritis destroy them. Only two instances of tuberculous tumor have been described.

Author.	How found.	Location.	Treatment.	Reference.
J. N. Mackenzie.	Autopsy.	Posterior membranous wall.	....	Archives of Medicine, 1882, p. 107.
H. von Schroetter.	Tracheal tube.	Irregular stenosis near bifurcation.	Curetted.	Deutsche med. Woch., 1901, No. 28.

In both Mackenzie's and Schroetter's cases the growths were first thought to be cancerous. In Mackenzie's case the lungs contained tuberculous cavities. In Schroetter's case there was clinically no demonstrable lesion of the lungs, and he therefore considered it a case of primary tracheal tuberculosis. He states that he saw the patient one year later, when she had gained in weight and the tubercle bacilli had disappeared from the sputum. He also mentions a similar case in a woman aged twenty years, but does not give a report of this case.

Syphilis sometimes causes extensive destruction of tissue, and by subsequent contraction of the cicatrices causes great distortion of the trachea. The edges of the syphilitic ulcer are sometimes the seat of papillary excrescences partly covered with stratified squamous epithelium.

Author.	How discovered.	Location.	Treatment.	Reference.
Hanszel	Laryngoscope.	Gumma of upper part.	Potassium iodide.	See Bibliography.
Bayer	Laryngoscope.	Almost complete closure of the trachea.	Mixed treatment.	" "
Glechsman . . .	Laryngoscope.	....	....	" "

3. *Vegetations.* These are granulomatous formations. Petel considers them exhaustively in a thesis written in 1879. Lemoine includes 11 of these in his list of benign tumors of the trachea, but incorrectly, as they are composed of granulation tissue. They form pedunculated polypoid growths, rarely larger than peas. They arise one to two months after the tracheotomy wound has been closed. They acquire an epithelial investment, sometimes covered with cilia.

4. *Intratracheal Thyroid Growths.* From a careful survey of the literature found, it is seen that these growths have occurred between the fifteenth and thirty-second years of age, slightly more often in women. They usually occur in the posterior and lateral wall, reaching from under the vocal cords, as far as the fourth tracheal ring. They were discovered in seven of the eleven cases with the laryngoscope. They form rather large, irregular tumors, with broad bases, firmly attached to the underlying structures. They consist of typical thyroid tissue, and in some the connective tissue is more abundant than in the normal thyroid structure.

Two views have been advanced to explain the presence of these growths in the trachea.

The first may be called the embryonal theory. According to this, they represent embryonic rudiments of the thyroid gland, which have been misplaced and begin to increase in size from the time of puberty. This view is taken by Heise, Radestock, Roth and Bruns. In favor of it is the location of the growth in most of the cases on the posterior wall, and in one case in a bronchus; the presence in one case of a fine membrane between the growth and the thyroid gland; the fact that in some cases there was no enlargement of the thyroid gland, and, lastly, that it is unusual for non-malignant growths to penetrate into foreign places.

The second: Ziemssen and Paltauf ascribed them to an abnormal activity on the part of the thyroid gland cells, which grow in between the thyroid and cricoid cartilages and a weakness of the cells of the tissue between the two. Paltauf materially strengthened Ziemssen's ideas through careful histological examinations. He found in his case that the thyroid gland was intimately connected with the tracheal rings and that it had grown through and was intimately mixed with the inner growths. Baurowicz accepts this explanation and notes that later on Bruns has also done the same.

SYMPTOMS. Symptoms of these various growths are only apparent when there is a considerable grade of narrowing of the trachea. They may therefore have existed for many years without having been

FIG. 1.

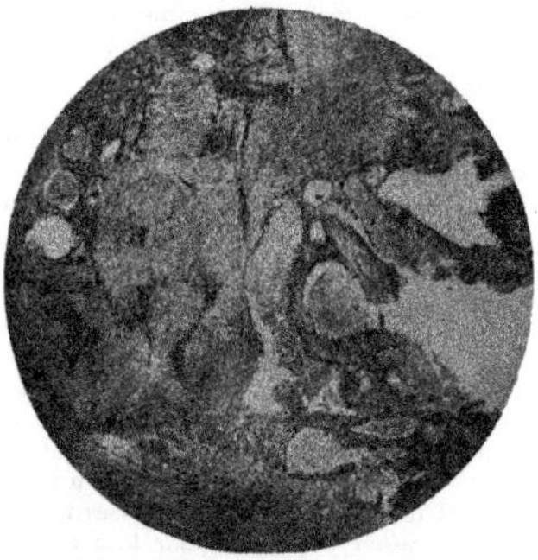

Photomicrograph, Dr. C. W. Potter. × 35. Zeiss planar, 20 mm. Gives a general idea of the structure of the tumor. The relative amounts of acini, fibrous tissue, and cell nests is shown. The central open space in the centre of the photograph is due to a tear in the section.

noticed by the patient. Usually shortness of breath is the first thing to attract the patient's attention. This may suddenly lead to an attack of suffocation to which the patient succumbs, as in the cases in which pedunculated polyps have closed the opening to a main bronchus or where a similar tumor is rent away by a fit of coughing and lodged in the glottis. Nicaise thinks that sudden and fatal suffocation can be explained by a spasm of the trachea.

The voice is usually enfeebled, rarely, however, to the point of aphonia. Hoarseness may or may not be present.

In cases of malignant growths there is also pain on deglutition.

Secondary symptoms are those of diffuse bronchiectasis, catarrhal bronchitis, and atelectasis following them.

Unless relieved death occurs (*a*) by suffocation, which may be sudden or gradual; (*b*) by pneumonia, lobar or lobular, (*c*) hemorrhage from the erosion of large arteries of the neck. At autopsy there has been noted dilatation of the large bronchi, congestion of the larynx and the trachea, emphysema of the lungs and dilatation of the heart.

DIAGNOSIS. The diagnosis of tracheal growths has been rendered much simpler by the inventions of the laryngoscope and tracheoscope.

We are concerned with (1) the presence of a tracheal growth; (2) the nature of the growth.

1. As a rule, this is very easy. Progressive dyspnœa with a pure voice would lead us to suspect it after the exclusion of tumor of the

FIG. 2.

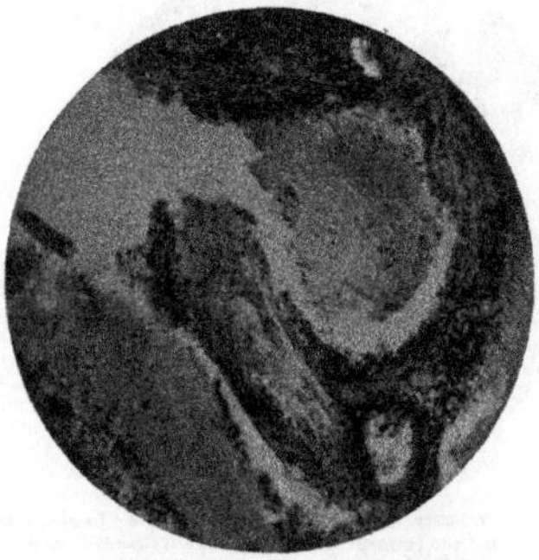

Photomicrograph, Dr. C. W. Potter. × 100. Zeiss planar, 20 mm. Acini, lined by a single layer of cells, some columnar, others irregularly shaped. The nuclei are well stained. Between the acini are strands of fibrous tissue. Section stained with hæmatoxylin and eosin.

thyroid gland and œsophagus or aneurysm of the aorta. With the laryngoscope, growths high up in the trachea, as in our case, are immediately recognized. Growths low down are much more difficult to see. However, by putting the patient in Killain's position, the lower parts of the trachea are usually very easily seen. Cases in which both these methods fail may be examined by introducing a tube directly into the trachea, after the method of Schroetter.

2. To help make a diagnosis of the nature of the tumor, we should determine the location, form, size, color, consistency, method of attachment and mobility of the growth. Even with these data it is

only rarely that a correct diagnosis of its nature is made. Papilloma, the most frequent growth, occurs usually on the anterior wall, as a pea-sized or larger growth, usually multiple, and of cauliflower-shape. It occurs at all ages. Clinically, primary tuberculous growths could not be differentiated from them. Fibroma, the next most frequent growth, occurs with equal frequency on the anterior and posterior walls, sometimes pedunculated, sometimes with broad base. It varies in size from a small berry to a walnut, is of a reddish color, and usually occurs in middle-aged persons. Adenoma or fibroadenoma, as well as sarcoma, would be very difficult to differentiate from the last-described group. To be distinguished from the adeno-

FIG. 3

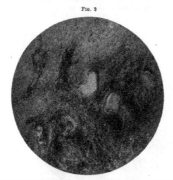

Photomicrograph, Dr. C. W. Potter. Zeiss planar, 20 mm. Ocular 3. Demonstrates the cell nests. These consist of round and polygonal cells, lying between strands of connective tissue. Several acini are also shown in this specimen. Section stained with hæmatoxylin and eosin. (Cramer's isochromatic plates used with all of these photographs.)

mata are the cystoadenomata occurring on the posterior surface of the trachea, as these originate from glands behind the muscular layer. Chondroma and chondro-osteoma appear as fine or coarse, irregular groups of nodules, scattered over the tracheal wall, usually only on the cartilaginous parts. They are very hard on palpation with the laryngeal probe. Intratracheal thyroid growths form large, irregular masses, firmly attached to the tracheal wall by a broad base. The presence of a struma of the thyroid gland will aid in making a correct diagnosis. Carcinoma forms, as a rule, a flat extensive infiltration of the mucous membrane and submucous tissues, but may occur as a circumscribed growth, or even as a single pedunculated polyp. It occurs more frequently in men and from the ages of forty to sixty years. Symptoms develop more quickly than in the non-malignant growths.

PROGNOSIS. The prognosis is, if not operated on, most unfavorable. When operated on, the growths higher up in the trachea offer a more favorable prognosis. Of 14 benign cases reported by Lemoine as having been operated on, 10 recovered; of 12 cases not operated on, 10 died. Carcinoma is, of course, the worst form. This runs its course if untreated in from one month to two years from the onset of the symptoms. It tends, however, to remain localized, rarely perforating the trachea, and has never penetrated to the thyroid gland. Metastases to the lymph glands and organs are rare. Sarcoma of the trachea may exist for a long time. Schroetter's case was observed for twenty years.

TREATMENT. The treatment may be palliative or radical. Palliative treatment is of use in cases which are inoperable on account of the extent of the growth, as in extensive carcinoma. It consists in the use of tracheal tubes (Schroetter's or O'Dwyer's) or in tracheotomy. If the tumor is in the upper part of the trachea the ordinary tracheal cannula will suffice. If lower down a long cannula (König's or Bruns') may be used.

Radical treatment consists in excising the growth. This may be done by an endotracheal operation or by a laryngotracheotomy. The endotracheal operation may be done with the aid of the laryngeal mirror or with the tracheoscope. It is suitable for pedunculated benign growths or for benign growths with not too broad a base. They can be removed with the cold or galvanocautery snare, with forceps, or with the ring knife. The extirpation of malignant tumors by this method, as in the cases reported by Koschier, is not good surgery where a complete extirpation is possible.

BIBLIOGRAPHY.

Balser. Virchow's Archiv, 1883, Bd. xci. S. 67.

Bayer. Abstract in Centralblatt f. Laryngologie, Rhinologie und Verwandte Wissenschaft., 1900, S. 271.

Brauer, L. Deutsche Archiv f. klinische Medicine, 1898–99, Bd. lxii. S. 4037.

Bruns, P. Heymann's Handbuch der Laryngologie und Rhinologie, 1898, Bd. i., Heft 2, S. 952.

Baurowicz. Fraenkel's Archiv f. Laryngologie und Rhinologie, 1898, Bd. viii.

Cohen. Ashhurst's Encyclopedia of Surgery, 1889, vol. v. p. 339.

Diamond, T. B. Abstract in Centralblatt f. Laryngologie, Rhinologie und Verwandte Wissenschaften, 1902, S. 252.

Freer, Otto. Journal of the American Medical Association, March 1, 1901, p. 876.

Gleitsmann, T. W. The Laryngoscope, February, 1902, p. 122.

Glechsman. Quoted by Lemoine.

Glockner. Virchow's Archiv, 1900, Bd. clx. S. 583.

Hanszel, F. Abstract in Centralblatt f. Laryngologie, Rhinologie und Verwandte Wissenschaften, 1900, S. 308.

Johanni and Kaufmann. Fraenkel's Archiv f. Laryngologie und Rhinologie, 1903, Bd. xiv.

Killain, G. Abstract in Year-book of Eye, Ear, Nose, and Throat, 1902.

Koschier, H. Wien. klinische Wochenschrift, 1897, Bd. xi. S. 1006.

Koschier, H. Wien. medicinische Wochenschrift, 1898, Bd. xlviii. S. 1673.

Kraus. Zeitschrift f. Heilkunde, Bd. vii. S. 245.
Lemoine. Étude sur les Tumeurs de la Trachée, thèse, Paris, 1900.
Levi, Ch. Abstract in Centralblatt f. Laryngologie, Rhinologie und Verwandte Wissenschaft., 1900, S. 98.
Mackenzie, J. N. Archives of Medicine, October, 1882, p. 107.
Manasse. Virchow's Archiv, 1900, Bd. clix. S. 117.
Prota. Abstract in the Centralblatt f. Laryngologie, Rhinologie und Verwandte Wissenschaft., 1900, S. 306.
Schmidt, Moritz. Die Krankheiten der oberen Luftweg, Berlin, 1903.
Schroetter, H. von. Deutsche medicinische Wochenschrift, 1901, No. 28.
Theisen, F. THE AMERICAN JOURNAL OF THE MEDICAL SCIENCES, 1902, p. 1051.
Ziegler. Special Pathological Anatomy, vol. ii. p. 781.

A CASE OF SUPPOSED SARCOMA OF THE CHEST WALL SYMPTOMATICALLY CURED BY MEANS OF THE X-RAY.

BY JAMES P. MARSH, M.D.,
SURGEON TO THE SAMARITAN HOSPITAL AND TROY ORPHAN ASYLUM, AND RADIOGRAPHER TO THE SAMARITAN HOSPITAL, TROY, N. Y.

THE general profession has accepted the efficacy of the x-ray therapy as regards external malignant conditions and certain diseases of the skin. The profession has also come to the conclusion that the x-rays are of no value in cases in which there is healthy tissue intervening between the growth and the impinging rays. This latter position seems to be very tenaciously held by the surgical cult. But perhaps the surgeons are excusable, inasmuch as the x-ray men themselves are very much divided as to the benefit to be derived in deep-seated malignant growths.

All of us who have had any experience have many failures to record. We have had many bitter disappointments, as we have seen the poor wretches sustained by a last flaring spark of hope gradually become worse as each treatment was given. Indeed, I doubt not that cases have occurred to all x-ray men in which the x-rays have seemed to stimulate the morbid process, to hasten metastasis.

Some of our good x-ray brethren appear to have nothing to show but enthusiasm, and others to be industriously trying to hide their light under a bushel. It seems, therefore, good and expedient, where we do have a success in deep-seated conditions, that it should be placed upon record for the encouragement of the x-ray fraternity, if for no other reason. Such reports ought to be in detail, so that everyone can tell at a glance just how the desired effect has been produced.

On December 27, 1902, R. F. entered my service at the Samaritan Hospital, having been referred by Drs. E. D. Ferguson and H. C. Gordinier. The patient is a schoolboy, aged sixteen years, very small for his age, white, and a native of the United States. He complains of a prominent tumor, which evidently takes its origin from the ribs, immediately beneath and just inside of the mid-portion of the left breast. This growth is not connected with the mammary gland.

The patient's father is dead; cause unknown. His mother and one sister are living and well.

R. F. has not had any of the diseases of childhood and has always enjoyed excellent health. He first noticed this tumor in May, 1902, and it has gradually increased in size until now it is about three inches in diameter and projects from the normal line of the chest about two inches. There has not been any pain in the growth and no particular inconvenience from it. His appetite has always been good and he has not lost flesh.

During the summer of 1902 he went to the Presbyterian Hospital, New York City. I understand Dr. A. J. McCosh saw him at that time and made a diagnosis of sarcoma. Dr. McCosh refused to operate, as he did not think that it would be of any service to the lad.

The patient is of fair complexion, and, although small for his age, well built and nourished. His expression is cheerful. The pupils are equal and react to light and distance. His tongue protrudes straight, no tremor, and it is covered with a thin, white coating. Examination of the lungs, heart, and arteries is normal. The liver dulness is normal and the spleen is not palpable. Abdomen, kidneys, genital organs, mental condition, cranial nerves, electric reactions, motion, and sensation are all normal.

Upon his left chest wall is found the tumor described above. This growth is quite firm and closely attached to the ribs.

Urine, 1022, acid; no albumin. There is no note as to whether Bence Jones' albumose was looked for or not. Hæmoglobin, 92 per cent. Reds, 4,440,000; whites, 9000.

Diagnosis. Sarcoma of the left chest wall.

The following detailed line of treatment was instituted: Queen, 12-inch coil. R. Friedländer tube, which had been gradually adapted to high penetration work.

Abbreviations. = 7 in. means the length of the spark backed up at the coil terminals when the tube was in operation. D. means the distance of the nearest point on the surface of the tube from the nearest point on the surface of the patient's body. T. means the length of exposure in minutes. The face was protected by two thicknesses of T-lead tin-foil.

December 29th. = 7 in. D., 10 in. T., 10 m.

30th. Complains of headache. = 7 in. D., 10 in. T., 10 m.

31st. This morning complains of headache, and the temperature, which had been normal, went up to 101° F. = 7 in. D., 10 in. T., 10 m.

January 1, 1903. Temperature fell to 97.2° F. Patient transferred to out-patient department.

Jan. 3d. = 7 in. D., 5 in. T., 10 m.

6th. = 5 in. D., 5 in. T., 10 m. The growth now measures $4\frac{1}{2}$ inches vertically by 3 inches transversely by $1\frac{3}{4}$ inches above the general surface at its highest point. It is quite hard to the touch and is firmly attached to the ribs and has enlarged veins running over its apex.

8th. = 8 in. D., 8 in. T., 10 m.

10th. = 8 in. D., 8 in. T., 10 m.

13th. = 8 in. D., 5 in. T., 10 m. The boy's mother thinks that the growth is smaller and softer. The patient begins to show an undoubted cachexia.

15th. = 8 in. D., 8 in. T., 10 m.

17th. = 8 in. D., 8 in. T., 10 m.

19th. = 8 in. D., 8 in. T., 10 m.

22d. = 8 in. D., 8 in. T., 10 m. Has had la grippe. In reaction. Growth smaller.

25th. = 8 in. D., 8 in. T., 10 m.

March 2d. = 8 in. D., 8 in. T., 10 m.

4th. = 8 in. D., 8 in. T., 10 m. Reaction marked. Looks very cachectic.

22d. = 8 in. D., 8 in. T., 10 m. Growth very much smaller.

25th. = 8 in. D., 8 in. T., 10 m.

27th. = 8 in. D., 8 in. T., 10 m.

30th. = 8 in. D., 8 in. T., 10 m.

April 1st. = 8 in. D., 8 in. T., 10 m.

3d. = 8 in. D., 8 in. T., 10 m.

6th. = 8 in. D., 8 in. T., 10 m. Reaction again appearing.

20th. = 5 in. D., 8 in. T., 10 m.

22d. = 5 in. D., 8 in. T., 10 m. Growth has entirely disappeared, and the patient has a good color and says that he feels perfectly well.

24th. = 5 in. D., 8 in. T., 10 m.

May 1st. = 5 in. D., 8 in. T., 10 m.

Capitulation. 26 treatments = $7\frac{7}{26}$ in. D., $7\frac{23}{26}$ in. T., 260 m.

On March 6, 1904, nearly one year after the disappearance of the growth, I heard indirectly, through his physician, that this boy was entirely well, without the slightest evidence of the tumor.

CHRONIC INTERSTITIAL NEPHRITIS IN THE YOUNG.

By Jose L. Hirsh, A.B., M.D.,

PROFESSOR OF PATHOLOGY IN THE UNIVERSITY OF MARYLAND.

It is true that chronic interstitial nephritis is no longer regarded as essentially a disease of old age, yet all authorities agree that it is an extremely rare condition in the young. As the disease is in the majority of instances associated with arteriosclerotic changes, we naturally expect to find the condition more frequent at the time of life when this alteration in the bloodvessels begins to appear. Osler[1] says, "The most common form of contracted kidney seen in this country is secondary to arteriosclerosis and seen in men over forty years who have worked hard, eaten freely, and taken alcohol in excess." Senator[3] asserts that the disease rarely begins before the thirtieth to fortieth year, and is most commonly observed in the fiftieth to sixtieth year. Flint[2] states that the disease is extremely rare in infancy and childhood, and that in an analysis of 102 cases, not a single one occurred under fourteen years of age. We find similar statements in all the text-books on the subject; still we do find some reference to it in some of the works on pediatrics.

It is not difficult to understand its rarity in childhood when we consider the chief causes leading to contraction of the kidney. Most common among them we find gout, chronic lead poisoning, alcoholism, overfeeding, chronic syphilis, and diabetes mellitus, conditions acting slowly and for the greater part associated with adult life. The relation of arteriosclerosis and kidney disease is still uncertain; either may be primary to the other; in a certain number of cases kidney disease may follow arteriosclerosis, on the other hand the arteriosclerosis may depend on the general rise of blood pressure due to the contracted kidney.

The causes cited are seldom met with in children: add to this the slow and insidious manner of the disease and its infrequency in children is readily explicable.

It is of interest to note that while in adults the proportion of cases of chronic interstitial nephritis in males to females is about 2½ to 1 (Senator), from the number of cases which I have been able to collect in the literature I find that a larger proportion of female than male children are affected.

That this form of chronic nephritis may occur in adolescence and even in childhood has been abundantly proven by clinical observations and autopsy records. Heubner[4] collected a series of 65 cases of nephritis in childhood from his private practice and hospital records, of these 4 were of the type of contracted kidney; while none of his cases came to autopsy, the urinary examinations with the associated cardiac and vascular changes leave little doubt as to the variety of the lesions. He further states that there were but 30 cases on record in which autopsies were made.

Of Dickinson's series of 308 cases, 1 occurred between eleven and twenty years.

Ashby and Wright[5] state that 5 cases have come under their personal observations, 3 cases in girls, aged eleven, ten, and seven years respectively, and 2 cases in boys, aged five and two years; all these cases came to autopsy and the clinical diagnosis was substantiated by the post-mortem findings. Gutherie[6] collected 7 cases, between five and fourteen years, all confirmed by autopsy. Steiner and Neuretter[7] report 6 cases with autopsy. It is highly probable, however, that several of the cases of Ashby and Wright, of Gutherie and Steiner are included in Heubner's series of 30 cases.

More recently Brill and Libman[8] have reported a case of primary chronic interstitial nephritis in a girl aged fourteen years, confirmed by autopsy. This case presents several points of interest, being associated with hemorrhages into the lungs, spleen, and mesentery, general chronic arteritis, with calcified deposits in the liver and probably cerebral hemorrhage (the brain was not removed). Heubner[9] calls attention to the fact that of the cases collected by him, only 7 were primary in nature, that is, were not preceded by an acute attack of the disease; and he is of the opinion that it is almost impossible in any individual case to know if there has been a pre-existing inflammation. We are to regard those cases only as primary which develop insidiously without any evidences of previons involvement; no matter when the symptoms first show themselves they are already those pertaining to the chronic forms.

That acute inflammation of the kidneys may occur in infancy and childhood, not only following scarlet fever but many other infectious diseases, is well known.

Both Epstein[10] and Koplik[11] have shown that acute nephritis not infrequently occurs in infants as the result of gastroenteritis.

Henoch[12] was the first to note the kidney complications occasionally following varicella. Holt[13] reports several cases of acute nephritis following pneumonia. Filia[14] reports 5 cases of post-impetiginous nephritis, the infectious material gaining access through the skin to the lymphatic circulation and thence the kidney through the blood current. Perl[15] notes a case of acute nephritis following vaccination. Mettenheimer[16] notes several cases following pertussis. Freeman[17] observes the comparative frequent complication of this disease in children following influenza.

The etiological factors underlying the contraction of the kidney of childhood are often as obscure as the disease is insidious.

Weigert,[18] Baginsky,[19] Westphal,[20] and Arnold[21] have described the condition as congenital. Sutherland and Walker[22] regard congenital syphilis as playing an important role in the etiology of the disease.

Heredity seems to play a part in certain cases, as in the remarkable instance cited by Dickinson,[23] Bright's disease appearing in one family for four generations. Pel[24] records an extremely interesting family history which showed in three generations of one family 18 cases of chronic nephritis. Almost all the members of the family affected had the disease for years, but reached an advanced age and almost without exception died in uræmic coma. It is also striking that one of the children died of acute nephritis following chicken-pox, an extremely rare complication of this mild affection.

This would seem to show that this child was congenitally subject to the disease. Romme[91] likewise relates a family history showing 18 cases of nephritis in one family in three generations. In the case of Brill and Libman the three oldest children had Bright's disease.

Two cases of contracted kidney in the young have recently come under my observation, both associated with alterations in the blood-vessels, though of an entirely different nature:

Case I.—C. W., white boy, aged fifteen years, was brought to the University Hospital on account of an uncontrollable hemorrhage from the gums following the extraction of a tooth the day previous. He complained of being short of breath and feeling very weak. He was put to bed and continuous pressure applied to the gum, which stopped the bleeding in a few hours. The following history was then obtained: The family history presents nothing of importance. As far as could be learned no other member of the family presented a history of kidney disease.

Patient had been a strong, robust child, had measles at six years, and chicken-pox at eight years, otherwise he had never been confined to bed. He attended school until his thirteenth year, after which he did light work about an office. About one year ago he began to complain of feeling very tired on slight exertion; his appetite began to fail and his sleep became restless. He noted that it was necessary to get up at night to empty his bladder, and this has continued up to the present time. Of late he has been having headache at irregular intervals, and the day previous to his entrance to the hospital he had an attack of especial severity which was associated with pain in the upper jaw and for which the tooth had been extracted. He had never had hemorrhage before and there were no bleeders in his family.

Present Condition. Patient is pale; the mucous membranes are almost colorless. The pupils are slightly irregular, but respond to light and accommodation. The neck is short and there is visible pulsations of the carotids. The chest is well formed; the lungs are normal, except a slight rale occasionally heard at the base of both lungs. The heart is rather tumultuous; the apex beat is noted most prominent in the fifth intercostal space, and just without the nipple line. The area of cardiac dulness is increased both toward the right and left; there is a soft systolic blow at the apex, and the second aortic is markedly accentuated. The radial pulse is full, of moderate tension, though compressible, but is completely cut off with some difficulty; there are 80 beats to the minute.

The liver extends one finger's breadth below the costal margin; the spleen is not palpable. There is no œdema about the extremities. Temperature, 99; respiration, 24.

Urinary examination showed the urine to be increased in quantity, though the exact amount was not noted. Color, light; specific gravity, 1012; no sugar; albumin, a very small amount by Heller's ring test. Casts: a few hyaline and an occasional granular cast were noted. Repeated examinations during patient's stay in the hospital gave about the same results, although on several examinations albumin was absent.

Blood examination showed 3,700,000 red blood corpuscles, 6500 white. The coagulation time was not diminished.

After rest in bed for a few days, patient's condition seemed to improve; however, after being about the wards for a week there was noted beginning œdema about the ankles, this gradually increased though at no time was it sufficient to cause any inconvenience. Dyspnœa became more marked and patient died five weeks after entering hospital.

Autopsy, Four Hours after Death. Body length 120 cm. Muscles flabby, skeletal development good. Rigor mortis absent. Œdema of the lower extremities. Both pleural cavities contain about 200 c.c. of a straw-colored fluid. The lungs are congested and on pressure a large amount of frothy serum exudes from the cut surface. The heart is markedly enlarged; this is chiefly due to hypertrophy of the left ventricle, which measures 2 cm. in thickness; the right ventricle measures 9 mm. The valves show no decided changes; both coronaries are somewhat thicker than normal. Weight of heart 300 grams.

The left kidney is smaller than normal; it weighs 68 grams; size 8 x 4 x 2 cm. The capsule is adherent, and when removed the outer surface of the cortex is seen to be granular; cysts are scattered over the surface. The substance of the kidney is firm, the cortex is reduced in size, and the entire section has a clouded appearance. The right kidney presents the same general appearance; weighs 80 grams; size, 8 x 6 x 3 cm.

The liver shows evidences of passive congestion; weighs 1200 grams. The gastrointestinal tract shows a few punctate hemorrhages throughout the mucosa. Spleen and pancreas normal.

The aorta is decidedly atheromatous; there are several calcareous plates in the dorsal and lumbar regions, spots of fatty degeneration are present throughout its whole extent.

Anatomical Diagnosis. Chronic passive congestion of the lungs and liver; hypertrophy of the heart; chronic interstitial nephritis; arteriosclerosis of the aorta.

Microscopic examination of the kidneys shows a great increase of the interstitial connective tissue; many of the glomeruli are shrunken and the capsule of Bowman thickened; some of the glomeruli are completely replaced by fibrous tissue; the cells of the tubules are degenerated, and the walls of the bloodvessels are much thickened. The sections show an advanced stage of contracted kidney.

The chief point of interest in this case besides the marked interstitial nephritis is the marked arteriosclerosis of the aorta. Simnitzky[26] has made a careful study of arteriosclerosis in young individuals, and in a recent communication presents a series of 38 cases varying in age from four to twenty-four years. He states that he has found the condition present to some extent in 27.5 per cent. of all cases up to the twenty-fifth year. He believes the infectious diseases play an important role in the etiology of the disease.

Ballantyne[27] found decided atheromatous changes in the aorta and pulmonary arteries in an eight months' fœtus. Marfan[28] describes similar lesions in three boys, aged nine, twelve, and thirteen years respectively. Sanne[29] mentions a case of arteritis chronica in a child aged two years, and an aortic aneurysm in a boy aged thirteen years.

The influence of heredity must not be lost sight of in these cases. Just as contracted kidney may be found in one family for several generations, so may changes in the bloodvessels. Osler speaks of this as "a tendency which cannot be explained in any other way than that in the make-up of the machine bad material was used for the tubing."

Case II.—L. B., white, unmarried female, aged eighteen years, entered the University Hospital on July 12, 1903, complaining of inability to control her bladder and frequent micturition. The family history is bad. Her maternal grandmother, mother, and two maternal aunts died of cancer of the breast. Her father suffered with some stomach trouble for eighteen months prior to his death. Brothers and sisters are healthy, although one sister, aged twenty-three years, has never menstruated. There is no history of tuberculosis or kidney disease.

Patient was never a very strong child; has had measles, pertussis, and diphtheria. Began menstruating at ten years and has continued normal since. When fourteen years old patient fell from a tree, injured her back, and was unable to move about for one year; she has suffered now and then from this trouble to the present time. She says that her "kidney trouble" began two years ago.

Patient is anæmic, her general development corresponds to a girl of about fourteen years; breasts are but slightly developed. Pupils are regular and respond to light and accommodation. Diffused moist rales are present over both lungs. Area of cardiac dulness is increased, the apex beat is 1 cm. without the mammary line; no murmurs are to be heard, but the second aortic sound is accentuated. Abdominal organs are negative. Tension of radial pulse is not increased, soft and easily compressible, no evidences of sclerosis. Beats 80.

Ophthalmological examination is negative.

Urine is increased in quantity; specific gravity, 1010; light color; no sugar; small amount of albumin; few hyaline casts; some pus cells. In the lower dorsal region there is a protrusion of the spinal process, which is painful on pressure, and is probably an old Pott's disease. There is some anasarca of lower extremities. Patient's condition continued unaltered until July 25th, when she began to complain of headache, she gradually became dull, and two days later comatose, and died July 28th.

Autopsy, Twelve Hours after Death. Body length 175 cm. Very slight build. Skeletal development small, muscular development good. Rigor mortis well marked. The tenth and eleventh dorsal vertebræ are protuberant, and the skin over same is excoriated.

The heart is slightly enlarged; there is no abnormality about the valves; the wall of the left ventricle is hypertrophied, measures

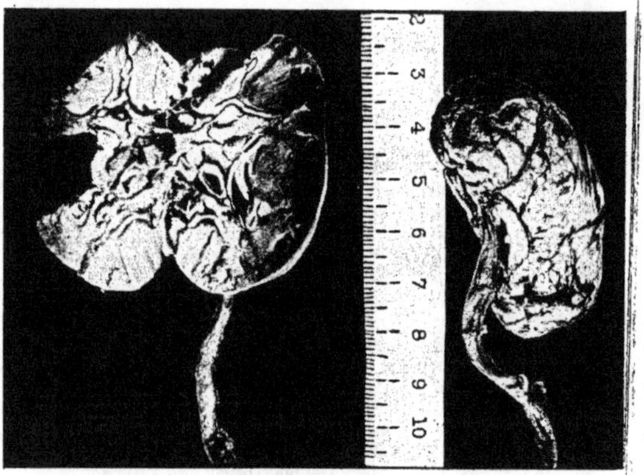

Kidneys in Case II. Actual size.

15 mm. in thickness; wall of right ventricle measures 7 mm. in thickness. Weight of heart 175 grams. The lungs are somewhat small, dark in color, much congested and crepitate throughout; there are no evidences of tubercle. The spleen and liver are somewhat smaller than normal, though normal in appearance. The gastrointestinal tract is normal.

The kidneys are extremely small. The right kidney measures 5 x 2.5 x 2 cm. and weighs 18 grams.; the left kidney measures 4.5 x 3 x 1.5 cm. and weighs 22 grams. Capsules of both kidneys are slightly adherent, and the cortex granular. On section the cortex is narrow, very firm and of a light color; there is no definite boundary line between the cortex and medulla; the pyramids are likewise contracted and have the appearance of scarred tissue.

The uterus appears somewhat smaller than normal; length 5½ cm., width at fundus 4 cm. The ovaries are well developed and show several false corpora lutea. Bladder normal.

The aorta is abnormally small; at its origin it measures 4.8 cm. in diameter; just below the diaphragm it measures 3.5 cm. in diameter. Throughout its entire extent it admits the small finger with some difficulty. There are no evidences of atheroma.

Both the renal arteries are small.

Examination of the inner surface of the 10th and 11th vertebræ shows a calcareous mass between them, an old tuberculous lesion.

Anatomical Diagnosis. Hypertrophy of the heart; congestion of the lungs; chronic interstitial nephritis; healed Pott's disease; congenital narrowness of the aorta and renal arteries.

Microscopic examination of all the organs with the exception of the kidneys exhibit nothing of especial interest. The alterations in the kidneys affect all the elements, the glomeruli, the tubules, the interstitial connective tissue and the bloodvessels. Many of the glomeruli are shrunken, some appear as a hyaline ball, the capsule of Bowman is thickened; other glomeruli are hypertrophied and congested. Scattered throughout the cortex in areas is seen a small-cell infiltration. In many parts the tubes are diminished in size or completely obliterated; in others they are dilated and filled with degenerated epithelial products. The intertubular connective tissue is thickened throughout, giving the medulla in places a fibroid appearance. The walls of the smaller bloodvessels are much thickened.

It may prove of interest to call attention to the size and weight of some of the reported cases of contracted kidney in the young.

No.	Author.	Age.	Sex.	Weight.	Size.	Combined weight of kidneys.
1	Barlow	6 years	F.	R. 13 grm. L. 21 "	5 × 4 × 0.5 cm. 6 × 3 × 1.5 "	38 grm.
2	Ashby and Wright . .	11 "	F.	R. 75 " L. 24 "	Not stated. " "	99 "
3	Ashby and Wright . .	12 "	M.	R. 38 " L. 37 "	" " " "	75 "
4	Bull	13 "	F.	R. 35 " L. 20 "	7.5 × 4 cm. 5 × 3 "	55 "
5	Hanford	13 "	F.	R. 60 " L. 15 "	8½ × 4½ × 2 cm. 5 × 4 × 2 "	75 "
6	Brill and Libman . .	14 "	F.	R. 59 " L. 34.5 "	9 × 4 × 3 cm. 6 × 3.5 × 2.5 cm.	93.5 "
7	Hirsh	18 "	F.	R. 22 " L. 18 "	5 × 2½ × 2 cm. 4½ × 3 × 1.5 cm.	40 "
8	Weigert	6 weeks	...	R. .... L.	1.7×1.0×0.5 cm. 2.0×1.1×0.4 "	Congenital.

The relationship between congenital narrowness of the aorta and arterial system and primary atrophy of the kidney has been noted by Lancereaux,[30] and by Besancon and Poillon.[31]

Bizot gives the average diameter of the aorta at its origin as 7 cm. in males and 6.4 cm. in females. Beneke gives the average in youth as 6 cm. The authors mentioned found in the narrow aortas a circumference of 4.2 to 5.2 cm.

Bibliography.

1. Osler. Practice of Medicine.
2. Flint. Practice of Medicine, 1886.
3. Senator. Die Erkrankungen d. Nieren, Nothnagel's Pathologie und Therapie.
4. Heubner. Ueber Chronische Nephritis im Kindersalter, Berlin, 1897.
5. Ashby and Wright. Text-book, 1900.
6. Gutherie. Chronic Interstitial Nephritis in Childhood, Lancet, 1897, vol. i.
7. Steiner and Neuretter. Prager Vierteljahr., Bd. cv. p. 74.
8. Brill and Libman. A Contribution to the Subjects of Chronic Interstitial Nephritis in the Young, Journal of Experimental Medicine, 1889, vol. iv.
9. Heubner. Loc. cit
10. Epstein. Prager med. Wochenschr., 1881, No. 33.
11. Koplik. Nephritis Complicating Gastroenteritis of Infants, Medical Record, April, 1899.
12. Henoch. Vorlesungen über Kinderkrank., Berlin, 1895.
13. Holt. Archives Pediatrics, April, 1892.
14 Filia. Review, Medical Record, May, 1903.
15. Perl. Berl. klin. Wochenschr., 1893, No. 28.
16. Mettenheimer. Jahrb. f. Kinderheilk., Bd. xxxii., S. 383.
17. Freeman. Nephritis of Influenza, Transactions of the Pediatric Society, 1892.
18. Weigert. Volkmann's Saml. klin. Vorträge, 1879, Nos. 162, 163.
19. Baginsky. Lehrbuch der Kinderkrank., Berlin, 1896.
20. Westphal. Berl. klin. Wochenschr., 1890, No. 29.
21. Arnold. Ziegler's Beiträge, Bd. viii.
22. Sutherland and Walker. British Medical Journal, 1903, vol. i. p. 959.
23. Dickinson. Diseases of Kidney, London, 1877, vol. ii.
24. Pel. Zeitschr. f. klin. Med., 1899.
25. Romme. Le presse médical, December 23, 1899.
26. Simnitzky. Ueber haufigkeit von Arterio-sclerotischen Veranderung in der Aorten junglicher Individuen, Zeitschr. f. Heilkunde., 1903, Bd. xxiv.
27. Ballantyne. Manual of Antenatal Pathology, 1902.
28. Marfan. Semaine méd., 1901, No. 13.
29. Sanne. Jahrb. f. Kinderheilk., Bd. xxv. p. 221.
30. Lancereaux. Monograph, Paris. Cited by Senator.
31. Besancon and Poillon. Paris, 1889. Cited by Senator.

KERNIG'S SIGN:

WITH REPORT OF CASES WHERE THE ANGLE HAS BEEN ACCURATELY DETERMINED.

By Joseph L. Miller, M.D.,
of Chicago.

Kernig, on September 21, 1882, read a paper before the St. Petersburg Medical Society on the presence of a sign which he considered pathognomonic for meningitis and which has since been known as Kernig's sign. This sign consists in inability to extend the leg fully when the thigh is at right angles to the trunk. Kernig made the test by having the patient sit on the edge of the bed with legs overhanging and then attempting to extend the legs. Osler first called attention to the fact that the sign could be elicited by having the patient lie on his back, and then, after flexing the thigh on the trunk to a right angle, an attempt is made to extend the leg on the thigh. This is a more satisfactory position, as it enables us to determine the angle with greater ease, and even very sick patients are not inconvenienced. Rudolph recommended making the test by first fully extending the leg, then flexing the thigh on the pelvis and measuring the angle at the hip, as by doing this only one angle need be gauged, while in the original method the thigh must first be placed at right angles to the trunk and then extend the leg. This I believe is an unnecessary refinement, as it is not essential that the angle of the thigh to the trunk be exactly a right angle, but approximately so, a point which can be sufficiently gauged by the eye; and, second, on account of the more irregular contour of the parts at the hip, it is more difficult to measure the angle with an instrument than it is at the knee. In the normal individual the leg can be almost completely extended when the thigh is at right angles to the trunk. Kernig reported that in case the sign was positive, the angle was about 135 degrees, but might reach 90 degrees, and since then the generally accepted view has been that an angle of 135 degrees or less is a positive Kernig. He called especial attention to the fact that in a patient with positive signs the leg could be completely extended, if the precaution was not taken to place the thigh at approximately a right angle to the trunk. He also reported that the sign might be present in the arms. He considered that this was an early and constant sign in meningitis, often persisting until the patient was well along in convalescence. His conclusions were based upon the examination of 15 cases of meningitis, the diagnosis being confirmed in 8 by autopsy. Thirteen of these cases were of the cerebrospinal form, 1 tubercular, and 1 suppurative. He also obtained the sign in spinal caries, pachymeningitis hemorrhagica, localized meningitis from otitis media, 1 case of hyperæmia of the meninges which he reports was possibly a beginning tuberculosis, chronic leptomeningitis, and a slight Kernig in a case of œdema of the pia.

Kernig's paper did not excite much attention. The first published confirmation of his results was made by Friis, in 1887, and again in 1892. Since then numerous reports have been made. All of these have emphasized the diagnostic value of the sign, and yet many of the recent works on medicine, neurology, or diagnosis fail to mention the sign; others merely refer to it without commenting on its value. None of these works report the various conditions, besides meningitis, where the sign is present or give accurate information as to what degree of flexor contraction constitutes the sign.

The lack of general knowledge of the subject is due, in part, to its unreliability. However, we have comparatively few signs which can be looked upon as pathognomonic, and lack of constancy merely lessens the value of the test, provided we are familiar with the source of error, and thus give it the proper weight.

Herrick reported 19 cases of meningitis: 9 cerebrospinal, 2 pneumococcus, 7 tubercular, 1 syphilitic. In 2 cases, 1 probably tubercular, the other following a pneumonia and associated with otitis media, the sign failed. Both of these cases were children, aged three and four years respectively, and the test was only made shortly before death, which may account for the result, as it has been noted that the rigidity of the neck may disappear or be much lessened just before death. In 1 case of probable tubercular meningitis, it was present in one leg, but not in a typical manner in the other. He examined 25 healthy individuals, in all of whom the sign was absent. In 100 cases of various troubles, the Kernig was present in only 2, 1 a gonorrhœal rheumatism of the knee, the patient having remained in bed with the legs flexed for several weeks, the other a subdural hemorrhage.

Netter has published two series of cases of meningitis, in all 72 in number, with positive Kernig in 91 per cent. In 1 of the negative cases the child had an advanced tuberculosis, in another the test was made only once.

Friis, of Copenhagen, in 1887, reported it present in 53 out of 60 cases. In 2 of the negative cases the test was doubtful, in 3 the examination could not be properly made, and in 2 it was absent.

In a later series in 1892, all of which were of the epidemic type, it was present in 21 out of 26 cases. He considered that there was no relation between the sign and the rigidity of the neck.

Bull found the sign present in a case of tuberculous meningitis, in a solitary tubercle of the cerebellum, with a few miliary tubercles in the overlying pia, and in a case of otitis media, with thrombosis of the transverse sinus and basal ecchymosis.

Blumm reports it present in 7 out of 9 cases of cerebrospinal meningitis.

Thyne, in a case with hemorrhage into the right lateral lobe of the cerebellum and the fourth ventricle.

Packard reported several negative cases: 1, a child, aged sixteen months, with general miliary tuberculosis, the membranes of brain and cord being involved, where daily examination gave negative results. In a second case of leptomeningitis following pneumonia, the sign was always absent. In a third case with miliary tubercles over the motor area of the cortex, repeated examinations were negative. He did not attach much importance to the sign in infants.

Magri refers to cases where, in uncomplicated typhoid and pneumonia, the sign was present, and to a case of his own where the patient had sciatica.

Sailer found the sign present in a case of focal encephalitis of the ascending parietal lobe with the overlying meninges congested, and in a patient where the diagnosis of unilateral lesion of the medulla was made.

Clark, in 2 cases of tubercular meningitis, never found the angle less than 150 degrees, and the sign was absent in a case of acute cerebrospinal meningitis of undetermined bacterial nature, where there was marked exudate over the thoracic cord.

Rudolph, by means of an instrument, measured the angle in 162 cases, found it less than 180 degrees in 60 per cent. of cases; 165 degrees or less in 0.4 per cent.; 135 degrees or less in 6 per cent. As above mentioned, his method was to measure the angle at the hip. Shields measured the angle in 100 cases, both febrile and afebrile, and in 5 found an angle of 120 degrees or less. Two of these were typhoid; in 1 unilateral, 100 degrees; the other bilateral, 110 degrees. In the former it did not disappear during convalescence. One case of uræmia, angle 110 degrees. The other 2 were hemiplegics, with angles of 115 degrees and 120 degrees respectively.

My own observations were confined chiefly: first, to acute infections—mainly typhoid and pneumonia; second, various forms of meningitis; third, central and peripheral nervous troubles; fourth, patients who had been confined to bed for several weeks, chiefly convalescents from acute infections and surgical cases. The material was obtained from the Cook County Hospital. The angle was measured by means of an inclinometer, an instrument of accuracy. On account of the irregular contour of the parts, it is, of course, impossible to obtain very exact measurements, even with an accurate instrument. All the tests were made with the patient in the dorsal position. The thigh was first placed at right angles to the trunk, then the leg was extended on the thigh until it either caused pain or could not be farther extended without using considerable force. Babinski's reflex was observed in most of the cases, and the results of this test are placed in the table.

In none of the cases examined was there an angle of 180 degrees, and in several healthy individuals it was impossible to obtain this angle without either allowing the thigh to recede from its position at right angles to the trunk, or using sufficient force to cause discomfort, the average angle being about 165 degrees.

An angle of 115 degrees or less has been considered a positive Kernig. This I believe is better than 135 degrees, as suggested by Kernig, as it excludes very few cases of meningitis, and an angle of 135 degrees is not infrequent in other conditions. A bilateral test was made in all cases. In the following table are summaries of the results:

Disease.	Total cases.	Kernig presents 115° or less.	Angle 120°.	Angle 125°.
Typhoid	48	4	5	9
Transverse myelitis	4	1		
Hemiplegia	17	7	2	2
Syphilitic spastic paraplegia	7	4	1	
Primary spastic paraplegia	1	1		
Carcinoma of spine	1	1		
Infantile paralysis	1	1		
Multiple neuritis	16	3	3	3
Sciatica	12	2	1	1
Delirium tremens	3	1		
Hysteria	3	...	...	1
Tetany	1	1		
Uræmia	2	2		
Illuminating-gas poisoning	1	1		
Cerebrospinal meningitis	6	4	1	
Tuberculous meningitis	3	3		
Diplococcus pneumoniæ meningitis	1			
Cerebrospinal syphilis	4	3		
Thigh fracture	3	1	1	
Pneumonia	22	3	...	5
Locomotor ataxia	6	1		
Lumbago	1			
Pericarditis	1			
Tetanus	1			
Status epilepticus	1			
Chronic chorea	1			
Acromegaly	1			
Paralysis agitans	4			
Syringomyelia	1			
Multiple sclerosis	2			
Typhoid spondylitis	1	...	...	1
Landry's paralysis	1			
Trichinosis	2	...	1	
Gonorrhœal myalgia	2			
Progressive muscular atrophy	1			
Amyotrophic lateral sclerosis	1			
Brain abscess	1	...	1	
Surgical cases exclusive of thigh fractures	8			

A Kernig was present in 45 of the 190 cases. Four of the 10 cases of meningitis failed to give the reaction, although 1 of these had an angle of 120 degrees. This was an epidemic cerebrospinal. One epidemic cerebrospinal had an angle of 150 degrees in the second week. The other negative cases were 1 each of pneumococcus and tuberculous meningitis, the latter giving an angle of 125 degrees. Strictly speaking, in only 2 cases of meningitis was there an absolute absence of the Kernig sign. In 1 of the cases the sign only appeared late, several days after a lumbar puncture, demonstrating the specific micro-organism. The diagnosis in all of these cases was verified either by lumbar puncture or autopsy.

Positive results were obtained in 7 of the 17 hemiplegias, and 4 others had an angle of 125 degrees or less. The sign was bilateral in 4 cases. One of these proved to be a hemorrhage into the ventricle. One was a double hemiplegia, with an interval of several weeks between the attacks. The other 2 were apparently uncomplicated hemiplegias, with no especial evidence indicating a ventricular or basal meningeal process.

Seven cases of Erb's syphilitic spastic paraplegia were examined: 4 gave the Kernig bilaterally, 1 had an angle of 120 degrees, the other 2 were completely negative. A case of primary spastic paraplegia was positive.

Of interest is the positive test in 3 of 16 cases of multiple neuritis, and 3 cases with an angle of 120 degrees, and 3 with an angle of 125 degrees. The sign was bilateral in all the cases. The majority of the cases examined were of several weeks' standing; 1 of the positive was of two months' duration, another one week. Only 3 cases of this series had an angle greater than 145 degrees.

Twelve sciaticas were examined, with 2 positive results. One of the negative cases had an angle of 125 degrees; another 120 degrees. The positive cases were both of a severe type. The patient with an angle of 125 degrees had a very mild attack.

Several have reported the sign present in uræmia. Only 2 cases were examined for the sign, and both were positive; 1 bilateral, the other unilateral.

Three out of 4 cases of cerebrospinal syphilis gave a bilateral positive test, the other was completely negative.

With a view of ascertaining whether the sign might develop in patients who had been confined to their bed for several weeks, the uninjured extremity in 3 cases of thigh fracture was examined, with 1 positive result and 1 with an angle of 120 degrees. Two patients who had been in bed for three weeks following a herniotomy were negative. Two patients in bed for four and six weeks, respectively, with fractured ribs were negative.

The pneumonias examined were the severe cases that entered the hospital. In all 22 cases were tested. Three gave a positive Kernig, 5 gave an angle of 125 degrees, and the remainder were negative. In those who gave the test there were no signs or symptoms of meningitis. The typhoids examined included those in the active stage of the disease and convalescents—the latter for the purpose of determining whether a prolonged stay in bed was a causative factor in the sign. In all 48 cases were examined: 4 were positive, 5 had an angle of 120 degrees, 9 an angle of 125 degrees. Twenty-four were in the active stage of the disease, 19 of these at least moderately severe cases. None of these gave a Kernig, all of the positive cases being in the convalescents. Those giving an angle of 120 degrees, 5 in number; 3 were in the active stage of the disease, 5 convalescents. Those giving an angle of 125 degrees, 5 were in the active stage of the disease, 4 convalescents. Only 1 of the convalescents had lain in bed with the knees drawn up.

Two cases of trichinosis were examined. In both of these the diagnosis was confirmed by finding the unencapsulated parasite in a piece of excised muscle and by the presence of an eosinophilia. One patient was in the very acute stage with intense muscular rigidity and soreness, sufficient, at least, to suggest a meningeal process, and the angle was 120 degrees. The other patient was in early convalescence, and the sign was negative.

The patient with the illuminating-gas poisoning died, and, as an autopsy was not obtained, it would be impossible to exclude a chronic cord or cerebral lesion which might have been responsible for the sign.

The results of these tests agree quite well with the investigations of others, and Henoch was first to call attention to the unreliability of the sign. Its frequency in other conditions, some of which may resemble meningitis, as an illustration, trichinosis and uræmia, lessen its diagnostic value. Its not infrequent absence in meningitis, especially in the tubercular form, and its often late and transitory appearance, lessens its significance. On account of its late or transitory appearance, daily or at least repeated examinations should be made. The presence or degree of sign is no index of the severity of the symptoms or gravity of the case.

Several theories have been advanced to explain the cause of the Kernig phenomena.

Netter considered that on account of inflammation the roots of the spinal nerves were irritated, and in extending the leg on the thigh the sacral nerves are stretched, causing reflex contraction of the flexors.

Friis suggested it was due to irritation of the cauda equina by the infected cerebrospinal fluid.

Chauffard considered it an exaggerated normal phenomena due to hypertonicity of the muscle.

Sailer would explain the sign by an irritative lesion of the pyramidal tract that diminishes but does not destroy its functional activity.

Rudolph believes the increased muscular tone, probably due to cerebellar irritation, is responsible for the sign in meningitis, and that recumbency may be the cause in some cases.

Several have explained the phenomena by increased intracerebral pressure, but Roglet's experiments show that in animals increased intracerebral pressure does not cause a muscular contraction of this nature. Rudolph reports slight decrease in the Kernig after spinal puncture.

From a clinical standpoint, it would appear that the various disease conditions in which the sign may be found excludes the probability of a common origin. Netter's view of nerve irritation might explain its frequency in meningitis, neuritis, and sciatica. Pyramidal-tract involvement offers the most plausible explanation of its presence in hemiplegia and spastic paraplegia.

Babinski's reflex was examined in most cases, in quite a number of patients contractions either negative or positive could not be obtained. In those who gave a positive reaction, repeated tests were made in order to be certain the reaction was not accidental, and any case that showed a single plantar flexion was classed as negative. In 17 cases of hemiplegia 11 gave a positive reaction, 5 negative, and 1 not tested. A case of illuminating-gas poisoning gave a typical positive reflex. As the patient died, we were unable to exclude a possible pre-existing cord lesion. Two typhoids gave the reflex; it differed, however, from the cases with lateral tract involvement by being slow and of very moderate degree, but always getting a dorsum flexion; neither of these cases had any other signs of involvement of the lateral tract. One of 4 cases of cerebrospinal syphilis was positive, and it is not improbable that the substance of the cord was involved. One case of gonorrhœal myalgia gave a slight positive reaction. A case of progressive muscular atrophy without any other signs of lateral-tract involvement gave the test in a very typical manner. The reaction was characteristic in a case of amyotrophic lateral sclerosis. One of 4 cases of transverse myelitis gave a positive test, and 1 case of carcinoma of spine. Seven of the 8 cases of spastic paraplegia were positive.

SUMMARY. 1. A maximum angle of 115 degrees gives more valuable results than does an angle of 135 degrees, as proposed by Kernig.

2. The angle obtained in any individual case depends, in part, upon the force used in extending the leg, and for this reason actual measuring of the angle is not essential.

3. The sign is present in a large percentage of the cases of meningitis; it is, however, not constant, may be transitory, or only appear late; therefore, daily examination should be made for its presence.

4. It is present in a typical manner, occasionally in a number of widely different disease conditions, and for this reason it is probable that there is not a uniform cause for the sign.

5. The sign is occasionally unilateral, exclusive of cases of hemiplegia or local trouble, which might explain its unilateral presence.

6. The presence of the sign in cases of suspected meningitis is merely another factor favoring the diagnosis. Its absence, especially early, is not infrequent, and should not be allowed to outweigh the positive findings.

BIBLIOGRAPHY.

Kernig. Berlin klin. Woch., December 29, 1884.
Osler. Lancet, June 24, 1897.
Rudolph. American Medicine, November 8, 1902.
Friis. Copenhagen Thesis, 1887. Quoted by Netter.
Herrick Journal of the American Medical Association, 1889, p. 35.
Netter. La semaine médical, 1898, p. 281.
Bull. Berlin. klin. Woch., 1895, p. 772.
Blumm. Munch. med. Woch., 1889. p. 446.
Thyne. Lancet, 1901, p. 397.
Packard. Archives of Pediatrics, April, 1900, p. 259.
Magri. Cent. f. innere Med., No. 46.
Sailer. THE AMERICAN JOURNAL OF THE MEDICAL SCIENCES, 1902.
Clark. Ibid.
Chauffard. La presse médical, 1901, p. 153.

REPORT OF TWO CASES OF VOLVULUS OF THE ENTIRE MESENTERY.[1]

BY A. D. WHITING, M.D.,
ASSISTANT SURGEON, GERMAN HOSPITAL, PHILADELPHIA, PA.

THE privilege of reporting the following case has been granted me by Dr. John B. Deaver. P. K., male, aged five years, was admitted to the Mary J. Drexel Home with a history of having been sick for five days, during which time he had suffered with nausea and vomiting and inability to expel flatus or fecal matter. When admitted he was shocked, being very weak, with cold, clammy skin and a rapid, running pulse. The abdomen was markedly distended. Rectal enemata were retained, being recovered through a rectal tube, not discolored. The patient did not react under treatment and died twelve hours after admission.

Partial post-mortem examination revealed the following: Peritoneal effusion of a serosanguineous character was present in large amount. The omentum was small, irregular in shape, and contained a small amount of fat. There were no peritoneal adhesions and no inflammatory exudate. The stomach was normal in size, but was pushed upward by the distended small bowel. The duodenum was normal, but slightly congested. The remainder of the small bowel was markedly distended and of a dusky hue. The bowel was drawn out of the abdomen when it was discovered that the root of the mesentery was so twisted on itself that it appeared like a cord. The turns of the mesentery were from right to left. The number of turns was not noted. By lifting the small bowel *en masse* the mesentery was readily untwisted.

The doctor who made the necropsy became infected during the examination, the infection being so virulent that, in spite of most active treatment, he suffered from general septicæmia, from which it was feared he could not recover. This unfortunate termination was, however, happily replaced by a perfect recovery after a tedious illness.

The second case was C. B., male, aged thirty-four years. He had had an attack of acute appendicitis in October, 1902, for which he was operated on in the German Hospital. The appendix was gangrenous; the intestine was injected, inflated, and covered with lymph. There was a local collection of pus at the base of the appendix. The abdominal cavity was cleansed as thoroughly as possible, after removal of the appendix, and four pieces of gauze were inserted for drainage, no attempt being made to close the wound. A fecal fistula developed which closed without operative interference before the patient left the hospital. After his discharge the patient suffered from intermittent pains in the right iliac

[1] Read before the Philadelphia Academy of Surgery.

fossa and along the line of the cicatrix. He was examined on May 2, 1903, at which time he complained of constipation, loss of appetite, and dull pain in the right iliac fossa. The scar was firm, the abdomen soft, with no points of tenderness. At 5 P.M., May 29, 1903, while walking up stairs, the patient was suddenly doubled up with most severe pain at the site of the cicatrix. He was nauseated, but did not vomit. He had had a bowel movement in the morning, but from the time of the onset of the violent pain until after a subsequent operation he was unable to pass either flatus or fecal matter. He was admitted to the German Hospital about 8 P.M. of the same day, at which time I saw him. He was in great distress, with severe cramp-like pains over the entire abdomen, but most marked in the right iliac fossa. The abdomen, which was slightly distended, was very tender. The rectus muscles were rigid. There was a large hernial opening at the site of the cicatrix which had not been present one week before. The temperature was 97.2°, pulse 58, respirations 26. I made a diagnosis of acute intestinal obstruction and advised immediate operation, to which consent was given.

Operation about 9 P.M., four hours after the onset of pain. Under ether anæsthesia an elliptical incision was made around the cicatrix, and the peritoneum was opened to the inner side of the cæcum. In dissecting the latter from the anterior abdominal wall, to which it was firmly adherent, it was unintentionally opened but immediately closed with two rows of Lembert sutures. Inspection showed the intestine near the ileocæcal junction to be bound together by dense adhesions, some of which were as large as the little finger. There was partial obstruction at the ileocæcal junction. With the exception of the last portion of the ileum and the duodenum, the entire small intestine was partially collapsed, lustreless, dusky red in color, and of a doughy feel. All adhesions were separated, the denuded surfaces being covered with cargile. The small intestine was drawn out of the wound in a search for the cause of the peculiar condition of the gut, when it was found that the entire mesentery was twisted upon itself, about a three-quarter turn, from left to right. The bowel was lifted up in a towel and the entire mass turned from right to left. This relieved the twist in the mesentery and returned it to its normal position. The circulation of the bowel was immediately re-established, the normal color and lustre rapidly returning. The separate layers of the abdominal wall were dissected out and the wound closed with tier sutures of silk; 500 c.c. of salt solution were injected into the rectum before the patient left the operating table. He reacted well. Flatus was passed through a rectal tube six hours after the operation, and voluntarily six hours later. The bowels moved freely on the second day. With the exception of slight infection in the lower part of the wound, the patient had no unfavorable symptoms and was discharged from the hospital on the 17th day after operation.

These two cases demonstrate the value of early operative interference in cases of suspected intestinal obstruction. The first case was brought to the surgeon when the patient was practically moribund, and of course no relief could be afforded. It is probable that the perfect recovery made by the second patient was largely due to the short interval which elapsed between the onset of the acute symptoms and the time of operation. The second case also shows the value of thorough inspection of the abdomen in cases of obstruction. I expected to find nothing but an occlusion of the bowel due to adhesions or bands. Had the real cause of the trouble been overlooked, the patient would necessarily have died.

In a very interesting article published in THE AMERICAN JOURNAL OF THE MEDICAL SCIENCES for May, 1903, Dr. George Tully Vaughan cites twenty-one cases of volvulus of the entire mesentery. Seventeen of these were operated, with four recoveries, a mortality of about 76 per cent. This mortality, as stated by Dr. Vaughan, is due to three causes: First, the serious nature of "a condition which strangulates almost the entire small intestine, injures the sympathetic plexus, and perhaps produces a rapidly fatal toxæmia." Second, the delay in operating. Third, "the difficulty in recognizing the true condition in order to act intelligently, four of the operators cited confessing their inability to do so after opening the abdomen. The patients died without relief, the true condition being at last disclosed at the necropsy."

A SIMPLE METHOD FOR THE REDUCTION OF LUXATIONS OF THE HUMERUS.

BY ELEANORE BOULTON, A.B., M.D.,
OF PHILADELPHIA, PA., U.S.A.

THOUGH the range of motion through movement of the humerus is great, the scapula normally admits of but little motion when the humerus is held in a fixed position. In luxations of the joint, however, the range of passive scapular motion is considerable, and it has been through studies of the possibilities due to this fact that the following methods have been evolved. They are, of course, susceptible to various modifications, according to the dexterity of the surgeon. The studies have extended over a period of four years' time, and include fifteen cases of the author's and nine cases which were referred to her; this number comprising only such cases as were uncomplicated by fracture of the scapula or clavicle, or of the necks of the humerus.

I. This method is applicable to subspinous dislocations, as well as to downward and forward luxations.

The surgeon stands behind the patient, who may sit or stand, as is convenient. In performing the manipulations the writer uses the hand corresponding to the side upon which the lesion exists.

The hand of the operator is partially closed, the thumb extended, and the wrist pronated. The ball of the thumb is placed below, against, and parallel to the lower margin of the scapula on the axillary border, just external to the inferior angle.

Firm pressure is exerted, and the wrist is slowly and steadily supinated, pressure upward and inward being exerted at the same time. This manipulation, if properly performed, pushes the lower angle of the scapula upward and toward the median line, depressing the lower lip of the glenoid cavity, and usually results in the prompt reduction of any variety of humeral dislocation.

In the subspinous variety, should reduction not occur, and a repetition of the manipulations bring no better result, pressure with the other thumb upon the head of the dislocated humerus, in the direction of the long axis of the bone, should be added, inserting the digit as deeply upon the head as is possible.

II. In subcoracoid or subglenoid dislocations, the operator stands behind the patient, as before, and places his hands on the patient's shoulders, with the palm of the hand at the base of the ring finger resting upon the acromion process of the scapula, the ball of the finger being placed below the clavicle. The ball of the middle finger is placed just above the clavicle, and that of the thumb beneath the spine of the scapula as far toward the inner end of the spine as is compatible with stability of position. The fingers should be slightly flexed, but not enough so as to interfere with firm pressure on the acromion process, nor so much so as to substitute the tips for the balls of the digits. The elbows should be extended. Quick but steady pressure should then be exerted in a downward, inward, and backward direction, considerable force being used.

This method has proven prompt and efficacious, even in cases in which the parts were greatly swollen from contusions sustained at the time of injury.

The following advantages are claimed for both methods:

1. There is little risk of further damage, since a short lever is used instead of a long one.

2. In cases in which fractures of the humerus, or of the bones of the forearm are present, the surgeon is enabled to effect reduction in a manner which does not necessitate the handling of the limb.

3. The patient does not suffer any great amount of pain during the procedure.

4. The patient is apt to be docile, since he does not expect redue-tion to be effected from the rear, and without manipulation of the arm.

Under the second method, if the patient offers resistance, he ordinarily starts forward, or, if sitting, he attempts to rise, thus assisting the surgeon.

REVIEWS.

International Clinics. Edited by A. O. J. Kelly, A.M., M.D., with the assistance of collaborators and correspondents. Vol. IV., pp. 321. Thirteenth series. Philadelphia: J. B. Lippincott Co., 1904.

This volume presents many subjects of importance and interest to practitioners, even though they are working within narrow lines. The treatment of Ulcer of the Stomach (Tyson), Infectious (rather than croupous) Pneumonia (Musser), Chronic Bronchitis (Claytor), and Syphilis (Julien) leave nothing to be desired so far as these topics are concerned. In Medicine, Duckworth pleads for a broader view for the student in the Physiognomical Diagnosis; Favill and Bishop concern themselves with the Kidneys; Duncan presents a practical paper on Tropical Dysentery; Satterthwaite continues his work on the heart in presenting well-reasoned-out remarks on Palpitation, Abnormal Rhythm, and the Frequent Pulse; Poynton endeavors to show how far there is a Parallelism between Clinical Symptoms and Pathological Lesions in Rheumatic Fever; Burnet gives a short paper on Angioneurotic Œdema (the literature might have been more profitably studied), and Syphilis as causing Aortitis is the subject chosen by Preble. Thus we find more than a third of the book devoted to Medicine and the subjects well and adequately presented from the standpoint of the physician.

In Surgery there is indeed a surfeit of the rare and recent. Keen and Da Costa, Senn, Albarran, Coomes, Battle, and Dugan, offering real advances on many topics, should satisfy the surgeon.

In Gynecology and Obstetrics four papers by Davenport, Wiggin, Pinard, and Frank, on both minor and major matters, possess much interest. James takes up Hemiplegia; Brewer reports an instance of Cerebral Hemorrhage and Right-sided Hemiplegia without Aphasia, and discusses Multiple Sclerosis and Delirium Tremens, offering much that will interest the general practitioner.

Orthopedics is represented by a single article by Porter on Congenital Dislocation of the Hip, Infantile Cerebral Paralysis, and Congenital Clubfoot.

In Ophthalmology, Wood on the Preparation of the Patient for Cataract Extraction, and Nolude on the Diagnosis and Treatment of Acute Glaucoma, furnish substantial information.

Of great present interest is the last paper, by McFarland, on the Present State of our Knowledge of Immunity, in which he endeavors to reconcile, imperfectly, as it seems to us, the theories of Metchnikoff and Ehrlich. Nor do we find the clearness and conciseness which has marked other contributions. Further, the diagram on page 298, borrowed from Grünbaum, needs further explanation than that vouchsafed by the writer for complete comprehension by those not familiar with the original. However, as a statement of our present notions regarding what has been the *crux* of both laboratory and clinical workers in this field, we may regard this as satisfactory. As each volume comes before us we are more and more impressed by the energy of the editor and his assistants in gathering really good work by distinguished men. In marked contrast to the deluge of communications which we are obliged to read and in reading know that their value can be but ephemeral, these contributions to medicine and surgery are distinctly grateful.

R. W. W.

Infectious Diseases: Their Etiology, Diagnosis, and Treatment. By G. H. Roger. Translated by M. S. Gabriel, M.D. Illustrated with 43 engravings. Philadelphia and New York: Lea Brothers & Co., 1903.

Amidst the great mass of stereotyped text-books it is truly refreshing to find a treatise upon the infectious diseases designed so as "to harmonize any seeming antagonism between experimental research and clinical observations, and to reduce the theories of infection and immunity to the basis of practical utility." The idea is enticing, and one is led to expect so much that an actual perusal of the book is somewhat disappointing. The classification of infections is itself rather artificial, and it is difficult to see upon what grounds yellow fever should be classed as a specific bacterial infection localized in the liver.

In the portion devoted to "nodular infections," the discussion on tuberculosis is in the main good, but the rest of the chapter, which deals with pseudotuberculosis, oidiomycosis, and actinomycosis, leaves certain points unexplained. Under the bacterioscopical examination of the blood one is surprised to find the statement that in typhoid fever the typhoid bacillus "is only very exceptionally encountered in the blood of the general circulation." Again, the conclusions which the author draws upon the etiology of dysentery are not at all in accord with the results of the latest researches upon this subject made in Japan, Germany, the Philippine Islands, and in this country.

A large portion of the book is devoted to a discussion of the "influence of infections upon the organism." Many of these chapters are excellent, and the general conception and treatment of this portion of the book is noteworthy. The sections upon the hæmopoietic organs, nervous system, and development of arteriosclerosis contain much that is new and valuable. The subject of fever in general is ably dealt with, and the author's original researches upon appendicitis, variola, and bone-marrow lend special interest to these subjects.

Of the 850 pages almost 300 are devoted to the treatment of infectious diseases. Naturally much space is given to serum-therapy. The book is valuable and worthy of careful study.

W. T. L.

CLINICAL TALKS ON MINOR SURGERY. By JAMES G. MUMFORD, M.D., Assistant Visiting Surgeon to the Massachusetts General Hospital, and Instructor in Surgery, Harvard University Medical School. Boston: The Old Corner Bookstore.

THIS little volume of *Clinical Talks on Minor Surgery* is most readable and is full of valuable information. It tersely presents the up-to-date treatment of minor surgical conditions. It is composed of ten lectures, each of which presents a number of important lessons for the student, and even the experienced surgeon can read them with profit. In the recent unparalleled advancement of surgery too little attention has been paid by teachers and writers to the lesser surgical ailments, and yet these conditions are those which fall to the general practitioner for treatment. Every student and every general practitioner will find in these few pages the recent advances in minor surgery delightfully presented. We can heartily endorse what the author has to say about the treatment of sprains, fractures, and dislocations.

J. H. G.

HANDATLAS DER ANATOMIE DES MENSCHEN. Mit Unterstützung von WILHELM HIS, Professor der Anatomie an der Universität, Leipzig. Bearbeitet von Werner Spalteholz, ao. Professor an der Universität Leipzig und Custos der Anatomischen Sammlungen. Dritter, Band 2. Abtheilung. Leipzig: Verlag von S. Hirzel, 1903.

THIS portion of Spalteholz's *Hand Atlas of Human Anatomy* deals with the nervous system and organs of special sense. We had not the pleasure of reviewing the former portions of this work, but of the present volume we can speak in the highest praise. It consists of beautiful illustrations of the entire nervous system, of the eye, the ear, and the nose. The text is full and descriptive. The illustrations are among the best which we have had the pleasure of seeing, and as an atlas the work can be highly commended. It is, however, to be regretted that so fine a piece of work should be found in a paper binding. J. H. G.

CRUSADE AGAINST CONSUMPTION. By LAWRENCE F. FLICK, M.D. Philadelphia: David McKay, 1903.

THIS little volume is, according to the author, offered to the public for the purpose of bringing about a clearer understanding of consumption. It is divided into forty-six chapters, each dealing with important questions which relate to the disease. As examples may be mentioned: What Consumption is; Diseases which Predispose to Consumption; How Tuberculosis is Spread by Contact with the Consumptive; Public Conveyances in the Spread of Tuberculosis; The Prevention of the Spread of Tuberculosis; Should Consumptives Marry?

The arrangement is simple and the terms popular, so that the subject-matter is quite within the grasp of the average layman and would certainly render him far more capable of aiding the medical profession in combating the disease.

While we may not agree with Dr. Flick in some minor statements, the work as a whole is an excellent one for the purpose, and we hope it may be widely circulated. T. A. C.

DISEASES OF THE NOSE AND THROAT. By CHARLES HUNTOON KNIGHT, A.M., M.D. Philadelphia: P. Blakiston's Son & Co., 1903.

THIS work, based upon Dr. Knight's lectures to students at Cornell University, can be consulted with profit not only by the undergraduate, for whom it is intended, but also by those who are doing more advanced work in the treatment of diseases of the nose and throat. Dr. Knight is well known as one of the most progressive workers in this special field in this country, and these lectures, embodying his own personal experiences and observations, are consequently possessed of great value to the specialist in laryngology. The author has wisely omitted going into the detailed anatomy of the nose and throat, referring the reader to larger works or to anatomical writings for the minutiæ of the subject. Throughout the entire work the author's effort at conciseness is visible, and its results have been most happy. Everywhere he utilizes his space to the fullest extent to bring out valuable practical points to the exclusion of unnecessary details. The illustrations, probably because many of them are taken from standard works, are above reproach. Taken as a whole the book may be regarded as a thoroughly up-to-date, concise presentation of the most important facts in laryngology and rhinology. F. R. P.

A TEXT-BOOK OF CLINICAL ANATOMY FOR STUDENTS AND PRACTITIONERS. By DANIEL N. EISENDRATH, A.B., M.D., Professor of Clinical Anatomy in the Medical Department of the University of Illinois (College of Physicians and Surgeons); Attending Surgeon to the Cook County Hospital, Chicago; Professor of Surgery in the Post-Graduate Medical School, Chicago. Philadelphia, New York, and London: W. B. Saunders & Co., 1903.

THE teaching of anatomy has during recent years undergone considerable improvement, but none is more notable than the teaching of applied anatomy to advanced students. It is a great mistake to allow a student to think that when he has passed his examinations in descriptive anatomy at the end of his second year that he is then possessed of all the anatomical knowledge necessary for the practice of medicine and surgery.

The object of the author of this book is to present to these advanced students and to practitioners the anatomical knowledge necessary to the successful practice of general medicine, surgery, or any of the specialties. Consequently, the book deals largely with topographical and relational anatomy. Such a work, in order to meet the demand of the reader, must present numerous and good illustrations, and with these the present work is well supplied. The longitudinal and transverse sections of the various regions of the body are well reproduced and serve a good purpose.

A criticism which might be offered on the illustrations is that there are a number of them repeated several times in the book. This is supposedly done for the convenience of the reader, and on this ground may be excused.

The text is lucid and its arrangement well adapted to the study of clinical anatomy. The profession, and particularly the teaching profession, should welcome the issue of books of this kind, and the present volume meets with our hearty commendation, as it is sure to be a great aid to both the student and the practitioner.

J. H. G.

The Diagnosis of Diseases of Women. A Treatise for Students and Practitioners. By Palmer Findley, B.S., M.D., Instructor in Obstetrics and Gynecology, Rush Medical College, in affiliation with the University of Chicago; Assistant Attending Gynecologist to the Presbyterian Hospital, Chicago. Illustrated with 210 engravings in the text and 45 plates in colors and monochrome. Philadelphia and New York: Lea Brothers & Co., 1903.

This is a well-written and beautifully illustrated book of about 500 pages. It should be in the hands of all who are making a special study of gynecological pathology. Special stress is laid upon microscopic diagnosis of the various lesions in Part II., and here the subject of the diagnosis of malignant processes is particularly well handled. The author has collected the thought of the best authorities, to whom credit is given, and has presented in a comprehensive and practical manner a great deal of information which cannot be obtained from general text-books on gynecology. While the book is handsomely illustrated, it contains many illustrations which are superfluous. Some of those of sounds, curettes, specula, dilators, tenacula, sponge tents, operating tables, etc., are unnecessary, and the views illustrating the different positions, etc., might with propriety be omitted in a book designed for advanced students.

J. B. S.

An Atlas of Human Anatomy for Students and Physicians. By Carl Toldt, M.D., Professor of Anatomy in the University of Vienna, assisted by Alois Dalla Rosa, M.D. Translated from the Third German Edition and adapted to English and American and International Terminology by M. Eden Paul, M.D. Brux., M.R.C.S., L.R.C.P. First Section: A. The Regions of the Human Body; B. Osteology. Second Section: C. Arthrology. New York and London: Rebman Company, 1903.

Under the head of Regional Anatomy, Toldt presents an atlas of human anatomy för students and physicians. The work is a translation by M. Eden Paul from the third German edition. The first two parts of this work are before us for review.

The first part deals with Osteology and is preceded by about ten pages of illustrations representing the various regions of the human body. There is no text, the anatomical points of interest being indicated on each bone. The cross-sections of the bones are particularly good. We feel, however, that this section of the work could be greatly improved by having the muscular and ligamentous attachments indicated on the bones, as is done in colors in so many of the recent works on anatomy.

The second part of this work presents the various articulations of the human frame. Its style is exactly that of the first part of the work, but in this some coloring of muscular attachments is presented.

The illustrations are so numerous and so good that it would be impossible for a student reading a description of a bone to fail to understand it with these cuts before him.

The volumes are of convenient size, and certainly must prove of great value to the student in the study of anatomy. J. H. G.

A TEXT-BOOK OF SURGERY FOR STUDENTS AND PRACTITIONERS. By GEORGE EMERSON BREWER, A.M., M.D., Lecturer on Clinical Surgery at the College of Physicians and Surgeons, Columbia University, New York; Attending Surgeon to the City Hospital; Junior Surgeon to the Roosevelt Hospital, etc. New York and Philadelphia: Lea Brothers & Co., 1903.

ALTHOUGH it is difficult for an author who undertakes to write a limited single-volume text-book on general surgery to avoid criticism at the hands of reviewers, we feel that Brewer has in this work presented as generally satisfactory a treatise as possible. He has called to his assistance several authorities on special subjects, such as surgical pathology, genito-urinary diseases, and orthopedics. The work was not prepared for the instruction or guidance of the surgeon, but for the student and the medical man who is obliged to occasionally treat surgical conditions, and the author is to be congratulated upon the accomplishment of his object.

One thing which especially strikes us in this book is its thorough up-to-date character. It is well written, very comprehensive, and a reliable guide. It is of necessity brief in many respects, but the author's terseness does much to forestall criticism in this respect. The illustrations are well chosen and good.

The chapter on Fractures meets with our hearty approval, though we cannot refrain from criticising the author for not urging early and continuous passive movements of the fingers in fractures of the lower end of the radius. This criticism, however, is applicable to a large number of text-books on general surgery.

We can commend this work very heartily to all medical students, since it is one of the best books of its size on the general surgery of to-day which we have seen. J. H. G.

BERICHT UEBER DIE LEISTUNGEN AUF DEM GEBIETE DER ANATOMIE DES CENTRALNERVENSYSTEMS IN DEM JAHREN 1901 UND 1902. Von PROF. DR. L. EDINGER und DR. A. WALLENBERG. Leipzig: S. Hirzel, 1903.

THIS valuable book is arranged as an extensive and comprehensive critical review of recent investigations upon the central nervous system, with special regard to anatomy. The bibliography, composed of over 600 references, includes articles published from all parts of the world, but these are so arranged that within a few pages one can readily find most of the work which has been done on any one subject. All references are given with full titles.

The work is divided into a number of sections. These deal with "Text-books," "Methods of Investigation," "Histology of the Nerve Cell," etc. The main anatomical divisions of the brain and spinal cord are considered under separate headings, and under these main sections subdivisions are again made. The book ends with a section upon the nervous system of the lower vertebrates.

The general method of abstracting the articles is that adopted in the critical reviews of Schmidt's *Jahrbuch*. All the reviews are clear, concise, and very satisfactory. W. T. L.

THE PRACTICAL MEDICINE SERIES OF YEAR BOOKS. Comprising Ten Volumes on the Year's Progress in Medicine and Surgery. Issued monthly, under the general editorial charge of GUSTAVUS P. HEAD, M.D., Professor of Laryngology and Rhinology, Chicago Postgraduate Medical School. Vol. IX.: Physiology, Pathology, Bacteriology, Anatomy. Dictionary edited by W. A. EVANS, M.S., M.D.; ADOLPH GEHRMANN, M.D.; and WILLIAM HEALY, A.B., M.D. Chicago: The Year Book Publishers, 1903.

THE second volume of the Year Books devoted to Physiology, Pathology, etc., is arranged in much the same manner as the first volume, but perhaps shows an improvement in certain particulars.

Investigations upon subjects which have attracted most attention during the year are brought together and reviewed in single paragraphs or sections, so that a general idea gathered from many authorities is given of the advance made in one particular line of research. Many of the reviews are quite long and illustrations from the original articles are sometimes reproduced. Although a uniform method of reference is not adopted, still the references are, as a rule, sufficiently complete to be of use. The addition of an author's index and short dictionary of new words is certainly in place. It is to be regretted that foreign literature is so glaringly neglected. American and English journals are quoted extensively, but the work from French, German, Italian, and Russian authorities receives but little recognition. W. T. L.

Practical Handbook of the Pathology of the Skin. An Introduction to the Histology, Pathology, and Bacteriology of the Skin, with Special Reference to Technique. By J. M. H. MacLeod, M.A., M.R.C.P., with eight colored and thirty-two black and white plates. Philadelphia: P. Blakiston's Son & Co., 1903.

Although the skin presents greater opportunities than any other organ or tissue of the body for the study of the processes of disease, the pathologist has made but comparatively limited use of these opportunities. The student of dermatology, therefore, finds but scanty and incomplete information in most text-books of pathology concerning the tissue-changes characteristic of cutaneous disease. The appearance of manuals like the one before us is to be hailed with satisfaction, not only because it is an indication of the scientific spirit with which the study of diseases of the skin is being pursued to-day, but still more because such books will teach the student as he has never been taught before the real nature of the pathological processes taking place in the skin.

The first few chapters of this handbook are devoted to the consideration of microscopic technique, more particularly to the special methods of fixation and staining useful in the study of normal and diseased skin. In the subsequent chapters the general pathology of the several anatomical divisions of the skin—the epidermis, the corium, and the appendages of the skin—is carefully described, special diseases being referred to only as they afford examples of the many lesions peculiar to diseases of the skin. A chapter is given to the technique of blood examinations and the blood changes found to accompany certain diseases of the skin, and to the significance of these changes. In the concluding chapters of the book the bacteriology of the skin is considered at some length. The various pathogenic fungi found in and upon the skin are described, together with the numerous staining and culture methods best adapted for their demonstration and study.

Numerous well-made illustrations, most of which are original, are scattered throughout the book, which materially add to its value as a text-book.

The plan of preceding the descriptions of the morbid anatomy of a part by a succinct account of its normal histology seems to us a most excellent one; as a matter of course, a knowledge of the normal structure of a tissue *must* precede an understanding of the alterations produced by disease.

In conclusion, we have only words of praise for this handbook, which we believe ought to be in the hands of every student of dermatology.

M. B. H.

TRAITE DE RADIOLOGIE MEDICALE. Edited by CHARLES BOUCHARD, Professeur de l'Institut, Professeur de Pathologie générale à la Faculté de médecine. Paris: G. Steinheil, 1904.

THIS treatise is in two large quarto volumes, containing almost 1100 pages of text and illustrations, and deals with the subject in great detail. Chapters have been written by numerous writers from the most prominent faculties of France. The opening chapters consider the sources and variety of electricity and of electric apparatus, a large space being devoted to the consideration of the Crookes tube and the physical and chemical properties of x-rays.

Book II. deals with the practical application of x-rays in medicine and surgery. The question of radiographic plates, their preparation, exposure, and development, is minutely treated.

The technique of fluoroscopic examinations and of skiagraphic procedures receives a thorough discussion, with numerous well-executed illustrations of apparatus, and next follows a treatise on "Stereometry and Stereoscopy." A large space is devoted to the study of the practical application of the x-rays in surgical conditions —fractures, osteitis, myelitis, acromegaly, orthopedics—and tumors of bone, luxations, arthritis, gout, rheumatism, and the arthropathies are thoroughly investigated. Following these are the examinations of the viscera, the vascular and nervous systems, the special senses, and obstetrical and fetal radiography. An interesting and instructive chapter follows on the accidents of radiology, and particularly of x-ray dermatitis and of burns. A remarkable feature of this enormous work is that only eleven pages are devoted to "Radiotherapy." No attempt has been made to describe methods of procedure, but a résumé of some diseases treated and the general results reported are mentioned. Other diseases the writer declines to discuss, on the ground that they are still in too experimental a stage for conclusions.

The book is an interesting exposition of a vast amount of investi gation, but it is not presented in a form that would render it available for the ordinary practitioner. F. F.

THE PRINCIPLES OF "OPEN-AIR" TREATMENT OF PHTHISIS AND OF SANATORIUM CONSTRUCTION. By ARTHUR RANSOME, M.D. London: Smith, Elder & Co., 1903.

THE present agitation for a more rational treatment of tuberculosis has called out a crop of semi-popular literature, of which this little book is a fair sample. While the author aims to set forth the principles upon which the open-air treatment—chiefly in sanatoria —should be based, and addresses himself to physicians, the style of the book is such as to make it appeal rather to the general public than to the medical profession. Except that it contains useful practical directions about hygiene, clothing and the like, and for the construction of a sanatorium, it has no special interest for practitioners. But anything that tends to popularize the knowledge of what has already been achieved by modern methods of treatment and what there still remains to be done, not only by the profession, but by municipalities and the general public also, deserves cordial commendation. R. M. G.

THE EXACT SCIENCE OF HEALTH BASED UPON LIFE'S GREAT LAW. By ROBERT WALTER, M.D. New York: Edward S. Werner Publishing Co. London: Kegan Paul, Trench, Trubner & Co., Ltd.

THE best that can be said of this publication is that the writer's purpose is probably sincere and that its practical teaching, which resolves itself into the principle of non-interference in disease, is not actively harmful. The style reminds one forcibly of that of Mrs. Eddy's book, and the matter is scarcely more intelligible. It bristles with scientific inaccuracies and still more mischievous perversions and misinterpretations of facts. The author is, no doubt, a conscientious carer for the sick, and has some practical notions on treatment, especially the methods collectively known as physiologic therapeutics; but for the comfort of the reading public we trust he will stick to his practice and leave the writing of books to those who are better versed in the craft. R. M. G.

PROGRESS

OF

MEDICAL SCIENCE.

MEDICINE.

UNDER THE CHARGE OF

WILLIAM OSLER, M.D.,

PROFESSOR OF MEDICINE, JOHNS HOPKINS UNIVERSITY, BALTIMORE, MARYLAND,

AND

W. S. THAYER, M.D.,

ASSOCIATE PROFESSOR OF MEDICINE, JOHNS HOPKINS UNIVERSITY, BALTIMORE, MARYLAND.

Studies in Pneumonia and Pneumococcus Infections.—ROSENOW (*Journal of Infectious Diseases*, March 19, 1904, p. 280), in a review of the literature on the frequency of pneumococcus septicæmia in pneumonia, emphasizes the fact that the results of different investigators show the greatest possible variation. These range from the total failure of the Klemperer brothers to isolate the pneumococcus from the blood in any of their cases to Prochaska's successful isolation of the organism in every one of 50 cases of pneumonia. The latter investigator laid no stress on the degree of dilution of the blood. Of his 50 cases, only 12 ended fatally.

Rosenow found a pneumococcæmia in 132 out of a total of 145 cases of pneumonia in which he took blood cultures. The pneumococcus was demonstrated in the blood in 4 cases before a positive diagnosis could be made, and in obscure cases of pneumococcus infection he thinks that blood cultures may be a diagnostic method of positive value. He is rather inclined to the view that in certain instances lobar pneumonia may be a secondary localization of a primary blood invasion. Rosenow agrees with Fraenkel, Prochaska, and others that the presence of pneumococci in the circulating blood is of no special prognostic value in pneumonia, because he holds with them that a pneumococcæmia occurs in practically all cases. There was a mortality of 40 per cent. in his series. He holds that the higher percentage of successful cultivations of the pneumococcus from the blood is due to recent improvements in technique, namely, the use of large quantities (5 c.c. to 7 c.c.) of blood in liquid media, especially bouillon, and of high concentration of blood instead of high dilutions to overcome the so-called bactericidal action of the blood.

The number and viability of the pneumococci in the blood at the time of the crisis is lessened. Rosenow believes that a leukocytosis is a favorable sign, as the number of leukocytes is a measure of the power of resistance of the individual. A leukopenia following a leukocytosis is an unfavorable indication, pointing as it does to an exhaustion of the resisting powers. The leukocytosis is probably incited by soluble substances liberated by the pneumococci.

Pneumonic blood and serum behaves as fresh normal blood does in having no bactericidal influence on the pneumococcus. The writer found that agglutination of the pneumococcus by pneumonic serum was constant. He demonstrated that the pneumococcus grown in pneumonic serum produces an acid, and offers the suggestion that some of the toxic symptoms of pneumonia may be due to acid intoxication. The viability and virulence of the pneumococcus are preserved for a very long period upon blood-agar, the hæmoglobin being the constituent most likely responsible for this effect. Rosenow finds that blood-agar plates are valuable for the differentiation of pneumococci and streptococci.

Paralysis Agitans.—Hart (*Journal of Nervous and Mental Diseases* March, 1904, p. 177) has made a clinical study of 219 cases of paralysis agitans occurring in Dr. M. Allen Starr's clinic since 1888. There were 139 men and 80 women. The earliest case was in a male, aged twenty-two years; the latest in a male, aged seventy-eight years. The largest number of cases, 40 per cent., began in the decade between fifty and sixty years. Occupation seemed to have no etiological bearing. Direct hereditary transmission can rarely be traced. In only 16 per cent. of the cases could paralysis agitans be found to have existed in relatives. Emotional influences were believed to have been the exciting cause in 40 of the cases. Next to emotion, traumatism seemed the most conspicuous predisposing factor, such a history being obtained in 31 cases. Other contributory causes given are certain acute infectious diseases, overwork, and alcoholism. Syphilis apparently played an unimportant part, and was admitted in only 2 cases. The writer states that the true etiology of the disease is not at all well understood.

Tremor was noted in 203 of the cases. The onset was seven times as frequent in the upper as in the lower extremity, and was more frequent on the right side of the body. In 3 cases it began in the head. It is usually lessened by voluntary motion. Muscular rigidity was present in 142 cases. Contractures were noted in 28 cases. In 173 instances the tendency of the patient to fall was tested. It was absent in 68 and present in 105 cases. The deep reflexes were investigated in 188 cases. Of these, 90 were normal; in 30 they were present but diminished; and in 68 they were more active than normal. There were definite voice changes of varying character noted in 120 cases. Pain in some part of the body was present in most of the cases. Paræsthesias were present in 120 cases also. These consisted usually of "prickling," "numbness," "tingling," "flushing," and "heat and cold." Hyperidrosis was present in 57 instances. The complications varied and could not be said to be dependent on the nervous disease. Two of the cases had hemiplegia.

The treatment was unsatisfactory and there were no cures. An effort in all cases was made to remove sources of anxiety and worry; to place the patient on a simple diet and to improve the general nutrition. The cases which showed most improvement were given massage, passive movements, and hydrotherapy. Medicinally, hydrobromate of hyoscine and sulphate of duboisine gave the best results. For a time at least they diminished the tremor and relieved insomnia.

On Black Urine.—A. E. GARROD (*Practitioner*, March, 1904, p 383) prefaces an interesting paper on the above subject, with an historical account of the condition. Black urine was described by Hippocrates and others before him. The data in these early cases are too meagre to afford a plausible explanation for their causes. In some of the later cases the descriptions are sufficiently full to conclude that hæmoglobin or admixture of blood, bile pigments, coloring matters from eating certain fruits, and the abnormal constituents of the urine in alkaptonuria were the causes of the discoloration.

Garrod states that in the following conditions the urine is dark-colored on voiding or becomes black on standing: (1) in cases of jaundice, especially when of long standing; (2) hæmaturia; (3) hæmoglobinuria; (4) hæmatoporphyrinuria; (5) melanotic sarcoma; (6) alkaptonuria; (7) ochronosis; (8) in cases in which abundance of indican (indoxyl sulphate) is present; (9) in certain cases of phthisis, only after standing for some time; (10) in certain rare cases of undetermined nature; (11) after the taking of certain drugs and articles of diet (including carboluria). In only a few conditions, such as alkaptonuria and melanuria, does the urine become actually black, and then only on standing.

Some of the above conditions are deserving of special comment. In hæmatoporphyrinuria the urine is usually of a port-wine color, but may be actually black. The color is only in part due to the hæmatoporphyrin. There are other dark abnormal pigments present. The great majority of the cases of this condition are due to the toxic action of overdoses of sulphonal and its allies. Hæmatoporphyrin is recognized by certain characteristic absorption bands on spectroscopic examination.

The melanuria of melanotic sarcoma is rare, and Garrod supports the observation of others, that it does not occur when the growth is limited to its primary seat or to a neighboring group of lymphatic glands, but only when the internal viscera, particularly the liver, are involved. The urine is usually of a normal color when passed, but darkens from the surface downward on exposure to the air. The addition of nitric acid to the cold urine at once produces blackness. Ferric chloride also causes immediate blackening and a gray precipitate which forms is redissolved by an excess of the reagent.

The urine in alkaptonuria behaves in the same way as that in melanuria does on exposure to the air. The darkening is hastened by the addition of an alkali. The urine reduces Fehling's solution and ammoniacal silver nitrate solution in the cold. It does not reduce bismuth solutions and does not ferment, and is thus distinguishable from diabetic urine. The abnormal substance which produces the characteristic reaction is homogentisic acid, first discovered by Baumann and Wolkow.

In the rare condition known as ochronosis, or pigmentation of the cartilages, first described by Virchow in 1866, the urine may be dark in color. Of 7 cases reported, the urine darkened in 3. In 2 additional cases recently reported by Osler the patients were also shown to be alkaptonurics. Garrod thinks, however, that homogentisic acid is not the only substance causing blackening of the urine in ochronosis.

The writer states that although the dark urine of indicanuria is not of infrequent occurrence, it is not so well recognized as it should be. He believes that many cases are mistaken for other conditions, and particularly for melanuria. The color is not due to the indigo pigments nor to indoxyl sulphates, which are colorless substances, but, as Baumann and Brieger showed, to higher oxidation products of indol. These urines blacken when warmed with nitric acid, but there is no such immediate blackening in the cold, as with true melanuria. They do not blacken with ferric chloride, and by this test they may be at once distinguished from those containing melanogen. Any morbid process which leads to abundant excretion of indican may give rise to such urine, as, for example, intestinal obstruction from any cause, excessive bacterial activity in the intestine, or putrefactive changes in collections of pus.

SURGERY.

UNDER THE CHARGE OF

J. WILLIAM WHITE, M.D.,

JOHN RHEA BARTON PROFESSOR OF SURGERY IN THE UNIVERSITY OF PENNSYLVANIA; SURGEON TO THE UNIVERSITY HOSPITAL,

AND

F. D. PATTERSON, M.D.,

SURGEON TO THE X-RAY DEPARTMENT OF THE HOWARD HOSPITAL; CLINICAL ASSISTANT TO THE OUT-PATIENT SURGICAL DEPARTMENT OF THE JEFFERSON HOSPITAL.

The Significance of the Zoological Distribution, the Nature of the Mitoses, and the Transmissibility of Cancer.—BASHFORD and MURRAY (*The Lancet*, February 13, 1904) state that within the past year specimens of malignant new-growths have accumulated from all the domesticated animals and from many other vertebrates. The clinical, pathological, anatomical, and microscopic characters of these new-growths are identical with those found in man in all essential features, although the animals themselves are drawn from the different classes of the vertebrate phylum. Stated generally, it may be said that malignant new-growths are frequent according as animals are carefully examined, and are unrecorded in forms which are difficult to examine or do not reach old age in considerable numbers. The figures are not sufficiently extensive to determine accurately the age incidence of the various types of new-growths in different animals, but a relatively higher incidence in old age is apparent.

In regard to the phenomena of cell division in malignant new-growths the following points are of great importance: A complicated sequence of cell changes has been found to be characteristic of carcinoma and sarcoma alike. This sequence is the same as that which initiates the origin of the sexual generation in plants from the asexual, and is terminal in the history of the sexual cells in animals. It must be noted also that all the cells of the malignant new-growths do not undergo the reducing division; a certain number differentiate in the direction of the tissue among which they have arisen, and in the secondary growths, when present, somatic mitoses occur in the growing margin, which, it will subsequently be shown, is also a feature in the growth of cancer when transferred to a new host.

The transmission of cancer from man to animals, or from one animal to another of a different species, has never been successfully performed. Successful transplantation experiments have been made, however, from animals suffering from malignant new-growths to others of the same species. Careful microscopic examination has clearly demonstrated that the new tumors which develop arise from the actual cells introduced. Transplantation is, in fact, identical with the process of metastasis, as it occurs in the individual providing the tumor. It is remarkable, however, that the tumor used in these experiments does not produce metastases naturally, and its malignancy is only evidenced by its progressive growth and the undifferentiated character of the cells. The process is in no sense an infection, the tissues of the new host not participating in the formation of the new parenchyma. The origin of the stroma has not been accurately determined. The experimental transmission of carcinoma shows that we must distinguish between the problem of the genesis of a malignant new-growth and that of the conditions which permit of its continued existence.

The wide zoological distribution of malignant new-growths—its limits are not yet determined—indicates that the cause of cancer is to be sought in a disturbance of those phenomena of reproduction and cell life which are common to the forms in which it occurs. Our observations on animals show that malignant new-growths are always local in origin and of themselves produce no evident constitutional disturbances whatsoever. These facts are in full accord with accumulated clinical experience in man. In connection with diagnosis and statistics one must emphasize the importance of the absence of specific symptoms. The evidence we have advanced that cancer is an irregular and localized manifestation of a process otherwise natural to the life cycle of all organisms probably explains why it is that malignant new-growths, and their extensive secondary deposits *qua* cancer, are devoid of a specific symptomatology.

Remarks on Extensive Carcinoma of the Œsophagus, with Unusual Nervous Complications.—SAUNDBY and HEWETSON (*British Medical Journal*, March 12, 1904), after reporting in detail this case, state that it is of special interest because it appears to constitute an exception to "Simon's Law": The occurrence of an isolated paralysis of the abductor filaments of the recurrent laryngeal nerve in cases in which the roots or trunks of the spinal accessory, pneumogastric, and recurrent nerves are injured or diseased is not an isolated pathological curiosity. There is a distinct proclivity of the abductor fibres to become affected in such cases, either at an earlier period than the adductor fibres or even exclusively." In this case, both physiologically and pathologically, the adductor disablement was earlier and more intense in degree than the abductor. The clinical evidence showed that this adductor paralysis was an early and constant feature of the laryngeal condition during the whole of the patient's life in hospital. The abductor muscles, on the other hand, appeared to act well until a few days before death, when a slight narrowing of the previously wide-open glottis was noticed.

The most reasonable explanation of this is that the nerve fibres going to the adductors of the vocal cords were disabled earlier and in much larger proportion than the nerve fibres going to the abductor muscles. This explanation, of course, takes for granted that the nerve fibres of the trunk of the recurrent laryngeal nerve are differentiated into special fibres for special muscles, though not necessarily arranged in any special position within the epineurium of the nerve.

Reflex Disturbances Associated with Adherent Prepuce.—SIMON (*British Medical Journal*, March 12, 1904) notes briefly three interesting cases in which marked symptoms were produced by an adherent prepuce, or narrowed urethral meatus. The first case was a boy, aged eighteen months, who suddenly became unable to walk. Any attempt to make him walk caused very severe pain. Careful examination failed to show any coxalgia, but the prepuce was found to be long and adherent. The child was circumcised, and recovery was immediate and complete. The second case, a boy aged fourteen years, had obstinate and severe intestinal colic, which was not relieved by medical treatment. An adherent prepuce being discovered, this was treated, and all the symptoms disappeared. In the last case, a boy aged three years, there was a history of his wakening at night, screaming and complaining of pain in the abdomen. No other cause being discovered, the penis was examined, and the prepuce found adherent and the meatus narrow. Under appropriate surgical treatment the symptoms disappeared.

Experimental Nephritis Followed by Decapsulation of the Kidney.—HALL and HERXHEIMER (*British Medical Journal*, April 9, 1904) state that when Edebohls first suggested the decapsulation of the kidney as a reasonable method of treatment in chronic nephritis he based his proposal upon the urinary and general improvements which followed the fixation of a movable kidney by the removal of its capsule. In one of his cases which died four months after decapsulation, he observed "enormously dilated and enlarged bloodvessels which penetrated from the fatty capsule through the capsule proper into the kidney substance." This access of additional blood he considered would provide increased nutrition, stimulate an extensive regeneration of the secreting cells, and consequently produce a more efficient excretion of waste products. Whether decapsulation yields better results than the simpler reni-puncture of Reginald Harrison, which has been so widely and successfully employed, is a question which the available clinical data have not yet satisfactorily answered. We must wait from two to five years before making any definite conclusions as to the value of this operation. Meanwhile, we may with advantage investigate the anatomical aspect of the procedure, and thus the present inquiry has for its main object the observation of the tissue changes which follow the decapsulation of kidneys in which nephritis has been induced.

While we must clearly admit that artificial animal nephritis cannot be too closely compared with nephritis in a human subject, yet we submit that the changes produced by metallic poisons are somewhat similar in each case, and the experiments provide at least some grounds for the probable occurrence of like processes in the human kidney.

We must, of course, for the moment only deal with the forms of degenerative nephritis, as it is yet impossible to induce an interstitial nephritis in animals. From the anatomical standpoint yielded by our experiments and those previously reported, decapsulation does not appear to offer any advantages. And if there exists no anatomical basis for the operation in acute degenerative nephritis, it is surely impossible that in chronic nephritis the capsular changes will be less marked. If indeed the changes are at all analogous, we should imagine that the laceration, the hemorrhage, and the new formation of the capsule would rather tend to accelerate the interstitial inflammation; while in the event of any concomitant arteriosclerosis there would be no possibility of much vascular anastomosis or even of a satisfactory replacement of the channels ruptured during the removal of the capsule.

But if there is no anatomical basis for the operation, there may be another explanation of the rapid flow of urine—the increased excretion of urea, the disappearance of the albumin and casts which have been observed to follow decapsulation. By some the results are ascribed to the relief of congestion, but in our experiments the intense hyperæmia persisted after the capsule had reformed. Pel, Jaboulay, and others suggest that the improvement is due to the action upon the sympathetic ganglia, and that the decapsulation should be considered in the same light as those operations which, undertaken to remove a renal calculus, lessen the pain and improve the general condition of the patient, although no calculus is found.

If the latter be the correct explanation, the question naturally then arises as to the necessity for the entire denudation of the renal cortex. Would not reni-puncture, or one longitudinal and several transverse incisions, while avoiding the main anatomical disadvantages, afford a sufficient stimulus to the sympathetic centres? We cannot at present offer any experimental evidence upon this point. That it would provide a sounder anatomical basis is probable; at all events, it would more locally limit the interstitial and capsular processes in kidneys, the seat of chronic nephritis.

Guiteras has recently compiled the results of some 120 cases in which the diagnoses of chronic nephritis were fairly well established before decapsulation and their postoperative courses followed for some months. Regarding the results from their most favorable standpoint, 16 per cent. of the total number may be said to be "cured," 40 per cent. thought to be improved, 11 per cent. unimproved, and 33 per cent. followed by early death. Suker reports 15 cases of nephritis in which retinal changes had occurred and which were submitted to decapsulation; 14 died within the "two-year" period, and the history of the remaining one was somewhat questionable.

The value of these statistics is, however, minimized by several considerations. First, the operation has been necessarily restricted to the latest stages of the disease, and has often been only performed as a last hope; secondly, the exact stages and extent of chronic nephritis do not permit of accurate diagnosis; thirdly, chronic nephritis is, as a rule, characterized by acute exacerbations and frequent remissions, its anatomical course is in the main a progressive one, and the remittent stages often occur under treatment other than that of decapsulation.

Of the above 33 per cent. mortality, 26 per cent. died from chronic interstitial nephritis; and of the remainder, in 25 per cent. death occurred from the so-called chronic parenchymatous nephritis, and in 75 per cent. "diffuse"(?) nephritis was assigned as the cause.

In acute nephritis, anuria, hæmaturia, puncture, and decapsulation of the kidney is said to yield relief and to favorably affect the function of the other kidney. In these cases it is suggested that the improvement is due simply to the relief of tension.

From the standpoint of pathology we may not make an excursion into the field of surgery, and therefore we must not discuss the possibilities of the operation. We feel, however, that the purpose of the paper would not be served unless we mentioned that, while many American and some French surgeons regard the procedure as one that has come to stay and as possessing much promise in the treatment of degenerative and interstitial nephritis, such operators as Israel, Nicolayson, and others have already abandoned the method in chronic conditions. It is, of course, a matter of common knowledge that the simpler reni-puncture relieves tension and promotes renal functions; so perhaps the description of the changes observed after decapsulation may give more prominence to the method of simple incision, may emphasize the probability of rapid local reparation when the temporary obstruction is removed, and may suggest the earlier surgical treatment of those post-febrile and acute renal manifestations which, when unrelieved, often terminate fatally.

THERAPEUTICS.

UNDER THE CHARGE OF

REYNOLD WEBB WILCOX, M.D., LL.D.,

PROFESSOR OF MEDICINE AND THERAPEUTICS AT THE NEW YORK POST-GRADUATE MEDICAL SCHOOL AND HOSPITAL; VISITING PHYSICIAN TO ST. MARK'S HOSPITAL.

Treatment of Infantile Diarrhœa by Gelatin.—Dr. Weil treats this condition with a 10 per cent. solution of gelatin prepared by adding 10 parts of yellow or white gelatin to 100 parts of boiling water. This is filtered, and while still warm put in test-tubes, into each of which is poured 10 c.c. of the solution. The contents of a tube can easily be added to the patient's feeding, and thus he may get 6 to 8 grams of gelatin per day. The contents of two tubes may be given with each feeding if necessary. In practice it is well to begin with three tubes on the first day and add one each day following. The effects of this treatment are excellent; the stools diminish in frequency, their consistence becomes better, and they gradually come back to the normal type. The color changes from green to yellow, the bad odor disappears, and their reaction becomes alkaline. As the stools become more normal the temperature declines and the general condition is improved. This treatment is not always applicable to acute and chronic types of the disease. It produces regularly good results in the simple gastroenteritis, but when, in addition to the digestive, there are lung, spleen, and liver involvement with albuminuria, the gelatin, while it modifies the stools, does not influence the other conditions.—*Journal de médecine de Paris*, 1904, No. 3, p. 22.

Gymnastics or **Massage in Therapeutics.**—Dr. Saquet holds that massage is preferable to active movements, especially in joint troubles. In muscular atrophy of so-called articular origin, but which is more likely the result of disuse, massage produces results after several weeks; gymnastics are less important and less rapidly curative when employed alone. It is necessary to remember that in massage normal movements are utilized and these are responsible for the cure. In the paralyses of children massage is found to be more rapid in producing good results than re-education. The results in the aged are less successful. Massage also is to be preferred to re-education in ataxic patients. In general, therefore, massage should be employed in preference to gymnastics, though the latter are successful in a limited number of cases. It is essential, however, that the masseur be a physician.—*Gazette médicale de Nantes*, 1904, No. 2, p. 21.

Ichthargan.—Dr. A. Kronfeld has found that this drug, which is a combination of ichthyol and silver (containing 30 per cent. of the latter and 15 per cent. of sulphur), is a valuable addition to the antiblennorrhagics now in use. Ichthargan is a brown powder, easily soluble in water, glycerin, and dilute alcohol. In acute gonorrhœa, in addition to prescribing rest and proper diet, the author prescribes the introduction once or twice a day of a drainage-tube impregnated with a 0.02 per cent. solution of ichthargan in gelatin. This tube is allowed to remain in the urethra until the gelatin has become dissolved. This usually takes from five to ten minutes. Then the tube is withdrawn. Such treatment is painless and produces good results. In chronic gonorrhœa a 0.02 per cent. solution of ichthargan is used as an injection. The qualities possessed by this drug, which should commend it to use, are its ability to act deep in the tissues, due to its ichthyol content and its astringent and antiseptic properties which it owes to the silver.—*Thérapeutische Monatshefte*, 1904, No. 1, p. 32.

Adrenalin in Gynecology.—M. H. Cramer considers that adrenalin 1:3000 applied upon tampons is efficacious in *pruritus vulvæ*. In endometritis solutions of a strength of 1:1000 or 1:2000 applied before cauterization causes an anæmia of the tissues and increase the efficacy of the treatment. The hæmostatic action of the substance makes its application before curettement or the use of the actual cautery useful in inoperable cancer of the cervix. When ap lied to the ulcerated surface for five minutes upon a tampon saturated with a 1:1000 solution or by an injection into the diseased tissues of about forty-five minims, renders the operation comparatively bloodless. Swabbing the uterine cavity with a 1:2000 solution immediately after curettage produces a complete hæmostasis, which renders inspection through the dilated cervix an easy matter.—*Revue française de médecine et de chirurgie*, 1903, No. 8, p. 184.

Treatment of Ozæna by Injections of Paraffin.—Dr. E. J. Moure employs the following technique in the treatment of this affection. The material used melts at 60° C., although others advocate paraffin of a lower melting point. The syringe has a capacity of forty-five minims, and if its cylinder is of ivory it will be found to conduct the heat less than if of metal. The syringe properly sterilized and heated is filled with the paraffin, which is injected at a temperature of 55° C. Holding the nasal speculum in place with the left hand, the mucous membrane is punctured and the paraffin slowly injected. Only one puncture should be made, lest the paraffin exude from the one first made. Rarely is it necessary to inject more than fifteen or thirty minims. The posterior portion of the inferior turbinate is the place of election for the puncture, although in certain cases other situations may be employed. Usually a single sitting only is necessary to bring the nasal fossa to its normal calibre, but supplementary injections may be made, if indicated, a few weeks later. In all cases the injection should be made from behind forward. After the operation the odor of the nasal secretion soon becomes less foul and the crusts disappear, although in some cases nasal irrigations may be necessary as an adjunct to the treatment, and in cases of not too long standing complete cure results. The paraffin treatment seems to be superior to any other at present employed. —*La semaine médicale*, 1904, No. 8, p. 61.

Aristochine in Whooping-cough.—DR. HERMANN KITTEL sums up his observations in regard to the employment of this drug in whooping-cough thus: He has treated thirty-four patients, of which he considers twenty-five entirely cured. Seven others were improved and in two instances the treatment had not been of sufficient length for inference to be drawn. The duration of the treatment varied from six days to four weeks, and in infants less than a year old the results were particularly startling, the cure taking place very quickly. In older children recovery was less rapid, due, perhaps, to the employment of too small dosage. To achieve the best results treatment should be begun early in the disease. The children under one year old received three times a day one and one-half grains for each month of their age, with fifteen grains as a maximum. Older children were given thirty grains three times a day. In no case was any untoward effect noticed.—*Journal de médecine de Paris*, 1903, No. 52, p. 520.

Collargol.—DR. AUGUSTE GUERIN summarizes various reports upon this drug, as follows: When given by inunction in scarlet fever and measles the patients recover without complications. In fevers it causes an amelioration of the general state and seems to exercise certain resorptive powers. It causes the joint effusion of rheumatism and the effusion of pleurisy to disappear in an extraordinarily short time. In infectious endocarditis it has brought about recovery and seems to modify for the better the course of pneumonia. In typhoid fever and tuberculosis, unfortunately, it has not seemed to give benefit, but in erysipelas, puerperal fever, osteomyelitis, phlebitis, and other pus infections it seems to have a field of usefulness. It may be employed as an intravenous injection in 1 per cent. solution, as a 15 per cent. ointment for inunction, or it may be given internally. The author inclines to the opinion that observers have been, perhaps, oversanguine concerning the drug and concludes that further and scientific observations upon it are needed.—*Journal de médecine de Bordeaux*, 1903, No. 52, p. 845.

Marmorek's Serum in Tuberculosis.—M. DIEULAFOY reports upon seven cases treated by this serum. Four of these were patients affected with pulmonary tuberculosis in different stages; two others had in addition laryngeal involvement, and the seventh was suffering from tuberculous pleurisy with effusion. From seventy-five to one hundred and fifty minims of the serum were injected at each dose, and the injections were given every day, every two days, or at longer intervals. The results were as follows: (1) the serum did not appear to affect the rise of temperature favorably; (2) the sputum often was doubled or tripled in quantity after an injection; (3) in several of the patients neighboring lesions in lungs or pleura seemed to be caused by the treatment; (4) the patients emaciated rapidly in spite of overfeeding. For these reasons the treatment was discontinued. Two of the pa i s were living at the time of the report, but the others have died. t The injections of the serum into inoculated animals seems to produce as unfavorable results as upon human beings.—*Bulletin de l'Académie de Médecine*, 1903, No. 39, p. 365.

Treatment of Croupous Pneumonia with Creosote Carbonate.—DRS. J. A. SCOTT AND CHARLES M. MONTGOMERY claim that while our methods of treatment of this disease are more humane and founded on a better therapeutie basis, the mortality has not been reduced if we take large numbers of cases into consideration. This report is based upon sixty-seven patients, of whom ten died, a mortality of 14.9 per cent. The amount of the remedy employed was ten to fifteen minims in capsules for adults every four hours. Their conclusions are that (1) creosote carbonate causes no irritability of the stomach; in no case was there vomiting or any disturbance of the digestion; no disturbance of the urine was noted. (2) The degree of toxæmia in all cases, barring the fatal ones, was mild; this is a difficult point to estimate, the extent of lung involved, temperature, etc., having little or nothing to do with it. (3) In the cases treated pseudocrises were common (fifteen), but bore no relation to the crises or to the mortality. (4) The mortality percentage does not corroborate the unusually low figures reported by various observers, nor does it prove that the results were due to the treatment, as equally good results have been secured in past years by other methods in the same hospital. (5) The study of the clinical effects of this remedy should be continued; the dosage should be increased, and the effects on the toxæmia should be carefully watched. —*Therapeutic Gazette*, 1903, No. 12, p. 793.

[The fifth paragraph of these conclusions contains at once a suggestion as to the cause of failure and the method whereby the reporters may lessen their mortality percentage. Attention is directed to the fact that the dose is to be that required, and inasmuch as apparently no harm results from doses many times larger than those cited and the degree of toxæmia is difficult to estimate, larger rather than smaller doses are advised.—R. W. W.]

Adrenalin in Typhoid Hemorrhage.—DR. GRAESER reports the history of a female patient, aged thirty-six years, who had a typical attack of typhoid fever, associated with a bronchopneumonia, or diffuse bronchitis. This patient recovered from the pneumonia, but developed a typhoid-like rash and a typical typhoid temperature. Two weeks after the onset of the typhoid and one week after the appearance of the roseola, an intestinal hemorrhage took place, which was treated with ice, opium, bismuth, and ergot. Bleeding was so extensive as to threaten death, and adrenalin was used, 30 minims, in saline solution, every three hours, with the result of a sudden cessation of the bleeding, either as coincidental or as causative.—*Münchener medicinische Wochenschrift*, 1903, vol. l. p. 1294.

Effect of Bismuth Preparations in Therapy.—Dr. B. Laquer writes that bismuth preparations act, not only mechanically on catarrhal and ulcerative conditions of the mucous membrane of the stomach and intestines, but also chemically, as antiseptics. Bismuth and its preparations, particularly bismuth protoxide, has a marked catalytic power and is capable of diminishing the proteid putrefactive processes in the intestinal tract. Bismuth subnitrate is reduced in the intestine by the action of the intestinal juices to bismuth protoxide, which, in part, explains its beneficial action.—*Archives de médecine des enfants*, 1903, No. 6, p. 340.

Diet in Constipation.—Dr. Henry F. Hughes, as a result of his experience in the Out-patient Department of the Massachusetts General Hospital, discusses this question and presents the following table of diet: Breakfast: Cereal, with cream and sugar—preferably corn meal, or rye and oats; two soft-boiled or scrambled eggs; bread—preferably black bread or pumpernickel, or rye bread, with much butter; fruit, apples or grapes. Dinner: Soup—preferably vegetable soup; fish or meat, or both, with salad; vegetables, at least two kinds—preferably spinach, cabbage, beets, turnips, potatoes, beans or peas, if desired; dessert of rice or bread pudding or custard, including daily a saucer of prunes. Supper: Bread and butter; cocoa; cold meat and vegetable salad; dessert of stewed fruit, apples or pears or figs. If necessary, include a saucer of prunes. Drink at least three pints of water daily.—*Boston Medical and Surgical Journal*, 1903, vol. cxlix. p. 317.

OBSTETRICS.

UNDER THE CHARGE OF

EDWARD P. DAVIS, A.M., M.D.,

PROFESSOR OF OBSTETRICS IN THE JEFFERSON MEDICAL COLLEGE; PROFESSOR OF OBSTETRICS AND DISEASES OF INFANCY IN THE PHILADELPHIA POLYCLINIC; CLINICAL PROFESSOR OF DISEASES OF CHILDREN IN THE WOMAN'S MEDICAL COLLEGE; VISITING OBSTETRICIAN TO THE PHILADELPHIA HOSPITAL, ETC.

Septic Infection during Labor and the Puerperal State.—Jardine (*Journal of Obstetrics and Gynecology of the British Empire*, March, 1904) draws attention to the fact that between the years 1875 and 1895 the number of deaths from puerperal septic infection in Scotland was greater than the mortality had been in what are called pre-antiseptic times. He accounts for this from the fact that at that time anæsthetics were misused and that the free employment of anæsthesia led to the performance of many unnecessary and injurious operations. Antiseptics were also misused, and indiscriminate douching did great harm. At the present time with aseptic precautions, with as little interference with the uterus as possible, and with the restriction of operations to cases in which they are clearly demanded, the mortality rate is again diminishing.

The Anatomy of Twin Monsters.—BERRY (*Journal of Obstetrics and Gynecology of the British Empire*, March, 1904) describes two cases of twin monsters, with their dissection, in which a study was made of the specimens to determine their mode of development. It was interesting to find that the livers were fused into one and that the hearts were also partially merged into one. In tracing the development of this monstrosity the writer believes that evidences are found to show that bilateral segmentation of a single ovum is necessary for the production of twins, and that so far as the liver is concerned it is developed from a middle portion of the intestine.

Vaginal Cæsarean Section: Three Cases.—MUNRO KERR (*Journal of Obstetrics and Gynecology of the British Empire*, March, 1904) publishes notes of three cases of vaginal Cæsarean section.

The first was in a primipara who had been twenty-four hours in labor. In spite of opium and hot douching, the cervix refused to dilate. In these cases Duhrssen's deep incision was selected, delivery was readily accomplished, and the cervix was closed by catgut stitches. The patient made a very good recovery, with good union. In a case of eclampsia the same method of deep incision of the cervix was successful, the patient recovering with good union. In this instance vaginal Cæsarean section was declined in favor of deep incision.

In the case of a multipara, five months pregnant, suffering from pernicious nausea, the patient suddenly became very ill with continuous vomiting and a very feeble pulse. The cervix was rigid and firmly contracted. Vaginal Cæsarean section was performed by separating the bladder from the uterus. The cervix was then split beyond the internal os and the fœtus and placenta readily removed. The uterus was then irrigated, the womb closed by sutures, the bladder brought down again and held in place by a few stitches. The vagina was packed with gauze. The patient made an uninterrupted recovery.

Kerr also reports a case of eclampsia in a woman in a very critical condition on whom he performed vaginal Cæsarean section. The child was dead when delivered by forceps. There was little bleeding after delivery; the uterus contracted firmly. Injury occurred to the bladder in this case, and the patient recovered with a vesicovaginal fistula.

Retention of the Fetal Skeleton in Utero.—POLANO (*Zentralblatt für Gynäkologie*, 1904, No. 14) reports the case of a multipara, aged thirty-six years, who had had seven normal labors, the last three years before. Menstruation had been interrupted for four months, and there had been repeated hemorrhage. Five days before admission to the hospital amniotic liquid was discharged. In spite of rest in bed and the use of opium, hemorrhage continued without much pain. On the eighth day after admission there was a foul discharge, and the femur of a fœtus was found in the vulva. The uterus was then dilated and the remaining bones of the skeleton were removed.

The Correction of Face Presentation by External Manipulation.—OSTRCIL (*Zentralblatt für Gynäkologie*, 1904, No. 14) reports a number of cases in which he has used either the method of Schatz or that of Thorn to correct face presentation early in labor. He was successful in most of these cases. In one of contracted pelvis, the amniotic liquid having escaped twenty hours previously, the chin was behind in the anteroposterior diameter of the pelvis. The effort to correct face presentation was unsuccessful, and the patient was delivered by embryotomy.

Shock or Hemorrhage.—LOMER, at a recent meeting of the Obstetrical Society of Hamburg (*Zentralblatt für Gynäkologie*, 1904, No. 14), described a case of extirpation of the uterus through the vagina at six months' pregnancy for carcinoma. Two-and-a-half hours after operation the patient collapsed, and abdominal section showed a small bleeding vessel, which was secured. The patient recovered.

In another case myomotomy was performed by a rapid and easy operation, the patient suffering from collapse one hour afterward. No sign of hemorrhage could be found, and the patient recovered under a moderate dose of morphia. A case of ruptured ectopic gestation was operated upon without especial difficulty, and the operation was followed by a very brief shock, from which the patient soon rallied.

He also reports the case of a patient, aged thirty-four years, who was taken in labor during the night and who gave birth to a large child fifty-five minutes after she awoke from sleep. There was hemorrhage, which was controlled by gauze packing and ergot. The uterus contracted firmly and the pulse was good, but the patient manifested every sign of fatal shock. Two hours after the packing was removed and replaced and hemorrhage was found to be absent. She slowly recovered.

In discussion, attention was drawn to the fact that in some of these cases no definite reason can be found for the production of the shock which is present.

Depressed Fracture of the Skull Caused by Labor and Its Treatment.—An interesting case of successful treatment for this dangerous complication is reported in the *British Medical Journal*, April 16, 1904, by Ross. The patient was a multipara. Labor had been in progress for fourteen hours without much improvement. The os was fully dilated, the head presented normally and was engaged. Delivery was effected by axis-traction forceps, there being considerable resistance at first, which suddenly yielded. The pelvis was slightly contracted.

There was a deep, almost circular depression, measuring about two inches in each direction across the left frontal bone. The edge of the bone at the anterior fontanelle was slightly tilted up. An effort to raise the depression by a i g the head between the knees and making pressure failed. Two days after birth operation was done at the Glasgow Maternity Hospital. An incision one inch long was made through the scalp near the anterior fontanelle, and the bone was cut through. An elevator was then inserted and passed forward between the bone and the dura mater. To avoid injury to the dura mater the incision in the bone was made one-quarter of an inch away from the suture to which it adheres. The inner portion of the bone was raised without difficulty and a sound and sensation were produced as if a dent in a celluloid ball were being pushed out. A fracture was found and the other fragment was also raised. There was little bleeding and the wound was closed readily with two stitches. The scalp wound healed in four days, the head becoming normal. The child had shown no symptoms following the injury.

GYNECOLOGY.

UNDER THE CHARGE OF

HENRY C. COE, M.D.,

OF NEW YORK.

ASSISTED BY

WILLIAM E. STUDDIFORD, M.D.

Position of the Arms during Narcosis.—Rothe (*Zentralblatt für Gynäkologie*, 1904, No. 12) comments on the comparative frequency of paralyses of the brachial plexus after operations in Trendelenburg's posture, which, he believes, are due to pressure exerted on the plexus at a point between the clavicle and the first rib. Some of these cases resist treatment for months. In addition to these he has noted a number of cases in which minor disturbances followed, such as temporary numbness, crawling sensations, etc.

He has found that all these unpleasant phenomena can be avoided by arranging the arms in a proper manner and at the same time noting the amount of compression to which the arteries are subjected. The pulse at the wrist is a valuable guide. He tried the plan of elevating only one arm, turning the head to the side, but found the same tendency to paralysis of the median nerve as before. Then he tried fastening the arms at the sides, below the table, with a cushion under each arm. This procedure has given the best results.

Prophylaxis of Postoperative Cystitis.—Baisch (*Zentralblatt für Gynäkologie*, 1904, No. 12) finds that two factors are present in the etiology of this condition: Disturbance of the innervation of the bladder leading to paralysis of the viscus, and interference with the nutrition of the organ, caused by extensive dissection. In addition, staphylococci and bacteria coli present in the urethra are apt to be introduced on the catheter.

In consequence the writer employed irrigation of the bladder after every catheterization, with the best results. Only 1 patient was able to urinate spontaneously after 31 abdominal hysterectomies. Of the 25 patients who survived, 22 were catheterized for twenty-two days without developing cystitis.

The most careful asepsis is necessary in using the catheter, and irrigations (with boric acid or protargol solution) should be continued until the patient is perfectly able to pass her water. In the case of minor operations the ischæmia is transient and less marked.

[In our experience the patient is less apt to suffer from permanent vesical inflammation than from urethritis and irritation at the neck of the bladder, due to the rough or unskilful use of glass catheters.—H. C. C.]

Removal of Ureteral Calculus per Vaginam.—GRADENWITZ (*Zentralblatt für Gynäkologie*, 1904, No. 12) reports the following case: The patient, aged forty-three years, had suffered for three years with colicky pains, beginning in the right kidney and radiating over to the left. She had passed two phosphatic calculi. On vaginal examination a small stone was felt in the bladder, which was easily removed per urethram after moderate dilatation. Four weeks later the patient re-entered the hospital on account of a return of the colicky pains. It was now possible to palpate a stone, the size of a cherry-pit, impacted near the left ureteral orifice. Cystoscopic examination was negative, and the daily excretion of urine was about two pints. Three months later only half this quantity was excreted, and catheterization of the left ureter showed that no urine escaped from that kidney, though the fact of hydronephrosis could not be established.

Under narcosis the usual transverse incision anterior to the cervix was made, the bladder was dissected upward, and the lower portions of the broad ligaments were divided between ligatures, although the uterine arteries were not tied. The stone was fixed by pressure through the abdominal wall, and after further blunt dissection the ureter was drawn down into view, incised, the calculus (uric acid) was removed, and the incision was closed with fine sutures. The patient's convalescence was afebrile, the daily amount of urine at once became normal, and four months later there was no evidence of further trouble.

Histology of Parametritis.—BUSSE (*Monatsschrift für Geb. u. Gyn.*, Band xviii., Heft 1) calls attention to the fact that so-called pelvic exudates differ widely anatomically. In some cases there is a simple œdema of the parametric tissues, in others fibrinous inflammation without marked increase in the leukocytes, such as is noted in the more acute forms. Suppuration follows, with later hypertrophy of the connective tissue and accompanying degenerative changes, especially fatty.

The Action of Oophorin.—MATHES (*Monatsschrift für Geb. u. Gyn.*, Band xviii., Heft 2) asserts that ovarian extract causes an excretion of the phosphates, which is less marked in women whose ovaries have been removed. In general, castration appears to diminish the salts in the body.

Leukocytosis in Diseases of the Pelvic Organs.—DUTZMANN (*Monatsschrift für Geb. u. Gyn.*, Band xviii., Heft 1), continuing his studies of this subject, presents the results in 2000 blood-counts, made in 223 patients. His conclusions are as follows: Leukocytosis is a valuable guide to the presence of pus in the case of pelvic exudates, and furnishes an indication for incision. The iodine reaction of the white cells serves to confirm the diagnosis in a doubtful case of supposed abscess.

In diseases of the adnexa the leukocyte-count not only assists the diagnosis, but guides the surgeon in his choice of the abdominal or vaginal route. In cases of fibromyoma, carcinoma and ectopic gestation leukocytosis is often the only indication of complicating purulent disease of the adnexa, or possible suppuration of an hæmatocele. Tubercular pus does not cause an increase in the number of leukocytes, and gonorrhœal only moderate, a fact explained by the greater resistance of the peritoneum to the specific organisms of those diseases. A high leukocytosis attends torsion of the pedicle of ovarian cysts, though pus may be absent; the iodine reaction is absent, however.

In septic infection the leukocyte count is especially valuable as regards prognosis, a persistent high leukocytosis being favorable, while a decline is to be regarded in the contrary light. In puerperal sepsis the proper time for interference may be judged accordingly. In eclampsia with hyperleukocytosis the attacks are less frequent, while a decline is noted in a less favorable case. The writer infers from this that in eclampsia there is a true infection (?)

Ovarian Hemorrhage.—ROUSSEAU (*Jour. méd. de Bruxelles*, 1903, No 50) reports 6 cases, the following being the most interesting:

Case I.—Three days after the beginning of menstruation the patient was seized with a severe pain in the right groin radiating down the thigh. Similar attacks followed at intervals of two months, and a tumor the size of the first developed in the cul-de-sac, which, on opening the abdomen, proved to be a large hæmatoma of the ovary.

Case II.—The patient had a sudden attack of pain, with tenderness and resistance over McBurney's point. Bilious vomiting and elevation of temperature. Several similar attacks followed during the next few months, the diagnosis of recurrent appendicitis was made, and on section a small hemorrhagic ovarian cyst was found with a twisted pedicle, the appendix being normal.

Case III.—The patient had a violent attack of abdominal pain, with vomiting and rapid increase of a pre-existing ovarian neoplasm. On section the abdomen was found to be full of blood which had escaped from a cancerous cyst. All the patients made a good recovery.

Operation for Prolapse of the Ovary.—MAUCLAIRE (*Semaine Gynécol.*, 1903, Nos. 35 and 36) describes the following operation for the relief of retroversion associated with prolapse of the ovaries which resists ordinary treatment: After opening the abdomen a slit is made in the upper part of either broad ligament midway between the uterus and the pelvic wall, the fimbria ovarica divided in order to free the prolapsed ovary, and any adhesions are separated. Any necessary conservative work is done. The ovary is drawn through this opening, which is contracted with sutures, so that the gland cannot slip back again, and, finally, the end of the tube is sutured to the anterior surface of the broad ligament near the ovary. Hysteropexy is performed to keep the uterus in an anterior position.

[Barrows, of New York, describes a similar operation, which he calls "shelfing" the ovary. Both seem to be open to the objection that the gland is not left in its normal relations and that its blood supply may be consequently interrupted.—H. C. C.]

Cancer of the Ovary in a Child.—KUSNETZKI (*Jour. Akuschi Shensk. bolesnej*; *Zentralblatt für Gynäkologie*, 1904, No. 13) reports the case of a girl, aged fourteen years, who had never menstruated. She had an abdominal tumor of a year's standing, accompanied with severe pains. It was larger than the fist, nodular, and movable. On section it was discovered to be pedunculated and was easily removed. The patient was examined nearly two years after operation and there was no evidence of recurrence.

OPHTHALMOLOGY.

UNDER THE CHARGE OF

EDWARD JACKSON, A.M., M.D.,
OF DENVER, COLORADO,

AND

T. B. SCHNEIDEMAN, A.M., M.D.,
PROFESSOR OF DISEASES OF THE EYE IN THE PHILADELPHIA POLYCLINIC.

Observations on Renal Retinitis.—Nettleship (*Royal London Ophthalmic Hospital Reports*, October, 1903), based upon the study of quite a large number of cases of this disease, comes to the following conclusions which, however, are confirmatory of what had been previously known rather than in themselves very novel.

It is, of course, in the chronic interstitial and chronic parenchymatous forms of nephritis that albuminuric retinitis so commonly occurs. A few cases are recorded in connection with lardaceous disease and with nephritis due to inflammation of the bladder, ureter, or pelvis of the kidney; but additional cases in connection with any of these maladies are deserving of careful record. The same may be said of retinitis due to acute nephritis of previously healthy kidneys; such cases are said to occur occasionally, especially after scarlet fever.

The chief exception to this rule that the retinal changes depend upon chronic nephritis is seen in the albuminuric retinitis of pregnancy. The renal condition here is not a true acute inflammation but a rapid degeneration of the epithelium such as is found in some forms of acute blood poisoning. Kidneys so affected may rapidly pass into a state of chronic nephritis and contraction. It is very important in every case of pregnancy retinitis that the condition of the kidney before pregnancy should be known when possible. The prognosis for life in pregnancy retinitis is better than in the ordinary cases; thus, of 22 cases recorded by Nettleship only 5 are known to have died and only one of these within two years. On the other hand, of 42 non-pregnancy cases only 9 lived more than two years, and no less than 25 died within one year. The pregnancy retinitis occurs only once as a rule, and in the majority of cases after several pregnancies. There are certain cases of failure of sight *after* confinement in which the vision remains bad for several weeks and then returns more or less. The condition of the fundus during the active period is not known.

A large excess (if the pregnancy cases are omitted) are males; in the writer's series of cases the age ranged from thirty to sixty years, the most prolific decade being from fifty to fifty-nine years. In these cases, between 80 and 90 in number, the prognosis for life seemed better when the retinitis came on after fifty-five years than before.

There are two principal factors in the production of renal retinitis, a morbid state of the blood and disease of the retinal arteries; in most cases both conditions are present. The ophthalmoscopic observer may fairly suspect an early stage of granular kidney whenever he finds decided hyaline thickening of the retinal arteries, especially in young subjects. This hyaline fibroid thickening of the retinal arteries is now well known to be indicated by intensification of the bright streak and compression of the veins where they are crossed by arteries. This condition is not always symmetrical in the two eyes nor evenly distributed in the same eye. After middle age hyaline thickening is less useful as a diagnostic sign of granular kidney. We must still take it, however, as a sign of danger of cerebral hemorrhage.

The general opinion is that the particular characters of the retinitis do not afford any guide to the kind of chronic kidney disease present. The more violent cases are chiefly toxic and the milder more chronic ones chiefly vascular in origin.

Nettleship thinks it certain that there is only one sort of renal retinitis and the many varieties of change seen during life indicates only different stages and degrees of (*a*) general œdema; (*b*) exudation into the nerve-fibre layer; (*c*) spots or patches of opacity in the deeper layers due to degeneration of fibrinous or albuminous effusion in the inner granule layers and perhaps to changes in Muller's fibres.

The optic neuritis and retinal hemorrhages so often present in varying degrees are not characteristic, though they increase the difficulty in interpreting the morbid appearances.

Other constitutional or local conditions produce retinitis resembling and sometimes indistinguishable from that caused by disease of the kidneys, of which the retinitis associated with glycosuria is particularly to be dwelt upon. In some of these cases the urine also contains albumin, and here the disease may be the ordinary albuminuric retinitis, but this is not true of others. The life prospects in the retinitis of diabetes seems better than in ordinary renal retinitis.

The typical retinitis of renal disease is nearly always symmetrical though not always equally so, and rarely the affection is confined to one eye. It is doubtful whether relapses occur, but we have proof that retinal hemorrhages are repeated in eyes that have passed through albuminuric retinitis.

Albuminuric choroiditis is mentioned by many writers. Iritis in renal disease has been seen in two cases by Knies.

Influence of Resection of the Cervical Sympathetic in Optic Nerve Atrophy, Hydrophthalmos, and Exophthalmic Goitre.—Ball (*Journal of the American Medical Association*, January 30, 1904), from personal experience and a review of reported cases by others, comes to the following conclusions: 1. Excision of the superior cervical ganglion of the sympathetic nerve is worthy of a trial in those cases of simple atrophy of the optic nerve which resist measures less heroic. 2. It is yet impossible to say whether the bilateral operation is advisable in unilateral optic nerve atrophy. 3. The value of sympathectomy in congenital hydrophthalmos has not been demonstrated. 4. In exophthalmic goitre complete excision of the cervical sympathetic is followed by a larger percentage of cures than is any other procedure. Thus far no deaths have been recorded. The number of operations, however, is small, and final conclusions can be announced only after a large number of cases shall have been treated by this method.

A Hitherto Undescribed Membrane of the Eye and its Significance.—VERHOEFF, Boston (*The Royal London Ophthalmic Hospital Reports*, October, 1903), after a careful study of many sections arrives at the following conclusions: In the pigment layer of the retina there is a fenestrated membrane identical in structure and staining reactions with the membrana limitans externa.

The rods and cones are not nervous elements, but modified ependymal cells, and are analogous to sensory epithelium.

The limiting membrane of the rosettes of the glioma retinæ is a fenestrated membrane similar in every way to the membrana limitans externa, and the rosettes correspond to the neuroepithelium of the normal retina.

The structure of the limiting membrane of rosettes explains why they assume their spherical and spiral-like forms.

"Neuroepithelioma retinæ" is no more suitable than "glioma retinæ" for the class of tumors to which these terms have been applied.

Enucleation and its Substitutes.—GRIMSDALE (*Medical Times and Hospital Gazette*, December 19, 1903) advocates a modified form of Mules' operation. The modification consists in leaving the cornea in place and making a large curved incision above it in the sclera. The cosmetic result is excellent. There is no sinking of the artificial eye. The movements of the latter are very good, as much as one-half inch laterally and vertically almost the normal. The objections to enucleation are not only cosmetic, but the irritation caused by the prothesis is to be considered also because of the large space between it and the concave stump, in which secretion accumulates, and decomposition gives rise to chronic conjunctivitis, and finally changes in the subconjunctival tissue, so that bands are formed which render the retention of an artificial eye difficult and sometimes impossible. Attempts at improving such a stump are not likely to be successful.

The injection of paraffin into the space of Tenon is certainly not devoid of its own special risks; it has been followed in some instances by thrombosis of the neighboring veins and may thus cause blindness in the other eye.

The attempt has been made to transplant a rabbit's eye whole into the empty orbit, but it has not been successful. Even where the transferred tissues have lived, they have softened and left a very imperfect stump.

As regards the comparative safety from sympathetic ophthalmia, the advantage seems to be with enucleation; although, as is well known, many cases have followed even enucleation. Still, these, like those which have followed Mules' operation, have been of a mild type. There is no case in which sympathetic ophthalmia has followed a Mules' operation for any other condition but injury—*i. e.*, not when the operation has been performed for staphyloma or similar condition.

When enucleation is decided upon it would, perhaps, be best to use Frost's method of inserting a large glass sphere in the hollow of Tenon's capsule after enucleation and stitching it in.

DISEASES OF THE LARYNX AND CONTIGUOUS STRUCTURES.

UNDER THE CHARGE OF

J. SOLIS-COHEN, M.D.,

OF PHILADELPHIA.

Topographical Anatomy of the Crypts of Hypertrophied Tonsils.—Under this title DR. A. COURTADE presents an elaborate and illustrated paper (*Archives internationales de laryngologie, d'otologie et de rhinologie, Mars-Avril*, 1903) showing that the crypts, which are more numerous than they are supposed to be, exist upon the top and the bottom of the tonsil as well as in the sides and front, and that they all converge toward the interior instead of having an indefinite or irregular course. He was led to this study by finding caseous masses expressed from the tonsil beneath the anterior pillar, and so minute that they could not be penetrated by an ordinary probe.

Foreign Body in the Œsophagus Removed by Gastrotomy.—At a meeting of the Clinical Society of London (*British Medical Journal*, October 31, 1903) DR. PATTERSON exhibited an inhaler removed by gastrotomy from the œsophagus of a male phthisical patient. It measured four and one-half inches in length and almost three-quarters of an inch in diameter. Inside the metal case was a glass inhaler containing a drachm of creosote. A skiagraph showed the case lying to the left of the spinal column and almost parallel to it. It produced no symptoms whatever, as after swallowing it the patient had not taken food. When the stomach was opened, one inch of the case was projecting from the œsophagus into the stomach, whence it was removed. The patient made an uninterrupted recovery.

Removal of Nasal Polypi.—DR. ALBERT RUAULT describes and depicts (*Annales des maladies de l'oreille, du larynx, etc.*, February, 1904) his improved intranasal polypotome, in which, by pressure of the thumb, the guard is pushed down over the wire loop. This instrument would appear to be much steadier than other forms of polypotome.

Vascular Rhinopharyngeal Fibroma.—At a meeting of the Clinical Society of London (*British Medical Journal*, October 31, 1903) DR. HERBERT TILLEY showed a lad, aged sixteen years, from whose rhinopharynx he had removed a fibro-angioma by various operations. When first seen, two years before, the patient had complete nasal obstruction, with blood-stained discharge from the left nostril of five months' duration. A large, sloughy, easily bleeding mass completely filled the left nasal fossa. In November, 1901, but half the growth could be removed by Ollier's method. In December, after a preliminary laryngotomy, division of the soft palate and removal of the left side of the hard palate, all visible growth was removed, also in March, 1902, after recurrence. In July, 1902, there was again extensive recurrence, and after preliminary laryngotomy the soft parts of the nose and face were turned upward; a large opening was made in the left canine fossa, and the lower half of the ascending process of the left superior maxilla was removed. The growth was seen to arise from the external surface of the antrum and ethmoidal region, and was completely removed. There had been no further recurrence. The boy had grown four inches, and early in the year the soft palate had been sutured.

Mucocele of the Ethmoid.—GUIZEZ reports (*Annales des maladies de l'oreille, du larynx, etc.*, February, 1904) an interesting case of ethmoidal mucocele of very large dimensions—say 3 cm. in every direction. It did not communicate with the nasal passage, and probably developed from one of the anterior cells of the prefrontal group. It was exposed by external excision and resection of the greatest part of the anterior wall, and found filled with a viscous, yellowish-brown liquid, rich in cholesterin. After curetting and careful scraping of the entire internal face of the osseous walls a solution of chloride of zinc one part to ten was applied and a drain left at the inferior angle of the wound. Recovery was prompt, without deformity, and with very little cicatrix.

Maxillary Sinusitis Due to a Dental Ectopia.—GUIZEZ reports (*Annales des maladies de l'oreille, du larynx, etc.*, February, 1904) a case in which the suppuration of the maxillary sinus was found to be due to a large molar tooth in its interior, the roots being implanted partly in the alveolus and partly in the floor of the sinus itself. This tooth was carious at the union of the neck and roots. For its liberation it was necessary to resect a portion of the alveolar process and the palatine vault. A slight buccal fistula presented for several weeks, but the purulent discharge and the subjective odor completely disappeared.

Chronic Suppuration of the Maxillary Sinus.—DR. CLAOUÉ, of Bordeaux, describes (*Annales des maladies de l'oreille, du larynx, etc.*, March, 1904) his new operation for gaining access to the sinus through the nasal passage in order to secure a thorough drainage, which he considers the chief feature of surgical treatment, more important even than careful curettage of the cavity. The operation is performed without general anæsthesia and consists of three stages, the last two of which may follow after the first immediately, or be postponed for a day or two, according to requirements.

1. The anterior two-thirds of the lower turbinated bone is removed close to the nasal wall with scissors, and the section is completed with the cold snare.

2. With a hand trephine, which is preferred to the motor, two perforations are made in the wall of the sinus about 2 cm. from the anterior extremity of the turbinate which had been removed; the intervening bridge is removed with the punch. The orifice thus made is then enlarged until it is nearly the size of the pulp end of the thumb.

3. The sinus is copiously washed out and then explored. If any diseased tissue exist sufficient to have kept up the suppuration, it is scraped with a curette with a flexible handle. A minute curettage is not

the aim of the operation. The sinus is then sponged out with chloride of zinc and tamponed for forty-eight hours with iodoform gauze.

Subsequent treatment consists in daily washing and the insufflation of non-irritant powders upon the whole interior surfaces.

The details of twelve cases are given, nine of which were cured. One remained content with this condition, and the two others were permanently relieved by opening the sinus at the canine fossa and then thoroughly curetting the interior. The place for drainage left by the first operation greatly favored this result.

Necrosis of Sphenoidal Sinus and Ethmoidal Cells.—A fatal case of necrosis of the sphenoidal and posterior ethmoidal cells, phlebitis of the cavernous sinus, pyæmia, is reported (*Journal of Laryngology, Rhinology, and Otology*, April, 1904) by Dr. A. L. Whitehead. The patient was a well-nourished woman, aged forty-seven years, who had enjoyed good health up to the time of the fatal illness, except for a purulent discharge from the left side of the nose, said to have followed an attack of facial erysipelas two years previously. For five weeks there had been frequent and very severe headaches and attacks of vertigo; for three days occasional attacks of vomiting, slight rigors, fever, and a general sense of malaise; for one day an uncomfortable sensation of tension in the left eye, with diplopia. There was some proptosis in this eye, and movements of the globe were restricted in all directions. In the nose, thick, creamy pus was seen descending between the septum and the middle turbinate of the left side.

Under ether the left middle turbinate was removed. The anterior wall of the sphenoidal sinus was found soft and carious, and the cavity full of pulpy material, pus, granulation tissue, and blood, the immediate posterior ethmoidal cells being similarly affected. The anterior wall of the sphenoidal sinus and the inner walls of the ethmoidal cells were removed, and the cavities were cautiously but thoroughly curetted, and then lightly packed with iodoform gauze to check hemorrhage.

Staphylococcus aureus was found in pure culture in the material removed.

The patient went from bad to worse and died of the pyæmia on the third day.

The condition was clearly one of chronic suppuration in the sphenoidal sinus and in the posterior ethmoidal cells, with an acute staphylococcic infection three or four days before she was operated upon.

Syphiloma of the Larynx.—Dr. Marcel Lermoyez reports (*Annales des maladies de l'oreille, du larynx, etc.*, February, 1904) a case of subglottic concentric syphiloma of the larynx just beneath the vocal bands in which tracheotomy seemed urgent. It resolved completely under semi-weekly injections of eight to twelve drops of gray oil and daily doses of more than six grams of potassium iodide.

Intralaryngeal Extirpation of Epithelioma.—Prof. Arslan, of the University of Padua, reports (*Annales des maladies de l'oreille, du larynx, etc.*, February, 1904) two cases in which recovery had remained permanent for four and five years respectively. He likewise details two more recent cases in which similar results have been maintained twenty months and nearly four years after operation. It will be understood, as a matter of course, that these cases must have presented especially favorable conditions for such success. It likewise shows that a radical operation from the exterior is not necessary in every instance of malignant neoplasm of the interior of the larynx.

Paralysis of the Vocal Cords.—Dr. L. Revol reports (*Annales des maladies de l'oreille, du larynx, etc.*, February, 1904) a case of bilateral recurrent paralysis of the larynx due to dilatation of the aorta as verified by radioscopic examination.

HYGIENE AND PUBLIC HEALTH.

UNDER THE CHARGE OF

CHARLES HARRINGTON, M.D.,

ASSISTANT PROFESSOR OF HYGIENE, HARVARD MEDICAL SCHOOL.

Notes on Disinfectants.—*Green Soap.* An elaborate series of experiments with various mixtures of carbolic acid and the official green soap of the German Pharmacopœia, free from free alkali and containing 44.02 per cent. of water, has been made by Dr. O. Heller (*Archiv für Hygiene*, Bd. xlvii. p. 213), who employed cultures of bacillus typhosus as test objects. His conclusions are as follows: Green soap possesses but slight disinfectant power, but it increases that of pure carbolic acid, and most markedly when the two substances are present in equal amounts. While typhoid bacilli are destroyed in twenty minutes by a 5 per cent. solution of carbolic acid, the same result is obtained by the employment of a 4 per cent. solution of equal parts of the two agents; that is, with less than half the required amount of carbolic acid alone. By analogy, one may conclude that the employment of soap in the preparation of disinfectants containing cresols insoluble in water not only brings about their solution to the required extent, but increases their bactericidal properties. This increase in power must be attributed either to the feebly disinfectant power of the soap or to the formation of a new complex compound of greater power, or the solution of the phenol (or cresol) experiences an increase in its rate of dissociation through the presence of the soap, and with it an increase in efficiency. But soap increases the bactericidal power of phenol to an extent out of all proportion to its own power in the same direction, and the mere fact of increasing solubility can have little or no influence.

Creolin. The term "creolin," says Dr. Samuel Rideal (*Public Health*, December, 1903, p. 156), seems to have been invented many years ago as a fancy name for an emulsion of cresols and neutral tar oils in a soap solution, and disinfectants under this name have been sold in different parts of the world and manufactured by several firms, who have from time to time modified the nature and the proportions of the various constituents without warning to the public. Samples of creolin, purchased in Brussels, Hamburg, and London, have been tested by him and found to have a disinfectant value varying from one and five-tenths to sixteen times that of pure carbolic acid. Chemical examination showed very wide differences in composition, which, however, furnishes no information as to their probable bactericidal value. Some specimens contain appreciable amounts of pyridine bases, which impart a very strong and characteristic odor, without contributing to the germicidal properties. He is of the opinion that if the name is to remain in the literature of the subject, a statement of the germicidal value in terms of some standard should be insisted upon in all cases.

Lysoform. Experiments with lysoform, a soft soap containing about 8 per cent. of formaldehyde and a small amount of volatile oil, conducted by GALLI-VALERIO (*Therapeutisches Monatsheft*, 1903, Bd. xvii. p. 452), bear out the findings of Symanski, Seydewitz, and others that it is slower in action than many other better-known agents. He found that a 5 per cent. solution required four hours' contact to destroy staphylococcus aureus, and that a 3 per cent. solution was ineffective against bacillus coli communis in less than forty-five minutes. SYMANSKI (*Zeitschrift für Hygiene und Infectionskrankheiten*, Bd. xxxvii. p. 393) killed staphylococci in pus with a 2 per cent. solution in five hours, and SEYDEWITZ (*Centralblatt für Bakteriologie und Parasitenkunde, I. Abth. Originale*, 1904, Bd. xxxii. p. 222) sterilized brushes infected with staphylococcus aureus and bacillus coli communis with a 5 per cent. solution in six hours, but cultures of these organisms by themselves were destroyed much more quickly. According to Symanski, lysoform is not irritant to the skin and mucous membranes, but Galli-Valerio asserts that solutions stronger than 3 per cent. cause too much irritation for local application in abdominal surgery.

Mercuric Cyanide. A series of tests of the bactericidal properties of mercuric cyanide, which is advocated in some quarters as an agent superior in some respects to corrosive sublimate, led HARRINGTON (*Boston Med. and Surg. Journal*, January 14, 1904) to conclude that this agent can hardly be classed among efficient germicides for surgical purposes. A 1 : 1000 solution was found to require more than three hours' contact to destroy staphylococcus aureus, and one of 1 : 500 exerted no bactericidal influence whatever against the same organisms at the end of a half-hour, beyond which time the experiments were not continued.

Hypochlorous Acid. Recent investigation having shown that, in solutions of chlorine containing about 0.05 per cent. of the gas, more than 90 per cent. of the chlorine exists in the form of hypochlorous and hydrochlorie acids, and it appearing not improbable that chlorine exerts its disinfectant action as hypochlorous acid, DRS. F. W. ANDREWES and K. J. P. ORTON (*Centralblatt für Bakteriologie und Parasitenkunde, I. Abth. Originale*, 1904, Bd. xxxv. p. 645) undertook a research to determine the germicidal action of the acid in a pure state. Accordingly, pure preparations of the acid were made and tested, and although the results obtained were at times conflicting, owing to the instability of the preparations when exposed to light and in the presence of traces of organic matter, the germicidal activity of the acid appeared to be of the most intense character. In filtered suspension in pure water, anthrax spores were killed by a 1 : 10,000 strength of hypochlorous acid in the total mixture in thirty seconds. Watery suspensions of the spores, dried on thick silk threads, were destroyed by a 7 : 1000 solution in five minutes, but spores of bacillus subtilis required twenty minutes. Staphylococcus aureus in suspension in pure distilled water was sterilized by a 1 : 100,000 solution in one minute, but not in fifteen seconds. A 1 : 250,000 solution just failed to kill a watery suspension of staphylococcus aureus in five minutes, but it killed a similar suspension of bacillus coli communis in between thirty and sixty seconds. In the presence of organic matter, and especially of proteids, it was anticipated that so unstable an acid would rapidly be decomposed and rendered inert; that it would prove almost devoid of inhibiting power in such a medium as bouillon; and that, up to a certain point, it would be rendered inert by the organic matter present, and, beyond it, it would kill quickly, with no extensive intermediate stage, such as is seen with phenol or corrosive sublimate, in which growth is restrained without actual death of the bacteria. Such was found to be the case, for while staphylococci in distilled water were killed immediately by 1 : 100,000, their growth in veal bouillon was restrained only by 1 : 5000, but they were destroyed within thirty minutes by 1 : 3000. Having satisfied themselves as to the intense germicidal activity of the pure acid and to the extent to which its power is impaired by the presence of organic matter, they investigated the principal methods by which it is or may be actually employed in practical disinfection, as in the form of chlorine water, bleaching-powder solutions, and mixtures of hydrochloric acid with oxidizing agents. They found that chlorine water is even more potent than is indicated by the figures of Krönig and Paul, for a watery suspension of anthrax spores, dried on quartz pebbles, was killed usually in between thirty and sixty seconds by a 0.015 per cent. solution, and in filtered suspension in distilled water by a 0.010 per cent. solution in ten seconds. The addition of hydrochloric acid to the extent of 0.4 per cent. by weight of the gas was found not to increase the germicidal power of the chlorine, but rather to weaken it. On the other hand, the germicidal power of bleaching-powder solution is increased by the addition of a weak acid (acetic and carbonic are the best) to liberate free hypochlorous acid (a strong acid liberates free chlorine). A saturated solution of bleaching-powder, containing 5 per cent. of calcium hypochlorite and so strong as to disintegrate a marine sponge in a minute, took between seven and ten minutes to destroy dried anthrax spores; but the same solution, diluted with twice its volume of 1.25 per cent. acetic acid, destroyed them in less than a minute. Hence, in employing bleaching-powder as a germicide, the addition of vinegar, or even free exposure to the carbon dioxide of the air, will be found of much value. Krönig and Paul's combination of potassium permanganate and hydrochloric acid was found to be slow (nearly four hours) in destroying anthrax spores dried on silk threads. As a substitute they tried a mixture of 1.1 c.c. hydrochloric acid, 3.7 grams ammonium persulphate [$(NH_4)_2S_2O_8$] and 95 c.c. water, in which, even after many weeks' keeping, the amount of chlorine and hypochlorous acid present amounts only to 0.008 per cent. At first the mixture is absolutely odorless, but in half an hour it has an extremely faint chlorous odor, which increases hour by hour until after three to four days it is very strong, indeed, and is that of hypochlorous acid rather than that of free chlorine. Its disinfectant value is at first very slight, but when six days old it will destroy anthrax spores in less than a minute. The mixture has the great advantage that it is colorless, transparent, and wholly devoid of staining power. Although both mixtures act at a great disadvantage in the presence of organic matter, the persulphate mixture is considerably the more effective in the presence of moderate amounts of albuminous material. The chief use appears to lie in the disinfection of the skin, in which role it proved experimentally to be quite successful. Thus, hands well scrubbed with soap and hot water and soaked in the solution for five minutes were found to give no growths from serapings from beneath the nails and about their roots; but it blackens and spoils metallic instruments, with which it should not be brought in contact.

PATHOLOGY AND BACTERIOLOGY.

UNDER THE CHARGE OF

SIMON FLEXNER, M.D.,

DIRECTOR OF THE ROCKEFELLER INSTITUTE FOR MEDICAL RESEARCH, NEW YORK.

ASSISTED BY

WARFIELD T. LONGCOPE, M.D.,

RESIDENT PATHOLOGIST, PENNSYLVANIA HOSPITAL, PHILADELPHIA.

Ascending Renal Infection; with Special Reference to the Reflux of Urine from the Bladder into the Ureters as an Etiological Factor in its Causation and Maintenance.—Combining experimental investigations with careful clinical observations, Sampson (*Johns Hopkins Hosp. Bull.*, 1903, vol. xiv. p. 334) has brought out many interesting facts concerning the anatomy and physiology of the ureters and urinary bladder, and has done much to explain the origin of ascending renal infections. He finds that the vesical portion of the ureter changes under various degrees of dilatation and of intravesical tension of the bladder, and in each of these conditions there is special provision for guarding the lumen of the ureter and thus preventing a reflux of urine from the bladder into the ureter. Under all conditions of the bladder the direction of the current of urine from the kidney to the bladder is a constant factor in the prevention of ascending infection. In addition, if the bladder is distended the ureteral orifice is protected by the oblique course of the ureter, the long ureteral valve, the lateral walls of the labia of the ureteral orifice, and the mucosa of the ureter. But if the bladder is contracted the course of the ureter is not so oblique, the ureteral valve is shorter, and these factors play a less important part. On the other hand, additional protection is afforded by a puckering of the ureteral orifice, for the ureteral labia come together, and the ureteral mucosa is thrown into folds. The anatomical structure and physiological action of the ureters, as well as clinical experience, would indicate that the function of the ureters is not only to carry urine away from the kidneys to the bladder, but also to prevent fluid from passing into the ureters from the bladder, and under normal conditions it is impossible for the latter to take place. It was practically impossible, when experimenting with dogs, to cause a reflux of urine from the bladder into the ureter with either an intact or injured ureteral orifice, or even with implanted ureters. Cases have been reported which contradict these observations, but the fact that an occasional case has been reported in which apparently a reflux has occurred, especially when nothing is known of the condition of the ureteral orifice in these instances, cannot be regarded as sufficient evidence for supposing that it may occur in all cases. In the production of pyonephrosis it is possible that organisms may be conveyed from the bladder to the kidney through the general circulation, the venous and arterial communication known as the vesico-utero-ovario-renal anastomoses, the bloodvessels of the ureter, the lymphatics, or the lumen of the ureter.

As regards blood infections, injections of culture of staphylococcus pyogenes aureus into the veins of animals demonstrated that for the development of pyonephrosis a stricture of the ureter was of great importance. It is well known that in general bacterial infections the organisms are eliminated by the kidneys, and if under such circumstances there should be a slight stricture of the ureter, infected urine would be dammed back into the kidney and produce pyonephrosis. Experimentally, this series of events does actually take place. In cystitis direct infection of the kidney through the lumen of the ureter is dependent in the vast majority of cases upon an extension of the inflammatory process from the bladder through the ureteral walls or along the lumen of the ureter. If, through inflammation or any other cause, the urine from the kidney is intercepted by a stricture or something occluding the lumen of the ureter, organisms may reach the urine which is dammed back, and rapidly travel up the ureter. Other modes of infection are possible by injury to the intravesical portion of the ureter, or possibly by a reflux of urine from the bladder into the ureter.

The reflux of urine from the bladder into the ureter may be considered an etiological factor in the causation and maintenance of renal infection only when the intravesical portion of the ureter is diseased, thus impairing its function, or when some ureteral abnormality exists.

On the Appearances and Significance of Certain Granules in the Erythrocytes of Man.—Since Kölliker, in 1846, first upheld the view that in the transition of the nucleated red cell to the fully developed normal erythrocyte the nucleus gradually disappears within the cell, this subject has been widely discussed and variously interpreted. Recent observations made upon fresh unfixed blood stained by neutral red have brought out certain facts concerning peculiar granules which appear in the erythrocytes treated by this method, and which may have some bearing upon nuclear changes. Vaughan (*Jour. of Med. Research*, 1903, vol. x. p. 342), using polychrome methylene blue as a stain, has studied fresh blood from normal individuals and persons suffering from various diseases. In normal blood most of the red cells remain unstained, but a few show small granules which are colored a decided purplish red, showing a definite affinity for the chromatin staining principle of polychrome methylene blue (methylene azure). The number of these granulated cells varies under normal conditions between very narrow limits, and averages about 1 per cent. of the total number of red blood corpuscles. In cases of anæmia it was discovered that when the number of nucleated red blood cells was high, the granular erythrocytes were proportionately increased, and in a case of pernicious anæmia during a blood crisis the granulated cells reached 18.8 per cent. The blood of newly born infants contained sometimes as much as 7 per cent. of granulated cells, but after several days they decreased to about 3 per cent. In various acute infections the granulated cells were seen in about the same proportion as in normal blood. Thus, their increase seemed always dependent upon the presence of nucleated red cells. The blood of embryo pigs contained about 17 per cent. of granulated erythrocytes. A study of the blood of geese and pigeons showed that as the nucleus of the erythrocytes degenerated, granules staining in the same manner as the chromatin of the nucleus appeared in the protoplasm and became scattered through the cell. The changes above described could not be demonstrated so readily in fixed specimens colored by Wright's, Jenner's, or Leishman's stains, and it is possible that during fixation the granules seen in the fresh preparations are broken up, and produce in the stained specimen the well-known appearance of polychromatophilia. The author after careful study does not believe that these granules are artefacts, but considers them as the remnants of the nuclear chromatin which has been set free in the red cells during the dissolution of the nucleus. Observations upon the blood platelets carried along the same lines go to show that these bodies react toward stains in precisely the same manner as do the granules in the red cells. This suggests that they too are derived primarily from the nucleus of the nucleated erythrocytes.

The Casuistry of Placental and Congenital Tuberculosis.—Warthin and Cowie (*Journal of Infectious Diseases*, 1904, vol. i. p. 140) discuss this important and interesting question. They report a case, together with abstracts of those cases from the literature which bear upon the subject. They show that the question of congenital tuberculosis, although definitely proved, has but 6 cases, including their own, to support it, in which the diagnosis is based upon anatomical changes and the presence of tubercle bacilli; in which the development of the lesion occurred so shortly after birth as to preclude the possibility of extrauterine infection, and in which syphilis was definitely excluded.

They also give abstracts of 35 probable or doubtful cases from the literature, which do not fulfil all the foregoing requirements, 8 undoubted and 1 probable case of placental tuberculosis, and 16 undoubted and 8 doubtful cases in which tubercle bacilli were found in the fœtus and placenta without histological changes.

In their own case the authors found miliary tuberculosis of the mother in the fifth month of pregnancy, tuberculosis of the placenta, and agglutination thrombi, containing many tubercle bacilli in the placenta and in the fœtus. As a result of their study, they conclude that the conditions of the circulation in the placental and uterine sinuses favor the collection of tubercle bacilli when present in the maternal blood, and that when the organisms are capable of multiplication, the first step in the development of tuberculosis of the placenta appears to be an agglutination and coagulation thrombosis of the maternal blood in the intervellous spaces. They believe that the syncytium possesses a certain degree of resistance against tubercle bacilli, and, although the passage of the tubercle bacilli through an apparently normal syncytium is still an open question, the senile degenerative changes in it during the later half of pregnancy favor the passage of the organism through the syncytium. Their findings show that tubercle bacilli, virulent to guinea-pigs, may be found in the chorionic villi and fetal blood without marked pathological changes in these structures. They assume that the fetal tissues are relatively immune to the action of tubercle bacilli, and that a true latent congenital tuberculosis is, therefore, both possible and probable.

The authors believe that the commonly accepted dicta regarding congenital tuberculosis are probably extreme, and that it is not at all unlikely that it is of much more common occurrence than is generally supposed.

Islands of Gastric Mucous Membrane Having the Structure of the Glands of the Cardiac Zone and Region of the Fundus and Glands Simulating the Lower Œsophageal Cardiac Glands in the Upper Portion of the Œsophagus.—SCHRIDDE (*Virchow's Archiv*, 1904, Bd. clxxv. p. 1) has found certain gland structures in the mucous membrane of the œsophagus in 21 out of 30 cases examined. They are usually bilateral and occur in the upper portions of the œsophagus. They are difficult to find macroscopically in the fresh state, but after the œsophagus has been fixed in Müller formal solution the glands assume a deep-brown color, while the mucous membrane of the œsophagus is bright yellow. Three varieties of glands can be distinguished: one type is like the lower œsophageal cardiac glands; it appears as branched tubules situated in the mucosa and opening out by ducts upon the surface between the pavement epithelium covering the papillæ. The tubules are lined by columnar epithelium possessing nuclei placed near the basement membrane. In the ampullæ there are cells which give a definite reaction for mucus. Finally, the presence of isolated covering cells can be made out. The second type of gland resembles very closely the glands in the cardiac region of the stomach. The third type, which appears important and rather rare, practically reproduces the gastric mucous membrane, and contains glands similar to those found both in the cardiac region and in the fundus. Small lymph follicles may be found, and the entire structure seems to be identical in its histological appearance and secretory functions with the normal mucous membrane of the stomach.

The author believes that the epithelial covering of the œsophagus and of these gland structures takes its origin from two absolutely different sources. The glands are thought to develop from the entoderm, while the œsophagus is covered by ectoderm extending down from the pharynx.

Notice to Contributors.—All communications intended for insertion in the Original Department of this Journal are received only *with the distinct understanding that they are contributed exclusively to this Journal.*

Contributions from abroad written in a foreign language, if on examination they are found desirable for this Journal, will be translated at its expense.

A limited number of reprints in pamphlet form will, if desired, be furnished to authors, *provided the request for them be written on the manuscript.*

All communications should be addressed to—

DR. FRANCIS R. PACKARD, 1831 Chestnut Street, Philadelphia, U. S. A.

INDEX.

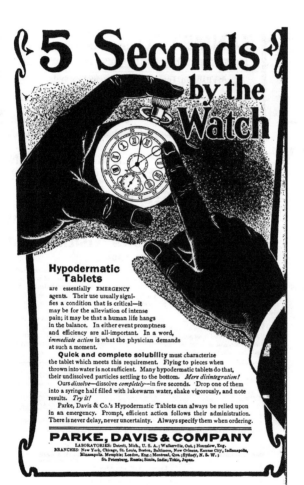

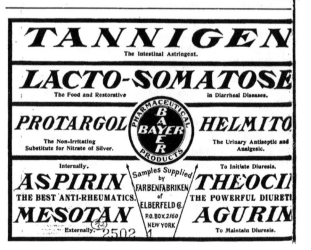

CPSIA information can be obtained
at www.ICGtesting.com
Printed in the USA
BVHW04*1224200818
525056BV00025B/2322/P

9 780260 138262